# Anesthesiology

Basavana G. Goudra
Michael Duggan • Vidya Chidambaran
Hari Prasad Krovvidi Venkata
Elizabeth Duggan • Mark Powell
Preet Mohinder Singh
Editors

# Anesthesiology

A Practical Approach

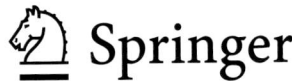

*Editors*
Basavana G. Goudra
Hospital University Pennsylvania
Perelman School of Medicine
Philadelphia, PA
USA

Vidya Chidambaran
Department of Anesthesiology,
Cincinnati Children's Hospital
Medical Center
Cincinnati, OH
USA

Elizabeth Duggan
Emory University Hospital
Atlanta, GA
USA

Preet Mohinder Singh
All India Institute of Medical Sciences
(AIIMS)
New Delhi, Delhi, India

Michael Duggan
Department of Anesthesiology
Emory University
Atlanta, GA
USA

Hari Prasad Krovvidi Venkata
University Hospitals Birmingham
Birmingham, United Kingdom

Mark Powell
University of Alabama at Birmingham
Birmingham, AL
USA

ISBN 978-3-319-74765-1   ISBN 978-3-319-74766-8   (eBook)
https://doi.org/10.1007/978-3-319-74766-8

Library of Congress Control Number: 2018942332

© Springer International Publishing AG, part of Springer Nature 2018
This work is subject to copyright. All rights are reserved by the Publisher, whether the whole or part of the material is concerned, specifically the rights of translation, reprinting, reuse of illustrations, recitation, broadcasting, reproduction on microfilms or in any other physical way, and transmission or information storage and retrieval, electronic adaptation, computer software, or by similar or dissimilar methodology now known or hereafter developed.
The use of general descriptive names, registered names, trademarks, service marks, etc. in this publication does not imply, even in the absence of a specific statement, that such names are exempt from the relevant protective laws and regulations and therefore free for general use.
The publisher, the authors, and the editors are safe to assume that the advice and information in this book are believed to be true and accurate at the date of publication. Neither the publisher nor the authors or the editors give a warranty, express or implied, with respect to the material contained herein or for any errors or omissions that may have been made. The publisher remains neutral with regard to jurisdictional claims in published maps and institutional affiliations.

This Springer imprint is published by Springer Nature, under the registered company Springer International Publishing AG
The registered company address is: Gewerbestrasse 11, 6330 Cham, Switzerland

# Foreword

There are an increasing number of textbooks published over the last several decades in the field of anesthesiology. Each of them has attempted to fill a particular niche. *Anesthesiology: A Practical Approach* fills the niche of practical textbooks which help the reader in providing daily care to their patients. It is also geared to provide a pragmatic approach to patient care that helps train the reader as a consultant anesthesiologist and is therefore an excellent resource to prepare for oral examinations. Dr. Goudra, a clinical associate professor of anesthesiology and critical care at the Perelman School of Medicine at the University of Pennsylvania, has been a prolific academic and has already published several textbooks. He has assembled an international group of section editors and authors to ensure a broad perspective of best practices from the preoperative through postoperative care. The readers of this text will clearly be enlightened and prepared to care for patients on a daily basis and demonstrate proficiency on any oral examinations.

Philadelphia, PA, USA                                                                                         Lee A. Fleisher

# Preface

By virtue of being the cornerstone of medical practice, the specialty of anesthesiology continues to expand into areas few ever thought possible. As anesthesia providers, we evolve at a faster rate than any other specialty, especially when presented with new and more complex challenges. Surgeons continue to test our versatility and adaptability, but the demands posed by nonsurgical specialties continue to grow at an ever-increasing pace. In fact, in many major university teaching hospitals, including the Hospital of the University of Pennsylvania, the number of procedures performed outside the operating rooms exceeds traditional surgeries. Whereas there is a decline in surgeries like lung resections, there has been an increase in procedures performed in interventional bronchoscopy suites. While the face of gastrointestinal surgery has changed, endoscopic procedures continue to grow at an astronomical pace. The neuroradiologists and cardiologists continue to displace the surgeons and defy the anesthesia providers.

There is no dearth of good textbooks in the field of anesthesiology. In fact, subspecialty books abound including my own, *Out of Operating Room Anesthesia*. Though online availability of books/chapters has revolutionized the way we access information, there is still a need for a book that is subspecialty-focused. More specifically, the need for a book that incorporates anesthesia management of various surgical and medical procedures under one roof has been long awaited.

The current book, *Anesthesiology: A Practical Approach*, is designed to be useful for both the everyday anesthesia practitioner and the resident preparing for their exam. The book is divided into seven sections: The first six sections address specific procedures pertaining to cardiothoracic surgeries, out of operating room procedures, pediatric including neonatal and fetal surgeries, and obstetrics, vascular, and neurosurgeries. The last section deals with many surgeries that either cross into multiple specialties or are entirely unique.

Each chapter has information that will assist the anesthesia provider to tailor the anesthetic to the specific procedure. We attempt to summarize and present information in the form of tables whenever possible, so that residents or postgraduate students can efficiently extract information when preparing for exams. We also attempt to be as thorough as possible, so that the 83 chapters discuss almost every situation that could be tested. Every chapter can also be read in isolation.

I thank my section editors from the USA, the Great Britain, and India for shouldering this mammoth task. Michael Duggan, MD, and Elizabeth Duggan, MD, from Emory University Hospital have contributed and edited the sections on cardiothoracic and vascular anesthesia, respectively. The section on neuroanesthesia is edited by Hari Krovvidi, FRCA, from the Birmingham University Hospital, UK. Vidya Chidambaran, MD, from the Cincinnati Children's Hospital has edited the challenging section of pediatric anesthesia. Mark Powell, MD, from the University of Alabama at Birmingham, Birmingham, Alabama, provided his valuable input into the obstetric anesthesia section. Finally, I would like to thank Preet Mohinder Singh, MD, from AIIMS, India, for his assistance with the section "Out of Operating Room Anesthesia."

I am extremely grateful to the contributors from across the world. The invaluable insight and unique expertise brought by each contributor made this project possible. I also thank Joanna Renwick, editor of the clinical medicine section, and Abha Krishnan, project coordinator (Books) of Springer Nature, for their unrelenting support in ensuring the timely production of the book.

Finally, I would like to thank Lee A. Fleisher, MD, the Robert D. Dripps professor and chair of anesthesiology and critical care and professor of medicine at the University of Pennsylvania and the champion of evidence-based anesthesia, for his continued support.

| | |
|---|---|
| Philadelphia, PA, USA | Basavana G. Goudra |
| Atlanta, GA, USA | Michael Duggan |
| Cincinnati, OH, USA | Vidya Chidambaran |
| Birmingham, UK | Hari Prasad Krovvidi Venkata |
| Atlanta, GA, USA | Elizabeth Duggan |
| Birmingham, AL, USA | Mark Powell |
| New Delhi, Delhi, India | Preet Mohinder Singh |

# Contents

**Part I  Cardiothoracic Anesthesia**

1. **Anesthesia for Coronary Artery Bypass Grafting with and Without Cardiopulmonary Bypass** .................. 3
   Michael A. Evans and Mark Caridi-Scheible

2. **Anesthesia for Valve Replacement and Repair** ............... 15
   Terence Wallace

3. **Anesthesia for Congenital Heart Diseases in Adults** .......... 21
   Korrin Scott and Sarah Burke

4. **Anesthesia for Heart and Lung Transplantation** .............. 31
   Blaine E. Farmer and Igor O. Zhukov

5. **Anesthesia for Pulmonary Endarterectomy** ................... 41
   Cara Iorianni and Ellen Richter

6. **Anesthetic Management for Minimally Invasive Cardiac Surgery** ......................................... 49
   Julius Hamilton and Mark Caridi-Scheible

7. **Anesthesia for Transcatheter Aortic Valve Replacement (TAVR) and Other Catheter-Based Intracardiac Procedures** .................................. 59
   Ratna Vadlamudi

8. **Anesthetic Considerations in the Patient with an Implanted Cardiac Device** ....................... 67
   Keyur Trivedi and Kinjal M. Patel

9. **Anesthesia for Aortic Surgery** ............................. 75
   Mario Christopher DeAngelis and Michael Stuart Green

10. **Anesthesia for Lung Resection** ............................ 85
    Allison Bechtel

11. **Anesthesia for Video-Assisted Thoracoscopic Surgery** ........ 97
    Jared Roussel and Susan Smith

12. **Anesthesia for Mediastinoscopy and Mediastinal Surgery** ..... 107
    Philip L. Kalarickal and Chai-Lin Winchester

| 13 | **Anesthesia for Tracheal Surgery** .......................... 113
Philip L. Kalarickal and Stephanie Opusunju Ibekwe |
| --- | --- |
| 14 | **Anesthesia for Esophageal Surgery** ....................... 119
Christopher Ma and J. Kirk Edwards |
| 15 | **Anesthesia for Pleural and Chest Wall Surgery** .............. 131
Jonathan Rost, Jeffery Gerritsen, and Talia K. Ben-Jacob |
| 16 | **Anesthetic Implications for Management of Thoracic Trauma** .......................... 141
Abimbola Faloye |
| 17 | **Anesthesia for Thymectomy** ............................. 147
Christopher R. Hoffman and Michael Stuart Green |
| 18 | **Anesthesia Issues in Patients with VADs Presenting for Noncardiac Surgery** ................................ 155
Ahmed Awad, Alann Solina, Theresa Gerges, and Muhammad Muntazar |

## Part II  Out of Operating Room Anesthesia

| 19 | **Anesthesia for ERCP** .................................. 175
Basavana G. Goudra and Preet Mohinder Singh |
| --- | --- |
| 20 | **Anesthesia for Colonoscopy** ............................ 189
George A. Dumas |
| 21 | **Anesthesia for Bronchoscopic Procedures** .................. 199
Mona Sarkiss |
| 22 | **Anesthesia for Cardioversion** ............................ 215
Michele L. Sumler and McKenzie Hollon |
| 23 | **Anesthesia for Dental Procedures** ........................ 221
Carolyn Barbieri and Meghan Whitley |
| 24 | **Anesthesia for Electroconvulsive Therapy** .................. 229
Paul Su and Jonathan Z. Pan |
| 25 | **Anesthesia for MRI and CT** ............................. 239
Gregory E. R. Weller |
| 26 | **Radiotherapy and Anesthesia** ........................... 255
Bharathi Gourkanti, David Mulvihill, Jill Kalariya, and Yue Li |
| 27 | **Anesthesia for Office Based Cosmetic Procedures** ........... 265
Sally S. Dawood and Michael Stuart Green |
| 28 | **Anesthesia for Upper GI Endoscopy Including Advanced Endoscopic Procedures** ................................ 273
Mary Elizabeth McAlevy and John Levenick |

## Part III  Pediatric Anesthesia

**29** **Anesthesia for Fetal Intervention and Surgery** ............... 287
Jagroop Mavi

**30** **Anesthesia for Neurosurgical Procedures**................... 293
Jaya L. Varadarajan

**31** **Anesthesia for Thoracic Surgery**........................ 305
David S. Beebe and Kumar G. Belani

**32** **Anesthesia for Specific Cardiac Lesions: Right-to Left Shunts**................................... 311
J. R. Paquin, J. E. Lam, and E. P. Lin

**33** **Aortic Stenosis: Anesthesia Considerations** .................. 323
Benjamin Kloesel and Kumar Belani

**34** **Anesthesia for Spinal Surgery in Children**................... 329
Ali Kandil, Deepika S. Rao, and Mohamed Mahmoud

**35** **Anesthesia for Pediatric Plastic and Craniofacial Surgery**..... 341
Shelley Joseph George and Michael Stuart Green

**36** **Anesthesia for Ears, Nose, and Throat Surgery**.............. 349
Edward Cooper, Tobias Everett, James Koziol, and Rajeev Subramanyam

**37** **Anesthesia for Ophthalmological Procedures** ................ 363
Charlotte Walter

**38** **Anesthesia for Neonatal Emergencies: General Principles**..... 369
Jakob Guenther and Kumar G. Belani

**39** **Anesthesia for Tracheoesophageal Fistula** ................... 381
Pornswan Ngamprasertwong

**40** **Anesthesia for Congenital Diaphragmatic Hernia**............ 387
Bobby Das, Nathaniel Lata, and Ximena Soler

**41** **Omphalocele and Gastroschisis**.......................... 395
Wendy Nguyen and Kumar Belani

**42** **Anesthesia for Hypertrophic Pyloric Stenosis** ................ 403
Trung Du

**43** **Anesthesia for Intestinal Obstruction**...................... 413
Ilana Fromer and Kumar G. Belani

**44** **Anesthesia for Epidermolysis Bullosa**...................... 421
Eric Wittkugel and Ali Kandil

**45** **Anesthesia for Children with Cerebral Palsy**................ 429
Ilana Fromer and Kumar Belani

| 46 | **Anesthesia for Nuss Procedures (Pectus Deformity)** ......... 435 |
|---|---|
| | Vanessa A. Olbrecht |

| 47 | **Pediatric Pain Management** ............................. 445 |
|---|---|
| | Jennifer Hickman and Jaya L. Varadarajan |

| 48 | **Pulmonary Hypertension** ............................... 457 |
|---|---|
| | Benjamin Kloesel and Kumar Belani |

| 49 | **Anesthesia Considerations in a Premie** ..................... 463 |
|---|---|
| | Arundathi Reddy and Edwin A. Bowe |

| 50 | **Anesthesia for Ex-Utero Intra-Partum Procedures** ............ 473 |
|---|---|
| | Magdy Takla, Irwin Gratz, and Bharathi Gourkanti |

### Part IV   Obstetric Anesthesia

| 51 | **Anesthesia for Cesarean Delivery** ......................... 487 |
|---|---|
| | Carrie M. Polin, Ashley A. Hambright, and Patrick O. McConville |

| 52 | **Anesthesia for Non-delivery Obstetric Procedures** ........... 497 |
|---|---|
| | John C. Coffman, Blair H. Herndon, Mitesh Thakkar, and Kasey Fiorini |

| 53 | **Anesthesia and Major Obstetric Hemorrhage** ................ 517 |
|---|---|
| | Tekuila Carter, Yasser Sakawi, and Michelle Tubinis |

| 54 | **Anesthesia for Medical Termination of Pregnancy** ........... 527 |
|---|---|
| | Patricia Dalby and Erica Coffin |

| 55 | **Anesthesia and Hypertensive Emergencies** .................. 535 |
|---|---|
| | Oksana Klimkina |

### Part V   Neuroanesthesia

| 56 | **Supratentorial Masses: Anesthetic Considerations** ........... 547 |
|---|---|
| | Marc D. Fisicaro, Amy Shah, and Paul Audu |

| 57 | **Anesthetic Management for Posterior Fossa Surgery** ......... 555 |
|---|---|
| | Naginder Singh |

| 58 | **Anesthetic Management of Cerebral Aneurysm Surgery (Intracranial Vascular Surgeries)** ......................... 563 |
|---|---|
| | Mohammed Asif Arshad and Paul Southall |

| 59 | **Anesthetic Considerations for Surgical Resection of Brain Arteriovenous Malformations** ........................... 573 |
|---|---|
| | Catalin Ezaru |

| 60 | **Awake Craniotomy** ..................................... 581 |
|---|---|
| | Ronan Mukherjee and Mohammed Al-Tamimi |

| 61 | Functional Brain Surgery (Stereotactic Surgery, Deep Brain Stimulation) | 589 |

Ilyas Qazi and Hannah Church

| 62 | Perioperative Management of Adult Patients with Severe Head Injury | 597 |

Adam Low

## Part VI Vascular Anesthesia

| 63 | Anaesthesia for Endovascular Aortic Aneurysm Repair (EVAR) | 607 |

Milad Sharifpour and Salman Hemani

| 64 | Anesthesia for Open AAA | 615 |

Jimmy C. Yao and Milad Sharifpour

| 65 | Anesthesia for Lower Extremity Bypass | 625 |

Jay Sanford and Brendan Atkinson

| 66 | Anesthesia for Nephrectomy with Vena Cava Thrombectomy | 635 |

Michael A. Evans and Francis A. Wolf

| 67 | Anesthesia for Carotid Endarterectomy | 645 |

Abigail Monnig and Gaurav Budhrani

| 68 | Anesthesia for AV Fistulas (Upper Extremity) | 657 |

Kavitha A. Mathew and Joseph V. Schneider

| 69 | Trauma Anesthesia | 667 |

Michael A. Evans and Richard B. Johnson

| 70 | Anesthesia for Pheochromocytoma and Glomus Jugulare | 679 |

Courtney C. Elder and Kavitha A. Mathew

| 71 | Anesthesia for TIPS | 689 |

Ricky Matkins and W. Thomas Daniel III

| 72 | Anesthesia for Liver Transplantation | 697 |

Philip L. Kalarickal and Daniel J. Viox

| 73 | Anesthesia for Kidney Transplantation | 707 |

Ellen Cho and Gaurav P. Patel

## Part VII Others

| 74 | Anesthesia Issues in Patients with Obstructive Sleep Apnea | 719 |

Amélie Dallaire and Mandeep Singh

| 75 | Anesthesia for Major Orthopedic Surgeries | 729 |

George Pan and Bradley Reid

| 76 | Anesthesia for Urological Procedures | 741 |

Hussam Ghabra and Susan A. Smith

| 77 | **Organ Harvesting and the Role of Anesthesiologist** .......... 755 |
|---|---|
| | Michael R. Schwartz and Erin W. Pukenas |

| 78 | **Anesthesia and Burns**................................. 765 |
|---|---|
| | Clare R. Herlihy and Cassandra Barry |

| 79 | **Anesthesia for Robot Assisted Gynecological Procedures**...... 777 |
|---|---|
| | Eilish M. Galvin and Henri J. D. de Graaff |

| 80 | **Anesthesia Issues in Geriatrics** .......................... 795 |
|---|---|
| | Nalini Kotekar, Anshul Shenkar, and Adarsh A. Hegde |

| 81 | **Anesthesia for Weight Reduction Surgery** .................. 827 |
|---|---|
| | Angelo Andonakakis and Kathleen Kwiatt |

| 82 | **Anesthesia for TURP** .................................. 845 |
|---|---|
| | Maimouna Bah and Michael Stuart Green |

| 83 | **Anesthesia for Major Joint Surgery** ...................... 851 |
|---|---|
| | Scott R. Coleman and Michael Stuart Green |

**Index**..................................................... 859

# About the Editors

**Basavana G. Goudra, M.D., F.R.C.A., F.C.A.R.C.S.I.** the principal editor of the book *Anesthesiology: A Practical Approach*, is a clinical associate professor of anesthesiology and critical care medicine at the Hospital of the University of Pennsylvania, Philadelphia, USA. He is an internationally recognized expert in the area of out of operating room anesthesia, specifically in the field of gastrointestinal endoscopy. Dr. Goudra graduated from Bangalore Medical College, Bangalore, India, and completed his residency at the Jawaharlal Nehru Institute of Medical Education and Research, Pondicherry, India. After further training in the Republic of Ireland and Cincinnati Children's Hospital, Cincinnati, USA, he was appointed as a consultant anesthetist at the Russells Hall Hospital, UK. In 2008, he was appointed as a member of the faculty in the Hospital of the University of Pennsylvania. He has over 60 PubMed-indexed publications that include scientific papers, case reports, meta-analysis, reviews, and editorials on a wide range of anesthesia- and pain-related topics. He lectures at the American Society of Anesthesiology annual meetings on a regular basis. He has invented airway devices including the "Goudra Bite Block" and "Goudra Mask Airway," which will improve the safety of upper gastrointestinal endoscopy in the years to come. He is also working on a number of other projects in the area of graduate medical student and resident education. The book *Out of Operating Room Anesthesia: A Comprehensive Review*, edited by Dr. Goudra, has been acclaimed by reviewers and is popularly used in the field.

**Michael Duggan, M.D., F.A.S.E.** is an assistant professor at Emory University Department of Anesthesiology, where he is the director of cardiothoracic anesthesiology and perioperative echocardiography. He gained his Primary ABA Certification in Anesthesiology and NBE Advanced Perioperative TEE Certification in 2011. He had previously completed an internship in internal medicine at Virginia Commonwealth University Health System and a residency and fellowship at the University of Pennsylvania Health System. He then became clinical assistant professor at Thomas Jefferson University Department of Anesthesiology prior to his appointment at Emory University.

**Vidya Chidambaran, M.B.B.S., M.D.** is an associate professor of anesthesia and perioperative pain at Cincinnati Children's Hospital Medical Center and University of Cincinnati College of Medicine. She completed her medical degree at Bangalore Medical College, India in 1996 and her MD in Anesthesia from Kasturba Medical College, India in 2000. She then completed an internship, residency and fellowship in the USA, at Jackson Memorial Hospital, Brookdale University Hospital and John Hopkins Hospital, respectively. She became Anesthesia Board certified in 2008 and Pediatric Anesthesia Board certified in 2014.

**Hari Prasad Krovvidi Venkata, M.B.B.S., M.D., F.R.C.A.** gained his medical degree from Gandhi Medical College, Hyderabad, India, in 1996 and his MD in anesthesia from the Postgraduate Institute of Medical Education and Research, Chandigarh, India, in 1999. He completed various senior house office roles in India and the UK, before becoming a specialist registrar at Birmingham School of Anaesthesia, UK, where he is now a consultant in neuroanesthesia.

**Elizabeth Duggan, M.D.** is an assistant professor at Emory University School of Medicine in Atlanta, Georgia. She completed her internship at Duke University Medical Center and residency training at the University of Pennsylvania. Additionally, she spent an additional postgraduate training year as a liver transplant fellow at the University of Pennsylvania. Dr. Duggan joined the faculty of Thomas Jefferson University as the director of hepatobiliary anesthesia and later transitioned to Emory SOM. While on staff at Emory University Hospital, she has held the roles of director of vascular anesthesia and medical director of the PACU and, most recently, has been appointed the chief of service for the general, vascular, neuroanesthesia, and kidney/liver transplant service. Her primary clinical roles are as a member of the liver transplant and vascular teams; her research focus lies within perioperative outcomes specifically in obstructive sleep apnea and stress hyperglycemia.

**Mark Powell, M.D.** gained his medical degree from the University of Alabama at Birmingham in 2008, where he also completed his internal medicine internship, anesthesiology residency, and obstetric anesthesiology fellowship. He gained his American Board of Anesthesiology certification in 2013. He is now an assistant professor at this institution and program director of the Obstetric Anesthesiology Fellowship.

**Preet Mohinder Singh, M.D.** is an assistant professor of anesthesiology, pain medicine, and critical care at the All India Institute of Medical Sciences (AIIMS), New Delhi, India. After completing his residency from AIIMS, Delhi, he joined the Department of Anesthesia as a faculty. His main area of focus is outcomes research, statistics in medicine, and out of operating room anesthesia. He has been a part of many research projects and published extensively in the above areas. He is also the co-editor of the book *Out of Operating Room Anesthesia: A Comprehensive Review*.

# Part I
# Cardiothoracic Anesthesia

# Anesthesia for Coronary Artery Bypass Grafting with and Without Cardiopulmonary Bypass

Michael A. Evans and Mark Caridi-Scheible

CABG and OPCAB patients have very similar demographics. The average patient is 66 years old, male, and Caucasian. Approximately 45–50% of patients present electively for surgery with both approaches. In-hospital mortality does not appreciably differ between CABG and OPCAB, at 3.0% and 3.2% respectively. OPCAB may be associated with a minor but statistically significant increase in hospital days (0.6 of a day) and overall cost ($1497) [1].

## Indications for Surgery Versus Percutaneous Coronary Intervention (PCI)

There has been substantial research regarding the selection of appropriate candidates for surgical revascularization in the presence of coronary artery disease (CAD). Table 1.1 is dedicated to the clinical trials comparing outcomes in PCI versus CABG. In multi-vessel disease, CABG and OPCAB often provide superior outcomes to PCI. In low-complexity lesions, PCI is often non-inferior to CABG. Overall, in comparison to PCI, CABG and OPCAB show a decreased need for repeat revascularization procedures but often have a higher rate of cerebrovascular accidents (CVA).

## Preoperative Risk Reduction

The cardiac surgical population has been one in which preoperative "preconditioning" has been shown to decrease morbidity and mortality. A 2012 Cochrane review showed that preoperative physical therapy decreased postoperative pulmonary complications in elective cardiac surgery [6]. Cessation of tobacco use four or more weeks prior to cardiothoracic surgery is likely to reduce complications [7]. In elective cases, a multidisciplinary approach involving a patient's cardiologist, cardiothoracic surgeon, and anesthesiologist must include preoperative optimization that comprehensively evaluates and identifies predictors of intra- and postoperative complications and seeks to correct them. In addition to a standard pre-anesthetic evaluation (history, physical, interpretation of existing diagnostic testing), bypass surgery patients require an evaluation specifically focusing on: myocardial ischemia and the potential for re-vascularization, ventricular function with notable regional wall motion abnormalities and the carotid arteries for atherosclerotic burden. In non-elective surgeries, such as in patients with recent myocardial infarction who remained hemodynamically stable, other factors such as systemic hepariniza-

M. A. Evans, M.D.
Department of Anesthesiology, Emory University School of Medicine, Emory University Hospital, Atlanta, GA, USA
e-mail: michaelevans@emory.edu

M. Caridi-Scheible, M.D. (✉)
Department of Anesthesiology, Emory University School of Medicine, Atlanta, GA, USA
e-mail: mscheib@emory.edu

Table 1.1 Selection of ideal candidates for operative revascularization: CABG/OPCAB versus PCI

| Name of trial | Year | Study design | Summary |
|---|---|---|---|
| SYNTAX [2] | 2009 | 1800 patients with 3-vessel or left main CAD. Randomized to PCI or CABG. Multicenter, parallel-group, randomized, controlled trial | Major cardiovascular events more frequent in PCI arm. Main contributor was need for repeat procedure for revascularization in PCI patients. CABG patients had more CVAs. Data suggested PCI and CABG were equivalent in low-complexity lesions |
| FREEDOM [3] | 2012 | 1900 patients with diabetes mellitus and angiographically-confirmed multi-vessel CAD. Open-label, multicenter, randomized controlled trial | Among the study population, CABG decreases death rate and rate of myocardial infarction when compared to PCI. Increased rate of CVA in the CABG arm |
| BEST [4] | 2015 | 880 patients with multi-vessel CAD. Randomized to PCI with second generation DES or CABG. Prospective, open-label, randomized controlled trial | PCI with drug-eluting stents (second generation) instead of CABG in the study population yielded 4.7% absolute increase in death, myocardial infarction (MI), or need for revascularization at study endpoint |
| EXCEL [5] | 2016 | 1905 patients with left main CAD. Randomized to PCI with second generation DES or CABG. Multicenter, open-label, randomized controlled trial | PCI found to be non-inferior at 3 years with regard to death, myocardial infarction, and stroke |

tion and antiplatelet therapy must be examined. These patients have a higher risk of surgical complications, some of which depend on timing of surgery. In patients that have surgery within three days of ST-elevation myocardial infarction (STEMI), there is a 33% reoperation rate, whereas when surgical revascularization occurs after three days, the reoperation rate is 3% [8]. In emergent cases, such as patients with cardiogenic shock after STEMI that have surgery within 6 h of presentation, in-hospital mortality has been shown to be 10.8%. Female sex, preoperative cardiogenic shock, preoperative troponin-I level, and timing of surgery have all been shown to predict morbidity and mortality in this population [9]. Performing an emergent procedure is indicated in active non-correctable ischemia, cardiogenic shock, failure or complication of PCI, and mechanical complications of ischemia such as left ventricular rupture and acute mitral regurgitation.

## Principles of Management

The dominant management principle for these patients rests with the fact that they are in need of revascularization and as such, strategies to increase oxygen supply and decrease demand are of paramount importance. Standard induction strategies are modified, and pre-induction monitors differ from patients that do not possess inducible ischemia. Maintenance of consistent perfusion pressure is critical to ensuring oxygen supply to susceptible myocardium. Avoidance of tachycardia allows the anesthesiologist to minimize cardiac demand, and proper depth of anesthesia and analgesia prior to airway instrumentation helps to avoid demand ischemia.

## Monitoring

All cardiac surgery is performed utilizing standard American Society of Anesthesiologists (ASA) monitors. Additionally, invasive arterial and central venous access are required, along with a central and peripheral site for temperature monitors, and a catheter to drain the bladder. Often, processed electroencephalography is utilized, and select patients may benefit from cerebral oximetry (near-infrared spectroscopy, NIRS) if concern for intraoperative cerebral hypoperfusion may arise. Point-of-care blood testing is also required, which allows the anesthesiologist and perfusionist to obtain both serial activated clotting times (ACTs) and arterial blood gas analysis. In select patients, transesophageal echocardiography (TEE) and/or a pulmonary artery catheter will be utilized for additional monitoring.

Coronary artery bypass surgeries necessitate these invasive monitors because critical coronary artery disease can lead to myocardial ischemia and beat-to-beat hemodynamic monitoring allows for the ability to rapidly correct any perfusion deficits. Surgical re-vascularization also involves manipulations of the heart and great vessels that lead to drastic changes in hemodynamics which may not be experienced in other procedures.

An intra-arterial catheter is typically placed prior to the induction of anesthesia. The radial artery is commonly chosen for cannulation for several reasons: a dual blood supply to the hand also includes the ulnar artery, and the course of the radial artery is relatively straight and superficial leading to a relative ease of insertion. Communication with the surgical team is paramount prior to placing a radial arterial line, as the radial artery is often utilized as a vascular conduit in coronary artery bypass surgery.

The type of central venous catheter used in these surgeries varies, but placing an introducer sheath will allow for the optional placement of a pulmonary artery catheter (PAC) into the same vein if deemed appropriate. If a pulmonary artery catheter is not needed, a separate infusion catheter may be placed through the sheath. It is often acceptable to place a central venous line after induction of anesthesia, unless a patient would be more safely anesthetized with central access in place. Patients with poor peripheral access may qualify for a pre-induction central line, along with patients in cardiogenic shock or exhibiting preoperative hemodynamic instability.

There is no clear method in choosing which patients might benefit from placement of a pulmonary artery catheter. A recent retrospective observational study of patients receiving primary CABG at a single center showed no harm nor benefit in managing CABG patients with a PAC when undergoing a primary CABG [10].

However, it did show that utilization of a PAC added significant cost to the patient's hospitalization. Randomized controlled trials in high risk surgical patients have repeatedly shown no benefit to ICU management directed by PACs, but these studies were not exclusive to cardiac surgical patients [11, 12]. Many anesthesiologists choose to utilize a PAC in patients with a reduced ejection fraction or valvular heart disease though supporting data for this approach is lacking.

The ASA and the Society of Cardiovascular Anesthesiologists (SCA) recommend utilization of transesophageal echocardiography (TEE) in all open-heart and thoracic aortic surgical procedures, and suggests that TEE be considered for all coronary artery bypass graft surgeries [13]. Additionally, the American College of Cardiology supports this recommendation, as CABG is a class IIa indication for TEE monitoring [14].

## Oxygen Supply and Demand

Table 1.2 includes a summary of modifiable hemodynamic aspects that contribute to optimization of oxygen delivery and minimization of demand.

Based on the variables listed in Table 1.2, several conclusions can be made. Tachycardia is perhaps the most detrimental hemodynamic parameter that can be modified by the anesthesiologist, as it both decreases oxygen supply and increases oxygen demand. Within a standard range, cardiac output depends linearly on heart rate such that severe bradycardia is harmful as it sacrifices oxygen delivery. A slow to normal heart rate is therefore optimal. Normotension is

**Table 1.2** Modifiable aspects in myocardial ischemia

| Hemodynamic variables that decrease myocardial oxygen demand | Hemodynamic variables that increase myocardial oxygen supply |
|---|---|
| Decreased heart rate | Decreased heart rate |
| Decreased contractility | Increased coronary blood flow [multifactorial] |
| Decreased afterload/decreased LV wall stress in systole [multifactorial] | Increased $CaO_2$ [increase in Hgb & $SaO_2$] |

also desired, as diastolic blood pressure strongly influences coronary perfusion pressure along with left ventricular end-diastolic pressure. Supra-normal blood pressure often cause harm because increases in afterload and systolic blood pressure contribute to left ventricular wall stress and subsequently increase oxygen demand in the myocardial tissue at risk.

## Coronary Artery Bypass Grafting Utilizing Cardiopulmonary Bypass (CABG)

Historically, the first successful utilization of cardiopulmonary bypass for surgery in humans was in 1953 when surgeon John Gibbon closed an atrial septal defect [15]. The techniques and technology have evolved greatly since that time, and CPB has been utilized for a plethora of cardiac and noncardiac surgeries. CPB is typically performed via midline sternotomy, but peripheral or alternative cannulation is possible in the presence of complicating anatomic factors.

## Preoperative Anesthetic Management

For elective CABG patients, special care should be taken to perform a physical exam on the day of surgery, as patients' comorbid conditions should be optimized for their procedure. Some anesthesiologists may prefer placement of central access preoperatively depending on patient factors and institutional preference. All patients generally will receive a preoperative arterial line and large-bore intravenous access. All patients should be screened for contraindications to TEE placement, even if intraoperative TEE is not initially planned. Lastly, expectations regarding postoperative management, such as extubation occurring in the operating room or the ICU, should be discussed with the patient and their family if applicable. Patients requiring heparin or nitroglycerin infusions for active or dynamic myocardial ischemia should not have these infusions stopped prior to induction.

## Induction and Maintenance of Anesthesia

There are several approaches to safe induction of anesthesia in patients with known coronary artery disease. Historically, an opioid-heavy induction technique was utilized, as opioids alone don't routinely depress myocardial function and blood pressure is usually preserved. Opioids also blunt the sympathetic response to laryngoscopy and intubation of the trachea. If opioids are chosen as the primary induction agent, a second agent that contains amnestic properties must also be administered to reduce the chance of recall. However, current trends for rapid post-operative emergence and neurologic evaluation, along with known complications of rapid high-dose opioid administration (chest wall rigidity and bradycardia), make the classic opioid-dominant method less common.

A multimodal approach to induction is typically utilized including judicious use of propofol, etomidate, or ketamine combined with a moderate dose of opioid and lidocaine. Throughout the perioperative period and specifically during induction, titration of a vasoactive agent such as phenylephrine or norepinephrine helps ensure appropriate coronary perfusion pressures. A beta-blocking agent such as esmolol should also be readily available to control the critical variable of heart rate, as discussed earlier. Neuromuscular blockade is typically utilized to facilitate tracheal intubation.

Typically, anesthesia is maintained with a volatile inhalational anesthetic although there is no absolute contraindication to total intravenous anesthetic (TIVA) if preferred. There is some data to suggest that volatile anesthetics may be cardio-protective [16], however the TIVA styles in the meta-analysis were variable and it appears that propofol-based TIVA may be protective as well [17]. Surgical stimulation varies tremendously throughout the procedure, and depth of anesthesia along with anticipatory analgesia must be titrated continuously prior to cardiopulmonary bypass. A baseline TEE evaluating regional myocardial performance, volume status, valvular heart disease, presence of intracardiac shunts and atherosclerotic disease of the aorta is performed prior to initiation of CPB.

## Intraoperative Anesthetic Management: Pre-bypass Period

Because of the length of surgery, hypothermia, and non-pulsatile flow, cardiac surgery patients may be at increased risk of nerve and other positioning injuries. Extreme care should be taken to pad and position a patient appropriately prior to skin preparation and draping by the surgical team, as the anesthesiologist will have limited access to extremities with the patient in the supine position with arms tucked at their sides. This includes the lower extremities which are often prepped and draped for saphenous vein harvest.

The most important goal for an anesthesiologist in the pre-bypass period is to prevent and treat myocardial ischemia. The tools utilized for ischemia monitoring include continuous electrocardiogram, transesophageal echocardiogram, and surveillance of changes in central pressures via transduction of a central venous line or PAC. ST-segment changes in the electrocardiogram is a non-invasive and easily-visualized monitor for new-onset cardiac ischemia. Intraoperative TEE monitoring is a valid diagnostic tool for ischemia associated with left ventricular systolic dysfunction or regional wall motion abnormalities (RMWAs). Lastly, abrupt increases in central venous or pulmonary artery pressures may signify that ischemia is affecting systolic or diastolic performance.

Fluid restriction prior to CPB is a key concern. Prior to initiation of CPB, the circuit requires a priming volume which will dilute the patient's hematocrit. Thus, further hemodilution of a patient's circulating red cell mass before initiation may drive the hematocrit lower than desired. As mentioned earlier, oxygen content is of critical importance in these patients with myocardium at ischemic risk. If the patient's hematocrit is sufficiently low preoperatively, several units of blood may need to be added to the bypass circuit priming solution. Hydroxyethyl starch and other non-albumin colloids should be avoided, as they have been shown to increase blood loss, postoperative acute kidney injury (AKI), reoperation due to bleeding, and blood product transfusion requirements [18, 19].

## Surgical Principles

Prior to cardiopulmonary bypass, the surgical team must perform sternotomy, expose the heart and harvest any arterial and venous conduits required to bypass diseased coronary vessels. Sternotomy provides direct access to the heart and great vessels, facilitating cannulation and access to the internal mammary artery (IMA) if it is to be utilized. Close communication with the surgical team during this time is essential as the anesthesiologist may be required to pause ventilation and temporarily deflate the lungs in order to avoid inadvertent lung injury. During takedown of the IMA, surgical exposure may be ameliorated by decreasing the patient's tidal volumes and reducing positive end expiratory pressure (PEEP). Small doses of heparin (typically 5000 units) are generally administered during harvest to prevent fibrin deposition in the bypass conduits. Some surgeons may prefer to avoid any heparinization during sternotomy in order to minimize blood loss and prevent excessive bleeding from complicating their exposure.

## Initiation of Cardiopulmonary Bypass

Before going on CPB, cannulae must be inserted by the surgeon to drain venous blood to the pump and reinfuse it into the arterial system. To prevent coagulation of blood within the cannulae, bypass machine and oxygenator (a catastrophic event), the patient must be systemically anticoagulated. Typically, 300–400 units of heparin per kilogram of body weight is bolused after dissection and exposure of the heart is completed. Argatroban or bivalirudin are alternative agents in the case of heparin allergies. Point of care (POC) activated clotting time (ACT) is generally used to monitor and re-dose anticoagulation. Goal ACT may vary by institution, however greater than 400 s is a common goal. Initiation of an antifibrinolytic infusion such as of tranexamic acid (TXA) or aminocaproic acid is currently recommended [20, 21]. Heparin resistance should be suspected if goal ACT is not achieved and administration of antithrombin III should be considered [22].

Traditionally, an aortic cannula is placed into the ascending aorta proximal to the innominate artery and distal to the planned location of the aortic cross-clamp (Fig. 1.1). In order to avoid unintended aortic dissection or intramural hematoma (IMH), the blood pressure is lowered via pharmacologic means or positioning (reverse Trendelenburg) prior to aortic cannulation. After the cannula is secured, the perfusionist will test the arterial flow to ensure proper line pressure and verify placement. Following a successful line test the arterial pressures can be normalized. Venous cannulation typically proceeds with atriotomy via the right atrium and insertion of the venous cannula into the inferior vena cava (IVC). Retrograde autologous priming (RAP) then commences, which consists of permissive backbleeding into the CPB circuit to reduce the amount of fluid needed to prime the circuit. This drainage rapidly decreases intravascular volume, so positioning manipulations (Trendelenburg) or temporary pharmacologic support with pressors may be indicated at this time. The pump is then activated and the flow is gradually increased until acceptable output is achieved (typically a cardiac index >2.2 L/min/m$^2$). Maintenance of anesthesia is generally achieved by a vaporizer attached to the oxygenator of the bypass circuit, so it is important to confirm with the perfusionist that their vaporizer is delivering the desired amount of anesthetic. The anesthesiologist will stop the ventilator and turn off their own vaporizer once the full transition of flow from the bypass machine is confirmed by the perfusionist.

Several other steps take place after achieving full flow on CPB. A means of cardioplegia administration must be provided, most commonly via an antegrade cannula placed in the aortic root. However, as delivery of antegrade cardioplegia relies on some forward patency of the coronaries, in some cases the surgeon may also choose to place a retrograde catheter into the coronary sinus to deliver cardioplegia through the coronary venous system. Next, the mean arterial pressure is lowered and the aorta is cross-clamped by the surgeon. Immediately following placement of the cross-clamp, cardioplegia is given to arrest the heart. An empty heart with complete and rapid cardiac arrest is crucial to ensure optimal myocardial protection.

The basic steps of the operation proceed in the following order:

- Patient is cooled to a target temperature (typically 32–34 °C)
- Diseased coronaries are opened distal to the blockages
- Grafts are sewn to target coronary vessels ("distal anastomoses")
- Patient Rewarmed
- Aorta Unclamped
- Partial Clamp Applied to Ascending Aorta
- Free end of grafts sewn to proximal aorta ("proximal anastomoses")
- De-airing of Ascending Aorta and Grafts
- Partial Clamp Removed
- Weaning of CPB

## On-Pump Anesthetic Management

While on pump, the perfusionist is generally managing acute changes in hemodynamics by manipulating pump flows and bolusing vaso-

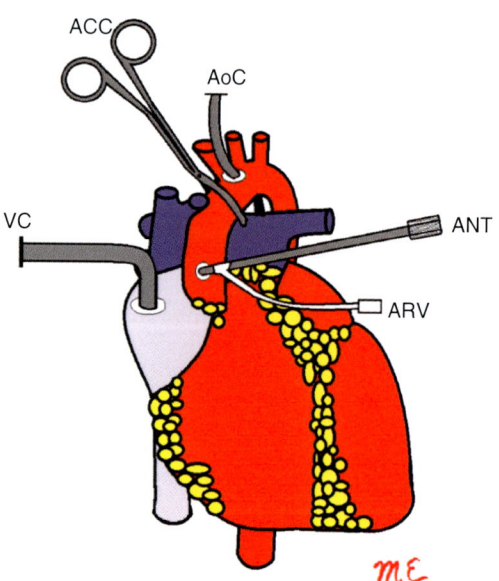

**Fig. 1.1** Cardiac instrumentation. *ACC* aortic cross clamp, *AoC* aortic cannula, *ANT* antegrade cardioplegia cannula, *ARV* aortic root vent, *VC* venous cannula

pressors directly into the circuit. Variability in blood pressure is to be expected as a result of requested pump flow alterations and delivery of cardioplegia which is often vasodilatory. It should be noted that despite improvements in circuit materials and pump technology, the bypass machine can induce a significant inflammatory response in the patient that results in persistent vasoplegia. For these less acute hemodynamic changes, the anesthesiologist may be required to titrate background infusions of vasopressors. The anesthesiologist must continue to monitor the patient carefully and maintain good communication with the perfusionist and surgeon to manage these issues. Hyperglycemia is often induced as part of the inflammatory response and should be managed via an insulin infusion. Preparation for the separation from bypass, including the setup of inotropic infusions and the future need for hemostatic blood products, should be accomplished during this period. As the bypass circuit and cell-conservation systems consume platelets and plasma-circulating factors, these factors should be considered in the assessment for necessary hemostatic blood products post-bypass. Algorithms for this are highly institution and patient-population dependent and beyond the scope of this chapter. Management of anticoagulation is generally done by the perfusionist, but the anesthesiologist should remain aware of the total dose of heparin administered.

## Separation from CPB

Prior to separating from bypass, the heart must be adequately recovered and prepared to resume full circulatory support for the body. The criteria for this are that the patient be completely rewarmed, that the heart has resumed normal rate and rhythm and that adequate time (generally at least 10 min) has elapsed since release of the cross-clamp for adequate coronary reperfusion. Drugs such as lidocaine and esmolol are typically given by the perfusionist before release of the clamp to prevent malignant arrhythmias, but sometimes defibrillation is required. Despite adequate reperfusion time, significant myocardial stunning may still be present either from residual cardioplegia or prior ischemia. This stunning can be overcome with use of inotropic agents, the selection of which include norepinephrine, dobutamine, epinephrine or milrinone. Epicardial pacing should also be considered if the heart is unable to achieve acceptable rate.

Once criteria are met, separation from bypass can begin. Depending on institution, this may be directed by the anesthesiologist or the surgeon, but in all scenarios clear communication amongst perfusion, surgery and anesthesia is critical for success. The process of weaning from CPB involves slowly impeding venous drainage to allow pre-load to return to the heart while slowly reducing pump flows. The heart's tolerance of this process should be monitored by direct visualization, by TEE when possible and by close observation of filling pressures on central line or PAC. For a closed-chamber procedure such as coronary bypass, residual air in the heart is not typically expected so excessive de-airing maneuvers are not required unless air is visualized on TEE. Once it is clear the heart is tolerating minimal circulatory support, the pump flow is stopped completely. The venous cannula is typically removed first and any residual blood volume left in the pump reservoir is slowly reinfused via the arterial cannula. The blood pressure is then lowered to a systolic pressure of 90–100 mmHg and the aortic cannula is removed. Heparin reversal with protamine is accomplished, the dosing for which is also institution dependent but is based on total heparin administered and should achieve ACT level close to baseline. Slow administration is important to avoid a protamine reaction and hypotension.

Following acceptable hemostasis at all anastomoses and surgical sites in the thorax, the chest is then closed. In most cases, the patient will then be transported directly to the ICU intubated. However, for uncomplicated surgeries where the patients are not on significant support, extubation in the OR is being increasingly considered. This decision should be made following close communication with the surgical team.

## Postoperative Management and Complications of CABG

For isolated CABG's, current Society of Thoracic Surgeons (STS) metrics call for rapid wake-up and extubation within 24 h of leaving the operating room. The anesthesiologist should be mindful of these goals when administering additional paralytic, analgesic or amnestic agents towards the end of the case.

A multitude of complications of CABG must be surveilled in the immediate postoperative period. Complications include post-cardiotomy ventricular failure, post-operative bleeding and need for emergent re-exploration, post-perfusion syndrome, atrial and ventricular arrhythmias, stroke, pleural effusions and infection. Initial monitoring for these complications is recommended to occur in the ICU setting where 1:2 nurse to patient ratio and continuous central monitoring of vital signs is available. This is changing with minimally invasive procedures that may be fast-tracked to standard surgical ward care, but for procedures requiring sternotomy ICU recovery remains recommended.

## Off-Pump Coronary Artery Bypass Grafting (OPCAB)

### Surgical Principles

Many of the details of pre-, intra- and postoperative management are similar between on-pump and off-pump procedures. We will discuss the relevant differences (summarized in Table 1.3), but otherwise it should otherwise be assumed that management is the same as described above. The core principle of the OPCAB is to avoid the complications of vasoplegia, myocardial stunning and ventricular failure that result from CPB. Additional benefits may include reduced bleeding due to less hemodilution and lower level of heparinization, along with bypass-induced consumptive coagulopathy. The overall benefit of the OPCAB is controversial although there is data to demonstrate improved outcomes in certain high-risk patients [23].

The technique for OPCAB involves positioning the beating heart to allow exposure of the affected vessel and stabilizing the small portion of the beating heart required to make an individual distal anastomosis. A variety of commercial devices are available, but fundamentally utilize external suction on the heart to position the apex in any permutation—including lifted up and out of the chest to expose the back of the heart. The vessel is then exposed and a suction device placed on either side of the vessel to hold that small portion of the heart in place. The distal end of the graft is then sewn to the vessel. Because blood is still being supplied to the coronary, a tourniquet is placed proximal to the anastomosis to prevent bleeding when the artery is opened. This tourniquet may induce ischemia in the supplied territory. Holding the heart in abnormal positions as

**Table 1.3** Major differences in anesthetic management of CABG and OPCAB

| Item | CABG on CPB | OPCAB |
| --- | --- | --- |
| Temperature management | Passive hypothermia pre-bypass, active hypothermia on pump, aggressive active re-warming just before and after separation | Maintain normothermia with active warming through entire case |
| Fluid management | Minimize fluid administration to minimize hemodilution prior to bypass run | Maintain euvolemia early in case, often patients require additional preload before manipulating heart |
| Anticoagulation | Heparinization titrated to ACT >400 s. Loading of antifibrinolytic | Reduced heparin administration titrated to ACT goal usually >300 s |
| Monitoring | TEE useful for multiple phases, especially for separation from CPB. PAC only for low EF, high risk of post-bypass dysfunction, or pulmonary morbidities | TEE valuable for initial volume assessment, but limited utility during manipulation of heart. PAC may help manage pre-load during manipulations |
| Pressors and inotropes | Expect higher pressors and inotrope requirements post-bypass due to stunning and vasoplegia | After revascularization, pressor and inotrope requirements often rapidly reduced/weaned. Infrequent need for inotropes |

is required to expose target coronaries may also impede inflow or outflow through the great vessels. The management of these often-encountered complications is discussed later in this chapter. Generally, the free end of the IMA (if it is used) is anastomosed first, usually to the LAD, which allows for early re-perfusion of a critical portion of the myocardium before continuing with the rest of the procedure.

Once the distal ends of all grafts are sewn, the heart is returned to its normal position and the surgeon will ask for the blood pressure to be reduced for work on the aortic (proximal) anastomoses. In order to gain a bloodless field, the surgeon may place a partial aortic clamp ("J-clamp"). An alternative to this clamp is the Maquet Heartstring™ device which allows puncture of the aorta and anastomosis around the hole without bleeding via a removable occluder on the luminal side of the hole. Once all proximal anastomoses are made, any clamps are removed restoring flow through the grafts, and all distal and proximal anastomoses are re-examined for integrity. This may involve lifting the heart manually for inspection of posterior anastomoses.

## Selection of Ideal Surgical Candidates

As previously stated, the differences in outcome between techniques are generally equivocal although there is some benefit in high-risk patients with multiple co-morbidities. Patients in whom aortic cross-clamp is also risky due to high-grade atherosclerotic disease of the aorta may also benefit from OPCAB.

There might be a trend towards reduced stroke with OPCAB. A multitude of comparative studies have been performed, but even recent studies have reached different conclusions. In a randomized controlled trial published in 2009 that enrolled 2203 patients (VA population), there was no significant difference in neuropsychological outcomes between the techniques, and on-pump CABG showed better graft survival and overall outcomes [24]. Conversely, a 2016 meta-analysis of randomized controlled trials analyzed 16,904 patients in 51 studies and concluded that on-pump surgery was associated with an increased occurrence of stroke [25]. Because there may be a higher likelihood that grafts will be patent years out from surgery with on-pump CABG [24, 26], older patients may be the population that benefits most from OPCAB both because they are at a higher risk of perioperative stroke and postoperative cognitive dysfunction, and because the grafts do not need to survive as long as in younger patients.

Predictably, manipulating the heart with non-anatomic positioning will significantly affect heart filling and function. This positioning is usually tolerated with appropriate management assuming that the heart has sufficient reserve to tolerate the hemodynamic swings. Generally, those with preserved ejection fraction (>40–45%) tolerate this well, but occasionally conversion to CPB is required if attempts to reposition the heart fail. Thoughtful consideration about who is likely to tolerate this manipulation is important as emergent conversion to CPB is associated with an increased mortality rate [27].

Additionally, despite the stabilization devices, movement at the anastomosis site can still make sewing difficult, and small or tortuous vessels may be especially difficult for the surgeon to find and adequately stabilize. Placing a tourniquet on vessels with high-grade or very proximal lesions (e.g. left main) may also be contraindicated. Finally, surgeon experience and comfort with the technique are variable and given the generally equivocal differences in outcome, many continue to prefer on-pump techniques.

## Intraoperative Anesthetic Management

Most steps in the surgical procedure are the same as with CABG until the administration of heparin. The purpose of administering heparin in OPCAB is to prevent blood from coagulating in grafts and low-flow vessels during the anastomotic period. This approach requires a lower level of anticoagulation than that needed to prevent clotting within a bypass circuit. Typically, half the dose of heparin is given with a target ACT typically greater than 300 s. It is the role of the anesthesiologist to manage ongoing dosing of anticoagulation, typically by measurement of an ACT every half hour. Antifibrinolytic infusions are generally not utilized. Prevention of hypothermia can be challenging given the operating room environment and the large exposure of an open chest so active warming devices should be utilized.

Unique anesthetic management of OPCAB principally consists of mitigating the hemodynamic swings induced by heart repositioning and monitoring for ischemia which can be induced by tourniquet placement on the coronary vessels. Anticipating hemodynamic swings and pre-emptively managing these changes are more successful than reacting to severe hemodynamic dysfunction. It is therefore critical that the anesthesiologist be in constant communication with the surgeon. Because of this, OPCAB can be much more labor-intensive for the anesthesiologist.

In preparation for lifting the heart, the anesthesiologist should assess circulating volume via arterial waveform analysis (PPV), TEE, and central/pulmonary filling pressures. If needed, judicious volume should be administered. Some anesthesiologists advocate for the prophylactic administration of 1–2 L boluses of IV fluids, however there is also significant risk of complications with volume overload including heart failure and pulmonary edema, so a goal-directed approach may be more prudent. The patient should also be placed in Trendelenburg position to passively increase pre-load to the heart. The MAP should be maintained higher than baseline with the use of a pressor in order to maintain perfusion pressure in face of reduced cardiac output. Inotropic agents should be considered for patients with borderline function. Finally, cardiac output can be increased despite reduced filling by means of epicardial pacing, especially in this population which frequently presents significantly beta-blocked. A heart rate of 70–80 should be targeted. The efficacy of these measures can be tested by the surgeon with a brief "test lift" of the heart to ensure tolerance. If lifting the heart causes dramatic drops in MAP, it may be necessary to administer additional volume or increase pressors before trying again.

Once the target vessel is stabilized and the surgeon occludes the vessel, the anesthesiologist should vigilantly monitor for signs of worsening ischemia in the affected territory. This evidence of ischemia is most likely to appear on EKG with either ST-changes or arrhythmias. TEE may detect new wall motion abnormalities depending on the target vessel, but TEE windows are often worsened when the heart is lifted away from firm contact against the esophagus.

If signs of ischemia develop, it is important to notify the surgeon immediately. Ischemia may resolve if MAP is elevated to increase flow through collaterals. This intervention must be balanced against the need to minimize afterload on the heart. Another option is for the surgeon to place an intra-luminal shunt in the target vessel. Shunting allows blood to flow past the tourniquet and into the distal vessel without introducing blood onto the field. The majority of the anastomosis is sewn, and the shunt is removed just prior to placement of the final sutures.

The surgeon will re-position the heart after each distal anastomosis, so swings in hemodynamics should be anticipated and pre-emptively treated. The most significant changes occur when the target vessels are the marginals or posterior descending artery (PDA) as these require either torqueing the heart or lifting the heart straight up. Asking the surgeon to give warning before these maneuvers will allow pressor to be bolused pre-emptively to minimize changes in MAP. Once all distal anastomoses are complete, the heart is returned to its anatomic position, so hemodynamics can return to baseline. After completion of proximals and restoration of blood flow, function may actually improve over baseline, so rapid weaning of pressors and inotropes is expected. The patient may still require ongoing volume resuscitation due to expected surgical bleeding until protamine is given. The surgeon may place a fine needle in the graft before restoring blood flow in order to de-air the graft. If there is retained air in the graft when flow is re-established, this may push further into the coronary artery causing occlusion of the vessel and resultant regional ischemia. This coronary air can usually be treated with bolus of pressor to maintain supra-normal MAP in an effort to push the air through.

After protamine is given, chest closure proceeds as in on-pump procedures and post-operative management is likewise similar.

# References

1. Chu D, Bakaeen FG, Dao TK, LeMaire SA, Coselli JS, Huh J. On-pump versus off-pump coronary artery bypass grafting in a cohort of 63,000 patients. Ann Thorac Surg. 2009;87(6):1820–6; discussion 1826–7. https://doi.org/10.1016/j.athoracsur.2009.03.052.
2. Serruys PW, Morice MC, Kappetein AP, Colombo A, Holmes DR, et al. Percutaneous coronary intervention versus coronary-artery bypass grafting for severe coronary artery disease. N Engl J Med. 2009;360(10):961–72.
3. Farkouh ME, Domanski M, Sleeper LA, Siami FS, Dangas G, et al. Strategies for multivessel revascularization in patients with diabetes. N Engl J Med. 2012;367(25):2375–84.
4. Park SJ, Ahn JM, Kim YH, Park DW, Yun SC, et al. Trial of everolimus-eluting stents or bypass surgery for coronary disease. N Engl J Med. 2015;372(13):1204–12.
5. Stone GW, Sabik JF, Serruys PW, Simonton CA, Genereux P, et al. Everolimus-eluting stents or bypass surgery for left main coronary artery disease. N Engl J Med. 2016;375(23):2223–35.
6. Hulzebos EHJ, Smit Y, Helders PPJM, van Meeteren NLU. Preoperative physical therapy for elective cardiac surgery patients. Cochrane Database Syst Rev. 2012;(11). https://doi.org/10.1002/14651858.CD010118.pub2.
7. Institute for Quality and Efficiency in Health Care (IQWiG). Complications after surgery: can quitting smoking before surgery reduce the risks? In PubMed Health: https://www.ncbi.nlm.nih.gov/pubmedhealth/PMH0072740/. Accessed 14 June 2017.
8. Gu YL, van der Horst IC, Douglas YL, Svilaas T, Mariani MA, Zijlstra F. Role of coronary artery bypass grafting during the acute and subacute phase of ST-elevation myocardial infarction. Neth Heart J. 2010;18(7–8):348.
9. Thielmann M, Neuhauser M, Marr A, Herold U, Kamler M, Massoudy P, Jakob H. Predictors and outcomes of coronary artery bypass grafting in ST elevation myocardial infarction. Ann Thorac Surg. 2007;84(1):17.
10. Xu F, Wang Q, Zhang H, Chen S, Ao H. Use of pulmonary artery catheter in coronary artery bypass graft. Costs and long-term outcomes. PLoS One. 2015;10(2):e0117610. Epub 2015 Feb 17.
11. Harvey S, Harrison DA, Singer M, Ashcroft J, Jones CM, Elbourne D, et al. Assessment of the clinical effectiveness of pulmonary artery catheters in management of patients in intensive care (PAC-Man): a randomised controlled trial. Lancet. 2005;366(9484):472.
12. Sandham JD, Hull RD, Brant RF, Knox L, Pineo GF, Doig CJ, et al. A randomized, controlled trial of the use of pulmonary-artery catheters in high-risk surgical patients. N Engl J Med. 2003;348(1):5.
13. American Society of Anesthesiologists and Society of Cardiovascular Anesthesiologists Task Force on Transesophageal Echocardiography. Practice guidelines for perioperative transesophageal echocardiography. An updated report by the American Society of Anesthesiologists and the Society of Cardiovascular Anesthesiologists Task Force on Transesophageal Echocardiography. Anesthesiology. 2010;112(5):1084–96.
14. Hillis LD, Smith PK, Anderson JL, Bittl JA, Bridges CR, Byrne JG, et al. 2011 ACCF/AHA guideline for coronary artery bypass graft surgery: a report of the American College of Cardiology Foundation/American Heart Association Task Force on Practice Guidelines. Circulation. 2011;124(23):e652–735.
15. Gibbon JH Jr. Application of a mechanical heart and lung apparatus to cardiac surgery. Minn Med. 1954;37:171–85; passim.
16. Uhlig C, Bluth T, Schwarz K, Deckert S, Heinrich L, et al. Effects of volatile anesthetics on mortality and postoperative pulmonary and other complications in patients undergoing surgery: a systematic review and meta-analysis. Anesthesiology. 2016;124:1230–45.
17. Ansley DM, Raedschelders K, Choi PT, Wang B, Cook RC, Chen DD. Propofol cardioprotection for on-pump aortocoronary bypass surgery in patients with type 2 diabetes mellitus (PRO-TECT II): a phase 2 randomized-controlled trial. Can J Anaesth. 2016;63(4):442–53.
18. Navickis RJ, Haynes GR, Wilkes MM. Effect of hydroxyethyl starch on bleeding after cardiopulmonary bypass: a meta-analysis of randomized trials. J Thorac Cardiovasc Surg. 2012;144(1):223–30.
19. Lagny MG, Roediger L, Koch JN, Dubois F, Senard M, Donneau AF, et al. Hydroxyethyl starch 130/0.4 and the risk of acute kidney injury after cardiopulmonary bypass: a single-center retrospective study. J Cardiothorac Vasc Anesth. 2016;30(4):869.
20. Koster A, Faraoni D, Levy JH. Antifibrinolytic therapy for cardiac surgery: an update. Anesthesiology. 2015;123(1):214–21. https://doi.org/10.1097/ALN.0000000000000688.
21. Ferraris VA, Brown JR, Despotis GJ, Hammon JW, Reece TB, et al. 2011 update to the society of thoracic surgeons and the society of cardiovascular anesthesiologists blood conservation clinical practice guidelines. Ann Thorac Surg. 2011;91:944–82.
22. Finley A, Greenberg C. Review article: heparin sensitivity and resistance: management during cardiopulmonary bypass. Anesth Analg. 2013;116(6):1210–22.
23. Hemmerling TM, Romano G, Terrasini N, Noiseux N. Anesthesia for off-pump coronary artery bypass surgery. Ann Card Anaesth. 2013;16(1):28–39.
24. Shroyer AL, Grover FL, Hattler B, Collins JF, McDonald GO, Kozora E, et al. On-pump versus off-pump coronary-artery bypass surgery. N Engl J Med. 2009;361(19):1827–37. https://doi.org/10.1056/NEJMoa0902905.
25. Deppe AC, Arbash W, Kuhn EW, Slottosch I, Scherner M, Liakopoulos OJ, et al. Current evidence of coronary artery bypass grafting off-pump versus on-pump: a systematic review with meta-analysis of over 16,900

patients investigated in randomized controlled trials. Eur J Cardiothorac Surg. 2016;49(4):1031–41; discussion 1041. https://doi.org/10.1093/ejcts/ezv268. Epub 2015 Aug 13.

26. Chivasso P, Guida G, Fudulu D, Bruno V, Marsico R, Sedmakov H, et al. Impact of off-pump coronary artery bypass grafting on survival: current best available evidence. J Thorac Dis. 2016;8(Suppl 10):S808–17. https://doi.org/10.21037/jtd.2016.10.13.

27. Chowdhury R, White D, Kilgo P, Puskas JD, Thourani VH, Chen EP, et al. Risk factors for conversion to cardiopulmonary bypass during off-pump coronary artery bypass surgery. Ann Thorac Surg. 2012;93:1936–41; discussion 42.

# Anesthesia for Valve Replacement and Repair

Terence Wallace

## Introduction

Over 100,000 procedures are performed on heart valves in the United States and this common surgical procedure has been increasing as the population ages [1]. The pathology causing either regurgitation or stenosis of these valves is diverse and includes calcium deposits, degradation, perforation, vegetation, and torn chordae (Table 2.1). Traditionally, a median sternotomy has been utilized to gain access to the heart, but mini-sternotomy, thoracotomy, and now percutaneous femoral access are increasing in popularity. As the population ages the amount of cardiac interventions in the operating room, hybrid operating room, and the catheterization lab are likely to increase as well. The hemodynamic consequences of the various valvular lesions causing the patient to present for surgery vary and can change quickly during the course of the anesthetic.

## Physiologic Consequences of Valvular Heart Disease

The anesthesiologist should have a basic knowledge of cardiac anatomy as it relates to the effects of valvular pathology on cardiac physiology and overall hemodynamics. Specifically, valvular pathology that leads to ventricular hypertrophy requires a higher perfusion pressure to ensure adequate myocardial perfusion. Recognizing wall motion abnormalities following valve surgery can alert the surgeon that there could be compromised blood flow in a particular coronary distribution. In addition, the cardiac conduction system can be affected by valve repairs and replacements due to suture location, or large valve sizes that stretch or compress the conduction pathways. While stenotic lesions tend to lead to pressure overload, regurgitant lesions often lead to volume overload. There can also be interplay between valvular pathology. For example, mitral valve stenosis can cause pulmonary hypertension and right ventricular dysfunction and ultimately tricuspid regurgitation. The anesthetic management must adjust for optimal management of the specific valvular pathology being addressed.

## Preoperative Evaluation

The goal of the preoperative evaluation is to assess the end-organ effects of valvular heart disease as well as the overall health risks of the patient. While the patient's valvular abnormality has likely been delineated by a preoperative echocardiography, many will also have a cardiac catheterization performed to determine if a concomitant coronary bypass surgery is

T. Wallace, M.D.
Clinical Assistant Professor of Anesthesiology, Sidney Kimmel Medical College of Thomas Jefferson University, Chief of Cardiac Anesthesiology, Christiana Care Health System, Anesthesia Services, P.A., Newark, DE, USA

Table 2.1 Common etiologies of valvular lesions

| | Etiologies |
|---|---|
| Aortic stenosis | Calcification<br>Bicuspid AV<br>Rheumatic fever |
| Aortic regurgitation | Endocarditis<br>Trauma<br>Connective tissue disease (Marfan's)<br>Rheumatic fever<br>Aortic dilation/dissection |
| Mitral stenosis | Rheumatic heart disease<br>Annular calcification<br>Infective endocarditis |
| Mitral regurgitation | Rheumatic heart disease<br>Degeneration<br>Mitral cleft<br>Myxomatous disease<br>Ischemic<br>Ruptured chordae<br>Infective endocarditis<br>Annular calcification |

indicated. Given that patients will be anticoagulated during valve surgery it is important to identify potential bleeding risks in the preoperative setting. Gastrointestinal (GI) endoscopic procedures are performed prior to elective valve surgery if there is a suspicion of bleeding from the GI tract. Pharyngeal, esophageal, and gastric abnormalities are teased out during the preoperative process to ensure there are no contraindications to transesophageal echocardiography (TEE).

The 2014 American Heart Association/American College of Cardiology guidelines delineate valvular heart disease into stages based on symptoms, hemodynamic severity of disease, and the impact of ventricular function [2].

- Stage A—presence of risk factors
- Stage B—asymptomatic valvular heart disease of mild to moderate severity
- Stage C1—severe asymptomatic valvular heart disease with compensated biventricular function
- Stage C2—severe valvular heart disease with decompensated right and/or left ventricular function
- Stage D—hemodynamically severe consequences

Routine blood testing including electrolytes, complete blood count, and coagulation profiles are obtained. Preexisting chronic kidney disease increases the risk for acute kidney injury so any interventions to modify this risk should be undertaken [3]. It is important to realize that many patients may be on newer anticoagulants or other medications, such as fish oil, that may not be evident on routine blood work. This underscores the importance of a thorough history when determining when medications and supplements were stopped by the patient.

Preoperative anemia is important to identify because of the increased morbidity and mortality in patients that receive blood transfusions. Preoperative iron supplementation and iron infusions can be given preoperatively [4]. If the patient has no objections to blood transfusions, a type and screen should be done. The presence of antibodies may delay surgery until the blood bank can secure an adequate amount of blood products for the case.

Patients may also have certain radiographic studies performed such as chest x-ray, CT scans, and ultrasounds that should be reviewed by the anesthesiologist prior to the procedure. Patients at high risk for carotid artery disease or those with prior stroke should be screened with Doppler ultrasound as the perioperative risk of stroke is increased in these patients [5]. These studies may help predict complications that may arise during the perioperative period.

## Anesthesia Monitoring

General anesthesia with endotracheal intubation is used for median sternotomy valve procedures. Patients remain intubated immediately postoperatively so 7.5 or 8.0 mm endotracheal tubes may be used so that bronchoscopy can be performed later if needed. While the standard ASA monitors are used, valvular surgery requires additional invasive monitoring. Arterial lines are placed prior to induction due to the rapid change in hemodynamics than can occur during anesthetic induction. Radial arterial lines are the most common, but brachial, axillary, and femoral arteries can be cannulated depending on the patient's anatomy and circulation [6].

In addition to large-bore peripheral intravenous access, central venous access is obtained. The right internal jugular vein is the most common site but the location may vary depending on the patient anatomy and circumstances. Whether to use a pulmonary artery catheter through the central venous access depends on the clinical situation and is often institution-specific. If one is placed then cardiac index, pulmonary artery pressures, and mixed venous oxygenation are all readily available to aid in perioperative management.

Transesophageal echocardiography (TEE) is used to evaluate the valvular pathology. Confirmation of the preoperative studies should be done as well as a comprehensive exam to assess if there is any new or unnoticed pathology that should be addressed [7]. Traditional two-dimensional and three-dimensional imaging, if available, can delineate the degree of regurgitation and/or stenosis present. Equally important is the identification of the underlying mechanism causing valvular dysfunction to enable best surgical correction. TEE is also quite valuable during weaning and separation from cardiopulmonary bypass. The degree of success in repair or replacement of the valve is evaluated as well as the presence of intracardiac air. Biventricular function and volume status are also evaluated with TEE throughout the intraoperative course.

Urinary catheters with temperature monitoring capabilities help monitor renal perfusion and fluid status. Temperature is monitored in two places generally consisting of a core temperature and more peripheral site. Cerebral oximetry is employed more selectively depending on the patient's history and risk of compromised cerebral perfusion.

## Intraoperative Physiologic Considerations

### Aortic Stenosis

*Pre-correction:* Maintaining normal sinus rhythm is especially important in aortic stenosis. The concentric hypertrophy of the left ventricle requires higher perfusion pressures or it can result in ischemia or arrhythmias, most commonly supraventricular tachycardias. Heart rate should be kept in a normal range of 60–80 beats per minute because tachycardia or bradycardia can lead to decreased cardiac output. To support blood pressure, the systemic vascular resistance should be maintained which makes phenylephrine a suitable choice with vasopressin or norepinephrine being other alternatives if the patient is not responsive to phenylephrine. Drugs that often increase chronotropy such as epinephrine or dobutamine are best avoided. Normovolemia is another goal of the anesthetic management, as the left ventricle can become very preload sensitive (Table 2.2).

*Post-correction:* With the underlying stenotic lesion successfully corrected, the left ventricle typically responds favorably and easily weans from cardiac bypass. The primary focus should remain on maintaining a high coronary perfusion pressure as the underlying hypertrophy still requires a higher pressure gradient to maintain adequate coronary blood flow.

### Aortic Regurgitation

*Pre-Correction:* Normal sinus rhythm is the ideal rhythm, but supraventricular tachycardias are better tolerated with aortic regurgitation. A normal to increased heart rate is warranted because it

**Table 2.2** Goals of hemodynamic management in patients with valvular lesions

|  | Rhythm | Preload | Afterload |
|---|---|---|---|
| Aortic stenosis | Sinus rhythm | Normal | Increased |
| Aortic regurgitation | Sinus/atrial fibrillation tolerated | Normal/decreased | Decreased |
| Mitral regurgitation | Sinus/atrial fibrillation tolerated | Normal/decreased | Decreased |
| Mitral stenosis | Sinus rhythm | Normal/decreased | Mildly increased |

decreases the time the heart spends in diastole while the regurgitation is occurring. Hypotension should be treated with drugs to increase contractility as opposed to increases in systemic vascular resistance alone as this will worsen the aortic regurgitation. Preload should be kept normal or even slightly reduced to avoid pulmonary congestion.

*Post-Correction:* The eccentric hypertrophy and left ventricular (LV) dilation that typically occurs in long-standing aortic regurgitation may cause the left ventricle to struggle immediately after surgical correction. It is not uncommon to utilize inotropic agents such as epinephrine, milrinone or dobutamine to assist ventricular function in the post-bypass period. Assuming a competent aortic valve was restored, over time the LV dilation typically regresses and patients have significant symptomatic improvement.

## Mitral Stenosis

*Pre-Correction:* Many patients with mitral stenosis tolerate the chronic atrial fibrillation (Afib) that is often present. However, if a patient initially in sinus rhythm converts to Afib they may suffer from an acute reduction in LV preload and in the absence of thrombus cardioversion should be strongly considered. Heart rate control is most paramount in these patients and should be maintained in the slow to normal range of 50–70 beats per minute. Tachycardia decreases the amount of time for the left atrium to empty into the left ventricle. Intravascular volume should be preserved, but fluid overload can lead to pulmonary edema. Similar to aortic stenosis, drugs that increase systemic vascular resistance are preferred though there is little left ventricular hypertrophy present. A primary concern is right ventricular failure due to elevated pulmonary vascular resistance at baseline so hypoxia, hypothermia, and acidosis should be avoided as this can contribute to acute right ventricular failure.

*Post-Correction:* Many patients do not require hemodynamic support much beyond baseline needs following a successful isolated mitral stenosis intervention. Once the pressure gradient between the left atrium and ventricle has been corrected these patients tend to respond quite well.

## Mitral Regurgitation

*Pre-Correction:* While normal sinus rhythm is ideal, many patients with mitral regurgitation will have atrial fibrillation, which is generally tolerated from a hemodynamic standpoint. Normal to slightly elevated heart rates reduce the amount of time for regurgitation to occur. Abrupt increases in systemic vascular resistance can worsen mitral regurgitation, so increasing contractility is the primary option for hypotension. Mitral regurgitation causes volume overload so preload should be maintained or reduced. Avoidance of hypoxia with the resultant increase in pulmonary vascular resistance is important as well (Table 2.2).

*Post-Correction*: A long-standing combination of left ventricular dilation and regurgitation flow into the left atrium causes LV function to initially appear worse than baseline after surgical correction. Transesophageal echocardiography can be vital post-correction to delineate left ventricular outflow tract obstruction either caused by a strut from a prosthetic valve or from systolic anterior motion of the anterior leaflet after a repair. It is common to utilize inotropic support for the LV depending on baseline function, duration of surgery and responsiveness of myocardium. Epinephrine, milrinone and dobutamine are common agents employed.

## Intraoperative Management

As mentioned earlier, a large-bore peripheral intravenous line and a radial arterial line are placed prior to induction. Induction is achieved with a combination of midazolam, fentanyl, and propofol or etomidate depending on the patient and desired hemodynamics. The medications selected and their exact dosing should take into consideration the physiologic variables mentioned above as well as baseline biventricular function. After loss of consciousness and mask ventilation is established, a non-depolarizing muscle relaxant is given and followed by endotracheal intubation. An internal jugular central line is then placed. Pulmonary artery catheters may be utilized and if so a baseline cardiac index and mixed venous saturation should be recorded. A transesophageal echocardiography probe is inserted if there is no contraindication and a baseline exam is performed. As mentioned above, a complete echocardiographic examination should be performed in addition to a focused interrogation of the underlying mechanism(s) causing the pathology of the valve in question. Anesthesia is maintained with inhalational agents while additional doses of fentanyl and muscle relaxants are given as needed. Additionally, many centers utilize anti-fibrinolytic medications such as aminocaproic acid or tranexamic acid.

While on cardiopulmonary bypass, the perfusionist generally uses boluses of phenylephrine to maintain mean arterial pressure (MAP), but may request additional help from the anesthesiologist in the form of a constant infusion of either phenylephrine or vasopressin if they are finding it difficult to maintain the MAP to adequately perfuse end-organs. Urine output is recorded every 15 min and communicated to the perfusionist to assist in the determination of fluid status and renal perfusion.

The anesthesiologist typically directs separation from cardiopulmonary bypass. After the valve is repaired or replaced an echo exam is performed to evaluate for residual intracardiac air and the success of the initial valve intervention. It is critical that the anesthesiologist identify pathology specific to the valve in question such as an unstable sewing ring, paravalvular leak or an abnormally high gradient. Additionally, damage or alteration to surrounding valves and structures should be assessed at this time as well. Vasopressors and inotropic agents may or may not be needed during separation from cardiopulmonary bypass and the choice of agent(s) depends on which valve was fixed and the function of the heart (see intraoperative physiologic considerations above). The duration of cardiopulmonary bypass, degree of myocardial protection, and aortic cross-clamp time factor into the need for post-bypass support. Following protamine administration, the decision to transfuse hemostatic blood products should be made based on laboratory values and the observation of non-surgical bleeding from the field.

## Postoperative Management

Postoperatively the patients are transported intubated to the cardiac intensive care unit where they are weaned from ventilator support as well as circulatory support in the intensive care unit. The degree of successful repair, biventricular function and variations in vasopressor requirements should be well-communicated to the ICU team. In addition to common complications following cardiac surgery, there are a few select complications to consider in patients following valve surgery. The rate of stroke is as high as 5% following an aortic valve intervention so an anesthetic tailored for a rapid neurologic examination is often warranted [8]. Complications following mitral valve interventions include heart block and dynamic left ventricular outflow tract obstruction. The presence of epicardial pacing wires and a meticulous echocardiographic examination can help mitigate these risks.

## References

1. Lee R, Li S, Rankin JS, et al. Fifteen-year outcome trends for valve surgery in North America. Ann Thorac Surg. 2011;91:677.
2. Nishimura RA, Otto CM, Bonow RO, et al. 2014 AHA/ACC guideline for the management of patients with valvular heart disease: a report of the American College of Cardiology/American Heart Association Task Force on Practice Guidelines. J Am Coll Cardiol. 2014;63:e57.
3. Thakar CV, Arrigain S, Worley S, et al. A clinical score to predict acute renal failure after cardiac surgery. J Am Soc Nephrol. 2005;16:162.
4. Society of Thoracic Surgeons Blood Conservation Guideline Task Force, Ferraris VA, Brown JR, et al. 2011 update to the Society of Thoracic Surgeons and the Society of Cardiovascular Anesthesiologists blood conservation clinical practice guidelines. Ann Thorac Surg. 2011;91:944.

5. Durand DJ, Perler BA, Roseborough GS, et al. Mandatory versus selective preoperative carotid screening: a retrospective analysis. Ann Thorac Surg. 2004;78:159.
6. Brzezinki M, Luisetti T, London MJ. Radial artery cannulation: a comprehensive review of recent anatomic and physiologic investigations. Anesth Analg. 2009;109:1763.
7. Hahn R, Abraham T, Adams M, et al. Guidelines for performing a comprehensive transesophageal echocardiographic examination: recommendations from the American Society of Echocardiography and the Society of Cardiovascular Anesthesiologists. J Am Soc Echocardiogr. 2013;26:921–64.
8. Kappetein AP, Van Mieghem NM, Reardon, MJ, et al. Neurological complications after transcatheter aortic valve implantation with a self-expanding bioprosthesis or surgical aortic valve replacement in patients at intermediate-risk for surgery. EuroPCR. Paris, France; 2017.

# Anesthesia for Congenital Heart Diseases in Adults

## 3

Korrin Scott and Sarah Burke

## Introduction

Congenital heart disease (CHD) is a broad spectrum representing a wide range of conditions that have significant implications for the anesthesiologist in the perioperative period. In 2010, the prevalence of CHD was approximately 13 per 1000 children and 6 per 1000 adults, with the greatest increase in prevalence occurring among adolescents and young adults [1]. It is speculated that the incidence of adults with CHD will surpass that of children in 2020.

The cause of many congenital heart conditions is idiopathic; however, there are several recognized genetic and environmental risk factors. Congenital rubella infection has been associated with pulmonary artery stenosis and patent ductus arteriosus. Down syndrome is often accompanied by endocardial cushion defects, and 22q deletion (DiGeorge syndrome) can be correlated with interrupted aortic arch, truncus arteriosus, or Tetralogy of Fallot. Other risk factors implicated in CHD include alcohol and tobacco abuse and medication exposures including lithium (Ebstein's malformation), thalidomide, isotretinoin, and valproate.

With advances in surgical and medical management, more than 85% of children born with CHD now survive to adulthood [2]. Because of this growing trend, many of these patients require additional curative or palliative cardiac surgery as adults. This brings its own unique set of implications for the anesthesiologist managing these patients within the perioperative period. In general, heightened concern for arrhythmias, ventricular dysfunction, pulmonary hypertension, cyanosis, hypoxemia and reoperation must be considered.

Adult patients with CHD fall primarily into three major categories: those with prior complete correction of their congenital defect, those with partial or palliative correction, and those patients who are diagnosed in adulthood without any childhood surgical intervention. It is vital in caring for these patients to understand the type of surgical correction (if any) they have had in the past, their current symptoms and natural progression, as well as the resulting hemodynamic goals based on their current physiology. While the underlying anatomy may often be complex and the evolution of the disease from childhood to adulthood results in unique physiology, CHD can further be divided into several physiologic categories that can aid in the approach to perioperative management (Table 3.1).

## Shunt Lesions

Shunt lesions are some of the most commonly encountered congenital defects. While they predominately present in childhood, smaller lesions

K. Scott, M.D. (✉) · S. Burke, M.D.
Emory University Hospital, Atlanta, GA, USA
e-mail: kjscot3@emory.edu;
sarah.coyle.burke@emory.edu

**Table 3.1** Common lesions and their anesthetic considerations

| Lesion type | Example(s) | Anesthetic considerations |
|---|---|---|
| Shunt | ASD VSD | (Left to right shunts): Normal/slightly elevated PVR Low SVR Normal PaCO$_2$ Low FiO$_2$ (titrate to PaO$_2$/O$_2$Sat) |
| Stenotic | Aortic stenosis (valvular, subvalvular or coarctation) Pulmonic stenosis | Maintain preload Low normal HR Maintain SVR |
| Complex | Hypoplastic left heart (Fontan circulation) | Maintain preload Augment contractility as needed Low PVR (passive flow) Spontaneous ventilation if possible |

may remain asymptomatic into adulthood. Commonly encountered shunt lesions include ventricular septal defects (VSDs), atrial septal defects (ASDs) and patent ductus arteriosus.

Overall, shunts are defined by the direction of blood flow (right to left vs. left to right), the size of the defect and the effect of the shunt on the intrinsic structures of the heart. The ratio of pulmonary and systemic flow (Qp/Qs) is an objective and quantifiable way of measuring the degree of shunt present. The shunt fraction is determined either via cardiac catheterization or calculated using echocardiography. In a left to right shunt, the flow through the pulmonary circulation is increased resulting in a ratio greater than one (i.e. 2:1), whereas the reverse is true in a right to left shunt (i.e. 0.5:1).

## Atrial Septal Defects

Small atrial septal defects often go undetected and are the most common shunt lesions initially diagnosed in adulthood. ASDs can be divided into one of four categories: ostium secundum (defect at the level of the fossa ovalis, the most common ASD), ostium primum (defect within the AV septum), sinus venosus ASD, and an "unroofed" coronary sinus (rare). A left to right shunt through an ASD is proportional to the size of the defect with increasing physiologic significance as the size increases. Over time, the right atrium (RA) dilates and volume overload of the right ventricle (RV) eventually develops. This leads to RV hypertrophy and elevated right sided pressures. As RA pressure increases, the shunt will decrease and potentially even reverse to a right to left shunt. This is known as Eisenmenger's reaction. Once this occurs, surgical correction is no longer recommended. Physical exam findings of a patent ASD include a systolic ejection murmur and a fixed split second heart sound.

## Ventricular Septal Defects

VSDs are the most common congenital heart defect at birth and are present in 42 infants per 10,000 live births [3]. They are also divided into four primary categories based on their location within the interventricular septum: membranous or perimembranous (most common), inlet VSDs (part of an endocardial cushion defect between mitral and tricuspid leaflets), supracristal or infundibular VSD (immediately below the pulmonary and aortic valves) and muscular VSDs (frequently present in multiples or post-infarct). Similar to ASDs, VSDs create a left to right shunt which results in over-circulation through the pulmonary vasculature. Due to the location of most VSDs the shunted blood largely bypasses the right ventricular (RV) cavity. Therefore, while some volume overload is present in the RV, the ventricle is typically spared of hypertrophy until later in the disease process when pulmonary hypertension develops. These patients often present with symptoms of heart failure, as the left ventricle (LV) becomes volume overloaded due to the pulmonary over-circulation. Physical exam findings include a harsh holosystolic murmur at the lower left sternal border. Surgical correction is recommended if the shunt fraction (Qp/Qs) is greater than 1.5 (or 2 in some sources), if the defect is part of a complex syndrome, or if the defect is located in the left ventricular outflow tract (risking severe aortic insufficiency by a prolapsing aortic valve leaflet). For larger VSDs, surgical intervention within the first 2 years of life is associated with regular long term survival, preserved LV function and normal pulmonary pressures [4]. Complications of a VSD repair include disruption of the ventricular conduction system, which can lead to bundle branch blocks or complete atrioventricular (AV) block.

## Endocardial Cushion Defects

Endocardial cushion defects (AV canal) is a lack of central separation of the heart. A complete AV canal includes a large ostium primum ASD, a large membranous VSD and a common AV valve [5]. Partial AV canal is defined by the absence of a VSD and is predominantly characterized by a large ostium primum ASD. It can be associated with a cleft mitral valve and resultant mitral regurgitation. This spectrum of defects is frequently associated with Down syndrome and typically presents early in childhood due to the significant shunt. Early findings of RA and RV dilation with both RV and LV hypertrophy are common, and the development of pulmonary hypertension (PHTN) appears earlier in the setting of a large left to right shunt. While typically repaired in childhood, partial AV canal defects can occasionally be diagnosed later in life. Consequences of prior repairs include mitral regurgitation, subaortic stenosis, or AV conduction block.

## Patent Ductus Arteriosis

The ductus arteriosus is part of normal fetal circulation that connects the pulmonary artery to the proximal descending aorta, thus allowing a majority of the blood ejected from the right ventricle to bypass the non-functioning fetal lungs. Prostaglandins and high PVR (through the fetus's noncompliant fluid filled lungs) maintain the patency of the ductus during fetal developments. Shortly after birth, the combination of reduced PVR and significant drop in prostaglandin levels causes the ductus to close.

While a PDA is one of the most common congenital heart defects, most are diagnosed and treated in early infancy either with medical management (typically indomethacin) or surgical ligation. It is uncommon to find large PDAs in adults, but occasionally small shunts can be diagnosed later in life. Symptoms of an untreated PDA are consistent with a left to right shunt such as cardiomyopathy, heart failure, and pulmonary hypertension. Adult patients with a PDA are additionally at an increased risk for coronary ischemia due to ongoing pulmonary runoff during the diastolic phase.

## Anesthetic Considerations for Shunt Lesions

The direction and volume of the shunt as well as the presence of pulmonary hypertension are important factors in the anesthetic management of these patients. Overall, the operative goal is to reduce the volume of shunted blood.

For left to right shunts in the absence of elevated pulmonary pressures, hemodynamic goals include normal to slightly elevated PVR and low SVR. Normal to slight hypercarbia with low inspired $FiO_2$ (30–40%) will maintain slightly elevated PRV, and low SVR is easily achieved with a variety of anesthetic techniques (general anesthesia, intrathecal, epidural). Hypovolemia is poorly tolerated due to high baseline circulating volume; therefore, sustaining slightly elevated preload is ideal. These patients are usually not cyanotic, but deterioration in gas exchange may result from pulmonary congestion.

Right to left shunts can exist when SVR drops or PVR increases drastically. (Long-standing right to left shunts are part of Eisenmenger's reaction and are not amenable to surgery). Under anesthesia, hyper-cyanotic spells respond to volume and a goal to increase SVR with phenylephrine or small doses of vasopressin. Finally, high peak pressures or elevated PEEP can increase the proportion of right to left shunt and must be avoided. In all patients with shunt, the threat of shunt reversal should prompt the anesthesiologist to apply in-line air filters and be vigilant about de-airing all IV lines.

Hypoxemia in the setting of shunts may be a result of inadequate pulmonary blood flow and/or a mixture of deoxygenated blood with oxygenated blood in the systemic circulation. Persistent hypoxemia can lead to tachycardia, hyperventilation, potential myocardial ischemia and dysfunction. In general, the anesthetic management of intracardiac shunts includes adequate hydration, maintenance of systemic blood pressure, minimalizing vast increases in PVR, and avoiding sudden increases in oxygen demand.

## Stenotic Lesions

Congenital stenotic lesions represent a heterogeneous spectrum of valvular, subvalvular, and supravalvular conditions. While often isolated congenital conditions (most often the pulmonic and aortic valves), these lesions can be present in the setting of more complex syndromes or involve impaired ventricular development.

## Congenital Aortic Stenosis

Aortic stenosis in adults is typically thought of as an age-related disease with calcification and sclerosis of the valve resulting in a decreased effective area for LV cardiac output. In the congenital population, which is estimated to be about 10% of all patients with aortic stenosis [6], valvular stenosis is typically the result of varying degrees of valve mal-development resulting in mild to severe obstruction and may be associated with other disorders or LV hypoplasia. The most common abnormality is a bicuspid aortic valve which is present in 1–2% of the population. Today, bicuspid aortic valve (BAV) is recognized as a syndrome incorporating aortic valve disorders and aortic wall abnormalities including aortic dilation, dissection, or rupture. Additionally, congenital defects such as VSDs, PDAs, coarctation of the aorta, Turner syndrome, and Marfan syndrome are commonly associated and require additional considerations when providing an anesthetic [6].

In children and adolescents with congenital aortic stenosis, balloon valvuloplasty is typically considered the initial treatment of choice with replacement reserved for patients who have failed valvuloplasty. For patients diagnosed later in life or early adulthood (as is common for BAV), traditional surgical valve replacement or transcatheter aortic valve replacement may be recommended. As with adult patients with acquired AS, maintenance of adequate preload and afterload with a normal to low heart rate are vital to maximize diastolic filling and coronary perfusion. Sinus rhythm should also be maintained since diastolic filling is often highly dependent on atrial kick. Recognition of any subvalvular stenosis including LVOT obstruction that would require intervention should also be addressed at time of valve replacement. Other anesthetic considerations revolve around associated aortic pathology (dissection vs. dilation) as well as associated acute or chronic aortic insufficiency (AI) that would further complicate hemodynamics when providing anesthesia for these patients.

## Coarctation of the Aorta

Coarctation of the aorta involves a segmental narrowing of the aorta, most often located just distal to the aortic arch near the origin of the ductus arteriosus. While severe coarctation typically presents with heart failure in the first few weeks of like, there is a bimodal age distribution for the development of symptoms [7]. Depending on the severity and location of the coarctation, the effects of supravalvular obstruction against the fixed orifice result in significant afterload on the LV leading to hypertrophy and eventual LV failure. Primary perioperative concerns relate to management of the fixed afterload and effects on the LV. Hypertension is present in the right arm, relative to the lower extremities (unless an anomalous origin of the right subclavian is present). The left arm may or may not be hypertensive based on the exact location of aortic narrowing. Prior to surgical correction, monitoring blood pressure and oxygen saturation with both an upper and lower body extremity is advised (i.e. right arm and left leg). Other considerations include risk of arrhythmia, premature coronary artery disease and bleeding in the setting of collateral circulation. While repair can occur in infancy, recurrent coarctation is a common problem seen in the adult population and may be managed with percutaneous treatment or reoperation. However, mortality can be as high as 5–10% with reoperation depending on comorbidities or LV dysfunction, as well as significant risk of morbidity including recurrent laryngeal nerve palsy, phrenic nerve injury, recoarctation, and aneurysm formation at the area of repair. Paraplegia (due to spinal cord ischemia) and arm claudication or subclavian steal are rare but significant possibilities. All patients (either surgical or interventional repair) should have close follow up and aggressive management of blood pressure control post-operatively [6].

## Pulmonary Stenosis

Congenital pulmonic stenosis is typically diagnosed in infancy with critical lesions or more complex lesions involving pulmonary atresia or tetralogy of Fallot. Presentation later in childhood or early adulthood manifests signs of RV hypertrophy, volume and pressure overload, and eventual RV failure. As in aortic stenosis, initial interventions to address the stenosis include percutaneous balloon valvuloplasty, with replacement reserved for complex pathology.

Perioperatively, hemodynamic goals include maintenance of RV preload and contractility while avoiding increases in PVR, which will worsen the already high afterload that the stenotic valve places on the RV. A careful balance of maintaining RV filling pressures and SVR while titrating fluids to avoid overload is key to preventing right heart volume overload which can precipitate arrhythmia and RV failure.

## Complex Lesions

### Ebstein's Malformation

Ebstein's malformation is a rare defect involving a wide spectrum of anatomic and functional abnormalities of the tricuspid valve and right ventricle. Clinical presentation of Ebstein's malformation depends on the severity of tricuspid valve leaflet distortion (most commonly an apicalized septal leaflet), size of the RV, and the presence of tricuspid regurgitation (TR) or shunt. The natural course of disease is for the leaflets to develop progressive restrictive motion from shortening and fibrosis of the chordae, which can result in either a regurgitant valve, stenotic valve, or both. When Ebstein's malformation presents in adults, common symptoms include exercise intolerance with dyspnea, fatigue, arrhythmias and right-sided heart failure. Mild to moderate tricuspid regurgitation is fairly well tolerated, but with increasing severity, symptoms of RV pressure and volume overload develop leading to RV dysfunction, hepatomegaly, ascites, peripheral edema, and cardiorenal syndrome. Indications for surgery also include cyanosis and paradoxical embolism as ASDs and PFOs are common associated conditions. Hemodynamic goals in this setting include maintaining adequate preload, supporting contractility and avoiding increases in PVR which place further strain on the RV. Postoperatively, these patients require lifelong surveillance for tricuspid valve dysfunction after repair, prosthetic valve degeneration, atrial and ventricular arrhythmias and ventricular dysfunction. Of note, AV block is common after tricuspid valve replacement [8].

### Tetralogy of Fallot

Tetralogy of Fallot (TOF) is the most common cyanotic congenital heart defect and involves a collection of four lesions including VSD (usually large and unrestrictive), RV outflow obstruction, RV hypertrophy and overriding aorta. Complete repair typically occurs in the first few years of life. While survival into adulthood now exceeds 90%, the repaired anatomy in patients with TOF can vary and it is crucial when caring for adults with history of TOF to determine the type of repair performed. Complete early surgical repair involves infundibular muscle resection, removal or dilation of pulmonary valve, and VSD closure. Some centers will intentionally create an ASD to serve as a "pop-off" to offset high right-sided pressures. Residual or recurrent pulmonary insufficiency or right ventricular outflow tract (RVOT) obstruction is typical and well tolerated; however, increased symptoms from arrhythmia, RV volume overload and failure can increase significantly in the third to fourth decade of life. Staging of reoperation on the pulmonic valve/RVOT in repaired TOF patients remains somewhat of a controversy with regards to optimal timing of the surgery. Asymptomatic patients may need reoperation early due to RV dilation, dysfunction or aneurysm, worsening TR, prolonged QRS interval or tachyarrhythmias. Subjective symptoms including exercise intolerance, heart failure symptoms, or syncope must also be considered. Late onset ventricular tachycardia (VT) is a problem in patients who have otherwise undergone successful TOF repair [9]. QRS prolongation (>180 ms) coupled with pulmonary regurgitation and RV dilation are the major risk factors for development of VT and risk of sudden death. Antiarrhythmic drug therapy has not been shown to increase survival; however, replacement of an incompetent pulmonary valve is associated with stabilization of the QRS and a reduction in arrhythmias [10]. Primary intraoperative considerations in redo PVR include concerns regarding RV volume overload or dysfunction, arrhythmia and significant bleeding in the setting of revision sternotomy and adhesions. Defibrillator pads should be placed prior to induction and blood should be immediately available prior to sternotomy. Furthermore, following surgical correction for pulmonic regurgitation, special attention should be paid to the function of the RV with the increased work required to pump across a competent valve.

## Single Ventricle Physiology

Single ventricle physiology, usually seen in the adult setting following a palliative surgical procedure, is one of the most intimidating conditions for the anesthesiologist to encounter. While there are numerous possible underlying physiologic conditions, essentially all patients share the common feature of only one ventricle of adequate size. Because of this, the plan for reconstruction is similar in nearly all of these anomalies, with the eventual goal of achieving Fontan circulation. Fontan circulation is characterized by passive, non-pulsatile flow through pulmonary circulation with the IVC and SVC draining directly into the pulmonary system, while the single ventricle pumps oxygenated blood systemically to the body. Factors that increase PVR will reduce pulmonary blood flow thus increasing CVP leading to inadequate filling of the single ventricle and decreased cardiac output.

The main physiologic consideration in these patients relates to the interdependence of pulmonary and systemic output as a result of a single functional ventricle with a goal of balanced circulation. Primary anesthetic considerations include maintaining adequate preload and contractility and avoiding factors that would increase PVR such as hypoxia, hypercarbia, or acidosis. Positive pressure alone can decrease venous return and result in decrease cardiac output, thus spontaneous ventilation is more hemodynamically favorable. If positive pressure is necessary, it should be initiated cautiously and with a goal of balancing low airway pressures with adequate minute ventilation. Similarly, insufflation for thoracic or abdominal procedures may be poorly tolerated and risks and benefits should be carefully weighed prior to surgery. Patients with Fontan circulation gradually develop congestive hepatic dysfunction accompanied by procoagulant and anticoagulant changes. Decreased levels of factors V and VII with prolonged PT are commonly the anticoagulant changes seen; while increased factor VIII and X are the procoagulant changes demonstrated. Additionally, decreased AT3, protein C and S further complicate the mixed picture, which can manifest as overt and covert thromboembolism [11, 12]. Other perioperative considerations involve significant risk of arrhythmia as loss of sinus rhythm can cause ventricular dysfunction leading to increased LA pressure and decreased pulmonary blood flow.

## Congenital Heart Disease in Non-cardiac Surgery

Apart from patients with prior correction or previously undiagnosed congenital heart disease requiring operative repair, the increased survival of patients with congenital heart disease into adulthood creates a significant increase in these patients undergoing noncardiac surgery. In the early 2000's there were estimated to be approximately 800,000 adults in the USA with congenital heart disease [13]; and this number continues to grow as childhood interventions improve.

While single lesions such as small ASDs and VSDs may have no long-term sequelae, those with a more complex history or anatomy have many considerations within the perioperative period. Most common long term complications include PHTN, risk of arrhythmia or conduction system defects (including the need for a pacemaker or defibrillator), LV or RV dysfunction, Fontan circulation, Eisenmenger syndrome, residual shunts, hypoxemia, and infective endocarditis.

Preoperatively, a thorough history and physical exam with recent imaging of the heart is imperative to caring for these patients. Identifying prior interventions, current symptoms, exercise tolerance, and any signs of heart failure or other end organ effects (impaired pulmonary function, cardiorenal syndrome, congestive hepatopathy) is crucial in devising an anesthetic plan. Furthermore, ascertaining current anatomy and physiology, including baseline pulmonary pressures, is important for establishing hemodynamic goals as well as to stratify risk. A multidisciplinary approach involving the anesthesiologist, surgeon, congenital cardiologist, and critical care teams should be employed to discuss pertinent patient and surgical specific concerns. Careful consideration of whether to stop or continue home anticoagulants, cardiovascular medications and diuretics should also occur. Anxiolytic premedication should be approached cautiously recognizing the significant implications of hypercarbia on pulmonary vascular resistance. Finally, antibiotic prophylaxis should be addressed based on current American Heart Association guidelines. Presently, the AHA recommends antibiotic prophylaxis for high and moderate risk patients when undergoing procedures that can be associated with bacteremia. The high risk group includes patients with previous infective endocarditis, prosthetic heart valves, complex congenital cyanotic heart disease, surgically constructed systemic or pulmonary shunts whereas the moderate risk group includes non-cyanotic heart disease not mentioned elsewhere, and mitral valve prolapse with valvular regurgitation [14].

Intraoperative management of patients with minimal residual pathology or low risk procedures may proceed with standard monitors including noninvasive blood pressure measurement. Invasive arterial pressure monitoring should be considered for the majority of patients with more than mild disease or those undergoing more complex procedures. Practitioners should have a low threshold for central venous access to trend central pressures and for administration of vasoactive agents. Additionally, a pulmonary artery catheter can be placed for enhanced monitoring and the utilization of intraoperative transesophageal echocardiography can be of significant benefit. These patients often have a history of difficult intravenous access given multiple surgical procedures and hospitalizations.

Arrhythmias are one of the most common reasons for hospitalization in patients with congenital heart disease and a represent a major concern in the operating room. Underlying pathophysiology and scarring from surgery make malignant arrhythmias significantly more common in the adult CHD population. One of the more common arrhythmias is intra-atrial re-entrant tachycardia (IART), which is frequently encountered in patients with Fontan circulation [15]. IART is generally resistant to pharmacotherapy and usually requires ablation or surgical intervention. Sudden cardiac death remains a grave concern for these patients with the highest risk seen in patients with underlying diagnoses of TOF, transposition of the great arteries, coarctation of the aorta, and aortic stenosis.

Pulmonary hypertension is defined as a mean pulmonary artery pressure greater than 25 mmHg. Most childhood lesions that precipitate pulmonary hypertension are now corrected early; however, there still exists a cohort of patients whose definitive surgery was performed after the development of PHTN. The aim of caring for these patients, even when undergoing noncardiac surgery, is to correct any reversible factors of increased pulmonary pressures as well as avoid any precipitating factors. For example, avoid sympathetic stimulation such as pain or light anesthesia, acidosis, hypoxia, hypercarbia, hypothermia, as well as increased intrathoracic pressure. Pharmacotherapy may need to be considered in the immediate perioperative period, and options include inhaled epoprostenol, inhaled nitric oxide as well as phosphodiesterase III inhibitors such as milrinone. In general, regional anesthesia is considered a more favorable choice for these patients, but if general anesthesia is required, controlled ventilation is usually mandatory.

Cyanosis can arise due to inadequate pulmonary blood flow or because of pulmonary hyperperfusion [16]. With inadequate pulmonary blood flow (usually R to L shunting), avoidance of perioperative dehydration, reduction of PVR, maintenance of SVR, and avoidance of increased oxygen consumption are crucial in perioperative management. Conversely, in patients with high pulmonary blood flow (left to right shunting), further increases in pulmonary blood flow may increase cardiac work and decrease systemic perfusion if the ventricular function is compromised. Chronic hypoxemia results in polycythemia as a compensatory response to improve oxygen transport; however, this comes with an increase in blood viscosity which can increase the risk of thrombosis and stroke [17]. Platelet count is often simultaneously decreased and platelet function may be abnormal. When combined with the coagulation abnormalities previously mentioned above for patients with cyanotic CHD, this creates a scenario when then patient is at risk for excessive perioperative bleeding as well as thrombosis.

Postoperatively, patients with complex CHD and some degree of decompensation or those undergoing high risk procedures should be monitored in an intensive care setting. Careful attention to dysrhythmias, bleeding, and potential thrombotic events is imperative in the immediate postoperative period. Additionally, serial arterial blood gas evaluation and management of pulmonary hypertension and respiratory status may be warranted. While a high oxygen saturation is generally considered ideal in ICU patients, it must be understood that in CHD patients with complete central mixing that there is a hyperbolic relationship between arterial saturation and the ratio of pulmonary and systemic flows. Checking blood gases regularly will allow closer control of PVR and therefore pulmonary blood flow in this subset of CHD patients. Because duration of inspiration has a greater effect than peak pressure in CHD patients on PPV, ventilator management that prioritizes a decreased duration of inspiration even in the setting of increased peak inspiratory pressures is usually the best strategy to improve pulmonary blood flow.

Given the heterogeneous population represented by congenital heart disease, a single approach to anesthetic management is not feasible and the aforementioned considerations must be in the forefront of the anesthesiologist's mind when caring for these patients. The care of adult patients with CHD is challenging and complicated. It is likely best approached with a multidisciplinary team familiar with the patient's unique physiology and comfortable managing these patients in the perioperative period.

## References

1. Marelli AJ, Ionescu-Ittu R, Macki AS, et al. Lifetime prevalence of congenital heart disease in the general population from 2000 to 2010. Circulation. 2014;130:749–56.
2. Warnes CA, Liberthson RR, Danielson GK, et al. Task force 1: the changing profile of congenital heart disease in adult life. J Am Coll Cardiol. 2001;37:1170–5.
3. Reller MD, Strickland MJ, Riehle-Colarusso T, Mahle WT, Correa A. Prevalence of congenital heart defects in metropolitan Atlanta, 1998–2005. J Pediatr. 2008;153:807–13.
4. Mongeon FP, Burkhart HM, Ammash NM, Dearani JA, Li Z, Warnes CA, Connolly HM. Indications and outcomes of surgical closure of ventricular septal defect in adults. JACC Cardiovasc Interv. 2010;3(3):290–7.
5. Chassot PG, Bettex DA. Anesthesia and adult congenital heart disease. J Cardiothorac Vasc Anesth. 2006;20(3):414–37.
6. Yuan S-M, Jing H. The bicuspid aortic valve and related disorders. Sao Paulo Med J. 2010;128(5):296–301.
7. Baum VC, Perloff JK. Anesthetic implications of adults with congenital heart disease. Anesth Analg. 1993;76:1342–58.
8. Warnes CA, Williams RG, Raushöre TM, et al. ACC/AHA 2008 guidelines for the management of

adults with congenital heart disease. Circulation. 2008;118:e714–833.
9. Gatzoulis MA, Balaji S, Webber SA, et al. Risk factors for arrhythmia and sudden cardiac death late after repair of tetralogy of Fallot: a multicenter study. Lancet. 2000;356:975–81.
10. Therrien J, Siu SC, Harris L, et al. Impact of pulmonary valve replacement on arrhythmia propensity late after repair of tetralogy of Fallot. Circulation. 2001;103:2489–94.
11. Jahangiri M, Kreutzer J, Zurakowski D, Bacha E, Jonas RA. Evolution of hemostatic and coagulation factor abnormalities in patients undergoing the Fontan operation. J Thorac Cardiovasc Surg. 2000;120:778–82.
12. Van Nieuwenhuizen RC, Peters M, Lubbers LJ, Trip MD, Tijssen JGP, Milder BJM. Abnormalities in liver function and coagulation profile following the Fontan procedure. Heart. 1999;82:40–6.
13. Warnes CA, Liberthson R, Danielson GK Jr, et al. Task force I: the changing profile of congenital heart disease in adult life. J Am Coll Cardiol. 2001;37:170–5.
14. Dajani AS, Taubert KA, Wilson W, et al. Prevention of bacterial endocarditis. Circulation. 1997;96:358–66.
15. Roos-Hesselink J, Perlroth MG, McGhie J, et al. Atrial arrhythmias in adults after repair of tetralogy of Fallot. Correlations with clinical, exercise, and echocardiographic findings. Circulation. 1995;91:2214–9.
16. Lovell AT. Anesthetic implications of grown-up congenital heart disease. Br J Anaesth. 2004;93:129–39.
17. Ammash N, Warnes CA. Cerebrovascular events in adult patients with cyanotic congenital heart disease. J Am Coll Cardiol. 1996;28:768–72.

# Anesthesia for Heart and Lung Transplantation

Blaine E. Farmer and Igor O. Zhukov

## Introduction

The first successful heart transplant took place in 1967; successful lung transplantation followed a decade later. Advances in diagnosis, prevention, and treatment of acute rejection led to these procedures becoming increasingly more common over the ensuing decades. Hearts and lungs now stand as the third and fourth most commonly transplanted organ in the United States [1]. These procedures significantly prolong survival and quality of life for thousands of patients suffering from advanced lung disease and heart failure with lung transplant survival reaching 70% and heart transplant 80% at the 3 year mark [2, 3]. However, as donor shortage continues to be the rate-limiting step, many patients are bridged with advanced support strategies while waiting for organ availability; this often makes transplantation and subsequent care even more challenging. Furthermore, successful transplantation can be compromised by several serious complications. Among the most dreaded are right ventricular (RV) failure for heart transplants and primary graft dysfunction (PGD) for the lung recipients. Emerging evidence emphasizes the role of meticulous anesthetic management in reducing the risk of PGD and other complications in heart and lung transplantation.

## Preoperative Management

### Donation Considerations

Preoperative assessment starts with selecting a suitable donor, matching not only the histological parameters of the recipient, but also their body size. In lung transplantation, the donor lungs should match the recipient within 20%. Though oversized grafts present technical challenges for the surgeons, recipients with undersized lung grafts have shown an increased risk of PGD, higher rates of tracheostomy, and greater resource utilization [4]. To possibly mitigate some of this risk, tidal volumes can be calculated using the ideal body weight of the donor to prevent inappropriately high volumes. Fortunately, in many cases the discrepancy created by using the recipient's weight may not be clinically significant [5]. In heart transplants the donor weight must match to within 30% of the recipient's, and similar to lungs, undersized grafts seem to be at greater risk for PGD [6].

Geographic location of the organ plays a role as increased travel prolongs the ischemic time. Warm ischemic time is kept to an absolute minimum, as grafts have been traditionally cooled to minimize metabolism and prolong the tolerated

B. E. Farmer, M.D.
Department of Anesthesiology, Emory University School of Medicine, Atlanta, GA, USA
e-mail: blaine.erickson.farmer@emory.edu

I. O. Zhukov, M.D. (✉)
University of Wisconsin, Madison, WI, USA
e-mail: zhukov@wisc.edu

period of ischemia. Lungs appear to be fairly tolerant of prolonged cold ischemic times, with similar recipient mortality between ischemic times of <4 h and >6 h [7]. Conversely, heart transplants appear at a greater risk of PGD and mortality after 210 min of cold ischemia [8]. A developing frontier is currently being explored by the makers of The Organ Care System (OCS) (TransMedics, Andover, Massachusetts), which utilizes a system very similar to an extracorporeal membrane oxygenation (ECMO) circuit to maintain a warm perfusion state of the organ. The device can be utilized by either allowing a longer transport time and acceptance of geographically distant organs, or by perfusing grafts considered to be of marginal function and ensuring suitability prior to transplantation. Early trials of OCS implementation are promising, indicating the possibility for significantly longer preservation of heart and lung grafts [9, 10]. This technology was also trialed for donation of hearts after cardiac death; although this subject is quite controversial, several remarkable successes stories have been published [11, 12].

**Table 4.1** Disease-specific intraoperative anesthetic considerations (from Slinger 2012)

| Recipient pathology | Intra-operative complications |
|---|---|
| Emphysema (COPD, Alpha-1 antitrypsin deficiency) | Hypotension with positive-pressure ventilation due to auto-PEEP |
| Cystic fibrosis | Profuse thick secretions. Difficult to maintain baseline $PaCO_2$ with positive pressure ventilation<br>Small stature, often difficult access in chest for surgeon. Chronic infections require specifically tailored antibiotics |
| Idiopathic pulmonary fibrosis | May have associated diseases (e.g., scleroderma)<br>Often older with coronary artery disease<br>May have severe pulmonary hypertension. May not tolerate one-lung ventilation and may require CPB |
| Primary pulmonary hypertension | Cardiovascular collapse secondary to hypotension on induction. CPB is considered standard |
| Bronchioalveolar carcinoma | Profuse watery secretions |

## Recipient Evaluation

The process starts with a thorough history and physical examination. Special attention should be given to both etiology and severity of the primary disorder that necessitates transplantation (Table 4.1). Potential lung recipients with sarcoidosis and idiopathic pulmonary hypertension are at the highest risk for graft dysfunction [13], as are congenital heart disease survivors and previously transplanted patients for consideration of heart transplant [14]. Secondary pulmonary hypertension portends poor outcomes and may even contraindicate lung transplantation in severe cases [13]. Any cardiac dysfunction, particularly right-sided, should be investigated in a potential lung recipient. Patients with prior intrathoracic surgery will likely have adhesions which may prolong the dissection phase of the operation and increase postoperative risk of bleeding; appropriate lead time and proper planning are essential to avoid excessive ischemic times. Similar accommodations may be needed for patients with a ventricular assist device (VAD), anticipated difficult airways, or difficult vascular access. The latter is frequently encountered in potential heart recipients due to repeated cannulation and/or underlying vascular disease.

Any recent history of infection is important given the recipient's high risk due to postoperative immunosuppression. Cystic fibrosis patients often have recurrent pulmonary infections, commonly with drug-resistant pathogens. Likewise, patients with mechanical circulatory support and externalized cannula or drivelines are susceptible to infection; open chest and infected ventricular assist devices are particularly vulnerable. In all cases, perioperative antibiotics are tailored to current or recent recipient pathogens, suspected donor pathogens, and those consistent with immunosuppressive therapy. Along with antibiotics, immunosuppressant doses and timing should be discussed with the surgical team beforehand to ensure proper timing and administration.

Preoperative blood work aids in the evaluation of co-existing organ dysfunction. Electrolyte abnormalities and renal failure are common in heart failure due to limited perfusion of the kidneys and alteration of the renin-angiotensin system. Liver function tests may be abnormal in right heart failure due to congestive hepatopathy. Coagulation studies are mandatory in any patient receiving anticoagulants or those at risk for coagulopathy. Blood products must be available with an active type and crossmatch prior to the start of surgery. Irradiated blood products may be preferred to lower the risk of graft vs. host disease due to the immunosuppression of recipients, though this complication is very rare following solid organ transplant. For cytomegalovirus (CMV) negative patients receiving CMV negative organs, leukoreduced blood should be utilized.

Preoperative cardiac echocardiography is commonly performed for both heart and lung transplant recipients to assess for ventricular dysfunction, valvular pathology, presence of shunting lesions, and pulmonary hypertension. If shunting is present, a right to left shunt can develop in the setting of RV pressure overload, and cause profound hypoxemia as well as paradoxical emboli. Right heart catheterization may be performed for patients with pulmonary hypertension to directly measure right sided pressures, cardiac output, and pulmonary vascular resistance (PVR). Additionally, left heart catheterization is usually performed for prospective lung transplant recipients with symptoms of coronary artery disease or with elevated risk due to medical comorbidities.

Preparation for advanced monitoring must occur in the preoperative period. The vast majority of transplant recipients will require at least one large bore peripheral IV, an arterial line, a multi-lumen central line with CVP monitoring, and a pulmonary artery catheter. Oximetry-enabled continuous cardiac output pulmonary artery catheters add oxygen delivery and utilization monitoring through the continuous display of central venous saturation. The pulmonary artery catheter must be placed with care due to the hemodynamic effects of arrhythmias in this tenuous patient population. It must be withdrawn to a safe depth prior to explant of the heart or lungs to ensure it is not accidentally cut or incorporated into the surgical anastomosis. Intraoperative transesophageal echocardiography is a requisite for heart and lung transplant: newly transplanted cardiac function, RV dysfunction and doppler interrogation of pulmonary vein anastomoses are examples of important TEE findings to relay to the transplant surgeon. Lastly, preoperative sedation should be given very judiciously, if at all, as it may further depress respiratory or cardiac function, and can lead quickly to decompensation.

## Lung Transplant Specific Evaluation and Management

All potential recipients should have recent pulmonary function testing (PFT) and lung perfusion scans done during their pre-transplant evaluation. The lung with the least perfusion is usually the first to be explanted, and PFTs can indicate disease severity and implicate the need for advanced support during the procedure [15]. Chronic bronchodilators, antibiotics, and pulmonary vasodilators should be continued. In the case of IV prostaglandins, they are typically continued until initiation of cardiopulmonary bypass (CPB). Placement of a thoracic epidural may be used to expedite extubation post-transplant, but this must be balanced against the chance of requiring CPB and the risk of epidural hematoma with systemic heparinization. If placement is deferred preoperatively, epidural placement may be revisited following surgery in select patients [16].

## Heart Transplant Specific Evaluation and Management

Implantable pacemakers and defibrillators are common in potential heart recipients and should be interrogated prior to surgery. If relevant, disable any ICD function prior to surgery and apply external defibrillator pads, especially in patients with a history of prior cardiac surgery, in whom a rapid sternotomy is not possible. Pacemakers may require switching to an asynchronous mode to avoid electrical interference during surgery, yet in patients with a minimal pacing burden the risk of precipitating an arrhythmia with asynchronous pacing also must be considered. These devices are typically explanted at the end of the procedure. Chronic inotropic therapy and mechanical support devices, including intra-aortic balloon pumps (IABP), VAD, and ECMO are usually maintained until CPB is initiated. Recent use of heparin products increases the risk for heparin-induced thrombocytopenia (HIT) or depletion of antithrombin III and heparin resistance. Patients with HIT and recent heparin exposure who can't have their transplant delayed will need anticoagulation with a direct thrombin inhibitor for CPB. Due to the lack of pharmacologic reversibility, patients receiving these agents are at a very high risk for bleeding complications [17].

## Intraoperative Management

### Induction

The key tenants of induction of anesthesia include maintenance of systemic vascular resistance (SVR), coronary perfusion, cardiac output, and avoidance of increased PVR. Inotrope dependent patients may need elevated support either with an increase from baseline support or addition of another agent prior to induction. Hypoxia, hypercarbia, acidosis, hypothermia, and increased sympathetic tone are the main precipitants of increased PVR, and should thus be avoided. A rapid sequence induction may be required for patients who are inadequately fasted due to emergent nature of transplant surgery. The surgical team should be present at induction in case emergent initiation of CPB is required.

Lung isolation using a left-sided double lumen endobronchial tube is typical for lung recipients, as it simplifies bronchoscopy inspection and clearance of secretions, ventilation of the graft lung independently from the native one, and rapid ability to switch ventilation between the lungs during initial dissection. Even in left single lung transplants, the short length of donor bronchus enables left-sided tube placement.

### Maintenance

The maintenance of anesthesia should follow the goals started at the induction of anesthesia. Either an inhaled volatile anesthetic or total intravenous anesthetic are acceptable choices, though nitrous oxide is not recommended due to its augmenting effect on PVR. Special attention should be paid to maintenance of normothermia, as reperfusion of the cold-stored graft(s), infusion of cold or room temperature blood products and intravenous fluids and massive pleura exposure with convective heat loss all contribute to recipient hypothermia. Hypothermia is not only concerning due to the increase in PVR, but can potentially precipitate arrhythmias and coagulopathy. In lung transplants, judicious volume replacement is paramount; lung grafts suffer from impaired permeability and thus are sensitive to pulmonary edema.

Conservative transfusion of blood products is also important for avoidance of transfusion associated lung injury or circulatory overload; PRBC transfusion of more than 1 L is an independent risk factor for PGD [13]. Vasoactive and inotropic support is universal in heart transplantation but is also frequently needed in lung transplantation and is tailored to each specific case, with epinephrine, norepinephrine, vasopressin, dobutamine, isoproterenol, and milrinone all having a defined role.

### Ventilation Strategy

Proper ventilation is a paramount concern in lung transplantation, but a lung protective ventilation strategy may also be beneficial during heart transplantation and transition of care into the recovery phase in the ICU. Pressure controlled modes may limit inflation pressures, reduce regional over distention, and provide more homogenous gas exchange in the lung [5]. Volume controlled modes on the other hand may deliver more consistent tidal volume in situations of dynamic compliance changes [18]. Tidal volumes less than or equal to 6ml/kg/IBW were advocated to improve outcomes in acute respiratory distress syndrome (ARDS) patients, and may increase the viability of lung grafts when adopted in potential donors [6]. If tolerated, consider further reducing tidal volumes during OLV. The increased cardiac output passing through a single lung during this period makes it more sensitive to ventilator-induced lung injury. Permissive hypercarbia during this period may help achieve tidal volume and inflation pressure goals. It is also postulated to improve cerebral perfusion, as many lung recipients are chronic $CO_2$ retainers and their cerebral autoregulation may be adapted to a higher $PaCO_2$. On the other hand, it could worsen pulmonary hypertension and precipitate right heart failure, particularly since lung grafts are more sensitive to hypercarbia-mediated vasoconstriction following reperfusion [18].

Ideally, peak inspiratory pressures and plateau pressures should be limited to less than 35 $cmH_2O$ and 30 $cmH_2O$, respectively. Higher inflation pressures in lung transplants are associated with increased mortality, poorer lung function at 72 h and 3 months, prolonged mechanical ventilation, increased ICU length of stay, and the need for renal replacement therapy. However, it's unclear if higher inflation pressures are truly the cause or are reflective of poor graft function [5]. The routine addition of 5–10 $cmH_2O$ of PEEP may improve bronchial microcirculation after reperfusion of lung grafts, as suggested by animal studies, though increased airway pressures can place increased stress on bronchial anastomoses. Lung recruitment maneuvers after periods of deflation or rewarming may be utilized, but should not exceed 30 $cmH_2O$. They should also be performed in communication with surgeons and while visually inspecting the lungs [18].

## Surgical Considerations: Lung Transplantation

Single lung transplant (SLT) has been associated with poorer outcomes and increased risk of PGD; it can also make post-transplant ventilation challenging due to a poorly functional native lung that will not be replaced in the near term. For these reasons, bilateral sequential single lung transplantation (BSSLT) is the most common transplant method. Often, the sequential nature of the procedure permits implantation without requiring CPB, which is an independent risk factor for PGD [13]. However, CPB is useful in patients with advanced lung disease and those with pulmonary hypertension due to the high risk of precipitating right ventricular failure during OLV. Some centers choose to use venoarterial (VA) ECMO in place of CPB, as it may reduce the risk of pulmonary and renal complications; there is no conclusive evidence to favor either approach at the present time [18].

Regardless of the chosen approach, the salient steps of the procedure are similar. A bilateral thoracosternotomy "clamshell" is commonly used for the bilateral lung transplant, while a single thoracotomy incision is sufficient for a unilateral lung transplant. In the case of the sequential bilateral lung transplants, both diseased lungs are mobilized to lessen the ischemia time of the graft prior to the graft arrival in the operating suite [15]. Bronchus, being the most posterior structure, is anastomosed first, followed by the pulmonary artery and pulmonary vein suture lines [15]. Application of the left atrial clamp during pulmonary venous anastomoses may produce arrhythmias, reduce left ventricular filling, or inadvertently occlude a coronary artery. De-airing is required prior to reperfusion and should be guided by TEE when available. Reperfusion is the most active time for the anesthesiology team, and is pivotal in the development of ischemia-reperfusion (IR) injury - a pattern of injury that occurs after reperfusion of a previously ischemic organ. The pathogenesis involves cell lysis and inflammation during the ischemic period, followed by formation of oxygen radicals and apoptosis after the return of oxygen and energy substrates to the cells [19]. To minimize the development of IR, the PA clamp is released gradually and $FiO_2$ is reduced to the minimum needed to achieve $SpO_2 > 92\%$ and $PaO_2 > 70$ mmHg. A $FiO_2 > 0.4$ at reperfusion is associated with an increased risk of severe PGD [13].

Other reperfusion complications include myocardial stunning due to return of cold, metabolite rich fluid from the graft. Arrhythmias such as atrial fibrillation or ventricular tachycardia can occur, warranting rapid treatment. It is common to have increased potassium and lactic acid immediately following reperfusion and therapy should be tailored to the most likely etiology. Air embolism can produce a multitude of problems, but most frequently affects the right coronary artery and right ventricular function. Vascular anastomotic imperfections may become apparent and can require rapid volume replacement.

Hypoxia after reperfusion should trigger suspicion for PGD, but another possibility during SLT is preferential ventilation of the remaining native lung due to differences in compliance. The resulting shunt can be temporarily corrected by clamping the PA while additional therapies are initiated. The lungs may need to be independently ventilated for a period of time, with the native lung receiving 100% oxygen while protecting the graft from hyperoxia at a lower $FiO_2$. Decubitus positioning may lessen the shunt fraction and improve oxygenation, but is of limited utility in the middle of the ongoing transplant [16].

## Surgical Considerations: Heart Transplantation

Orthotopic heart transplantation must be performed while on CPB, to permit anastomoses of right and left heart inflow and outflow in a bloodless field. In order to minimize ischemic time, the surgeon may elect to finish the most anterior anastomosis of pulmonary artery after releasing the aortic cross-clamp and reperfusion of the graft [20]. Whatever strategy is employed, the heart is de-aired prior to release of the aortic cross clamp while the patient is maintained in Trendelenburg position to minimize air traveling into the cerebral vasculature. Carotid occlusion to accomplish the same goal is controversial, though occasionally performed. Weaning from CPB can be attempted once the graft is allowed sufficient time for reperfusion, and myocardial stunning or other ill effects from return of metabolite rich fluid are less of a concern. Arrhythmias are common during this period, and restoration of sinus rhythm may require electrical cardioversion or defibrillation. Augmented contractility with inotropic support is standard at many centers. An ideal heart rate between 90 and 110 beats per minute is maintained to decrease excess preload and facilitate cardiac output, either with epicardial pacing or chronotropic agents.

Hemodynamic goals for the CPB wean are based on maintenance of systemic afterload and therefore coronary perfusion, while avoiding RV failure due to excessive preload. Biventricular function should be assessed visually and by TEE, along with monitoring of pulmonary and systemic pressures. If significant hypotension or dysfunction becomes apparent, CPB flows should be increased and preload volume taken back to the CPB reservoir as RV failure is the most common cause of failure to separate from the CPB. The use of mild hyperventilation, inhaled pulmonary vasodilators, and inotropes and vasopressors with favorable effects on the RV such as milrinone are often employed.

## Primary Graft Dysfunction: Lung Transplantation

In lung transplantation, PGD occurs in 10–30% of cases and is the leading cause of morbidity and mortality [13]. PGD is similar to acute respiratory distress syndrome (ARDS), both histologically and clinically [6]. The essential clinical features are impaired oxygenation and evidence of diffuse pulmonary edema on imaging occurring within 72 h of lung transplant and not attributable to other causes. The International Society of Heart and Lung Transplant (ISHLT) differentiate PGD grades primarily by $PaO_2/FiO_2$ ratio (Table 4.2) [21]. Multiple studies demonstrate that severe PGD worsens functional outcomes and increases early mortality, duration of mechanical ventilation, ICU length of stay, and the risk of later developing a form of chronic rejection, termed bronchiolitis obliterans [13].

**Table 4.2** Recommendations for grading primary graft dysfunction severity in lung transplantation (from Christie et al., 2004)

| Grade | $PaO_2/FiO_2$ | Radiographic infiltrates consistent with pulmonary edema |
|---|---|---|
| 0 | >300 | Absent |
| 1 | >300 | Present |
| 2 | 200–300 | Present |
| 3 | <200 | Present |

**Table 4.3** Recommended classification for primary graft dysfunction in heart transplantation (from Kobashigawa 2014)

| Type of primary graft dysfunction | Diagnostic criteria |
|---|---|
| Left ventricular (PGD-LV) | Includes isolated LV failure and biventricular failure |
| Mild | LVEF <40%, RAP >15 mmHg, PCWP >20 mmHg, CI < 2.0 L/min/m² (lasting >1 h), requiring low dose inotropes |
| Moderate | As in mild, but requiring either high dose inotropes or newly placed IABP |
| Severe | Dependence on MCS, excluding IABP |
| Right ventricular (PGD-RV) | Isolated RV failure only. Requires either a + b, or c<br>• RAP >15 mmHg, PCWP <15 mmHg, CI < 2.0 L/min/m² (lasting >1 h)<br>• TPG < 15 mmHg and/or PASP <50 mmHg<br>• Need for RVAD |

The first line of treatment is inhaled nitric oxide (iNO) or an inhaled prostaglandin, most commonly epoprostenol in this country. It has long been suggested that prophylactic iNO could potentially reduce IR injury and prevent the need for CPB in OLV, due to its favorable effects on reducing PVR, improving V/Q mismatch, ameliorating the systemic inflammatory process, and limiting oxidative stress [22]. However, a preponderance of evidence has failed to show any benefit in prophylactic use [23]. Therefore, it's use is primarily restricted to treatment of pulmonary hypertension, RV failure, and early PGD [24]. If hypoxia cannot be corrected through pulmonary vasodilators, veno-venous ECMO is typically employed to support oxygenation postoperatively; conservative ventilation is utilized while the lungs are recovering on this support [25].

## Primary Graft Dysfunction: Heart Transplantation

PGD occurs in an estimated 5–10% of heart transplantations and is considered the leading cause of early mortality after transplant [26]. According to the ISHLT, it can be classified based upon the affected ventricle, with left ventricular PGD being further graded by severity (Table 4.3). Clinically, it manifests as ventricular dysfunction without an obvious etiology that develops within 24 h of transplant. The development of PGD also increases the risk for coronary artery vasculopathy, which is a significant source of late graft failure with an incidence of approximately 50% after 10 years [14].

The mainstay of treatment for PGD is inotropic support. Epinephrine, milrinone, and dobutamine are commonly employed. Right-sided failure may benefit from pulmonary vasodilators such as iNO or epoprostenol, which reduce PVR to alleviate pressure overload. Mild to moderate dysfunction may improve with the placement of an IABP [27]. Inability to wean from CPB typically requires more significant mechanical circulatory support (MCS), including VA-ECMO or placement of a VAD (Tables 4.4 and 4.5).

## Right Ventricular Failure

Both heart and lung transplants are at high risk of acute RV failure and exhibit similar pathophysiology. Due to respiratory disease, lung transplant patients may already have some degree of pulmonary hypertension and right heart strain. During OLV, one of the main branches of the PA is clamped and the entire cardiac output must pass through one lung, which leads to a dramatic increase in PVR. Periods of hypoxia or hypercarbia are also common and increase PVR further. In heart transplants, the donor right ventricle is

**Table 4.4** Heart transplantation-important perioperative considerations

| Plan/preparation/adverse events | Reasoning/management |
|---|---|
| Preprocedural evaluation | |
| Cardiac structure, function, thrombus<br>Pulmonary hypertension<br>Pacemaker/AICD interrogation<br>Pulmonary, liver, or renal involvement<br>Recent infections | – Initially evaluated by TTE or TEE, heart catheterization<br>– Disable defibrillators and antitachycardia pacing, set pacemakers to asynchronous mode<br>– Frequently affected in advanced heart failure<br>– Guides antibiotic selection, informs risk of intraoperative sepsis |
| Preoperative support | |
| Chronic inotrope therapy<br>Intraaortic balloon pump<br>Ventricular assist device<br>Total artificial heart | – May need to increase prior to induction, continue until supported on CPB<br>– Continue until CPB<br>– May require reversal of anticoagulation. Allow extra time for explant |
| Positioning—Supine | Access for median sternotomy and CPB cannulas |
| Vascular access and invasive monitors | |
| 1+ large bore peripheral IV<br>1–2 arterial lines<br>Central line with side port (9F and larger)<br>   Pulmonary artery catheter<br>   Transesophageal echocardiography | – 16, 14, or 12G preferred with warmed fluids<br>– Hemodynamic monitoring and blood gas analysis<br>– Vasoactive infusions, PAC placement, and/or volume resuscitation. Additional central line may be required.<br>– Monitoring of PA pressures before explant of native heart and after reperfusion of graft, cardiac output measurement, $SvO_2$<br>– To assess cardiac function before, during, and after CPB, and diagnosis of intraoperative events |
| GA with controlled induction and standard ETT | Minimize increases in PVR, drop in SVR, and maintain coronary perfusion |
| Procedural adverse events<br>Hypoxemia<br>Hypercarbia<br>Hypotension<br>Bleeding<br>Air embolus<br>Primary graft dysfunction<br>RV failure | As indicated |
| Postoperative considerations<br>As described for procedural adverse events excepting air embolus<br>ICU transport and handoff | As indicated |

unaccustomed to the pre-existing pulmonary hypertension present in the recipient and has limited ability to increase its contractility to meet the demand. Therefore, in both cases, an acute increase in afterload contributes significantly to right ventricular failure. Inhaled pulmonary vasodilators are the first line of treatment as they attenuate RV afterload. Initiation of milrinone, a phosphodiesterase 3 inhibitor, increases contractility and further decreases PVR. The addition of epinephrine works synergistically to improve inotropy and helps counteract the systemic vasodilation seen with these agents. If additional support for systemic vascular resistance is needed, vasopressin may be used to increase the systemic pressure and therefore coronary perfusion with less effect on PVR. Medically refractory RV failure may be treated with an IABP, which is postulated to help by unloading interventricular septum and augmenting diastolic blood pressure and therefore coronary perfusion [27]. ECMO may be superior to VAD placement for treatment of both primary and secondary acute RV failure [28].

## Postoperative Management

Postoperatively, patients are usually transported to the ICU intubated, where they can be monitored closely for any complications. For lung

**Table 4.5** Lung transplantation-important perioperative considerations

| Plan/preparation/adverse events | Reasoning/management |
|---|---|
| Preprocedural evaluation | |
| PFTs and lung perfusion scanning<br>Pulmonary hypertension<br>Cardiac dysfunction<br>Intracardiac shunt<br>Liver or renal involvement<br>Recent infections | – Used to assess function and determination of first explanted lung<br>– Initially evaluated by TTE with bubble study, with heart catheterization and other testing as indicated<br>– Suggests possible right ventricular dysfunction and left ventricular dysfunction, respectively<br>– Guides antibiotic selection, informs risk of perioperative sepsis |
| Operative approach | |
| Single lung transplant<br>Bilateral sequential single lung transplant<br>CPB or ECMO | – Be prepared for independent ventilation of lungs due to potential differences in compliance<br>– Use lung protective ventilation and lowest possible $FiO_2$ during OLV with new graft<br>– Preferred for significant pulmonary hypertension due to high risk of acute RV failure with OLV |
| Position | |
| Lateral decubitus<br>Supine | – Improved V/Q matching during OLV<br>– Improved access for bilateral transplants and/or cannulation for CPB or mechanical support |
| Vascular access and invasive monitors | |
| 1+ large bore peripheral IV<br>Arterial line<br>Central line with side port (9F and larger)<br>Pulmonary artery catheter | – 16, 14, or 12G preferred with warmed fluids, however fluid administration should be kept to a minimum<br>– Hemodynamic monitoring and blood gas analysis<br>– Vasoactive infusions, PAC placement, and/or volume resuscitation. Additional central line may be required<br>– Monitoring of PA pressures before explant of native lung and after reperfusion of graft, cardiac output measurement, $SvO_2$ |
| GA with left-sided double lumen endobronchial tube (DLT) | DLT required for OLV, lung isolation, possible independent ventilation of lungs postoperatively |
| Procedural adverse events<br>Hypoxemia<br>Hypercarbia<br>Hypotension<br>Bleeding<br>Air embolus<br>Primary graft dysfunction<br>RV failure | As indicated |
| Postoperative considerations<br>As described for procedural adverse events excepting air embolus<br>ICU transport and handoff | As indicated |

recipients, the double lumen endobronchial tube is ideally replaced with a single lumen tube prior to transportation, unless independent lung ventilation is needed or additional airway concerns exist. Adequate sedation should be verified prior to transport to prevent difficulties with ventilation, increased sympathetic tone with hemodynamic swings, or dislodging of essential lines and support apparatus. Invasive blood pressure, ECG, and $SpO_2$ monitoring are required. Transporting with a portable ventilator may be considered to ensure proper ventilation, inflation pressures, and is particularly useful in patients receiving inhaled vasodilators and those where manual ventilation may otherwise prove difficult. Clamping of the endotracheal tube prior to switching ventilators will preserve alveolar recruitment and lessen the chance of hypoxia and unnecessary lung trauma. The transition of care to the ICU team should include description of intraoperative complications, required vasoactive and inotropic support, recent ventilator settings, and recommended titration parameters as agreed upon with the surgical team.

## References

1. 2016 Annual Report of the U.S. Organ Procurement and Transplantation Network and the scientific registry of transplant recipients. Rockville, MD: Department of Health and Human Services, Health Resources and Services Administration, Healthcare Systems Bureau, Division of Transplantation.
2. Scientific Registry of Transplant Recipients. Heart. https://www.srtr.org/document/pdf?fileName=\012017_release\pdfPSR\GAEMTX1HR201611PNEW.pdf.
3. Scientific Registry of Transplant Recipients. Lung. https://www.srtr.org/document/pdf?fileName=\012017_release\pdfPSR\GAEMTX1LU201611PNEW.pdf.
4. Beer A, Reed RM, Bolukbas S, Budev M, Chaux G, Zamora MR, et al. Mechanical ventilation after lung transplantation. An international survey of practices and preferences. Ann Am Thorac Soc. 2014;11(4):546–53.
5. Thakuria L, Davey R, Romano R, Carby MR, Kaul S, Griffiths MJ, et al. Mechanical ventilation after lung transplantation. J Crit Care. 2016;31(1):110–8.
6. Costanzo MR, Taylor D, Hunt S, et al. The International Society of Heart and Lung Transplantation guideline for the care of heart transplant recipients. J Heart Lung Transplant. 2010;29:914–56.
7. Lannon JD, Ball A, RBC YN, Clark S, Mascaro J, et al. The effect of cold and warm ischemia time on survival after lung transplantation in a large national cohort. J Heart Lung Transplant. 2014;32(4S):S94.
8. Wagner FM. Donor heart preservation and perfusion. Appl Cardiopulm Pathophysiol. 2011;15:198–206.
9. Warnecke G, Moradiellos J, Tudorache I, Kuhn C, Avsar M, Wiegmann B, et al. Normothermic perfusion of donor lungs for preservation and assessment with the organ care system lung before bilateral transplantation: a pilot study of 12 patients. Lancet. 2012;380(9856):1851–8.
10. Saez DG, Zych B, Sabashnikov A, Bowles CT, Robertis FD, Prashant NM, et al. Evaluation of the organ care system in heart transplantation with an adverse donor/recipient profile. Ann Thorac Surg. 2014;98(6):2099–106.
11. Boucek MM, Mashburn C, Dunn SM, Frizell R, Edwards L, Pietra B, et al. Pediatric heart transplantation after declaration of cardiocirculatory death. N Engl J Med. 2008;359(7):709–14.
12. Dhital KK, Iyer A, Connellan M, Chew HC, Gao L, Doyle A, et al. Adult heart transplantation with distant procurement and ex-vivo preservation of donor hearts after circulatory death: a case series. Lancet. 2015;385(9987):2585–91.
13. Diamond JM, Lee JC, Kawut SM, Shah RJ, Localio AR, Bellamy SL, et al. Clinical risk factors for primary graft dysfunction after lung transplantation. Am J Respir Crit Care Med. 2013;187(5):527–34.
14. Kobashigawa J, Zuckermann A, Macdonald P, Leprince P, Esmailian F, Luu M, et al. Report from a consensus conference on primary graft dysfunction after cardiac transplantation. J Heart Lung Transplant. 2014;33(4):327–40.
15. Hayanga JW, D'Cunha J. The surgical technique of bilateral sequential lung transplantation. J Thorac Dis. 2014;6(8):1063–9.
16. Slinger P. Anesthetic management for lung transplantation. Tx Med. 2012;24:24–32.
17. Wadia Y, Cooper JR, Bracey AW, et al. Intraoperative anticoagulation management during cardiac transplantation. Tex Heart Inst J. 2008;35:62–5.
18. Barnes L, Reed RM, Parekh KR, Bhama JK, Pena T, Rajagopal S, et al. Mechanical ventilation for the lung transplant recipient. Curr Pulmonol Rep. 2015;4(2):88–96.
19. Ferrari RS, Andrade CF. Oxidative stress and lung ischemia-reperfusion injury. Oxidative Med Cell Longev. 2015;2015:590987.
20. Fischer S, Glas KE. A review of cardiac transplantation. Anesthesiol Clin. 2013;31(2):383–403.
21. Christie JD, Carby M, Bag R, Corris P, Hertz M, Weill D, et al. Report of the ISHLT working group on primary lung graft dysfunction part II: definition. A consensus statement of the International Society for Heart and Lung Transplantation. J Heart Lung Transplant. 2005;24(10):1454–9.
22. Meade MO, Granton JT, Matte-Martyn A, McRae K, Weaver B, Cripps P, et al. A randomized trial of inhaled nitric oxide to prevent ischemia-reperfusion injury after lung transplantation. Am J Respir Crit Care Med. 2003;167(11):1483–9.
23. Tavar AN, Tsakok T. Does prophylactic inhaled nitric oxide reduce morbidity and mortality after lung transplantation? Interact Cardiovasc Thorac Surg. 2011;13(5):516–20.
24. Pasero D, Martin EL, Davi A, Mascia L, Rinaldi M, Ranieri VM. The effects of inhaled nitric oxide after lung transplanttation. Minerva Anestesiol. 2010;76(5):353–61.
25. Diamond JM, Ahya VN. Mechanical ventilation after lung transplantation. It's time for a trial. Ann Am Thorac Soc. 2014;11(4):598–9.
26. Chew HC, Kumarasinghe G, et al. Primary graft dysfunction after heart transplantation. Curr Transplant Rep. 2014;1:257–65. https://doi.org/10.1007/s40472-014-0033-6.
27. Arafa OE, Geiran OR, Andersen K, Fosse E, Simonsen S, Svennevig JL. Intraaortic balloon pumping for predominantly right ventricular failure after heart transplantation. Ann Thorac Surg. 2000;70(5):1587–93.
28. Taghavi S, Zuckermann A, Ankersmit J, Wieselthaler G, Rajek A, Laufer G, et al. Extracorporeal membrane oxygenation is superior to right ventricular assist device for acute right ventricular failure after heart transplantation. Ann Thorac Surg. 2004;78(5):1644–9.

# Anesthesia for Pulmonary Endarterectomy

Cara Iorianni and Ellen Richter

## Introduction

Pulmonary endarterectomy (PEA) is a complex surgical procedure involving the removal of obstructive material from the pulmonary arteries. It has become the preferred treatment for patients with chronic thromboembolic pulmonary hypertension (CTEPH) and is also more recently being considered in patients with chronic thromboembolic disease who exhibit persistent dyspnea in the absence of pulmonary hypertension (PH) [1]. PEA is a technically demanding procedure and requires a multidisciplinary team of pulmonologists, cardiothoracic surgeons, and cardiac anesthesiologists as well as sophisticated postoperative intensive care. The lowest mortality rates have been achieved at experienced centers, with the University of California, San Diego reporting the highest case volume (>3000 cases) to date [2, 3]. However, the number of institutions performing the procedure is expected to grow in congruence with the increased recognition and diagnosis of chronic thromboembolic pulmonary disease.

C. Iorianni, M.D.
Department of Anesthesiology, Emory University, Atlanta, GA, USA
e-mail: cara.ann.iorianni@emory.edu

E. Richter, M.D. (✉)
Division of Cardiothoracic Anesthesiology, Department of Anesthesiology, Emory University, Atlanta, GA, USA
e-mail: ellen.richter@emory.edu

## Epidemiology and Pathophysiology of Chronic Thromboembolic Pulmonary Hypertension

CTEPH is classified by the World Health Organization as Group 4 of disorders that cause PH [4] and is caused by recurrent or unresolved thromboemboli in the major pulmonary vessels. It is both a rare and under diagnosed condition, occurring in approximately 3% of acute pulmonary embolism (PE) survivors within 2 years of the event [5]. Without treatment, CTEPH results in persistently elevated pulmonary vascular resistance and pulmonary artery pressures, right heart failure, and death in 90% of patients within 3 years of diagnosis [6]. It is, however, a unique form of PH in that it is potentially curable with PEA surgery, making early diagnosis and surgical referral important to surgical success and patient survival.

CTEPH is a form of pre-capillary PH defined as a mean pulmonary arterial pressure (mPAP) >25 mmHg with a pulmonary capillary wedge pressure (PCWP) <15 in the setting of chronic thrombi and/or emboli limiting flow in the elastic pulmonary arteries (main, lobar, segmental, subsegmental) after at least 3 months of effective anticoagulation [7]. Incomplete dissolution of thrombus after acute or recurrent PE leads to thrombus organization and fibrosis as well as secondary changes in the more distal pulmonary vasculature. Persistent pulmonary vascular obstruction and resultant increased pulmonary arterial pressures induce reactive medial hypertrophy and intimal hyperplasia in vessels distal to obstruction. This occlusive vascular remodeling narrows the vessel lumens throughout the lung and further increases pulmonary vascular resistance (PVR). Microvascular changes occurring beyond the initial thrombus often generate pulmonary artery pressures greater than initially observed with acute PE and may be indistinguishable from idiopathic pulmonary artery hypertension [6].

There is no clear understanding as to why CTEPH develops in a minority of patients with acute PE. Exact mechanisms for incomplete thrombus resolution have been explored, including hypercoaguability, impaired fibrinolysis, and increased inflammation, but have been limited by the lack of a definitive animal model [8]. Elevated levels of factor VIII are found with higher incidence (around 40%) in patients with CTEPH compared to controls, and approximately 20% of CTEPH patients carry anticardiolipin antibodies, Lupus anticoagulant, or both [9]. Inflammatory states such as ventriculoatrial shunts for hydrocephalus therapy, infected pacemaker wires, inflammatory bowel disease, chronic osetomyelitis, splenectomy, and malignancy have been associated with increased incidence of CTEPH [8–10]. Despite advances in the understanding of underlying mechanisms of CTEPH, most patients who develop CTEPH do not have a recognized coagulation defect, fibrinolytic deficiency, or one of the associated medical conditions noted above. In fact, the European CTEPH Registry reports that only 74.8% and 56.1% of CTEPH patients have a previously diagnosed PE and deep vein thrombosis (DVT), respectively [10]. This suggests that a significant number of CTEPH cases will present following asymptomatic venous thromboembolism. There is no current consensus on how to predict who will develop CTEPH and who may benefit from closer surveillance [8].

## Clinical Manifestations and Pre-operative Evaluation

PEA candidates often present with some degree of right heart failure and hypoxemia along with their associated sequelae. Similar to other patients with PH, patients with CTEPH usually present later in the disease process with symptoms of fatigue and dyspnea on exertion. As the disease progresses and right heart function worsens, patients may also experience atypical chest pain, orthopnea, syncope, hemoptysis, abdominal distension, and lower extremity edema. On physical exam, patients may exhibit a loud P2, tricuspid regurgitation (TR) murmur, palpable right ventricular heave, jugular venous distention, hepatomegaly, ascites, peripheral edema, and pulmonary artery flow murmurs over the lung fields due to turbulent flow through narrowed vessels. Hypoxemia and hyperventilation with hypocarbia can occur as dead space ventilation increases and are accompanied by a balanced reduction in bicarbonate levels. Pre-operative testing for surgical consideration is extensive and includes echocardiography, a right heart catheterization, and pulmonary angiography. These studies provide information detailing the severity of PH, degree of right heart dysfunction, and distribution of disease and should be reviewed in addition to the patient's laboratory values prior to surgery [9].

Most patients being considered for PEA have significantly elevated mPAP and PVR, with mPAP generally >45 mmHg and PVR approximately 9 Wood units [8]. High mPAP and PVR, while associated with greater perioperative mortality, should not exclude patients from PTE candidacy, as these patients often achieve the greatest symptomatic and hemodynamic improvements after PEA [2, 9]. An important factor in determining operability is the surgical accessibility of disease. Significant hemodynamic compromise in the setting of relatively low clot burden on imaging is suggestive of more distal disease involving subsegmental arteries [8, 9]. This disease pattern is more difficult to approach surgically, is associated with residual PH, and portends a worse perioperative prognosis [11]. These patients may not be considered good candidates for PEA; however, determination of operability remains very center- and surgeon-dependent [8].

## Guiding Principles of PEA

Although unilateral PEA via thoracotomy has been described historically, the vast majority of cases today are bilateral and performed via median sternotomy using cardiopulmonary bypass (CPB) and deep hypothermic circulatory arrest (DHCA) [2]. Experts advise avoiding a unilateral approach to PEA because it necessitates a subsequent contralateral reoperation (most patients have bilateral disease), risks hemodynamic compromise with PA clamping, provides inadequate surgical exposure due to bronchial blood flow, and exposes patients to excessive blood loss from engorged collateral vessels in the thorax [9, 12]. Median sternotomy allows good bilateral surgical exposure without entering the pleural cavities and facilitates quick initiation of CPB in the event of instability. CPB is required not just to mitigate hemodynamic instability but also to allow cooling for DHCA. Periods of DHCA are generally required for a successful, complete endarterectomy; otherwise, bronchial bleeding can severely hamper identification of the endarterectomy plane [2]. A true endarterectomy, in the plane of the media and extending into the subsegmental vessels, must be completed; simple thrombectomy will not result in improvement in CTEPH and is associated with high perioperative morbidity and mortality [12].

## Pre-operative Preparation

Some patients, particularly those with a contraindication to later anticoagulation, may have an inferior vena cava (IVC) filter placed a few days prior to PEA to prevent recurrent PE from lower extremity DVT [3]. Prior to induction, patients typically have a large-bore peripheral IV and radial arterial line placed. Although CTEPH patients are thought to have a relatively fixed PVR, various factors can still worsen PH, so premedication should be titrated cautiously. Pain and anxiety can increase PVR, but excessive sedation and concomitant respiratory depression can cause hypercarbia and hypoxia, which may also raise pulmonary artery (PA) pressures. Some authors recommend sparing use of benzodiazepines and complete avoidance of opioids [2]. Patients who do receive premedication should have supplemental oxygen and full monitors applied [13]. Placement of a central line is usually deferred until after induction, because many PEA patients may not be able to tolerate lying flat. A pre-induction pulmonary artery catheter (PAC) is generally not required, because information about right heart function and pulmonary pressures is already available from the extensive preoperative diagnostic work-up [2].

## Induction and Pre-bypass Period

### Induction

After preoxygenation, patients are induced with standard monitors plus invasive arterial pressure monitoring. The primary concern during induction is the maintenance of right ventricular function. CTEPH patients typically have a hypertrophied, dilated right ventricle (RV) with some degree of dysfunction. In this setting, the coronary blood supply to the RV becomes more tenuous and is proportional to systemic pressures but inversely related to intracavitary RV pressures. Therefore, the hemodynamic goals for a successful induction are to maintain systemic vascular resistance (SVR), avoid further increases in PVR, and support RV contractility. Phenylephrine or norepinephrine may be used to maintain systemic blood pressures, but vasopressin is a reasonable alternative, since it appears to cause minimal rise in PVR [14]. Hypoxia, hypercarbia, and acidosis should be avoided. Most induction agents can be used successfully, provided the above goals are met [2]. The bulk of the induction dose of narcotics should be titrated in after a muscle relaxant has been given to avoid chest wall rigidity and resultant inadequate ventilation. Attempts to lower PVR using systemic vasodilators (e.g., nitroglycerin or sodium nitroprusside) may be quite harmful; they tend to have little effect on PVR in the setting of CTEPH, and the drop in systemic pressures can precipitate RV ischemia and rapid hemodynamic collapse [13].

It may be prudent to start an inotrope infusion just before induction, especially in patients at high risk of instability (i.e., those with severe PH or with significantly depressed RV function, as indicated by an RVEDP >15 mmHg, severe TR, PVR >1000 dynes s cm$^{-5}$, or a cardiac index <1.5 L/min/m$^2$) [2]. Epinephrine is a reasonable choice, since it supports contractility, bolsters SVR, and maintains an elevated heart rate. Drops in heart rate should be treated promptly, and sinus rhythm should be maintained if possible.

## Lines and Monitors

Intubation proceeds with a single-lumen endotracheal tube (ETT). A large end-tidal $CO_2$ to $PaCO_2$ gradient is present in CTEPH, so arterial blood gases must be monitored to evaluate the adequacy of ventilation [2]. A transesophageal echocardiography probe is introduced after intubation. This is done before central line and PAC insertion to guide PAC placement, monitor RV function, and look for right atrium (RA) or proximal pulmonary artery (PA) thrombus. Next, a central catheter is inserted in the right internal jugular vein under ultrasound guidance. Some authors recommend avoiding Trendelenburg position during line placement, because patients with RV dysfunction may become unstable with the increase in venous return. A PAC is introduced next. Placement may be difficult due to RV dilation and the presence of TR. It may be advisable to forego wedging the PAC due to a potentially increased risk of PA bleeding and rupture in CTEPH [15]. If intracardiac or pulmonary artery thrombus is present, the PAC should not be advanced further than the superior vena cava (approximately 20 cm depth) to avoid dislodging any clot. A femoral arterial line is inserted to monitor central arterial blood pressure.

Patients are often monitored with processed electrical encephalography (EEG) to assess anesthetic depth and to ensure isoelectricity prior to institution of DHCA. Cerebral oximetry measures the tissue saturation of the superficial frontal cortex and thus is helpful in evaluating the adequacy of oxygen delivery to this area [16]. It may also detect large-scale cerebral ischemic events, but should not be confused as a measure of global cerebral perfusion. Core temperature is monitored with bladder and rectal temperature probes, tympanic membrane or nasopharyngeal temperatures are used as surrogates for brain temperature, and blood temperature is followed with the PAC. A head wrap, which circulates cold water, can be applied to the head to augment cerebral cooling.

If the patient's hematocrit permits, one or 2 units of autologous blood are removed and stored in Citrate Phosphate Dextrose Adenine (CPDA) bags. CTEPH patients are often chronically hypoxic and commonly have some degree of polycythemia. Moderate hemodilution to a hematocrit of 18–25% is believed to be beneficial in patients undergoing DHCA, because it decreases blood viscosity and promotes uniform cooling [2, 17]. Autologous blood collection also saves valuable plasma coagulation factors and platelets from being diluted or destroyed during a long CPB run.

## Transesophageal Echocardiography (TEE)

TEE provides essential real-time information about cardiac function and other important parameters during PEA. Signs of chronic PH with right-sided volume and pressure overload include RA enlargement with right-to-left shift of the interatrial septum, RV dilation and hypertrophy, a D-shaped interventricular septum throughout the cardiac cycle, and tricuspid annular dilatation with resultant TR. The PA systolic pressure can be estimated using the peak tricuspid regurgitant jet velocity. The severity of TR should be determined to monitor for postoperative improvement. Pericardial effusions are common because elevated right-sided pressures impair pericardial lymphatic drainage [18]. High right atrial pressures may also impede thebesian drainage, causing the coronary sinus to be enlarged [9]. RV function should be evaluated thoroughly. A tricuspid annular systolic plane excursion (TAPSE) of <1.6 cm, a tissue Doppler

S′ of the basal RV free wall <10 cm/s, or an RV myocardial performance index (RMPI or Tei index) of >0.4 are all indicative of impaired RV function [9, 19]. Up to 35% of CTEPH patients have a patent foramen ovale (PFO), so the interatrial septum should be interrogated with color flow Doppler (CFD) [20]. A bubble study with agitated saline may be performed if CFD is inconclusive, but this maneuver should be done with caution and only after the patient is prepped and draped, because hemodynamic collapse has been reported during application of the Valsalva maneuver [9]. The baseline TEE exam should also evaluate left ventricular function, identify any other valvular abnormalities, and look for intracardiac and pulmonary thrombus.

## Bypass Initiation and Deep Hypothermic Circulatory Arrest

After median sternotomy, the pericardium is opened, and a bolus of IV heparin is given. The distended and depressed right heart may tolerate surgical manipulation poorly, so as soon as an activated clotting time (ACT) of >450 s has been achieved, ascending aortic and bicaval cannulation proceeds and CPB is initiated. Antifibrinolytics are often avoided because CTEPH patients tend to be hypercoagulable at baseline. A typical pump priming solution is used. Patients also typically receive a dose of methylprednisolone (for its anti-inflammatory and cell membrane stabilizing properties), mannitol (for free radical scavenging and osmotic diuresis), and phenytoin (for post-operative seizure prophylaxis) [2]. The patient is gradually cooled (over 60–90 min) to 20 °C with the CPB circuit and possibly cooling blankets and a head wrap. The left ventricle (LV) can distend with hypothermia-induced fibrillation, so an LV vent is placed via a pulmonary vein.

When core temperature reaches 20 °C and tympanic membrane temperature approaches 16–18 °C, the aorta is cross clamped, cardioplegia is administered to ensure diastolic arrest, and a cooling jacket may be placed on the heart for additional myocardial protection. The surgeon incises the right PA and begins exposing the endarterectomy plane. When bronchial bleeding obscures the field, a bolus of propofol is given to ensure an isoelectric EEG, and circulatory arrest is initiated. All monitoring lines are turned off to the patient during DHCA to prevent accidental entrainment of air. Circulatory arrest is limited to 20 min; if additional time is required to complete the endarterectomy, CPB is restarted for at least 10 min between DHCA periods [13]. An additional dose of steroid and mannitol can be given once CPB is restored as the arteriotomy is being closed. The process is repeated for the left-sided endarterectomy.

Antegrade cerebral perfusion is sometimes employed to avoid circulatory arrest to the brain, but a totally bloodless field cannot be guaranteed with this approach, and almost 10% of patients may require conversion to total circulatory arrest [21].

## Rewarming and Separation from CPB

Rewarming is done slowly, with no more than a 10 °C difference between blood and core temperature. This avoids gas bubble formation in blood, minimizes cerebral oxygen desaturation, and lowers the chance of incomplete warming which can contribute to a delayed fall in temperature after separation from bypass. Depending on patient size and systemic perfusion on CPB, rewarming to a core temperature of 36–36.5 °C usually takes 90–120 min. During this time, any other planned procedures (most commonly PFO closure or coronary artery bypass grafting) are completed. Tricuspid valve repair or replacement is only done if a structural leaflet abnormality is present, because TR tends to improve significantly once post-operative RV remodeling normalizes annular geometry [22]. Communication with the surgical team about the extent and perceived success of the endarterectomy should occur prior to weaning from CPB.

A substantial improvement in hemodynamics should be expected in most patients following a successful endarterectomy; CI often doubles,

PVR may fall to a quarter of its preoperative level, and RV function tends to improve quickly [23]. However, the long bypass and cross clamp times entailed by this procedure cause many patients to require inotropic support to wean from CPB. PA pressures should be evaluated, and RV function should be assessed on TEE. Some patients, particularly those with predominantly distal disease, have persistently elevated PVR and are at high risk of post-operative decompensation. These patients require aggressive inotropic support (the pulmonary vasodilating effects of milrinone makes it a good choice), and use of inhaled prostacyclin or nitric oxide should be considered. The heart is de-aired under TEE guidance and paced at 90–100 beats per minute with temporary epicardial pacing leads. As ventilation resumes a high $EtCO_2$ to $PaCO_2$ gradient may persist and may even worsen transiently after reperfusion [24]. At this point, the radial arterial pressure is often significantly lower than femoral pressure (a 20 mmHg gradient is typical). This phenomenon can occur after lengthy periods of CPB with DHCA and may be due to regional vasoconstriction and so-called "proximal shunting" of blood [25, 26].

As CPB flows are decreased and the heart ejects and generates pulmonary blood flow, the anesthesiologist should check for signs of pulmonary complications. The presence of prink frothy secretions in the ETT may indicate that reperfusion pulmonary edema (RPE), a high-permeability type of edema affecting endarterectomized lung segments, is occurring. Dark blood in the ETT indicates a surgical injury with disruption of the blood-airway barrier. Fiberoptic bronchoscopy can aid in locating the region of the injury. Minor bleeds can be managed conservatively with isolation of the affected lung segment via bronchial blocker or double lumen endotracheal tube placement, heparin reversal, topical vasoconstrictor application down the ETT, and correction of any coagulopathy present [2, 13]. Mild pulmonary edema can be managed by increasing positive end expiratory pressure (PEEP). Severe edema or bleeding can jeopardize oxygenation and ventilation and can result in hemodynamic instability. Extracorporeal membrane oxygenation (ECMO) may be needed in the most severe cases to support gas exchange and circulation.

## The Post-bypass Period and Post-operative Care

Despite the long CPB times, hemostasis is usually achieved with heparin reversal alone, and blood products are needed infrequently. At surgical conclusion, patients are transported to the ICU intubated and sedated. Some authors recommend using transport ventilators to ensure adequate ventilation en route to the ICU [2]. Patients are typically awakened briefly for a neurological exam before being re-sedated and observed on a ventilator overnight to monitor for RPE. Up to 40% of PEA patients develop this complication, and 90% of cases manifest within 48 h of surgery [2, 27]. Treatment is supportive; mainstays of therapy include PEEP, aggressive diuresis, avoidance of high cardiac output states, and minimization of $FiO_2$ where possible.

Another unique sequela of PEA is the phenomenon of pulmonary arterial "steal," wherein pulmonary blood flow is redistributed to newly reperfused segments that may not be contributing to gas exchange. The resulting V/Q mismatch can cause significant post-operative hypoxemia. Fortunately, pulmonary arterial steal tends to resolve over time in most patients [28].

Perhaps the most feared complication of PEA is residual PH, which afflicts 5–35% of patients and is the leading cause of perioperative mortality [29–32]. Residual PH is thought to occur in cases where endarterectomy fails to address distal chronic thromboembolic disease or where there is significant concomitant small-vessel pulmonary vasculopathy present [2]. Treatment includes RV support with inotropes, SVR maintenance, and preload optimization. Inhaled nitrous oxide or iloprost may be useful as well.

Other post-operative complications common to open heart procedures can occur and include pericardial effusions, atrial arrhythmias, mediastinal bleeding, wound infections, and pneumonia. Perioperative mortality has fallen over time and was reported to be 2.2% in the most recently described patient cohort from UCSD [29].

**Summary Table**

| Plan/preparation/adverse events | Reasoning/management |
|---|---|
| Pre-procedural evaluation: Hypoxemia, polycythemia, coagulopathy, TTE and RHC findings (RV function, TR, mPAP, PVR), distribution of thromboembolic disease on pulmonary angiography | Polycythemia generally require autologous blood collection prior to CPB/DHCA. Severe preoperative pulmonary hypertension and predominantly distal vessel involvement predict worse perioperative outcomes |
| Pre-medication: Consider low dosages of benzodiazepines with oxygen and standard monitoring applied, minimize opioids | Alleviate pain/anxiety but avoid respiratory depression with hypoxia/hypercarbia (and resultant increase in PVR/PAPs) |
| Access: Large bore peripheral IV, radial arterial line (pre-induction), CVC/PAC (post-induction) | Reliable IV access and cautious monitoring of systemic blood pressure is required during induction. Many patients do not tolerate pre-induction CVC placement |
| Monitoring: Standard ASA + arterial line + PAC + TEE + processed EEG + cerebral oximetry | Follow PAPs, TR, and RV function to guide intraoperative management and determine overall success of endarterectomy. Evaluate for PFO. Use processed EEG to assess anesthetic depth and to ensure isoelectricity prior to DHCA. Cerebral oximetry is used to assess cerebral blood flow |
| Induction: Maintain RV perfusion and function | Maintain SVR with induction agent/dosing selection and vasopressors as needed; prevent increases in PVR by avoiding hypercarbia, hypoxia, and acidosis; consider inotropes |
| Intubation: Single lumen tube | Placement of double lumen tube (DLT) or bronchial blocker may be required in the event of airway bleeding |
| Major intra-operative considerations: CPB, DHCA, reperfusion pulmonary edema (RPE), airway bleeding | Assess for pulmonary complications prior to separation from CPB<br>RPE—Provide supportive care with increased PEEP and diuresis<br>Airway bleeding—Consider DLT or bronchial blocker placement, heparin reversal, topical vasoconstrictor application down the ETT, and correction of any coagulopathy<br>Severe RPE or bleeding may require ECMO |
| Post-operative complications: Reperfusion pulmonary edema, pulmonary artery steal, residual pulmonary hypertension, pericardial effusions, atrial arrhythmias, mediastinal bleeding, wound infections, pneumonia | As indicated<br>Note that residual pulmonary hypertension is a sign of significant unresectable distal disease and poor prognosis |

# References

1. Taboada D, Pepke-Zaba J, Jenkins DP, Berman M, Treacy CM, Cannon JE, et al. Outcome of pulmonary endarterectomy in symptomatic chronic thromboembolic disease. Eur Respir J. 2014;44(6):1635–45.
2. Banks DA, Pretorius GV, Kerr KM, Manecke GR. Pulmonary endarterectomy: part II. Operation, anesthetic management, and postoperative care. Semin Cardiothorac Vasc Anesth. 2014;18(4):331–40.
3. Hoeper MM, Madani MM, Nakanishi N, Meyer B, Cebotari S, Rubin LJ. Chronic thromboembolic pulmonary hypertension. Lancet Respir Med. 2014;2(7):573–82.
4. Simonneau G, Galie N, Rubin LJ, Langleben D, Seeger W, Domenighetti G, et al. Clinical classification of pulmonary hypertension. J Am Coll Cardiol. 2004;43(12 Suppl S):5s–12s.
5. Ende-Verhaar YM, Cannegieter SC, Vonk Noordegraaf A, Delcroix M, Pruszczyk P, Mairuhu AT, et al. Incidence of chronic thromboembolic pulmonary hypertension after acute pulmonary embolism: a contemporary view of the published literature. Eur Respir J. 2017;49(2):pii: 1601792.
6. Shenoy V, Anton JM, Collard CD, Youngblood SC. Pulmonary thromboendarterectomy for chronic thromboembolic pulmonary hypertension. Anesthesiology. 2014;120(5):1255–61.
7. Lang IM, Madani M. Update on chronic thromboembolic pulmonary hypertension. Circulation. 2014;130(6):508–18.
8. Robbins IM, Pugh ME, Hemnes AR. Update on chronic thromboembolic pulmonary hypertension. Trends Cardiovasc Med. 2017;27(1):29–37.
9. Banks DA, Pretorius GV, Kerr KM, Manecke GR. Pulmonary endarterectomy: part I. Pathophysiology,

clinical manifestations, and diagnostic evaluation of chronic thromboembolic pulmonary hypertension. Semin Cardiothorac Vasc Anesth. 2014;18(4):319–30.
10. Lang IM, Pesavento R, Bonderman D, Yuan JX. Risk factors and basic mechanisms of chronic thromboembolic pulmonary hypertension: a current understanding. Eur Respir J. 2013;41(2):462–8.
11. Thistlethwaite PA, Mo M, Madani MM, Deutsch R, Blanchard D, Kapelanski DP, Jamieson SW. Operative classification of thromboembolic disease determines outcome after pulmonary endarterectomy. J Thorac Cardiovasc Surg. 2002;124:1203–11.
12. Madani MM, Jamieson SW. Pulmonary embolism and pulmonary thromboendarterectomy. In: Cohn LH, editor. Cardiac surgery in the adult. 4th ed. New York: McGraw-Hill; 2012.
13. Manecke GR. Anesthesia for pulmonary endarterectomy. Semin Thorac Cardiovasc Surg. 2006;18(3):236–42.
14. Sarkar J, Golden PJ, Kajiura LN, Murata LA, Uyehara CF. Vasopressin decreases pulmonary-to-systemic vascular resistance ratio in a porcine model of severe hemorrhagic shock. Shock. 2015;43(5):475–82.
15. Roscoe A, Klein A. Pulmonary endarterectomy. Curr Opin Anaesthesiol. 2008;21(1):16–20.
16. Green DW, Kunst G. Cerebral oximetry and its role in adult cardiac, non-cardiac surgery and resuscitation from cardiac arrest. Anaesthesia. 2017;72(Suppl 1):48–57.
17. Syvatets M, Tolani K, Zhang M, Tulman G, Charchaflieh J. Perioperative management of deep hypothermic circulatory arrest. J Cardiothorac Vasc Anesth. 2010;24(4):644–55.
18. Blanchard DG, Dittrich HC. Pericardial adaptation in severe chronic pulmonary hypertension. An intraoperative transesophageal echocardiographic study. Circulation. 1992;85(4):1414–22.
19. Rudski LG, Lai WW, Afilalo J, Hua L, Handschumacher MD, Chandrasekaran K, Solomon SD, Louie EK, Schiller NB. Guidelines for the echocardiographic assessment of the right heart in adults: a report from the American Society of Echocardiography endorsed by the European Association of Echocardiography, a registered branch of the European Society of Cardiology, and the Canadian Society of Echocardiography. J Am Soc Echocardiogr. 2010;23(7):685–713.
20. Dittrich HC, McCann HA, Wilson WC. Identification of interatrial communication in patients with elevated right atrial pressure using surface and transesophageal contrast echocardiography. J Am Coll Cardiol. 1993;21(Supp):135A.
21. Thomson B, Tsui SS, Dunning J, Goodwin A, Vuylsteke A, Latimer R, Pepke-Zaba J, Jenkins DP. Pulmonary endarterectomy is possible and effective without the use of complete circulatory arrest—the UK experience in over 150 patients. Eur J Cardiothorac Surg. 2008;33(2):157–63.
22. Menzel T, Kramm T, Wagner S, Mohr-Kahaly S, Mayer E, Mayer J. Improvement of tricuspid regurgitation after pulmonary thromboendarterectomy. Ann Thorac Surg. 2002;73(3):756–61.
23. Jamieson SW, Kapelanski DP. Pulmonary endarterectomy. Curr Probl Surg. 2000;37(3):165–252.
24. Manecke GR, Wilson WC, Auger WR, Jamieson SW. Chronic thromboembolic pulmonary hypertension and pulmonary thromboendarterectomy. Semin Cardiothorac Vasc Anesth. 2005;9(3):189–204.
25. Mohr R, Lavee J, Goor DA. Inaccuracy of radial artery pressure measurement after cardiac operations. J Thorac Cardiovasc Surg. 1987;94(2):286–90.
26. Baba T, Goto T, Yoshitake A, Shibata Y. Radial artery diameter decreases with increased femoral to radial arterial pressure gradient during cardiopulmonary bypass. Anesth Analg. 1997;85(2):252–8.
27. Levinson RM, Shure D, Moser KM. Reperfusion pulmonary edema after pulmonary artery thromboendarterectomy. Am Rev Respir Dis. 1986;134(6):1241–5.
28. Moser KM, Metersky ML, Auger WR, Fedullo PF. Resolution of vascular steal after pulmonary thromboendarterectomy. Chest. 1993;104(5):1441–4.
29. Madani MM, Auger WR, Pretorius V, Sakakibara N, Kerr KM, Kim NH, Fedullo PF, Jamieson SW. Pulmonary endarterectomy: recent changes in a single institution's experience of more than 2,700 patients. Ann Thorac Surg. 2012;94(1):97–103.
30. Mayer E, Jenkins D, Lindner J, D'Armini A, Kloek J, Meyns B, Ilkjaer LB, Klepetko W, Delcroix M, Lang I, Pepke-Zaba J, Simonneau G, Dartevelle P. Surgical management and outcome of patients with chronic thromboembolic pulmonary hypertension: results from an international prospective registry. J Thorac Cardiovasc Surg. 2011;141:702–10.
31. Bondermann D, Skoro-Sajer N, Jakowitsch J, Adlbrecht C, Dunkler D, Taghavi S, Klepetko W, Kneussl M, Lang IM. Predictors of outcome in chronic thromboembolic disease. Circulation. 2007;115:2153–8.
32. Dartevelle P, Fadel R, Mussot S, Chapelier A, Hervé P, de Perrot M, Cerrina J, Ladurie FL, Lehouerou D, Humbert M, Sitbon O, Simonneau G. Chronic thromboembolic pulmonary hypertension. Eur Respir J. 2004;23(4):637–48.

# Anesthetic Management for Minimally Invasive Cardiac Surgery

Julius Hamilton and Mark Caridi-Scheible

## Introduction

According to the American Heart Association, minimally invasive cardiac surgery is defined as "a small chest wall incision that does not include a full sternotomy" [1]. This description is inclusive of intra-cardiac (i.e., valve replacement, septal defect repair) and extra-cardiac (i.e., coronary bypass) procedures with or without the implementation of cardiopulmonary bypass. The development of minimally invasive approaches has been cultivated by the desire to improve value in cardiac surgery. This value can be achieved by decreasing costs by reducing the time of postoperative recovery and by improving cosmesis while maintaining or improving quality of care. Use of a minimally invasive approach introduces an added level of complexity which requires a skilled perioperative team and appropriate patient selection. For example, studies of minimally invasive cardiac bypass procedures (MIDCAB) have demonstrated lower cost of total care, shorter ICU length of stay [2], and decreased surgical stress [3]; yet this is often paired with longer cross clamp times [4] and the introduction of a prolonged period of one lung ventilation [5] to achieve these endpoints. This interplay of risks and rewards demands that the decision to use a minimally invasive approach be determined by carefully considering the right procedure by the right surgeon for the right patient, rather than just by the length of the incision [6].

## Minimally Invasive Coronary Bypass

Minimally invasive approaches to coronary bypass range from the use of a minithoracotomy (MIDCAB) to totally endoscopic coronary artery bypass (TECAB) (see Fig. 6.1). In comparison to intra-cardiac procedures, these extra-cardiac procedures provide an opportunity to avoid use of cardiopulmonary bypass. Studies have demonstrated many benefits of minimally invasive coronary bypass, including reduced ICU length of stay, shorter hospitalization, reduced transfusion requirements, reduced cost of total care [2], less surgical stress [3], less fluid shift, and fewer neuropsychiatric disturbances [7] when compared to CABG with a full sternotomy. The surgical approach often requires utilization of one lung ventilation to improve visualization and because of limited surgical exposure, minimally invasive bypass procedures are often limited to a single bypass. This makes minimally invasive coronary bypass less than ideal for the patient with signifi-

J. Hamilton, M.D.
Emory University School of Medicine,
Emory University Hospital, Atlanta, GA, USA
e-mail: jehami3@emory.edu

M. Caridi-Scheible, M.D. (✉)
Department of Anesthesiology, Emory University School of Medicine, Atlanta, GA, USA
e-mail: mscheib@emory.edu

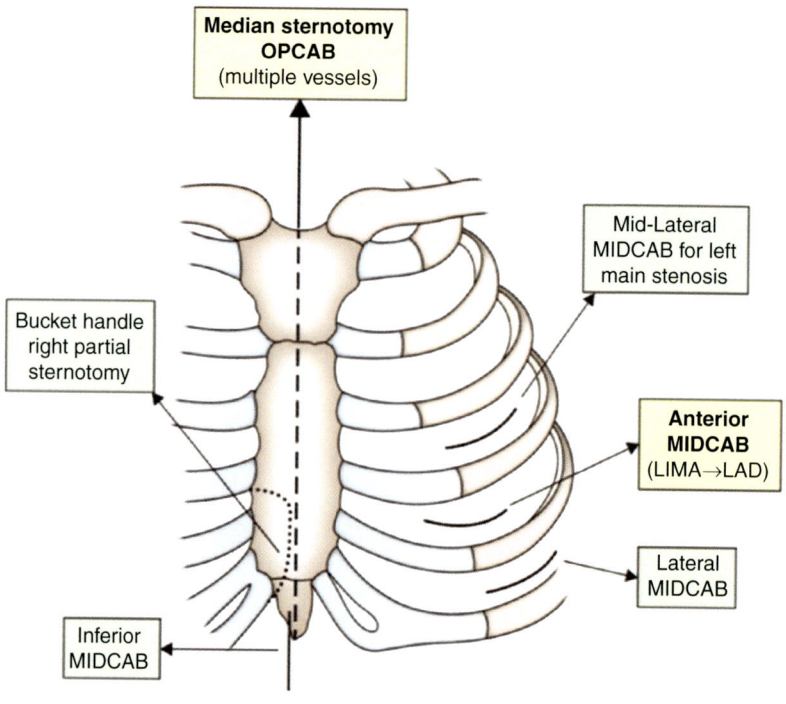

**Fig. 6.1** Various approaches for mini-thoracotomy

cant pulmonary disease or multi-vessel coronary disease. When cardiopulmonary bypass is utilized there is typically a longer aortic cross clamp time [4] and longer procedure duration when compared to conventional bypass procedures. A subset of MIDCAB includes the use of robotic assistance (such as the da Vinci® system) to harvest the internal mammary artery from the chest wall.

Totally endoscopic coronary artery bypass also employs the use of robotic technology and as the name suggests, the procedure is performed from start to finish via endoscopy. This approach requires peripheral cannulation for cardiopulmonary bypass, a pressurized capnothorax, and extensive use of transesophageal echocardiography [8]. Myocardial preservation can be achieved by performing the procedure on a beating heart or with the use of an endoaortic occlusion balloon catheter which functions as the aortic cross clamp as well as a conduit for the delivery of antegrade cardioplegia.

Table 6.1 summarizes important anesthetic considerations for minimally-invasive coronary bypass grafting surgery.

## Minimally Invasive Aortic Valve Surgery

First described in 1993, a minimally invasive approach to aortic valve replacement ("Mini"-AVR) has grown to a variety of approaches that avoid full sternotomy. These approaches have included port access, infra-axillary [9], parasternal [10], lower hemi-sternotomy [11], and transverse sternotomy [12]. Currently the most popular approaches are upper hemi-sternotomy and right anterior thoracotomy [13]. A meta-analysis performed by Brown et al., found that when compared to a conventional sternotomy, "Mini"-AVR was found to be equally efficacious without increased risk of death or other major complication, but found no other clinical benefits [14]. A subsequent meta-analysis comparing AVR to "Mini"-AVR demonstrated a significant reduction in ICU length of stay [15].

"Mini"-AVR, like other MICS techniques heavily depend on institutional practices and the experience of the perioperative team. Following the learning curve, improvement in outcomes is seen with growing expertise of the perioperative

**Table 6.1** Anesthetic considerations for minimally-invasive coronary bypass grafting

|  | MIDCAB | TECAB |
|---|---|---|
| Airway management | One lung ventilation (OLV) utilized<br>Double lumen endotracheal tube (DLT) or single lumen endotracheal tube (SLT) with bronchial blocker (BB) | Same as MIDCAB |
| Cannulation strategy | Off pump | ± CPB<br>Peripheral Cannulation (arterial and venous)<br>Endoaortic occlusion balloon (EAOB) for antegrade cardioplegia<br>Coronary sinus catheter for retrograde cardioplegia |
| Monitoring | Standard ASA<br>Arterial line<br>CVP<br>± TEE<br>± PA catheter | Standard ASA<br>Arterial line<br>CVP<br>TEE (used for correct placement of venous and arterial cannulae when CPB utilized) |
| Myocardial preservation | N/A | Beating heart<br>Cardioplegic arrest (antegrade and/or retrograde) |
| Pain management | Parenteral narcotics<br>Thoracic epidural<br>Regional techniques:<br>Paravertebral block/catheter<br>Intercostal block<br>Serratus anterior block/catheter | Same as MIDCAB |
| Special considerations | Proximal occlusion:<br>ST changes and new wall motion abnormalities should be expected with proximal occlusion of the left anterior descending coronary artery<br>Cardiac stabilizer:<br>Application of a cardiac stabilizer may cause cardiac dysrhythmias or the reduction of cardiac output. Mechanical (IABP), pacer, pressor or inotropic/chronotropic support may be necessary<br>Limited access:<br>Defibrillation may be difficult in situations of poor exposure for internal defibrillation. External defibrillator pads should be placed | Same as MIDCAB |

team. This is best displayed by Brigham and Women's implementation of "Mini"-AVR as routine practice. Following a 5 year learning curve, an analysis of 10 years of surgical outcomes was performed with use of propensity-scored matching. When compared to full sternotomy, the upper hemi-sternotomy (see Fig. 6.2) showed clinical benefits of shorter duration of mechanical ventilation, reduced ICU length of stay, shorter hospitalization, decreased incidence of new onset atrial fibrillation, and decreased transfusion requirements without any difference in short or long-term mortality [16]. Such positive results increase the value in cardiac surgery and strengthen the argument for widespread adoption of "Mini"-AVR.

Use of an upper hemi-sternotomy provides familiarity to the cardiac surgeon, as well as permits for fast conversion to a full sternotomy if necessary. The conversion of hemi-sternotomy to full sternotomy is infrequent and occurs at a rate of 3% [14] Bleeding, ventricular dysfunction, or poor exposure are common causes for conversion and although infrequent, conversion to a full

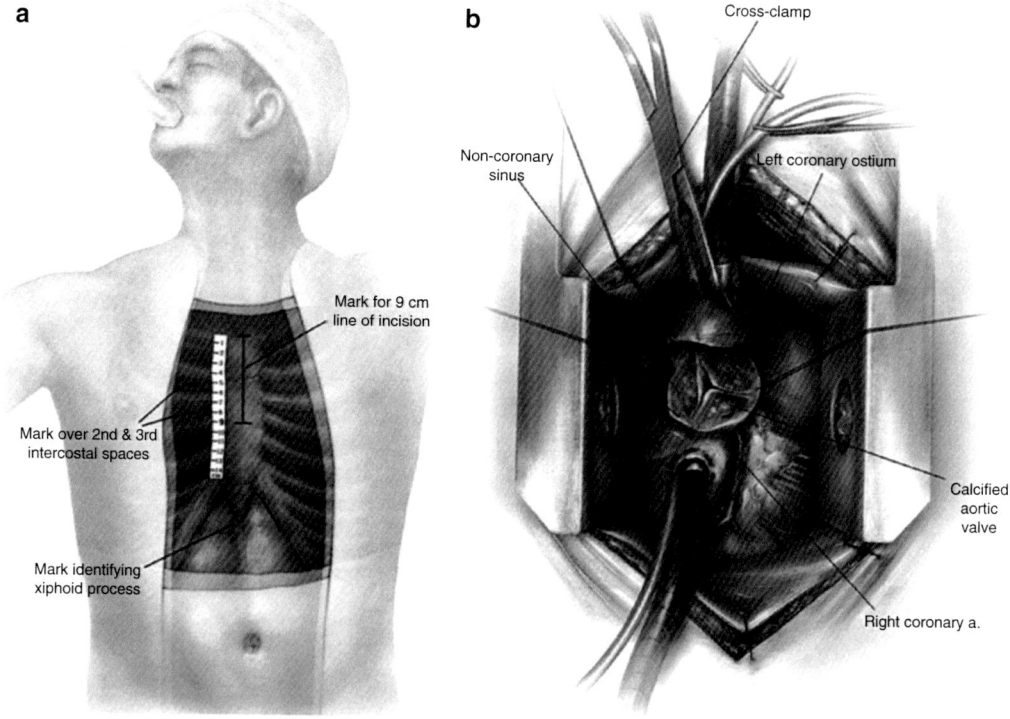

**Fig. 6.2** "Mini"-AVR via upper hemi-sternotomy approach

sternotomy has been accompanied by a significant increase in morbidity and mortality [14] Central arterial and venous cannulation can be used with this approach, though some centers prefer peripheral venous cannulation for a more accessible surgical field. Antegrade cardioplegia is utilized for myocardial preservation and direct ostial delivery can be used in the presence of aortic regurgitation.

Table 6.2 summarizes important anesthetic considerations for Mini-AVR.

## Minimally Invasive Mitral Valve Surgery

Popular approaches to minimally invasive mitral valve surgery (MIMVS) include approach via a right mini-thoracotomy ("Mini"-Mitral) and robotic mitral valve surgery. An analysis of the Society of Thoracic Surgeons National Database (STS database) from 2004 to 2008 found shorter hospitalization, fewer blood transfusions, and higher rates of repair rather than replacement when comparing minimally invasive mitral valve surgery to conventional full sternotomy. Unfortunately, these benefits were paired with increased duration of aortic cross clamp time, longer duration of cardiopulmonary bypass, and most prominently, an increased risk of permanent stroke [17]. Stroke and MIMVS has been a very controversial topic in the literature. Modi et al., found no increased risk of stroke in MIMVS versus a conventional approach in their 2008 meta-analysis [18]. The findings in the STS database are likely strongly influenced by their definition of MIMVS, "patients undergoing femoral arterial and femoral or jugular venous cannulation" [18]. Thus, these findings may be most contributed to cannulation strategy rather than surgical incision. In the subgroup analysis of the STS database, the risk of stroke was increased threefold in procedures without aortic cross clamp, such as beating heart or fibrillatory arrest. This data suggests incomplete de-airing as a likely contributor to perioperative stroke. Transesophageal

**Table 6.2** Anesthetic considerations for Mini-AVR

| | "Mini" AVR |
|---|---|
| Airway management | OLV utilized in mini-thoracotomy cases<br>DLT or SLT with bronchial blocker<br>SLT for hemi-sternotomy |
| Cannulation strategy | Typically central aortic and central or peripheral venous cannulation |
| Monitoring | Standard ASA<br>Arterial line<br>CVP<br>TEE<br>± PA catheter |
| Myocardial preservation | Cardioplegic arrest with direct aortic cross clamp<br>Antegrade cardioplegia<br>Direct ostial delivery can be utilized in presence of aortic insufficiency |
| Pain management | Parenteral narcotics<br>Regional techniques:<br>Hemisternotomy<br>Pecs blocks<br>Mini-thoracotomy<br>Paravertebral block/catheter<br>Intercostal block<br>Serratus anterior block/catheter |
| Special considerations | Limited access:<br>Defibrillation may be difficult in situations of poor exposure for internal defibrillation. External defibrillator pads should be placed<br>Poor exposure is the most common indication for conversion to full sternotomy |

echocardiography should be used to guide de-airing in these cases.

MIMVS via right mini-thoracotomy employs one lung ventilation to improve surgical exposure. Depending on surgeon preference, the mini-thoracotomy can be supplemented by endoscopic access ports with use of capnothorax. In cases employing cardioplegic arrest, use of a direct aortic cross clamp or an endoaortic occlusion balloon (EOAB) can be used to deliver antegrade cardioplegia. Percutaneous endocoronary sinus catheters may also be deployed under TEE guidance to provide retrograde cardioplegia. Additionally, a substitution for a left ventricular vent (traditionally placed in open procedures in a right pulmonary vein) is a pulmonary artery vent placed in a manner similar to a pulmonary artery (PA) catheter which functions to empty the pulmonary circulation (and therefore the left atrium) when on CPB. The pulmonary vent has the ability to measure pulmonary pressures when not being used as an active vent but should be removed from the central venous introducer prior to leaving the operating room. Venous cannulation is often accessed by a femoral venous cannula which requires TEE guidance for appropriate placement. In the 10-year experience of transitioning from conventional mitral valve surgery to routine MIMVS of Glauber et al., presence of severe left ventricular dysfunction, severe chronic obstructive pulmonary disease, pleural adhesions, and endocarditis with abscess involving the mitro-aortic continuity all led to utilization of a full sternotomy instead [19].

Robotic mitral surgery is limited to specialized centers with adequate surgical volume to develop and maintain expertise. Comparative outcome data of robotic mitral valve surgery versus conventional surgery is limited. In the meta-analysis by Cao et al., a mortality benefit was found in favor of robotic mitral surgery, but this analysis was confounded by heterogeneity of the cohorts of the largest study included [20] and its removal from the data analysis erased the mortality benefit [21]. However, individual institutional experiences have shown safe use of robotic mitral valve surgery in the hands of expert surgeons with specialized teams. Murphy et al., demonstrate the safety of their technique along with appropriate discrimination in patient selection. Patients excluded from undergoing robotic mitral valve surgery included those with severe aortoiliac atherosclerosis, right pleural scarring, or significant mitral annular calcification [22]. Conversely, patients presenting for redo operations or whom required tricuspid repair received a mini-thoracotomy approach instead.

The addition of robotic telemanipulation systems provide improved visualization with a three-dimensional console for the operating surgeon as well as increased degrees of movement. The right lung is deflated and one lung ventilation is maintained by capnothorax to provide adequate visualization. Arterial and venous cannulation are accessed peripherally via femoral vessels and often requires the use of vacuum assisted venous drainage. Myocardial preservation is achieved by antegrade cardioplegia delivered by endoaortic occlusion balloon. With TEE guidance, the anesthesiologist places a retrograde coronary sinus catheter to further aid myocardial protection. TEE-guided coronary sinus catheter placement is facilitated by the acquisition of a "deep" 4 chamber view or a modified bicaval view. Appropriate placement of the coronary sinus catheter can be confirmed by injection of dye under fluoroscopy or with inflation of the occlusion balloon with subsequent display of a ventricularized waveform [23] (Fig. 6.3).

Table 6.3 summarizes important anesthetic considerations for minimally invasive mitral valve surgery.

## Patient Selection and Optimization

Appropriate patient selection and optimization of comorbidities is essential to operative success. Many MICS procedures require prolonged one-lung-ventilation with or without capnothorax to increase surgical exposure, thus patients with significant pulmonary disease are poor candidates for this type of approach. One-lung-ventilation can lead to hypercarbia and hypoxemia with resultant increases in right ventricular afterload secondary to an increase in pulmonary vascular resistance [24]. This increase in pulmonary arterial pressure and decrease in cardiac output should be expected.

For the patient with pre-existing pulmonary disease, pulmonary function tests and an arterial blood gas on room air may provide additional information for risk stratification, as patients with resting hypercarbia ($PaCO_2 > 50$ mmHg) or hypoxemia ($PaO_2 < 60$ mmHg) are poor candidates for prolonged one-lung ventilation [24]. Smoking cessation should be strongly encouraged for at least 2 weeks prior to surgery. Preoperative bronchodilators should be considered in the patient with known reactive airway disease or a significant smoking history.

Presence of other cardiac lesions can lead to a significant change in the surgical plan and approach, thus perioperative transesophageal echocardiography is essential to appropriate management. For instance, presence of tricuspid regurgitation with tricuspid annular dilation in the patient scheduled for a robotic mitral valve repair will significantly modify the surgical plan with robotic surgery no longer being the ideal approach [21].

When considering approaches requiring peripheral arterial cannulation for cardiopulmonary bypass, the patient with a history of peripheral vascular disease may be at increased risk for distal ischemia. Data suggests use of peripheral arterial cannulation to lead to an increased risk of perioperative stroke [17], giving pause to use of peripheral cannulation in the patient with severe atherosclerotic disease.

**Fig. 6.3** Coronary sinus catheter and minimally invasive cardioplegia catheter placement

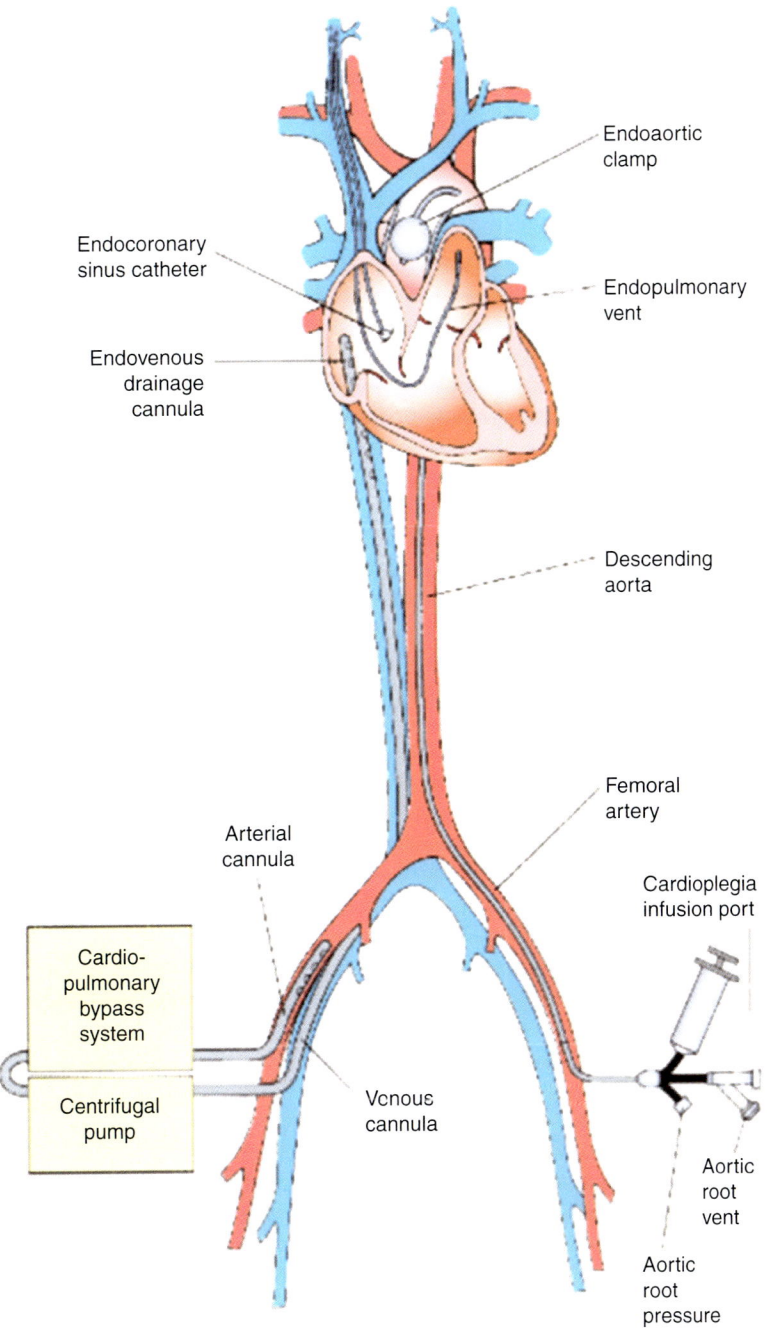

**Table 6.3** Anesthetic considerations for minimally invasive mitral valve surgery

|  | "Mini" MVR | Robotic MVR |
| --- | --- | --- |
| Airway management | OLV DLT or SLT with bronchial blocker | Same as mini MVR |
| Cannulation strategy | Central or peripheral cannulation | Peripheral cannulation |
| Monitoring | Standard ASA Arterial line CVP TEE PA catheter or PA vent | Standard ASA Bilateral radial arterial lines CVP TEE PA catheter or PA vent |
| Myocardial preservation | Cardioplegic arrest with direct aortic cross clamp or EAOB Possible use of retrograde cardioplegia by coronary sinus catheter | Cardioplegic arrest with antegrade cardioplegia, retrograde cardioplegia Antegrade cardioplegia by EAOB Retrograde cardioplegia by coronary sinus catheter |
| Pain management | Parenteral narcotics Regional techniques: Paravertebral block/catheter Intercostal block Serratus anterior block/catheter | Parenteral narcotics Regional techniques as indicated |
| Special considerations | Limited access: Defibrillation may be difficult in situations of poor exposure for internal defibrillation so external defibrillator pads should be placed Poor exposure is the most common indication for conversion to full sternotomy | Limited access: Total endoscopic access necessitates placement of external defibrillation pads TEE guidance: TEE-guided placement of EAOB and coronary sinus catheter |

# Bibliography

1. Rosengart TK, Feldman T, Borger MA, Vassiliades TA, Gillinov AM, Hoercher KJ, et al. Percutaneous and minimally invasive valve procedures: a scientific statement from the American Heart Association Council on Cardiovascular Surgery and Anesthesia, Council on Clinical Cardiology, Functional Genomics and Translational Biology Interdisciplinary Working Group, and Quality of Care and Outcomes Research Interdisciplinary Working Group. Circulation. 2008;117(13):1750–67.
2. Zenati M, Domit TM, Saul M, Gorcsan J, Katz WE, Hudson M, et al. Resource utilization for minimally invasive direct and standard coronary artery bypass grafting. Ann Thorac Surg. 1997;63(6 Suppl):S84–7.
3. Ganapathy S. Anaesthesia for minimally invasive cardiac surgery. Best Pract Res Clin Anaesthesiol. 2002;16(1):63–80.
4. Chaney MA, Durazo-Arvizu RA, Fluder EM, Sawicki KJ, Nikolov MP, Blakeman BP, et al. Port-access minimally invasive cardiac surgery increases surgical complexity, increases operating room time, and facilitates early postoperative hospital discharge. Anesthesiology. 2000;92(6):1637–45.
5. Ganapathy S. Thoracic epidural analgesia offers improved postoperative analgesa following midcab. Second meeting of ISMICS 1999.
6. Mihaljevic T, Gillinov M. Invited commentary. Ann Thorac Surg. 2012;93(5):1468.
7. Murkin JM, Boyd WD, Ganapathy S, Adams SJ, Peterson RC. Beating heart surgery: why expect less central nervous system morbidity? Ann Thorac Surg. 1999;68(4):1498–501.
8. Deshpande SP, Lehr E, Odonkor P, Bonatti JO, Kalangie M, Zimrin DA, et al. Anesthetic management of robotically assisted totally endoscopic coronary artery bypass surgery (TECAB). J Cardiothorac Vasc Anesth. 2013;27(3):586–99.
9. Ito T, Maekawa A, Hoshino S, Hayashi Y. Right infraaxillary thoracotomy for minimally invasive aortic valve replacement. Ann Thorac Surg. 2013;96(2):715–7.
10. Cohn LH, Adams DH, Couper GS, Bichell DP, Rosborough DM, Sears SP, et al. Minimally invasive cardiac valve surgery improves patient satisfaction while reducing costs of cardiac valve replacement and repair. Ann Surg. 1997;226(4):421–6; discussion 427–8
11. von Segesser LK, Westaby S, Pomar J, Loisance D, Groscurth P, Turina M. Less invasive aortic valve surgery: rationale and technique. Eur J Cardiothorac Surg. 1999;15(6):781–5.

12. Moreno-Cabral RJ. Mini-T sternotomy for cardiac operations. J Thorac Cardiovasc Surg. 1997;113(4):810–1.
13. Malaisrie SC, Barnhart GR, Farivar RS, Mehall J, Hummel B, Rodriguez E, et al. Current era minimally invasive aortic valve replacement: techniques and practice. J Thorac Cardiovasc Surg. 2014;147(1):6–14.
14. Brown ML, McKellar SH, Sundt TM, Schaff HV. Ministernotomy versus conventional sternotomy for aortic valve replacement: a systematic review and meta-analysis. J Thorac Cardiovasc Surg. 2009;137(3):670–679.e5.
15. Khoshbin E, Prayaga S, Kinsella J, Sutherland FWH. Mini-sternotomy for aortic valve replacement reduces the length of stay in the cardiac intensive care unit: meta-analysis of randomised controlled trials. BMJ Open. 2011;1(2):e000266.
16. Neely R, et al. Minimally invasive aortic valve replacement versus aortic valve replacement through full sternotomy: the Brigham and Women's Hospital experience. Ann Cardiothorac Surg. 2015;4(1):38–48. [cited 2017 Feb 13]. http://www.annalscts.com/article/view/5084/6300.
17. Gammie JS, Zhao Y, Peterson ED, O'Brien SM, Rankin JS, Griffith BP. Less-invasive mitral valve operations: trends and outcomes from the society of thoracic surgeons adult cardiac surgery database. Ann Thorac Surg. 2010;90(5):1401–10.
18. Modi P, Hassan A, Chitwood WR. Minimally invasive mitral valve surgery: a systematic review and meta-analysis. Eur J Cardiothorac Surg. 2008;34(5):943–52.
19. Glauber M, Miceli A, Canarutto D, Lio A, Murzi M, Gilmanov D, et al. Early and long-term outcomes of minimally invasive mitral valve surgery through right minithoracotomy: a 10-year experience in 1604 patients. J Cardiothorac Surg. 2015;10:181. [cited 2017 Feb 13]. http://www.ncbi.nlm.nih.gov/pmc/articles/PMC4672482/.
20. Stevens L-M, Rodriguez E, Lehr EJ, Kindell LC, Nifong LW, Ferguson TB, et al. Impact of timing and surgical approach on outcomes after mitral valve regurgitation operations. Ann Thorac Surg. 2012;93(5):1462–8.
21. Cao C, Wolfenden H, Liou K, Pathan F, Gupta S, Nienaber TA, et al. A meta-analysis of robotic vs. conventional mitral valve surgery. Ann Cardiothorac Surg. 2015;4(4):305–14.
22. Murphy DA, Miller JS, Langford DA, Snyder AB. Endoscopic robotic mitral valve surgery. J Thorac Cardiovasc Surg. 2006;132(4):776–81.
23. Miller GS. Coronary sinus catheter placement in minimally invasive cardiac surgery: tricks, tactics, and tribulations. Lecture presented at Texas; 2017.
24. Cryer HG, Mavroudis C, Yu J, Roberts AM, Cué JI, Richardson JD, et al. Shock, transfusion, and pneumonectomy. Death is due to right heart failure and increased pulmonary vascular resistance. Ann Surg. 1990;212(2):197–201.

# Anesthesia for Transcatheter Aortic Valve Replacement (TAVR) and Other Catheter-Based Intracardiac Procedures

Ratna Vadlamudi

## Transcatheter Aortic Valve Replacement

TAVR was initially performed in 2002 and to date, more than 50,000 valves have been implanted [1]. Valves can be classified into two major categories: balloon-expandable valves and self-expanding valves. Perhaps the best example of each is the Edwards SAPIEN valve (balloon-expandable) and the Medtronic CoreValve (self-expanding).

Anesthetic management of patients undergoing TAVR is complex for many reasons. TAVR remains a developing procedure for many cardiac surgeons, cardiologists and anesthesiologists due to the learning curve associated with novel techniques and prostheses. The patient population is also highly complex with multiple co-morbid conditions that must be managed in the perioperative period. Proper understanding of the implantation procedure as well as implications of co-morbidities is vital to safe and effective anesthetic care. TAVR is currently FDA approved for high and intermediate risk patients. Two independent cardiac surgeons are required to evaluate potential patients and determine their suitability for SAVR versus TAVR [2].

Minimum requirements for TAVR programs include an active multi-disciplinary heart team, comprised by cardiologists, cardiac surgeons, cardiac anesthesiologists, intensivists, and other staff. Active valve surgery and catheterization programs are also required before an institution can begin a TAVR program.

## Preoperative Assessment and Anesthetic Choice

The approach to care for a patient presenting for TAVR begins with a thorough pre-anesthesia consultation. As with any patient presenting for cardiac surgery, attention should be paid to identifying co-morbid conditions and quantifying their severity. Patients should be assessed for pulmonary disease, renal impairment, neurologic conditions, frailty, vascular disease, and other cardiac conditions, including coronary artery disease and other valvular disease. Management of these conditions is discussed in detail below.

Pertinent data should be reviewed, including echocardiography, computed tomography, left and right heart catheterization, pulmonary function tests and laboratory data. All current medications should be reviewed with attention to β-blockers, anticoagulants and therapy for chronic pain conditions.

Anesthetic management for TAVR can be achieved with general anesthesia (GA) or

---

R. Vadlamudi, M.D.
Emory University School of Medicine, Emory University Hospital, Atlanta, GA, USA
e-mail: rvadlam@emory.edu

monitored anesthesia care (MAC) with local anesthesia. Standard American Society of Anesthesiologists (ASA) monitoring is mandatory for both methods. Need for invasive monitoring is dependent on the patient's overall condition and planned approach. Most centers will utilize invasive blood pressure monitoring. Experience level of the proceduralists and institution should also be considered as initial procedures may have a higher risk for complications. If a patient is enrolled in a particular TAVR study, the study protocol may require specific monitoring. For example, a newer TAVR prosthesis may require prolonged transesophageal echocardiography (TEE) for sizing assessment and valve deployment, which requires GA. Several centers have reported success with sedation techniques for TAVR, and as valve systems become more refined, sedation and MAC techniques may be more feasible [3]. Advantages exist for both techniques and are summarized in Table 7.1.

There are multiple ways to achieve adequate sedation with a MAC technique. These include infusions of dexmedetomidine, propofol, remifentanil or ketamine. Alternatively, intermittent bolus doses of benzodiazepines and/or narcotics can be utilized. The risk of delirium and paradoxical reaction should be considered for elderly patients receiving benzodiazepines.

# Management of Co-morbid Conditions

Key to the formation of an appropriate anesthetic plan is an understanding of the roles of other chronic disease in the management of TAVR patients. This section will discuss the major co-morbid conditions frequently encountered in the TAVR patient population.

## Coronary Artery Disease

Coronary artery disease (CAD) is frequently present in TAVR patients. The majority of patients will have left heart catheterization (LHC) as part of preoperative planning. This is done to define the anatomy of the coronary arteries in relation to the aortic root and also to assess for obstructive CAD. If significant disease is present, percutaneous coronary intervention (PCI) may be performed. The type of coronary intervention is important for the anesthesiologist to consider as anti-platelet therapy may need to be continued in the perioperative period. Alternatively, PCI may be performed during the TAVR procedure.

In the setting of prior coronary artery bypass grafting (CABG), certain approaches to TAVR, which will be discussed in future sections, may be contraindicated.

**Table 7.1** Pros and cons of general anesthesia and monitored anesthesia care for transcatheter aortic valve replacement

|  | GA | MAC with local |
|---|---|---|
| Advantages | • TEE guidance for valve deployment and paravalvular leak assessment<br>• Patient immobility<br>• Controlled airway for periods of hypotension, rapid pacing or complications during the procedure<br>• Preferred for non-transfemoral TAVR approaches | • Potential for decreased hemodynamic instability<br>• Ability to monitor for neurologic complications if light sedation tolerated<br>• Potential for quicker recovery following the procedure |
| Disadvantages | • Potential hemodynamic compromise related to GA<br>• Requires emergence and extubation from GA | • Airway compromise necessitating conversion to GA mid-procedure<br>• Patient may not be fully cooperative or may be unable to remain supine or immobile |

## Mixed Valvular Disease

Patients with valvular disease in addition to aortic stenosis present a challenge for the anesthesiologist as they often have conflicting goals for hemodynamic management. For example, patients with structural mitral valve regurgitation often benefit from a higher heart rate and lower afterload which is counterproductive in the management of aortic stenosis. Being aware of the presence and severity of co-existing valvular disease to optimize cardiac output is vital to safe anesthetic care. Use of transesophageal echocardiography (TEE) can be critical in management of these patients as it allows for real time assessment of cardiac function and changes in severity of dynamic valvular disease throughout the procedure.

## Decreased Ejection Fraction (EF)

Low EF in the TAVR patient population can be secondary to multiple etiologies such as valvular, ischemic or dilated cardiomyopathies. Preoperative optimization is important in the care of these patients but rapid hemodynamic compromise during the procedure can occur. Addition of vasopressors and inotropes can be enough to stabilize most of these patients. In those that require additional support, intra-aortic balloon pump (IABP) counter pulsation or temporary ventricular assist device (VAD) may be needed.

## Pulmonary Disease

Some patients may be impaired by significant pulmonary disease such as chronic obstructive pulmonary disease, restrictive lung disease, pulmonary fibrosis, pulmonary hypertension or obstructive sleep apnea. These conditions demonstrate the importance of anesthetic planning in TAVR, as the major advantage of GA is control of ventilation and optimization of oxygenation. However, patients with severe disease may ultimately have difficulty weaning from mechanical ventilation, which make MAC with local techniques appealing. Achieving adequate sedation can be challenging, as $CO_2$ retention will worsen these underlying conditions. Non-invasive ventilation strategies such as bi-level positive airway pressure (BiPAP) or continuous positive airway pressure (CPAP) may be useful in these patients. Of particular importance is the intraoperative monitoring of end-tidal $CO_2$ and vigilant monitoring of respiratory function in the postoperative period. Preoperative discussion with the patient and the procedural team with regards to the level of expected sedation and advantages of controlled ventilation with GA will optimize outcomes for these patients.

## Renal Disease

Presence of renal impairment, including end stage renal disease (ESRD) is a challenge in the TAVR patient population primarily due to challenges in vascular access and the use of contrast dye during the procedure. Close monitoring of volume status and electrolytes, including potassium and bicarbonate, throughout the perioperative period is critical.

## Neurologic Disease

Due to the incidence of cerebrovascular accident (CVA) after TAVR, it is important to define the patient's baseline neurologic status prior to the procedure. Stroke rate after TAVR approaches 10% at 30 days and 14% at 1 year [4]. Although maintaining adequate perfusion pressure is warranted, many CVAs related to TAVR are thought to be embolic in nature due to the forced displacement of the calcified native aortic valve by the prosthetic TAVR valve.

## Vascular Disease

Presence of vascular disease can lead to vascular access deployment challenges and may require non-transfemoral approach to TAVR (discussed below).

As stated previously, total percutaneous TF deployment is the most common approach to TAVR. Given the frequent presence of peripheral arterial disease, the femoral vessels may not be of adequate caliber to allow the catheter and sheath placement necessary for valve deployment. Other approaches were subsequently developed to offer TAVR for that patient population. To date, transapical (TA), transaortic (TAo) or direct aortic, trans-subclavian, transcarotid and transcaval approaches will be described below.

## Transapical

Transapical approach to TAVR involves a left mini-thoracotomy for exposure of the left ventricular apex. Ventriculotomy is performed and valve deployment occurs in an antegrade fashion. Following deployment, the delivery catheter is removed and purse string sutures close the apical defect.

Anesthetic considerations for this approach:

- Intermittent pauses in respirations (typically one lung ventilation is not required)
- Significant bleeding from left ventriculotomy
- Coronary artery damage from left ventriculotomy
- Sub-mitral apparatus damage from deployment catheter

## Transaortic

Transaortic or direct aortic access involves a small upper sternotomy, usually in the second to fourth interspaces to expose the ascending aorta. The deployment catheter is placed and valve deployment is carried out retrograde from the ascending aorta.

Anesthetic considerations for this approach:

- Significant bleeding from aortotomy
- Aortic dissection

## Transcarotid

Transcarotid approach for TAVR is achieved with right common carotid artery access. The femoral artery is also accessed for shunting to the distal carotid artery to provide cerebral perfusion. Cerebral oximetry is utilized to monitor for cerebral hypoperfusion and ischemia.

Anesthetic considerations for this approach (Fig. 7.1):

- Cerebral malperfusion and stroke risk
- Bleeding from carotid access site
- Potential airway compromise if hematoma develops at carotid access site
- Central venous access should be placed at a site other than the right internal jugular vein

## Transcaval

Transcaval approach is a newer approach to TAVR deployment. Given the incidence of peripheral vascular disease in the TAVR patient population and presence of contraindications to the alternate approaches described above,

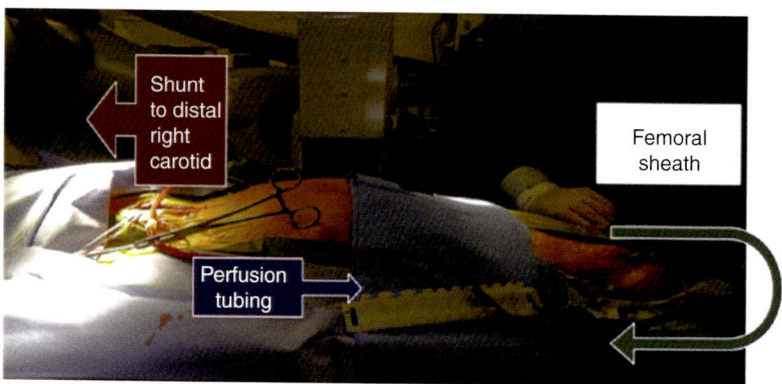

**Fig. 7.1** Transcarotid approach to TAVR

transcaval approach was developed as a method to deliver TAVR therapy in this population. Due to the increased compliance and size of ileofemoral veins when compared to ileofemoral arteries, access is obtained in the femoral vein and advanced into the inferior vena cava (IVC). A tract is then created between the IVC and the abdominal aorta and progressively dilated until the deployment catheter has been placed. Valve deployment is then carried out in a standard fashion. After deployment, an occluder device is placed to seal the tract and if residual leak remains, an aortic stent graft can be placed.

Anesthetic considerations for this approach:

- Retroperitoneal bleeding from IVC or abdominal aorta
- Residual bleeding from IVC-aorta tract requiring advanced intervention

### Subclavian or Axillary

This approach to TAVR is achieved via either direct subclavian or axillary artery access or access via a synthetic graft.

Anesthetic considerations for this approach:

- Compromised flow to LIMA graft if left subclavian artery is accessed

## Complications

### Neurologic

One of the more common complications of TAVR is CVA, presumed to be embolic secondary to the prosthesis forcibly displacing the native valve. Initial PARTNER (Placement of Aortic Transcatheter Valves) data demonstrated statistically significant rates of neurologic events (CVA or TIA) in both high risk and inoperable patient groups. One-year data in high risk PARTNER patients demonstrated a stroke rate of 6% in TAVR patients versus 3.2% in SAVR patients [5]. However, 5 year follow up PARTNER data confirmed that the increased risk of neurologic complication appears to be procedure-related and does not show continued increase post-procedure.

Five-year data in high risk PARTNER patients was 10.4% in TAVR patients versus 11.3% in SAVR patients [5]. Interestingly, initial CoreValve data did not demonstrate an increased risk of CVA in CoreValve patients (8.8% for CoreValve vs. 12.6% for SAVR) [6]. This may be due to specific characteristics of the prosthesis and the manner in which the prosthesis is deployed.

### Vascular

Rates of vascular complications are increased in TAVR compared to SAVR patients, regardless of prosthesis type, as they are greater than 10% in initial PARTNER data and approaching 6% in initial CoreValve data [7]. This is due to many factors, most importantly, size of deployment catheters and frequent incidence of vascular disease in the TAVR patient population. However, as TAVR techniques and deployment systems have become more refined, this increased incidence should more closely approach SAVR groups.

### Hemodynamic Instability

Given the frequent occurrence of co-morbid conditions, the high-risk patient population and the presence of severe aortic valve disease, it is not surprising that hemodynamic instability occurs during TAVR procedures:

- Rhythm disturbances
  - The presence of intracardiac wires and catheters frequently cause arrhythmias. Most of these are limited to the time the wires and catheters are manipulated and do not represent a new-onset arrhythmia.
  - Certain prostheses require rapid ventricular pacing to induce cardiac standstill during valve deployment. This is achieved by a percutaneous RV pacing lead, which is usually advanced from a femoral venous approach. Some patients may require defibrillation after pacing is ceased to restore a perfusing rhythm.

- Some prosthetic valves have a known risk for causing heart block, specifically those valves which occupy portions of the left ventricular outflow tract (LVOT) or those that continue to slowly expand after deployment, which can lead to overstretching of the LVOT. Due to the presence of conduction tissue in the LVOT, pressure exerted on that area by a valve prosthesis may lead to heart block. This can occur immediately after valve deployment or in the days to weeks after deployment. CoreValves in particular are known to have a ~30% risk of patients requiring permanent pacemaker (PPM) implantation post TAVR [8].
- An important step in defining this risk is identifying those patients who are at higher than normal risk; specifically those patients with underlying bundle branch delays. If those patients are to receive a valve prosthesis that places them at a higher risk for requiring post-procedure pacing, it is reasonable to place a temporary pacing wire during the procedure and transfer the patient to a telemetry setting for further monitoring.
- Coronary artery obstruction
  - Care is taken during SAVR to ensure the left and right coronary ostia are not occluded. However, during TAVR, the aorta is not opened and the valve is positioned via fluoroscopic and echocardiographic guidance. While contrast injections in the aortic root are performed to define the anatomy of the coronary ostia, valve deployment may obstruct flow to one or both coronary arteries. This will usually lead to significant hemodynamic instability and may require open coronary artery bypass grafting or percutaneous coronary intervention.
- Paravalvular leak
  - Rate of paravalvular leak (PVL) is higher in TAVR patients when compared to SAVR patients. In PARTNER trial patients, presence of even mild PVL is associated with decreased 5-year survival [5]. This stands in contrast to CoreValve patients, who although initially had higher rates of moderate or severe PVL when compared to SAVR patients, at 1 year follow up the majority of these patients had mild or no PVL. The difference is likely due to the continued self-expansion of the CoreValve prosthesis, which is a characteristic not found in the Edwards SAPIEN valve.
  - Significant PVL is usually addressed during the procedure, as it will lead to a low cardiac output state and heart failure if left untreated. This can be treated by attempting to further expand the valve, repositioning the valve in the case of a retrievable/repositionable prosthesis, or placing a new prosthesis in the existing one (valve-in-valve).
- Valve malposition
  - Poor position of the prosthesis is a severe complication that can lead to significant hemodynamic instability. The valve may be too low in the LVOT and not fully covering the native valve leading to poor prosthesis and native valve function. The valve may be too high in the annulus, leading to coronary artery obstruction as described above. Another feared complication is embolization of the valve, which can occur into the left ventricle (LV) or distally into the ascending aorta. Often an embolized valve will require open retrieval as current iterations of TAVR prostheses have limited retrievability after deployment.
  - Key to minimizing this risk is proper selection of valve size. Unlike SAVR, there is no ability for the surgeon to use valve sizers on an exposed aortic annulus. Proceduralists rely on pre-procedure CT and MRI measurements and echocardiographic data. Specifically, 3D transesophageal echocardiography (TEE) annulus measurements have been shown to better correlate with CT annulus measurements and are becoming standard guiding measurements for TAVR [9].
- Aortic Dissection or Rupture
  - Balloon valvuloplasty prior to valve deployment or valve expansion in the aortic annulus may lead to aortic trauma,

specifically localized dissection or frank rupture. These are devastating complications of TAVR and often lead to significant morbidity and mortality due to the need for open repair on high-risk patients. Great care and vigilance is required particularly during transaortic approach to TAVR as the ascending aorta is approached directly for valve deployment.

## Post-procedure Care

Initially, TAVR patients at most centers were transferred from the hybrid operating room or cardiac catheterization lab to an ICU setting for close hemodynamic and neurologic monitoring. As the experience of cardiologists, surgeons and anesthesiologists grows, prostheses and deployment systems become more refined, and patient selection improves, it is reasonable to treat each patient individually for their post-procedure care. Higher-risk patients will continue to require an ICU-level post-procedure monitoring. But more straightforward patients who had an uncomplicated percutaneous transfemoral TAVR may be appropriate for management on a standard ward unit prior to discharge home. As with any patient, input from all the services caring for the patient should be obtained prior to deciding where the patient should recover from their procedure.

## Other Percutaneous Valve Therapies

### Mitral Valve

Mitral regurgitation is the commonest valvular heart disease and a frequent indication for cardiac surgery. Advancements in medical management and an aging population have resulted in more high risk patients being considered for mitral valve interventions. Transcatheter mitral valve repair or replacement (TMVR) encompasses mitral valve repair, most commonly with MitraClip edge to edge repair. This has been the most popular TMV repair technique with greater than 40,000 repairs performed [10]. The approach for MitraClip placement is via femoral venous access with a trans-septal puncture to enter the left atrium and is generally associated with unchanged hemodynamics from the patient's baseline. It is important for the anesthesiologist to be aware of potential mitral stenosis post MitraClip placement and be prepared to manage the hemodynamic changes associated with mitral stenosis.

TMV replacement includes a TAVR prosthesis placed in the mitral position, either in a native annulus, a prior mitral ring repair or mitral valve bioprosthesis and the rarer valve in mitral annular calcification (MAC). The valve in MAC uses the severe calcification present in the patient's mitral annulus as an anchor for a TAVR prosthesis. Limited data is available for TMV replacement. Multiple TMV replacement prostheses are currently in development and early investigation.

Approach is generally via a transfemoral, trans-septal approach. Some techniques utilize a transapical approach. TMV replacement may require rapid ventricular pacing to induce cardiac standstill for valve placement.

### Tricuspid Valve

Regurgitation is the most common form of tricuspid valve disease, which is often secondary to left-sided valve disease. Transcatheter tricuspid valve repair or replacement (TTVR) can be performed in a prior valve repair, prior bioprosthesis or in a native valve. Newer techniques and prostheses are being developed to treat this challenging problem. It is known that patients with moderate or severe tricuspid regurgitation (TR) have increased morbidity and mortality. Recurrence of significant TR after prior tricuspid valve surgery may be >50% at 5 years [11].

TTVR may be approached via a transfemoral or transjugular technique. Rapid pacing may be required during the procedure but is used cautiously due to potential for trapping a temporary right ventricular pacing lead when a prosthesis is placed. Lack of significant annular support has proven challenging for the use of existing transcatheter prostheses in the tricuspid position. Case reports exist for use of Melody valve, a bovine jugular vein in a metal frame, in the tricuspid position.

Other emerging procedures include tricuspid annulus remodeling techniques, which act to reduce the dilated tricuspid annulus that is often the cause of secondary tricuspid regurgitation, and tricuspid valve coaptation devices.

## Pulmonic Valve

Transcatheter pulmonic valve replacement (TPVR) has been FDA approved since 2010 in the form of the Melody valve, a bovine jugular vein in a metal, radiopaque stent. SAPIEN valves have also been used in the pulmonic position, and are advantageous in patients with larger right ventricular outflow tracts, as Melody valves are only available in 20 and 22 mm sizes.

## Anesthetic Management

Due to the complex anatomy and newer applications of existing devices, TMVR, TTVR and TPVR can be technically challenging for proceduralists and anesthesiologists. Imaging guidance is often key to successful valve repair or replacement, therefore both TEE and fluoroscopy are used during these procedures. General anesthesia is preferred to ensure patient comfort and safety during the prolonged TEE needed for the procedure. Need for invasive monitoring is determined based on overall patient condition. Most centers will utilize arterial blood pressure monitoring in addition to ASA standard monitors. Central venous access may be indicated if patients have significant hemodynamic instability from their underlying valvular heart disease.

As these procedures are continuing to develop and evolve, there is a lack of data relating to complications and long-term outcomes. The heart team model, which gained popularity in many successful TAVR programs, is vitally important in these procedures. Effective communication regarding anesthetic technique, patient selection, procedure and patient-specific concerns, and a plan for post-procedure care should be done in a thoughtful and collaborative manner.

## References

1. Grover FL, Vemulapalli S, Carroll JD, et al. 2016 annual report of the Society of Thoracic Surgeons/American College of Cardiology Transcatheter Valve Therapy Registry. J Am Coll Cardiol. 2017;69(10):1215–30.
2. Decision memo for transcatheter aortic valve replacement (TAVR) (CAG-00430N). www.CMS.gov.
3. Babaliaros V, Devireddy C, Lerakis S, et al. Comparison of transfemoral transcatheter aortic valve replacement performed in the catheterization laboratory (minimalist approach) versus hybrid operating room (standard approach). J Am Coll Cardiol Intv. 2014;7:898–904.
4. Tsai MT, Tang GHL, Cohen GN. Year in review: transcatheter aortic valve replacement. Curr Opin Cardiol. 2016;31:139–47.
5. Mack MJ, Leon MB, Smith CR, et al. 5-year outcomes of transcatheter aortic valve replacement or surgical aortic valve replacement for high surgical risk patients with aortic stenosis (PARTNER 1): a randomized controlled trial. Lancet. 2015;385(9986):2477–84.
6. Adams DH, Popma JJ, Reardon MJ, et al. Transcatheter aortic-valve replacement with a self-expanding prosthesis. N Engl J Med. 2014;370(19):1790–8.
7. Horne A, Reineck E, Hasan RK, et al. Transcatheter aortic valve replacement: historical perspectives, current evidence, and future directions. Am Heart J. 2014;168:414–23.
8. Reardon MJ, Adams DH, Kleiman NS, et al. 2-year outcomes in patients undergoing surgical or self-expanding transcatheter aortic valve replacement. JACC. 2015;66(2):113–21.
9. Hahn RT. Guidance of transcatheter aortic valve replacement by echocardiography. Curr Cardiol Rep. 2014;16(1):442.
10. Gössl M, Farivar RS, Bae R, et al. Current status of catheter-based treatment of mitral valve regurgitation. Curr Cardiol Rep. 2017;19(5):38.
11. Bouleti C, Juliard JM, Himbert D, et al. Tricuspid valve and percutaneous approach: no longer the forgotten valve! Arch Cardiovasc Dis. 2016;109:55–66.

# Anesthetic Considerations in the Patient with an Implanted Cardiac Device

## 8

Keyur Trivedi and Kinjal M. Patel

## Introduction

The number of patients with cardiovascular implantable electronic devices (CIEDs) has grown significantly in recent years. Additionally, as technology has evolved, these devices are performing a multitude of complex functions. Anesthesiologists caring for these patients need to be aware of how these devices operate to best oversee them through the perioperative period.

Implantable devices that require anesthetic considerations include pacemakers (PMs), defibrillators (ICDs), and loop recorders. It is important to understand the different types of CIEDs, the standard CIED nomenclature, the management of these devices in the perioperative period and the approach to unknown devices.

## Devices and Nomenclature

### Pacemakers

Pacemakers are often permanently implanted devices, but can also be temporarily placed. They are commonly placed for bradycardia, sinus node dysfunction, atrioventricular (AV) node dysfunction, and for synchronous pacing in patients with interventricular conduction delay.

Pacemakers are powered by pulse generators that are usually placed below the left or right clavicle. These pulse generators are connected to individual leads that provide therapy to a specific chamber of the heart. Knowledge of the generator's location will help guide the perioperative management of the device.

Transvenous pacemaker leads can be placed in a single chamber or multiple chambers of the heart and controlled by the pulse generator to achieve the desired outcome. Commonly, pacemakers are classified as single chamber, dual chamber, or biventricular. Single chamber pacemakers provide therapy to either atrium or ventricle only. Dual chamber pacemakers provide therapy to both the atrium and ventricle. Transvenous atrial pacemaker leads are usually placed in the right atrial appendage and ventricular leads are placed in the right ventricular apex. The second ventricular lead of a biventricular pacemaker, usually placed for cardiac resynchronization therapy (CRT), is placed in a left ventricular epicardial vein via the coronary sinus. Epicardial leads can also be placed surgically on the external surface of the myocardium and connected to a pulse generator.

Pacemaker leads can sense the activity of a chamber, and either inhibit or trigger pacing in accordance with the device programming. If the intrinsic activity of the chamber is lower than the rate set on the device, the pulse generator will

K. Trivedi, M.D. (✉) · K. M. Patel, M.D.
Cooper Medical School of Rowan University,
Camden, NJ, USA
e-mail: Trivedi-keyur@cooperhealth.edu;
Patel-kinjal@cooperhealth.edu

trigger the lead to pace at the programmed rate. If the lead senses chamber activity at a rate higher than that set on the device, pacing will be inhibited. In a dual chamber pacemaker, pacing or inhibitory activity in each chamber is coordinated based on lead sensing in both chambers. This allows for a more physiologic pacing mode, promoting AV synchrony and decreasing AV valve regurgitation [1].

## Defibrillators

ICDs are capable of sensing a malignant tachyarrhythmia and subsequently delivering a targeted therapy to terminate the abnormal rhythm. Most ICDs are transvenous, however, newer subcutaneous models are becoming more commonplace. Transvenous ICDs deliver shocks through a ventricular lead connected to a pulse generator located below either clavicle. Subcutaneous ICDs deliver shocks via a pulse generator placed in the left axilla and an electrode tunneled toward the sternum. Transvenous ICDs possess additional PM functions that may be needed after defibrillatory therapy if profound bradycardia is detected. Like pacemakers, ICDs can contain only ventricular leads, both atrial and ventricular leads, or bi-ventricular leads. The pulse generator is programmed to sense both ventricular tachycardia (VT) and ventricular fibrillation (VF). If VT is sensed, depending on the rate and inherent programming of the ICD, the device may try to pace faster than the VT rate to terminate the arrhythmia. If VT continues, the ICD will defibrillate the patient. However, if VF is sensed, the ICD will immediately defibrillate the patient.

## Loop Recorders

Implantable loop recorders are small devices placed subcutaneously over the chest wall for longer-term surveillance of potential rhythm abnormalities. They continuously record and store electrocardiographic data that can be retrieved at a later date for analysis. As electromagnetic interference found in the operating room can erase stored data, this data should be retrieved when possible prior to any elective surgical procedures [2].

## Nomenclature

The North American Society of Pacing and Electrophysiology (NASPE)/British Pacing and Electrophysiology Group (BPEG) code for antibradycardia, adaptive rate and multisite pacing is universally accepted to describe pacemaker programming. Understanding the pacemaker programming codes allows the anesthesiologist to predict device behavior in the perioperative setting. The standard pacemaker code consists of four or five positions, though often only the first three positions are mentioned (Table 8.1). The first letter specifies the chamber(s) being paced. The second letter specifies the chamber(s) where electrical activity is sensed. The third letter specifies the pacemaker's response to sensed events. The fourth letter describes the presence or absence of rate modulation, and the fifth position points to the location or absence of multisite pacing.

Typically, only the first three positions are mentioned to create a designation such as DDD, DOO, AAI, or VVI. A pacemaker in the DDD

**Table 8.1** NASPE/BPEG code for pacemaker programming [4]

| Position I | Position II | Position III | Position IV | Position V |
|---|---|---|---|---|
| Pacing site | Sensing site | Response | Rate modulation function | Multisite pacing location |
| D—Dual (A and V)<br>A—Atrium<br>V—Ventricle | D—Dual (A and V)<br>A—Atrium<br>V—Ventricle<br>O—None | I—Inhibited<br>T—Triggered<br>D—Dual (triggered and/or inhibited)<br>O—None | R—Rate modulating<br>O—None | D—Dual (A and V)<br>A—Atrium<br>V—Ventricle<br>O—None |

mode can sense and trigger both chambers of the heart. Dual chamber pacemakers are typically set to this designation to maintain AV synchrony in patients. DOO pacing, also called asynchronous pacing, stimulates both chambers to be paced at the set rate regardless of underlying activity.

AAI can be used in patients with preserved AV conduction but with symptomatic sinus bradycardia. In these patients, the atria are both paced and sensed, with the pacemaker being inhibited when intrinsic atrial activity is sensed above the set rate.

VVI can be used in patients with chronic atrial fibrillation. The ventricular lead can both pace and sense, and the response to intrinsic activity above the set rate is inhibition of pacemaker activity.

Rate responsive PMs are specialized pacemakers developed to help increase cardiac output in response to increasing metabolic demands, such as exercise. These PMs depend on specific sensors (pH, body motion, minute ventilation, thoracic impedance, etc.) to guide therapy [3] and may need special attention in the perioperative period.

## Perioperative CIED Management

### Preoperative Considerations

Patients presenting for procedures with CIEDs need a thorough evaluation of their device and a plan for perioperative device management. Reviewing the patient history and medical record, as well as available chest radiographs and electrocardiograms should alert the provider that a CIED is present. Palpation of a subcutaneous foreign body or a scar below either clavicle may reveal the presence of a CIED [5].

Examining the manufacturer's identification card or the patient's chest radiograph can help identify the type of device implanted (ICD or Pacemaker). Most current CIEDs have an x-ray code that can help identify the device. The manufacturer's database and pacemaker clinic records are other resources that may help identify the type of device. Consulting a cardiologist or CIED team (physicians or physician extenders who monitor CIED function) is also a possibility if time permits [5].

If the implanted device has a pacing function, the patient's dependence on the pacing function must be determined. A history of bradyarrhythmia causing syncope or a history of AV node ablation would suggest a pacemaker dependent patient. The patient's underlying rate and rhythm can be uncovered by setting the CIED pacing function to VVI at a rate of 40 or by temporarily disabling the pacing function of the device [5]. Preoperative interrogation of the device by the CIED team will identify how often a patient relies upon the pacing function of the device.

Information regarding the device's function must be obtained prior to any elective procedure. Current recommendations are for pacemakers to be interrogated within 12 months of the procedure and ICDs to be interrogated within 6 months. While this information can be obtained from an interrogation report, it is recommended that physicians without experience managing CIEDs obtain guidance for perioperative CIED management from a CIED team. Industry-employed allied health professionals acting alone without supervision by a physician is inappropriate [5, 6].

The CIED team needs specific information from the perioperative team to provide a prescription for CIED management. The exact procedure, the anatomic location of the procedure, the surgical venue (i.e., operating room, interventional radiology, etc.), the patient's positioning and post-operative disposition (ICU, telemetry bed, discharge to home, etc.) should be communicated. Any potential risk of electromagnetic interference (EMI) also needs to be discussed [6].

The Heart Rhythm Society (HRS) and the American Society of Anesthesiologists (ASA) have identified key elements that are necessary in the communication from the CIED team to the procedural team [6]:

- The manufacturer, model number, type of device and indication for placement of the device.
- Device response to magnet placement over the pulse generator. Response can vary with different manufacturers.
- Date of the last interrogation.

- Battery life remaining in the pulse generator. Devices with less than 3 months of battery life are at an increased risk of damage from EMI.
- CIED leads in place for less than 3 months should also be noted. They are at increased risk of being dislodged by intracardiac catheters.
- The pacing mode, the programmed lower rate and the patient's dependency on the pacemaker.
- Specific to ICDs, the lowest heart rate threshold for a defibrillatory and/or anti-tachycardia pacing.
- Presence of rate responsive sensors. Modern devices have rate responsive sensors that can cause unintended changes in heart rate from motion artifact or increased minute ventilation during anesthesia.
- The presence of any alerts on the CIED or leads.
- The pacing threshold for each lead should be confirmed to ensure an adequate safety margin.

Additionally, the CIED team should provide guidance on the perioperative management of the device. This includes recommendations for programming of the pacing mode, inactivating ICD therapy and inactivating minute ventilation sensors. The CIED team should discuss the use of a magnet with the perioperative team along with appropriate post-operative management, especially if device reprogramming is required.

## Intraoperative Considerations

Electromagnetic interference (EMI) can affect CIED functionality. While electrocautery is the most frequent offender (monopolar ≫ bipolar), patient factors and specialized monitoring equipment can also disrupt normal CIED function. Shivering and fasiculations can also mimic electrical activity, inhibiting pacing or triggering a defibrillatory shock. Evoked potential monitoring in patients can also generate EMI, interfering with CIED operations [1].

Pacemakers generally respond to EMI by inhibiting pacing, which can be life threatening in pacemaker dependent patients. However, not every model responds the same way; reversion to a preprogrammed backup mode or a change to asynchronous mode can also be seen in pacemakers subjected to EMI. An ICD subjected to prolonged EMI can result in unwanted shock delivery. While modern CIEDs are equipped with several technologies to reduce the effect of EMI (bipolar leads, insulated pulse generator housing and cables, EMI noise protection algorithms etc.), anesthesiologists still need to be aware of the consequences of EMI-CIED interactions.

Intraoperative management of a patient with a CIED involves ensuring a stable cardiac rhythm and protecting the CIED from EMI. Achieving these goals requires appropriately monitoring patients, identifying and managing EMI in the operating room or procedure suite, and intervening as necessary to manage dysrhythmias [6].

Patients with CIEDs should have monitoring of a peripheral pulse and continuous EKG or rhythm strip. Peripheral pulse monitoring is best accomplished by pulse plethysmography or arterial pressure tracing. Palpation of a peripheral pulse, auscultation of heart sounds and ultrasound of a peripheral pulse are cumbersome alternative measures [5]. The patient's EKG tracing should be monitored in pacing mode to identify pacing stimuli. Patients with ICDs are required to have continuous cardiac monitoring and immediate access to defibrillation upon discontinuing tachyarrhythmia therapy, including the time prior to arrival in the operating room [6].

Monopolar electrocautery is the most common source of EMI in the operating room and its commonly used coagulation feature causes more EMI than the cutting feature [7]. When the current from the electrocautery unit is directed toward the generator-heart circuit, the CIED may experience more EMI. Use of electrocautery above the umbilicus also places the patient at higher risk for EMI-related CIED dysfunction. Other specific procedure related sources of EMI are noted in Table 8.2 [6].

Several steps can be taken to mitigate the risks of EMI in patients with CIEDs. Bipolar electrocautery and harmonic scalpel are generally considered safe unless applied directly to the CIED

**Table 8.2** Procedure related CIED considerations [6]

| Procedure | Special considerations | CIED needs to be evaluated prior to discharge from monitored setting? |
|---|---|---|
| Radiofrequency ablation | • Avoid direct contact between ablation catheter and CIED generator and leads<br>• If above umbilicus, need asynchronous mode for pacemaker dependent patients<br>• Tachycardia detection should be disabled<br>• Direct current path away from CIED | Yes |
| Lithotripsy | • Avoid focusing beam near pulse generator<br>• If lithotripsy triggers on the R-wave, consider disabling atrial pacing | Can be evaluated within 1 month of procedure |
| MRI | • Generally contraindicated—consult cardiologist for recommendations | |
| Radiation therapy | • Most likely source of EMI to result in CIED reset<br>• Can be safely performed if device is outside field of radiation | Within 24 h for high risk cases (direct beam to the chest or high energy photon radiation) |
| Electroconvulsive therapy | • ICD tachyarrhythmia therapy should be disabled<br>• Ventricular arrhythmia might occur due to hemodynamic effects of ECT<br>• Pacemaker dependent patients may require temporary pacing or asynchronous mode | Can be evaluated within 1 month of procedure |
| Ocular procedures | • Do not discontinue tachyarrhythmia therapy | Can be evaluated within 1 month of procedure if monopolar electrocautery is used |
| Cardiothoracic surgery | | Yes |
| Intraoperative cardiac arrest or external electrical Cardioversion | | Yes |
| Hemodynamically challenging surgeries (e.g., AAA repair) | | Yes |
| Emergency surgery above umbilicus with EMI exposure | | Yes |

generator [5, 6]. For monopolar electrocautery, the current return pad must be placed so the direction of current from the electrocautery device to the return pad does not cross the generator or leads of the CIED. For example, in procedures involving the head and neck, the current return pad is placed posteriorly on the shoulder, contralateral to the generator. Bursts of electrocautery for less than 5 s also reduce the risk of EMI. Despite taking all recommended precautions, EMI may affect the CIED. A pacemaker may erroneously sense the EMI as the patient's intrinsic rhythm and may result in pacemaker inhibition (termed "oversensing"). An ICD may erroneously sense EMI as a rapid arrhythmia and trigger the delivery of anti-tachycardia therapy [6].

A magnet placed over a CIED can help manage the effects of EMI on CIEDs and the success of this approach depends on the device's programmed response to a magnet. It is important to note that some CIEDs have a magnet mode that must be enabled for the magnet to have its desired effect; this underscores the knowledge gained from a preoperative CIED evaluation. All operating rooms where there is a possible interaction between EMI and CIEDs should have a magnet immediately available. Most pacemakers will go into an asynchronous mode with magnet application and most ICDs will have their anti-tachycardia therapy disabled with magnet application. It is important to note that combined pacemaker/ICDs will only have their anti-tachycardia therapy disabled by magnet application. For combined devices to have asynchronous pacing, they must be reprogrammed [6].

The decision to place a magnet on a device versus reprogramming the device should take the advantages and disadvantages of each approach into account. A magnet can be placed and removed by the anesthesia team. A magnet can be utilized to quickly turn off anti-tachycardia therapy and can also be removed to quickly restore ICD function. Reprogramming the device requires the presence of a third party with the appropriate equipment and can be more cumbersome. Placing a magnet requires the placement site, which may be limited by patient positioning or body habitus, to be accessible. Reprogramming a CIED eliminates the concern of maintaining a magnet in the proper position. A drawback of reprogramming a CIED is that the changes of reprogramming are not readily reversible. A programmer must be present to restore the CIED's original programming. Once an ICD is reprogrammed to suspend tachycardia detection (therefore suspending all ICD therapy), the patient must have continuous EKG monitoring and defibrillator pads placed. Reprogramming an ICD carries the risk that the cardiology team is not notified to reactivate the device following the procedure. The HRS suggests "tagging" these patients so they are not discharged with an inactive ICD [6].

The HRS/American Society of Anesthesiology (ASA) Expert Consensus Statement provides focused guidance for the perioperative management of devices. The anti-tachyarrhythmia therapy in ICDs does not need to be deactivated for all procedures. Procedures superior to the umbilicus requiring the use of monopolar electrocautery should indeed have tachyarrhythmia therapy disabled [6]. Note that the ASA practice advisory recommends deactivating the tachyarrhythmia therapy on all ICDs when monopolar electrocautery is used [5]. In pacemaker dependent patients, the asynchronous mode (via reprogramming or magnet placement) is only necessary when electrocautery is used superior to the umbilicus. Magnets may be used to render a pacemaker asynchronous to protect the device from inhibition. Magnets used on a combined pacemaker/ICD will only deactivate the tachyarrhythmia therapy for the device. If a patient with a combined device is also pacemaker dependent, a magnet will not affect the pacing function. The pacemaker function of the device will require reprogramming to enable asynchronous pacing [5, 6].

Occasionally, patients with CIEDs will require emergent cardioversion or defibrillation. In such cases, all sources of EMI should be discontinued. If a magnet is present on an ICD generator, it should be removed to enable anti-tachycardia therapy. If there continues to be a need for external cardioversion or defibrillation then advanced cardiac life support should dictate treatment. Patches or pads for cardioversion or defibrillation are placed in an anterior-posterior position to minimize the risk of damage to the CIED. All patients undergoing cardioversion/defibrillation must have their CIED interrogated prior to leaving a monitored environment [5].

## Post-operative Considerations

The postoperative management of patients with CIEDs involves appropriate interrogation of the device and restoring device function. Intraoperative hemodynamic instability, preoperative or intraoperative reprogramming of the device, or concerns about CIED function are all indications for postoperative interrogation of the CIED. Table 8.2 lists interrogation recommendations for patients undergoing specific procedures [6]. Patients who are low risk (no EMI exposure, no CIED problems during surgery, no blood transfusion and no reprogramming of the device) do not need an immediate postoperative interrogation. All patients awaiting ICD interrogation must be fully monitored in the PACU or ICU until anti-tachycardia therapy is restored [5, 6].

Equipment for back-up pacing, cardioversion and defibrillation must be immediately available.

## The Unknown Device

Emergent or urgent surgery necessitates proceeding to surgery without all desired information regarding the CIED. The type of device may be determined by a discussion with the patient focused on prior cardiac interventions, examining medical records, checking for a patient device card and calling the device manufacturer, and checking the chest x-ray for the presence of a thicker coil in the right ventricle. The thicker coil dictates that an ICD is present as pacemakers alone do not have these coils [6].

If the patient has a pacemaker, an EKG or rhythm strip should be examined for the presence of pacer spikes. The presence of spikes before most or all P waves and/or QRS complexes indicates the patient is likely to be pacemaker dependent. A magnet should be placed prior to surgery for procedures above the umbilicus, for procedures where electrocautery cannot be limited to short burst or for procedures where patient positioning will make access to the pacemaker difficult. If a patient is not pacemaker dependent, a magnet needs to be readily available but not necessarily placed prior to surgery. The waveform of either an arterial line or pulse oximetry should be monitored. A sudden loss of either waveform that coincides with a burst of electrocautery may indicate inhibition of pacemaker function. If the procedure allows, transcutaneous pacing pads should be placed in the anterior-posterior position and monopolar electrocautery should be used in short bursts. All patients should be monitored postoperatively until the device is evaluated [6].

Emergency surgical patients who will receive monopolar electrocautery with an ICD should proceed to surgery with a magnet placed over the device to deactivate the device. Transcutaneous pads for both pacing and defibrillation should be applied to the patient. If a patient with an ICD is also being paced, a magnet will not place the pacemaker into asynchronous mode. The EMI must be managed with short bursts of electrocautery. If a patient has bradycardia due to EMI pacing inhibition, the cardiology team may need to reprogram the device. Patients must remain in a monitored setting until the CIED is evaluated postoperatively [6].

### Conclusion

Patients with CIEDs are commonly managed by anesthesia teams in the perioperative setting. Successful oversight of these devices during this period requires careful assessment and appropriate planning. Consulting the hospital CIED team, the patient's cardiologist, or the device manufacturer can help the anesthesia team understand how a specific device functions. In urgent situations, a focused patient history, chest X-Ray and EKG may shed light on the nature of the CIED. Understanding how these devices operate, and their response to EMI or magnet placement is critical for successful patient management.

## References

1. Stone ME, Salter B, Fischer A. Perioperative management of patients with cardiac implantable electronic devices. Br J Anaesth. 2011;107(S1):i16–26. https://doi.org/10.1093/bja/aer354.
2. Costa A, Richman DC. Implantable devices: assessment and perioperative management. Anesthesiol Clin. 2016;34:185–99. https://doi.org/10.1016/j.anclin.2015.10.014.
3. Dell'Orto S, Valli P, Greco EM. Sensors for rate responsive pacing. Indian Pacing Electrophysiol J. 2004;4(3):137–45.
4. Bernstein A, Daubert J, Fletcher R, Hayes D, Luderitz B, Suttontt R, et al. The revised NASPE/BPEG generic code for antibradycardia, adaptive-rate, and multisite pacing. Pacing Clin Electrophysiol. 2002;25(2):260–4. https://doi.org/10.1016/j.aan.2016.07.008.
5. American Society of Anesthesiologists. Practice advisory for the perioperative management of patients with cardiac implantable electronic devices: pacemakers and implantable cardioverter-defibrillators: an updated report by the American Society of Anesthesiologists task force on perioperative management of patients with cardiac implantable elec-

tronic devices. Anesthesiology. 2011;114(2):247–61. https://doi.org/10.1097/ALN.0b013e3181fbe7f6.
6. Crossley GH, Poole JE, Rozner MA, Asirvatham SJ, Cheng A, Chung MK, et al. The Heart Rhythm Society (HRS)/American Society of Anesthesiologists (ASA) expert consensus statement on the perioperative management of patients with implantable defibrillators, pacemakers and arrhythmia monitors: facilities and patient management: this document was developed as a joint project with the American Society of Anesthesiologists (ASA), and in collaboration with the American Heart Association (AHA), and the Society of Thoracic Surgeons (STS). Heart Rhythm. 2011;8(7):1114–54. https://doi.org/10.1016/j.hrthm.2010.12.023.
7. Schulman PM, Rozner MA. The perioperative management of implantable pacemakers and cardioverter-defibrillators. Adv Anesth. 2016;34:117–41. https://doi.org/10.1016/j.aan.2016.07.008.

# Anesthesia for Aortic Surgery

Mario Christopher DeAngelis
and Michael Stuart Green

## Incidence

Approximately 2000 new aortic dissections are diagnosed each year. Each 10,000 admissions will have one estimated admission for aortic dissection. One series of autopsy reviews showed that a dissection could be found in 1 out of every 600 post mortem exams [1].

The most common ages for patients to present with an aortic dissection are aged 40–70 years, with Marfan syndrome patients presenting in their 30s and 40s. Aortic dissections occur approximately twice as common in men as in women [2, 3].

Thoracic aortic aneurysms are estimated to represent 1–4% of aneurysms found on autopsy. The ascending aneurysm is seen approximately twice as common as a localized descending aneurysm. Aortic arch aneurysms, without extension past the arch, can be found in less than 10% of the total number of aneurysms discovered on autopsy.

Though there have been widely varied findings from several autopsy series, the accepted incidence of a thoracic aortic aneurysm is 10/100,000 patients. This disease was responsible for 17,215 U.S. deaths in 2009 [4]; with the understanding that some fatal emergency department visits for chest pain are misdiagnosed as myocardial infarction (MI) but may be the result of an aortic rupture. The actual mortality of thoracic aortic aneurysms may remain an unknown value, as the diagnosis is not always considered in time for treatment or appropriate testing.

## Presentation, Classifications and Diagnosis

Aortic dissections can be fatal in the pre-hospital setting. Making this diagnosis even more difficult is that aortic dissections can present in several forms. Table 9.1 lists some of the presenting symptoms and diagnostic tests used in cases of suspected aortic dissection.

Once the diagnosis has been confirmed, the location of the involved portion of the aorta is used to classify the dissection. There are two major systems used to classify aortic dissections: the DeBakey and Stanford systems [5, 6].

The DeBakey System classifies aortic dissection into three types, as follows:

- Type I—The intimal tear occurs in the ascending aorta, but the descending aorta is also involved
- Type II—Only the ascending aorta is involved
- Type III—Only the descending aorta is involved; type IIIA originates distal to the left subclavian artery and extends as far as the diaphragm, whereas type IIIB involves the descending aorta below the diaphragm

M. C. DeAngelis, M.D.
M. S. Green, D.O., M.B.A. (✉)
Department of Anesthesiology and Perioperative Medicine, Drexel University College of Medicine, Philadelphia, PA, USA
e-mail: Michael.Green@Drexelmed.edu

**Table 9.1** Presenting signs/symptoms and diagnostic tests for thoracic aortic dissection

Signs/symptoms:
- Severe chest pain (most common, but not always present)
- MI-like symptoms: Jaw pain, chest pressure (from dissection into the coronaries)
- Tearing or ripping sensation in the chest
- New neurological symptoms (CVA, carotid dissection, hemiparesis, hemiplegia)
- CHF symptoms of dyspnea and orthopnea (from acute aortic insufficiency)
- Dysphagia from esophageal compression
- Recurrent laryngeal nerve compression with new voice hoarseness
- Can be painless, which is more common when Marfan syndrome or new neurological symptoms are present
- HTN from release of catecholamines or worsening of existing HTN
- Hypotension
- Blood pressure difference > 20 mmHg between upper extremities
- Cardiac tamponade with associated symptoms
- Dyspnea from possible hemothorax (if dissection ruptures into the pleural space)

Diagnostic laboratory tests:
- Elevated BUN/Cr: Possible renal artery involvement or pre-renal state from hypovolemia or cardiogenic shock
- Elevated troponin I and T: Ischemia from coronary dissection/hypotension
- Elevated LDH: Hemolysis from clots in false lumen
- Decreased hematocrit and hemoglobin: Aortic rupture or leak
- ABG: Evaluate for worsening acidosis, electrolyte disturbances and increasing lactate (possibly caused by bowel ischemia)
- EKG: May show acute ischemia if coronaries are involved, LVH common due to preexisting HTN, possible tamponade findings if aorta dissects/ruptures into pericardial space

Imaging studies
- CXR: First initial test usually obtained
- Contrast CT: Recommended as definitive test by American College of Radiology [35]
- MRA (with and without contrast): If CTA contraindicated
- TEE: More sensitive than TTE, evaluates valvular function, requires skilled operator present, able to be performed on unstable patients receiving treatment in critical care settings. TEE allows for aortic views in multiple planes (short and long axis views), allowing for identification of artifacts vs true pathology
- MRA without contrast
- Aortography: Former gold standard test
- TTE: A quick and non-invasive study to rule out tamponade and evaluate for aortic regurgitation in the setting of aortic dissection

The Stanford System splits dissections into two types, as follows:

- Type A—The ascending aorta is involved (DeBakey types I and II)
- Type B—The descending aorta is involved (DeBakey type III)

The Stanford system is designed to delineate treatment. Type A dissections require surgical intervention whereas type B dissections can be managed medically.

Aortic aneurysms can be identified by the portion of the aorta they involve (arch, ascending or descending) and by their shape. Aneurysms of the aorta can be classified as either saccular or fusiform. The more common saccular aneurysm involves a single portion of the wall which appears as an outpouching of the aorta. A fusiform aneurysm has a symmetrical shape which involves the full circumference of the aortic wall.

## Preoperative Assessment

The primary goal is to determine the urgency of the planned procedure; emergency cases require intense teamwork to enable optimal patient preparation in the minimum amount of time. Once the urgency of the case has been established, the surgical approach must be considered. Cases involving the aortic root, ascending aorta and proximal arch are usually approached by median sternotomy; while distal arch or descending aortic cases can be reached by a left thoracotomy, sometimes requiring an additional abdominal incision.

The general medical condition of the patient must be carefully evaluated, as each dysfunctional organ system adds a level of complexity to the anesthetic. A full review of preoperative testing is beyond the scope of this work, but specific recommendations will be given.

When patients present with a suspected aortic aneurysm or dissection, control of the blood pressure is paramount. Prior to diagnostic testing, these patients should have IV access established and be placed in a monitored setting. A systolic blood pressure (BP) goal of 100–120 mmHg will reduce aortic wall stress, while maintaining perfusion to vital organ systems [7]. Heart rate (HR) control is also recommended, with a target in the range of 60–70 bpm. If a measurement of cardiac output is available, a cardiac index between 2 and 2.5 is desirable. Higher cardiac index values increase the possibility of dissection extension or aneurysm rupture. Agents used to lower BP and HR can be divided into two main groups: ejection velocity reducers and vasodilators.

Lowering ejection velocity will decrease the force of blood exiting the aortic valve, hence lessening stress on the aneurysm or dissection point. Examples of the drugs used for this purpose are esmolol and labetalol.

Esmolol is the most titratable medication for this purpose. A loading dose of 500 µg/kg over 1–2 min, followed by a titrated infusion of 50–300 µg/kg/min, is recommended. Esmolol is an ultra-short acting beta blocker, which has a half-life of approximately 9 min. A benefit of using esmolol is that it can be rapidly titrated, or stopped, if the patient's condition changes. Patients with possible adverse reactions to beta blockade (heart failure or asthma) can be managed with esmolol with termination of the infusion if intolerance is noted.

Labetalol combines alpha and beta blockade, allowing some vasodilation with ejection velocity reduction. Labetalol can be administered as an IV bolus of 10–20 mg, with a short period of observation (5–10 min) to determine its effect. The dose can be escalated for the desired BP. Alternatively, a 1 mg/min labetalol infusion can be used for the same effect. The onset of action of IV labetalol is 2.5 min with a half-life of 5.5 h. Labetalol's longer half-life should be considered when choosing a beta blocker as the shorter half-live of esmolol enables more rapid titration.

Vasodilating medications directly affect vascular tone. The ideal vasodilator has not been identified, but several commonly used medications are listed below:

Nicardipine, an IV dihydropyridine calcium channel blocker, is available for infusions ranging from 5–15 mg/h. The main disadvantage to nicardipine is its long duration with prolonged infusions. There is a 2.7 min alpha half-life and intermediate beta phase of 44.8 min, followed by a terminal 14.4 h gamma half-life [8].

Clevidipine is a newer dihydropyridine calcium channel blocker. It decreases blood pressure by direct arterial vasodilation with no effect on venous capacitance. Compared to nicardipine, clevidipine has an alpha half-life of 1 min. It also has a faster onset of action, not needing the hepatic biotransformation required by nicardipine. As clevidipine does not cause venodilation like sodium nitroprusside and nitroglycerin, there is no preload reduction. This avoids the reflex tachycardia, blood pressure lability and abrupt hypotension seen with nitroprusside. Infusion rates are 0.4–3.2 µg/kg/min. The maximum recommended dose is 6–8 µg/kg/min, though higher doses have been used in studies [9].

Nitroprusside was formerly the preferred vasodilator for patients with aortic dissections and aneurysms, but is has since fallen out of favor due to the increase in maximal left ventricular force and reflex tachycardia noted with its administration [10]. Coronary steal and accumulation of cyanide metabolites have also been described with nitroprusside, making it a less than ideal first choice of antihypertensive. Typical dosing ranges from 0.3 to 10 µg/kg/min.

Fenoldapam is a selective dopamine-1 agonist, which causes arteriolar and renal dilation. It has a fast onset and 5 min half-life, making it an attractive choice for rapid BP control. Coronary steal is unlikely, due its selective renal action. Fenoldapam can improve creatinine clearance, which can be useful in patients with severe hemodynamic compromise. Doses of 0.01–1.6 µg/kg/min are recommended.

Nitroglycerin, at infusion ranges of 0.2–2 µg/kg/min, is useful if there are signs of myocardial ischemia. In general, nitroglycerin is less useful than other agents as its vasodilatory effects are more pronounced on the venous instead of the arterial system.

It should be noted that analgesic medications must not be withheld from the patients, as the discomfort will only worsen the hyperdynamic response which is to be avoided.

## Anesthetic and Surgical Management

Once the decision has been made to take the patient to the OR, a primary goal is to address any ongoing bleeding. When this has been achieved, the repair of the lesion can be considered. Aneurysm repairs commonly involve a synthetic tube graft which replaces the diseased section of aorta; this may require reimplantation of the major arterial branches of the aorta. Control of the dissection point is important with aortic dissections, as distal portions of the dissection are often compressed by the true lumen when it expands after surgery.

The anesthesiologist will continue preoperative BP control and monitor for signs of ischemia such as EKG changes, decreasing urine output and rising serum lactate levels. Comorbid conditions must also be considered and treated as many patients with aortic disease present with diabetes, COPD and side effects of chronic medical therapy (anticoagulants, for example). The anesthesiologist will be managing the initial and post cardiopulmonary bypass (CPB) bleeding associated with these cases, which can be profound. DHCA's effect on coagulation must also be considered, as hypothermia causes a progressive delay in the initiation of thrombus formation as well as a decrease in the speed of clot creation and growth. The effects of hypothermia are more pronounced when acidosis is present [11, 12]. A type and cross for 8–10 units of PRBCs and 4 units of FFP should be considered for the initial blood product orders, with further orders guided by clinical conditions and coagulation testing (Thromboelastagrophy (TEG) or standard PT/PTT/INR/Fibrinogen, for example).

Table 9.2 reviews the surgical approaches, CPB approach and placement of monitors used for ascending, arch and descending aortic repairs. Beyond standard monitors, it is common to utilize TEE for these cases assuming no contraindication exists. The TEE probe should be placed by the most skilled operator, with minimal force, as patients with dilated aortic pathology can have esophageal narrowing from the mass effect of the lesion. An oral gastric tube (OGT) can be carefully placed before TEE to evacuate gastric contents which may interfere with TEE imaging.

Arterial line placement is mandatory for these cases, but the location is determined by the aortic lesion site. Ascending cases require invasive monitoring distal to the great vessels, generally a left radial or femoral arterial line is preferred. Cases involving the arch often involve DHCA, and with the use of antegrade cerebral perfusion via right axillary artery cannulation a left radial or femoral arterial cannulation site should be utilized. In DHCA not involving right axillary artery cannulation arterial monitoring can be either left or right-sided. Descending aortic cases may involve the left subclavian origin, so right radial arterial line will provide adequate BP monitoring for the upper body.

**Table 9.2** Site of aortic surgery and considerations

| |
|---|
| **Ascending** |
| • Median Sternotomy |
| • CPB with aortic cannula distal to affected aortic segment/femoral arterial cannulation |
| • May involve aortic valve repair/replacement |
| • May involve coronary arteries |
| • Pericardium can be involved |
| • Arterial line placement in left upper extremity and/or femoral artery |
| • EEG/BIS/cerebral Oximeter often used |
| • Bleeding and post CPB cardiac dysfunction common |
| **Arch** |
| • Median Sternotomy |
| • CPB with/without DHCA |
| • Arterial line placement preferred in left upper extremity or femoral artery if ACP possible |
| • May use RCP/ACP for cerebral protection |
| • EEG/BIS/cerebral Oximetry often helpful diagnostic tools |
| • Monitor postoperatively for neurological deficits |
| **Descending** |
| • Left thoracotomy |
| • Single lung ventilation |
| • Thoracic epidural/epidural cooling possible |
| • Aorta cross-clamped |
| • Possible shunt, LA-FA CPB or partial CPB for distal perfusion |
| • CSF drainage with lumbar drain |
| • Arterial line placement in right upper extremity and femoral artery |
| • MEP/SSEP monitoring likely |
| • Bleeding, cardiac dysfunction, paralysis and renal failure possible |

Large bore and central intravenous access are mandatory for these cases. The amount of blood products transfused can be excessive and many of these patients require vasoactive infusions to manage contractility and BP derangements. Multiple central venous catheters may be necessary to accomplish these goals. Discussion with the surgical team is useful, as the femoral vessels on one side may be required for CPB access.

Pulmonary artery catheters (PAC) have historically been placed for these surgeries and many providers rely on a PAC for invasive hemodynamic management. The ability to measure and trend pulmonary artery pressures, cardiac output/index, mixed venous oxygen saturation and systemic vascular resistance is appealing for these patients. The data for PACs has been mixed; the general consensus is that patients should be selected carefully and only well trained operators should place/manage these patients. Chatterjee, et al. provides a review of indications for PAC use [13].

Temperature management is critical. Residual hypothermia can lead to coagulation disturbances, increased oxygen demand from shivering and increased wound infection. Hyperthermia has been associated with negative neurocognitive outcomes [14]. Core temperature is generally measured with a bladder catheter outfitted with a temperature probe. Urine output is tracked as a surrogate measure of renal perfusion. Cerebral temperature can be approximated with a nasopharyngeal (NP) probe, recognizing the potential for bleeding with NP probe placement/removal in patients with coagulation disturbances. Slowly rewarming, while minimizing the difference between core and cerebral temperatures, has been advocated in assisting with avoiding neurological injury [15].

Special monitoring or techniques often include:

EEG/BIS/Cerebral Oximetry: These diagnostic tools provide data on cerebral function and are almost always requested when DHCA is required. The goal of DHCA is to decrease the metabolic demand of the brain, therefore increasing the time the brain can be without blood flow. EEG monitoring allows for direct monitoring of cerebral activity and its suppression with hypothermia/anesthetics. As the brain temperature decreases, the EEG goes through several changes with electrocortical silence as the final signal detected. Amplitude decreases, as does frequency, before EEG burst suppression is noted. EEG detects cerebral ischemia within approximately 30 s of malperfusion, by displaying decreased amplitude and frequency [16].

Near infrared spectrophotometry (NIRS), or cerebral oximetry, can also be used as a measure of cerebral activity. NIRS only samples a small area 2–3 cm deep in the frontal cortex, so it is less likely to detect perturbations outside the distribution of the internal carotid artery. However, NIRS is non-invasive and easily applied. Normal cerebral oximetry values are 50–75% as there is a significant portion of venous blood measured. Bilateral decreased values can be seen with decreased oxygen delivery, such as low perfusion pressures or anemia. Unilateral decreases in NIRS values, especially after an intervention (e.g., carotid clamping when involved in aneurysm or dissection repair) may influence cerebral protection strategies used (use of ACP/RCP) [17].

Lumbar Cerebrospinal fluid (CSF) drainage/ monitors or Regional Epidural Cooling/ Motor or Somatosensory evoked potentials (MEP or SSEP): Spinal cord ischemia is a devastating complication of repairs of aortic aneurysm in the thoracic or thoracoabdominal sites. Open thoracoabdominal aneurysm repair (TAAA) carries a risk of 8–28% of spinal cord ischemia, while an endovascular approach (TEVAR) reduces the risk to 4–7% [18].

Increasing spinal cord perfusion pressure can be achieved by draining CSF through a subarachnoid catheter placed pre-operatively. Caution should be exercised during placement as a traumatic tap with bleeding can cause an elective case to be delayed due to concern for spinal hematoma formation given the coagulation disturbance seen with this surgery. The perfusion pressure of the spinal cord is estimated to be the

MAP minus the CSF pressure. Draining CSF will lower the CSF pressure, which is also measured using the spinal catheter. Caution should be exercised not to drain CSF too quickly for fear of intracranial bleeding. A CSF pressure target of 10 mmHg is often used [19].

SSEP and MEP can identify reversible spinal cord ischemic changes. A reduction in amplitude in either signal has been correlated with spinal cord ischemia, but it should be noted the sensitivity/specificity of these tests have not been fully determined. SSEP and MEP signals can be affected by many factors that are not spinal ischemia (anesthetic drugs, peripheral nerve damage, isolated limb ischemia, intraoperative stroke, for example), so not all changes in these signals are necessarily caused by spinal ischemia [20]. Volatile agents and muscle relaxants can have effects on SSEP and MEP monitoring, respectively. Some recommendations for optimal anesthetic agents appear below. Hypothermia has effects on SSEP monitoring, notably increased latencies and disappearance of the N13 wave and N20-P22 complex. SSEP monitoring is a sensitive detector of embolic stroke, as it monitors all sensory pathways and can be used to identify the distribution of the stroke [16].

Regional spinal cooling can be accomplished by placing a low thoracic (T11–12) epidural catheter, in addition to a L3-4 thermistor outfitted subarachnoid catheter. Once placed, cooled saline (4 °C) can be infused through the epidural and CSF temperature can be measured by the spinal catheter. This technique is not widely used, but one series examining this procedure noted a decrease in postoperative paraplegia after TAAA repair [21].

Cerebral Perfusion with anterograde or retrograde cerebral perfusion (ACP or RCP) plus DHCA: DHCA is used in cases where cerebral vessels are not able to be perfused using standard CPB aortic cannulation. These cases include aortic aneurysms or dissections involving the arch or great vessels of the head and neck. The CPB machine is used to cool the patient's core temperature, with a goal of an NP temp less than 24 °C, in an attempt to protect the brain when the pump is shut off to allow the surgeons a period of bloodless surgery on the affected vessels. Cerebral metabolic rate of oxygen consumption decreases 6–7% with each 1 °C cooled. This reduction in cerebral oxygen consumption does not solely explain DHCA's protective effect, but the mechanism is not fully understood at this time. The length of acceptable DHCA is controversial, but 30–40 min has been used as a goal to decrease the risk of cerebral injury [22]. Packing the patient's head in ice bags is also thought to provide regional cooling to enhance cerebral protection.

ACP involves perfusion of the some or all of the cerebral vessels, using an arterial cannulation site or sites. The right axillary artery is commonly used for this purpose. RCP uses retrograde perfusion via the venous system and SVC cannulation can be used for this purpose. Left ventricular venting can be accomplished with superior pulmonary vein cannulation. During circulatory arrest, cerebral perfusion utilizes cold blood (6–10 °C) flow to the cerebral vessels. Proposed benefits of ACP are the ability to run a greater flow at a higher pressure which increases perfusion to the cerebral circulation and enables a lesser degree of hypothermia when compared to RCP. RCP proponents have postulated that debris in the arterial circulation can be flushed out, reducing the possibility of embolic complications. There is currently no clear consensus on which vessels to cannulate, how many vessels to perfuse, or the use of RCP, ACP or DHCA alone [23].

Shunts/Cardiopulmonary Bypass: In cases where DHCA is not needed, standard CPB is used. Heparin coated shunts can be used in descending aortic cases to divert blood away from the affected segment. Partial CPB is sometimes used, with left atrial to femoral arterial (LA-FA) diversion of blood through an oxygenator.

Specific issues with Descending Aortic Surgery: Several techniques can be employed for the repair of a descending aortic lesion. The proximal aorta can be cross clamped, and the repair is completed as quickly as possible. Surgical speed is critical to reduce end organ damage especially if the renal arteries are included in the clamped segment. Cross clamping causes several changes in physiology, which should be anticipated and managed appropriately. Arterial hypertension, decreased venous capacity and shunting of blood away or towards the proximal circulation (dependent on location of cross clamp) have all been described [24]. Vasodilators are used to control the hypertension caused by cross clamping, but maintaining a higher SBP (180's) to encourage collateral flow to the compromised organs is a technique which has also been described.

Upon cross clamp removal there is reactive hyperemia, vasodilation, and decreased SVR and preload. The release of thromboxane and acidotic mediators, along with elevated filling pressures, further disrupt hemodynamic status. The surgeon should slowly remove the cross clamp, as profound hypotension may result from reperfusion. If the hypotension is life threatening, the clamp can be temporarily replaced until volume and hemodynamic status are improved.

As mentioned above, a heparinized shunt can be placed in the left atrium/proximal aorta, providing blood flow distal to the clamped segment. This method relies on the patient's natural cardiac output for perfusion, so patient selection is important if this technique is to be employed.

LA-FA bypass uses a CPB circuit to provide flow to the upper and lower parts of the body, excluding the clamped aortic segment. Constant communication with the perfusionist and surgeon is necessary to coordinate upper and lower body perfusion. The LA supplies both the left ventricle (LV) and acts as the "venous return" to the bypass circuit. This requires attention to LV volume status, usually accomplished with TEE. If LV flow is inadequate, as can be the case with high bypass flows, the upper body (coronaries and brain) will be inadequately perfused. The converse is also true, that if the bypass flow is too low, the lower body (viscera, extremities, spine) perfusion could be compromised. Placing a right radial and a femoral arterial line allows for simultaneous monitoring of upper and lower body perfusion pressures, which can help direct the bypass flow desired. An alternative to true LA-FA bypass is partial CPB, accomplished by placing a percutaneous femoral venous cannula to partially empty the right atrium and provide venous return to the bypass machine which is then delivered to the femoral artery.

Tracking arterial blood lactate levels and urine output are critical when utilizing this technique. Decreases in urine output and increases in lactate levels are often caused by ischemia and should be communicated to the surgical and perfusion team immediately. Reperfusion of the renal arteries should be accomplished as soon as surgically possible and adequate blood pressure and hemoglobin must be ensured to minimize long-term renal injury.

## Anesthesia Type

General anesthesia is required for open repairs of the aortic arch, ascending aorta and descending aorta. Patients presenting emergently are considered to have a full stomach, for which a rapid sequence induction (RSI) would be indicated. The need for rapid airway control must be balanced with adequate anesthetic depth during airway manipulation to prevent hypertension leading to extension of the dissection or aneurysm. A modified RSI is sometimes used, allowing for titration of medications with gentle bag mask ventilation with or without cricoid pressure. Endovascular repair of abdominal or thoracic aortic aneurysms (EVAR, TEVAR) have been performed with monitored anesthesia care and regional anesthesia and will be discussed later.

Induction medications are selected to accomplish the above goals. Propofol will assist in lowering BP, but may cause exaggerated hypotension in the setting of hypovolemia. Etomidate causes less hypotension, while ketamine can increase HR and BP. Opioids are used to blunt the response to laryngoscopy. Muscle relaxation is required for optimal surgical conditions as patient movement can be devastating with delicate surgical anastomoses. Anesthesia is usually maintained with volatile agents, opioids and benzodiazepines and non-depolarizing muscle relaxants. Cases with SSEP/MEP monitoring require agents which have minimal effects on the monitored signals. Using a total intravenous anesthesia (TIVA) technique can assist the neuromonitoring staff in obtaining the most accurate signals. Propofol and remifentanil infusions are often used, with partial or no volatile agents. In the case of MEP monitoring, muscle relaxation is limited to induction to preserve motor responses to the applied stimuli during critical portions of the surgery.

Airway management must be well thought out depending on the clinical situation. Single lumen endotracheal tubes (ETT) are used for repairs of the aortic arch and ascending aorta. A double lumen endotracheal tube (DLETT) or bronchial blocker (BB) is required for open repair of a descending aortic lesion, as a left thoracotomy is the typical surgical approach. The positioning of the DLETT/BB can be difficult, as the left mainstem bronchus may be narrowed by the aortic pathology. Aggressive manipulation of the DLETT/BB could result in aortic rupture. A right sided DLETT could be considered in extreme situations.

Intraoperative Phase: Other medications which can be administered during these cases include: corticosteroids, naloxone and barbiturates (where available):

Corticosteroid pre-treatment had been described to protect against spinal injury in dogs [25]. Another report did not show any protective effects of corticosteroid use in human traumatic spinal injury [26]. Large doses of steroids (1 g of Methylprednisolone) are commonly used for this procedure but this is often institution-dependent. Glycemic control with large doses of steroids will likely require inulin infusion treatment, especially in patients with diabetes. Glucose levels over 200 mg/dL have been associated with higher risks of mortality and morbidity [27]. However, "tight" control of glucose control (<140 mg/dL) was also associated with increased complications. The American College of Physicians recommends a glucose target between 140 and 200 mg/dL [28] and the Society of Thoracic Surgeons uses postoperative blood glucose <180 mg/dL as an outcome metric.

Barbiturates were shown to be protective in central nervous system (CNS) protection from ischemic insults [29]. The discontinuation of thiopental production has effectively removed this medication from practice. A dose of thiopental was given just prior to the onset of circulatory arrest. Propofol has been substituted, with effective EEG burst suppression, but without proven CNS benefit [30].

The levels of endogenous opiates measured in canine CSF, after spinal injury, were noted to be elevated. Opiates may decrease cerebral blood flow and increase cerebral vascular resistance. Acher et al. demonstrated that naloxone infusion with CSF drainage effectively lowered the incidence of spinal cord injury in patients undergoing TAAA [31]. Thoracic epidural anesthesia may be used in TAAA, which decreases the dependence on opioids for post-operative pain control and their possible deleterious effects on spinal cord function.

CPB Separation/Post CPB: The anesthesiologist will be called upon to provide hemodynamic support in the separation from CPB. This is accomplished by providing inotropic and vasopressor support, optimizing preload, and treating acid/base disorders. TEE can be invaluable in determining which therapies are required, as well as evaluating the possible repair/replacement of the aortic valve in ascending aortic cases. After rewarming above 32 °C, vascular resistance can decrease, requiring vasoconstrictors. The use of bicarbonate is controversial, with therapy generally reserved for pH less than 7.2 and need for vasopressors. However, the increase in pH has been shown to be transient and hemodynamics noted to be unchanged [32].

With fluid shifts and physiologic derangements following circulatory arrest it is common to transfuse a significant number of blood products during these procedures. While a full discussion of this topic is beyond the scope of this chapter, the use of point of care devices (TEG, ROTEM) as well as standard laboratory values should be factored in to hemostatic blood product management. Surgenor noted that a lower hematocrit (HCT) was associated with low output cardiac failure; transfusions did not decrease this risk. Interestingly, there may be an increased risk when transfusing for a HCT greater than 21 [33]. However, as many of these patients are critically ill and require significant oxygen delivery, a target HCT above 21 is often warranted.

Endovascular Approaches (TEVAR): This discussion of aortic anesthesia would be incomplete without mentioning the increasingly use of endovascular techniques for descending aortic aneurysm.

TEVAR involves obtaining femoral/iliac artery access to allow the operator to place a guidewire in true lumen of aorta, past the location of the aneurysm. If there is enough of a "landing zone" (normal aorta on either end of the aneurysm, which does not occlude branching vessels), a stent graft can be deployed to exclude the false lumen.

TEVAR has been successfully completed using general anesthesia, MAC and regional anesthesia. TEE is sometimes used in TEVAR for imaging guidance, making a general anesthetic most reasonable. Many of the spinal protective strategies described are used only in high-risk TEVAR procedures as procedures in the abdominal aorta alone carry an extremely low risk of paraplegia. There is data to suggest that infrarenal EVAR patients have an increased length of stay with general anesthesia [34].

Complications from TEVAR include the following: vascular injury, endograft collapse or migration, malperfusion of viscera, endoleaks, retrograde dissection and neurologic sequelae. Care must be taken to avoid side branch occlusion, especially of the renal arteries and artery of Adamkiewicz.

Conclusions: Diseases of the aorta can pose great challenges to the anesthesiologist. Knowledge of the physiology, location and surgical management of these diseases will guide effective anesthetic care of these patients.

## References

1. The Gale encyclopedia of medicine. 3rd ed. Stamford, CT; 2008.
2. Patel PD, Arora RR. Pathophysiology, diagnosis, and management of aortic dissection. Ther Adv Cardiovasc Dis. 2008;2(6):439–68.
3. Ramanath VS, Oh JK, Sundt TM, Eagle KA. Acute aortic syndromes and thoracic aortic aneurysm. Mayo Clin Proc. 2009;84(5):465–81.
4. Go AS, Mozaffarian D, Roger VL, Benjamin EJ, Berry JD, et al. Heart disease and stroke statistics—2013 update: a report from the American Heart Association. Circulation. 2013;127:e6–e245.
5. DeBakey ME, Henly WS, et al. Surgical management of dissecting aneurysms of the aorta. J Thorac Cardiovasc Surg. 1965;49:131.
6. Miller DC, Stinson EB, et al. Aortic dissections. J Thorac Cardiovasc Surg. 1979;78:367.
7. Ince H, Nienaber CA. Diagnosis and management of patients with aortic dissection. Heart. 2007;93: 266–70.
8. https://www.accessdata.fda.gov/drugsatfda_docs/label/2011/019734s017lbl.pdf.
9. https://chiesiusa.com/wp-content/uploads/Cleviprex-us-prescribing-information-nov-fda-approved.pdf.
10. Meretoja OA, Laaksonen VO. Hemodynamic effects of preload and sodium nitroprusside in patients subjected to coronary artery bypass grafting. Circulation. 1978;58:815–25.
11. Hanke AA, Dellweg C, Schöchl H, Weber CF, Jüttner B, Johanning K, Görlinger K, Rahe-Meyer N, Kienbaum P. Potential of whole blood coagulation reconstitution by desmopressin and fibrinogen under conditions of hypothermia and acidosis—an in vitro study using rotation thrombelastometry. Scand J Clin Lab Invest. 2011;71:292–8.
12. Hanke AA, Dellweg C, Kienbaum P, Weber CF, Görlinger K, Rahe-Meyer N. Effects of desmopressin on platelet function under conditions of hypothermia and acidosis: an in vitro study using multiple electrode aggregometry. Anaesthesia. 2010;65:688–91.
13. Chatterjee K. The Swan-Ganz catheters: past, present, and future. A viewpoint. Circulation. 2009;119(1):147–52.
14. Grigore AM, Grocott HP, Mathew JP, Phillips-Bute B, Stanley TO, Butler A, Landolfo KP, Reves JG, Blumenthal JA, Newman MF. The rewarming rate and increased peak temperature alter neurocognitive outcome after cardiac surgery. Anesth Analg. 2002;94:4–10.
15. Nathan HJ, Wells GA, Munson JL, Wozny D. Neuroprotective effect of mild hhypothermia in patients undergoing coronary artery surgery with cardiopulmonary bypass: a randomized trial. Circulation. 2001;104:I85–91.
16. Stecker MM, Cheung AT, Pochettino A, Kent GP, Patterson T, Weiss SJ, Bavaria JE. Deep hypothermic circulatory arrest: Effects of cooling on electroencephalogram and evoked potentials. Ann Thorac Surg. 2001;71(1):14–21.
17. Vretzakis G, et al. Cerebral oximetry in cardiac anesthesia. J Thorac Dis. 2014;6(Suppl 1):S60–9.
18. Greenberg RK, Lu Q, Roselli LG, et al. Contemporary analysis of descending thoracic and thoracoabdominal aneurysm repair. A comparison of endovascular and open techniques. Circulation. 2008;118:808–17.

19. Cheung AT, Weiss SJ, McGarvey ML, et al. Interventions for reversing delayed onset postoperative paraplegia after thoracic aortic reconstruction. Ann Thorac Surg. 2002;74:413–9.
20. Guerit JM, Witdoeckt C, Verhelst R, Matta AJ, Jacquet LM, Dion RA. Sensitivity, specificity and surgical impact of somatosensory evoked potentials in descending aortic surgery. Ann Thorac Surg. 1999;67(6):1943.
21. Black JH, Davison JK, Cambria RP. Regional hypothermia with epidural cooling for prevention of spinal cord ischemic complications after thoracoabdominal aortic surgery. Sem Thorac Cardiovasc Surg. 2003;15:345–52.
22. Yan TD, Bannon PG, Bavaria J, Coselli JS, Elefteriades JA, Griepp RB, et al. Consensus on hypothermia in aortic arch surgery. Ann Cardiothorac Surg. 2013;2:163–8.
23. Sugiura T, Imoto K, Uchida K, Minami T, Yasuda S. Comparative study of brain protection in ascending aorta replacement for acute type A aortic dissection: retrograde cerebral perfusion versus selective antegrade cerebral perfusion. Gen Thorac Cardiovasc Surg. 2012;60:645–8.
24. Gelman S. The pathophysiology of aortic cross clamping and unclamping. Anesthesiology. 1995;82:1026–60.
25. Laschinger JC, Cunningham JN, Cooper MM, Krieger K, Nathan IM, Spencer FC. Prevention of ischemic spinal cord injury following aortic cross-clamping: use of corticosteroids. Ann Thorac Surg. 1984;38:500–7.
26. Galandiuk S, Rapue G, Appel S, Polk HC. The two-edged sword of large does steroids for spinal cord trauma. Ann Surg. 1993;218:419–27.
27. Outtara A, Lecomte P, Le Manach Y, et al. Poor intraoperative blood glucose control is associated with a worsened hospital outcome after cardiac surgery in diabetic patients. Anesthesiology. 2005;103(4):687–94.
28. Qaseem A, Humphrey LL, Chou R, Snow V, Shekelle P. Use of intensive insulin therapy for the management of glycemic control in hospitalized patients: a clinical practice guideline from the American College of Physicians. Ann Intern Med. 2011;154(4):260–7.
29. Nylander WA Jr, Plunkett RJ, Hammon JW Jr, Oldfield EH, Meacham WF. Thiopental modification of ischemic spinal cord injury in the dog. Ann Thorac Surg. 1982;33:64–8.
30. Stone JG, Young WL, Marans ZS, et al. Consequences of electroencephalographic-suppressive doses of propofol in conjunction with deep hypothermic circulatory arrest. Anesthesiology. 1996;85:497–501.
31. Acher CW, Wynn MM, Hoch JR, Popic P, Archibald J, Archibald J, et al. Combined use of cerebral spinal fluid drainage and naloxone reduces the risk of paraplegia in thoracoabdominal aortic aneurysm repair. J Vasc Surg. 1994;19:236–48.
32. Cooper DM, et al. Bicarbonate does not improve hemodynamics in critically III patients who have lactic acidosis: a prospective, controlled clinical study. AIM. 1990;112:492.
33. Surgenor SD, et al. Intraoperative red blood cell transfusion during coronary artery bypass graft surgery increases the risk of postoperative low-output heart failure. Circulation. 2006;114(1S):I43–8.
34. Edwards MS, Andrews JS, Edwards AF, et al. Results of endovascular aortic aneurysm repair with general, regional, and local/monitored anesthesia care in the American College of Surgeons National Surgical Quality Improvement Program database. J Vasc Surg. 2011;54:1273–82.
35. American College of Radiology. ACR appropriate criteria for acute chest pain—suspected aortic dissection. https://acsearch.acr.org/docs/69402/Narrative/.

# Anesthesia for Lung Resection

Allison Bechtel

## Introduction

The most common indication for lung resection surgery is lung cancer which is the culprit for the majority of cancer-related deaths in the world. Surgical resection may yield a cure for patients with non-small cell carcinoma without metastases [1]. Other indications include resection of infected lung tissue, pleural cavity, and lung abscesses, pulmonary infarction, pulmonary hemorrhage, pleurodesis for persistent pulmonary edema/pleural effusion, and pulmonary bleb resection following pneumothorax. Advances in the field of thoracic surgery include minimally-invasive resections with video-assisted thoracoscopic techniques which are associated with decreased morbidity and mortality [2]. Anesthesia for these surgical procedures will be discussed in another chapter. Patients undergoing open lung resection require a thoracotomy incision for adequate surgical exposure of the lung tissue. Options for lung resection surgery include wedge resection, segmental resection, lobectomy, sleeve lobectomy, and pneumonectomy. The extent of the lung resection depends on the patient's lung disease as well as the patient's pulmonary and cardiovascular reserve. Perioperative mortality in patients who have a lobectomy and open thoracotomy is low at approximately 2% with a perioperative morbidity rate of 24.9% [3]. As expected, the mortality for patients requiring a pneumonectomy in indeed higher at 6.2% [4].

Patients presenting to the operating room for open thoracotomy and lung resection require general anesthesia and airway management that allows for one-lung ventilation. Lung protective ventilation strategies in the operating room before, during, and after one-lung ventilation are important in order to minimize damage to the operative and non-operative lung. There is an ongoing evolution in pain management strategies for open lung resection due to the use of liposomal bupivacaine for intercostal nerve blocks, intrathecal preservative-free morphine administration, and the trend towards decreased intravenous opioid use intraoperatively. Enhanced recovery following surgery is a growing area of interest in surgery and anesthesia and these strategies are beneficial for thoracic surgery patients as well.

## Surgical and Anatomical Considerations

Open lung resection requires a surgical incision, most commonly through a lateral or posterolateral thoracotomy with the patient positioned in the lateral decubitus position. The posterolateral thoracotomy is an S-shaped incision under the edge of the scapula to the 5th intercostal interspace anteriorly. In order to access both lungs, surgeons may perform a median sternotomy,

A. Bechtel, M.D.
Department of Anesthesiology, University of Virginia, Charlottesville, VA, USA
e-mail: As4sk@virginia.edu

bilateral anterior thoracotomies, or a clamshell incision (bilateral anterior thoracotomies combined with a transverse sternotomy). The clamshell incision is often used for bilateral lung transplantation to provide reliable exposure to both lungs fields. The median sternotomy approach is useful when there is tumor located in the anterior mediastinum. The posterolateral thoracotomy approach is traditionally performed by dividing the latissimus dorsi and serratus anterior muscles although muscle-sparing approaches with vertical or transverse incisions may be used to decrease postoperative pain at the expense of surgical exposure in appropriate patients [5]. One-lung ventilation is initiated prior to entry into the chest. The surgeons then mobilize the lung tissue and identify the bronchovascular structures. Both lungs have 10 bronchovascular structures as the main bronchus divides into the lobar bronchi which then further divides into the segmental bronchi. Blood supply initiates from the main pulmonary artery then divides to form segmental pulmonary arteries. Venous drainage occurs through intersegmental veins that travel in the subpleural plain to reach the pulmonary hilum and the main pulmonary vein. The right upper pulmonary vein drains the right upper and middle lobes while the right lower pulmonary vein drains the right lower lobe as well as a several branches from the right middle lobe. The left upper pulmonary vein is responsible for drainage of the left upper lobe and the left lower pulmonary vein drains the left lower lobe [6]. The surgical team must be familiar with the anatomy of the bronchovascular structures in order to maintain hemostasis during lung resection. A stapler is frequently used to transect the vascular branches and pulmonary parenchyma that is to be removed and close the lobar and segmental bronchi. Smaller bronchi and vascular branches may be closed with sutures. After resection, it is important to test for a significant air leak by administrating positive pressure to the operative lung. Adequate hemostasis is also vital given the extensive vascular supply through this area. The anesthesiologist must be prepared to resuscitate a patient in the case of inadvertent vascular injury. Injury to a main pulmonary artery will often lead to rapid blood loss requiring prompt recognition and coordination between the surgeon and anesthesiologist. The surgeon may need to hold pressure on or clamp the site of injury temporarily during resuscitation prior to definitive repair to obtain hemodynamic stability.

## Preoperative Evaluation

Prior to induction of anesthesia, it is important to perform a thorough preoperative evaluation of the patient's medical conditions and to anticipate possible difficulties throughout the perioperative period. The preoperative evaluation should certainly include a focus on airway management given the frequent need for one lung ventilation during lung resection surgery. As the most common indication for lung resection surgery is lung cancer, patients often have a history of tobacco abuse as well as chronic obstructive pulmonary disease. These patients will need to undergo risk stratification from a pulmonary and cardiovascular standpoint. The anesthesiologist is essential for the preoperative evaluation given their knowledge of the anesthetic options and surgical procedure as well as the patient's specific co-morbidities. The main goal is to identify patients at risk for perioperative morbidity and mortality in order to optimize a patient's functional status preoperatively and counsel patients about their risks before undergoing lung resection surgery [7].

As the majority of patients with lung cancer have a history of cigarette smoking, there is an increased prevalence of coronary artery disease in this patient population as evidenced by the 2–3% risk of a major cardiac complication following lung resection [8]. Major cardiac complications include myocardial ischemia, pulmonary edema, ventricular fibrillation, cardiac arrest, complete heart block, and cardiac-related death. In this setting, the revised cardiac risk index is useful to risk stratify patients with cardiac disease [9]. The revised cardiac risk index includes history of ischemic heart disease, congestive heart failure, cerebrovascular disease, insulin-dependent diabetes, preoperative creatinine >2 mg/dL, and patients undergoing high risk surgery including vascular, intraperitoneal, and intrathoracic surgeries [10]. Patients with more risk factors have a higher risk of a perioperative cardiac event such that greater than or equal to three risk factors is equal to a risk of 2.8–7.9 with 95% confidence intervals [10].

There is a cardiac risk stratification scheme for patients undergoing thoracic surgery specifically, the thoracic-RCRI created by Brunelli et al. [11] Using the thoracic-RCRI involves point allocation for certain surgeries and patient conditions including 1.5 points for pneumonectomy, history of ischemic heart disease, history of cerebrovascular disease, and 1 point for creatinine greater than 2 mg/dL. Patients with 0 points are low risk and patients with 1.5 points are intermediate risk. Patients with 2 or more points are high risk. Anesthesiologists can use the thoracic-RCRI to determine which patients require a cardiology consultation prior to surgery including patients with more than 2 points who are diagnosed with new cardiac disease or have a known cardiac history and are on medication. Patients with decreased functional status and more than 2 points will also require a preoperative cardiac consultation [11]. This risk stratification method may require further validation and should likely be used in conjunction with the patient's medical history and the revised cardiac risk index.

Patients presenting for lung resection often undergo pulmonary function testing prior to proceeding with the planned surgery. This testing helps to identify patients at risk for postoperative respiratory complications and poor functional outcome due to baseline pulmonary dysfunction. The anesthesiologist must evaluate the patient's functional status as well as the pulmonary function tests and recall that spirometry values depend on patient cooperation. Patients with excellent preoperative functional status and patients with FEV1 and DLCO >60% of predicted values are at low risk for postoperative respiratory complications. Intermediate risk patients have an FEV1 and DLCO values between 40–80% of predicted values. Patients who have an FEV1 < 30–40% are high risk and may not be candidates for surgery without further testing [8]. Another important parameter to evaluate is the postoperative predicted values for FEV1 and DLCO as well as exercise $VO_2$ max. The postoperative predicted values can be calculated by the preoperative value x (1-fraction of total perfusion of resected lung.) A decrease in the predicted postoperative FEV1 and DLCO increases the risk for postoperative respiratory complications such that for every 5% decrease in predicted postoperative values there is a 10% increase in risk for respiratory complications [8]. Exercise testing may be performed in order to determine the cardiorespiratory reserve in terms of stair climbing, the 6-min walk test, and the $VO_2$ max. Patients with a $VO_2$ max less than 10–15 mL/kg/min are high risk and may not be candidates for lung resection surgery [8]. Finally, preoperative arterial blood gas stratifies high risk patients as having a $PaO_2$ < 60 mmHg and/or a $PaCO_2$ > 50 mmHg. Table 10.1 describes the evaluation and determination of surgical candidates for lung resection.

**Table 10.1** Preoperative lung function assessment: evaluation strategy for patients with lung cancer [8]

| Surgical candidates: | FEV1 and DLCO >60% predicted | FEV1 and DLCO <60% predicted + Predicted postop FEV1 and DLCO > 40% | Predicted postop FEV1 and DLCO <40% + exercise $VO_2$ Max > 15 mL/kg/min | Exercise $VO_2$ max <15 mL/min + predicted postop exercise $VO_2$ max > 10 mL/kg/min |
|---|---|---|---|---|
| Surgical alternatives: | FEV1 and DLCO <60% predicted + Predicted postop FEV1 and DLCO <40% + Exercise $VO_2$ max <15 mL/kg/min + Predicted postop exercise $VO_2$ max < 10 mL/kg/min | | | |

## Maintenance of Anesthesia and Intraoperative Concerns

Patients who require a lateral or postero-lateral thoracotomy are positioned in the lateral decubitus position with the operative lung in the nondependent position after induction and intubation. Lateral positioning requires either a bean bag, hip positioners, or bolsters to support the patient on their side as well as an axillary roll to avoid axillary compression. The head and neck need to be maintained in the neutral position. The upper arm is often extended and placed on an arm board or sling which allows for access to the bilateral upper extremities throughout the surgery. It is often preferential to place the arterial line in the dependent arm in order to reduce compression of the catheter and tubing system with less signal disturbances due to arm positioning. The bed is flexed following lateral positioning to open the rib spaces and allow for maximal surgical exposure. After positioning, it is important to confirm correct placement of the double lumen tube (DLT) or bronchial blocker (BB) as tube migration may occur due to neck extension and positioning maneuvers. Positioning the DLT or BB while the patient is supine with the headrest removed may lead to less displacement following lateral positioning [12].

Hemodynamic management during open lung resection often requires placement of an intra-arterial line in order to closely monitor the patient's blood pressure and be vigilant for changes due to bleeding, surgical manipulation of the great vessels or other intraoperative complications. In addition, close monitoring of the electrocardiogram is important to evaluate for new arrhythmias, signs of myocardial ischemia, or tachycardia which is important to avoid especially in patients with coronary artery disease.

The goal for volume administration in lung resection surgery is to maintain euvolemia and hemodynamic stability while avoiding excessive volume administration. Excessive fluid administration has been implicated in the development of acute respiratory distress syndrome postoperatively while hypovolemia may lead to inadequate tissue perfusion [13]. It appears that maintenance of euvolemia combined with lung protective mechanical ventilation strategies will yield adequate tissue perfusion without increasing extravascular lung water [14]. There are challenges for assessing volume status in these thoracic patients since low tidal volumes, one lung ventilation, and open chest may yield the pulse pressure variation (PPV) and pulse variability index (PVI) less accurate for determining fluid responsiveness. Passive leg raise immediately after induction of anesthesia and placement of the arterial line is positive if there is an increase in mean arterial blood pressure (MAP) by 10–15% indicating that the patient is likely to be fluid responsive. This is not overly feasible during lung resection surgery. Intraoperatively, the use of pulse pressure variation with fluid responsiveness determined by PPV >12% during two-lung ventilation prior to thoracotomy allows for continuous assessment of volume status [15, 16]. PPV may not be accurate during OLV during open lung resection due to the lack of intrathoracic pressure changes from the non-ventilated lung, the decreased pressures in the ventilated lung from low tidal volume ventilation, and the open chest cavity during positive pressure ventilation [17]. PPV may still be a variable to consider during OLV keeping in mind that PPV >6% may indicate fluid responsiveness during OLV and that there will be decreased sensitivity and increased specificity of PPV to indicate fluid responsiveness [15–17]. For patients with hemoglobin greater than 7 g/dL with no surgical bleeding, administration of crystalloid or a colloid such as 5% albumin may be indicated when the PPV is >6%. Patients who are hypotensive and their PPV is less than the above stated values for fluid responsiveness likely require intravenous vasopressor support. It is also important to assess surgical blood loss and consider administration of packed red blood cells in hypotensive patients with ongoing bleeding and hemoglobin less than 7 g/dL.

The choice for anesthetic agents for induction and maintenance depends on the patient's co-morbidities, available agents, and the anesthesiologist's preference. The use of volatile anesthetic agents for maintenance of anesthesia with Sevoflurane, Isoflurane or Desflurane may be beneficial during lung resection due to the decreased release of inflammatory mediators in the ventilated lung compared to intravenous anesthesia with propofol infusion [18]. However, there is no evidence to support to the use of inhalational over intravenous anesthetic techniques with regards to outcome differences [19]. In addition, it is important to provide a balanced anesthetic. For pain management, thoracic epidural anesthesia with local anesthetic only, opioid only, or a combination of local anesthetic and opioid infusion may be administered intraoperatively and continued for postoperative pain management. Other adjuncts for a balanced anesthetic may include remifentanil, ketamine, dexmedetomidine, and lidocaine infusions. A discussion of enhanced recovery following thoracic surgery will be included in a separate section.

In addition to routine ASA monitors, patients often require intra-arterial access for hemodynamic monitoring as well as arterial blood gas assessment. Large-bore peripheral intravenous (IV) access is necessary for volume administration in the case of blood loss and vasopressor administration to treat hypotension. Central venous access is only required in patients who have poor peripheral access or significant co-morbidities including severe pulmonary hypertension or significant baseline cardiac dysfunction.

## Airway Management

Patients undergoing lung resection require one-lung ventilation (OLV) including isolation of the operative lung with ventilation of the non-operative lung. This can be accomplished with a left or right double-lumen endotracheal tube (DLT) as well as a single lumen endotracheal tube (SLT) with a bronchial blocker (BB) or a single lumen tube advanced into the right or left main stem bronchus. BB available for use include the Arndt blocker, Cohen flexitip blocker, Fuji Uniblocker, and Rusch EZ-Blocker [20]. DLTs and BB are both effective for providing lung isolation and one lung ventilation. Bronchial blockers may be advantageous in patients with a difficult airway who require an awake fiberoptic intubation with a single lumen tube. Placement of a bronchial blocker may take longer to position initially and be more likely to require re-positioning during the procedure [21]. Endobronchial cuff pressure on the bronchial wall of less than 30 mmHg is necessary with bronchial blockers and DLTs to prevent mucosal damage. The typical cuff volumes (2–6mLs for a DLT and 4–6mLs for a bronchial blocker) required to form an adequate seal up to 25 mmHg for positive pressure ventilation exert <30 mmHg pressure on the bronchial wall [22]. Risks associated with airway management for lung resection include airway edema, trauma, hoarseness, sore throat, and damage to the lips, teeth, gums, and oropharyngeal structures.

The choice of ideal DLT size has been debated and is important in order to facilitate safe placement of a correctly-sized DLT on the first attempt. The use of a DLT that is too small may lead to higher cuff pressures to prevent a leak and maintain appropriate lung isolation as well as ventilation and oxygenation. In addition, smaller DLTs may require intraoperative repositioning and may be difficult to suction secretions. On the other hand, the use of a DLT that is too large may lead to significant airway trauma, including tracheal rupture. Tracheal rupture following DLT placement is rare with an incidence of less than 1% [23]. This should be suspected in any patient that is difficult to oxygenate and ventilate following intubation in the presence of mediastinal and subcutaneous emphysema or a tension pneumothorax. These patients require tracheal repair and are at risk for postoperative mediastinitis and sepsis. The risk for airway trauma following placement or removal of a DLT is increased when the anesthesiologist is inexperienced, requires multiple blind attempts to place, and uses force to advance the DLT [23]. Extreme care should be taken when deciding on the size of the DLT depending on the patient's physical characteristics as well as the anesthesiologists experience since no clear guidelines exist. The anesthesiologist must use the appropriate size DLT and avoid over-inflation of the bronchial cuff. In addition, the stylet should be removed after the DLT is correctly positioned at the level of the glottis and the tube should be rotated correctly so that the memory bend follows the anatomy of the left and right main stem respectively. The use of an exchange catheter when changing between a DLT and a SLT has also been implicated in airway trauma and should be done cautiously. Patients risk factors for airway trauma include women, age >50 years old, short stature, obesity, COPD, coughing or movement during placement, tracheomalacia, chronic steroid use, and history of chest radiotherapy. Patients with these risk factors require a thorough preoperative airway evaluation and careful placement of an appropriately sized DLT by an experienced anesthesiologist [24].

The decision to use a right or a left DLT is also important and depends on the anesthesiologist's experience with placement of right-sided DLTs and familiarity with the fiberoptic bronchoscope as well as the patient's anatomy. A right-sided DLT needs to be placed just past the carina with a fiberoptic scope in order to place the additional side opening (Murphy eye) at the right upper lobe takeoff appropriately. The preference of a left DLT occurs due to the longer left main stem bronchus and ease of correct placement with the resultant appropriate lung isolation. A right DLT may need to be used for patients with left endobronchial tumors or history of prior left main stem surgery and reconstruction, but they are contraindicated for patients with a right upper lobe take-off above the level of the carina.

There are several techniques for deciding on size of left DLT. Using a patient's height is not an accurate technique for estimating left DLT size. A more accurate assessment of the patient's anatomy includes measuring the length and diameter of the left main bronchus on a postero-anterior chest radiography and taking into consideration that the chest radiography measurements are magnified by approximately 9% such that the actual length and diameter are less than measured on the radiograph. Most 37Fr and 39Fr left DLT can be used in patients with a left main bronchus diameter of 13 mm while 35Fr left DLTs should be used for patient with a diameter of 12 mm and a 41Fr left DLT can be used for patients with a diameter of 14 mm. Computed-tomography scans of the left main bronchus or tracheal width may also be useful to determine the size of left DLT. Another technique involves measuring the tracheal width at the level of the clavicles on postero-anterior chest radiography. For tracheal diameter greater than or equal to 18 mm, a 41Fr DLT may be used, for tracheal diameter greater than or equal to 16 mm, a 39Fr DLT may be used, for tracheal diameter greater than or equal to 15 mm, a 37 Fr DLT may be used and finally when the trachea measures less than 15 mm a 35Fr DLT may be used according to the Bodsky criteria. When these criteria were used, larger DLTs were placed with only minor difficulty advancing the DLT and only one postoperative complications possibly due to the DLT placement [25].

## One-Lung Ventilation

One-lung ventilation (OLV) strategies have evolved over the years. Historically, patients were administrated 10 mL/kg tidal volumes with high airway pressures during OLV in order to avoid hypercarbia. The current focus is on lung protective strategies during OLV as well as during two-lung ventilation (TLV) in order to minimize lung injury intraoperatively. This is especially important since patients requiring lung resection are at risk for respiratory complications due to chronic lung disease, lung resection surgery itself (surgical manipulation of lung tissue and loss of lung tissue from the resection) as well as the effects of mechanical ventilation with positive-pressure ventilation. Lung protective strategies to prevent ARDS with two lung ventilation include calculation of predicted body weight and delivery of 4–6 mL/kg tidal volumes with a respiratory rate <35 breaths/min that achieves an optimal minute ventilation and positive end-expiratory pressure (PEEP) applied whenever $FiO_2$ increased. Goals include plateau pressures less than 30 $cmH_2O$, $SpO_2$ 88–95%, $PaO_2$ 55–80 mmHg, and pH 7.3–7.45 [26]. Predicted body weight is determined by the following equation for men equal to

50 kg + 2.3 kg × [height (in.) − 60] and for women equal to 45.5 kg + 2.3 kg × [height (in.) − 60] [27].

Several studies have evaluated lung protective strategies in patients undergoing lung resection. In these studies, the lung protective strategies during OLV included lower tidal volumes of 4–6 mL/kg ideal body weight with the application of PEEP 3–10 mmHg, recruitment maneuvers, and the used of pressure-controlled ventilation compared to volume-controlled ventilation [28, 29]. Optimal PEEP is of upmost importance as excessive PEEP can increase pulmonary vascular resistance and shunt blood flow to the operative lung while inadequate PEEP will allow for de-recruitment of alveoli and impaired oxygenation. A PEEP decrement trial may be performed in order to optimize lung compliance and oxygenation. This may be performed following a recruitment maneuver with 40 cmH$_2$O opening pressure and 20 cmH$_2$O of PEEP for 20 breaths during which PEEP is decreased by 2 cmH$_2$O every 2 min until the maximal dynamic compliance is obtained. Each decrease in PEEP level required an alveolar recruitment maneuver prior to the change. The PEEP level at the maximal dynamic compliance reflects the optimal PEEP for the patient [30].

## Hypoxemia on One Lung Ventilation

Hypoxemia during one-lung ventilation (OLV) is common due to transpulmonary shunting. This is an important intraoperative concern in patients undergoing open lung resection. Patients who are at increased risk for hypoxemia during OLV include patients undergoing right lung resection, patients with lower arterial oxygen concentrations during two lung ventilation, patient with normal perfusion to both lungs, and patients positioned supine compared to lateral decubitus position due to effects of gravity on perfusion [31].

Hypoxic pulmonary vasoconstriction (HPV) describes the diversion of pulmonary blood flow away from hypoxic alveoli towards alveoli with higher oxygen tensions. HPV often plays a critical role in the maintenance of adequate oxygenation during OLV. Inhibition of HPV may occur due to systemic vasodilators, volatile anesthetics, high and low pulmonary artery pressures, hypocapnia, high and low mixed venous oxygen saturations, and lung infection. Optimization of oxygenation during OLV requires maintaining adequate blood flow to the ventilated lung by limiting airway pressures and avoiding high PEEP levels, hyperventilation, and high peak inspiratory pressures. HPV may occur in the ventilated lung if alveoli are not receiving adequate oxygenation. Patients with COPD are at risk for developing intrinsic PEEP if there is not enough expiration time. This will also decrease perfusion to the ventilated lung and place the patient at risk for hypoxemia.

For patients who desaturate during OLV, there are several steps that can be taken to improve oxygenation. First, while troubleshooting the underlying cause and associated treatment of hypoxemia, it is important to increase FiO$_2$. Some patients may require ventilation with an FiO$_2$ of 1.0 to prevent HPV from developing in the ventilated lung. The next step is to confirm that the pulse oximetry reading is correct and not a sign of poor plethysmography or poor perfusion due to hypotension that needs to be addressed. . In the case of an acute and severe drop in oxygen saturation, it is important to alert the surgeons and return to two-lung ventilation until the patient's oxygenation has improved. For a gradual decline in oxygen saturation, the next step is to confirm correct positioning of the double lumen tube or bronchial blocker. If the tube or blocker are too deep, then the resultant lobar ventilation may be the source of the hypoxemia. Repositioning will decrease transpulmonary shunt and improved oxygenation. If the tube or blocker are inappropriately withdrawn, the appropriate lung isolation may not be possible due to a significant leak around the bronchial balloon in the trachea. In addition, herniation of the bronchial balloon over the carina may prevent adequate oxygenation and ventilation of the non-operative lung due to obstruction of the contralateral main stem bronchus. After correct tube position is confirmed, the patient may require oxygen insufflation and

**Table 10.2** Treatment algorithm for hypoxemia during one-lung ventilation

| | Treatment options | Rationale |
|---|---|---|
| 1 | Increase FiO$_2$ to 100% | Prevent HPV in the ventilated lung |
| 2 | Confirm pulse oximetry measurement. | Poor pulse oximetry plethysmography may occur with significant hypotension |
| 3 | Check position of DLT or blocker | Tube malposition may lead to inadvertent lobar ventilation or inadequate oxygenation and ventilation |
| 4 | Administer oxygen insufflation and CPAP 2–10 mmHg to non-ventilated lung | Provide oxygen to the alveoli in the non-ventilated lung and decrease transpulmonary shunt |
| 5 | Recruitment maneuver to the ventilated lung | Recruit alveoli and decrease atelectasis in the dependent lung |
| 6 | Administer PEEP 5–10 mmHg to ventilated lung | Maintain open alveoli following recruitment maneuver and prevent atelectasis, especially with smaller tidal volume ventilation |
| 7 | Return to 2-lung ventilation | Decrease transpulmonary shunt |
| 8 | Clamp pulmonary artery to operative lung | Decrease transpulmonary shunt |

continuous positive airway pressure (CPAP) of 5–10 mmHg to the non-ventilated lung. This maneuver is effective for decreasing transpulmonary shunting and increasing oxygenation [32]. Low tidal volume with low pressure ventilation of the operative lung is also effecting for treating hypoxemia though it often interferes with surgical exposure. However, to provide differential ventilation, two ventilators are necessary and this is often difficult to obtain acutely in the OR when needed [33]. The next step for the treatment of hypoxemia during OLV is to increase PEEP to the ventilated lung. High PEEP levels need to be avoided to prevent shunting of blood away from the ventilated lung. Recruitment maneuvers and optimal PEEP is effective in decreasing atelectasis in the ventilated lung, preventing the development of further atelectasis and improving oxygenation. Some patients may experience a rapid decline in arterial oxygenation or a persistent hypoxemia despite the above therapies and will require a return to two-lung ventilation to improve oxygenation. Close communication with the surgeon is imperative. The final step in the treatment of hypoxemia during OLV is to eliminate transpulmonary by clamping or ligating the pulmonary artery that supplies the non-ventilated lung. This is a routine step for patients undergoing pneumonectomy, but surgeons do not do this during routine lung resections including lobectomies or wedge resections. Besides direct vascular injury, a major concern of unilateral pulmonary artery ligation is the precipitation of acute right ventricular failure. Recently, the use of adjunct dexmedetomidine has been studied in patients with severe COPD undergoing lung resection surgery. Dexmedetomidine use was associated with improved oxygenation and lung function compared to placebo that was thought to be due to decreased intrapulmonary shunt and less bronchoconstriction [34].

Table 10.2 summarizes various available options in the management of hypoxemia during one-lung ventilation.

## Pain Management

Patients who undergo thoracotomy for lung resection may experience severe pain postoperatively due to damage to the pleura, overlying muscles, and ribcage. In addition, there may be damage to the intercostal nerves that are located along the underside of the ribs. Therefore, adequate pain management is imperative to prevent a variety of postoperative complications including collapsed lung, pneumonia, blood clots due to decrease mobility and respiratory dysfunction. Pain management strategies for patient undergoing thoracotomy and lung resection include thoracic epidural with local anesthesia and/or opioid medications, paravertebral block, intercostal nerve block, single shot intrathecal opioids, systemic opioids, and intra-pleural local anesthetic administration. Thoracic epidural with local anesthetics, lipophilic opioid only, or combination of local anesthesia and opioid are effective strategies for intraoperative and postoperative pain management. Paravertebral blocks provide adequate pain control for patient and may be associated with less side effects including hypotension, nausea and vomiting, and urinary retention [35].

Chronic pain following thoracotomy is an important complication and includes patients who have persistent pain at the thoracotomy site for greater than 2 months postoperatively. This is a pain syndrome that is characterized by nociceptive and neuropathic pain that is more likely to occur in younger women with psychological vulnerability and intercostal nerve damage [36]. Multi-modal pain management including epidural anesthesia may help prevent the development of this chronic pain syndrome [37]. Preoperative oral Gabapentin administration is not effective for preventing chronic postthoracotomy pain syndrome, but when Gabapentin is continued postoperatively, it appears to be a safe and effective adjunct for acute and chronic pain management following thoracotomy [38]. Patients may suffer from postoperative anxiety and depression. Risk factors for postoperative depression include thoracotomy incision, shortness of breath, severe pain, and diabetes [39].

## ERAS

A recent development in anesthesia and surgery involves the Enhanced Recovery after Surgery (ERAS) protocols. The goals for an open lung resection ERAS protocol are to minimize intravenous opioid use and use a restricted, goal-directed fluid therapy technique to reduce perioperative morbidity. Prior to coming to the hospital, patients are instructed to consume clear fluid (Gatorade) up to 2 h prior to their surgical procedure. In the preoperative holding area, patients receive Celecoxib, Gabapentin, and Acetaminophen via oral administration. In the operating room, patients are administered 250 μg of intrathecal preservative-free morphine prior to induction followed by heparin SQ following the spinal. Induction includes propofol, ketamine 0.5 mg/kg, magnesium 30 mg/kg given over 10 min, and dexamethasone 4 mg. Intraoperative analgesia includes ketamine infusion at 0.3–0.6 mg/kg/h and liposomal bupivacaine (Exparel) intercostal nerve blocks performed by the surgeon. Other intraoperative management strategies on the ERAS protocol include use of lung protective ventilation with tidal volumes of 6–8 mL/kg ideal body weight during two-lung ventilation and 3–5 mL/kg ideal body weight during one-lung ventilation with a recruitment breath prior to initiation of OLV. PEEP 5 mmHg is utilized during OLV to the ventilated lung unless the patient has severe COPD, evidence of auto-PEEP, or there is a determination of another level for ideal PEEP based on a PEEP decrement trial or empirically to optimize oxygenation and prevent hypoxemia. In addition, the use of CPAP 0–5 mmHg to the operative lung may be considered after communication with the surgeon. The postoperative ERAS pathway includes monitoring in a thoracic step-down unit or intensive care unit as well as rescue opioids administered as needed, ketamine 0.15 mg/kg/h IV infusion and 2 doses of IV Tylenol. Oral pain medications include acetaminophen 975 mg BID, Celecoxib 100 mg PO BID, and Gabapentin 300 mg PO TID. This particular ERAS protocol no longer uses epidural analgesia for patients who are candidates for the full protocol and these patients do not receive an opioid PCA postoperatively. The use of liposomal Bupivacaine for multilevel intercostal nerve blocks performed by the surgeon may provide superior pain control compared to thoracic epidural anesthesia for up to 72 h following administration but requires further, prospective study [40].

## Postoperative Considerations

Following lung resection surgery and thoracotomy, patients are often transferred to the intensive care unit (ICU) in order to closely monitor their respiratory status and hemodynamics. There are several complications following lung resection surgery including respiratory failure, atrial fibrillation, and acute kidney injury. Respiratory failure contributes to significant morbidity and mortality. Early extubation in the operating room is preferred following open lung resection when patients meet extubation criteria. Respiratory complications following open lung resection may be due to airway or vocal cord injury, bleeding, air leak, pneumothorax, bronchopulmonary fistula, deep venous thrombosis or pulmonary embolism, infection, phrenic nerve injury, pulmonary edema, atelectasis, pleural effusions, pneumonitis, bronchospasm, and mediastinal emphysema [41]. Patients with more extensive open lung resections and comorbidities require postoperative ICU care including continuous monitoring of arterial blood pressure, heart rate and rhythm, oxygen saturation and chest tube drainage. Patients without significant comorbidities may be transferred out of the ICU on postoperative day 1. Younger patients (age <75 years old) without cardiac comorbidities and postoperative FEV1 greater than 60% may be candidates for postoperative care in the recovery room followed by the general surgical floor with continuous monitoring of electrocardiography and oxygen saturation. Audible alarms for tachycardia, bradycardia, and desaturation as well as vital signs and chest tube drainage checks every hour on postoperative day 0–1 are important for close respiratory monitoring [42].

Atrial fibrillation following lung resection surgery is a postoperative complication more frequently encountered in older, male, obese patients with chronic hypertension, congestive heart failure, chronic renal failure, COPD, or high alcohol consumption. In addition, patients undergoing more extensive lung resection surgery, open resection compared to video-assisted thoracoscopic surgery, and those who require packed red blood cell transfusion or inotropes are at an increased risk for postoperative atrial fibrillation [43]. The incidence of postoperative atrial fibrillation occurs in approximately 12% of patients likely due to sympathetic stimulation and catecholamine release as a result of pain, intravascular volume changes, or direct cardiac manipulation. Treatment involves replacing electrolytes including magnesium and potassium, pharmacological or electrical cardioversion, rate control, and anticoagulation if there are no contraindications [44].

Another important postoperative complication following open lung resection surgery is acute kidney injury (AKI). Patient who develop AKI are at increased risk for prolonged stay in the intensive care unit and hospital as well as increased morbidity and mortality. Preoperative risk factors for the development of AKI have been evaluated in several studies and likely include chronic hypertension, peripheral vascular disease, low glomerular filtration rate, and angiotensin receptor blocking medications (ARB) use. Other risk factors may include duration of anesthesia, hydroxyethyl starch infusion, ASA classification, and decreased forced expiratory volume in 1 s (FEV1). Patients undergoing thoracoscopic lung resection procedures may have a lower risk for postoperative acute kidney injury which may be due to surgical selection of lower risk patients for thoracoscopic procedures. It may also be due to decreased release of inflammatory mediators including C-reactive protein, interleukin-6, interleukin-8, and reactive oxygen species production during thoracoscopic lung resection compared to open resection. Increased levels of inflammatory mediators may contribute to the development of postoperative AKI [45]. At many institutions, patients are instructed to discontinue their ACE inhibitors and ARB medications for 24 h prior to surgery for patients undergoing lung resection surgery although the optimal time frame for discontinuing these medications prior to this surgery has likely not been determined.

### Conclusion

Anesthesia for lung resection is a challenging procedure that requires careful preparation as well as communication with the surgical team. As lung resection surgical procedures trend towards minimally invasive incisions, it is important to be knowledgeable about the important considerations for safe conduct of anesthesia for patients who require a thoracotomy for lung resection surgery.

# References

1. Rauma V, Salo J, Sintonen H, Räsänen J, Ilonen I. Patient features predicting long-term survival and health-related quality of life after radical surgery for non-small cell lung cancer. Thorac Cancer. 2016;7:333–9.
2. Desai H, Natt B, Kim S, Bime C. Decreased in-hospital mortality after lobectomy using video-assisted thoracoscopic surgery compared to open thoracotomy. Ann Am Thorac Soc. 2016;14(2):262–6. https://doi.org/10.1513/annalsats.201606-429oc.
3. Cao C, Manganas C, Ang S, Peeceeyen S, Yan T. Video-assisted thoracic surgery versus open thoracotomy for non-small cell lung cancer: a meta-analysis of propensity score-matched patients. Interact Cardiovasc Thorac Surg. 2012;16:244–9.
4. Boffa D, Allen M, Grab J, Gaissert H, Harpole D, Wright C. Data from the society of thoracic surgeons general thoracic surgery database: the surgical management of primary lung tumors. J Thorac Cardiovasc Surg. 2008;135:247–54.
5. Athanassiadi K, et al. Muscle-sparing versus posterolateral thoracotomy: a prospective study. Eur J Cardiothorac Surg. 2007;31(3):496–500. Web. 15 Mar 2017.
6. Van Der Spuy JC. The surgical anatomy of the pulmonary vessels. Thorax. 1953;8(3):189–94. Web.
7. Della Rocca G, Vetrugno L, Coccia C, Pierconti F, Badagliacca R, Vizza C, Papale M, Melis E, Facciolo F. Preoperative evaluation of patients undergoing lung resection surgery: defining the role of the anesthesiologist on a multidisciplinary team. J Cardiothorac Vasc Anesth. 2016;30:530–538de.
8. Brunelli A, et al. Physiologic evaluation of the patient with lung cancer being considered for resectional surgery. Chest. 2013;143(5):e166S–90S. Web. 15 Mar 2017.
9. Ford MK, Beattie WS, Wijeysundera DN. Systematic review: prediction of perioperative cardiac complications and mortality by the revised cardiac risk index. Ann Intern Med. 2010;152:26–35.
10. Roshanov PS, Walsh M, Devereaux PJ, et al. External validation of the revised cardiac risk index and update of its renal variable to predict 30-day risk of major cardiac complications after non-cardiac surgery: rationale and plan for analyses of the VISION study. BMJ Open. 2017;7(1):e013510. https://doi.org/10.1136/bmjopen-2016-013510.
11. Brunelli A, Cassivi SD, Fibla J, et al. External validation of the recalibrated thoracic revised cardiac risk index for predicting the risk of major cardiac complications after lung resection. Ann Thorac Surg. 2011;92:445–8.
12. Seo J-H, et al. Double-lumen tube placement with the patient in the supine position without a headrest minimizes displacement during lateral positioning. Can J Anesth. 2012;59(5):437–41. Web. 15 Mar 2017.
13. Alam N, Park BJ, Wilton A, et al. Incidence and risk factors for lung injury after lung cancer resection. Ann Thorac Surg. 2007;84(4):1085–91.
14. Assaad S, et al. Extravascular lung water and tissue perfusion biomarkers after lung resection surgery under a normovolemic fluid protocol. J Cardiothorac Vasc Anesth. 2015;29(4):977–83. Web. 15 Mar 2017.
15. Lee J, Jeon Y, Bahk J, Gil N, Hong D, Kim J, Kim H. Pulse pressure variation as a predictor of fluid responsiveness during one-lung ventilation for lung surgery using thoracotomy: randomised controlled study. Eur J Anaesthesiol. 2011;28:39–44.
16. Fu Q, et al. Evaluation of stroke volume variation and pulse pressure variation as predictors of fluid responsiveness in patients undergoing protective one-lung ventilation. Drug Discov Ther. 2015;9(4):296–302. Web. 15 Mar 2017.
17. Jeong D, Ahn H, Park H, Yang M, Kim J, Park J. Stroke volume variation and pulse pressure variation are not useful for predicting fluid responsiveness in thoracic surgery. Anesth Analg. 2017;125(4):1158–65.
18. Schilling T, et al. Effects of volatile and intravenous anesthesia on the alveolar and systemic inflammatory response in thoracic surgical patients. Anesthesiology. 2011;115(1):65–74. Web. 15 Mar 2017.
19. Módolo NSP, et al. Intravenous versus inhalation anaesthesia for one-lung ventilation. Cochrane Database Syst Rev. 2013: CD006313. Web. 15 Mar 2017.
20. Campos J. Lung isolation techniques for patients with difficult airway. Curr Opin Anaesthesiol. 2010;23:12–7.
21. Campos J. An update on bronchial blockers during lung separation techniques in adults. Anesth Analg. 2003;94(5):1266–74.
22. Roscoe A, et al. Pressures exerted by endobronchial devices. Anesth Analg. 2007;104(3):655–8. Web. 15 Mar 2017.
23. Liu H, Jahr JS, Sullivan E, Waters PF. Tracheobronchial rupture after double-lumen endotracheal intubation. J Cardiothorac Vasc Anesth. 2004;18.228–33.
24. Pedoto A. How to choose the double-lumen tube size and side. Anesthesiol Clin. 2012;30(4):671–81. Web.
25. Brodsky JB, Macario A, Mark JB. Tracheal diameter predicts double-lumen tube size: a method for selecting left double-lumen tubes. Anesth Analg. 1996;82:861–4.
26. Acute Respiratory Distress Syndrome Network, Brower RG, Matthay MA, Morris A, Schoenfeld D, Thompson BT, Wheeler A. Ventilation with lower tidal volumes as compared with traditional tidal volumes for acute lung injury and the acute respiratory distress syndrome. N Engl J Med. 2000;342(18):1301–8. Web. 15 Mar 2017.
27. Blank RS, et al. Management of one-lung ventilation. Anesthesiology. 2016;124(6):1286–95. Web. 15 Mar 2017.

28. Licker M, de Perrot M, Spiliopoulos A, et al. Risk factors for acute lung injury after thoracic surgery for lung cancer. Anesth Analg. 2003;97:1558–65.
29. Yang M, Ahn HJ, Kim K, et al. Does a protective ventilation strategy reduce the risk of pulmonary complications after lung cancer surgery?: a randomized controlled trial. Chest. 2011;139:530–7.
30. Ferrando C, Mugarra A, Gutierrez A, et al. Setting individualized positive end-expiratory pressure level with a positive end-expiratory pressure decrement trial after a recruitment maneuver improves oxygenation and lung mechanics during one-lung ventilation. Anesth Analg. 2014;118:657–65.
31. Karzai W, Schwarzkopf K. Hypoxemia during one-lung ventilation: prediction, prevention, and treatment. Anesthesiology. 2009;110(6):1402–11.
32. Hogue CW Jr. Effectiveness of low levels of nonventilated lung continuous positive airway pressure in improving arterial oxygenation during one-lung ventilation. Anesth Analg. 1994;79:364–7.
33. Chigurupati K, Raman SP, Pappu UK, et al. Effectiveness of ventilation of nondependent lung for a brief period in improving arterial oxygenation during one-lung ventilation: a prospective study. Ann Card Anaesth. 2017;20(1):72–5.
34. Lee S, Kim N, Lee C, Ban M, Oh Y. Effects of dexmedetomidine on oxygenation and lung mechanics in patients with moderate chronic obstructive pulmonary disease undergoing lung cancer surgery. Eur J Anaesthesiol. 2016;33:275–82.
35. Joshi G, Bonnet F, Shah R, et al. A systematic review of randomized trials evaluating regional techniques for postthoracotomy analgesia. Anesth Analg. 2008;107:1026–40.
36. Yeung J, Melody T, Kerr A, Naidu B, Middleton L, Tryposkiadis K, Daniels J, Gao F. Randomised controlled pilot study to investigate the effectiveness of thoracic epidural and paravertebral blockade in reducing chronic post-thoracotomy pain: TOPIC feasibility study protocol. BMJ Open. 2016;6:e012735.
37. Andreae MH, Andreae DA. Local anaesthetics and regional anaesthesia for preventing chronic pain after surgery. Cochrane Database Syst Rev. 2012;10:CD007105. https://doi.org/10.1002/14651858.CD007105.pub2.
38. Zakkar M, Frazer S, Hunt I. Is there a role for Gabapentin in preventing or treating pain following thoracic surgery? Interact Cardiovasc Thorac Surg. 2013;17(4):716–9. https://doi.org/10.1093/icvts/ivt301.
39. Park S, Kang C, Hwang Y, Seong Y, Lee H, Park I, Kim Y. Risk factors for postoperative anxiety and depression after surgical treatment for lung cancer. Eur J Cardiothorac Surg. 2015;49:e16–21.
40. Khalil K, Boutrous M, Irani A, Miller C, Pawelek T, Estrera A, Safi H. Operative intercostal nerve blocks with long-acting bupivacaine liposome for pain control after thoracotomy. Ann Thorac Surg. 2015;100:2013–8.
41. Sengupta S. Post-operative pulmonary complications after thoracotomy. Indian J Anaesth. 2015;59(9):618–26.
42. Park S, Park I, Hwang Y, Byun C, Bae M, Lee C. Immediate postoperative care in the general thoracic ward is safe for low-risk patients after lobectomy for lung cancer. Korean J Thorac Cardiovasc Surg. 2011;44:229–35.
43. Lee S, Ahn H, Yeon S, Yang M, Kim J, Jung D, Park J. Potentially modifiable risk factors for atrial fibrillation following lung resection surgery: a retrospective cohort study. Anaesthesia. 2016;71:1424–30.
44. Garner M, Routledge T, King J, Pilling J, Veres L, Harrison-Phipps K, Bille A, Harling L. New-onset atrial fibrillation after anatomic lung resection: predictive factors, treatment and follow-up in a UK thoracic centre. Interact Cardiovasc Thorac Surg. 2016;24(2):260–4.
45. Ishikawa S, Griesdale DEG, Lohser J. Acute kidney injury after lung resection surgery. Anesth Analg. 2012;114(6):1256–62. Web. 15 Mar 2017.

# Anesthesia for Video-Assisted Thoracoscopic Surgery

# 11

Jared Roussel and Susan Smith

## Introduction and History

Video-assisted thoracoscopic surgery (VATS) is a specific type of minimally invasive thoracic surgical (MITS) in the thoracic cavity. Historically, thoracic surgery was performed with open thoracotomy incisions leading to significant postoperative pain. However, VATs, much like laparoscopic procedures in the abdomen, offers patients the same surgical outcomes with less tissue injury and a quicker recovery time.

A VATs procedure utilizes a thoracoscope attached to a camera with the images from inside the thoracic cavity displayed on a video screen. As demonstrated below in Fig. 11.1, the surgeon's hands are not inside the body but instead are outside guiding the video scopes and various instruments to perform the surgical procedure.

The use of thoracoscopes to perform procedures within the thorax can be traced back as far as 1910 when used by Dr. Jacobaeus to diagnose and treat pleural effusions [1]. Thoracoscopes used during this era were constructed as a hollow cylinder with a small light on the end. This was of limited use given that only a single individual could visualize a small surgical field. However, in the 1990s the procedure made great advancements with the introduction of a small camera that could not only display the image on a video screen for the entire operative team but also enabled image magnification.

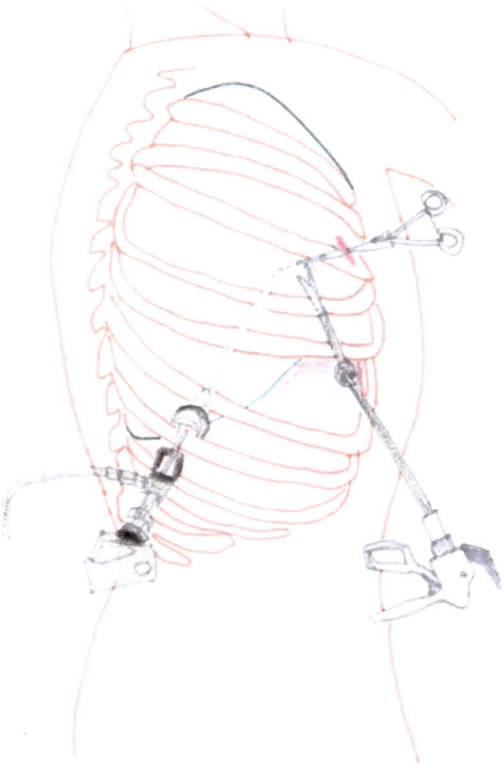

**Fig. 11.1** Video-assisted thoracoscopic surgery

The early approaches to VATS usually entails three small incisions created in the thorax to insert the camera and two different instruments

J. Roussel, M.D. · S. Smith, M.D. (✉)
Department of Anesthesiology, Ochsner Health System, New Orleans, LA, USA
e-mail: jared.roussel@ochsner.org; susan.smith@ochsner.org


B. G. Goudra et al. (eds.), *Anesthesiology*, https://doi.org/10.1007/978-3-319-74766-8_11

[2]. Evolution of the minimally invasive technique has progressed so that some practitioners are utilizing only two incisions. This developed even further when Dr. Gaetano Rocco developed a technique using only one port for the scope and instruments [3]. This technique is referred to as uniportal VATS and is considered an emerging technique of thoracic surgery [4, 5]. One of the more recent advances involves the use of wireless cameras that can be remotely controlled by a guidance system and yield a better three-dimensional view [5].

## Preoperative Evaluation

The preoperative evaluation for VATS should be approached in the same manner as the evaluation for an open thoracotomy as the postoperative effects of lung resection are the same and there exists the possibility that conversion to an open procedure becomes necessary. The focus of the preoperative evaluation for VATS, in addition to standard preoperative considerations, should be directed at the respiratory reserve of the patient and their likelihood to tolerate one lung ventilation and potential pulmonary resection. Published guidelines direct the utility of various pulmonary tests prior to lung resection surgery [6]. Typically, pulmonary function tests (PFTs) are only routinely utilized in patients undergoing larger resections (lobectomy or pneumonectomy) but can also be performed on patients with severe COPD as this is the only absolute contraindication to undergoing the VATS procedure for pulmonary resection [7, 8]. Several studies have shown a significant increase in postoperative complications when preoperative FEV1 is <40% of predicted and further studies have shown that a calculated postoperative FEV1 or DLCO <40% predicts not only an increased risk for perioperative complications but also an increase incidence of postoperative mortality after lung cancer resection [9].

A separate patient population with an important indication for preoperative imaging is the presence of an anterior mediastinal mass for thoracoscopic surgery. A CT scan will help determine the location and degree of airway compromise present. This is paramount in planning induction and maintenance of anesthesia in these patients. Another test modality to be considered is flow volume loops. However, it should be noted that studies have demonstrated that flow volume loops correlate poorly to the degree of airway compromise [10]. Therefore, clinical exam findings and imaging should take a higher priority.

Another modality utilized to evaluate patients undergoing thoracoscopic surgery is quantitative perfusion scanning which demonstrates the distribution of perfusion in the lungs. This modality has been shown to be particularly predictive in patients undergoing a pneumonectomy. However, in patients undergoing smaller resections (surgeries appropriate for VATS) the predicted postoperative function did not correlate as well [11, 12].

For patients with pre-existing lung pathology, the preoperative evaluation should assess the risk of postoperative pulmonary complications [13]. With the exception noted above, there is no delineated degree of lung pathology that prohibits surgery. Specifically, for patients with COPD, evaluation should delineate if the patient has had any recent exacerbations, infections or acute worsening from their baseline status [14]. Any patient with predictors for postoperative complications or who may require controlled ventilation after surgery requires a clear discussion of these risks in the preoperative setting.

Additional preoperative testing can include baseline pulse oximetry, ABGs, electrolyte and glucose testing, and a type and screen. For patients with FEV1 < 50% of predicted, a baseline ABG would be useful to delineate carbon dioxide retention with $PaCO_2$ > 45 mmHg. In addition, electrolytes and glucose testing would be useful in patients on bronchodilator/glucocorticoid therapy. Type and screen should be performed on all anatomical resections. Cross matching should be performed at the provider's discretion, considering the patient's preoperative hematocrit, proposed surgery, and input from the surgeon regarding potential for blood loss. In addition to screening for potential pulmonary complications, one must not ignore the potential for cardiac complications as well. We recommend following the American College of Cardiology (ACC) and American Heart Association (AHA) guidelines for cardiac risk stratification prior to non-cardiac surgery [15]. Routine preoperative screening ECGs should be performed on patients undergoing intrathoracic surgery as recommended by these guidelines [15].

Other considerations the anesthesiologist should be aware of relate to the underlying disease process. For example, patients exhibiting signs of upper extremity and facial edema should trigger a concern for thoracic outlet syndrome or SVC syndrome. Any tumor or mass that has imaging findings or symptoms of airway compression or obstruction command preemptive planning prior to the induction of anesthesia. Patients with severe pain related to malignancy or metastases are more likely to encounter pain in the immediate postoperative period and are at higher risk to develop chronic pain.

Another element of the preoperative evaluation is smoking status. It has been shown that smoking preoperatively increases risk for postoperative morbidity [16]. A common concern is trying to determine the optimal time interval between cessation and surgery. Analyses show that smoking cessation for at least 4 weeks decreases the risk of postoperative pulmonary complications, with a duration of 8 weeks being preferable [16, 17]. There is also the concern that smoking cessation for a time period less than the preferred 8 weeks can actually increase complications [18]. This concern stems from a single study done on patients undergoing CABG surgery [19]. Further meta-analyses have not reproduced this finding and even cessation from 24–48 decreases carboxyhemoglobin levels. Regardless of timing related to surgery, patients should be encouraged to quit smoking [20].

Finally, one additional aspect of preoperative evaluation to address is pulmonary rehabilitation prior to surgery. Preoperative incentive spirometry, respiratory muscle strengthening, and deep breathing is a cost effective and risk-free method of reducing post-operative pulmonary complications and should be pursued in as many patients undergoing thoracic surgery as possible, especially those with COPD [21]. Preoperative pulmonary rehabilitation has been shown to be beneficial in patients with COPD and non-small cell lung cancer (NSCLC) undergoing resection [22]. This has shown the greatest benefit in the patients with the worst pre-rehabilitation status and functional capacity.

## Intraoperative Management

Prior to induction of anesthesia, one must be sure adequate preparation has been undertaken for the various scenarios that can be encountered during VATS. Standard monitors should be placed including EKG, pulse oximetry, and non-invasive blood pressure monitors. Care should be taken with regards to EKG lead placement so as not to place them over the surgical field as well as on the dependent side where the patient will be laying while anesthetized. The use of an intra-arterial catheter should be considered on patients with comorbid diseases which would warrant closer monitoring of blood pressure as well as procedures such as a lobectomy requiring pulmonary vascular instrumentation. It is rare to utilize additional invasive monitors such as central venous catheters, pulmonary artery catheters and transesophageal echocardiography.

Induction agents should be chosen based on the patient's comorbid conditions. One unique consideration for both VATS and open thoracic cases is the potential for pre-incisional bronchoscopy by the surgical team. Open lines of communication between the anesthesia and surgical teams should be maintained to determine if this is necessary. If desired, initial intubation could proceed with a single lumen ETT (SLT) prior to the chosen method of lung isolation to facilitate the bronchoscopy. The risks added by multiple airway manipulations should be considered for each individual patient and discussed with the surgical team.

## Lung Isolation Techniques

A primary anesthetic consideration for patients undergoing VATs is one lung ventilation (OLV). This allows the operative lung to be isolated (not ventilated) to optimize the surgical field. As a result the patient will rely on a single lung for complete ventilation and oxygenation. The two primary ways to achieve OLV are either a double lumen endotracheal tubes (DLT) or a bronchial blocker (BB). Both of these techniques have shown to be effective in one lung ventilation during a VATs procedure.

Traditionally, DLTs were used to accomplish the task of lung isolation. However, there are some difficulties with using DLTs most commonly in patients with airway abnormalities or a difficult airway. Additionally, if patients require ventilator support postoperatively after the use of a DLT, a single lumen tube should replace the DLT which can be problematic in a swollen and edematous airway. There is also an association of an increase in airway trauma with DLT compared to BB. Knoll et al. prospectively randomized 60 patients to BB or DLT and found that hoarseness was more common and lasted longer in patients with DLTs [23]. Every patient in this study also had a post-surgical bronchoscopy and the incidence of vocal cord lesions was statistically higher in the DLT group compared to BB (44% vs. 17%, $p = 0.04$).

It has become accepted that BBs are quite reliable for left bronchial placement but can be more problematic for placement on the right side. In 2001 Bauer et al. prospectively randomized 35 patients undergoing VATS to one of three groups: left-sided DLT, left-sided BB, or right-sided BB. A left-sided BB averaged the longest of all devices to place (4.21 min LBB vs. 2.26 min DLT and 2.41 min RBB) and had a higher incidence of becoming dislodged requiring adjustment compared to the other two devices [24]. However, the quality of lung isolation was deemed excellent or fair by the surgical team in all DLT and LBB patients and poor in 44% of RBB placements [24]. In the largest randomized study examining this topic to date, Narayanaswamy et al. placed 104 patients having left-sided thoracic surgery into one of four groups: left-sided DLT and three left-sided BBs (Arndt, Cohen and Fuji) with the quality of lung deflation scored by a surgeon blinded to intervention [25]. There was no difference in lung collapse scores amongst any group up to 20 min after pleural opening. However, the average time to initial lung isolation was less for DLT (93 s) than for all BB (203 s, $p = 0.0001$) with no difference found amongst the BB themselves. The BB required significantly more repositioning after initial placement (35 incidents vs. 2 incidents, $p = 0.009$) with the Arndt device requiring the most repositioning in this study.

## Double Lumen Endotracheal Tubes

Left-sided DLTs are more frequently utilized as right-sided DLT presents unique challenges for placement. Indications for right-sided DLTs are generally when the surgical field involves an area where the left-sided DLT will reside. Examples of this would be left pneumonectomy, left sleeve resection, left tracheobronchial lesion and left-sided bronchial compression from tumor or lesion. Left-sided single lung transplants are often amenable to left-sided DLT as a relatively short segment of donor bronchus is maintained. The hesitancy by anesthesiologists to place right-sided DLTs lays in the difference in anatomy between the right and left bronchus. The right-sided bronchus is shorter than the left and the right upper lobe take off is inconsistent as to its exact location relative to the carina with an average distance of only 1.5–2 cm. This necessitates that the right sided DLT be designed to not only ventilate the right middle and lower lobes but account for the variable position of the upper lobe (Fig. 11.2). However, partially refuting this long-held belief was a 2000 study by Campos et al. which randomized 40 left-sided thoracic surgical patients to a right or left-sided DLT [26]. They did find that the R-DLT took just over 1 min longer to place (3.4 min vs. 2.1 min, $p = 0.04$) and though there was more malposition of the right-sided tube judged on fiberoptic bronchoscopy (5 vs. 2) it did not reach statistical significance. Intraoperative chest radiography in the lateral decubitus position in all 20 patients with a right-sided DLT did not show any incidence of right upper lobe collapse and the quality of left lung isolation was similar between the two groups.

**Fig. 11.2** Double lumen tubes for lung isolation

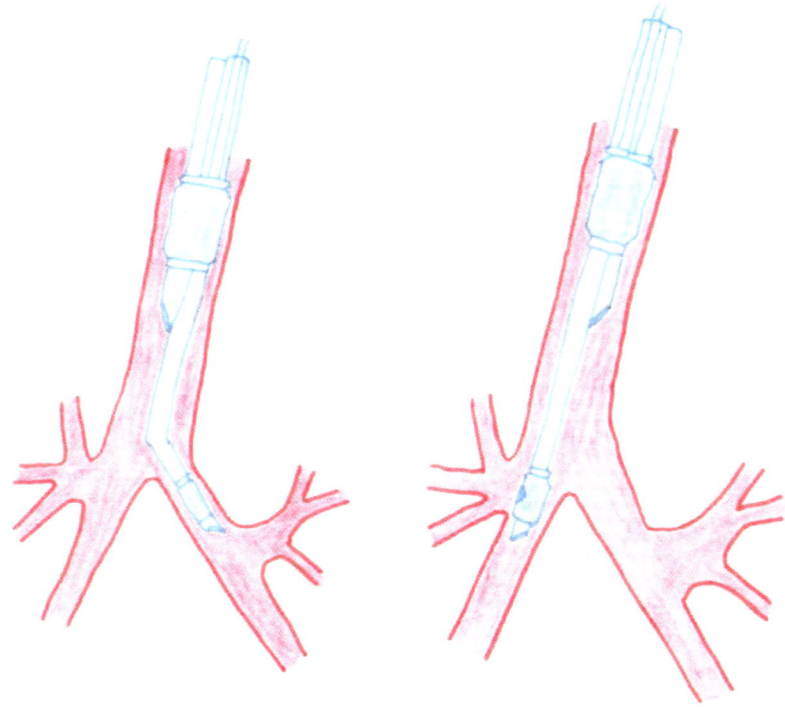

Selecting the size of the DLT has traditionally relied on few objective criteria. Routinely, female patients would receive either a 35 French (F) or 37 F tube while men received a 39 F or 41 F tube. However, it has been shown in a number of studies that tracheal and bronchial diameter are more predictive than sex, height and weight when selecting appropriate DLT size [27–29]. Selecting a DLT that is too small may require excessive bronchial cuff volume and pressure which can lead to bronchial injury as well as DLT migration and malposition. Conversely, selecting a DLT that is too large may directly lead to airway or bronchial injury. An appropriately-sized DLT should pass through the glottic opening and move easily down the trachea and into the intended bronchus. Further, it is believed that an appropriately sized DLT is one where the left bronchial segment outer diameter is approximately 1–2 mm smaller than the left bronchial width to be able to accommodate the cuff on the left bronchial segment of the DLT [28]. A complicating factor is that although DLTs are assigned French gauge sizes, the diameter and length of the bronchial segment is variable. In 2003 Russel and Strong independently measured the width of the deflated bronchial cuff portion of 174 left-sided DLTs from four manufacturers ranging in size from 28 to 41 F. They found a wide variety of bronchial cuff widths which did not decrease in size as the F size decreased and there was even greater than a 1 mm difference between the same size tube from the same manufacturer [30].

A number of studies have sought to define the easiest and most accurate way to measure both tracheal and bronchial width. Cadaver studies have shown a consistent ratio in the width of bronchus to trachea width [27]. However, cadaver anatomy can be distorted and as a result most studies have involved chest x-rays or CT scans for measurement. Because the left bronchus is easily seen on more than half of chest x-rays, the diameter of the left main stem bronchus as a predictive tool can be widely used. However, the tracheal diameter has also been taken into consideration as a predictive tool given its ease of visualization on nearly 100% of chest x-rays. In 2001, Brodsky et al. examined CT scans on both men and women presenting for thoracic surgery and found that bronchial and tracheal width were

**Table 11.1** Selection of double lumen endotracheal tubes

| Measured tracheal width (TW) in mm [51] | Predicted left bronchial diameter Men 0.75(TW) Women 0.77(TW) [29] | Outer diameter of Mallinckrodt DLT in mm [51] | | Outer diameter of Mallinckrodt left sided bronchial lumen in mm [29] | |
|---|---|---|---|---|---|
| 18 | M 13.5 W 13.9 | 41 | 13.7 | 41 | 10.6 |
| 16 | M 12 W 12.3 | 39 | 13.0 | 39 | 10.1 |
| 15 | M 11 W 11.6 | 37 | 12.3 | 37 | 10.0 |
| 14 | M 10.5 W 10.8 | 35 | 11.7 | 35 | 9.5 |

routinely larger in men versus women [31]. He went on to show that the even though there was a difference in the absolute measurement, the ratio of the left bronchial width to the tracheal width was quite consistent between men and women and suggested this as a tool to predict DLT size [29]. Table 11.1 below shows the relationship between the Mallinckrodt DLT and an individual patient's anatomical measurements to help select DLT size. As stated above, size of DLT can vary between manufacturers [30].

## Patient Positioning

VATs procedures routinely require the lateral decubitus position for optimal surgical exposure. Flexion of the bed is typically performed to help enlarge the intercostal spaces. For the anesthesia team, the transition to final surgical positioning is a critical time with several patient manipulations that require vigilance. Close attention must be paid to the endotracheal tube and the lung isolation device in use, whether a DLT or BB. Be sure to deflate any balloons that are placed in a bronchus prior to patient movement to reduce the risk of bronchial injury. Neutral position of the neck after bed flexion is critical to avoid injury to the cervical spine and should be routinely checked throughout the procedure. In addition to the airway, vascular access must be monitored to ensure IVs flow well and the arterial pressure tracing is acceptable. No lines, ports, or monitors should be placing any pressure on the patient as they could potentially remain there for some time causing unnecessary harm. The most common site of peripheral nerve injury seen for these procedures is the brachial plexus. Neutral positioning of the upper extremities with use of proper padding helps to reduce this risk. Once the proper positioning is achieved and all the above steps are verified, fiberoptic bronchoscopy confirms accurate position of the DLT or BB and one lung ventilation is initiated.

## One Lung Physiology

VATs surgical procedures bring a set of unique physiologic challenges to the anesthesiologist. Consideration should not only be given to the change in pulmonary physiology that occurs with induction of general anesthesia but also changes that occur from switching to the lateral decubitus position and the initiation of one lung ventilation. As general anesthesia is induced, a reduction in functional residual capacity occurs and an increase in dead space largely due to an increase in West zone 1 from positive pressure ventilation. As the patient is moved into the lateral decubitus position the dependent lung (non-operative lung closest to the OR table) generally receives more perfusion of blood while the non-dependent receives more ventilation. The dependent lung not only has the weight of the mediastinum pushing on it but the paralyzed diaphragm allows a greater compressive force from the abdominal contents. A further insult comes from flexion of the table and the sum of these forces creates more resistance to ventilation than the non-dependent lung. When the non-dependent lung portion of the DLT is clamped and opened to atmosphere, the non-dependent lung should collapse creating an acceptable surgical field with minimal motion.

**Table 11.2** Drugs effects of hypoxic pulmonary vasoconstriction (HPV)

| Drugs NOT known to decrease HPV | Drugs known to decrease HPV |
|---|---|
| IV Anesthetics | Calcium channel blockers |
| Inhaled $B_2$ agonists | Nitroglycerin |
| Low dose IV $A_1$ agonists | ACE inhibitors |
| | Phosphodiesterase inhibitors |
| | Inhaled anesthetics—though not significantly until above 1 MAC |

However, this forces the dependent lung to be fully responsible for ventilation and oxygenation. This is largely accomplished with hypoxic pulmonary vasoconstriction (HPV), a phenomenon that causes vasoconstriction of the pulmonary vascular tree in areas of hypoxia. Receptors known to be in the pulmonary capillaries detect the low oxygen tension and as a result pulmonary vasculature vasocontricts effectively shunting blood to the dependent lung. Human studies show that approximately half of blood is shunted from the non-dependent to the dependent lung following isolation [32]. The anesthesiologist should be aware of medications including vasodilators the inhibit HPV see Table 11.2. Also, understanding that although IV anesthetics do not inhibit HPV, inhaled anesthetics greater than 1 MAC decrease HPV [33].

## Maintenance

Maintenance goals for these surgeries require that the patient remain anesthetized, still, and mechanically ventilated to ensure the best possible surgical visualization. Typically, IA are used to achieve this goal as their anti-inflammatory and bronchodilatory effects can be beneficial and they are rapidly eliminated on emergence. Total IV anesthesia (TIVA) can also be used for these surgeries as it does offer less inhibition of HPV. One retrospective study has shown a survival benefit for a wide variety of cancer patients using TIVA versus patients using IA; however, this study was not specific for lung cancer and cannot presently be applied to this patient populations [34]. Typically, opioids and neuromuscular blockade are added to either volatile or intravenous anesthetic for a balanced anesthetic approach. Consistent neuromuscular blockade is typically utilized during the procedure but must be judiciously reversed prior to emergence in this group of patients at high risk of postoperative respiratory compromise.

There are also several approaches to pain control in this surgical group. Options include IV opiates, non-narcotic analgesia (ketorolac, acetaminophen, etc.), thoracic epidural catheters, and regional anesthetic blocks including paravertebral and intercostal nerve blocks [35–37]. Regarding ketorolac, an abstract published in 2006 randomized thoracic surgical patients to receive preemptive ketorolac, postoperative ketorolac or control. There was no statistical difference in blood loss between all three groups with both ketorolac groups decreasing postoperative morphine consumption in a statistically significant manner (preemptive a 36% reduction and postoperative a 17% reduction) [35]. As there is risk of renal impairment with the use of non-steroidal anti-inflammatory agents (NSAIDs), attention should be paid to the patient's baseline renal function, urine output and risk for renal injury prior to administering NSAIDs. A study published in the European Journal of Cardio Thoracic Surgery looked at 30 patients undergoing thoracotomies and showed that intercostal blocks were more beneficial during the first 24 h, but at 48 h patients with thoracic epidurals had better pain scores. This study was limited by its small size and the fact that VATS was not specifically studied but does highlight an important difference in patient comfort [36].

Fluid management trends on the more restrictive side for large pulmonary resections to reduce the risk of postoperative acute lung injury(ALI). Larger resections carry a greater risk of ALI and tend to have more scrutiny on fluid balance. Postoperative ALI carries a high morbidity and in several studies, excessive fluid resuscitation has been a predictor of postoperative ALI [38–40]. In the 2003 study looking at 879 pulmonary resection patients, the difference in intraoperative fluid administration between those who suffered ALI vs. controls was 1.68 L vs. 1.22 L ($p = 0.005$) [38].

While a difference of less than 500 mL does not seem impressive, the authors go on to stress that the rate of postoperative fluid administration also plays a role and suggest that greater than 4 L of fluid administration in the first 24 h is a likely contributor to ALI. There must be a balance between avoiding fluid overload and avoiding decreased perfusion to end organs caused by hypovolemia. Quantification of euvolemia is difficult, as a recent analysis of 80 patients in Anesthesia & Analgesia concluded that pulse pressure variation and stroke volume variation are not accurate in thoracic surgical patients [41]. Although there is insufficient data to promote crystalloid over colloid, Hydroxyethyl starches should be avoided for their dose dependent increase in coagulopathy as well as AKI [42–45]. As further data specific to fluid management in the thoracic surgical patient population grows, anesthesiologists must incorporate it into their management strategy.

## Emergence

Prior to emergence and extubation, there should be communication with the surgical team regarding any particular concerns or risks for the patient following their VATS. Included in this discussion would be any potential need for the surgical team to perform bronchoscopy prior to extubation. Although this is rare, anesthesia providers may be under the impression this requires a single lumen tube. However, a simple screening bronchoscopy can often be performed using a pediatric scope through a DLT and does not portend the increased risk and difficulty of an additional extubation and reintubation in close proximity to full emergence. As stated earlier, full reversal of neuromuscular blocking agents should be ensured prior to extubation. The vast majority of thoracic surgical patients are able to extubated in the operating room with close attention paid to ongoing oxygenation and ventilation. Deciding to keep a patient intubated must factor in the severity of the patient's pre-existing lung disease, the extent of surgery performed, and the patient's current respiratory status. It is preferred to transfer care of an intubated patient to the ICU with a single lumen tube in place but the risk of a difficult DLT extubation and reintubation from swelling and length of surgery must be considered.

## Outcomes Using Vats Procedures

The Society of Thoracic Surgeons General Thoracic Surgery Database (STS GTSD) reports that the use of VATS for lobectomy and segmentectomy increased from 8% in 2003 to 43% in 2009 [46]. However, a concern from the oncology community is the effectiveness of the surgery and any effect on postoperative outcomes. A 2016 study by Yang et al. utilizing the National Cancer Data Base (NCDB), found that VATS was associated with a reduction in the length of stay and not associated with increased perioperative mortality or reduced short-term survival [47]. In addition, other studies have shown long-term survival is no different in VATS vs. patients who receive open procedures for Stage 1 NSCLC [48] while postoperative pain and quality of life are improved [49, 50]. Additional studies have shown similar outcomes not only in more advanced cancers but also in patients with poor pulmonary function [46, 51]. However, Medberry et al. examined almost 17,000 patients in the NCDB and found that upstaging of early stage lung cancer via nodal sampling was observed more frequently in lobectomies performed via open thoracotomy versus VATS [52]. However, these results were not significant in the subset of procedures completed in academic institutions where it was postulated there is a greater level of expertise in performing VATS. Finally, a systematic review published in 2016 reports that lymph node dissection especially in N2 and greater disease is better in open versus VATS procedures [53]. As the utilization of VATS continues to grow in thoracic surgery, the area of nodal sampling will likely be a topic of further study.

## References

1. Luh SP, Liu HP. Video-assisted thoracic surgery—the past, present status and the future. J Zhejiang Univ Sci B. 2006;7(2):118–28. Review. PMID: 16421967.

2. Sihoe AD, et al. The evolution of minimally invasive thoracic surgery: implications for the practice of uniportal thoracoscopic surgery. J Thorac Dis. 2014;6(Suppl 6):S604–17.
3. Rocco G, Khalil M, Jutley R. Uniportal video-assisted thoracoscopic surgery wedge lung biopsy in the diagnosis of interstitial lung diseases. J Thorac Cardiovasc Surg. 2005;129(4):947–8. PMID: 15821673.
4. Reinersman JM, Passera E, Rocco G. Overview of uniportal video-assisted thoracic surgery (VATS): past and present. Ann Cardiothorac Surg. 2016;5(2):112–7. PMID: 27134837.
5. Ng CS, Rocco G, Wong RH, Lau RW, Yu SC, Yim AP. Uniportal and single-incision video-assisted thoracic surgery: the state of the art. Interact Cardiovasc Thorac Surg. 2014;19(4):661–6. PMID: 24994696.
6. Society of Cardiothoracic Surgeons of Great Britain and Ireland Working Party. BTS guidelines; guidelines on selection of patients with lung cancer for surgery. Thorax. 2001;56(2):89–108.
7. Brunelli A, Kim AW, Berger KI, Addrizzo-Harris DJ. Physiologic evaluation of the patient with lung cancer being considered for resectional surgery: diagnosis and management of lung cancer, 3rd ed: American College of Chest Physicians evidence-based clinical practice guidelines. Chest. 2013;143(5):e166s–90s.
8. Alam NZ. Lung resection in patients with marginal pulmonary function. Thorac Surg Clin. 2014;24(4):361–9.
9. Colice GL, Shafazand S, Griffin JP, Keenan R, Bolliger CT, American College of Chest Physicians. Physiologic evaluation of the patient with lung cancer being considered for resectional surgery: ACCP evidenced-based clinical practice guidelines (2nd edition). Chest. 2007;132(3 Suppl):161S–77S.
10. Torchio R, Gulotta C, Perboni A, Ciacco C, Guglielmo M, Orlandi F, Milic-Emili J. Orthopnea and tidal expiratory flow limitation in patients with euthyroid goiter. Chest. 2003;124(1):133–40.
11. Ali MK, Mountain CF, Ewer MS, Johnston D, Haynie TP. Predicting loss of pulmonary function after pulmonary resection for bronchogenic carcinoma. Chest. 1980;77(3):337–42.
12. Fields AC, Divino CM. Surgical outcomes in patients with chronic obstructive pulmonary disease undergoing abdominal operations: an analysis of 331,425 patients. Surgery. 2016;159(4):1210.
13. Smetana GW, Lawrence VA, Cornell JE. Preoperative pulmonary risk stratification for noncardiothoracic surgery: systematic review of the American College of Physicians. Ann Intern Med. 2006;144(8):581.
14. Milledge JS, Nunn JF. Criteria of fitness for anaesthesia in patients with chronic obstructive pulmonary disease. Br Med J. 1975;3(5985):670.
15. Fleisher LA, Fleischmann KE, Auerbach A, Barnason S, Beckman J, Bozkurt B, Davila-Roman V, Gerhard-Herman M, Holly T, Kane G, Marine J, Nelson T, Spencer C, Thompson A, Ting H, Uretsky B, Wijeysundera D. 2014 ACC/AHA guideline on perioperative cardiovascular evaluation and management of patients undergoing noncardiac surgery. J Am Coll Cardiol. 2014;64(22):e77–137.
16. Gronjaer M, Eliasen M, Skoy-Ettrup LS, Tolstrup JS, Christiansen AH, Mikkelsen SS, Becker U, Flensborg-Madsen T. Preoperative smoking status and postoperative complications: a systematic review and meta-analysis. Ann Surg. 2014;259(1):52–71.
17. Wightman JA. A prospective survey of the incidence of postoperative pulmonary complications. Br J Surg. 1968;55(2):85.
18. Mastracci TM, Carli F, Finley RJ, Muccio S, Warner DO. Effect of preoperative smoking cessation interventions on postoperative complications. J Am Coll Surg. 2011;212(6):1094–6.
19. Warner MA, Divertie MB, Tinker JH. Preoperative cessation of smoking and pulmonary complications in coronary artery bypass patients. Anesthesiology. 1984;60(4):380–3.
20. Gourgiotis S, Aloizos S, Aravosita P, Mystakelli C, Isaia EC, Gakis C, Salemis NS. The effects of tobacco smoking on the incidence and risk of intraoperative and postoperative complications in adults. Surgeon. 2011;9(4):225–32.
21. Valkenet K, van de Port IG, Dronkers JJ, de Vries WR, Lindeman E, Backx FJ. The effect of preoperative exercise therapy on postoperative outcome: a systematic review. Clin Rehabil. 2011;25(2):99–111.
22. Mujovic N, Mujovic NE, Subotic D, Marinkovic M, Milovanovic A, Stojsic J, Zugic V, Grajic M, Nikolic D. Preoperative pulmonary rehabilitation in patients with non-small cell lung cancer and chronic obstructive pulmonary disease. Arch Med Sci. 2014;10(1):68–75.
23. Knoll H, Ziegeler S, Schreiber JU, Buchinger H, Bialas P, Semyonov K, Graeter T, Mencke T. Airway injuries after one-lung ventilation: a comparison between double-lumen tube and endobronchial blocker: a randomized, prospective, controlled trial. Anesthesiology. 2006;105(3):471–7.
24. Bauer C, Winter C, Hentz JG, Ducrocq X, Steib A, Dupeyron JP. Bronchial blocker compared to double-lumen tube for one-lung ventilation during thoracoscopy. Acta Anaesthesiol Scand. 2001;45(2):250–4.
25. Narayanaswamy M, McRae K, Slinger P, Dugas G, Kanellakos GW, Roscoe A, Lacroix M. Choosing a lung isolation device for thoracic surgery: a randomized trial of three bronchial blockers versus double-lumen tubes. Anesth Analg. 2009;108(4):1097–101. https://doi.org/10.1213/ane.0b013e3181999339.
26. Campos JH, Massa FC, Kernstine KH. The incidence of right upper-lobe collapse when comparing a right-sided double-lumen tube versus a modified left double-lumen tube for left-sided thoracic surgery. Anesth Analg. 2000;90(3):535–40.
27. Brodsky JB, Lemmens HJ. Tracheal width and left double-lumen tube size: a formula to estimate left-bronchial width. J Clin Anesth. 2005;17(4):267–70.
28. Kaplan J, Slinger P. Lung separation techniques. Thoracic anesthesia, 3rd ed. Javier H. Campos. Elsevier Science; Copyright 2003.

29. Brodsky JB, Macario A, Mark JB. Tracheal diameter predicts double-lumen tube size: a method for selecting left double-lumen tube size. Anesth Analg. 1996;82(4):861–4.
30. Russell WJ, Strong TS. Dimensions of double-lumen tracheobronchial tubes. Anaesth Intensive Care. 2003;31(1):50–3.
31. Brodsky JB, Malott K, Angst M, Fitzmaurice BG, Kee SP, Logan L. The relationship between tracheal width and left bronchial width: implications for left-sided double-lumen tube selection. J Cardiothorac Vasc Anesth. 2001;15(2):216–7.
32. Morrell NW, Nijran KS, Biggs T, Seed WA. Magnitude and time course of acute hypoxic pulmonary vasoconstriction in man. Respir Physiol. 1995;100(3):271–81.
33. Lumb AB, Slinger P. Hypoxic pulmonary vasoconstriction: physiology and anesthetic implications. Anesthesiology. 2015;122(4):932–46. https://doi.org/10.1097/ALN.0000000000000569.
34. Wigmore TJ, Mohammed K, Jhanji S. Long term survival for patients undergoing volatile versus IV anesthesia for cancer surgery: a retrospective analysis. Anesthesiology. 2016;124(1):69–79.
35. Boussofara M, Mtaallah MH, Bracco D, Sellam MR, Raucoules M. Co-analgesic effect of ketorolac after thoracic surgery. Tunis Med. 2006;84(7):427–31.
36. Wurnig PN, Lackner H, Teiner C, Hollaus PH, Pospisil M, Fohsl-Grande B, Osarowsky M, Pridun NS. Is intercostal block for pain management in thoracic surgery more successful than epidural anesthesia? Eur J Cardiothorac Surg. 2002;21(6):1115–9.
37. Mukherjee M, Goswami A, Gupta S, Sarbapalli D, Pal R, Kar S. Analgesia in post-thoracotomy patients: comparison between thoracic epidural and thoracic paravertebral blocks. Anesth Essays Res. 2010;4(2):75–80.
38. Licker M, de Perrot M, Spiliopoulos A, Robert J, Diaper J, Chevalley C, Tschopp J. Risk factors for acute lung injury after thoracic surgery for lung cancer. Anesth Analg. 2003;97(6):1558–65.
39. Alam N, Park BJ, Wilton A, Seshan VE, Bains MS, Downey RJ, Flores RM, Rizk N, Rusch VW, Amar D. Incidence and risk factors for lung injury after lung cancer resection. Ann Thorac Surg. 2007;84(4):1085–91.
40. Yao S, Mao T, Fang W, Zu M, Chen W. Incidence and risk factors for acute lung injury after open thoracotomy for thoracic diseases. J Thorac Dis. 2013;5(4):455–60.
41. Jeong DM, Ahn HJ, Park HW, Yang M, Park J. Stroke volume variation and pulse pressure variation are not useful for predicting fluid responsiveness in thoracic surgery. Anesth Analg. 2017;125(4):1158–65.
42. Ashes C, Slinger P. Volume management and resuscitation in thoracic surgery. Curr Anesthesiol Rep. 2014;4:386–96.
43. Chau EH, Slinger P. Perioperative fluid management for pulmonary resection surgery and esophagectomy. Semin Cardiothorac Vasc Anesth. 2014;18(1):36–44.
44. Ahn HJ, Kim JA, Lee AR, Yang M, Heo B. The risk of acute kidney injury from fluid restriction and hydroxyethyl starch in thoracic surgery. Anesth Analg. 2016;122(1):186–93.
45. Kozek-Langenecker SA. Fluids and coagulation. Curr Opin Crit Care. 2015;21(4):285–91.
46. Ceppa DP, Kosinski AS, Berry MF, Tong BC, Harpole DH, Mitchell JD, D'Amico TA, Onaitis MW. Thoracoscopic lobectomy has increasing benefit in patients with poor pulmonary function: a Society of Thoracic Surgeons Database analysis. Ann Surg. 2012;256(3):487–93. PMID: 22868367.
47. Yang CF, Sun Z, Speicher PJ, Saud SM, Gulack BC, Hartwig MG, Harpole DH Jr, Onaitis MW, Tong BC, D'Amico TA, Berry MF. Use and outcomes of minimally invasive lobectomy for stage I non-small cell lung cancer in the National Cancer Data Base. Ann Thorac Surg. 2016;101(3):1037–42. PMID: 26822346.
48. Yang HX, Woo KM, Sima CS, Bains MS, Adusumilli PS, Huang J, Finley DJ, Rizk NP, Rusch VW, Jones DR, Park BJ. Long-term survival based on the surgical approach to lobectomy for clinical stage I nonsmall cell lung cancer: comparison of robotic, video-assisted thoracic surgery, and thoracotomy lobectomy. Ann Surg. 2016;265(2):431–7. PMID: 27011367.
49. Bendixen M, Jørgensen OD, Kronborg C, Andersen C, Licht PB. Postoperative pain and quality of life after lobectomy via video-assisted thoracoscopic surgery or anterolateral thoracotomy for early stage lung cancer: a randomised controlled trial. Lancet Oncol. 2016;17(6):836–44. https://doi.org/10.1016/S1470-2045(16)00173-X. PMID: 27160473.
50. Handy JR Jr, Asaph JW, Douville EC, Ott GY, Grunkemeier GL, Wu Y. Does video-assisted thoracoscopic lobectomy for lung cancer provide improved functional outcomes compared with open lobectomy? Eur J Cardiothorac Surg. 2010;37(2):451–5. PMID: 19747837.
51. Chen K, Wang X, Yang F, Li J, Jiang G, Liu J, Wang J. Propensity-matched comparison of video-assisted thoracoscopic with thoracotomy lobectomy for locally advanced non-small cell lung cancer. J Thorac Cardiovasc Surg. 2016;153(4):967–976.e2. pii: PMID: 28088426.
52. Medbery RL, et al. Nodal upstaging is more common with thoracotomy than with VATS during lobectomy for early-stage lung cancer: an analysis from the National Cancer Data Base. J Thorac Oncol. 2016;11(2):222–33.
53. Zhang W, Wei Y, Jiang H, Xu J, Yu D. Thoracotomy is better than thoracoscopic lobectomy in the lymph node dissection of lung cancer: a systematic review and meta-analysis. World J Surg Oncol. 2016;14(1):290. PMID: 27855709.

# Anesthesia for Mediastinoscopy and Mediastinal Surgery

## 12

Philip L. Kalarickal and Chai-Lin Winchester

## Introduction

Since its introduction in 1959, mediastinoscopy has been a widely-used procedure for the diagnosis and staging of bronchogenic carcinoma and other diseases of the mediastinum [1]. The procedure can be performed as a sole entity or as part of a multi-tiered approach involving video-assisted thoracoscopy or open thoracotomy. Despite advances in noninvasive imaging studies, mediastinoscopy remains essential for the pre-operative staging of bronchogenic carcinoma with a procedural sensitivity of greater than 90% and a specificity of 100%. Other modalities are less predictive: the sensitivity and specificity for computerized tomography (CT) is 55% and 81% compared to positron emission tomography (PET) with 80% and 88%, respectively [2]. A summary of anesthetic considerations for medstinal surgery is presented in Table 12.1.

## Anatomy

The mediastinum is the space between the two pleural cavities extending from the thoracic inlet (superior border) to the diaphragm (inferior border). The sternum and the anterior surface of the vertebral bodies comprise the anterior and posterior borders, respectively. The mediastinum is divided into a superior and inferior mediastinum by the transverse thoracic plane, which extends horizontally from the sternal angle to the inferior border of the T4 vertebra. The inferior mediastinum itself is divided into anterior, middle, and posterior compartments by the heart and pericardium.

The anterior compartment of the inferior mediastinum contains the thymus and anterior mediastinal lymph nodes. It is bound by the sternum, pericardium, ascending aorta and great vessels.

The middle compartment of the inferior mediastinum contains the pericardium, heart, ascending and transverse portions of the aorta, trachea, main bronchi, superior and inferior vena cava, phrenic nerve, vagus nerves, brachiocephalic vasculature and the main pulmonary vasculature.

The posterior compartment of the inferior mediastinum lies between the pericardium and the vertebral column. It contains the descending aorta, esophagus, thoracic duct, azygos vein, sympathetic chain and posterior group of lymph nodes.

There are no anatomical or fascial planes that separate the different compartments. Intrathoracic lymphatic drainage is from the pulmonary periphery towards the central lymph nodes (one of the first stations for metastatic

P. L. Kalarickal, M.D., M.P.H. (✉)
C.-L. Winchester, M.D.
Emory University School of Medicine,
Atlanta, GA, USA
e-mail: pkalari@emory.edu;
chai-lin.winchester@emory.edu

**Table 12.1** Summary of the anesthesia considerations for mediastinoscopy and mediastinal surgery

| Plan/preparation/adverse events | Reasoning/management |
|---|---|
| Preoperative evaluation | Assessment and optimization of comorbidities<br>Review of imaging and physical exam for the presence of a mediastinal mass and it's secondary effects<br>Laboratory evaluation for comorbid conditions<br>Type and screen |
| Position | Supine, operating room table may be turned 90 degrees per surgical preference |
| Access | Large-bore peripheral access is usually sufficient<br>Arterial line—right radial to assess for compression of innominate artery by mediastinoscope. Place NIBP in opposite arm to assess adequacy of systemic perfusion in cases of innominate compression |
| GETA | Consideration for ventilation effects of anterior mediastinal masses<br>Consider awake intubation or maintenance of spontaneous ventilation if necessary<br>Consideration for judicious use of neuromuscular blockade in setting of Eaton Lambert syndrome or myasthenia gravis with thymoma |
| Procedural adverse events | |
| Compression of innominate artery | Pulse oximeter or arterial catheter in right radial artery for monitoring. NIBP in opposite arm |
| Hemorrhage | Rare, but potentially catastrophic requiring close communication with surgical team |
| Recurrent laryngeal nerve injury | Monitor closely in post anesthetic care unit for signs of respiratory distress |
| Postoperative and post-discharge considerations | |
| Disposition | Following reassuring postoperative chest radiograph and satisfactory respiratory & hemodynamic function discharge to home or standard floor bed |

spread), thus making lymph node sampling indispensable to the establishment of diagnosis and staging. Access to the upper and lower paratracheal as well as subcarinal lymph nodes is provided by cervical mediastinoscopy. Access to the aortopulmonary lymph nodes is provided by anterior mediastinoscopy via an incision in the second intercostal space (Chamberlain's procedure). A thorough understanding of the anatomy is essential for understanding the surgeon's perspective on the procedure and to anticipate the anesthetic considerations and potential complications.

## Indications

The most common indication for mediastinoscopy is for staging and determination of the resectability of bronchogenic carcinoma. Lymphadenopathy with associated with lymphoma, sarcoidosis, infectious granulomatous diseases, and other diseases of the mediastinum are additional indications.

## Contraindications

Prior mediastinoscopy has been touted as a relative contraindication for repeat mediastinoscopy. Scar tissue from the previous procedure will eliminate the plane of dissection, making it difficult to recognize the normal tissue. However, in a group of 101 patients from 1975 to 1989, no mortality was observed [3]. There were a significantly higher number of complications in repeat versus. primary mediastinoscopies (23% vs. 2%), though the authors make note that the higher percentage is partly accounted for by the inclusion of minor complications. In smaller series, no mortality or morbidity has been mentioned. Thus, Veughs et al. conclude that an earlier mediastinoscopy is not necessarily an absolute contraindication for repeat mediastinoscopy.

Other relative contraindications include superior vena cava syndrome (increased risk of bleeding from distended veins), severe tracheal deviation, severe cervical spine disease (poor neck extension may limit adequate surgical exposure), previous chest radiotherapy, and thoracic aortic aneurysms. All of these entities have the potential to distort anatomy and increases risk of vascular puncture with the mediastinoscope.

## Mediastinoscopy Procedure

The patient is typically positioned in the supine position. The head of the bed may be elevated, increasing risk of venous air embolism if the venous vasculature is compromised. A roll may be placed behind the shoulders to maximize neck extension and surgical exposure. For cervical mediastinoscopy, a transverse incision is made above the suprasternal notch. The strap muscles are then dissected and the pre-tracheal fascia is raised and opened to reveal the trachea. Further blunt dissection exposes the mediastinal lymph nodes. For anterior mediastinoscopy, the second or third costal cartilage is resected and the mediastinum is explored without entering the pleural space (limited anterior thoracotomy). For both approaches, visualization is often limited and lymph nodes are often aspirated prior to biopsy.

## Preoperative Considerations

As with all surgical procedures, the presence of co-existing disease states should be evaluated preoperatively. In cases of bronchogenic carcinoma, a smoking history may coexist with other morbidities such as hypertension, coronary artery disease, peripheral vascular disease, and pre-existing pulmonary disease. In patients with pre-existing carotid arteriosclerosis or cerebrovascular disease, diminished blood flow to the right carotid artery from compression of the innominate artery by the mediastinoscope may precipitate acute stroke.

Patients with anterior mediastinal masses should have an extensive preoperative evaluation as such pathology has the potential for catastrophic cardiovascular collapse or airway obstruction upon induction of anesthesia [4]. Preoperative imaging, such as a chest X-ray or CT may reveal an incidental mass as most these patients are asymptomatic. CT would give information on the location and extent of the mediastinal mass, as well as possible invasion of surrounding structures. If there is a question of invasion or obstruction of vascular structures, angiography may provide valuable information.

Symptoms of airway compromise include dyspnea, particularly postural dyspnea in the supine position, stridor, cough, unilateral wheeze, or persistent respiratory tract infection. General anesthesia exacerbates the compressibility of large airways by decreasing lung volumes and by relaxing bronchial smooth muscle [5]. Maintenance of spontaneous ventilation may be desired to avoid precipitating complete obstruction in these patients.

Superior vena cava syndrome may result from enlarged lymph nodes or an obstructing mediastinal mass. The clinical manifestations include but are not limited to dyspnea, edema of the face and arms, stridor, engorged and distended veins in the neck, and dysphagia. Edema of the larynx and tongue from poor venous drainage can make intubation challenging, as visualization may be obstructed and the patients are at risk of bleeding from relatively minor trauma secondary to increased venous pressures. Pre-operative interventions in the management of SVC syndrome may include head elevation, steroids, diuretics and even percutaneous vascular interventions.

Paraneoplastic manifestations are well-known complications of lung cancer. Secretion of various substances with significant hormonal activity may mimic hyperparathyroidism and SIADH. Lambert-Eaton Syndrome is a paraneoplastic syndrome most often seen with small cell carcinoma. It is associated with muscle weakness that improves with exercise and is not mitigated by acetyl cholinesterase inhibitor therapy. Patients with Lambert-Eaton Syndrome show an increased sensitivity to both non-depolarizing and depolarizing muscle relaxants. Thirty percent of patients with a thymoma will have myasthenia gravis, an auto-immune condition characterized by weakness and fatigability that worsens with exercise and is treated with acetyl cholinesterase inhibitor therapy [4]. These patients are typically sensitive to non-depolarizing neuromuscular blockers and are often resistant to depolarizing neuromuscular blockers. Both of these conditions mandate judicious use of these drugs [5]. Although the availability of sugammadex allows for complete reversal of aminosteroid neuromuscular blocking agents, the patient's underlying muscle weakness must still be considered after sugammadex utilization.

## Anesthetic Management

### Access and Monitoring

The proximity to vital structures such as the aorta, superior vena cava, azygous vein, pulmonary arteries and veins makes surgical complications, though rare, potentially devastating. Large-bore peripheral venous access should be obtained given the possibility of massive hemorrhage. A type and screen for possible transfusion should be performed. Pulse oximetry should be obtained on the right upper extremity to provide information of compression of the innominate artery by the mediastinoscope leading to cerebral and extremity ischemia. Invasive arterial blood pressure monitoring in the right extremity is preferred for more rapid detection of hemodynamic compromise and compression of major vessels with the mediastinoscope. Pulse oximetry may be unable to detect innominate artery compression until ischemia is already present [6]. Noninvasive blood pressure cuffs should be on the left arm to avoid inappropriately treating hypotension from vessel compression.

### Induction

Mediastinoscopy is usually done under general endotracheal anesthesia (GETA). Induction for GETA is dependent upon the patient's symptoms and degree of airway obstruction, if any. If no evidence of obstruction is present, intravenous induction can be performed after adequate preoxygenation. If there is concern for airway obstruction during induction of general anesthesia, awake fiberoptic intubation in the supine or sitting position depending on symptomatology should be considered. A reinforced endotracheal tube should be considered in cases of possible airway obstruction. Inhalational induction may also be pursued to maintain spontaneous ventilation to prevent airway collapse on induction. If ventilation becomes difficult, a rigid bronchoscope should be available. Given the possibility of intraoperative gas exchange impairment in patients with severe airway compromise and pulmonary vasculature involvement, it may be prudent to have cardiopulmonary bypass standby in the operating room on very select patients.

Another option, however uncommon, is to perform the procedure under local anesthesia. Local anesthesia would be used for the cervical incision. With this option, spontaneous ventilation is preserved. The level of consciousness can also be continuously monitored in patients with impaired cerebral circulation. There are risks of patient movement leading to vascular damage and excessive sedation leading to airway compromise. This would necessitate emergent conversion to general anesthesia and the possibility of immediate surgical exploration.

### Maintenance

Muscle relaxation may be advantageous to aid in ventilation and prevent coughing and other sudden movements, thereby decreasing the risk of complications. However, in patients with thymoma, Lambert-Eaton syndrome and possibly pre-existing neuromuscular disease, the use of neuromuscular blockade should be judicious. For maintenance of anesthesia, either inhaled volatile anesthetics or intravenous anesthetics may be utilized.

## Management of Intraoperative Complications

### Major Hemorrhage

One of the most feared complications of mediastinoscopy is major hemorrhage. Major hemorrhage, defined as that requiring surgical exploration for definitive control, is an uncommon but potentially fatal event, with a reported incidence of 0.4% [7]. Other series report rates between 0 and 0.6%. The most common site of biopsy resulting in major hemorrhage is that of the lower right paratracheal region. The most frequently injured vessels are the innominate vein, azygos vein, and pulmonary arteries. Bleeding encountered intra-operatively is initially treated with compression. Factors that may increase the risk of a major bleeding complication include induction chemotherapy agents, prior radiation to the mediastinum, prior surgical procedure, and repeat mediastinoscopy [7]. Packing is used initially to control bleeding. If the patient demonstrates persistent hemodynamic instability, surgical exploration is required either through median sternotomy or thoracotomy. Large bore venous access should be obtained in the lower extremities, as bleeding may be from vessels that drain into the SVC. If thoracotomy is necessary, one-lung ventilation may be required. In a recent case series, mortality for major hemorrhage was 7% [7].

**Venous Air Embolism**

Venous air embolism may occur once venous bleeding develops. If patients are spontaneously breathing, the risk is higher given the development of negative intrathoracic pressure during inspiration. Positioning of the patient with the patient's head above the level of the heart also increases risk of venous air embolism. Manifestations include arrhythmias, reduced lung compliance, hypoxemia, hypercarbia, sudden decrease in end-tidal carbon dioxide, and cardiovascular collapse. Although various monitoring devices can help detect the presence of venous air embolism, such as transesophageal echocardiography, end-tidal nitrogen, and precordial Doppler, these are often not feasible with mediastinoscopy. Treatment involves prevention of further entrainment of air by covering the field with saline soaked gauze, tilting the table if possible, administering 100% oxygen to reduce embolus volume by eliminating nitrogen, and treating right sided heart failure while maintaining hemodynamic support as possible. Mortality of VAE ranges from 48 to 80% [8].

**Other Complications**

1. Stroke is a rare complication of mediastinoscopy. Strokes are usually located in the right hemisphere and occur because of compression of the innominate artery, resulting in diminished flow through the right carotid and subclavian arteries. Invasive arterial blood pressure monitoring in the right extremity enables continuous monitoring for vascular compression to prevent this complication.
2. Autonomic reflexes may occur as a result of compression or stretching of the great vessels or the vagus nerve. Bradycardia may be profound and may necessitate pharmacologic treatment and temporary cessation of surgical manipulation [9].
3. Entry into the pleural cavity can result in a pneumothorax which is often not apparent until the postoperative period where chest radiograph should be routinely performed. Tension pneumothorax is a rare but significant complication that may manifest acutely as increased peak inspiratory pressures, tracheal shift, and hypotension.
4. Phrenic or recurrent laryngeal nerve injuries are also possible complications. The rate of vocal cord palsies is <1%. In a study evaluating the use of recurrent laryngeal nerve monitoring during mediastinoscopy, 14 out of 15 patients demonstrated intense recurrent nerve stimulation during digital dissection along the anterior trachea. This suggests that the recurrent laryngeal nerve injuries occur more from traction than direct stimulation [10]. In a series of patients undergoing mediastinoscopy, a 6% rate of at least temporary vocal cord paralysis was noted when all patients underwent preoperative and postoperative laryngoscopy [11].
5. Esophageal injury and chylothorax are rare complications following mediastinoscopy.

**Postoperative Care**

Postoperatively, the patient should be monitored for hemodynamic stability and dyspnea. Unilateral recurrent laryngeal nerve injury often presents with hoarseness, raspy voice and dyspnea though may not be present immediately following extubation. Though rare, bilateral nerve damage would present with stridor, increasing respiratory insufficiency and patient discomfort including significant use of accessory muscle for respiration. This condition demands rapid diagnosis and often necessitates emergent reintubation. Pneumothorax may often present postoperatively and a chest radiograph should be routinely performed. Most patients with a small asymptomatic pneumothorax can be managed conservatively without the need for a chest tube. Pain management can be managed with intravenous or oral opioids as thoracic neuraxial anesthesia is rarely performed for mediastinoscopy. Other nerve blocks, such as intercostal injections can provide analgesia [9]. Depending on pre-existing morbidity and course of surgery, patients are often able to be discharged the same day [12].

## References

1. Carlens EL. Mediastinoscopy: a method for inspection and tissue biopsy in the superior mediastinum. Dis Chest. 1959;36:343–52.
2. Hammoud ZT, Anderson RC, Meyers BF, Guthrie TJ, Roper CL, Cooper JD, Patterson GA. The current role of mediastinoscopy in the evaluation of thoracic disease. J Thorac Cardiovasc Surg. 1999;118:894–9.
3. Vueghs PJM, Schurink GA, Vaes L, Langemeyer JJM. Anesthesia in repeat mediastinoscopy: a retrospective study of 101 patients. J Cardiothorac Vasc Anesth. 1992;6(2):193–5.
4. Gothard JW. Anesthetic considerations for patients with anterior mediastinal masses. Anesthesiol Clin. 2008;26:305–14.
5. Attar AS, Taghaddomi RJ, Bagheri R. Anesthetic management of patients with anterior mediastinal masses undergoing chamberlain procedure (anterior mediastionostomy). Iran Red Crescent Med J. 2013;15(4):373–4.
6. Ahmed-Nusrath A, Swanevelder J. Anesthesia for mediastinoscopy. Continuing education in anaesthesia. Critical Care Pain. 2007;7:6–9.
7. Park BJ, Flores R, Downey RJ, Bains MS, Rusch VW. Management of major hemorrhage during mediastinoscopy. J Thorac Cardiovasc Surg. 2003;126:726–31.
8. Shaikh N, Ummunisa F. Acute management of vascular air embolism. J Emerg Trauma Shock. 2009;2(3):180–5.
9. Thomsen RW. Mediastinoscopy and video-assisted thoracoscopic surgery: anesthetic pitfalls and complications. Semin Cardiothorac Vasc Anesth. 2008;12(2):128–32.
10. Roberts JR, Wadsworth J. Recurrent laryngeal nerve monitoring during mediastinoscopy: predictors of injury. Ann Thorac Surg. 2007;80:288–92.
11. Sayar A, Çitak N, Büyükkale S, Metin M, Kök A, Çelikten A, Gürses A. The incidence of hoarseness after mediastinoscopy and outcome of video-assisted versus conventional mediastinoscopy in lung cancer staging. Acta Chir Belg. 2016;116(1):23–9.
12. Vallières E, Pagé A, Verdant A. Ambulatory mediastinoscopy and anterior mediastinotomy. Ann Thorac Surg. 1991;51:1122–6.

# Anesthesia for Tracheal Surgery

Philip L. Kalarickal
and Stephanie Opusunju Ibekwe

## Introduction

Tracheal resection and reconstructive surgeries are advanced procedures that require coordination and communication between anesthesiology and surgery teams as the airway is shared between the two services. The anesthesiologist must have an understanding of the airway anatomy as well as the pathological process that necessitates tracheal resection and reconstruction. In addition, the anesthesiologist must be knowledgeable of the surgical procedure, preoperative evaluation, appropriate patient selection and the intra- and post-operative management of these complicated patients.

## Applied Anatomy and Physiology of the Trachea

An understanding of tracheal anatomy is important when planning for surgical resection and reconstruction. The trachea extends from the cricoid cartilage to the carina. It consists of semicircular cartilaginous rings that span the anterior and lateral aspects allowing for tracheal flexibility and mobility. The posterior portion of the trachea consists of fibro-muscular tissue which abuts the esophagus posteriorly [1]. The recurrent laryngeal nerve lies between the trachea and esophagus on the postero-lateral aspects of the trachea.

The adult trachea is approximately 11 cm in length [1]. It is unique in having both intrathoracic and extrathoracic components with the neck in a neutral position. Due to its inherent flexibility, extension and flexion of the neck can make the trachea more extrathoracic or intrathoracic, respectively [2]. The mobility of the trachea becomes important with surgical positioning—exaggerated extension of the neck is utilized to advance as much of the trachea out of the mediastinum for improved exposure and manipulation. Factors such as obesity, body habitus, and flexibility of the neck must be considered prior to surgical intervention [3].

Tracheal perfusion is an important factor in surgical resection and reconstruction. The blood supply of the trachea is derived from the inferior thyroid artery, bronchial arteries, and smaller contributions from the subclavian, internal mammary, innominate, internal thoracic and supreme intercostal arteries [2]. Although it has a rich blood supply, the trachea is vulnerable to vascular disruption during surgical manipulation and circumferential dissection should be avoided [3].

Indications for surgical resection or reconstruction of the trachea are often benign. The most common cause of tracheal injury necessitating surgical revision is prolonged intubation or

P. L. Kalarickal, M.D., M.P.H. (✉) · S. O. Ibekwe, M.D., M.P.H., M.S.
Emory University School of Medicine, Atlanta, GA, USA
e-mail: pkalari@emory.edu; sopusun@emory.edu

tracheostomy resulting in subglottic stenosis [3]. Other indications for tracheal resection are tracheal trauma (from steering wheel injuries during motor vehicle collisions or suicide attempt by hanging), tracheal masses, tracheolmalacia, and congenital tracheal abnormalities [4].

## Preoperative Evaluation

### History and Physical Exam

Preoperative evaluation for tracheal resection requires a detailed review of the patient's airway history and a thorough physical exam concentrating on the patency of the airway and physiologic degree of obstruction (Fig. 13.1). Review of imaging including computed tomography (CT) scans and evaluation of pulmonary function tests (PFT) are also of importance in this patient population. A review of the patient's comorbid conditions is critical in forming a comprehensive anesthetic plan.

The history and physical exam are the most important part of the preoperative evaluation of the patient. The typical history of a patient with tracheal obstruction is that of progressive dyspnea of unknown source, found to be independent of cardiac function and not improved with bronchodilator therapy [3]. Dyspnea and more ominously, stridor at rest, is an indication of advanced tracheal obstruction necessitating urgent or emergent intervention. These symptoms are often not noted until the airway has been narrowed to 5–6 mm in diameter [5]. On physical exam, the "birthday candle test" may be employed to elucidate the degree of tracheal obstruction [1]. In order to employ this test, the patient should take a maximal inspiration and blow into the clinician's outstretched hand as if they are blowing out a candle. The examiner can feel the power of the expired airflow and make a coarse estimation of the degree of tracheal obstruction [1].

Coexisting medical conditions should be evaluated and considered in the anesthetic plan. Relative contraindications to tracheal resection include severe pulmonary dysfunction necessitating ventilator dependence, daily steroid use, and history of head and neck radiation therapy. These conditions introduce a threat to already vulnerable tracheal anastomoses and increase the risk of dehiscence [6].

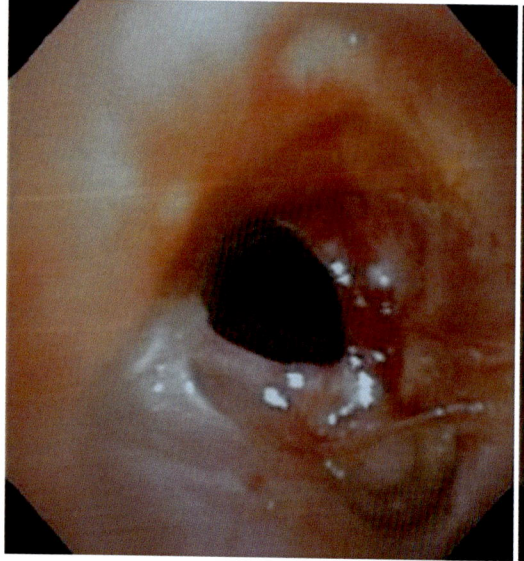 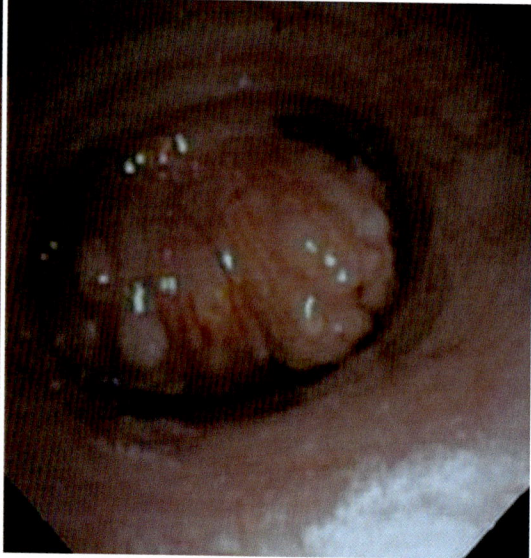

**Fig. 13.1** (Left) Circumferential tracheal stenosis from endotracheal tube cuff. (Right) a benign cartilaginous tumor in the proximal tracheal. Reproduced from: Kaiser LR, Kron IL, Spray TL eds. Tracheal Resection and Reconstruction. In: Mastery of cardiothoracic surgery 2nd ed

## Imaging

As mentioned earlier, CT is the most informative imaging test for tracheal anatomy [1]. In order to increase the sensitivity of the CT scan, 3D reconstruction may be used [7]. Evaluation of the preoperative CT scan demonstrate the level and degree of tracheal obstruction present when planning initial airway management.

Flexible bronchoscopy is utilized in tracheal resection evaluation to provide information regarding the character of the lesion obstructing the trachea. It can also provide information about the extent of the lesion, the patency of the airway, and the presence of malacia in a spontaneously breathing patient [2]. Findings from imaging and bronchoscopy must be paired with a thorough history and physical exam prior to clinical decision making.

## Functional Testing

Pulmonary function tests are especially important for patients with carinal involvement of their tracheal anomaly [2] (Fig. 13.2). The most important feature of the pulmonary function test is the ratio between the peak expiratory flow to the forced expiratory volume in 1 s ($FEV_1$). A ratio that is >10:1 is suspicious for obstruction [2]. PFTs can also provide information about the character of the obstruction: extrathoracic, intrathoracic and variable lesions can be diagnosed by observing the flow volume loops [8].

## Anesthetic Considerations

### Monitoring and Intravenous Access

Two bilateral large bore intravenous lines should be placed preoperatively as the arms are usually tucked for this procedure. Central venous access is usually not required. In addition to standard ASA monitors, an arterial line should be placed to closely monitor blood pressure. In order to allow for accurate measurement of systemic blood pressure during brachiocephalic compression, the arterial line should be placed in the left radial artery. Placement of the pulse oximeter and non-invasive blood pressure (NIBP) cuff on the right extremity can help identify brachiocephalic trunk compression [4] (Tables 13.1 and 13.2).

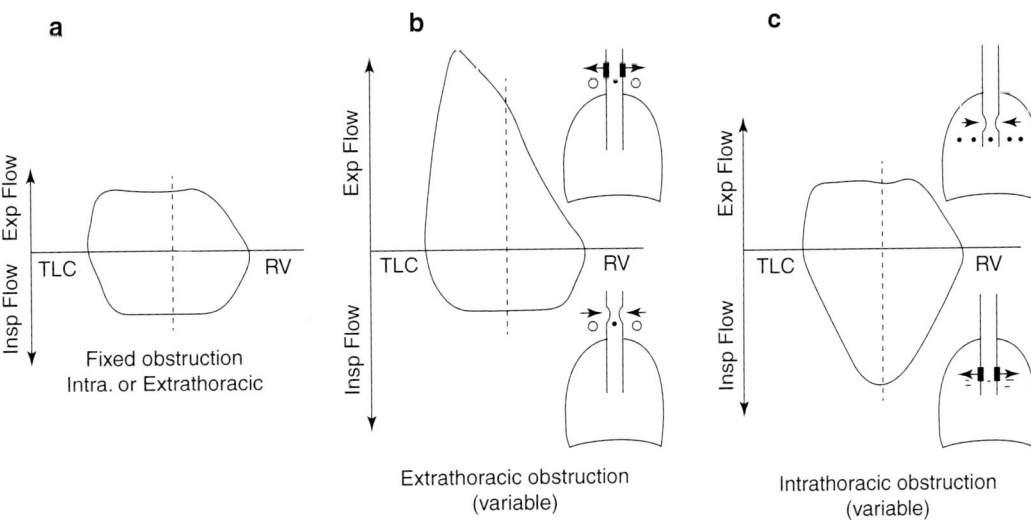

**Fig. 13.2** Flow-volume loops demonstrating fixed, extrathoracic and intrathoracic obstructions. Reproduced from: McRae, K. Anesthesiology Clinics of North America. 2001; 19: 497–541

Table 13.1 Anesthesia setup in patients undergoing tracheal surgery

| Equipment on the anesthesia set-up | Equipment on the surgical set-up |
|---|---|
| Long, flexible endotracheal tubes | Rigid bronchoscopes |
| Jet ventilator | Tracheostomy instruments |
| Dedicated $O_2$ supply for jet ventilator | Sterile airway hoses |
| Jet ventilation catheters | Sterile Y-piece |
| Fiberoptic bronchoscope(s) | Sterile wire-bound (flexible) endotracheal tubes |
| High flow anesthesia machine | |
| Second anesthesia machine or second ventilator | |

## Airway

Preoperative sedation should be titrated judiciously to avoid inadvertent obstruction of the airway. Patency of the airway dictates the plan for induction of anesthesia. If the patient's airway would be irreversibly compromised by airway relaxation and collapse, intubation while maintaining spontaneous ventilation or an awake tracheostomy should strongly be considered.

It is important to have the correct equipment readily available prior to induction of anesthesia (Table 13.1) [3]. Multiple sized reinforced endotracheal tubes (ETT) starting from 5.0 mm internal diameter and larger are important to ensure the appropriate ETT can be inserted into the trachea after rigid bronchoscopy. Trans-tracheal jet ventilation should be immediately available. Mechanical support, in the form of extracorporeal membrane oxygenation (ECMO) or cardiopulmonary bypass (CPB) may be necessary in situations of extreme difficulty of oxygenation and/or ventilation [4].

Patients that have been deemed appropriate for induction of anesthesia can be given a typical induction dosage of intravenous anesthetic medications (propofol 1–2 mg/kg, fentanyl 1–1.5 mcg/kg and rocuronium 0.7–1 mg/kg). After induction, rigid bronchoscopy is used to examine the trachea and the extent of tracheal disease. During rigid bronchoscopy, dilatation of the trachea can be performed to ensure accommodation of the largest ETT feasible [9].

To decrease the need for surgical dissection, the patient is positioned to optimize the portion of the trachea extended out of the mediastinum and into the cervical region. The neck is hyperextended, and a roll is placed beneath the scapula. Lesions lower in the tracheobronchial tree may require a median sternotomy or right thoracotomy incision and one lung ventilation (Fig. 13.3). This may require placement of a double lumen ETT, bronchial blocker, or advancement of the single lumen ETT into the left main stem bronchus [3]. As mentioned above, CPB or ECMO may be necessary if oxygenation is compromised.

## Maintenance

During the dissection phase of tracheal resection and reconstruction, anesthesia can be maintained with inhaled volatile anesthetics. However, after the airway is open, the surgeon will place a sterile ETT into the trachea and sterile ventilator tubing is passed onto the surgical field [9]. In order to ensure effective anesthesia and to minimize OR pollution of anesthetic gases, total intravenous anesthesia should be utilized [3]. The preoperative placement of a processed EEG monitor such as the bispectral index (BIS) can aid in maintaining an appropriate depth of anesthesia during the TIVA.

Hemodynamic goals are to maintain adequate blood pressure for end organ perfusion. The surgical team will work to preserve vascular flow to the remaining trachea. The lack of significant vascular anastomoses typically places no restrictions on the use of mild vasopressors. Fluid goals are to attempt to ensure euvolemia and minimize tracheal and oropharyngeal edema by judiciously replacing deficits from NPO status, exposure and blood loss. Estimated blood loss for this procedure is usually less than 500 cc but may become significant.

## Extubation

It is desirable to extubate the patient in the operating room following tracheal resection and

**Table 13.2** Summary of the anesthetic considerations in patients undergoing tracheal surgery

| Plan/preparation/adverse events | Reasoning/management |
|---|---|
| The plan for tracheal resection will be general anesthesia with endotracheal tube or tracheostomy tube. Emergency airway equipment such as jet ventilation, multiple ETTs available as small as 5.0 mm, and a surgeon should be present at induction. The potential need for ECMO or CPB should be considered preoperatively | Patients in need of tracheal resection and reconstruction are at heightened risk for airway collapse on induction of anesthesia. One must anticipate the need for advanced airway manipulation and intervention prior to induction, as a delay of just minutes can result in anoxic brain injury or death |
| Preprocedural evaluation<br>  Imaging<br>  PFTs<br>  Detailed airway history<br>  Airway exam, sitting and supine<br>  Comorbidities | If the airway is so fragile that induction of general anesthesia could cause irreversible collapse, the patient should have a tracheostomy placed in the position in which he/she can easily oxygenate and ventilate spontaneously |
| Position—typically supine with neck extended and shoulder roll applied | This brings the trachea into a more cervical position and out of the mediastinum which decreases the amount of surgical dissection required |
| IV access—2 large bore IV catheters in bilateral upper extremities | The arms are typically tucked, and with a planned TIVA it is wise to have an IV in the contralateral extremity [6] |
| Standard ASA monitors with invasive arterial pressure | Left radial artery is preferred for arterial catheter because surgical compression of the innominate artery will cause imprecise measurements [6]. Pulse oximetry and NIBP on the right extremity can help monitor for the presence of compression |
| Maintenance | Volatile anesthesia is reliable until the airway is dissected. When the airway is open, TIVA is preferable because the open airway increases the risk of OR pollution of volatile anesthetics and unreliable delivery of the gases to the patient |
| Procedural adverse events<br>  Injury to neck structures such as the superior and recurrent laryngeal nerves, the major vessels in the neck and thoracic duct.<br>  Trauma to new anastomosis on extubation<br>  Tracheal edema | Intraoperative dexamethasone IV can help decrease tracheal edema.<br>Extubate the patient with 'guardian suture' between the patient's chin and chest. Smooth awake extubation without coughing |
| Postoperative and post-discharge considerations<br>  Tracheal disruption<br>  Recurrent laryngeal nerve injury<br>  Severe pain and discomfort | Tracheal disruption may be fatal, immediate re-exploration is vital.<br>Recurrent laryngeal nerve injury may cause airway obstruction necessitating immediate reintubation [9]. Reintubation should be approached with extreme caution |

reconstruction as the presence of the ETT postoperatively puts the patient at risk for re-injury to the trachea as well as anastomotic dehiscence. The patient is maintained in partial flexion by the application of sutures between the under-surface of the chin and the skin on the upper chest [7]. A controlled, non-noxious extubation is vital to the success of the tracheal resection and reconstruction. One described technique utilized titration of propofol and remifentanil to a level of cooperative sedation; the trachea was then extubated under bronchoscopic guidance [10].

## Postoperative Considerations

The patient should be closely monitored in an intensive care unit for postoperative complications. Disruption of the tracheal anastomosis is a serious and potentially fatal complication. Additional complications include tracheal edema and recurrent laryngeal nerve injury. Any necessary attempts to reintubate these patients postoperatively should proceed with an experienced clinician in the most controlled setting allowable such as the operating room.

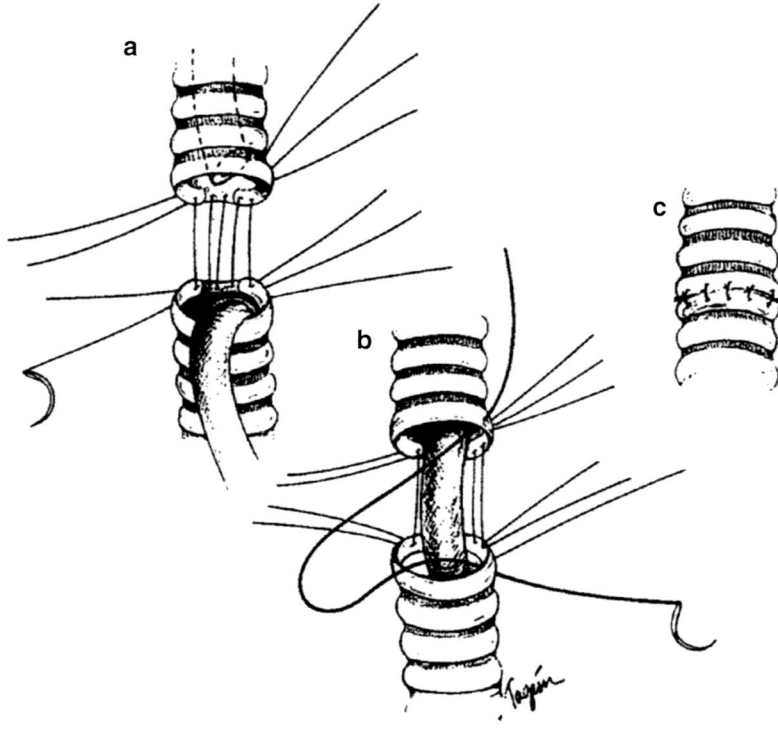

**Fig. 13.3** During dissection, the patient is ventilated via an ETT in the distal trachea (a). After the sutures are placed, an ETT is advanced from above and cuff inflated (b). Lastly, the patient is placed in a neck flexion position and the sutures are tied (c). Reproduced from: Grillo HC. Curr Prob Surg. 1970; 7: 3–59

## References

1. Hobai IA, Changani SV, Alfille PH. Anesthesia for tracheal resection and reconstruction. Anesthesiol Clin. 2012;30:709–30.
2. Pinsonneault CCA, Fortier J, Donati F. Tracheal resection and reconstruction. Can J Anesth. 1999;46:439–55.
3. Sandberg W. Anesthesia and airway management for tracheal resection and reconstruction. Int Anesthesiol Clin. 2000;38:55–75.
4. Roman PE, Battafarano RJ, Grigore AM. Anesthesia for tracheal reconstruction and transplantation. Curr Opin Anaesthesiol. 2013;26:1–5.
5. Geffin B, Bland J, Grillo HC. Anesthetic management of tracheal resection and reconstruction. Anesth Analg. 1969;48:884–90.
6. Mathisen DJ. Complications of tracheal surgery. Chest Surg Clin N Am. 1996;6:853–64.
7. Kaiser LR, Kron IL, Spray TL. Tracheal resection and reconstruction. In: Mastery of cardiothoracic surgery. Philadelphia: Lippincott, Williams & Wilkins; 2007. p. 85–90.
8. McRae K. Anesthesia for airway surgery. Anesthesiol Clin North Am. 2001;19:497–541.
9. Waddell TK, Uy KFL. Techniques of Tracheal Resection and Reconstruction. In: Sugarbaker DJ, Bueno R, Colson YL, Jaklitsch MT, Krasna MJ, Mentzer SJ eds. Adult Chest Surgery, 2nd ed. China: McGraw-Hill Education; 2015.
10. Saravanan P, Marnane C, Morris EAJ. Extubation of the surgically resected airway—a role for remifentanil and propofol infusions. Can J Anesth. 2006;53:507–11.

# Anesthesia for Esophageal Surgery

## 14

Christopher Ma and J. Kirk Edwards

## Introduction

This chapter covers the three major esophageal surgical categories: esophagogastroduodenoscopy (EGD) with stenting, fundoplication/hiatal hernia repair, and esophagectomy. For each surgery, a brief review of the inciting pathology and procedure technique is followed by preoperative and intraoperative anesthetic considerations. At the end of this chapter, postoperative anesthetic considerations relevant to all surgical types are discussed.

## The Esophagus

### Anatomy

The esophagus is a muscular tube usually around 20–25 cm in length that descends from the inferior pharynx at the C6 spinal level. It passes through the anterior and posterior mediastinum posterior to the trachea and left mainstem bronchus, pierces the hiatus in the right diaphragm, and ends at the gastro-esophageal junction (GEJ) around T11. At the GEJ, the phrenoesophageal ligament stabilizes the esophagus to the diaphragm. Embryologically, the esophagus develops from the postpharyngeal foregut and differentiates itself from the stomach at around 4 weeks of age [1, 2].

Anatomically, the muscular esophagus is comprised of four primary layers: mucosa, submucosa, muscularis propia, and adventitia. The mucosa is further subdivided into epithelium, lamina propia, and muscularis mucosa layers. The cells lining the lumen of the upper and mid-esophagus are predominantly stratified squamous epithelium. This transitions into more acid-resistant, simple columnar epithelium as you approach the GEJ. The muscularis propia of the upper third of the esophagus is predominantly striated, whereas the muscularis propia of the lower two thirds of the esophagus is smooth muscle [3].

### Function

Functionally, the esophagus can be divided into three parts: the upper esophageal sphincter (UES) or cervical esophagus, the mid esophagus or thoracic esophagus, and the lower esophageal sphincter (LES) or abdominal esophagus. The LES is a 2–4 cm zone of higher pressure within the diaphragmatic hiatus with a denser composition of connective and muscular tissue. It is the primary physical barrier to prevent the reflux of gastric contents back into the esophagus. At rest, LES tone is about 15 mm Hg. During swallowing, the oropharynx elevates to occlude the naso-

C. Ma, M.D. · J. K. Edwards, M.D. (✉)
Emory University School of Medicine,
Atlanta, GA, USA
e-mail: cmma@emory.edu;
jkedwar@emory.edu

pharynx and the epiglottis drops to occlude the larynx. The UES and LES then relax in coordination with esophageal peristalsis to allow for passage of food [1, 2].

## Neurovascular Supply

The upper esophagus is supplied by branches of the superior and inferior thyroid artery, which come from the thyrocervical trunk off of the subclavian artery, and is drained by the inferior thyroid veins. Parasympathetic innervation to this area comes from branches of the recurrent laryngeal nerve, while sympathetic fibers arise from the T4-T6 chain.

The thoracic esophagus or mid esophagus is supplied by bronchial and esophageal branches of the thoracic aorta. Blood from this region is drained by the azygos and hemiazygos veins predominantly. The parasympathetic innervation here transitions from branches of the recurrent laryngeal nerve to the esophageal plexus.

The lower esophagus is supplied by branches of the left phrenic, left gastric, and splenic arteries which come off the abdominal aorta and celiac trunk around T12-L1. Blood supplying the abdominal esophagus is drained primarily by the lower esophageal veins into the left gastric vein. This region is innervated parasympathetically by the vagal esophageal plexus, and sympathetically by the thoracic sympathetic chain.

Of note, the azygos and gastric veins draining the mid and lower esophagus, respectively, form a network between the portal and systemic venous system and are the site of esophageal varices in patients with portal hypertension [1].

## Common Esophageal Surgeries

The majority of esophageal surgeries and procedures are targeted at interventions to treat gastroesophageal reflux, repair congenital lesions, and resect neoplasms. The following sections reviews anesthetic concerns and management concepts that apply to the most common esophageal procedures.

## Esophagogastroduodenoscopy (EGD) with Stenting Surgery

EGDs can be performed to diagnose or treat a variety of different GI pathologies, including reflux, bleeding, strictures, and dysphagia. This section will focus on EGD with stent placement, the subtype most frequently performed in the thoracic surgical population and most frequently requiring general anesthesia.

### Baseline Considerations
**Pathology**: EGD stent placement is typically performed to treat obstruction from tumors, strictures, and fistulas in the esophagus or stomach. It can also be utilized as an initial stabilizing therapy in the acute treatment of esophageal perforation. The stents are made of either a metallic mesh or plastic silicon. The material of the stent chosen depends on the underlying pathology and goal of therapy.

**Procedure technique**: Once the patient is anesthetized, the endoscopy probe is inserted into the oropharynx and advanced, under visualization, towards the esophagus. Upon identifying the lesion of interest, a guidewire is typically first passed distal to the lesion. Fluoroscopy may also be utilized in combination with video visualization at the discretion of the proceduralist. Strictures often require balloon dilation, depending on the degree of stenosis. A properly-sized stent is then advanced over the wire, positioned to overlap the proximal and distal margins of the lesion, and subsequently deployed. After the stent is placed, a post-procedural esophagram may be performed to evaluate placement and resolution of obstruction or fistula.

### Preoperative Evaluation and Concerns; Operating Room Preparation
A full history and physical exam should be conducted with special attention paid to the airway and any signs or symptoms of dysphagia or gastric regurgitation. These patients will be positioned supine. The bed may also be either turned 90° and/or moved away from the anesthesia machine, to allow the proceduralist access to the patient's mouth.

Patients with gastric tubes should have their stomachs vented in order to avoid excessive gastric distention that may be caused by either non-invasive positive pressure ventilation, prior to intubation, or carbon dioxide insufflation during the EGD.

These patients typically present with signs or symptoms suggestive of esophageal narrowing or dysmotility, both of which would put them at higher risk for aspiration. Standard "nil per os" (NPO) guidelines should be followed, with the American Society of Anesthesiology(ASA) recommending the procedure to be performed no sooner than 6 h following a light meal or 2 h following clear liquids [4]. Conservative NPO management and prophylactic pharmacotherapy, if appropriate (i.e., ranitidine), may be especially beneficial in patients with significant esophageal obstruction or dysmotility. Uncommonly, poor PO intake can result in electrolyte abnormalities (i.e., critical hypomagnesemia or hypernatremia) that should be corrected before the procedure. One peripheral intravenous line (IV) should be adequate access for the case, and blood typing is not typically indicated.

## Intraoperative Management

**Induction and airway**: While most screening EGDs may be performed under monitored anesthesia care, the majority of patients presenting for an EGD with stent placement will likely require general anesthesia. These patients typically present with signs or symptoms suggestive of esophageal narrowing or dysmotility, both of which put them at higher risk for aspiration. As a result, for those airways predicted to be non-difficult, induction of general anesthesia will usually comprise of a rapid sequence induction (RSI) and single lumen endotracheal tube (ETT) placement. In patients with a history of difficult intubation or predicted difficult airway based on physical exam, it is important to consider an awake fiberoptic intubation.

**Anesthetic management**: EGD with stent placements are typically short cases, rarely lasting longer than 60 min. General anesthesia may be maintained with either inhaled volatile agents or a total IV anesthetic technique (TIVA). The mean arterial pressure (MAP) should generally be maintained close to preoperative values. Though supporting data is poor, this is classically defined as within 20% of baseline blood pressure values.

Due to their underlying disease, these patients frequently have difficulty with oral intake, which may result in malnourishment or a greater degree of dehydration than typical fluid deficit calculations would suggest. Assuming hemodynamic stability, fluid management goals for EGD stent placements are to replace any deficits and maintain euvolemia. If the patient becomes hypotensive despite adequately replenishing preoperative fluid deficits, however, a 10 mL/kg crystalloid fluid bolus may be considered, assuming no relative contraindications or preexisting conditions that may be exacerbated by more volume (i.e., congestive heart failure (CHF)). Persistent hypotension is commonly a result of a reduced systemic vascular resistance (SVR) secondary to the pharmacologic effects of general anesthetic drugs, which can be mitigated by titrated doses of a pure vasopressor (phenylephrine) or combination vasopressor/inotrope (ephedrine, norepinephrine).

Just as these patients are at higher risk for aspiration during induction, they are also at high aspiration risk on emergence and should therefore be extubated awake and following commands, to ensure adequate airway protection. Recovery in a post-anesthesia recovery unit (PACU) is indicated.

**Analgesic management**: For cases in which multiple stents are placed or the esophagus, a deep anesthetic and/or judicious use of short acting opioids (remifentanil) can counteract the acute but short-lived intraoperative sympathetic stimuli. These cases typically do not cause significant postoperative pain or discomfort. Adequate postoperative analgesia can usually be provided with opioid sparing therapies such as intravenous ketorolac or acetaminophen, though low dose opioid administration may also be of benefit.

# Fundoplication/Hiatal Hernia Surgery

## Baseline Considerations

**Pathology**: Gastroesophageal reflux disease (GERD) is a fairly common disorder that affects up to 25% of the U.S. population [5]. While diet, lifestyle changes, and pharmacotherapy will typically improve symptoms, surgical therapy may be indicated for individuals with GERD symptoms: refractory to other therapies, causing pulmonary symptoms from reflux (chronic cough or inflammation), or causing severe esophagitis. Patients with GERD frequently have an associated hiatal hernia. Hiatal hernias are defined as a weakening of the supportive phrenoesophageal ligament that attaches the esophagus to the diaphragm. This weakening results in displacement of the LES, and potentially other abdominal organs, into the thoracic cavity. Hiatal hernias are classified into 4 types [2]:

Type I: Most common type (95% of all hiatal hernias). These are also known as a "sliding" hiatal hernia, as the GEJ and gastric stomach are able to herniate upward through the phrenoesophageal ligament. There is a strong association with GERD and surgical treatment is primarily reserved for refractory GERD.

Type II: These are also known as the paraesophageal hernia. The LES is fixed in the correct anatomic location, while the gastric fundus herniates into the thoracic cavity through a defect in the phrenoesophageal ligament. As the risk of this incarceration or strangulation is high, surgical repair is therefore warranted.

Type III: Has elements of both sliding and paraesophageal hernias. The GEJ and greater curve of the stomach can herniate through the phrenoesophageal ligament into the chest. The stomach can eventually rotate on itself within the thorax, a condition known as organoaxial rotation or gastric volvulus, which is associated with vascular insufficiency, bleeding, necrosis, obstruction, and perforation. Risk of incarceration or strangulation is high, and therefore surgical repair is warranted.

Type IV: Type III hiatal hernias where other abdominal organs such as spleen or colon also herniate into the chest.

**Procedure technique**: The approach for surgical repair of hiatal hernias, and therefore the anesthetic considerations and management for these procedures, largely depends on the severity of disease and presence of other concomitant diseases (i.e., esophageal dysmotility). There are many different named fundoplication techniques (e.g., Nissen, Belsey, Hill, Toupet, Mark IV, Collis-Belsey) all of which may employ a different combination of open versus laparoscopic abdominal, and possibly even transthoracic, approaches. A randomized control trial comparing laparoscopic versus open Nissen fundoplication has found no significant difference at 10 years in effectiveness of either approach with a lower reoperation rate for incisional hernia in patients with laparoscopic repair [6]. Patients selected for fundoplication via an open left posterolateral thoracotomy typically either have a much larger hiatal hernia, concern for pleural adhesions, esophageal perforation, and/or esophageal dysmotility. These patients will also necessitate left lung isolation for surgical exposure, and they will have higher postoperative analgesic requirements.

The goal of the fundoplication, regardless of approach, is to repair the hiatal defect and provide a wrap of the stomach around the lower esophagus in attempt to restore LES tone and function. The degree and location of the gastric wrap around the lower esophagus can vary greatly depending on the indication. Of the classic named wraps, a Nissen provides a 360° circumferential wrap, Toupet a 270° posterior wrap, Thal a 270° anterior wrap, Dor a 180–200° anterior wrap, and Lind a 300° posterior wrap [7].

## Preoperative Evaluation and Concerns; Operating Room Preparation

A full history and physical exam should be conducted with special attention paid to the airway and any signs or symptoms of dysphagia or gastric regurgitation. As with EGD for stent placement patients, standard NPO guidelines should be followed, with the ASA recommending the procedure to be performed no sooner than 6 h following a light meal or 2 h following clear liquids [4]. Most patients presenting for a fundoplication or hiatal hernia surgery also typically have some degree of GERD or esophageal dysmotility disease, thus putting them at higher risk for aspiration. Conservative NPO management and prophylactic pharmacotherapy, if appropriate (i.e., ranitidine), may be beneficial in patients with significant esophageal obstruction or dysmotility. Uncommonly, poor PO intake can result in electrolyte abnormalities (i.e., critical hypomagnesemia or hypernatremia) that should be corrected before the procedure.

As there is typically minimal blood loss from this procedure, one to two peripheral IVs 18 g or larger will likely be sufficient. Similarly, a blood type and screen will suffice for laparoscopic procedures, though a type and crossmatch should be considered for open approaches or for patients with baseline anemia. An arterial line for blood pressure monitoring is usually unnecessary, but may be indicated in the setting of either certain baseline comorbid conditions (i.e., CHF, valvular pathology) or more complicated approaches leading to higher blood loss.

Patients receiving a fundoplication via the laparoscopic abdominal approach will have five abdominal ports and be positioned in lithotomy with steep reverse Trendelenburg. In this position, with the subsequent caudal shift in body fluid, care should be taken to ensure adequate perfusion pressure intraoperatively. Those receiving a fundoplication with a transthoracic approach will be placed in the right lateral decubitus with the bed flexed to expand the thoracic cage, enabling a posterolateral thoracotomy. When positioning the patient laterally, the uppers arms should rest at or below the level of the shoulders, and pressure points should be padded. These interventions will reduce the chances of brachial plexus or other upper extremity nerve injury. The bed should not require rotation but may be moved away from the anesthesia machine if more space is needed by the surgical team.

For patients undergoing a fundoplication via the transthoracic or thoracotomy approach, lung isolation will necessitate the use of either a double lumen endotracheal tube (DLT) or bronchial blocker through a standard ETT, as well as a fiberoptic bronchoscopy setup to assess proper positioning of this equipment.

## Intraoperative Management

**Induction and airway**: For patients with airways not predicted to be difficult, induction of general anesthesia will typically consist of a RSI with insertion of a single lumen ETT or a DLT depending on the approach described above. In patients with a history of difficult intubation or predicted difficult airway based on physical exam, it is important to consider an awake fiberoptic intubation.

**Anesthetic management**: General anesthesia may be maintained with either inhaled volatile agents or a TIVA. The MAP should generally be maintained close to preoperative values (classically defined as within 20% of baseline).

For those undergoing a fundoplication via a transthoracic or thoracotomy approach, the patient will likely need to be on one lung ventilation (OLV) for left lung isolation. Appropriate positioning of the bronchial blocker or DLT is critical.

Due to their underlying disease, these patients also may have difficulty with PO intake which may result in malnourishment or a greater degree of dehydration than typical fluid deficit calculations would suggest. Assuming hemodynamic stability, fluid management goals for fundoplications are to replace any deficits and maintain euvolemia. If the patient becomes hypotensive despite adequately replenishing preoperative fluid deficits, however, a 10 mL/kg crystalloid fluid bolus may be considered assuming no relative contraindications or preexisting conditions that may be exacerbated by more volume (i.e., CHF). Persistent hypotension is commonly a result of a reduced SVR secondary to the pharmacologic effects of general anesthetic drugs, which can be mitigated by titrated doses of a pure vasopressor (phenylephrine) or combination vasopressor/inotrope (ephedrine, norepinephrine).

Just as these patients are at higher risk for aspiration during induction, despite attempted surgical repair they are also at a high aspiration risk on emergence and should therefore be extubated awake and following commands. A nasogastric tube is usually placed for postoperative decompression, which will effectively reduce the risk of significant aspiration. Recovery in the PACU is usually adequate, followed by transfer to a floor unit for further management.

**Analgesic management**: Multimodal analgesia techniques have been shown to be beneficial in speeding recovery and decreasing length of stay in patients recovering from many different types of surgical procedures including colorectal, urologic, and hepatobiliary surgeries [8–10]. Interventions such as preoperative gabapentin, preoperative and intraoperative acetaminophen, and intraoperative ketamine and ketorolac may reduce the opioid requirements and improve patient comfort. Additionally, intraoperatively, a balance of long (hydromorphone) and short acting (fentanyl, sufentanil) opioids can be titrated for surgical stimuli and early postoperative comfort. For patients receiving an open abdominal approach, an epidural or bilateral transverse abdominis plane (TAP) blocks can greatly reduce the need for parenteral analgesics. For patients receiving a posterolateral thoracotomy for fundoplication, neuraxial anesthesia is highly recommended either by thoracic epidural, a paravertebral catheter, or single shot paravertebral blocks. Indeed, neuraxial analgesia will promote post-anesthetic lung expansion, ambulation, comfort, and wound healing [11, 12].

The following Table 14.1 summarizes the important considerations, from an anesthetic perspective, for fundoplication/hiatal hernia surgery.

## Esophagectomy Surgery

### Baseline Considerations

**Pathology**: Esophagectomy is most commonly performed to resect neoplastic disease. Occasionally, it may also be indicated for intractable esophageal stricture, severe recurrent GERD, or achalasia [13]. Depending on the target location of the intervention (upper, middle, or lower esophagus), esophagectomy may be performed through a variety of incisions and surgical techniques. In all approaches, the stomach is mobilized into the thorax and anastomosed with the remaining esophageal tissue to form a neotube.

**Procedure technique**: There are several approaches for an esophagectomy, each with a different incision profile and each ideal for specific pathologic regions. The following Table 14.2

**Table 14.1** Surgical approaches for fundoplication/hiatal hernia surgery, with important considerations for each technique

| Approach | Abdominal laparoscopic | Abdominal open | Transthoracic |
|---|---|---|---|
| Surgical incision/ports | 5 abdominal ports | Midline laparotomy | Left posterolateral thoracotomy |
| Positioning | Supine versus lithotomy; steep reverse Trendelenburg | Supine | Right lateral decubitus; hip flexion |
| Access | 1–2× IVs (at least one 18 g or larger) | 1–2× IVs (at least one 18 g or larger) | 2× IVs (at least one 18 g or larger) |
| Airway | Single lumen ETT | Single lumen ETT | DLT or single lumen ETT with bronchial blocker |
| Induction | Consider RSI and aspiration precautions | Consider RSI and aspiration precautions | Consider RSI and aspiration precautions |
| Maintenance | Inhaled balanced anesthetic or TIVA | Inhaled balanced anesthetic or TIVA | Inhaled balanced anesthetic or TIVA |
| Fluid management | Euvolemia | Euvolemia | Euvolemia |
| Analgesic | Multimodal | Multimodal; consider neuraxial or regional | Multimodal; consider neuraxial |
| Emergence | Awake extubation | Awake extubation | Awake extubation |

**Table 14.2** The standard approaches for esophagectomies with associated incision sites, surgical targets, and specific considerations [14, 15]

| Esophagectomy approach | Incision(s) | Target | Advantages/disadvantages and considerations |
|---|---|---|---|
| Transhiatal | • Midline laparotomy<br>• L cervical incision | • Lower esophagus | • No thoracotomy<br>• Blind mid thoracic dissection |
| Transthoracic (Ivor Lewis) | • Midline laparotomy<br>• R thoracotomy | • Middle esophagus<br>• Lower esophagus | • Direct visualization<br>• Thoracotomy<br>• One lung ventilation |
| Three hole (McKeown) | • Midline laparotomy<br>• R thoracotomy<br>• L cervical incision | • Middle esophagus | • Direct visualization<br>• Thoracotomy<br>• One lung ventilation |
| Minimally invasive | • 4 thoracic ports<br>• 5 laparoscopic ports<br>• ± L cervical incision | • Variable targets | • Thoracoscopy<br>• One lung ventilation<br>• Long procedure<br>• Improved, morbidity, mortality, and quality of life |
| Thoracoabdominal | • L Thoracoabdominal | • GE junction<br>• Lower, esophagus | • Thoracotomy<br>• One lung ventilation |

lists the common approaches. Importantly for the anesthesiologist, the Ivor Lewis and McKeown approaches involve a thoracotomy incision and OLV.

## Preoperative Evaluation and Concerns; Operating Room Preparation

A full history and physical exam should be conducted with special attention paid to the airway, cardiac function, and pulmonary function. In these cases, there are many perioperative factors that cause increased stress on the cardiovascular system including one lung ventilation, hypoxemia, hemorrhage, dysrhythmias, and pain. These patients should therefore be evaluated for cardiovascular risk in accordance to the ASA and the American College of Cardiology/American Heart Association (ACC/AHA) guidelines [16, 17]. For potential thoracotomy or thoracoscopy cases, patients with significant morbid obesity or chronic lung disease may also benefit from preoperative pulmonary function testing to gauge the ability to tolerate the one lung ventilation likely to be employed for extended periods of time.

Those with esophageal malignancies typically receive adjuvant or neoadjuvant chemotherapy and radiation therapy in the perioperative period. Careful evaluation of the airway should be a priority in these patients given the friability and change in tissue compliance of the upper airway in the setting of radiation therapy [18]. Additionally, chemotherapy agents may cause bone marrow suppression and immunosuppression, which by effect can result in significant frailty and a reduced tolerance to the vasodilating and myocardial depressant effects of general anesthetics.

The degree of intravenous access obtained for the surgery depends, in part, on approach. Due to the esophagus' proximity to the major thoracic vessels, two peripheral intravenous catheters are recommended (18 gauge or larger) to ensure the ability to quickly administer volume in the event of heavy bleeding. Complex dissections and thoracotomy incisions also increase the potential for volume loss and bleeding, necessitating good intravenous access. A central venous line provides more definitive access, the ability to deliver vasopressors and inotropes not suitable for peripheral administration and provides the ability to trend a central venous pressure. It should be noted that a central venous pressure has not been shown to consistently correlate with total blood volume. The decision to insert a central venous line is patient and provider-dependent. An arterial line is recommended to gauge the response to volume loss and volume administration, and to immediately quantify systemic hypotension from great vessel compression that can occur with manual dissection and manipulation of the esophagus. A blood type and screen is a minimum requirement, and more extensive procedures (those with a heavy thoracic component) or patients with baseline anemia should have a preoperative type and crossmatch performed.

An epidural is frequently placed for intraoperative and postoperative analgesia, especially when a thoracotomy incision will be utilized. Furthermore, decreased inflammation and increased capillary flow at the anastomotic site are potential positive effects from epidural local anesthetic [19].

### Intraoperative Management

**Induction and airway**: With the operative indication commonly being neoplasm rather than reflux, an RSI is not always indicated but should be considered if the latter is present. As noted above, a difficult airway should be anticipated with extensive neck radiation, especially with fixed submental tissues or decreased neck range of motion. These patients may warrant video laryngoscopy, emergency airway preparations, and/or an awake fiberoptic intubation. For the transhiatal approach, a single lumen, appropriately-sized ETT should be sufficient, whereas approaches involving thoracotomy or thoracoscopy typically require lung isolation, thus warranting placement of a DLT or a single lumen ETT with a right-sided bronchial blocker.

**Anesthetic and analgesic management**: General anesthesia may be maintained with either inhaled volatile agents or a TIVA. The MAP should generally be maintained close to preoperative values (classically defined as within 20% of baseline).

For those cases necessitating a thoracotomy or thoracoscopy, the patient will likely need to be on one lung ventilation (OLV) for right lung isolation. Appropriate positioning of the bronchial blocker or DLT is critical.

Hemodynamic, fluid, and analgesic management goals for esophagectomy cases are interrelated and to some extent are affected by the notion that iatrogenic vasopressor administration will impede blood flow to a tenuous surgical anastomosis. While published data is not robust, animal and human studies suggest the following [20–22]:

- In the setting of euvolemia, a normal dose range of vasopressor or vasopressor/inotrope, to counteract either vasodilating general anesthetics or a sympathectomy from a local anesthetic epidural, does not affect anastomosis integrity.
- High dose administration of vasopressor or vasopressor/inotrope, in the setting of volume depletion and/or anemia, may reduce anastomotic perfusion.
- Intraoperative epidural local anesthetic infusion has not been shown to affect anastomosis integrity.

Additionally, the literature speculates that local anesthetic epidurals reduce inflammation and increase capillary blood flow at the anastomotic site [19]. Based on these results, euvolemia, multimodal analgesia that includes epidural infusion, and titrated vasopressor to maintain systemic vascular resistance would seem most effective. The disputable practice at many centers is to avoid all use of vasopressors in lieu of volume, which can result in significant positive fluid loads resulting in postoperative respiratory failure and volume overload-induced heart failure [23]. Also confounding conservative management is the oftentimes incomplete understanding of the patient's volume status to gauge the need for fluid. Specifically, chronic beta blockade, abdominal insufflation, and one lung ventilation will affect heart rate, urine output, and pulse pressure variation, respectively. Additionally, central venous pressures do not solely trend volume status and can also vary from one lung ventilation. Stroke volume variation and stroke volume index, as measure from arterial waveform analysis, may prove useful in a goal directed approach, but data is needed specifically for the esophagectomy surgical population [24].

Care should be taken to extubate the patient awake and upon confirmation of solid unassisted pulmonary mechanics and gas exchange, since noninvasive positive pressure support can damage the anastomosis site. A nasogastric tube is usually placed and secured for postoperative decompression, which will reduce the risk of any significant aspiration. Immediate recovery in a PACU versus intensive care unit (ICU) is institution specific, but most patients will ultimately transfer to an ICU for 1–2 days postoperatively.

## Postoperative Management for Common Esophageal Surgeries

### Postoperative Complications and Considerations

The postoperative considerations and management for patients after esophageal surgery are broad and largely dependent on the specific procedure performed. As with any patient who receives general anesthesia, global considerations and complications in the postoperative esophageal surgery patient include monitoring for early postoperative surgical complications (i.e., bleeding), ensuring adequate respiratory effort, providing analgesic support, and screening for common post-anesthetic issues (nausea, vomiting, delirium). Some caveats of postoperative care are listed below.

**Hemodynamic and fluid management**: Typically, patient blood pressure should be maintained near the preoperative baseline and fluid resuscitation should target euvolemia. Hypotension is not uncommon postoperatively for patients receiving major esophageal surgery and has a broad differential including the common etiologies of residual anesthetic agents, hypovolemia, and sympathectomy from neuraxial local anesthesia. In the case of residual sedation and neuraxial blockade, after euvolemia has been achieved, low dose vasopressor can be used to increase vascular tone. As stated previously, a discussion should be had regarding the use of vasopressors or combination vasopressor/inotropes in the setting of a fresh esophagostomy anastomosis. If volume is desired over vasopressor, care should be taken not to incite the side effects of volume overload such as heart failure and pulmonary edema. Invasive arterial line monitoring and urine output are often helpful in fluid status assessment, coupled at some centers with trending stroke volume variation/indices, central venous filling pressures, venous oxygen saturations, serum lactates, and/or cardiac outputs.

**Respiratory insufficiency**: For those patients with respiratory insufficiency postoperatively, the differential is broad but includes more generic post-anesthetic etiologies like residual neuromuscular blockade, upper airway obstruction, splinting from pain or excessive opioid administration. Thoracotomy pain, particularly inhibitory to inspiratory effort, should be treated appropriately to allow for adequate re-expansion of collapsed alveoli and prevention of atelectasis. Due to the location of these surgeries, the differential diagnosis should also include bronchospasm, aspiration, pneumothorax, and pneumomediastinum.

Persistent respiratory insufficiency usually necessitates a chest radiograph and arterial blood gas analysis to rule out gross pathology and quantify the derangement in gas exchange. If respiratory failure requires assistance, positive pressure mask ventilation should be minimized or avoided in those patients who contain esophageal anastomotic sites as this can strain the suture lines. If reintubation is necessary, the risk of an unintentional esophageal intubation following an esophagectomy can result in anastomotic disruption. The decision to reintubate a patient following an esophagectomy should be made prior to the onset of full respiratory distress and should be managed by the most experienced provider available.

**Nausea/vomiting**: Baseline risk factors for postoperative nausea and vomiting include young age, female sex, and history of postoperative nausea and vomiting. Beyond these elements, patients with previous esophageal stricture or obstruction may have acute worsening of reflux after EGD with stent placement. Fortunately, suctioning of the stomach, coupled with decompression via a nasogastric tube, lowers the risk of significant aspiration or emesis. Rescue treatment for postoperative nausea and vomiting should be in accordance with the Society of Ambulatory Anesthesia and ASA guidelines [25, 26]. Prophylactic preoperative and intraoperative

**Table 14.3** Summary of anesthetic considerations for common esophageal surgeries

| Procedure | EGD stenting | Fundoplication | Esophagectomy |
|---|---|---|---|
| Surgical approach/incision | Oral | • Laparoscopic abdominal<br>• Open abdominal<br>• Transthoracic | • Transverse cervical + laparotomy + R thoracotomy<br>• Laparotomy + neck<br>• Laparotomy + R thoracotomy<br>• Thoracoabdominal |
| Positioning | Supine | • Supine<br>• Lithotomy<br>• Right lateral decubitus | • L lateral decubitus<br>• Supine |
| Access | 1× IV | 1–2× IVs (at least one 18 g or larger) | 2× IVs (at least 18 g or larger), consider arterial and central venous lines |
| Airway | Single lumen ETT | Single lumen ETT versus DLT or single lumen ETT with bronchial blocker, depending on approach | Single lumen ETT versus DLT or single lumen ETT with bronchial blocker, depending on approach |
| Induction | Consider RSI and aspiration precautions | Consider RSI and aspiration precautions | Consider difficult airway in the setting of extensive radiation therapy |
| Maintenance | Inhaled balanced anesthetic or TIVA | Inhaled balanced anesthetic or TIVA | Inhaled balanced anesthetic or TIVA |
| Fluid/blood management | Euvolemia/no blood typing | Euvolemia/usually type and screen | Euvolemia/usually type and cross |
| Analgesic | Balanced and multimodal with minimal requirements | Multimodal; consider neuraxial for open procedures | Multimodal with neuraxial anesthesia |
| Emergence | Awake extubation | Awake extubation | Awake extubation |
| Surgery specific postoperative concerns | • Nausea/vomiting<br>• Stent collapse or malpositioning<br>• Dysphagia<br>• Esophageal perforation<br>• Pneumomediastinum | • Nausea/vomiting<br>• Dysphagia | • Analgesic management<br>• Respiratory insufficiency<br>• Hemodynamic instability<br>• Pulmonary Edema |

therapies include singular or combination use of scopolamine, propofol, aprepitant, ondansetron, dexamethasone, and/or acetaminophen, as well as minimizing pro-emetic drugs (i.e., etomidate, volatile anesthetics). Rescue therapies in the recovery room include ondansetron, diphenhydramine, low dose propofol, haloperidol, and promethazine.

## Summary

The perioperative considerations for anesthetic management of esophageal surgery patients can vary widely depending on the patient's underlying pathology, surgical approach, and other comorbidities. As with any patient scheduled to receive anesthesia, a full history and physical should be performed. In this patient population, it is imperative that the anesthesiologist assess and identify the severity and extensiveness of the patient's disease process(es), particularly those affecting the airway, ability to swallow, or pertaining to gastroesophageal reflux. As with any surgical patient, decisions regarding anesthetic management ultimately depends on weighting the risks and benefits of a multitude of factors, as described above in more detail. The following is a summary Table 14.3 highlighting some of the considerations for the common esophageal surgical procedures discussed in this chapter.

## References

1. Kuo B, Urma D. Esophagus—anatomy and development. Part 1 Oral Cavity, pharynx and esophagus. GI Motility online. 2006. doi: https://doi.org/10.1038/gimo6.
2. Linden PA. Chapter 29. Overview. In: Sugarbaker DJ, Bueno R, Krasna MJ, Mentzer SJ, Zellos L, editors. Adult chest surgery. New York, NY: McGraw-Hill; 2009. http://accesssurgery.mhmedical.com.proxy.library.emory.edu/content.aspx?bookid=427&sectionid=40372668. Accessed 30 Mar 2017.
3. Krasna M, Ebright M. Chapter 10. Overview. In: Sugarbaker DJ, Bueno R, Krasna MJ, Mentzer SJ, Zellos L, editors. Adult chest surgery. New York, NY: McGraw-Hill; 2009. http://accesssurgery.mhmedical.com.proxy.library.emory.edu/content.aspx?bookid=427&sectionid=40372647. Accessed 30 Mar 2017.
4. American Society of Anesthesiologists Committee. Practice guidelines for preoperative fasting and the use of pharmacologic agents to reduce the risk of pulmonary aspiration: application to healthy patients undergoing elective procedures: an updated report by the American Society of Anesthesiologists Committee on Standards and Practice Parameters. Anes. 2011;114(3):495–511. https://doi.org/10.1097/ALN.0b013e3181fcbfd9.
5. El-Serag HB, Sweet S, Winchester CC, Dent J. Update on the epidemiology of gastro-oesophageal reflux disease: a systematic review. Gut. 2014 Jun;63(6):871–80. https://doi.org/10.1136/gutjnl-2012-304269.
6. Broeders JA, Rijnhart-de Jong HG, Draaisma WA, Bredenoord AJ, Smout AJ, Gooszen HG. Ten-year outcome of laparoscopic and conventional nissen fundoplication: randomized clinical trial. Ann Surg. 2009 Nov;250(5):698–706. https://doi.org/10.1097/SLA.0b013e3181bcdaa7.
7. Du X, Hu Z, Yan C, Zhang C, Wang Z, Wu J. A meta-analysis of long follow-up outcomes of laparoscopic Nissen (total) versus Toupet (270°) fundoplication for gastro-esophageal reflux disease based on randomized controlled trials in adults. BMC Gastroenterol. 2016;16(1):88. https://doi.org/10.1186/s12876-016-0502-8.
8. Spanjersberg WR, Reurings J, Keus F, van Laarhoven CJ. Fast track surgery versus conventional recovery strategies for colorectal surgery. Cochrane Database Syst Rev. 2011;2:CD007635. https://doi.org/10.1002/14651858.CD007635.pub2.
9. Azhar RA, Bochner B, Catto J, Goh AC, Kelly J, Patel HD, Pruthi RS, Thalmann GN, Desai M. Enhanced recovery after urological surgery: a contemporary systematic review of outcomes, key elements, and research needs. Eur Urol. 2016;70(1):176–87. https://doi.org/10.1016/j.eururo.2016.02.051.
10. Melloul E, Hübner M, Scott M, Snowden C, Prentis J, Dejong CH, Garden OJ, Farges O, Kokudo N, Vauthey JN, Clavien PA, Demartines N. Guidelines for perioperative care for liver surgery: enhanced recovery after surgery (ERAS) society recommendations. World J Surg. 2016;40(10):2425–40. https://doi.org/10.1007/s00268-016-3700-1.
11. Giménez-Milà M, Klein AA, Martinez G. Design and implementation of an enhanced recovery program in thoracic surgery. J Thorac Dis. 2016;8(Suppl 1):S37–45. https://doi.org/10.3978/j.issn.2072-1439.2015.10.71.
12. Li W, Li Y, Huang Q, Ye S, Rong T. Short and long-term outcomes of epidural or intravenous analgesia after esophagectomy: a propensity-matched cohort study. PLoS One. 2016;11(4):e0154380. https://doi.org/10.1371/journal.pone.0154380.
13. Madenci AL, Reames BN, Chang AC, Lin J, Orringer MB, Reddy RM. Factors associated with rapid progression to esophagectomy for benign disease. J Am Coll Surg. 2013;217(5):889–95. https://doi.org/10.1016/j.jamcollsurg.2013.07.384.
14. Peyre CG, Sugarbaker DJ. Three-hole esophagectomy: the brigham and Women's hospital approach. In: Sugarbaker DJ, Bueno R, Colson YL, Jaklitsch MT, Krasna MJ, Mentzer SJ, Williams M, Adams A, editors. Adult chest surgery. 2nd ed. New York, NY: McGraw-Hill; 2014.
15. Zeng J, Liu JS. Quality of life after three kinds of esophagectomy for cancer. World J Gastroenterol. 2012;18(36):5106–13. https://doi.org/10.3748/wjg.v18.i36.5106.
16. Committee on Standards and Practice Parameters, Apfelbaum JL, et al. Practice advisory for preanesthesia evaluation: an updated report by the American Society of Anesthesiologists Task Force on preanesthesia evaluation. Anes. 2012;116(3):533–8. https://doi.org/10.1097/ALN.0b013e31823c1067.
17. Fleisher LA, Fleischmann KE, Auerbach AD, Barnason SA, Beckman JA, Bozkurt B, Davila-Roman VG, Gerhard-Herman MD, Holly TA, Kane GC, Marine JE, Nelson MT, Spencer CC, Thompson A, Ting HH, Uretsky BF, Wijeysundera DN. 2014 ACC/AHA guideline on perioperative cardiovascular evaluation and management of patients undergoing noncardiac surgery: executive summary: a report of the American College of Cardiology/American Heart Association Task Force on Practice Guidelines. Circulation. 2012;130(24):2215–45. https://doi.org/10.1161/CIR.0000000000000105.
18. Iseli TA, Iseli CE, Golden JB, Jones VL, Boudreaux AM, Boyce JR, Weeks DM, Carroll WR. Outcomes of intubation in difficult airways due to head and neck pathology. Ear Nose Throat J. 2012;91(3):E1–5.
19. Ng JM. Update on anesthetic management for esophagectomy. Curr Opin Anaesthesiol. 2011;24(1):37–43. https://doi.org/10.1097/ACO.0b013e32834141f7.
20. Al-Rawi OY, Pennefather SH, Page RD, Dave I, Russell GN. The effect of thoracic epidural bupivacaine and an intravenous adrenaline infusion on gastric tube blood flow during esophagectomy. Anesth Analg. 2008;106(3):884–7. https://doi.org/10.1213/ane.0b013e318164f153.

21. Klijn E, Niehof S, de Jonge J, Gommers D, Ince C, van Bommel J. The effect of perfusion pressure on gastric tissue blood flow in an experimental gastric tube model. Anesth Analg. 2010;110(2):541–6. https://doi.org/10.1213/ANE.0b013e3181c84e33.
22. Theodorou D, Drimousis PG, Larentzakis A, Papalois A, Toutouzas KG, Katsaragakis S. The effects of vasopressors on perfusion of gastric graft after esophagectomy. An experimental study. J Gastrointest Surg. 2008;12(9):1497–501. https://doi.org/10.1007/s11605-008-0575-y.
23. Wei S, Tian J, Song X, Chen Y. Association of perioperative fluid balance and adverse surgical outcomes in esophageal cancer and esophagogastric junction cancer. Ann Thorac Surg. 2008;86(1):266–72. https://doi.org/10.1016/j.athoracsur.2008.03.017.
24. Hand WR, Stoll WD, McEvoy MD, McSwain JR, Sealy CD, Skoner JM, Hornig JD, Tennant PA, Wolf B, Day TA. Intraoperative goal-directed hemodynamic management in free tissue transfer for head and neck cancer. Head Neck. 2016;38(Suppl 1):E1974–80. https://doi.org/10.1002/hed.24362.
25. Gan TJ, Diemunsch P, Habib AS, Kovac A, Kranke P, Meyer TA, Watcha M, Chung F, Angus S, Apfel CC, Bergese SD, Candiotti KA, Chan MT, Davis PJ, Hooper VD, Lagoo-Deenadayalan S, Myles P, Nezat G, Philip BK, Tramèr MR, Society for Ambulatory Anesthesia. Consensus guidelines for the management of postoperative nausea and vomiting. Anesth Analg. 2014;118(1):85–113. https://doi.org/10.1213/ANE.0000000000000002.
26. Apfelbaum JL, Silverstein JH, Chung FF, Connis RT, Fillmore RB, Hunt SE, Nickinovich DG, Schreiner MS, Silverstein JH, Apfelbaum JL, Barlow JC, Chung FF, Connis RT, Fillmore RB, Hunt SE, Joas TA, Nickinovich DG, Schreiner MS, American Society of Anesthesiologists Task Force on Postanesthetic Care. Practice guidelines for postanesthetic care: an updated report by the American Society of Anesthesiologists Task Force on Postanesthetic Care. Anes. 2013;118(2):291–307. https://doi.org/10.1097/ALN.0b013e31827773e9.

# Anesthesia for Pleural and Chest Wall Surgery

## 15

Jonathan Rost, Jeffery Gerritsen, and Talia K. Ben-Jacob

## Introduction

As the incidence of lung cancer increases, the frequency with which chest wall and pleural cavity surgery occurs is likely to increase as well. Tumor invasion of the chest wall requiring resection and reconstruction, pleurodesis and drainage of malignant effusions will also rise in synchrony with cancer incidence [1]. The rise in these surgeries is in addition to the number of congenital chest wall diseases already being repaired regularly.

While pleurodesis is on the rise as the incidence of lung cancer increases, there has been a reduction in the amount of pleural cavity surgery performed to treat tuberculosis and empyema due to improvements of medical management and minimally invasive techniques. Decortication is the most commonly performed pleural cavity surgery and it involves excision of an empyema sac and/or thickened pleura from the lung and chest wall and can be done with a minimally invasive approach. However, anesthesiologists need to be aware of the Clagett procedure, rib resections and Eloesser flaps, because while these procedures are decreasing in frequency, they will still be performed when all other options are exhausted and for patients too ill to undergo surgery for thoracotomy, surgical decortication or muscle flap transposition [2, 3].

The Eloesser flap and Claggett's procedure are two surgical treatment options for patients with tuberculosis and pleural space infections associated with bronchopleural fistulae. The purpose of the aforementioned surgeries is to create a one-way valve that would allow the infected fluid from the chest cavity to passively drain without trapping air. The greatest differences between the Eloesser flap and a Clagett window is that the Clagett window is considerably larger and was designed to be a temporary measure to allow decontamination of the pleural space with a subsequent closure.

Chest wall and pleural cavity cases can be very challenging for even the most experienced anesthesiologist. Given the variety of surgical and physiologic derangements that may occur with these surgeries, extensive perioperative communication between the surgeon and the anesthesiologist is required for improved outcomes. Discussion should focus on intraoperative and post-operative physiologic changes, highlighting the mechanics of ventilation and the degree of surgical intervention needed. Additional discussion centered on surgical stimulation and postoperative pain management are warranted.

J. Rost, M.D. · J. Gerritsen, M.D.
Department of Anesthesiology,
Cooper University Hospital, Camden, NJ, USA
e-mail: Rost-Jonathan@cooperhealth.edu;
Gerritsen-Jeffrey@cooperhealth.edu

T. K. Ben-Jacob, M.D. (✉)
Division of Critical Care, Department of Anesthesiology, Cooper Medical School of Rowan University, Cooper University Hospital, Camden, NJ, USA
e-mail: ben-jacob-talia@CooperHealth.edu

## Preoperative Considerations

Patient who present for chest wall and/or pleural cavity surgery may often be weak and debilitated and they may often have difficulty at their pre-surgical baseline with oxygenation or ventilation. Severe chest wall deformities are often associated with restrictive lung defects. These patients may also be at risk for arrhythmias and outflow tract obstructions given heart location and displacement [4]. The preoperative evaluation should focus on the extent and severity of pulmonary disease and cardiovascular involvement. Patients in poor general health, at extremes of age, or with chronic obstructive pulmonary disease are known to be at increased risk for postoperative complications [4].

A thorough history and physical exam should be performed. In addition to the standard questions asked, areas of focus should include: quantitation of dyspnea, characteristics of cough and sputum, smoking status, and exercise tolerance. Also, if a patient is presenting for resection of chest wall cancer, investigation into chemotherapy regimen is important as agents such as adriamycin can be cardiotoxic and bleomycin will affect the lungs [5, 6]. Included in the physical exam should be a focus on the respiratory system. Patients need to be evaluated for breathing pattern and rate, baseline oxygen saturation, breath sounds, presence of pulmonary hypertension and cardiac murmur. Presence of wheezing, abnormal breath sounds, rales, or tracheal deviation suggest the need for further work up [7].

Preoperative studies that may need to be performed before thoracic wall and pleural surgery include: chest X-Ray (CXR), electrocardiogram (ECG), arterial blood gas (ABG), pulmonary function tests (PFTs), chest computerized tomography (CT) scan, cardiac stress test and/or evaluation of exercise function [8, 9]. CXR is required for evaluation of preexisting lung disease and the pre-op CXR can serve as a comparison study following empyema or other drainage procedures. Often times a CXR is not sufficient and CT scan may be required. Chest CT also provides information with regard to airway obstruction and chest wall deformities [8]. It aids the anesthesiologist in determining whether or not they can safely pass an endotracheal tube into the trachea, especially in the case of airway or anterior chest wall tumors. Pulmonary function tests (PFTs) are performed to aid in the assessment of baseline respiratory function. Severe chest wall deformities are often associated with restrictive lung defects; the implication for intraoperative management may be significant depending on the surgery planned. Pleural effusions or empyema often affect diffusion capacity of the lungs. Preoperative PFTs allow the anesthesiologist to determine the likelihood a patient will tolerate one lung ventilation and can help predict whether or not the patient is at increased risked for postoperative pulmonary complications. They can also predict the degree to which the pre-existing conditions may compromise the ability to ventilate adequately during the procedure [10, 11]. Patients with known COPD, asthma and emphysema should undergo baseline PFT testing. PFT results showing forced expiratory volume in 1 s (FEV1) $\leq 50\%$ normal or $\leq 600$ mL, Vital capacity (VC) $\leq 1700$ mL and hypoventilation of large part of the lungs expressed as a FEV1/VC ratio $\leq 32–58\%$ inform the anesthesia provider who is at risk for hypoventilation, hypercapnia, and other respiratory complications in the intraoperative and postoperative period.

A preoperative ABG will allow the anesthesiologist to determine the severity of the patient's underlying lung disease and also help predict if the patient is at increased risk for postoperative respiratory complications. Patients with a low PO2 and oxygen saturation of less than 90% on room air at baseline are at higher risk for postoperative complications including prolonged ventilation. In addition, patients who are hypercapnic (PaCO2 > 50 mmHg) on baseline ABG are at increased risk for poor outcomes as anesthesia can worsen hypercapnia leading to somnolence and prolonged intubation postoperatively.

Cardiac testing includes EKG, exercise stress testing and cardiac ultrasound [9]. Many of the patients presenting with chest wall deformities and large volumes in the pleural cavity are at increased risk for arrhythmias and outflow tract obstruction. This is due to cardiac displacement from the underlying disease and may require evaluation [4, 9]. Asymptomatic patients with no signs of concerning pathology on CXR or CT need no further evaluation than an EKG while preoperative cardiac testing should increase as symptoms or radiologic findings worsen. Further testing can include an echocardiogram or nuclear stress test.

Pulmonary and cardiac complications continue to be the major sources of morbidity and mortality for these patients [9]. Therefore, as with any surgical patient, patients should be evaluated and medically optimized by their primary care physician, cardiologist and/or pulmonologist prior to surgery. However, in the setting of emergent Eloesser flap and Claggett's procedures, patients are often unable to undergo testing given the acuity of the underlying illness and should be managed with the preoperative data that is available.

## Intraoperative Considerations

### Monitoring

Routine monitoring during chest wall and pleural cavity surgery should include pulse oximetry, end-tidal capnography, electrocardiogram, invasive or noninvasive blood pressure, and temperature. A Foley catheter is necessary during long procedures and in unstable patients; it may also be necessary when epidural analgesia is planned. Bispectral index or processed EEG can be considered. Arterial line placement is not required but should be considered for patient-specific factors or if surgical intervention may result in excessive blood loss or cause rapid hemodynamic changes. In certain procedures such as pectus excavatum repair (Nuss procedure), the anesthesiologist must be prepared for the possibility of hemorrhage, with appropriate intravenous (IV) access planned [12]. Invasive hemodynamic monitors such as central venous pressure (CVP) and pulmonary artery (PA) catheter are not indicated unless there are significant patient-specific factors such as severe lung disease, myocardial ischemia or anatomic vascular restrictions. A dynamic index such as stroke volume variation or other similar monitor may be used if blood loss is expected to be significant. The Nuss procedure also includes a risk of arrhythmia and hemodynamic disturbances from cardiac compression, requiring vigilance in monitoring hemodynamics during key portions of the case.

### Choice of Anesthetic

There are a variety of anesthetic options for pleural cavity procedures depending on the method and extent of surgery necessary, the need for lung isolation and the preference of the patient. Though most cases do not require lung isolation, when needed, general anesthesia with double lumen tube placement or bronchial blocker placement is utilized. Smaller procedures without lung isolation may be performed under epidural or regional anesthesia such as thoracic paravertebral block. Some procedures such as pleural effusion drainage, pleural biopsy, drainage of empyema, evacuation of hematoma, chest wall biopsy or lung biopsy may be performed under local anesthesia with monitored anesthesia care [13].

For patients having general anesthesia, choice of anesthetic agent involves the usual concerns including need for anesthesia, analgesia, and paralysis to facilitate mechanical ventilation and surgical exposure. Intravenous induction will typically involve administration of propofol, ketamine or etomidate, an opiate, and likely a muscle relaxant to facilitate intubation. Maintenance can be provided by inhaled or intravenous methods. Nitrous oxide should be avoided whenever pneumothorax might occur and as it will also expand the volume of blebs or endotracheal tube cuffs it should generally be discouraged in this population. Additional concerns in some instances include maintenance of hemodynamic stability and effects of agents on hypoxic pulmonary vasoconstriction. Generally, the intravenous anesthesia agents have less effect on hypoxic pulmonary vasoconstriction than do volatile agents [14]. In practice, the differences between the newer inhaled and intravenous agents effect on arterial oxygenation are minimal at clinically effective doses [15]. Avoidance of coughing and straining on emergence may be important in some chest wall surgeries to avoid development of subcutaneous emphysema. Administration of opiate, lidocaine, or dexmedetomidine may be useful to reduce coughing and straining during emergence.

## Lung Isolation

Lung isolation may be required in chest wall surgery that also involves the thoracic cavity. It is typically not required in the Nuss procedure as $CO_2$ insufflation during thoracoscopy is adequate. If lung isolation is needed, it can be achieved using a bronchial blocker or double lumen endobronchial tube after interdisciplinary discussion with the surgical team and evaluation of the patient's particular situation.

A double lumen endobronchial tube has many advantages in that it allows better suctioning and CPAP to the deflated lung and better facilitates intermittent ventilation if needed. If a patient will require awake fiberoptic intubation, needs to remain intubated postoperatively or starts with a pre-existing endotracheal tube or tracheostomy with small stoma a bronchial blocker may be the preferred option. Placement of bronchial blocker or double lumen tube should be confirmed by fiberoptic bronchoscopy immediately prior to initiation of lung isolation and one lung ventilation. As with any case where one lung ventilation is employed, the anesthesiologist should remain vigilant for early detection and treatment of hypoxemia and hypercarbia.

Of particular interest are patients requiring one lung ventilation for pleural cavity surgery to treat bronchopleural fistula (BPF). A bronchopleural fistula is an opening between the pleural space and the central bronchial tree. This can occur due to trauma, infection, carcinoma, rupture of a bleb or most commonly after lung resection or pneumonectomy. Lung isolation in BPF cases is critically important to avoid significant air leak with positive pressure ventilation or more concerning, the development of tension pneumothorax. The patient should either have a pre-existing chest tube on the affected side or have one placed prior to induction of anesthesia and attached to active suction. An ideal scenario to avoid air leak from the affected bronchus is for an awake intubation with a double lumen tube with the bronchial tip placed into the healthy bronchus under direct visualization with fiberoptic bronchoscopy. However, awake intubation with a double lumen tube is quite challenging even with excellent topicalization and a cooperative patient. An alternative is for an inhalational induction with preservation of spontaneous respiration, standard laryngoscopy with initial placement of the bronchial cuff high in the trachea, then proceeding with fiberoptic bronchoscopy to guide the tip into the desired bronchus. Once the correct bronchus has been entered, one lung ventilation can ensue. The above maneuvers may not be necessary in a patient known to have a small BPF with a pre-existing chest tube on suction where a small air leak following standard induction and double lumen intubation is tolerated.

## Positioning

Positioning for chest wall surgery will depend on the location of the surgery and exposure required. Pressure points should always be checked, and positioning should always minimize the risk of nerve injury. Many of these patients will require surgery on the lateral chest wall and standard positioning precautions should help reduce the risks associated with the lateral decubitus position. Of note, the Nuss procedure for pectus excavatum often requires abduction of the left arm to obtain surgical access which has resulted in case reports of brachial plexus injury. Placing the left arm in an arthroscopy sling may reduce this occurrence [16].

## Intraoperative Complications

Serious complications can occur during chest wall surgery. During tumor resection of the chest wall there can be complications depending on the location and size of the tumor and involvement of surrounding structures. Bleeding may be extensive, and injury to the diaphragm or lung can occur. Resections involving three or more contiguous ribs may result in flail chest, leading to respiratory compromise during spontaneous ventilation if chest wall rigidity is not adequately restored during reconstruction. Respiratory complications are common after chest wall tumor resection and respiratory failure is the most common cause of postoperative mortality [17].

During the Nuss Procedure, complications include hemorrhage, pneumothorax, hemothorax, right ventricular puncture, cardiac compression and arrhythmia. The risk of pneumothorax and mediastinal and subcutaneous emphysema following the Nuss procedure continue into the postoperative period [18].

During pleurodesis and decortication surgeries there are infrequent complications of hemorrhage, subcutaneous emphysema and persistent air leak. Greater amounts of infection and scarring will lead to greater risk of hemorrhage. Complicated effusions or empyemas may require conversion from VATS to open thoracotomy on occasion [19]. Patients with active infections may develop sepsis before, during or after surgery and this should always remain high on the differential diagnosis of the anesthesiologist. During open window thoracostomy surgery for bronchopleural fistula there may be difficulty ventilating due to large air leak or development of a tension pneumothorax. Infectious material can spread via bronchopleural fistula to the lungs, compromising respiratory function.

There are a variety of complications that may occur during initiation of one lung ventilation, including airway trauma to teeth, pharynx, larynx, trachea or bronchus. Malposition of the tube tends to occur during surgical manipulation and cause trauma or airway obstruction and a fiberoptic bronchoscope must be available throughout the surgery. Depending on the severity, some complications may require prolonged intubation and hemodynamic support.

## Postoperative Pain Control

Chest wall surgery can be variable in the amount of pain experienced postoperatively depending on the extent of surgery. No matter which type of surgery is performed, pain in this region can be difficult to control because of the constant movement, tension and strain placed on the chest wall required for respiration. The dynamic nature of the chest wall increases nerve irritation after an incision, leading to increased pain. Muscle weakness from deconditioning, changes in chest wall mechanics, and pain can lead to significant post-operative pulmonary complications including atelectasis, pneumonia, and increased hospital stay [20]. The severity of these complications suggests the need to adequately control pain and actively encourage early postoperative pulmonary conditioning. Given the difficulty in controlling pain for a dynamic system, a multi-modal pain control approach is recommended to allow patients maximum relief while limiting adverse effects of individual therapies [21]. Regional anesthesia as a part of this multi-modal pain control approach is highly recommended for its low systemic adverse effect profile and patient comfort with pulmonary conditioning. Anesthesia providers should work closely with their surgical colleagues to determine the extent and exact location of the surgical procedure to determine if regional anesthesia is possible.

Pectoralis plane infiltration, also known as PEC blocks I and II, directly target thoracic wall innervation, specifically the medial and lateral pectoral nerves. Blocking of these nerves would adequately cover pain on the anterior to lateral chest wall which is ideal for superficial or soft-tissue anterior chest wall surgery. These blocks do not adequately cover the lateral or posterior chest wall or pleura, and are not recommended for use with surgeries focused on those areas. These techniques are relatively safe and easy to perform using ultrasound guidance, directly visualizing the pectoralis major, pectoralis minor, and serratus anterior, and their fascial planes. Visualization for placement of the local anesthetic of choice varies between the blocks but may easily be performed in tandem to accomplish the widest block. When used appropriately, these blocks decrease the dose of post-operative narcotic used and decrease VAS pain scores [22]. However, these blocks may be limited both by anatomical coverage and efficacy, as PEC blocks were shown to be inferior to paravertebral block when directly compared in breast surgery, requiring earlier and higher doses of narcotic rescue medication [23].

Thoracic epidural analgesia (TEA) is another popular technique for chest wall surgeries. TEA has a broader range of coverage, encompassing the posterior chest wall and often pleural innervation in addition to the anterior and lateral chest wall. The epidural spread of local anesthetic will also cover the thoracic sympathetic chain at similar levels to spinal nerves, which allows more visceral coverage as well as decreasing autonomic stress response and spinal nerve wind-up response to pain. Leaving an epidural catheter in place allows for an increased duration of pain control. This added pain coverage makes thoracic epidural analgesia an option for a broader range of surgeries including surgery requiring thoracotomy incision, posterior thoracic wall, intrathoracic, or axial skeletal surgery. In at least one study published in the Journal of Pediatric Anesthesia comparing TEA to chest wall catheters, thoracic epidural catheters were more successful for initial pain control after surgery in children undergoing Nuss procedure for pectus excavatum, with pain scores lower on postoperative day 1 [24]. In another study on the same procedure in a similar patient population, thoracic epidural catheters were shown to have lower pain scores to PCA-morphine, and had less incidence of post-operative urinary incontinence and nausea and vomiting [25].

TEA may exert some visceral effect by blocking the thoracic sympathetic chain. Sympathetic block with local anesthetic may lead to both arterial and venous dilation from decreased sympathetic smooth muscle tone, thereby decreasing systemic afterload and preload and reducing systemic blood pressure. For patients without adequate hydration, hypotension can be severe. Tachycardia associated with decreased preload may be undesirable in the patient with vascular or coronary disease or with outflow tract obstruction from anatomical defects. However, the sympathetic blockade may also be associated with decreased systemic catecholamine response and lead to fewer cardiovascular events when compared to traditional IV analgesia [26]. This suggests that patients with significant risk for perioperative cardiac morbidity secondary to increased systemic catecholamines, notably arrhythmia or ischemia, may benefit from TEA analgesia in the postoperative period.

Since the epidural spread of anesthetic is related to the volume infused, continuous TEA catheters allow the dose of anesthetic to be titrated to desired effect. Local anesthetic administered in the thoracic epidural space tends to stay fairly local, as negative thoracic inspiratory pressure keeps the medication from spreading inferiorly to the lumbar level by gravity. This lower volume of infiltration in combination with low concentration decreases the risk of local anesthetic systemic toxicity, though inadvertent intravascular injection may still occur. Given a continuous infusion and possible catheter migration, a high level of monitoring is required throughout the postoperative period. A multidisciplinary discussion with the surgical and medical teams regarding anticoagulation in the perioperative period is warranted if TEA catheter placement is planned.

Paravertebral nerve blocks (PVB) can have similar analgesia coverage to TEA, but because of laterality of placement, these blocks can be used to achieve unilateral blockade. These blocks can be extremely effective for analgesia [23, 27]. However, two studies published in 2017 examined patients receiving thoracotomy for lung tumor resection suggest TEA analgesia can be superior to PVB likely due to the wider block effect possible with TEA [28, 29]. An advantage of PVB compared to TEA is that the anesthesiologist can directly determine which levels are blocked, not relying on spread of medication through the epidural space which is variable. Furthermore, PVB may be possible when TEA may be contraindicated as in spinous process injuries, or the severely intravascularly depleted patient at risk for hypotension or tachycardia with TEA [27]. There also exists the option to leave a paravertebral catheter in place following initial injection for increased duration of analgesia.

Intercostal nerve blocks are similar in both technique and advantages to a paravertebral block, as similar individual thoracic nerves can

**Table 15.1** Table showing the anatomical coverage of each type of nerve block discussed

| Nerve block type | Anatomic coverage for analgesia | | | | | Associated hypotension |
|---|---|---|---|---|---|---|
| | Anterior chest wall | Posterior chest wall | Pleura | Viscera | Unilateral/directional | |
| PEC I and II | + | − | − | − | + | − |
| TEA | + | + | + | + | − | + |
| PVB | + | + | + | + | + | +/− |
| ICNB | + | + | − | − | + | − |
| Intrapleural catheter | − | − | + | + | + | − |

*PEC* pectoralis fascia infiltration, *TEA* thoracic epidural analgesia, *PVB* paravertebral nerve block, *ICNB* intercostal nerve block

be targeted for analgesia which can decrease the need for post-operative narcotic doses [30]. The major theoretical advantage to this technique is a more lateral or peripheral block, allowing for more accurate medication placement as local anesthetic spread is less likely to occur medially to the contralateral side or craniocaudally [31]. This also decreases the risk of inadvertent dura puncture, high spinal, and sympathetic block. The risk of inadvertent pleural puncture and pneumothorax remain present with this technique. Unfortunately, the duration of these blocks is limited by the excellent perfusion of the intercostal area.

Local infiltration of local anesthetics can be prolonged with safe continuous infusion pumps. The surgeon can infiltrate local anesthetic medication, liposomal bupivacaine or insert medication delivery catheters directly into the pleural or surgical plane. This allows for direct analgesia to the site. In a study from the Mayo Clinic, pleural On-Q pumps with low-dose continuous bupivacaine had equal analgesic effects to thoracic epidural catheter after minimally invasive repair of petus excavatum, and even had some implicit patient preference, though this latter measure was not directly measured [32]. The study out of Nemours Children's Hospital at DuPont noted that while TEA catheters had better pain scores on POD 1 of the Nuss procedure, every subsequent day the chest-wall catheters has equal analgesic effect to the TEA group [22]. The On-Q pump allows for continuous low-dose analgesic medication delivery in a safely secured method. This combination allows for maximal safety profile, though is not without theoretical risks; a catheter can always migrate and safety mechanisms must be properly initiated to avoid overdose. There is minimal risk for spinal or nerve injury, hypotension, or inadvertent pneumothorax with direct placement by the surgeon. Table 15.1 shows the anatomical coverage of each type of nerve block discussed.

Opiate medications are unlikely to be avoided entirely in these painful surgeries given their efficacy for analgesia. However, their side-effect profile can be severe and every effort at a balanced analgesic approach is recommended. As some patients cannot tolerate any of the regional techniques listed above, whether from allergy, refusal, or practicality of placement, total parenteral analgesia may occasionally be necessary. Opiate medications are the mainstay of this treatment as their Mu and Kappa agonist activity effectively dulls pain recognition in the central nervous system. The practical anesthesiologist should be aware of the most common and the most dangerous adverse effects of these medications. The most common adverse effects are constipation, post-operative ileus, urinary retention, and sedation. The more dangerous adverse effects are primarily related to respiratory depression at higher doses, which may be necessary to treat the severity of pain these patients experience, yet this population remains at particular risk for complications related to hypoventilation in the postoperative period. As such, other systemic non-opiate adjuncts should be considered: acetaminophen, NSAIDs, neuropathic pain medication such as gabapentin, and/or ketamine. There is also role for non-medication adjuncts, including patient education, music therapy, a TENS device, or hot-cold temperature therapy [21]. It is important to note, however, that a study published in a 2011 Journal of Anesthesia noted that a single dose of perioperative ketamine prior to incision intended to prevent inflammatory cascade response showed no improvement in post-operative pain scores or plasma levels of inflammatory markers in thoracic surgical patients [33].

## Postoperative Complications

The risk for post-operative complications after chest wall surgery is related to the type of surgery and extent of surgical correction of thoracic wall defects. Anesthesiologists need to be aware of these potential complications as often times these patients will need to return the operating room. The most common complications include device malfunction (such as a broken wire in the Nuss Bar placement), pneumothorax, hemothorax, wound infection, hypoxemia, severe pain, post-thoracotomy pain syndrome, pleural effusion and failure of surgical goal [34, 35]. A major concern for patients recovering from chest wall surgery is undertreated pain causing splinting and respiratory insufficiency. When planning an anesthetic and analgesic approach to these cases, the patient's risk for postoperative respiratory failure must be of paramount concern. The decision to recover a patient in the ICU versus a ward bed should take into account the patient's baseline respiratory function, extent of surgical involvement, concern for respiratory insufficiency and additional co-morbidities. The incidence of postoperative hypoxemia related to hypoventilation can be higher after thoracic surgery than for major abdominal surgery, though this is less commonly monitored [35]. Post-Thoracotomy Pain Syndrome (PTPS) is unfortunately common, having an incidence of 25–60% of thoracotomy incisions [36]. Longer hospital stay and increased post-operative opiate use in the first three days after surgery were indicative of patients later diagnosed with PTPS, though no major or modifiable risk factors are currently known for preventing PTPS [37].

In summary, patients presenting for pleural cavity and chest wall surgery have variable pathologies and are often high risk for complicated procedures. A detailed discussion with the surgical team is of the utmost importance in order to tailor the anesthetic appropriately to allow for the best possible outcome.

## References

1. Neustein SM, Eisenkraft JB, Cohen E. Anesthesia for thoracic surgery. In: Barash PG, Cullen BF, Stoelting RK, Cahalan MK, Stock MC, editors. Clinical anesthesia. Philadelphia: Lippincott Williams and Wilkins; 2009. p. 1032–72.
2. Vallieres E. Management of empyema after lung resections (pneumonectomy/lobectomy). Chest Surg Clin N Am. 2002;12:571–85.
3. Zanotti G, Mitchell JD. Bronchopleural fistula and empyema after anatomic lung resection. Thorac Surg Clin. 2015;25(4):421–7.
4. Maagaard M, Tang M, Ringgaard S, Nielsen HH, Frokiaer J, Haubuf M, et al. Normalized cardiopulmonary exercise function in patients with pectus excavatum three years after operation. Ann Thorac Surg. 2013;96:272–8.
5. Chatterjee K, Zhang J, Honbo N, Karlinerb JS. Doxorubicin cardiomyopathy. Cardiology. 2010;115(2):155–62.
6. Patil N, Paulose RM, Udupa KS, Ramakrishna N, Ahmed T. Pulmonary toxicity of Bleomycin—a case series from a Tertiary Care Center in Southern India. J Clin Diagn Res. 2016;10(4):FR01–3.
7. Slinger PD. Perioperative respiratory assessment and management. Can J Anaesth. 1992;39:115–31.
8. McHugh MA, Poston PM, Rossi NO, Turek JW. Assessment of potential confounders when imaging pectus excavatum with chest radiography alone. J Pediatr Surg. 2016;51(9):1485–9.
9. Gerson MC, Hurst JM, Herrtzberg VS, et al. Prediction of cardiac and pulmonary complication related to elective abdominal and non-cardiac surgery in thoracic surgery in geriatric patients. Am J Med. 1990;88:101–7.
10. Ivanov A, Yossef J, Tailon J, Worku BM, et al. Do pulmonary function tests improve risk stratification before cardiothoracic surgery? J Thorac Cardiovasc Surg. 2016;151(4):1183–1189.e3.
11. Kurlansky P. Preoperative PFTs: the answer is blowing in the wind. J Thorac Cardiovasc Surg. 2016;151(4):918–9.
12. Mavi J, Moore DL. Anesthesia and analgesia for pectus excavatum surgery. Anesthesiol Clin. 2014;32(1):175–84.
13. Katlic MR. Video-assisted thoracic surgery utilizing local anesthesia and sedation. Eur J Cardiothorac Surg. 2006;30(3):529–32.
14. Lumb AB, Slinger P. Hypoxic pulmonary vasoconstriction: physiology and anesthetic implications. Anesthesiology. 2015;122(4):932–46.

15. Pruszkowski O, Dalibon N, Moutafis M, Jugan E, Law-Koune JD, Laloë PA, Fischler M. Effects of propofol vs sevoflurane on arterial oxygenation during one-lung ventilation. Br J Anaesth. 2007;98:539–44.
16. Fox ME, Bensard DD, Roaten JB, Hendrickson RJ. Positioning for the Nuss procedure: avoiding brachial plexus injury. Paediatr Anaesth. 2005;15(12):1067–71.
17. Mansour KA, Thourani VH, Losken A, et al. Chest wall resections and reconstruction: a 25-year experience. Ann Thorac Surg. 2002;73(6):1720–6.
18. Hebra A, Swoveland B, Egbert M, Tagge EP, Georgeson K, Othersen HB Jr, Nuss D. Outcome analysis of minimally invasive repair of pectus excavatum: review of 251 cases. J Pediatr Surg. 2000;35(2):252–7; discussion 257–258.
19. Luh S-P, Chou M-C, Wang L-S, Chen J-Y, Tsai T-P. Video-assisted thoracoscopic surgery in the treatment of complicated parapneumonic effusions or empyemas. Chest. 2005;127(4):1427–32. https://doi.org/10.1016/s0012-3692(15)34497-4.
20. Ambrosino N, Gabbrielli L. Physiotherapy in the perioperative period. Best Pract Res Clin Anaesthesiol. 2010;24(2):283–9.
21. Christine P-A, Gupta S. Choices in pain management follow thoracotomy. Chest. 1999;115(5):122S–4S.
22. Li N-L, Yu B-L, Hung C-F. Paravertebral block plus thoracic wall block versus paravertebral block alone for analgesia of modified radical mastectomy: a retrospective cohort study. PLoS ONE. 2016;11(11):e0166227.
23. Hetta R. Pectoralis-serratus interfascial plane block versus thoracic paravertebral block for unilateral radical mastectomy with axillary evacuation. J Clin Anesth. 2016;34:91–7.
24. Choudry B, Sacks R. Continuous chest wall ropivacaine infusion for analgesia in children undergoing Nuss procedure: a comparison with thoracic epidural. Paediatr Anaesth. 2016;26(6):582–9.
25. Frawley G, Frawley J, Crameri J. A review of anesthetic techniques and outcomes following minimally invasive repair of pectus excavatum (Nuss procedure). Paediatr Anaesth. 2016;26(11):1082–90. https://doi.org/10.1111/pan.12988; Epub 2016 Aug 11.
26. Waurick VA. Update in thoracic epidural anaesthesia. Best Pract Res Clin Anaesthesiol. 2005;19(2):201–13.
27. Kosinski S, et al. Comparison of continuous epidural block and continuous paravertebral block in postoperative analgaesia after video-assisted thoracoscopic surgery lobectomy: a randomised, non-inferiority trial. Anaesthesiol Intensive Ther. 2016;48(5):280–7. https://doi.org/10.5603/AIT.2016.0059.
28. Tamura T, et al. A randomized controlled trial comparing paravertebral block via the surgical field with thoracic epidural block using ropivacaine for post-thoracotomy pain relief. J Anesth. 2017;31(2):263–70. https://doi.org/10.1007/s00540-017-2307-5; Epub 2017 Jan 23.
29. Soniya B, et al. Comparison between thoracic epidural block and thoracic paravertebral block for post thoracotomy pain relief. J Clin Diagn Res. 2016;10(9):UC08–12.
30. Ahmed Z, Samad K, Ullah H. Role of intercostal nerve block in reducing postoperative pain following video-assisted thoracoscopy: a randomized controlled trial. Saudi J Anaesth. 2017;11(1):54–7. https://doi.org/10.4103/1658-354X.197342.
31. Hord AH, Wang JM, Pai UT, Raj PP. Anatomic spread of India ink in the human intercostal space with radiologic correlation. Reg. Anesth. 1991;16(1):13–6.
32. Jaroszewski DE, Temkit M, Ewais MM, et al. Randomized trial of epidural vs. subcutaneous catheters for managing pain after modified Nuss in adults. J Thorac Dis. 2016;8(8):2102–10. https://doi.org/10.21037/jtd.2016.06.62.
33. Dale O, Somogyi AA, Li Y, Sullivan T, Shavit Y. Does intraoperative ketamine attenuate inflammatory reactivity following surgery? A systematic review and meta-analysis. Anesth Analg. 2012;115(4):934–43.
34. Shah M, Frye R, Marzinsky A, et al. Complications associated with bar fixation following Nuss repair for pectus excavatum. Am Surg. 2016;82(9):781–2.
35. Kawai H, Tayasu Y, Saitoh A, et al. Nocturnal hypoxemia after lobectomy for lung cancer. Ann Thorac Surg. 2005;79(4):1162–6. https://doi.org/10.1016/j.athoracsur.2004.09.063.
36. Wildgaard K, Ravn J, Kehlet H. Chronic post-thoracotomy pain: a critical review of pathogenic mechanisms and strategies for prevention. Eur J Cardiothorac Surg. 2009;36(1):170–80. https://doi.org/10.1016/j.ejcts.2009.02.005.
37. Kinney MA, Jacob AK, Passe MA, Mantilla CB. Increased risk of postthoracotomy pain syndrome in patients with Prolonged Hospitalization and increased postoperative Opioid use. Pain Res Treat. 2016;2016:7945145. https://doi.org/10.1155/2016/7945145; Epub 2016 Jun 2.

# Anesthetic Implications for Management of Thoracic Trauma

Abimbola Faloye

## Introduction

Injury to the thoracic organs may be from blunt force or penetrating missiles and can result in obvious or subtle injuries. Penetrating injuries tend to be more straightforward to diagnose and manage, as the offense is clear and obvious. They are often managed surgically. Blunt force trauma tends to result in multiple, less obvious injuries, can require more studies for diagnosis, and is often treated medically rather than surgically.

The leading causes of death from thoracic trauma are hypoxia and hypoventilation. The primary survey is a targeted examination to identify, rule out or treat life-threatening injuries and it appropriately places airway and ventilation as top priorities (Table 16.1). A quick examination of the face, oropharynx, neck and chest should be performed by looking, palpating, and listening for breath sounds. On first glance a patient with difficulty breathing may be easily identified. However, patients who appear comfortable may quickly deteriorate.

A. Faloye, M.D.
Emory University School of Medicine,
Atlanta, GA, USA
e-mail: aopanug@emory.edu

## Airway and Ventilation

The airway should be assessed for patency, chest wall examined for breath sounds, step offs, and deformities that would indicate multiple broken ribs or flail chest. Unstable or unconscious patients require an immediate and definitive airway which is usually accomplished by orotracheal intubation. Some patients with obvious and extensive maxillofacial deformities, airway lacerations, profound edema or profuse airway hemorrhage benefit from a cricothyrotomy or tracheostomy. Universally, all trauma patients are assumed to have "full stomachs" and are at risk for regurgitation and aspiration. Hence a rapid sequence induction (RSI) is standard in these scenarios. In cases of a known or highly-suspected difficult airway, RSI is more dangerous and other modes of induction should be undertaken. The traditional approach to RSI is to use succinylcholine as muscle relaxant. In cases in which succinylcholine is contraindicated, such as allergy, recent burns >24 h, myopathies, or hyperkalemia,

Table 16.1 ABCDE of trauma

| Airway | Assess patency of airway |
|---|---|
| Breathing | Assess breathing pattern, chest movement, breath sounds |
| Circulation | Assess pallor, pulses, blood pressure, bleeding |
| Disability | Assess neurological status. |
| Exposure | Remove all clothing |

© Springer International Publishing AG, part of Springer Nature 2018
B. G. Goudra et al. (eds.), *Anesthesiology*, https://doi.org/10.1007/978-3-319-74766-8_16

rocuronium can be used. The dosage given for RSI is based on the $ED_{95}$ of the drug with RSI dosing typically 4× the $ED_{95}$ of the drug [1].

## Circulation

Quick examination of neck veins, peripheral pulses and blood pressure should be done. Hypovolemic shock typically presents with flat neck veins, weak peripheral pulses and low blood pressure.

Distended neck veins and low peripheral circulation usually indicates a myocardial restriction or failure; the differential includes five things: (a) Myocardial infarction, (b) Myocardial contusion, (c) tension pneumothorax (d) cardiac tamponade, (e) acute air embolism.

Most trauma centers and emergency rooms are now equipped with ultrasound machines used for *FAST* (Focused Assessment with Sonography for Trauma) exams. The FAST exam is useful for the evaluation of the torso and abdomen for the presence of free fluid after traumatic injury. Classically, FAST utilizes the subxiphoid window to evaluate for fluid around the heart. Large pneumothorax may also be seen on FAST.

Myocardial infarction from coronary occlusion is more likely in elderly trauma patients.

Myocardial contusion is commonly seen in cases of blunt chest trauma and presents with depressed cardiac function, arrhythmia, and increase in cardiac enzymes [2]. Intracardiac injuries may also be present.

Cardiac tamponade can be seen in all cases of blunt and penetrating chest trauma. In cases of blunt trauma the source may be myocardial rupture, dissection of the proximal ascending aorta or laceration of pulmonary veins. Distended neck veins may not be present in cases of severe blood loss. Pulsus paradoxus is only present in a fraction of cases and is rarely seen in the emergency department [3] whereas a pericardial effusion is often apparent on FAST examination. Rapid fluid resuscitation should begin to restore circulating volume to the heart as sudden hemodynamic collapse may ensue with the institution of positive pressure ventilation. Prior to induction, the patient should be prepped and draped with the surgeon at the bedside ready to perform an emergent pericardial window. The patient may be kept spontaneously ventilating to maintain negative intrathoracic pressures and promote venous return (see Sect. Anesthetic Considerations for Specific Conditions).

## Neurological Status

Level of consciousness and arousal is the simplest, most reliable measure of neurologic injury. The Glasgow Coma scale (Table 16.2) should be recorded on arrival. Computed Tomographic scan of the head is the primary tool to assess for head injury and should be done as soon as possible in cases of decreased level of consciousness. Spinal cord injuries typically present with focal neurological deficits in an extremity. Injuries above T6 usually result in complete loss of sympathetic innervation below the level of injury. It manifests as hypotension and bradycardia which is commonly referred to as spinal shock. Typically, spinal shock resolves within 3–6 weeks. Supportive therapy with vasopressors and inotropes is needed in the interim.

**Table 16.2** Glasgow Coma scale

| | | |
|---|---|---|
| I. Eye opening | | |
| | Spontaneously | 4 |
| | To voice | 3 |
| | To pain | 2 |
| | None | 1 |
| II. Verbal response | | |
| | Oriented | 5 |
| | Confused | 4 |
| | Inappropriate words | 3 |
| | Incomprehensible words | 2 |
| | None | 1 |
| III. Motor response | | |
| | Obeys commands | 6 |
| | Purposeful movements (pain) | 5 |
| | Withdraws from (pain) | 4 |
| | Flexion (pain) | 3 |
| | Extension (pain) | 2 |
| | None | 1 |

## General Considerations

The mechanism of injury often determines the cluster of injuries noted. Most patients with blunt chest trauma also have associated extra-thoracic injuries [4].

The initial examination of the thorax should be targeted towards excluding life threatening injuries.

- Tension pneumothorax
- Massive hemothorax
- Open pneumothorax
- Cardiac tamponade
- Flail chest
- Cardiac rupture
- Aortic rupture

Radiographic imaging is often needed to assess presence of pulmonary contusions, simple pneumothorax, or hemothorax, blunt aortic injury, blunt myocardial injury.

## Fractures of the Bony Thorax

Sternal and scapula fractures occur after high energy trauma and are often associated with deeper injuries. Fractures of multiple ribs can lead to flail chest.

Flail chest is a condition caused by fracture of multiple ribs often leading to "floating" ribs. During spontaneous inhalation, the thorax is sucked in by the negative intra-thoracic pressure, and the abdomen pushes out. The reverse occurs with exhalation. Flail chest leads to inefficient gas exchange.

## Other Injuries

Pulmonary contusion
Cardiac contusions
Ruptured diaphragm
Tracheobronchial injury
Pulmonary laceration
Great vessel injury

## Anesthetic Management

Thoracic injury often results in emergent surgical interventions. It is important for anesthesia providers to maintain calmness and equanimity, and to rapidly assess the patient on arrival to the operating room. A quick examination assessing airway, breathing patterns and obvious deformities should be conducted. Often the surgeon(s) or emergency personnel must be relied upon for patient history and pertinent information. Verifications of what radiological/ultrasonography procedures have been performed and their results can be very helpful.

Induction of anesthesia and institution of positive pressure ventilation can lead to rapid deterioration and catastrophic results in previously compensated patients who have suffered massive blood loss, or who have cardiac tamponade or tension pneumothorax.

Anesthesia care providers should seek to exclude the presence of the latter two in cases of thoracic trauma prior to induction of anesthesia.

## Airway

Establishment of a definitive airway is a priority. It may be simple and straightforward with direct laryngoscopy. Patients with cervical trauma or with cervical spine precautions require maintenance of in-line stabilization of the neck to protect against flexion and extension.

In cases of severe injury to a unilateral hemithorax the need for lung isolation should be assessed. Absolute indications for lung isolation include, but are not limited to, prevention of contamination from spillage from the other lung or control of distribution of ventilation such as seen in cases of an open pneumothorax (see Table 16.3). A double lumen tube is best for lung isolation in these cases because of the ease of suctioning [5].

Intubation should be accomplished using a larger endotracheal tube, size 8.0 mm and above, where possible. This is done in case the patient needs to remain intubated for an extended period of time. It is easier to perform bronchoscopy through larger tubes and the work of breathing is decreased in spontaneously ventilating patients with the wider diameter.

**Table 16.3** Indications for lung isolation and/or single lung ventilation

| Absolute |
| --- |
| 1. Isolation of one lung from the other to avoid spillage or contamination<br>　(a) Infection<br>　(b) Massive hemorrhage |
| 2. Control of distribution of ventilation<br>　(a) Bronchopleural fistula<br>　(b) Bronchopleural cutaneous fistula<br>　(c) Surgical opening of a major conducting airway<br>　(d) Giant unilateral lung cyst or bulla<br>　(e) Tracheobronchial tree disruption<br>　(f) Life threatening hypoxemia caused by unilateral lung disease |
| Relative |
| 1. Surgical exposure—high priority<br>　(a) Thoracic aortic aneurysm<br>　(b) Pneumonectomy<br>　(c) Thoracoscopy<br>　(d) Pulmonary resection via median sternotomy<br>　(e) Upper lobectomy<br>　(f) Mediastinal exposure |
| 2. Surgical exposure—medium (lower priority)<br>　(a) Middle and lower lobectomies and subsegmental resections<br>　(b) Esophageal resection<br>　(c) Procedures on the thoracic spine |
| 3. Post-cardiopulmonary bypass after removal of a totally occluding chronic unilateral pulmonary emboli |
| 4. Severe hypoxemia caused by unilateral lung disease |

## Ventilation

There are four key ventilatory principles to adhere to in thoracic trauma patients:

- Avoid nitrous oxide: nitrous rapidly fills small spaces and can turn a simple pneumothorax into a life threatening one.
- Continuously track peak airway pressures: Increasing peak airway pressures is often an early sign in acute lung injury (ALI/ARDS) as it signals decreasing pulmonary compliance. It is also a sign of acute obstruction. Troubleshoot this by moving from the machine to the patient, checking for kinks. Suction the endotracheal tube. Direct visualization with a pediatric fiberoptic bronchoscope may be necessary.
- Monitor end-tidal CO2: Decreasing end-tidal $CO_2$ may be an indication of decreased pulmonary perfusion, acute obstruction or dislodgment of the endotracheal tube, or a tracheoesophageal fistula.
- Blood Gases: Adequacy of oxygenation and ventilation can be assessed using serial arterial blood gases. Calculation of the P:F ($PaO_2$:$FiO_2$) ratio is helpful to assess development of ALI/ARDS. Wean from 100% oxygen as soon as possible as these patients are at increased risk of developing ALI.

## Monitors

Standard monitors include pulse oximetry, 5 lead ECG, NIBP, and in-line capnography. An arterial line is often indicated for continuous hemodynamic monitoring and access for frequent blood draws. Central venous pressures may be monitored with the caveat that trends should be integrated with other variables instead of treating a single value.

There is a growing use of intraoperative transesophageal echocardiography (TEE) to monitor cardiac function and volume status. TEE should always be considered in cases of refractory or persistent hypotension to assess global cardiac function, presence of wall motion abnormalities, exclude intracardiac shunts, severe regurgitant valve lesions, or aortic dissections. TEE is contraindicated in any case with known or suspected esophageal injury.

## Anesthetic Agent

With extensive lung injury, intravenous anesthetics should be considered to maintain stable anesthetic depth and to decrease the risk of intraoperative awareness. Drugs like midazolam, ketamine and dexmedetomidine may be used as adjuncts as they have a more favorable hemodynamic profile than propofol. Etomidate has been shown to cause temporary adrenal suppression and has been linked to an increase in mortality in septic patients [6]. It should be used with caution.

## Fluid Management and Resuscitation

The goal of resuscitation is establishment of euvolemia. Resuscitation in cases of massive blood loss should be accomplished using red blood cells and blood components. Excessive use of crystalloids should be avoided as these increase the risk of lung injury the and need for prolonged postoperative mechanical ventilation [7, 8].

## Anesthetic Considerations for Specific Conditions

### Cardiac Tamponade

Cases of severe tamponade can be rapidly managed with a subxiphoid incision and drainage under local anesthesia. However, in trauma, the effusion is usually blood and results from a ruptured or lacerated myocardium, aorta, or great vessel. In such cases, relieving the pressure may result in continued hemorrhage and resultant exsanguination. For this reason, pericardial effusions in the setting of trauma are surgically managed. In tamponade, intracardiac pressures are deceptively elevated due to increased extracavitary pressures. Cardiac chamber collapse (atria and right ventricle) in diastole contributes to limited filling and decreased stroke volume. Cardiac output is heavily dependent on the heart rate, and blood pressure is dependent mostly on peripheral vasoconstriction. Hence, induction of anesthesia can cause rapid cardiovascular collapse. Drugs for induction and maintenance of anesthesia should be chosen with the goal of preserving cardiac contractility and maintaining systemic vascular resistance. Vasodilators and negative inotropic agents should be avoided. Ketamine has sympathomimetic effects and may be helpful in preserving heart rate and blood pressure however it should be noted that it is a direct myocardial depressant and should be avoided in patients under maximal sympathetic stress. Patients with cardiac tamponade should be induced only after the surgeon is ready to make an incision as rapid hemodynamic deterioration may ensue. Significant blood loss should be expected and at least two large bore IVs and an arterial line should be obtained prior to induction of anesthesia with a low threshold for placement of central venous access. Assuming no contraindications, TEE is helpful in monitoring volume status, biventricular function and to assess for residual pericardial effusion and the presence of additional cardiovascular pathology.

### Cardiac Contusion

Blunt force trauma to the heart can cause minor bruising or hemodynamically significant cardiac dysfunction such as arrhythmias, free wall rupture, septal rupture, or valve rupture. It can be caused by direct impact of a missile to chest, or compression between the sternum and the vertebral column. Treatment depends on the symptoms and severity of injury. Ruptures of the free wall, septum, and valves necessitate surgical repairs conducted on cardiopulmonary bypass.

### Aortic Transection/Dissection

True aortic rupture is highly lethal. The majority of these patients die at the scene of trauma, and mortality continues to rise rapidly within the first hour [4]. Partial dissections, contained ruptures, and true dissections may enable survival long enough for surgical therapy. Presenting symptoms vary and range from shock, to cold, ischemic extremities, decreased urine output, and ischemic organs below the level of injury. The most common location of injury is the aortic isthmus. Hypertension is likely to lead to increased bleeding and increase the risk of further rupture or extension of an intimal tear. Hypotension is usually a sign of decreased intravascular volume secondary to blood loss and should be treated with blood administration. The location of the injury determines the accuracy of blood pressure measurements. Injuries that occur distal to the innominate artery may result in different blood pressure readings in both arms. When feasible, a right radial arterial line should be obtained as it will give the most proximal BP readings. In centers which utilize right axillary artery cannulation for surgical management of aortic dissection a left radial arterial line should instead be placed. Central line access and large bore IVs should be obtained for rapid volume infusion.

### Tension Pneumothorax

Early recognition of tension pneumothorax is of critical importance for a favorable outcome. The classic signs are hypotension, distended neck veins, cyanosis, tachypnea, diminished breath sounds on the affected side and tracheal deviation. Distended neck veins may be absent in hypovolemic patients.

Although definitive confirmation is done by chest radiograph (CXR), if it is suspected immediate treatment should be undertaken without waiting for a CXR. A 14 gauge IV catheter should be inserted in the second intercostal space in the mid-clavicular line. A loud gush of air is confirmation of diagnosis. A tube thoracostomy should then be inserted prior to instituting positive pressure ventilation. Simple pneumothorax may become tension pneumothorax after institution of positive pressure ventilation. Signs include elevated airway pressures, hypoxia, and hypotension.

## Air Embolism

Air embolism occurs when there is an interruption of the bronchopulmonary barrier. It is often seen in cases of injury near the hilum of the lung where pulmonary veins are in close proximity to their bronchi. Early consideration of air embolism when working through a differential diagnosis is extremely helpful in identifying this condition. Air embolism usually presents as rapid and intractable hemodynamic deterioration that may present or worsen with the institution of positive pressure ventilation. Air can embolize into the cerebral circulation causing acute stroke symptoms, and into the coronary circulation causing arrhythmias, AV block, ST segment elevations, and asystole. The treatment is immediate thoracotomy with the patient in a steep head down, and clamping of the hilum to prevent further entrainment of air along with supportive hemodynamic treatment with fluids and vasopressors.

## Chest Wall Fractures (Flail Chest)

Flail chest is often associated with pulmonary contusions and pneumothorax and often results in inefficient gas exchange. The paradoxical movement of the chest with spontaneous respiration results in hypoxemia and hypercarbia. Gas exchange is improved with muscle relaxation and controlled ventilation.

## Tracheobronchial Disruption

A defect in the trachea or bronchus manifests as loss of tidal volumes in the context of a bloody airway. Unfortunately, the injury is often not suspected until after intubation. Isolating the defect is often a painstaking process done by careful surgical dissection and inspection. The fiberoptic bronchoscope is of limited utility when significant bleeding is present. For surgical repair, lung isolation is often needed. The decision to switch from a single lumen tube to a double lumen tube is fraught with risk. It may be dangerous to attempt an intraoperative exchange in the presence of bleeding, limited respiratory reserve and any difficulty encountered with initial intubation. Depending on the location of the injury, the use of a bronchial blocker can facilitate lung isolation. Alternatively, an attempt may be made to advance a single lumen endotracheal tube into the contralateral mainstem bronchus to improve ventilation and enable surgical repair.

## References

1. Francois Donati DRB. Neuromusclular blocking agents. In: Clinical anesthesia. 6th ed. Philadelphia: Wolters Kluwer Lippincott Williams and Wilkins; 2009. p. 504–5.
2. Bertinchant JP, Polge A, Mohty D, Nguyen-Ngoc-Lam R, Estorc J, Cohendy R, et al. Evaluation of incidence, clinical significance, and prognostic value of circulating cardiac troponin I and T elevation in hemodynamically stable patients with suspected myocardial contusion after blunt chest trauma. J Trauma. 2000;48(5):924–31.
3. Burlew CC, Moore EE. Chapter 14. Emergency department thoracotomy. In: Mattox KL, Moore EE, Feliciano DV, editors. Trauma. 7th ed. New York, NY: McGraw-Hill; 2013.
4. Wall MJ, Tsai P, Mattox KL. Chapter 26. Heart and thoracic vascular injuries. In: Mattox KL, Moore EE, Feliciano DV, editors. Trauma. 7th ed. New York, NY: The McGraw-Hill Companies; 2013.
5. Benumof JL. Separation of the two lungs (double lumen tube and bronchial blocker intubation). In: Anesthesia for thoracic surgery. 2nd ed.; 1995. p. 331–6.
6. Chan CM, Mitchell AL, Shorr AF. Etomidate is associated with mortality and adrenal insufficiency in sepsis: a meta-analysis*. Crit Care Med. 2012;40(11):2945–53.
7. Kasotakis G, Sideris A, Yang Y, de Moya M, Alam H, King DR, et al. Aggressive early crystalloid resuscitation adversely affects outcomes in adult blunt trauma patients: an analysis of the Glue Grant database. J Trauma Acute Care Surg. 2013;74(5):1215–21; discussion 21–2.
8. Chang R, Holcomb JB. Optimal fluid therapy for traumatic hemorrhagic shock. Crit Care Clin. 2017;33(1):15–36.

# Anesthesia for Thymectomy

Christopher R. Hoffman and Michael Stuart Green

## Introduction

Thymomas are an uncommon pathology, thus subsequent thymectomies are infrequently encountered. The National Cancer Institute's Survalence, Epidemiology, and End Results (SEER) program projected the incidence of thymomas to be 0.13 per 100,000 person-years, or an estimated 390 cases per year in the United States [1]. The European Association for Cardio-Thoracic Surgery (EACTS) designates a "high-volume center" for thymectomy to be one performing the procedure ten times annually [2]. Realistic epidemiology of thymomas is difficult to assess due to the variety in their clinical presentation. One third present with symptoms consistent with myasthenia gravis. One third present with localized symptoms of tumor growth such as a palpable mass or superior vena cava (SVC) syndrome. The remaining cases are incidental radiographic findings and it is likely in this category where true prevalence is underreported [3]. Thymectomy is typically indicated in candidates with classes of generalized myasthenia gravis. The goal is remission or reduced need for immunosuppressive or myasthenia medications. Severe cases of SVC syndrome due to invasive thymoma necessitating thymectomy have also been reported [4].

## Myasthenia Gravis

Myasthenia gravis is an autoimmune disorder of the neuromuscular junction. The characteristic weakness is due to an antibody mediated destruction or inactivation of postsynaptic acetylcholine receptors at this junction. Population based epidemiology of myasthenia gravis estimates its prevalence at 20 per 100,000 people. Disease progression is insidious, typically presenting in the third and fifth decades of life in women and men, respectively [5]. Presenting symptoms commonly involve ocular muscles, causing ptosis and diplopia. If the disease progresses, symptoms become more generalized to involve bulbar and peripheral musculature. Weakness classically worsens with repeated motor stimulation, a hallmark of concern when muscles of respiration become involved (Table 17.1).

In myasthenia gravis, circulating antibodies trigger complement-mediated lysis or blockade of acetylcholine receptors, evidenced by the abundance of IgG and complement deposits in neuromuscular junctions [6]. The nidus for the antibody is not definitively proven, but a correlation of myasthenia gravis to thymus gland irregularities is well studied. Myasthenia gravis is

---

C. R. Hoffman, D.O. · M. S. Green, D.O. (✉)
Department of Anesthesiology and Perioperative Medicine, Drexel University College of Medicine, Philadelphia, PA, USA
e-mail: Michael.Green@Drexelmed.edu

**Table 17.1** Summary of the considerations for providing anesthesia to patients undergoing thymectomy

| Perioperative stage | Management |
|---|---|
| Physical evaluation | • Assess SVC/tumor compression symptoms—edema, dyspnea, dysphagia, headache<br>• Assess myasthenia symptoms—extent of motor and respiratory involvement, medical therapy, cardiovascular exam<br>• Conduct complete airway exam<br>• Evaluate in seated, supine, semi-supine positions |
| Radiographic assessment | • Chest radiography is likely insufficient data<br>• Inspect chest CT for airway deviation and potential for intrathoracic compression<br>• Possible role for flow/volume loops in extensive disease or to evaluate dynamic airway collapse/tracheomalacia |
| Risk optimization | • Evaluate short and long-term therapies and interventions<br>• Risk stratify likelihood to remain intubated post procedure<br>• Review need for premedications (e.g. steroid, anticholinesterase) |
| Room preparation | • Alert blood bank for potential massive resuscitation<br>• Prepare for rigid bronchoscopy and cardiopulmonary bypass to be immediately available<br>• Identify surgical approach |
| Invasive lines | • Evaluate SVC symptoms for potential lower extremity venous cannula<br>• Assess need for peripheral vs. central venous access<br>• Assess need for preinduction arterial cannula<br>• Discuss with surgery need for preinduction bypass cannulation if high risk anticipated |
| Induction | • Evaluate any possibility for neuraxial anesthesia<br>• Optimize patient positioning for induction based on preoperative assessments<br>• Maintain spontaneous respiration if possible<br>• Proceed with awake or inhalational fiberoptic bronchoscopy to intubate<br>• Limit need for paralytic if possible |
| Maintenance | • Maintain spontaneous respiration<br>• Limit positive intrathoracic pressure<br>• Ensure adequate anesthetic depth<br>• Monitor for vascular insult necessitating resuscitation |
| Emergence | • Review risk stratification for likelihood to remain intubated<br>• Ensure optimal neuromuscular blockade reversal if applicable |
| Postoperative | • Review with neurology any requirement for postoperative continuation of myasthenia gravis therapies (e.g. anticholinesterase, plasmapheresis)<br>• Observe respiratory mechanics with caution<br>• Monitor for surgical complications |

present with concomitant presence of thymic hyperplasia in 70% of cases and thymoma in 15% of cases. Long-term follow-up for myasthenia patients receiving thymectomy also supports the association, with a 44% remission rate and 91% palliation rate [7].

## Thymoma

The most common type of thymoma involves neoplastic epithelial cells responsible for T-cell maturation. Abnormal proliferation of cells responsible for immune cell development is unsurprisingly associated with multiple autoimmune disorders. Myasthenia gravis is the most common presentation but other conditions associated with thymoma include cytopenia, hypogammaglobulinemia, polymyositis, and systemic lupus erythematosus [8]. As the thymus gland is anatomically located posterior to the sternum and anterior to the great vessels and pericardium, the other major concern is compression of surrounding structures in the setting of invasive thymoma. In this location the surgical removal of a thymoma presents the same perioperative concerns involved in the manipulation of any anterior mediastinal mass (e.g. teratoma, bronchogenic cyst, lymphoma).

## Preoperative Evaluation

### Physical Evaluation

As with all mediastinal masses, primary concerns focus on symptoms associated with tumor size and positioning. The principal concerns are airway and respiratory exam regarding derangements in anatomical structure and patency. A structural and functional evaluation should be conducted in seated and supine positions to observe for sudden changes in presentation. Patient history should include past radiation therapy as an additional concern when evaluating the airway. Symptoms consistent with SVC syndrome should also be assessed and include face or chest wall edema, dyspnea, dysphagia, headache, and stridor. Acute and chronic changes should be noted. Myasthenia gravis specifically presents with periods of exacerbation and remission over time. An assessment of motor strength is required along with a thorough history of frequency and severity of symptomatic episodes. The extent of extraocular, pharyngeal, laryngeal, and truncal musculature is of particular importance. Respiratory muscle impairment warrants auscultation of lung fields to evaluate possible recent aspiration. An uncommon association with myasthenia gravis and cardiomyopathy necessitates a focused cardiovascular exam.

### Radiographic Evaluation

The physical exam only partially addresses concerns regarding tumor size, position, and subsequent impact on intrathoracic deviation. The concern is the potential for airway or major cardiovascular compression by the tumor mass and its manipulation. This potential obstruction may not be fully realized in awake patients, spontaneously breathing and protecting their own airway. Life-impending compression may present upon administered anesthetics or paralytics. Preoperative evaluation typically includes computed tomography (CT) of the chest. Considering all potential mediastinal pathologies, thoracic CT shows superiority in detecting abnormal masses and staging carcinoma when chest radiography was equivocal [9]. Evaluating thymic abnormality specifically, CT has been found to be more accurate in differentiating benign cyst from solid tumor and the extent of tumor invasion [10]. From an airway perspective, radiographical assessment can miss subclinical compression. Evidence of such a finding via CT has been shown as a predictor for airway obstruction on induction or emergence [11]. There is a possible role for flow-volume loops to detect variable intrathoracic obstruction potentially consistent with tracheomalacia, defined as the flaccidity of the supporting tracheal cartilage, widening of the posterior membranous wall, and reduced anterior-posterior airway caliber. The use of flow-volume loops is not routinely mandated and is likely only part of preoperative testing in the presence of substantial warning signs during symptom assessment [12].

### Risk Assessment and Optimization

The severity of clinical presentation of myasthenia combined with recent changes in therapies should allow one to determine the adequacy of preoperative optimization. A stable exam on a long-term anticholinesterase medication dose reassures potential under or over-treatment (excess dosing can lead to cholinergic crisis). An unstable exam may lead to dosing changes and surgical delay. Severe disease progression may warrant plasmapheresis or intravenous immunoglobulins, removing or binding circulating antibodies to temporary improve symptoms and decrease perioperative complications. Chemo or radiotherapy typically follows tumor resection and debulking. However it may be utilized preoperatively in the setting of recurrent disease or severe SVC obstruction and warrants concern [13].

Premedications typically include steroid stress dosing in the setting of chronic supplementation. Morning administration of chronic anticholinesterase dose varies. Decreasing the dose weighs patient respiratory discomfort or compromise and possible postoperative motor weakness against potentially decreasing interaction with intraoperative cholinergic and anticholinergic medications. In general morning doses may be held or halved in the setting of mild disease and maintained at regular dosing if severe disease is present [14]. Preoperative sedation is typically avoided due to concerns for airway obstruction. An antisialagogue may be administered to help facilitate fiberoptic intubation if severe disease is suspected or airway compromise likely.

In addition to the aforementioned perioperative concerns to be addressed, one also must consult with the patient regarding the risk of needing postoperative ventilation. Risk factors for postoperative ventilatory support include pyridostigmine dose >750 mg/day, vital capacity <40 mL/kg (or 2.9 L), peak inspiratory pressure <−25 cmH$_2$O, disease duration >6 years, and concomitant pulmonary disease (e.g. COPD). These risk factors do not take surgical approach into account [14].

## Anesthetic Management

Prior to the start of the anesthetic one should ensure the availability of both cardiopulmonary bypass and a rigid bronchoscope. If such resources are required time will be of the essence and delay could gravely impact outcome. Patients at high risk for airway or cardiovascular compression are identifiable with aforementioned testing. However, even asymptomatic thymomas have been complicated by acute compression, necessitating rigid bronchoscopy to establish a definitive airway or cardiopulmonary bypass to ensure oxygen delivery [15]. Surgical approach also contributes to potential risk. Traditional approach is via median sternotomy, permitting total exposure of large-sized tumor at the risk of increased postoperative ventilatory assistance. When appropriate, similar surgical outcomes with less respiratory compromise have been reported with less invasive transcervical and video-assisted mediastinoscopy. Nevertheless, potential for acute cardiopulmonary compromise is present both during sternotomy or insertion of a mediastinoscope [16].

Site selection for intravenous access relies on severity of SVC syndrome, if present. Severe edema or compression may warrant lower limb vessel cannulation to avoid poor drug circulation or infiltration and subsequent worsening of edema. The decision to include central venous access depends on extent of tumor and level of concern for massive resuscitation. A need for cardiopulmonary bypass may interfere with femoral cannulation. Severity of symptoms, tumor size, or likelihood of compression may also necessitate pre- or post-induction arterial catheterization. If mediastinoscopy is the surgical approach, there is consideration to cannulate the right radial artery to monitor potential brachiocephalic artery compression immediately. If clinical presentation reflects high likelihood of intrathoracic compression there is consideration for preinduction femoral bypass cannulation. Utilization of this invasive anticipatory preparation is not routine and requires thorough education and cooperation from the patient.

The anesthetic management for thymectomy typically involves intubation due to the respiratory involvement of the disease progression and the risks for intrathoracic compression. In specific settings there are cases of thymectomy performed under neuraxial anesthesia. Limited generalized symptoms, less extensive tumor invasion, and minimized surgical approach may allow for thymectomy under a thoracic epidural. Employing an epidural high enough to block upper thoracic dermatomes risks respiratory compromise in a setting where function may already be limited. Cardiovascular compromise should also be monitored, as cardioaccelerator fibers will undergo sympathectomy. SVC compression leading to epidural vein engorgement may complicate epidural placement. If these risks are understood and controlled, there is potential benefit to this modality as induction and intubation can be avoided [17].

Patient positioning for induction of anesthesia is limited if significant symptoms present. Dyspnea exacerbated by supine position may require induction and intubation in an upright or semi-upright position. Maintaining spontaneous respiration during induction is essential to avoid airway obstruction. Awake fiberoptic bronchoscopy with judicious sedation and airway topicalization should be implemented. If this is intolerable (e.g. pediatric population, ineffective topicalization) then spontaneous respiration should be maintained via inhalational induction.

Induction medication should also preserve spontaneous respiration. Ideally limited supplementation with ketamine, dexmedetomidine, or midazolam may help facilitate awake fiberoptic bronchoscopy. If necessary, nitrous oxide and sevoflurane can be implemented for inhalational induction. Avoidance of muscle relaxant entirely is ideal. If unavoidable, administering succinylcholine may be used. Myasthenia gravis patients develop a resistance to succinylcholine and larger doses may be required. This resistance results from fewer functional nicotinic receptors at the motor end plate for succinylcholine to act upon. Additionally, myasthenia patients are at an increased risk of developing a phase II block, particularly with repeat dosing [18]. Concomitant anticholinesterase therapy or depletion of cholinesterase due to plasmapheresis may prolong the action of succinylcholine.

Myasthenia gravis patients are sensitive to nondepolarizing muscle relaxants and should be avoided when possible. Sensitivity exists in patients with only minimal disease, those in remission, or even in undiagnosed myasthenia cases. When considering muscle relaxant selection and administration, the primary goal is to attempt to return to spontaneous ventilation expeditiously. Should severe obstruction occur, positioning the patient lateral or prone may temporarily improve symptoms while more invasive measures to resolve compression are implemented.

Ensuring adequate anesthetic depth in a spontaneously breathing patient reduces concerns during the maintenance phase. Inhaled anesthetics may cause muscle relaxation in healthy individuals. In the myasthenia patient this additional weakness may be profound and needs consideration. Coughing or fighting the endotracheal tube due to light anesthetic will substantially alter intrathoracic pressure and lends to mass shift in the cavity. High suspicion for potential vascular complications and subsequent blood loss is essential during dissection. SVC compression can lead to elevated central venous pressure and exacerbate venous blood loss. Aberrant anatomy may lead to unanticipated arteriotomy. The potential for massive resuscitation should always be anticipated and communicated with blood bank with cross-matched blood available.

If neuromuscular blockade was established and requires reversal at the conclusion of the procedure, titrate anticholinesterase with caution. Inexact dosing may result in inadequate reversal or cholinergic crisis. Cholinergic crisis results from an excess of acetylcholine at the nicotinic and muscarinic receptors. This leads to further muscle weakness. To differentiate cholinergic crisis from myasthenic crisis, an edrophonium test may be administered. Maintain a low threshold to remain intubated postoperatively in the setting of substantial preoperative disease, aforementioned risk factors, or pharmacologic neuromuscular blockade. Inappropriate reversal and extubation can lead to agitated breathing and coughing, disrupting the surgical closure and potentially necessitating reintubation in a typically difficult airway.

The timing and degree of resolution of preoperative symptoms varies, and myasthenia medication may be continued in full or limited doses in the postoperative setting. Postoperative recovery should be observed in an intensive care setting to trend improvement in respiratory mechanics. Hypoventilation-induced atelectasis, pneumothorax, pneumomediastinum, air embolism, recurrent laryngeal nerve injury, and tracheomalacia/airway collapse may necessitate reintubation. Episodes of re-expansion pulmonary edema after mediastinal surgery have been reported [19]. Inadequate hemostasis may lead to cardiac tamponade, hemothorax, or cardiovascular instability.

## Outcomes

The incidence of thymectomy lends to empirical perioperative management, with evidence-based treatment guidelines difficult to establish. Surgical intervention for thymomatous myasthenia gravis with severe generalized symptoms is the general recommendation. Meta-analyses of studies addressing postoperative outcome shows superiority of surgical versus non-surgical treatment, in which the median relative rates were 2.1 in complete remission, 1.6 in asymptomatic status, and 1.7 in symptom improvement [20]. The effectiveness of this approach is unclear in non-thymomatous myasthenia gravis, as reported outcomes vary widely. Reported remission rates for non-thymomatous thymectomy are between 38 and 72% at 10 year follow up [21]. Clinical course also varies, as one review reported the mean time required to reach remission was 10.6 months versus 23.5 months for thymomatous and non-thymomatous thymectomy, respectively. The duration of remission was 43.1 months versus 30.8 months in thymoma and non-thymoma groups, respectively. Despite poorer remission onset and length, these groups had no statistically significant difference in remission rate or adverse outcome [22]. Results are less definitive but are substantial enough to consider surgical intervention on an individual basis. Limited data supports or refutes repeat thymectomy in post-surgical refractory myasthenia gravis. The procedure is uncommon and the varied nature of the perioperative course limits statistical review. Reported cases vary in initial symptom presentation, operative approach, postoperative therapies, and length of time between initial and repeat procedures. Residual thymic tissue is not reliably identified radiographically in these cases. The risks associated with a second mediastinal surgery, especially in the setting of a potential redo-sternotomy, are not benign and warrant consideration. Repeat complete remission is rarely reported, but 52–95% of patients experienced improved symptoms [23]. These risks and benefits also require stratification on an individual basis.

## References

1. Engels EA. Epidemiology of thymoma and associated malignancies. J Thorac Oncol. 2010;5(10 Suppl 4):S260–5.
2. Lucchi M, Van Schil P, Schmid R, Rea F, Melfi F, Athanassiadi K, Zielinski M, Treasure T. Thymectomy for thymoma and myasthenia gravis. A survey of current surgical practice in thymic disease amongst EACTS members. Interact Cardiovasc Thorac Surg. 2012;14(6):765–70.
3. Couture MM, Mountain CF. Thymoma. Semin Surg Oncol. 1990;6:110–4.
4. Rosa GR, Takizawa N, Schimidt D, Sugita M. Surgical treatment of superior vena cava syndrome caused by invasive thymoma. Rev Bras Cir Cardiovasc. 2010;25(2):257–60.
5. Phillips LH. The epidemiology of myasthenia gravis. Ann N Y Acad Sci. 2003;998:407–12.
6. Tuzun E, Christadoss P. Complement associated pathogenic mechanisms in myasthenia gravis. Autoimmun Rev. 2013;12(9):904–11.
7. Bril V, Kojic J, Ilse WK, Cooper JD. Long-term clinical outcome after transcervical thymectomy for myasthenia gravis. Ann Thorac Surg. 1998;65(6):1520–2.
8. Souadjian JV, Enriquez P, Silverstein MN, Pepin JM. The spectrum of diseases associated with thymoma: coincidence or syndrome? Arch Intern Med. 1974;134(2):374–9.
9. Crowe JK, Brown LR, Muhm JR. Computed tomography of the mediastinum. Radiology. 1978;128(1):75–87.
10. Baron RL, Lee JK, Sagel SS, Levitt RG. Computed tomography of the abnormal thymus. Radiology. 1982;142:127–34.
11. Azizkhan RG, Dudgeon DL, Buck JR, et al. Life-threatening airway obstruction as a complication to the management of mediastinal masses in children. J Pediatr Surg. 1985;20:816–22.
12. Pravash UBS, Abel MD, Hubmayr RD. Mediastinal masses. A case report and review of the literature. Anaesthesia. 1984;39:899–903.
13. Giannopoulou A, Gkiozos I, Harrington KJ, Syrigos KN. Thymoma and radiation therapy: a systematic review of medical treatment. Expert Rev Anticancer Ther. 2013;13(6):759–66.
14. Dillon F. Anesthesia issues in the perioperative management of myasthenia gravis. Semin Neurol. 2004;24(1):83–94.
15. Neuman GG, Weingarten AE, Abramowitz RM. The anesthetic management of the patient with an anterior mediastinal mass. Anesthesiology. 1984;60:144–7.
16. Shrager JB, Deeb ME, Mick R, et al. Transcervical thymectomy for myasthenia gravis achieves results comparable to thymectomy by sternotomy. Ann Thorac Surg. 2002;74:320–6.
17. Tsunezuka Y, Oda M, Matsumoto I, Tamura M, Watanabe G. Extended thymectomy in patients with myasthenia gravis with high thoracic epidural anesthesia alone. World J Surg. 2004;28(10):962–5.
18. Baraka A, Baroody M, Yazbeck V. Repeated doses of suxamethonium in the myasthenic patient. Anaesthesia. 1993;28:782–4.

19. Yanagidate F, Dohi S, Hamaya Y, Tsujito T. Reexpansion pulmonary edema after thorascopic mediastinal tumor resection. Anesth Analg. 2001;92(6):1416–7.
20. Gronseth GS, Barohn RJ. Practice parameter: thymectomy for autoimmune myasthenia gravis (an evidence-based review): report of the Quality Standards Subcommittee of the American Academy of Neurology. Neurology. 2000;55(1):7–15.
21. Lin M, Chang Y, Huang P, Lee Y. Thymectomy for non-thymomatous myasthenia gravis: a comparison of surgical methods and analysis of prognostic factors. Eur J Cardiothorac Surg. 2010;37:7–12.
22. Kim HK, Park MS, Choi YS, et al. Neurologic outcomes of thymectomy in myasthenia gravis: comparative analysis of the effect of thymoma. J Thorac Cardiovasc Surg. 2007;134(3):601–7.
23. Ng JK, Ng CS, Underwood MJ, Lau KK. Does repeat thymectomy improve symptoms in patients with refractory myasthenia gravis. Interact Cardiovasc Thorac Surg. 2014;18(3):376–80.

# Anesthesia Issues in Patients with VADs Presenting for Noncardiac Surgery

Ahmed Awad, Alann Solina, Theresa Gerges, and Muhammad Muntazar

## Introduction

Heart Failure (HF) is the inability of the heart to pump blood at a rate adequate to fulfill the metabolic requirements of the tissues and organs. The American Heart Association (AHA) and the American College of Cardiology Foundation (ACCF) have developed a HF staging system, in which stage D is advanced HF that is refractory to medical therapy [1]. Table 18.1 summarizes the four stages of HF.

Heart failure is further classified based on the presence of left ventricular (LV) functional abnormalities. Patients range from those with normal LV function and a preserved ejection fraction (EF) to those with a markedly reduced EF. Thus, two categories of patients exist: those with heart failure and a preserved ejection fraction (HF$p$EF) and those with heart failure and a reduced ejection fraction (HF$r$EF).

According to the 2016 AHA Heart Disease and Stroke Statistics Update, about 5.8 million people in the United States are currently diagnosed with HF. Of this number, 2.9 million people have HF$r$EF, and about 10% (200K–250K) of those with HF$r$EF have stage D [2]. Stage D has a very poor prognosis despite maximal medical treatment and cardiac synchronization therapy, which includes the use of pulmonary vasodilators, diuretics, inotropic agents, systemic vasopressors, biventricular pacemakers, and/or automated implantable cardioverter-defibrillator (AICD) placement.

Cardiac transplantation remains the standard of care for patients with refractory HF. However, with limited heart donors, only 2000–4000 heart transplantations are performed per year. Thus, a growing population of patients with stage D HF has created the need to consider alternative therapies. The use of ventricular assist devices (VADs) has emerged as a viable treatment option for these patients.

The Randomized Evaluation of Mechanical Assistance for the Treatment of Congestive Heart Failure (REMATCH) trial and the Investigation of Nontransplant-Eligible Patients Who Are

A. Awad, M.D., M.B.A., C.B.A. (✉)
Cardiac Anesthesiology, Cooper Medical School of Rowan University/Cooper University Health Care, Camden, NJ, USA
e-mail: Awad-Ahmed@CooperHealth.edu

A. Solina, M.D.
Department of Anesthesiology, Cooper Medical School of Rowan University/Cooper University Health Care, Camden, NJ, USA

T. Gerges, M.D.
Cooper Medical School of Rowan University/Cooper University Health Care, Camden, NJ, USA

M. Muntazar, M.D., F.A.C.M.Q.
Cardiac Anesthesiology, Deborah Heart and Lung Center, Browns Mills, NJ, USA

**Table 18.1** ACCF/AHA stages of heart failure (Hunt et al., Circulation. 2009)

| Stage | ACCF/AHA stages of HF description |
|---|---|
| A | At high risk for HF but without structural heart disease or symptoms of HF |
| B | Structural heart disease but without signs or symptoms of HF |
| C | Structural heart disease with prior or current symptoms of HF |
| D | Refractory HF requiring specialized interventions |

*ACCF* American College of Cardiology Foundation, *AHA* American Heart Association, *HF* heart failure

Inotrope-Dependent (INTREPID) trial demonstrated a substantial reduction in any cause mortality and showed improved survival rates for patients with LV assist devices (LVADs) [3, 4]. Figures 18.1 and 18.2 show the survival curves for medical therapy and LVADs.

LVAD therapy continues to develop and grow. In 2015, there were more LVADs implanted annually than cardiac transplantations, with 2973 devices implanted versus 2819 heart transplants performed [5].

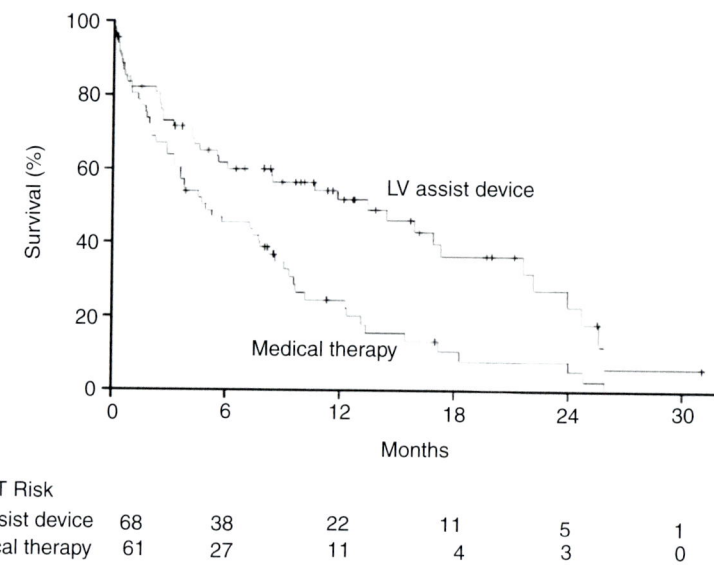

**Fig. 18.1** *REMATCH trial results, Rose et al. NEJM 2001*: Kaplan–Meier analysis of survival in the group that received LVADs and the group that received optimal medical therapy. (Reproduced with permission of NEJM)

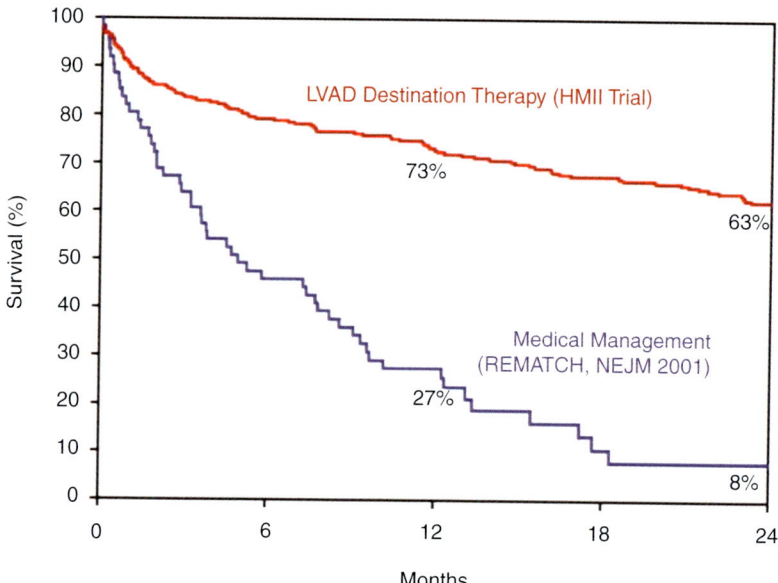

**Fig. 18.2** *REMATCH trial results, Park et al. Circ: Heart Failure 2012*: The survival benefit of destination therapy with continuous-flow left ventricular assist device (CF-LVAD) compared with medical management. HMII: HeartMate II (Reproduced with permission of Circulation: Heart Failure)

## The Devices

The ventricular assist device (VAD) is a man-made pump that replaces the damaged patient's ventricle, which is implanted surgically or percutaneously to help decompress the ventricle, restore circulation, and provide adequate organ perfusion, thus preventing the development of multiple organ failure [6]. It is important to have a good understanding of the anatomy of these devices as it will enable the provider to anticipate complications and plan for their management.

## Anatomy of VADs

Most of these assist device systems are comprised of an inflow cannula, a pump, an outflow cannula, a power supply, and a display/control console. The inflow cannula drains and unloads the assisted ventricle. The pump receives the inflow cannula return and pumps the blood to either the pulmonary artery (right ventricular assist) or the proximal aorta (left ventricular assist). The pump is attached by a driveline that exits the body and connects to an external controller console. A power supply attaches to the console. The screen of the controller console can display pump flow (liters/minute), pump speed, pulse index, and pump power. Some devices like the Heartware HVAD will also show waveforms that depict the rate of blood flowing through the pump (Fig. 18.3).

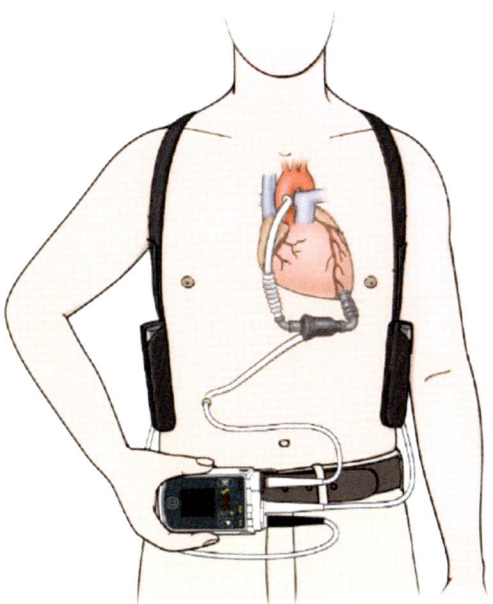

**Fig. 18.3** Implanted HeartMate II (Reproduced courtesy of Thoratec Corporation)

## Indications for VADs: Who Gets Them?

The latest report (seventh report) by the Interagency Registry for Mechanically Assisted Circulatory Support (INTERMACS) stated that 15,745 adult patients had received primary implants of VADs since June 2006. This report summarizes the first 9 years of patient enrollment [7]. Per the report, at the time of implantation most patients (85%) that have received the implant lie within INTERMACS levels 1–3. INTERMACS levels classify the different degrees of clinical severity of HF into seven levels [8] (Table 18.2). Patients with ACC/AHA stage D ventricular HF, in which maximum medical management and cardiac resynchronization therapy have been deemed unsuccessful for at least 45 of the last 60 days, or patients requiring an intra-aortic balloon pump for 7 of the last 14 days are patients currently authorized to receive VADs by the Centers for Medicare and Medicaid Services. Other inclusion criteria include a LVEF <25% and a peak oxygen consumption of 14 mL/kg/min [9]. Although the device was initially developed as a transitional treatment prior to a definitive heart transplant, the increased need for transplantation together with the lack of a heart transplant supply has driven the VAD therapy to be used for a broader array of clinical applications. A recent observational study examined the benefit of targeting a less critically ill population to receive VADs. In the Risk Assessment and Comparative Effectiveness of Left Ventricular Assist Device and Medical Management in Ambulatory Heart Failure Patients (ROADMAP) study, LVADs were utilized for those in the ambulatory class

**Table 18.2** INTERMACS (Interagency Registry for Mechanically Assisted Circulatory Support) scale for classifying patients with advanced heart failure

| Profiles | Definition | Description |
|---|---|---|
| INTERMACS 1 | 'Crash and burn' | Hemodynamic instability in spite of increasing doses of catecholamines and/or mechanical circulatory support with critical hypoperfusion of target organs (severe cardiogenic shock) |
| INTERMACS 2 | 'Sliding on inotropes' | Intravenous inotropic support with acceptable blood pressure but rapid deterioration of kidney function, nutritional state, or signs of congestion |
| INTERMACS 3 | 'Dependent stability' | Hemodynamic stability with low or intermediate, but necessary due to hypotension, doses of inotropics, worsening of symptoms, or progressive kidney failure |
| INTERMACS 4 | 'Frequent flyer' | Temporary cessation of inotropic treatment is possible, but the patient presents frequent symptom recurrences and typically with fluid overload |
| INTERMACS 5 | 'Housebound' | Complete cessation of physical activity, stable at rest, but frequently with moderate water retention and some level of kidney dysfunction |
| INTERMACS 6 | 'Walking wounded' | Minor limitation on physical activity and absence of congestion while at rest. Easily fatigued by light activity |
| INTERMACS 7 | 'Placeholder' | Patient in New York Heart Association (NYHA) functional class II or III, with no current or recent unstable water balance |

of refractory heart failure INTERMACS patient profiles 4–7. Although the study showed better survival with an improved functional status in the LVAD group, this was offset by an increase in adverse effects compared with patients in the optimal medical management group [10].

## Types of Ventricular Assist Devices

There are many different types of VADs. VADs can be classified, depending on the ventricle being supported, into right ventricular assist devices (RVADs), left ventricular assist devices (LVADs), or biventricular assist devices (BVADs). VADS are mostly used to support the left ventricle; less frequently they are used to support the right ventricle and even less frequently, both ventricles. From this point forward, we will mostly discuss LVADs, as they are the most commonly used VADs and probably the most likely devices to be encountered by a non-cardiac anesthesiologist.

VADs also can be classified, depending on their durability and the purpose of usage, into short-term circulatory support devices and long-term circulatory support devices. Patients with cardiogenic shock are frequently started on short-term or temporary mechanical support devices and are then assessed for recovery, eligibility to receive a transplant or long-term mechanical support devices.

1. *Short-Term circulatory support devices*: This section describes the use of mechanical support devices on a short-term basis as an acute rescue strategy. These devices can be utilized as a bridge to transplantation, as a bridge to candidacy, or a bridge to recovery.
   - Bridge to Transplantation (BTT): For current transplant candidates who need assist devices to sustain life until cardiac transplantation.
   - Bridge to Candidacy (BTC): For non-transplant candidates in the hope of making the patient a candidate via a change in a modifiable risk factor (noncompliance, BMI greater than 35, recent cancer diagnosis, or poor social support).
   - Bridge to Recovery (BTR): For approved candidates who may show ventricular improvement with only temporary use of an assist device. Tables 18.3 and 18.4 and Figs. 18.4, 18.5, 18.6, 18.7, and 18.8 summarize the devices that are used on a short-term basis.

**Table 18.3** Short-term, percutaneous cannulation, mechanical circulatory support systems

| Device name | Manufacturer | Description and position of the pump | Duration |
|---|---|---|---|
| Intra-aortic balloon pump | Maquet cardiovascular Fairfield, New Jersey | Distal aortic arch and descending aorta balloon-filled helium counterpulsation. The pump lies outside the body pumping helium to a balloon mounted on a catheter situated inside the aorta | Days |
| Extracorporeal membrane oxygenation (ECMO) | Multiple manufacturers for different parts | It has a continuous flow centrifugal pump and inflow and outflow cannula, oxygenator. Venoarterial extracorporeal membrane oxygenation (ECMO) provides circulatory support and oxygenation for a short period of time until the primary problem is fixed | Days-weeks |
| TandemHeart | Cardiac Assist, Pittsburgh, Pennsylvania | It is an external centrifugal pump that drains blood from the left atrium and pumps it into the femoral artery. Extracorporeal with the venous cannula inserted via the femoral vein and positioned in the left atrium through an atrial septal puncture, and outflow cannula placed into the femoral artery. The pump itself is strapped to the thigh close to the femoral cannula | Days |
| Impella recover | ABIOMED Danvers, Massachusetts | It is a small axial flow pump placed in the ascending aorta with the inlet inside the left ventricle across the aortic valve and the outlet part in the ascending aorta, so blood is pumped from the left ventricle across the aortic valve, leading to decompression of the left ventricle and improved forward flow | Days |

**Table 18.4** Surgically implanted, mechanical, circulatory support systems

| Device name | Manufacturer | Description and position of the pump | Duration |
|---|---|---|---|
| ABIOMED BVS 5000 and AB 5000 | ABIOMED Danvers, Massachusetts | It is a pulsatile, extracorporeal, asynchronous ventricular assist device. It has a pneumatically driven pump that converts compressed air into hydraulic power and is compromised of dual chambers, one for passively filling with blood by gravity and no vacuum applied and the other chamber for pumping blood to deliver 5-6 L/min | Weeks |
| CentriMag ventricular assist | Thoratec Pleasanton, California | It has a continuous flow centrifugal pump and inflow and outflow cannula with the possibility to add an oxygenator. It provides circulatory support and potential oxygenation for short period until the primary problem is fixed | Hours-Weeks |

2. *Intermediate or long-term circulatory support devices*: Intermediate-term circulatory support can be used as a BTT for patients requiring mechanical assistance or as a Destination Therapy (DT). Patients that do not qualify for cardiac transplantation who require long-term circulatory support can be placed on an assist device as a DT. VADs also can be classified depending on the type of technology into first generation, second generation, and third generation LVADS (Table 18.5).
   - The first generation LVADs attempted to resemble the native ventricle via its pumping ability and, therefore, resulted in blood flow that was pulsatile. However, they did not come without disadvantages, including their requirement of a large device surface area due to the large pumping chamber and frequent exchanges needed due to wear and tear.
   - The second generation LVADs sought to mitigate the disadvantages of the first generation LVADs by shifting to continuous-flow devices. These continuous-flow devices utilize axial flow which directs outflow from the pump parallel to the axis of rotation. The continuous-flow pumps draw blood from the patient's left ventricle into the device, which is propelled continuously around the impeller and subsequently ejected into the patient's aorta.

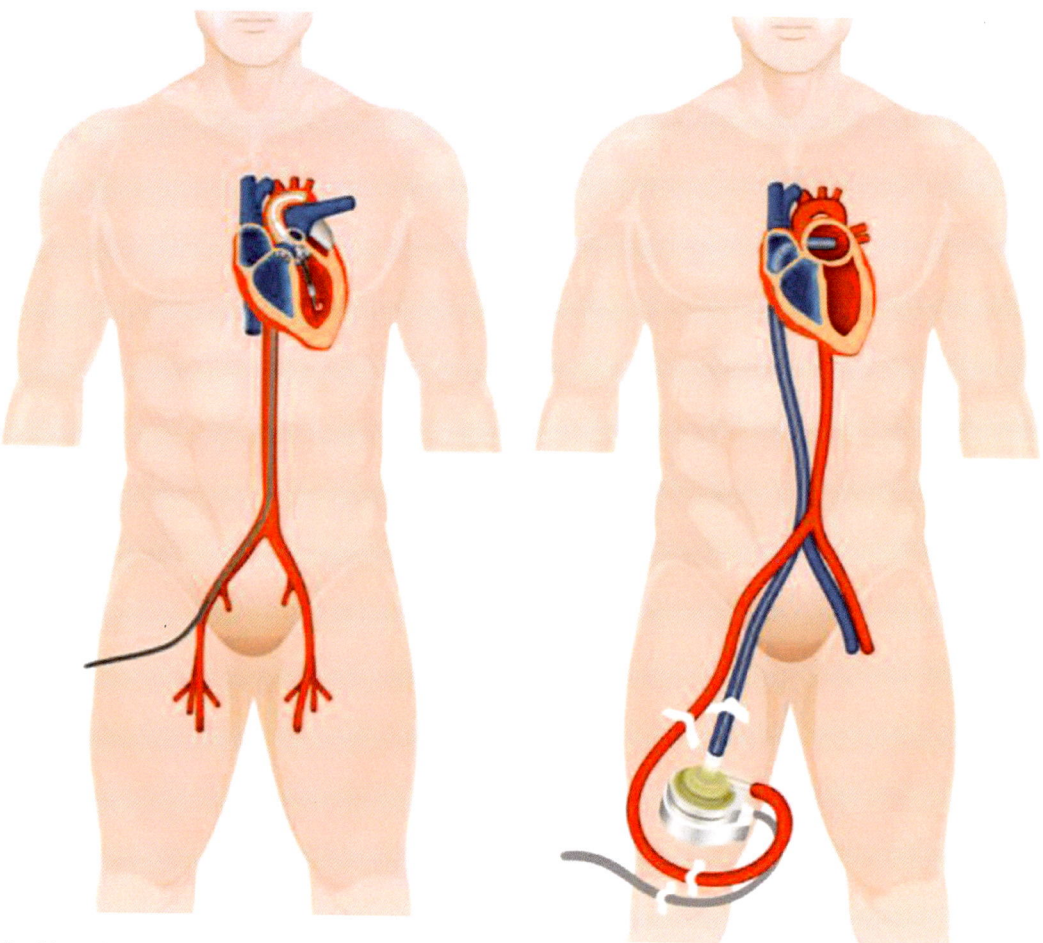

**Fig. 18.4** Illustration showing Intra-aortic balloon pump (Reproduced with permission of Springer)

**Fig. 18.5** Illustration showing veno-arterial ECMO (Reproduced with permission of Springer)

- The third generation LVADs are continuous-flow centrifugal pumps which directs outflow from the pump perpendicular to the axis of rotation. These devices emerged with new unique technology to prevent pump thrombosis. They have a magnetically levitated, more efficient centrifugal, continuous-flow pump, with smaller size, limited blood contact with fewer moving parts, and the absence of mechanical bearings and seals. These technological advances proved that pump thrombosis could be alleviated, as seen in the recently published MOMENTUM III trial [11]. The third generation LVADs were compared against the second generation LVADs in the treatment of refractory HF in the ENDURANCE trial [12]. This trial showed that continuous-flow centrifugal pumps are noninferior to axial-flow pumps with regard to survival free from disabling stroke or device removal for malfunction or failure. A common problem for continuous-flow second generation pumps was the development of pump thrombosis. Table 18.5 examines the three generations of VADs and their pumps. Figure 18.9 shows continuous axial-flow and centrifugal-flow pumps.

The technological advances in circulatory support devices are evident. Not only are these devices becoming miniaturized and suitable for intrapericardial insertion, but they also are better

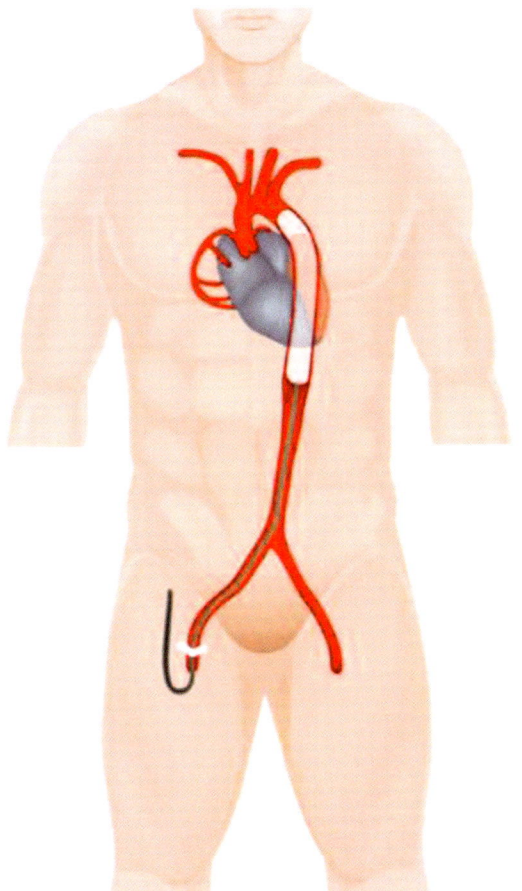

**Fig. 18.6** Illustration showing Impella Recover (Reproduced with permission of Springer)

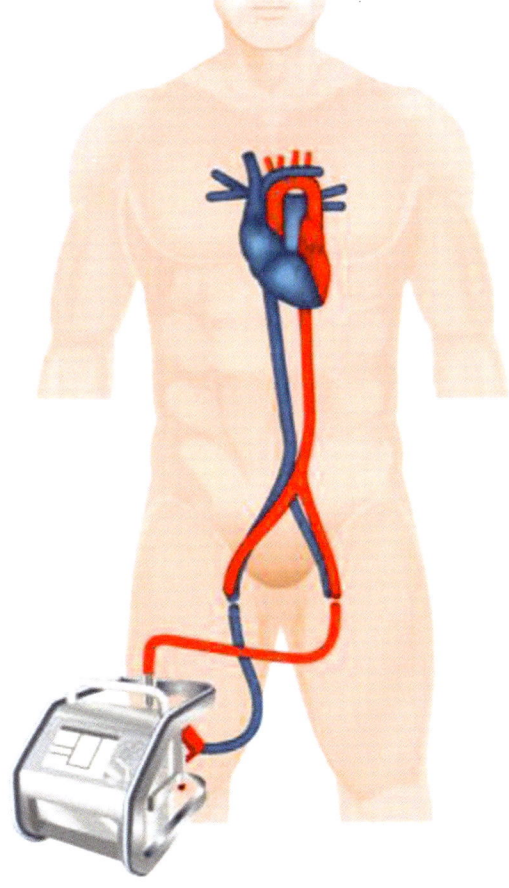

**Fig. 18.7** Illustration showing TandemHeart (Reproduced with permission of Springer)

designed to decrease rates of complications (Figs. 18.10 and 18.11).

## Physiological Changes That Occur After VAD Implantation

How do these devices change the patient's physiology?

- Implantation of a VAD and restoration of the systemic circulation leads to improvements in end organ function and normalization of serum kidney and liver markers [13].
- Unloading of the left ventricle in the immediate period and for a short time after implantation will lead to a reduction in LV size and a slight improvement in the EF. Additionally, unloading the ventricle will lead to a reduction in wall tension and improved myocardial energetics.
- The first generation VADs used pulsatile pneumatic pumps. However, the second generation devices are continuous-flow devices with non-pulsatile pumps, so the pulse is often less palpable. The third generation devices also use non-pulsatile pumps. However, they allow for some pulsatility that can be monitored.
- Blood flow depends on ventricular loading conditions and is estimated from power consumption. The venous return fills the right ventricle which must function to fill the left ventricle. The RV outflow is the LVAD inflow.

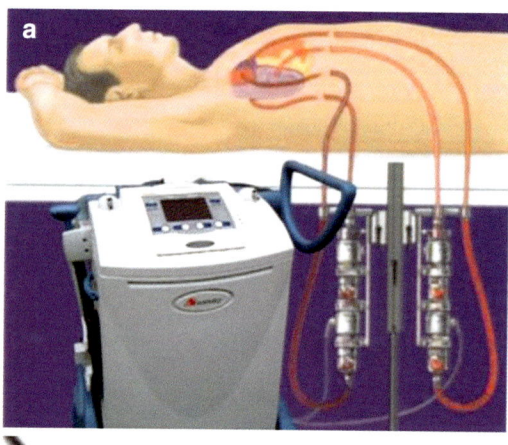

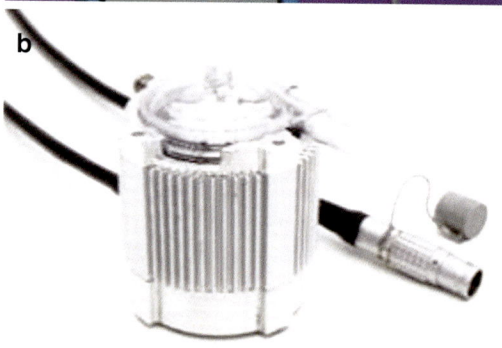

**Fig. 18.8** (**a**) Illustration showing Abiomed BVS 5000 pump and console ventricular assist (Reproduced with permission of Springer). (**b**) CentriMag ventricular assist (Reproduced courtesy of Thoratec)

- The continuous-flow LVAD is sensitive to changes in preload and afterload. Reduced LV volume will decrease flow through the pump as will acute increases in LV afterload.

## Common Complications Associated with VADs

Although INTERMACS data show that VADs prolong survival and improve the quality of life of patients with end-stage heart failure, real and life threatening complications are still a problem for these patient populations. The risk and kind of complications after VAD therapy depend largely on which generation of device is used, the length of time the device has been inserted, and the patient's clinical status. Postoperative complications after VAD implantation can be divided into early (less than 30 days from implantation) and late (greater than 30 days from implantation). The frequency of complications is much higher with pulsatile pumps than continuous-flow VADs. Here, we describe some of the most common complications that occur in patients implanted with VADs, as described in the INTERMACS 7 database [7].

## Early Complications

### Bleeding

Bleeding is the most common complication in the early postoperative period after the implantation of VADs. Multiple factors contribute to this complication including the use of anticoagulation, hepatic dysfunction from hepatic congestion that leads to a decrease in circulating coagulation factors, and platelet dysfunction [14, 15].

### Infection

Although the risk of infection has fallen because of technological advancement of VADs, it remains an important complication and can be divided into driveline-related infections (DLIs) and non-DLIs, for example, pneumonia, endocarditis, peritonitis, and urinary tract infections. Multiple factors contribute to a higher rate of infection in this patient population including malnourishment, blood transfusions, foreign body-related infections, and the presence of comorbidities such as diabetes [16–18].

### Arrhythmias

Cardiac arrhythmias are not uncommon complications in patients with VADs. Arrhythmias may be atrial arrhythmias such as atrial fibrillation or atrial flutter. Ventricular arrhythmias may be in the form of ventricular tachycardia or ventricular fibrillation. Ventricular arrhythmias, although not fatal, can cause right ventricular compromise. Right ventricular dysfunction also can lead to ventricular arrhythmias. These patients can present with syncope due to a ventricular arrhythmia [19].

**Table 18.5** Examples of the three generations of mechanical circulatory support systems with the types of their corresponding pumps (Images reproduced courtesy of Thoratec Corporation and HeartWare)

| First generation | Second generation | Third generation |
| --- | --- | --- |
| – Pulsatile flow<br>– Large pumping chamber → only in select patients<br>– Easily worn out; frequent exchanges. These are volume displacement pumps<br>– Examples:<br>  • HeartMate XVE LVAD more than 5 L<br>  • Thoratec PVAD<br>  • Thoratec IVAD more than 3 L<br>  • Novacore LVAD<br>  • CardioWest total artificial heart (TAH) | – Continuous flow<br>– Axial flow<br>– Smaller in size with fewer complications than first-generation devices, and improved efficiency and durability<br>– Examples:<br>  • HeartMate II<br>  • The Jarvik 2000<br>  • MicroMed-DeBakey<br>  • Incor Berlin Heart | – Continuous flow but demonstrate increased pulsatility<br>– Centrifugal flow<br>– Examples:<br>  • HeartWare, HVAD<br>  • Thoratec, HeartMate III<br>  • DuraHeart |
| Thoratec PVAD | HeartMate II | HeartWare, HVAD |
| Pulsatile-flow pump | Continuous axial-flow pump | Continuous centrifugal-flow pump |

## Right Ventricular Failure

Right ventricular (RV) failure after VAD implantation is associated with a significant increase in mortality. Unloading the LV with an LVAD will reduce LV size. The LV-RV geometric relationship may be further disturbed by LVAD induced increase in RV preload, and a leftward bowing/shift of the interventricular septum. These geometric changes may compromise RV function and lead to the development of RV failure. A significant blood transfusion can also lead to RV compromise from released leukotrienes and inflammatory mediators [20].

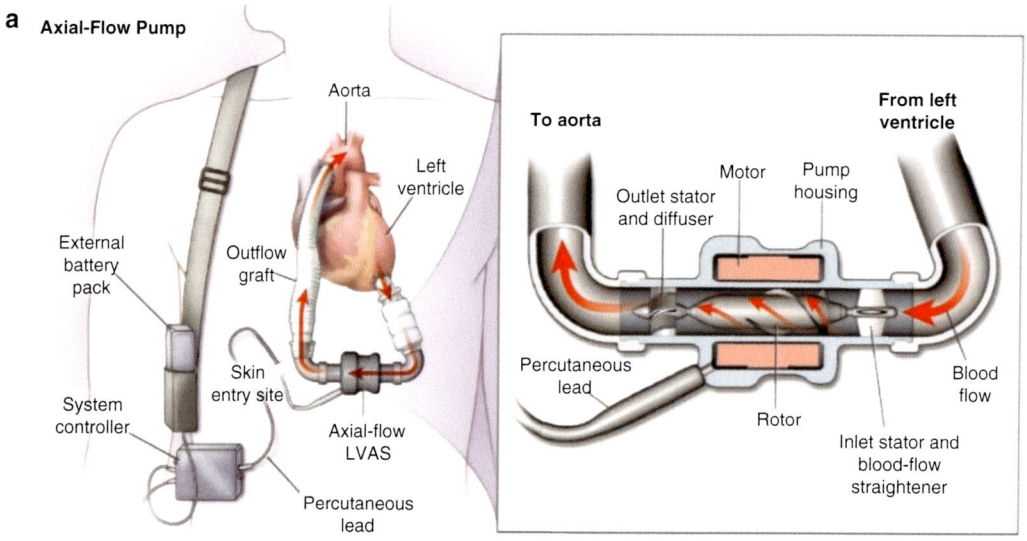

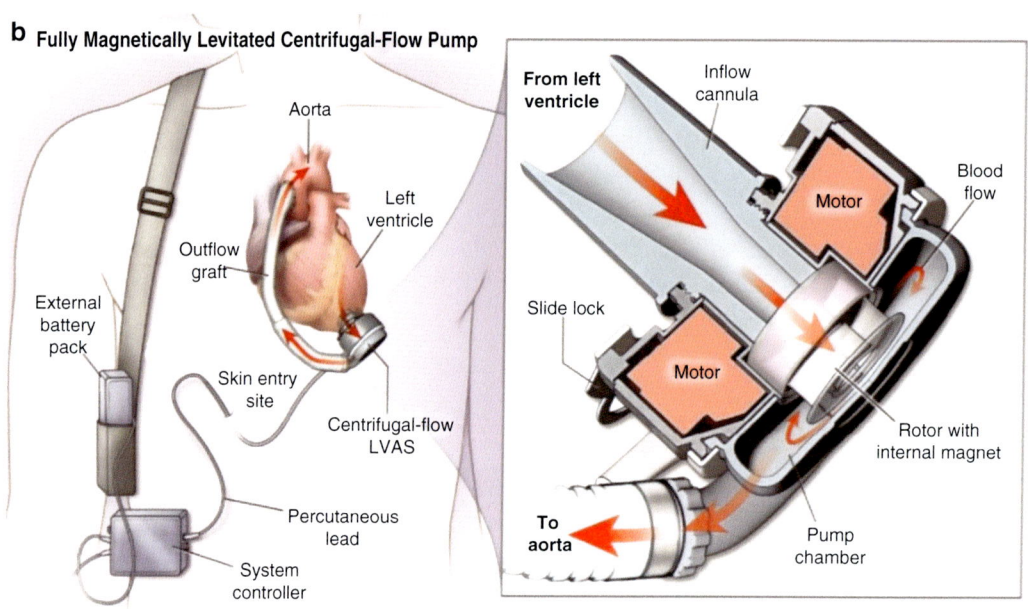

**Fig. 18.9** Diagrams of continuous-flow axial-flow pump (**a**) and centrifugal-flow pump (**b**) (Reproduced with permission Mehra et al. NEJM 2017)

### End-Organ Failure

Although renal and hepatic function typically improves after VAD implantation, renal and hepatic failure can occur. Pre-existing organ dysfunction, the development of RV failure, malnutrition, infection, and the use of nephrotoxic and hepatotoxic drugs all contribute to renal and hepatic damage. Once developed, hepatic or renal dysfunction is associated with worse outcomes in VAD-supported patients.

### Suction Events

A reduction in LV preload, and an increase in the negative pressure within the left ventricle, may result in part of the LV wall being sucked into and covering the opening of the pump's inlet cannula. The pump then sounds an alarm, and the speed will decrease to relieve the suction. Suction events are usually initiated by a low intracardiac volume, which may be due to RV failure or tamponade. Suction events can lead to occurs because of thromboembolic events. Exposure of the circulating blood to VADs coupled with turbulent flow precipitates thrombus formation. Moreover, inadequate blood pressure control and non-therapeutic anticoagulation further increase the potential for thromboembolic complications. There is no difference in stroke rates between patients with pulsatile-flow versus continuous-flow VADs [7].

## Late Complications

Late complications are either those that continue from the early postoperative period or are new types of complications that develop in the late postoperative period.

### Aortic Valve Degeneration

The aortic valve usually does not open in patients with continuous-flow VADs. Hence, valves in these patients are continuously subjected to high pressure that leads to aortic valve degeneration and the development of aortic regurgitation [22–24].

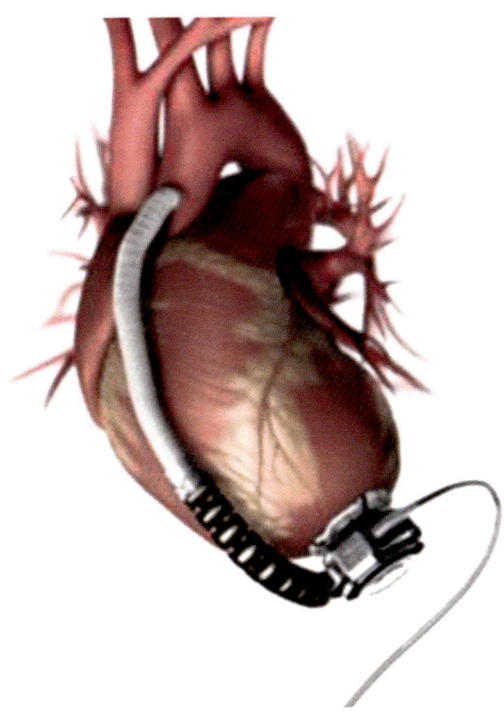

**Fig. 18.10** Implanted HeartMate II (Reproduced courtesy of Thoratec Corporation)

### Severe Gastrointestinal Bleeding

Gastrointestinal bleeding in patients with continuous-flow VADs is common. Causes include the development of an arteriovenous malformation (AVM), excessive anticoagulation, and acquired von Willebrand factor (vWF) deficiency type II [25].

### Device Thrombosis

According to the INTERMACS 7 data, the axial-flow pump had a 10% incidence of device thrombosis, while the third-generation centrifugal-flow pump had a 0% incidence of device thrombosis. With improvements in technology, this complication is less of a problem than before. Because device thrombosis and replacement of the device is associated with a very high mortality and morbidity, properly adjusted anticoagulation is of paramount importance. An increase in signs of hemolysis, including elevated levels of lactate dehydrogenase (LDH) above 750, or a haptoglobin level less than 7 are associated with a high incidence of device thrombosis [26]. The Protocol

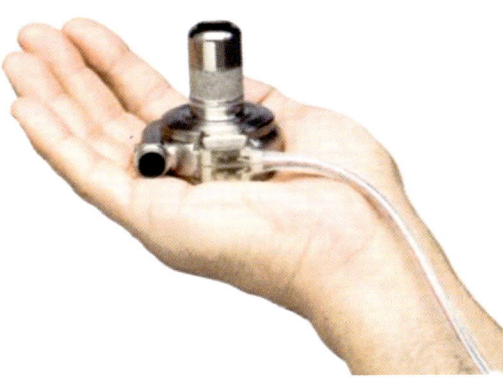

**Fig. 18.11** The HeartWare HVAD Pump comparing its size to the palm of a hand (Reproduced courtesy of The HeartWare™)

low LVAD flows and can prompt ventricular arrhythmias [21].

## Neurological Complications

Hemorrhagic and ischemic strokes in patients with VADs are uncommon, but devastating complications. Hemorrhagic stroke occurs because of vigorous anticoagulation, while Ischemic stroke

Lowers Pump Thrombosis in HeartMate II (PREVENT) trial is an ongoing trial designed to determine recommended clinical practices to decrease device thrombosis in patients with axial-flow circulatory assist devices.

## Preoperative Evaluation and Considerations

Communication with the VAD team at your institution should precede the development of an in-depth anesthetic plan. If no such team exists at your institution, then contact the VAD team at the center that placed and currently manages the VAD. The VAD team usually includes a cardiac surgeon, a cardiologist, a perfusionist, and an LVAD coordinator or nurse. If you are not able to communicate with a VAD team, then contact the emergency number of the VAD company. Valuable information obtained from the VAD team includes knowledge of the duration of implantation, the current pump settings, and any complications that the patient may have endured. It is also important to obtain information about whether the device insertion site is intrapericardial or intraperitoneal. Knowledge about its driveline location may help guide the surgical approach, so the site may be avoided during the proposed procedure. A review of previous anesthesia records, if available, is very helpful. The next step in the preoperative evaluation is to assess patient's risks based on the standard risk evaluation, as defined by the ASA classification. This risk evaluation includes obtaining a history from the patient and reviewing all of the patient's systems. This is usually followed by performance of a thorough physical exam. Finally, one should request and review all biochemical investigations and imaging studies based upon associated comorbidities [27, 28].

## Airway Assessment/Aspiration Risk

A meticulous airway assessment is necessary for patients with VADs undergoing any surgical procedure. A few questions need to be answered in this assessment. How difficult is it to intubate this patient? Does the patient have a previous tracheostomy that may require a smaller endotracheal tube? Is the aspiration risk significant and is blood present in the upper GI tract? Does the patient have obstructive sleep apnea and how difficult will it be to ventilate this patient? Are they an appropriate candidate for monitored anesthesia care (MAC) anesthesia? A standardized assessment should involve use of the four-point modified Mallampati scoring, with assessment of the width of the mouth opening and the presence or absence of a short neck and/or limited neck mobility. The anesthesia strategy will be built on the answers to these questions, so precautions can be taken to prepare for managing a difficult airway or difficult ventilation and preventing aspiration during induction of anesthesia [29, 30].

## Cardiovascular Assessment

Cardiovascular assessment of the patient should also be performed as per the standard protocols. Optimization of the patient's clinical condition by a HF cardiologist is preferable. Knowledge about the status of the right ventricle prior to surgery is key to properly planning for intraoperative management [9, 31]. If any questions exists as to current right ventricular function, a preoperative echocardiogram is indicated. It is also important to know if the patient has an AICD or pacemaker and if the patient is dependent on the pacemaker. An AICD should be suspended and the pacemaker may need to be reprogrammed to an asynchronous mode should be done if electrocautery will be used.

## Hepatic/Renal Assessment

Determination of the patient's hepatic and renal function is critical, as hepatic congestion will often impair liver function and result in a dysfunctional coagulation status. Therefore, one should consider analysis of synthetic liver function laboratory studies such as albumin and coagulation parameters. The co-existence of renal disease with heart failure necessitates evaluation of renal function and electrolyte studies prior to elective anesthetic management of these patients.

## Hematology: Anticoagulation Requirements

Patients who receive VADs are anticoagulated with warfarin and an antiplatelet medication (aspirin or clopidogrel). Most centers will typically target an INR of 2-3, though this will vary by patient, device and institution. Management of anticoagulation should factor the risk of bleeding versus the risk of thrombosis in the upcoming procedure. Decisions regarding reversal of anticoagulation should involve members of the VAD and surgical team in conjunction with the anesthesiologist. In addition to the preoperative coagulation profile testing, the patient should have a type and screen with blood available for more than minor procedures [9, 28, 30–32]. In the event of an emergent procedure with significant bleeding risk, the anesthesiologist may consider partial reversal of the anticoagulation. This should be a team-based decision and may be accomplished by giving fresh frozen plasma but vitamin K or prothrombin complex concentrates are not recommended. Complete and persistent reversal of anticoagulation will increase the risk of device thrombosis and embolic stroke [9].

## Medications

A thorough review of all medications that the patient is taking is important to identify possible anesthesia implications. For example, treatment with sildenafil, milrinone, or midodrine implies right ventricular failure. As mentioned above, these patients are maintained on anticoagulation. The patient is often admitted prior to an elective procedure to transition from warfarin to heparin and optimize the patient's coagulation status prior to the procedure [31].

## Intraoperative Anesthetic Considerations

### Power

When the patient arrives in the operating room or the procedure room, the control console should be plugged into wall power outlet as soon as possible to make sure that the batteries are not consumed. Also, backup batteries should be available [31].

### Infection Prophylaxis

Often, the driveline and pump pocket are significant sources of infection that must be considered prior to any procedure. Sepsis and infections in patients with VADs not only increase the length of hospitalization, but more importantly, increase mortality rates. Antibiotic prophylaxis should be selected to treat gram-positive and gram-negative bacteria, with antibiotics for anaerobes in the case of intra-abdominal surgery. Antifungals such as fluconazole are often utilized in higher-risk patients [9, 31].

### Hemodynamic Monitoring

As with all anesthetic techniques, it is crucial for the anesthesiologist to be able to monitor the blood pressure, pulse, and oxygen saturation which can be challenging with continuous flow VADs.

First-generation VADs provide pulsatile flow, so patients will have a pulse. Second- and third-generation VADs provide continuous flow. Therefore, the patient usually presents with a reduced pulse, however noninvasive blood pressure determination and pulse oximetry is usually often possible. This should be determined preoperatively, and the use of an arterial line should be considered prior to the induction of anesthesia. Although turning the pump speed down might help capture better pulsatility, this should not be a commonly used perioperative strategy. Complete absence of a pulse generally indicates a significant reduction in LV preload, which could be from true hypovolemia or from RV failure and indicates further investigation. As mentioned earlier, preoperative and intraoperative echocardiography should be considered a definitive study in answering volume and RV inquiries. Because noninvasive blood pressure monitors rely on variations in pulsations to calculate a patient's blood pressure, manual measurement with the aid of Doppler may be used. Applying the Doppler probe over the brachial artery while deflating the cuff and listening for a continuous sound does correlate with mean arterial blood pressure [33, 34]. However, this technique is cumbersome and not well-tailored to intraoperative use. An arterial catheter line for invasive arterial blood pressure monitoring should be considered in VADs patients undergoing procedures associated with blood loss or significant fluid shifts [9]. The use of ultrasound or Doppler with a micro-puncture wire may facilitate the arterial line placement. As mentioned earlier, patients with VADs are susceptible to driveline and pump infections. Therefore, any invasive monitoring should be performed using a meticulous aseptic technique. Cerebral oximetry can be utilized when the pulse oximeter readings are not reliable and serial arterial blood gas measurements should be undertaken [9].

## Anesthetic Techniques

There are a range of anesthetic techniques that can be employed depending on factors such as the patient's comorbidities, the attending anesthesiologist's skills, the anticipated duration of the procedure, and the location of the procedure in the hospital. Ready availability and the quality of expert help are other factors to consider.

### Neuraxial Anesthesia

Neuraxial anesthesia is typically contraindicated in these patients due to potential complications from residual anticoagulation.

### Regional Anesthesia

Regional anesthesia may be appropriate depending on numerous factors such as anticoagulation, the type of surgery, the adaptability of the surgeon and patient comfort and preference.

### Monitored Anesthesia Care (MAC)

MAC is certainly an option for VAD patients in the operating room and procedural suites. Goudra et al. [33] showed that MAC can be safely used to perform the majority of gastrointestinal endoscopy procedures in patients with LVADs.

## General Anesthesia with Endotracheal Intubation

General endotracheal anesthesia (GETA) is most commonly used in this patient population. If there any concerns regarding the airway, ability to maintain adequate spontaneous ventilation, or aspiration risk, the use of an endotracheal tube (ETT) is advisable.

- *Induction*
  A deliberate and graded induction of anesthesia is crucial to prevent any drop in cardiac output which is dependent upon the RV to drive the preload to the LVAD. All invasive monitors should be placed prior to induction. Any preexisting automated internal cardiac defibrillators should be inactivated prior to electrocautery use, and external defibrillator pads should be placed prior to induction [9]. If a "full stomach" is suspected or if the patient has a gastrointestinal bleed and the possible presence of blood in the stomach, a rapid sequence induction is warranted. In addition, the patient should be adequately anesthetized before instrumentation of the airway. Stimulation by direct laryngoscopy may cause an increase in the systemic vascular resistance, and consequentially, a drop in cardiac output [9, 34].
- *Maintenance*
  A balanced anesthesia technique with monitoring of the anesthetic depth using the Bispectral index should be considered. The anesthetic technique should be consistent with maintenance of

> preload, afterload, and the function of the non-assisted ventricle.
> - *Emergence*
>   Extreme caution during emergence and extubation is vital to avoid abrupt changes in the blood pressure and heart rate, which may decrease the patient's cardiac output.

## Hemodynamic Management

### Preload and Right Ventricular Function

As mentioned earlier, RV failure may be challenging to manage intraoperatively. The anesthesiologist may choose to use a central venous catheter or pulmonary artery catheter to monitor the patient's hemodynamic status. Central venous cannulation, as used by Nelson et al., will allow monitoring of the patient's preload throughout the case and attempt to reduce septal shift and suction events, especially in the case of anticipated large shifts of intravascular volume [1, 2]. Low dose milrinone may be of therapeutic utility to maintain RV function, especially in the setting of pulmonary hypertension. Milrinone is usually the selected inotrope due to its additional ability to decrease RV afterload through pulmonary arterial vasodilation. However, one must consider that milrinone must be loaded or have reached a steady-state equilibrium over several hours for maximum effect. Epinephrine should be considered when an immediate rescue of the RV is necessary. The systemic vasodilation accompanying milrinone can be offset by titration of phenylephrine or vasopressin. Vasopressin tends to have a greater effect on increasing the SVR while sparing PVR increases to assist the right ventricle. The mean arterial pressure (MAP) should be maintained at a level equal to 70–80 mm Hg to help support RV perfusion. Inhaled Nitric oxide or Epoprostenol may be used in the situation of low SVR because of its specificity for the pulmonary vasculature. Hypothermia, hypercarbia and hypoxia, high ventilation pressures, or use of excessive PEEP can cause an increase in PVR. These factors can further compromise the functional reserve of the right ventricle and should be avoided. Development of arrhythmias can have damaging effect on the RV function and should be treated immediately [35].

### Intraoperative Patient Position

Reverse Trendelenburg position will decrease venous return and will diminish the preload for the right ventricle. Trendelenburg position will increase preload initially, however, the preload will ultimately equilibrate. One lung ventilation and the lateral decubitus position can easily lead to hypercarbia, hypoxia, and an increase in PVR, eventually causing RV stress. The prone position can lead to increased intra-abdominal pressure and decreased venous return. Compression of the RV outflow tract can occur by pressure exerted from the VAD's outflow cannula which lies anterior to the pulmonary artery. Sometimes the only way to recover an adequate hemodynamic status is to return the patient to the supine position [34].

### VAD Function

It is essential to maintain visual contact with the VAD monitor to be able to continuously monitor the Flow, RPM, Power (Watts), and Pulse Index, throughout the duration of the procedure. It is important to realize that flow is not an absolute number but is estimated from a relationship with pump power at a given pump speed.

## Crisis Management

### 1. Hypotension

In case of sudden hypotension, one can utilize the VAD monitor and displayed values to work through a differential diagnosis. Pulse index is a dimensionless number which tends to fall as the native LV contributes less to cardiac output. Pump power falls as less red blood cells come into contact with the pump impeller and vice versa. Therefore, one can utilize the trend of these two variables to help troubleshoot intraoperative hypotension. The combination of a low pulse index with falling pump power indicates decreased LV preload, which could represent low circulating volume or RV failure. Following the trend of a CVP or monitoring RV function on TEE can help differentiate these two causes. The combination of a low pulse index with rising pump power typically indicates reduced LV afterload as the underlying cause of hypotension [36].

### 2. Cardiac Arrest

Diagnosing cardiac arrest in LVAD patients may be difficult, but Ozmete et al., have shown it to be possible via observation of a decrease in LVAD flow, fixed arterial and CVP traces, and disappearance of capnography traces [37]. It may also be confirmed with intraoperative TEE. It is well established that BLS and ACLS guidelines do not recommend performing chest compressions in LVAD patients due to fear of shearing a thinned ventricular apex via the metallic inflow cannula, damaging hardware, changing device localization, or causing a bleed in an already anticoagulated patient [37]. Although chest compressions are not ACLS or BLS recommended, as Ozmete et al., have shown via their successful resuscitative experience, in addition to a few other reports, chest compressions can be effectively and safely performed. There is no contraindication to external cardioversion or defibrillation for patients with a VAD [37, 38].

### 3. Suction Event

The sudden onset of hypotension with ventricular arrhythmias may indicate a suction event where the LVAD inflow cannula is partially or completely occluded by the ventricular septal wall. This often results in pump alarms and slowing of pump speed to enable the provider to resuscitate with volume and medications to support RV function as appropriate.

## Postoperative and Post-discharge Considerations

Recovery of these patients can occur in the recovery room or intensive care unit (ICU), depending on the patient's condition. Resuming anticoagulation after an elective procedure usually depends on the type of surgery performed. Monitoring the patient for bleeding should be done by following the hemoglobin, platelet count, and coagulation profile.

## References

1. Hunt SA, Abraham WT, Chin MH, et al. 2009 focused update incorporated into the ACC/AHA 2005 guidelines for the diagnosis and management of heart failure in adults: a report of the American College of Cardiology Foundation/American Heart Association Task Force on Practice Guidelines. Circulation. 2009;119:e391–479.
2. Mozaffarian D, Benjamin EJ, Go AS, Arnett DK, Blaha MJ, Cushman M. Heart disease and stroke statistics—2016 update. Circulation. 2016;133:e38–e360.
3. Rose EA, Gelljns AC, Moskowrtz AJ, Heitjan DF, Stevenson LW, Dembitsky W, et al. Long-term use of a left ventricular assist device for end-stage heart failure. N Engl J Med. 2001;345(20):1435–43.
4. Rogers JG, Butler J, Lansman SL, Gass A, Portner PM, Pasque MK, et al. Chronic mechanical circulatory support for inotrope-dependent heart failure patients who are not transplant candidates: results of the INTrEPID trial. J Am Coll Cardiol. 2007;50(8):741–7.
5. Current Status of the Intermacs Registry. https://www.uab.edu/medicine/intermacs/reports/public-statistical-reports.
6. Park SJ, Milano CA, Tatooles AJ, Rogers JG, Adamson RM, et al. Outcomes in advanced heart failure patients with left ventricular assist devices for destination therapy. Circ Heart Fail. 2012;5:241–8.
7. Kirklin JK, et al. Seventh INTERMACS annual report: 15,000 patients and counting. J Heart Lung Transplant. 2015;34(12):1495–504.
8. Stevenson LW, Pagani FD, Young JB, Jessup M, Miller L, Kormos RL, et al. INTERMACS profiles of advanced heart failure: the current picture. J Heart Lung Transplant. 2009;28:535–41.
9. Slininger KA, Haddadin AS, Mangi AA. Perioperative management of patients with left ventricular assist devices undergoing noncardiac surgery. J Cardiothorac Vasc Anesth. 2013;27(4):752–9.
10. Estep JD, Starling RC, Horstmanshof DA, Milano CA, Selzman CH, Shah KB, Loebe M, Moazami N, Long JW, Stehlik J, et al. Risk assessment and comparative effectiveness of left ventricular assist device and medical management in ambulatory heart failure patients: results from the ROADMAP study. J Am Coll Cardiol. 2015;66(16):1747–61.
11. Mehra MR, Naka Y, Uriel N, Goldstein DJ, Rogers JC, Slaughter MS, et al. Intrapericardial left ventricular assist device for advanced heart failure. N Engl J Med. 2017;376:451–60.

12. Rogers JG, Pagani FD, Antone J, Mehra MR, Naka Y, Uriel N, Goldstein DJ, Cleveland JC Jr, Colombo PC, Walsh MN, Salerno C, et al. Intrapericardial left ventricular assist device for advanced heart failure. N Engl J Med. 2017;376(5):440–50.
13. Hasin T, Topilsky Y, Schirger JA, et al. Changes in renal function after implantation of continuous-flow left ventricular assist devices. J Am Coll Cardiol. 2012;59(1):26–36.
14. Schaffer JM, Arnaoutakis GJ, Allen JG, Weiss ES, Patel ND, Russell SD, Shah AS, Conte JV. Bleeding complications and blood product utilization with left ventricular assist device implantation. Ann Thorac Surg. 2011;91(3):740–7.
15. Eckman PM, John R. Bleeding and thrombosis in patients with continuous-flow ventricular assist devices. Circulation. 2012;125(24):3038–47.
16. Gordon RJ, Quagliarello B, Lowy FD. Ventricular assist device-related infections. Lancet Infect Dis. 2006;6(7):426–37.
17. Topkara VK, Kondareddy S, Malik F, Wang IW, Mann DL, Ewald GA, et al. Infectious complications in patients with left ventricular assist device: etiology and outcomes in the continuous-flow era. Ann Thorac Surg. 2010;90(4):1270–7.
18. Katugaha SB, Gibreal M, Carter AC, Cowger JA, Salerno CT, Maltais S, Dunlay S, Dardas TF, Aaronson KD, Pagani FD, Stulak J, Shah P. The effect of infections in VAD recipients on survival and risk of thromboembolism. J Heart Lung Transplant. 2017;36(4):S38.
19. Anderson M, Videbaek R, Boesgaard S, et al. Incidence of ventricular arrhythmias in patients on long term support with a continuous-flow assist device (HeartMate II). J Heart Lung Transplant. 2009;28:733–5.
20. Kormos RL, Teuteberg JJ, Pagani FD, Russell SD, John R, Miller LW, et al. Right ventricular failure in patients with the HeartMate II continuous-flow left ventricular assist device: incidence, risk factors, and effect on outcomesJ. Thorac Cardiovasc Surg. 2010;139(5):1316–24.
21. Vollkron M, Voitl P, Ta J, Wieselthaler G, Schima H. Suction events during left ventricular support and ventricular arrhythmias. Anesth Analg. 2007;26(8):819–25.
22. John R, Mantz K, Eckman P, Rose A, May-Newman K. Aortic valve pathophysiology during left ventricular assist device support. J Heart Lung Transplant. 2010;29(12):1321–9.
23. Slaughter MS, Pagani FD, Rogers JG, et al. Clinical management of continuous-flow left ventricular assist devices in advanced heart failure. J Heart Lung Transplant. 2010;29(4):S1–39.
24. Rajagopal K, Daneshmand MA, Patel CB, Ganapathi AM, Schechter MA, Rogers JG, Milano CA. Natural history and clinical effect of aortic valve regurgitation after left ventricular assist device implantation. J Thorac Cardiovasc Surg. 2013;145(5):1373–9.
25. Malehsa D, Meyer AL, Bara C, Struber M. Acquired von Willebrand syndrome after exchange of the HeartMate XVE to the HeartMate II ventricular assist device. Eur J Cardiothorac Surg. 2009;35(6):1091–3.
26. Starling RC, Moazami N, Silvestry SC, Ewald G, Rogers JG, Milano CA, et al. Unexpected abrupt increase in left ventricular assist device thrombosis. N Engl J Med. 2014;370(1):33–40.
27. Riha H, Netuka I, Kotulak T, et al. Anesthesia management of a patient with a ventricular assist device for noncardiac surgery. Semin Cardiothorac Vasc Anesth. 2010;14(1):29–31.
28. Stone ME. Current status of mechanical circulatory assistance. Semin Cardiothorac Vasc Anesth. 2007;11:185–204.
29. Sheu R, Joshi B, High K, Thinh Pham D, Ferreira R, Cobey F. Perioperative management of patients with left ventricular assist devices undergoing noncardiac procedures: a survey of current practices. J Cardiothorac Vasc Anesth. 2015;29:17–26.
30. Stone M, Hinchey J, Sattler C, Evans A. Trends in the management of patients with left ventricular assist devices presenting for noncardiac surgery: a 10-year institutional experience. Semin Cardiothorac Vasc Anesth. 2016;20:197–204.
31. Hessel EA 2nd. Management of patients with implanted ventricular assist devices for noncardiac surgery: a clinical review. Semin Cardiothorac Vasc Anesth. 2014;18:57–70.
32. Goudra BG, Singh PM. Anaesthesia for gastro intestinal endoscopy inpatients with left ventricular assist devices: initial experience with 68 procedures. Ann Card Anaesth. 2013;16:250–6.
33. Myers TJ, Bolmers M, Gregoric ID, Kar B, Frazier OH. Assessment of arterial blood pressure during support with an axial flow left ventricular assist device. J Heart Lung Transplant. 2009;28(5):423–7.
34. Oleyar M, Stone M, Neustein SM. Perioperative management of a patient with a nonpulsatile left ventricular-assist device presenting for noncardiac surgery. J Cardiothorac Vasc Anesth. 2010;24(5):820–3.
35. Morgan JA, Paone G, Nemeh HW, Murthy R, Williams CT, Lanfear DE, Tita C, Brewer RJ. Impact of continuous-flow left ventricular assist device support on right ventricular function. J Heart Lung Transplant. 2013;32(4):398–403.
36. Chung M, Sobol J, Sladen R. Ventricular assist device classification and basic functional mechanics. In: High K, editor. Mechanical circulatory support: ventricular assist devices (VADs) and extracorporeal membrane oxygenation (ECMO); 2014.
37. Ozmete O, Bali C, Ergenoglu P, Suner HI, Aribogan A. Resuscitation experience in a patient with left ventricular assist device. J Clin Anesth. 2016;34:253–4.9.
38. Nelson EW, Hdnke T, Finley A, et al. Management of LVAD patients for noncardiac surgery: a single-institution study. J Cardiothorac Vasc Anesth. 2015;29(4):898–900.

# Part II

# Out of Operating Room Anesthesia

# Anesthesia for ERCP

Basavana G. Goudra and Preet Mohinder Singh

## Introduction

The developments in the field of advanced gastrointestinal (GI) endoscopy are evident. Endoscopic retrograde Cholangiopancreatography (ERCP) is one of the most prominent and challenging advanced endoscopic procedure. An estimated 500,000 ERCPs were performed annually in the United States in 2004 [1, 2]. Choledocholithiasis, pancreatic Stones, ampullary/papillary abnormalities (sphincter of Oddi dysfunction, ampullary cancers/adenomas), biliary and pancreatic ductal abnormalities (leaks, benign and malignant strictures) are some of the indications. A major limitation of ERCP is the two-dimensional fluoroscopic view of the biliary tree [3, 4]. As a result, delineation of the etiology of biliary strictures becomes a challenge. This poses difficulties when attempting to delineate the etiology of biliary strictures. Additionally, even in expert centers, the removal of bile duct stones with standard ERCP-guided maneuvers fails in approximately 10% of patients. Use of SpyGlass® system (Boston Scientific, Natick, MA, USA), addresses some of the limitations of the conventional mother-daughter system. It is a single-operator cholangioscopy system with four-way steering and separate working and irrigation channels. The technology is used for both diagnostic and therapeutic purposes.

We addressed some of the issues pertaining to the airway management of ERCP few years ago [5]. However, sufficient new knowledge has accumulated in the intervening period and a complete review is overdue. The annual ERCP procedures performed in the USA alone is more than 500,000 per year [6]. Biliary complications remain one of the most outstanding factors influencing long-term results after orthotopic liver transplantation [7]. Fully covered self-expanding metal stents employed in the management of distal malignant biliary strictures may be advantageous and prolong survival [8]. The benefits of ERCP are yet to reach the developing world, where sedation for advanced endoscopic procedures is rudimentary. Although, deep sedation with propofol remains the standard approach, other techniques are attempted. The drive by some of the gastroenterologists to perform these procedures under moderate propofol sedation has produced mixed results [9].

## Applied Anatomy and Physiology of Hepato-Pancreato Biliary Tract

### Pancreaticobiliary Drainage System

An understanding of the anatomical basis of ERCP is important for an anesthesiologist. It will

B. G. Goudra, M.D., F.R.C.A., F.C.A.R.C.S.I. (✉)
Hospital University Pennsylvania Perelman School of Medicine, Philadelphia, Pennsylvania, USA
e-mail: goudrab@uphs.upenn.edu

P. M. Singh, M.D., D.N.B.
Department of Anesthesia, All India Institute of Medical Sciences, New Delhi, India

better equip us to predict complications and prepare for their management. Anatomically, the procedure targets to cannulate the ampulla of Vater using a side viewing endoscope. Ampulla of Vater is the protrusion seen on the luminal side of the second part of duodenum. The ampulla is internally bound by a muscular valve-the sphincter of Oddi, that controls the flow of biliopancreatic secretions from the common bile duct. As a result, the ampulla of Vater behaves as a receptacle for the openings of the common bile duct and the ventral pancreatic duct into the lumen of the gut. Physiologically, the secretions of the pancreas (lipase and trypsinogen) and the gall bladder (bile) have a unique function and are capable of auto-digestion if inadvertently activated. Trypsinogen once activated in the duodenal lumen by the enteropeptidase cleaves proteins into peptides, while pancreatic lipase assisted by the bile degrades the dietary fats. Any anatomical obstruction to the drainage of these secretions can thus initiate the process of auto-digestion with serious consequences. The ensuing inflammation will further narrow the cannulating lumen. Thus, an otherwise uncomplicated cannulation in conditions like impacted stone might become particularly challenging.

Bile secreted by the liver traverses the left and right hepatic ducts, before draining into the common hepatic duct. The common hepatic duct is joined by the cystic duct to form the common bile duct that drains into the duodenum [Fig. 19.1]. Pathological obstruction can occur in any of the above ducts and ERCP allows one to localize the site of obstruction/pathology [Fig. 19.2]. Nonetheless, successful cannulation is a necessary prerequisite for delineation of the pancreatic and biliary tree. Occasionally, anatomical variations in these structures can render the procedure technically challenging, thus necessitating prolonged anesthesia support. A history of difficult or failed cannulation should draw attention to this possibility and guide the anesthesia plan accordingly.

Normally the diameter of the common bile duct is less than 6 mm [10] and that of the main pancreatic duct (also called the duct of Wirsung) is about 3 mm [11]. Larger stones should alert the anesthesiologist to the possibility of procedural difficulties. Anesthesiologists must also be aware of the fact, that obstructed bile flow acts as a nidus for growth of gram negative organisms. Patients with carcinoma head of pancreas presenting with painless jaundice or patients with painful jaundice (suspected cholangitis) or patients with obstructed stents are associated with biliary stasis [12]. As long as the biliary tree is obstructed, the infection remains fairly contained. These patients need immediate symptomatic relief and are frequently referred to gastroenterologists for ERCP. The insertion of stent in these patients allows biliary decompression; however, can also trigger systemic

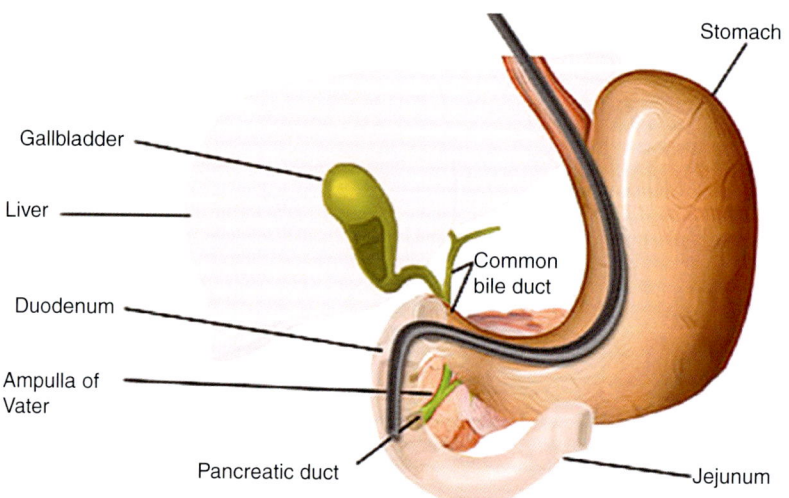

**Fig. 19.1** Diagram showing normal anatomy of the hepatobiliary system. The image schematically shows an endoscope in the second part of duodenum (the site of cannulation of papilla)

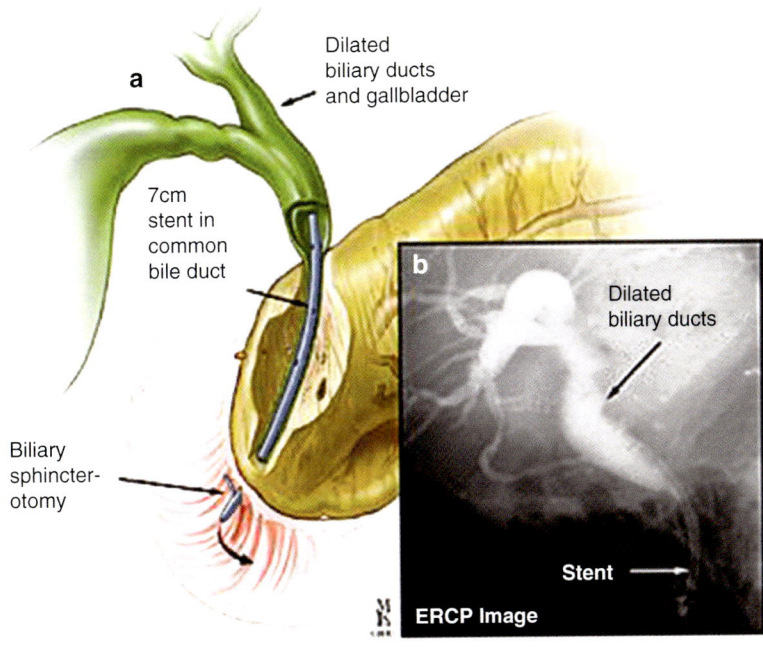

**Fig. 19.2** Figure showing radiocontrast injected into the biliary system during therapeutic ERCP where a stent was inserted to relive the biliary obstruction. Biliary tree proximal to previous obstruction is dilated

spread of the gram-negative organisms or endotoxins. Thus, presenting as immediate onset unexplained pyrexia, tachycardia and hypotension [13]. In fact this is a very realistic problem and the incidence of this has been reported to be varying from 1.8 to 15% [14]. The commonest organism to colonize and requiring antibiotic therapy include Escherichia coli, Pseudomonas spp., Klebsiella spp. and Enterobacter spp. [15]. Infective complications should be kept in mind where prolonged obstruction (carcinoma pancreas) or recurrent obstruction (infected stones) are present. Appropriate antibiotic prophylaxis and a high index of suspicion may prevent ERCP related sepsis, that carries high mortality.

Occasional pancreatic developmental anomalies like pancreatic divisum (where dorsal and ventral pancreatic buds fail to fuse) may necessitate the cannulation of minor duodenal papilla as well. In fact, the above anatomical correlations are indirectly evident in the procedural difficulty grading for ERCP as proposed by the American Society of Gastroenterologists (ASGE) [16]. A brief form of this grading and its relevance to anesthesiologist is presented in Table 19.1. This classification is primarily based upon anatomical issues related to the pancreatobiliary system and is independent of other associated medical comorbidities that may also be relevant to the anesthesiologist. Higher grades reflect increasing procedural complexity and likely to pose greater challenges to the anesthetic provider. Yet another anatomical aspect that an anesthesiologist should consider prior to conduct of anesthesia is history of upper GI surgery. Such complexities are seen often in post-bariatric surgery patients. Even in the early days of bariatric surgery it was recognized that incidence of biliary stones amounts up to nearly 36% after surgery. Thus these patients would frequently be planned for an ERCP eventually [17]. Careful planning based upon the anatomy of the surgical procedure is important. In addition to technical difficulties in the endoscopy especially cannulation, one might have to delay the procedure until complete healing of the recent anastomotic staple lines has occurred. In patients where gastric banding is used, these bands must be deflated prior to initiation of the endoscopy for ERCP. As a general rule anesthesiologist, must be prepared for longer and technically challenging procedures in post-bariatric surgery patients [18]. Evidence suggest that after the biliopancreatic diversion procedures, the endoscopic access into the biliary tree is virtually

**Table 19.1** Grading system proposed by the American Society of gastrointestinal endoscopy to predict ERCP difficulty and possible anesthetic implications

| Grade | Pre-procedure findings | Anesthesia implication/expectation |
|---|---|---|
| I | • Deep cannulation of main papilla—for sampling<br>• Biliary stent removal/exchange | • Short procedure<br>• Less complex/patient discomfort<br>• Moderate to deep sedation |
| II | • Biliary stone <10 mm—extraction<br>• Pancreatic duct stent placement<br>• Therapeutic dilatation of extrahepatic strictures<br>• Biliary leak treatment | • Slightly increased procedure time<br>• Moderate to deep sedation |
| III | • Biliary stone >10 mm—extraction<br>• Pancreatic divisum-minor papilla cannulation<br>• Migrated stents removal<br>• Procedures with acute inflammatory conditions<br>• Pancreatic strictures<br>• Pancreatic stone <5 mm—removal | • Prolonged procedure time<br>• High patient discomfort possible<br>• May need general anesthesia rarely |
| IV | • Internally migrated pancreatic stent removal<br>• Pancreatic stone >5 mm—removal<br>• Necrosectomy/pesudocyst drainage<br>• Post Whipples or Roux-en-Y surgery<br>• Intrahepatic stone removal<br>• Ampulectomy | • Prolonged procedure<br>• High level patient discomfort<br>• Low threshold for general anesthesia |

impossible because of the length of the interposed intestinal segment and thus such patients should be planned for open procedures rather than endoscopy [18]. Needless to say that these challenges would be compounded by already anticipated anesthetic difficulties seen in obese patients.

## Neurovascular Supply

Developmentally, the second part of the duodenum determines the junction between the foregut and the midgut. Thus, it receives blood supply from sub-divisions of the coeliac truck (via gastroduodenal artery) and the superior mesenteric trunk (via inferior pancreatico-duodenal branches). Both anesthesia providers and endoscopists are well aware and prepared to deal with the commonly recognized adverse events like bleeding, perforation, infection, and those resulting from the sedative medications. Air embolism is a very rare endoscopic complication; however, can be severe and occasionally fatal. Air embolism is most commonly associated with ERCP; although, may also result from any endoscopic procedure including an EGD, an enteroscopy, an EUS, a colonoscopy, and a sigmoidoscopy. Both the above arterial systems can be the entry point of air embolus (or the insufflated $CO_2$) during ERCP. A high index of suspicion should be maintained for the possibility of air embolism in patients presenting with unexplainable sudden hemodynamic collapse during the procedure. Known air embolism risk factors in patients undergoing ERCP include—surgeries or previous interventions of biliary tract, transhepatic portosystemic shunts, blunt or penetrating trauma to liver, sphrincterctomy, metallic stent placement and hepatic abscess/tumor [19].

Another reason to understand the vascular supply is to localize the source of bleeding during complications resulting from the ERCP. Most post ERCP bleeds are intraluminal. Proximal to the major papilla any procedural injury results in bleeding from superior pancreaticoduodenal vessels. Distal injuries often cause bleeding from the inferior pancreaticoduodenal vessels. ERCP with sphincterctomy is considered as a high risk procedure for bleeding and considerations should be given to adjustment of anti-thrombotic medications in these patients prior the procedure [20].

For an anesthesiologist it is important to recognize that (being a derivative of the foregut and the midgut) the nerve supply of the duodenum, biliary tree and the pancreas originates from the vagus nerve. The post ganglionic cholinergic fibers increase the duodenal mobility and also increase the tone of the sphincter Oddi. As a result, anticholinergic medications like hyoscine-N-butyl bromide (HBB, 20 mg i.v. in increments, up to 40 mg) are commonly used as a duodenal relaxant. It can relax the sphincter and thus assist in cannulation during ERCP [21, 22]. However, ventricular tachycardia can occur immediately following the administration of HBB during ERCP, that can cause severe hypotension and myocardial ischemia. Due to vagal innervation, vasovagal cardiac arrest has been reported during sphincter manipulation [23]. Further, studies have demonstrated that opioids can enhance the tone of myenteric cholinergic system and thus contribute to an increase in bile duct pressure noted during the ERCP [24]. Studies have shown that fentanyl, morphine, and meperidine significantly increase pressure in the common duct [25, 26]. Moreover, naloxone administered 20 min later can decrease such pressure increases. In contrast, butorphanol produces insignificant changes. Meperidine has no effect on Oddi's sphincter motility, while tramadol has an inhibitory effect on the motility of the sphincter of Oddi and decreases levels of basal pressure of Oddi's sphincter and amplitude of phasic contractions.

## Preoperative Evaluation

### Risk Estimation Strategies

In order to have an anesthetic plan, patients should be evaluated based on the standard risk assessment scales as per the ASA classification. In a very large retrospective review comprising patients from 74 centers in the United States, Enestvedt et al. revealed that increasing ASA grade was a reliable predictor of peri-procedural complications in patients undergoing upper GI endoscopy. Further they noted that when similar grading system is used for all upper GI endoscopies, the odds ratio for adverse effects was highest during ERCP. Nevertheless, the association between the two in the multivariate model (that accounted for factors like age etc.) failed to achieve statistical significance [27]. Unlike patients presenting for surgeries, patients undergoing ERCP pose additional challenges during risk stratification. Some of the patients presenting for ERCP can have pancreaticobiliary system related acute metabolic derangements. The present ASA grading system unfortunately does not accommodate/quantify these metabolic derangements in its risk classification strategy [28]. Thus, one should keep in mind that these patients are likely to be placed in a lower risk category based upon standard risk assessment scales. Despite this, the proportion of ASA III/IV patients undergoing ERCP compared to ASA I/II patients is notable. Contrasting from other preoperative evaluations where most patients planned for elective procedures can be optimized prior to surgery to lower their ASA status (thereby lowering the perioperative risks). These options are somewhat limited in patients undergoing ERCP. They particularly might have secondary ailments resulting from hepatobiliary derangement. Patients frequently have high bilirubin values, primary hepatic enzyme/functional derangement and secondary systemic involvement due to liver/pancreas involvement. In all these cases ERCP is in fact therapeutic and thus needs to be performed without alternative options to further optimize patients. Thus, the proportion of ASA III/IV patients for non-emergency (elective procedures) is higher. In fact, our own and many other retrospective reviews have time and again demonstrated the same. It is likely that many patients presenting for ERCP might fall into higher ASA grades than assigned and every effort should be made to study the associated metabolic derangements.

Cardiovascular assessment of the patient should also be performed as per the standard protocols. A well-established tool for cardiovascular risk assessment for patients undergoing non-cardiac surgery that can be used in these patients is the "Revised cardiac risk index" (RCRI). It however should be pointed out that even RCRI underestimates the risks involved during ERCP. RCRI incorporates the nature of procedure as one of the six predictors it uses. As per the recently defined term "major adverse cardiac event" (MACE), Endoscopy falls into a *low-risk* procedure where the combined surgical and patient characteristics predict a risk of death or myocardial infarction (MI) (combined as MACE) is <1% [29]. In a recent meta-analysis Day et al. concluded that the incidence rates of cardiac morbidity/mortality in older adults undergoing ERCP (baring other endoscopic procedures) amounts to nearly 3.7% [30]. However, the MACE incorporated into the RCRI assumes all endoscopic procedures low risk (i.e. MACE <1%). Thus, especially in case of ERCP the RCRI would rather underscore a patient on risk assessment scales. ERCP is associated with a high risk of inducing both infective (cholangitis) and non-infective inflammation (pancreatitis). Both can result in a wide variety of cardiovascular perturbations which are not accounted during present classification. As a result, a combined approach using the above indices and the patient's functional status should play the pivotal role in defining peri-procedure risk of systemic complications.

## Biochemical Investigations

Most of the biochemical investigations routinely ordered prior to ERCP are intuitive rather than evidence based. Controversy surrounds the use of routine coagulation profile testing. In 2008 British guidelines advocated to include routine pre-procedural coagulation profile performed within 3 days of ERCP [31]. However, the "American Society for gastrointestinal endoscopy" (ASGE) guidelines on the contrary suggest that prothrombin time (PT) fails to predict or poorly correlates with intra-procedural hemorrhage and thus is an un-necessary investigation [32]. Supporting this notion, randomized trial by Egan et al. also demonstrated that routine coagulation profile is associated with poor cost benefit ratio. Coagulation testing may however be useful in patients with high bilirubin or in patients with history of bleeding diathesis [33].

ASGE recommends that the use of routine blood biochemical testing (electrolytes, blood glucose and renal functional testing) in patients undergoing ERCP should be guided by the medical history. Interestingly, unsuspected abnormalities are found in only 0.2–1.0% of patients undergoing routine preoperative chemistry screening and thus would not be cost effective [34, 35]. We suggest resorting to these investigations with a low threshold (after clinical history) and adhering to local hospital protocols thus keeping a balance between cost benefit and eventual medicolegal implications. Laboratory workup of the patient (including Chest roentgenogram, electrocardiogram etc.) prior to anesthesia/sedation for ERCP should be based upon associated co-morbidities and follow the standard protocols/statements released by the ASA on preoperative evaluation [36].

## Airway

Beyond the systems evaluation, a careful airway assessment is pertinent in patients undergoing ERCP. With an increasing number of anesthesia providers providing deep sedation without endotracheal intubation, the airway evaluation assumes special significance. The unplanned intubation rates during ERCP have been reported to be around 3% [37]. Thus, ability and preparedness to manage an unexpected "difficult airway" especially at the time of emergency can prevent a possible catastrophe. In a recent evaluation of 3041 ERCP procedures, there were 843 (28%) hypoxic events requiring airway manipulation, while 49 (1.6%) patients required unanticipated endotracheal intubation as a result of food in the stomach. Eight (0.3%) procedures were terminated early due to sedation-related hypotension ($n = 5$) and refractory laryngospasm ($n = 3$), whereas, six patients were admitted after the ERCP for aspiration pneumonia as a result of sedation. Patients who developed sedation related adverse events (SAE) were older, had a higher mean BMI, and had longer mean procedure durations [38].

A standardized evaluation should include Modified Mallampati (MMP) scoring, mouth opening, short neck, limited neck movement or any airway related abnormalities. ERCP procedures most often do not need paralysis and air insufflation of the stomach and intestines during the endoscopy can predispose to aspiration. Presence of a significant aspiration risk might change the planned deep sedation in favor of general anesthesia with endotracheal intubation, thereby reducing the possibility of aspiration. The immediate rescue at the time of airway related event is bag and mask ventilation. As a result, all patients must also be evaluated for signs of difficult mask ventilation (beard, edentulous, facial abnormalities, geriatric etc.). Presence of snoring at night or history of obstructive sleep apnea can be a red flag with an increased risk of airway obstruction during deep sedation. In our own study we were able to demonstrate that in obese patients the frequency hypoxic events correlated more with history of OSA rather than BMI alone [39]. Often, hypoxia can preset without sufficient notice and the severity could be alarming, even to a skilled clinician. Traditional teaching entail turning these patient's supine. However, maintaining ventilation should take precedence over other measures. If it requires intubation in the lateral position, one might attempt, if it is safe to do so.

## Anesthetic Considerations: Safety Issues

Belief exists among both patients and the gastroenterologists that (GI) endoscopic procedures are safer than surgical procedures performed in the comfort of the operating room under general anesthesia. However, the evidence is contrary to this belief. In 1961, Dripps et al. highlighted the role of human factors in the cause of deaths during anesthesia [40]. In fact, the incidence of major adverse events including cardiac arrest is higher in patients undergoing GI endoscopic procedures than surgical procedures [41]. While examining the role of sedation morbidity and mortality at out of OR locations, Metzner et al. [42] concluded that providing sedation in remote locations poses a significant risk to the patient, particularly related to oversedation and inadequate oxygenation/ventilation. The proportion of respiratory events for remote location claims was double that of operating room claims (44% versus 20%, $P < 0.001$), with issues related to oxygenation and (or) ventilation being the most common reasons for the claim. These events occurred seven times more frequently in remote locations than in operating room claims (21% versus 3%, $P < 0.001$). However, even though some researchers have cited closed claims studies as evidence of anesthesia risk trends, the nature of the data makes it inappropriate for calculation or comparison of risk [43].

Our own data of 73,029 GI endoscopic procedures, revealed an incidence of cardiac arrest and death (all causes, until discharge) of 6.07 and 4.28 per 10,000 in patients sedated with propofol, compared with non-propofol-based sedation (0.67 and 0.44). The incidence of cardiac arrest during and immediately after the procedure (recovery area) for all endoscopies was 3.92 per 10,000; of which, 72% were airway related. About 90.0% of all periprocedural cardiac arrests occurred in patients who received propofol and many were hypoxemia related [41]. Using regression modeling, we found a strong association between the type of sedation along with various patient factors and the frequency of adverse events [44]. ERCP along with other advanced endoscopic procedures was responsible for the majority of sedation related adverse events. However, a note of caution is advised in the interpretation of these results. Although, the denominator consisted of 73,029 GI endoscopic procedures, demographic data was only available for the numerator. It is unlikely that such data is available in retrospective studies. Yet, the fact remains that the incidence of hypoxemia was a significant contributor to both death and cardiac arrests in peri-procedural period.

## Anesthetic Considerations: Anesthesia Providers

Utilizing a small pool of dedicated anesthesia providers is known to increase both safety and efficiency of ERCP procedures [45]. In an analysis of data from 1167 ERCP procedures (where 653 (56%) were assisted by regular and 514 (44%) were assisted by non-regular anesthesiologists), it was discovered that, across all ASA classes, regular anesthesiologists were safer and more efficient than non-regular anesthesiologists. Overall, mean anesthesia time was 24.82 ± 12.96 in the procedures cared by the same smaller pool versus 48.63 ± 21.53 min. Safety as determined by higher mean oxygen saturations was higher with regular anesthesiologists. Although, the regular anesthesiologists tended to intubate more frequently, this factor did not decrease the efficiency. Had all the ERCP procedures were performed by the regular anesthesiologists, the hospital could have saved US $ 758536.00 over 2 years with ERCP associated anesthesia cost alone. As a result, it is important to consider the use of appropriately trained and dedicated anesthesia providers in an ERCP suite. One of the limitation of this study was the fact that non-regular anesthesiologists were involved in a disproportionate number of in-patient ERCPs. It is likely that these ERCPs are complicated and the patient population was less healthy.

## Anesthetic Considerations: Prone/Semi Prone Positioning

Patients undergoing endoscopic retrograde cholangiopancreatography (ERCP) are typically examined in the left lateral or prone position [46]. Both these positions are believed to decrease the risk of aspiration pneumonia and to permit easier introduction of the scope through the pharynx, and they are usually considered by the endoscopists to be more comfortable. It is suggested to start the procedure with the patient in a semi lateral position and continue with the patient prone once the duodenum has been reached. Supine position may be preferred in examining patients with suspected hilar biliary strictures, those with previous Billroth II gastrectomy, and those whose pancreatic duct anatomy is already known to be difficult to interpret. Better interpretation of the biliary and pancreatic anatomy: with the liver and the pancreas lying on the spine under the force of gravity is an advantage of supine ERCP.

Nevertheless, from the anesthesia provider's perspective, prone positioning segregates ERCP into a separate category among all GI endoscopic procedures. It is partly due to our long-held belief regarding the consequence of airway loss in an unintubated patient undergoing procedure in prone position. However, distinction needs to be made between surgical procedures versus ERCP procedure conducted in prone position. Unlike surgical procedures, endoscopic procedures can be aborted rapidly to facilitate airway management. Yet, frequent interruptions to provide adequate oxygenation including ventilation are not appreciated. In order to limit such stoppages, sedation must be titrated to a level where adequate spontaneous ventilation is preserved. In view of variable stimulation and a 300–400% pharmacokinetic and pharmacodynamic variability associated with the use of propofol, this goal is difficult to achieve on a consistent basis [47, 48]. Airway manipulations (without procedure interruptions) are often required to achieve the goal. The second and more important requirement is to be observant and get involved for any airway compromise with measures including bag-mask ventilation or emergency endotracheal intubation. Although endoscopists understand the risks of hypoxemia, they need to be told clearly that the ERCP scope needs to be withdrawn to facilitate airway intervention, when deemed necessary. Regarding the pros and cons of an unintubated airway management during ERCP, the readers are referred to one of our earlier publication [5].

## Procedure/Operating Room Preparation

Deep sedation without a definitive airway is the technique adapted by majority of anesthesia providers during ERCP. It is beyond any doubt that these patients experience depths seen during general anesthesia [49]. As a result, the degree of monitoring during these procedures should be similar to general anesthesia in an operating room. The American Society of Anesthesiology (ASA) guidelines on standards for basic anesthetic monitoring (Committee of Origin: Ambulatory Surgical Care, Approved by the ASA House of Delegates on October 21, 2009, and last amended on October 15, 2014) [50, 51] mandates end tidal carbon dioxide monitoring in patients undergoing deep sedation. With regards to end tidal carbon dioxide as a mode of ventilation monitoring, the statement on respiratory monitoring during endoscopic procedures reads.

> "Monitoring for exhaled carbon dioxide should be conducted during endoscopic procedures in which sedation is provided with propofol alone or in combination with opioids and/or benzodiazepines, and especially during these procedures on the upper gastrointestinal tract. Careful attention to airway management must be provided during endoscopic retrograde cholangiopancreaticography (ERCP) procedures performed in the prone position where ventilatory monitoring, airway maintenance, and resuscitation may be especially difficult."

Reliable sample is not always obtainable during an unintubated ERCP. Yet, this should not preclude using the method as a monitor for ventilation. Moreover, in the event of unexpected endotracheal intubation, it becomes a mandatory monitoring tool.

Standards and practice parameters committee of ASA issued their most recent guidelines in 2013 and these should be adhered to in all non-operating room settings including ERCP rooms [52]. Although, unsubstantiated by class 1 evidence, sufficient data exists to support these recommendations. Considering that most of the adverse events are airway related, it makes perfect sense to have a portable breathing system, capable of delivering at least 90% oxygen, A mapleson breathing system can be used both as a primary oxygen administration tool in some cases or a rescue apparatus [53]. Anesthesia workstation may not be required during every case. However, at least one unit should be available and be properly checked and serviced. Need for inhalational anesthesia cannot be ruled out in any endoscopy suite.

Mobile anesthesia carts are valuable, although a dedicated anesthesia machine might be preferable. Need for unanticipated endotracheal intubation and endotracheal anesthesia is highest in ERCP rooms. As a result, these rooms should be equipped accordingly. A typical mobile anesthesia cart used in the nonoperating room anesthesia (NORA) suite should contain emergency drugs (phenylephrine, ephedrine, atropine, glycopyrrolate, succinylcholine), propofol, nasal airways, endotracheal tubes, laryngoscopes, Intravenous cannulae, tourniquets, oropharyngeal airways, assorted syringes, needles, extension tubing, filters, oxygen cannulae, face masks, intravenous fluids, propofol administration sets, and Mapleson C breathing systems [54]. The institutional standards should be met both in the design and maintenance of procedure rooms meant for ERCP.

## Authors Preferred Technique

We recognize that the anesthesia technique employed depends on factors such as patient co-morbidity, attending endoscopist skills, anticipated duration and the geographical location of the procedure rooms. Speed and the quality of expert help available is another factor. The technique described below takes into consideration both safety and efficiency. We do not believe that all ERCP procedures need endotracheal intubation (ETT). Moreover, as we have discussed elsewhere, routine endotracheal intubation is associated with its share of complications and shortcomings [5]. Endotracheal intubation negatively impacts efficiency metrics in an interventional endoscopy unit. As a result, careful assessment for the need for intubation should be emphasized [55]. Although, secure airway is the major advantage of ETT, only a small minority would benefit it. In our experience, need for unexpected intubation during ERCP is extremely rare. During 653 consecutive ERCPs, the need for emergent ETT or procedure interruption was zero [56]. Thus, with appropriate sedation titration and patient selection, unintubated ERCP can be performed safely. At the end of the proposed technique, attention is drawn to the situations where ETT approach is preferable.

Whenever deep sedation is attempted, it is of supreme importance to be prepared to both support and secure the airway at minimum notice. Confusion exists as to the nomenclature of the anesthesia provided for ERCP or any endoscopic procedure. Our own study involving patients undergoing colonoscopy with either non-propofol based sedation or propofol sedation, showed that the depth of sedation achieved with propofol often exceeds those employed during surgical procedures [49]. As measured by Sedline (Masimo Corp., Irvine, CA), a brain function monitor, the depth of sedation during propofol administration was in the range of general anesthesia or deep general anesthesia in about 50% of patients for varying periods of time. However, unlike, colonoscopy, during ERCP the airway is neither easily accessible nor can be supported easily. As a result, if the anesthesia practitioner has any doubts, ETT might be preferable. Providing deep sedation for an ERCP needs to be approached with the same diligence as a major surgery in an operating room. Preoperative evaluation, especially airway and aspiration risk factors, need to be sought, explained and documented. A breathing system (e.g., Mapleson C), laryngoscope, facemasks, various oral and nasal airways, laryngeal mask airways, endotracheal tubes of varying sizes, and emergency drugs should be readily available. Additional airway adjuncts like bougies, stylets, and a video laryngoscope could be lifesaving. It is important to check both the availability and functionality of these before the start of the day and at the start of every procedure. Often airway emergencies like laryngospasm and intractable airway obstruction occur with little warning during these procedures. Readiness to address unanticipated airway emergencies could be the difference between apnea-related cardiac arrest and death or a safe discharge.

In our practice, induction is typically with propofol. The dose is variable and depends on the patient's age, weight, height, comorbidity, and medication history, all of which influence the pharmacokinetics and pharmacodynamics. We typically proceed with 1–1.5 mg/kg, although the dose may need to be drastically reduced in elderly patients. Propofol may be preceded (1–2 min before) with fentanyl 25–50 μg for analgesic, propofol sparing and antitussive effects. This is followed by an infusion of propofol at about 120–150 μg/kg/min for most procedures. Preserving the patency of the upper airway and maintenance of spontaneous ventilation along with suppression of the cough reflex are important. At the peak clinical effect of propofol, signaled by loss of eyelash reflex, unresponsiveness, and sometimes apnea, a nasal trumpet is typically inserted and connected to a Mapleson C breathing system (Fig. 19.3). At the peak of sedation depth, ERCP scope is introduced, which also provides sufficient stimulation to initiate (if patient

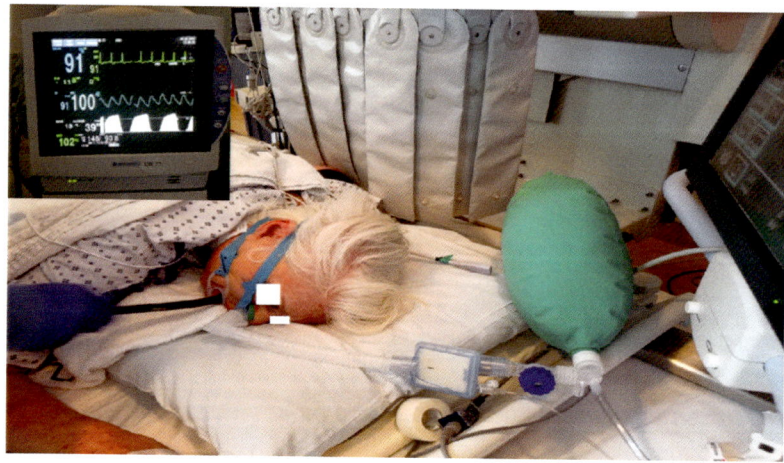

**Fig. 19.3** Mapleson C connected to a nasal airway with real time monitor and ETCO$_2$ tracing in the corner

was apneic) and sustain spontaneous ventilation. Post procedure discomfort is rare, other than mild throat irritation; therefore, we limit the dose of fentanyl to about 100 μg, unless the patient is on chronic opioid therapy or other reasons.

We employ endotracheal intubation rarely, even for prolonged and challenging endoscopic retrograde cholangiopancreatography (ERCP). The experience of the anesthesiologist in the area seems to play a major part in this decision [5, 45, 56]. Anesthesiologists unfamiliar with this practice are advised to employ general anesthesia with endotracheal intubation. Indeed, it is a challenge to render patients unresponsive, yet spontaneously breathing. Apnea lasting 30–45 s is not uncommon; however, stimulation produced by timely insertion of the endoscope aids resumption of spontaneous ventilation. The nasal trumpet allows some degree of controlled ventilation, if necessary. More notably, it delivers 100% oxygen at the laryngeal inlet. The gastroenterologist may request glucagon for GI relaxation. Glucagon is usually supplied as a vial with 1 mg powder and a vial with 1 mL solvent; the usual initial dose is between 0.2 and 0.5 mg intravenously. It may affect blood glucose; therefore, it should be used with caution in patients with diabetes or insulinoma. Endotracheal intubation is the airway management of choice for drainage of a pancreatic pesudocyst.

We recognize that depending on individual experience, a clinician adapts and modifies his/her own technique. Among the many techniques administration of propofol in combination with ketamine [57] is popular. Reduced pain and apnea is an advantage of this technique. In this study, 0.5 mg/kg of propofol was injected followed by 0.5 mg/kg of ketamine for bolus injection. Further sedation was provided by propofol alone. A similar study documented fewer sedation related events in the propofol-ketamine group, although recovery time was longer [58].

Topical anesthetics such as Benzocaine 20% (Hurricaine®) spray are occasionally employed to reduce the sedation requirements and suppress gag reflex [59]. Methemoglobinemia is a real danger with such practice. The cardinal sign of methemoglobinemia is a "brownish" cyanosis which does not respond to administration of 100% oxygen. Despite reversal of all sedatives. $O_2$ saturation ($SaO_2$) by pulse oximetry will not rise above 80s, even with administration of 100% oxygen. Multi-wavelength oximeters can determine the true oxygen saturations, unlike pulse oximeters that typically use two wavelengths.

## General Anesthesia with Endotracheal Intubation

As stated earlier, if the anesthesia provider has any concern regarding the airway or ability to maintain adequate spontaneous ventilation, ETT is advisable. Any increased risk of sedation related adverse events should be considered as a red flag [60]. Some of these factors include previous problems with sedation/anesthesia, cardiac disease (e.g., aortic stenosis), obstructive sleep apnea, difficulties with positive pressure ventilation or endotracheal intubation and advanced osteoarthritic cervical spine disease. Similarly, presence of a short neck with limited neck extension, decreased hyoid-mental distance (<3 cm in adults), trismus, macroglossia, tonsillar hypertrophy, micrognathia, morbid obesity and presence of full beard might lower the threshold for administering general anesthesia with ETT. Causes of increased risk of aspiration include large pseudo cyst of pancreas, gastric outlet obstruction and bleeding. Gastric ultrasonographic measurement of the gastric antral cross-sectional area has been proposed to estimate preanesthetic residual gastric contents volume [61, 62]. The measurement of antral area may allow a more accurate estimate of the presence or absence of gastric contents at risk of lung injury in the event of regurgitation and aspiration (gastric volume >0.8 mL/kg and/or with solid particles), defining the "risk" stomach. The technique may help the anesthesiologist to assess the risk of pulmonary aspiration according to clinical history of the patient, in order to choose an appropriate strategy including rapid sequence induction with ETT, thereby minimizing the occurrence of this complication. Spyglass cholangioscopy is a relatively newer technique; however, the anesthesia related factors remain the same.

Endoscopic retrograde cholangiopancreatography (ERCP) in patients with surgically altered upper gastrointestinal anatomy, such as Roux-en-Y gastric bypass (RYGB), can be more challenging compared to those with a normal anatomy [18, 63]. RYGB, which is performed for medically complicated obesity, is the most commonly encountered altered anatomy in patients presenting for ERCP procedure. In addition, ERCP in these patients is further challenging due to the oblique orientation of the papilla relative to the forward viewing endoscope and the limited enteroscopy-length therapeutic accessories that are currently available. Overall, reported therapeutic success is approximately 70–75% with a complication rate of 3–4%. Obesity and the metabolic disorders induced by it are risk factors for gallstones formation and their complications and these patients may present for related conditions. In view of these complexities, it is advisable to perform these procedures under general anesthesia with ETT.

## Postoperative and Post-discharge Considerations

Often the post procedure complications are extensions of expected or unexpected intraprocedural adverse events-both sedation and procedure related. As per our own analysis the red flags for possible complications predictors include-high pre-procedure ASA class, high MMP grade, high BMI, patient age at surgery and use of propofol based sedations [44]. Hypoxemia resulting from aspiration of gastric contents is uncommon, although a serious complication. Cardiac arrhythmias, hyper/hypo glycemia, hyper/hypotension and severe pain and discomfort might require immediate attention. Patients typically present for outpatient ERCP procedures with an expectation to be discharged home within 30–60 min after the procedure. As a result, any delay in discharge will be difficult to understand. An explanation of the events and the reasons for delayed discharge would greatly assist the patients and the family in coping with such events. Such an approach might ward off a potential complaint/litigation.

**Conflicts of Interest** Funding and Conflicts of interest—none.

## References

1. Silviera ML, Seamon MJ, Porshinsky B, Prosciak MP, Doraiswamy VA, Wang CF, et al. Complications related to endoscopic retrograde cholangiopancreatography: a comprehensive clinical review. J Gastrointestin Liver Dis. 2009;18(1):73–82.
2. Puig I, Calvet X, Baylina M, Isava Á, Sort P, Llaó J, et al. How and when should NSAIDs be used for preventing post-ERCP pancreatitis? A systematic review and meta-analysis. PloS One. 2014;9(3):e92922.
3. Tieu AH, Kumbhari V, Jakhete N, Onyimba F, Patel Y, Shin EJ, et al. Diagnostic and therapeutic utility of SpyGlass (®) peroral cholangioscopy in intraductal biliary disease: single-center, retrospective, cohort study. Dig Endosc. 2015;27(4):479–85.
4. Siiki A, Rinta-Kiikka I, Koivisto T, Vasama K, Sand J, Laukkarinen J. Spyglass single-operator peroral cholangioscopy seems promising in the evaluation of primary sclerosing cholangitis-related biliary strictures. Scand J Gastroenterol. 2014;49(11): 1385–90.
5. Goudra B, Singh PM. ERCP: the unresolved question of endotracheal intubation. Dig Dis Sci. 2013; 59(3):513–9.
6. Branch null. ERCP-induced pancreatitis. Curr Treat Options Gastroenterol. 2000;3(5):363–70.
7. Nemes B, Gámán G, Doros A. Biliary complications after liver transplantation. Expert Rev Gastroenterol Hepatol. 2015;9(4):447–66.
8. Sampaziotis F, Elias J, Gelson WTH, Gimson AE, Griffiths WJH, Woodward J, et al. A retrospective study assessing fully covered metal stents as first-line management for malignant biliary strictures. Eur J Gastroenterol Hepatol. 2015;27(11):1347–53.
9. Buxbaum J, Roth N, Motamedi N, Lee T, Leonor P, Salem M, et al. Anesthetist-directed sedation favors success of advanced endoscopic procedures. Am J Gastroenterol. 2016;112(2):290–6.
10. Bowie JD. What is the upper limit of normal for the common bile duct on ultrasound: how much do you want it to be? Am J Gastroenterol. 2000;95(4): 897–900.
11. Hadidi A. Pancreatic duct diameter: sonographic measurement in normal subjects. J Clin Ultrasound. 1983;11(1):17–22.
12. Westphal JF, Brogard JM. Biliary tract infections: a guide to drug treatment. Drugs. 1999;57(1):81–91.
13. Motte S, Deviere J, Dumonceau JM, Serruys E, Thys JP, Cremer M. Risk factors for septicemia following endoscopic biliary stenting. Gastroenterology. 1991;101(5):1374–81.
14. Bae S, Kim T, Kim M-C, Chong YP, Kim S-H, Sung H, et al. Clinical characteristics and outcomes of spontaneous bacterial peritonitis caused by Enterobacter

15. Palabiyiko I, Tekeli E, Aysev D, Sirlak M, Kaymakci S, Ozturk S. ERCP related sepsis. Am J Infect Dis. 2005;1(2):87–9.
16. Cotton PB, Eisen G, Romagnuolo J, Vargo J, Baron T, Tarnasky P, et al. Grading the complexity of endoscopic procedures: results of an ASGE working party. Gastrointest Endosc. 2011;73(5):868–74.
17. Shiffman ML, Sugerman HJ, Kellum JM, Moore EW. Changes in gallbladder bile composition following gallstone formation and weight reduction. Gastroenterology. 1992;103(1):214–21.
18. Iorgulescu A, Turcu F, Iordache N. ERCP after bariatric surgery—literature review and case report. J Med Life. 2014;7(3):339–42.
19. Donepudi S, Chavalitdhamrong D, Pu L, Draganov PV. Air embolism complicating gastrointestinal endoscopy: a systematic review. World J Gastrointest Endosc. 2013;5(8):359–65.
20. ASGE Standards of Practice Committee, Anderson MA, Fisher L, Jain R, Evans JA, Appalaneni V, et al. Complications of ERCP. Gastrointest Endosc. 2012;75(3):467–73.
21. Lynch CR, Khandekar S, Lynch SM, Disario JA. Sublingual L-hyoscyamine for duodenal antimotility during ERCP: a prospective randomized double-blinded study. Gastrointest Endosc. 2007;66(4):748–52.
22. Ozaslan E, Karakelle N, Ozaslan NG. Hyoscine-N-butylbromide induced ventricular tachycardia during ERCP. J Anaesthesiol Clin Pharmacol. 2014;30(1):118–9.
23. Vallakati A, Reddy M, Olayee M, Lakkireddy D. Cardiac arrest from asystole during endoscopic retrograde cholangiopancreatography: a rare but fatal complication. J Atr Fibrillation. 2013;6(4):47–9.
24. Thompson DR. Narcotic analgesic effects on the sphincter of Oddi: a review of the data and therapeutic implications in treating pancreatitis. Am J Gastroenterol. 2001;96(4):1266–72.
25. Radnay PA, Duncalf D, Novakovic M, Lesser ML. Common bile duct pressure changes after tentanyl, morphine, meperidine, butorphanol, and naloxone. Anesth Analg. 1984;63(4):441–4.
26. Wu S-D, Zhang Z-H, Jin J-Z, Kong J, Wang W, Zhang Q, et al. Effects of narcotic analgesic drugs on human Oddi's sphincter motility. World J Gastroenterol WJG. 2004;10(19):2901–4.
27. Enestvedt BK, Eisen GM, Holub J, Lieberman DA. Is ASA classification useful in risk stratification for endoscopic procedures? Gastrointest Endosc [Internet]. 2013 Mar [cited 2016 Jun 3];77(3). http://www.ncbi.nlm.nih.gov/pmc/articles/PMC3816502/.
28. Sankar A, Johnson SR, Beattie WS, Tait G, Wijeysundera DN. Reliability of the American Society of Anesthesiologists physical status scale in clinical practice. Br J Anaesth. 2014;113(3):424–32.
29. Devereaux PJ, Sessler DI. Cardiac complications in patients undergoing major noncardiac surgery. N Engl J Med. 2015;373(23):2258–69.
30. Day LW, Lin L, Somsouk M. Adverse events in older patients undergoing ERCP: a systematic review and meta-analysis. Endosc Int Open. 2014;2(1):E28–36.
31. Williams EJ, Green J, Beckingham I, Parks R, Martin D, Lombard M, et al. Guidelines on the management of common bile duct stones (CBDS). Gut. 2008;57(7):1004–21.
32. ASGE Standards of Practice Committee, Levy MJ, Anderson MA, Baron TH, Banerjee S, Dominitz JA, et al. Position statement on routine laboratory testing before endoscopic procedures. Gastrointest Endosc. 2008;68(5):827–32.
33. Egan RJ, Nicholls J, Walker S, Mellor K, Young WT, Stechman MJ. Routine coagulation screening is an unnecessary step prior to ERCP in patients without biochemical evidence of jaundice: a cross-centre study. Int J Surg Lond Engl. 2014;12(11):1216–20.
34. Kumar A, Srivastava U. Role of routine laboratory investigations in preoperative evaluation. J Anaesthesiol Clin Pharmacol. 2011;27(2):174–9.
35. Kaplan EB, Sheiner LB, Boeckmann AJ, Roizen MF, Beal SL, Cohen SN, et al. The usefulness of preoperative laboratory screening. JAMA. 1985;253(24):3576–81.
36. Committee on Standards and Practice Parameters, Apfelbaum JL, Connis RT, Nickinovich DG, American Society of Anesthesiologists Task Force on Preanesthesia Evaluation, Pasternak LR, et al. Practice advisory for preanesthesia evaluation: an updated report by the American Society of Anesthesiologists Task Force on Preanesthesia Evaluation. Anesthesiology. 2012;116(3):522–38.
37. Berzin TM, Sanaka S, Barnett SR, Sundar E, Sepe PS, Jakubowski M, et al. A prospective assessment of sedation-related adverse events and patient and endoscopist satisfaction in ERCP with anesthesiologist-administered sedation. Gastrointest Endosc. 2011;73(4):710–7.
38. Yang JF, Farooq P, Zwilling K, Patel D, Siddiqui AA. Efficacy and safety of propofol-mediated sedation for outpatient endoscopic retrograde cholangiopancreatography (ERCP). Dig Dis Sci. 2016;61(6):1686–91.
39. Goudra BG, Singh PM, Penugonda LC, Speck RM, Sinha AC. Significantly reduced hypoxemic events in morbidly obese patients undergoing gastrointestinal endoscopy: predictors and practice effect. J Anaesthesiol Clin Pharmacol [Internet]. [cited 2016 Jun 3]. http://www.joacp.org/article.asp?issn=0970-9185;year=2014;volume=30;issue=1;spage=71;epage=77;aulast=Goudra
40. Dripps RD, Lamont A, Eckenhoff JE. The role of anesthesia in surgical mortality. JAMA. 1961;178:261–6.
41. Goudra B, Nuzat A, Singh PM, Gouda GB, Carlin A, Manjunath AK. Cardiac arrests in patients undergoing gastrointestinal endoscopy: a retrospective analysis of 73,029 procedures. Saudi J Gastroenterol. 2015;21:400–11.
42. Metzner J, Domino KB. Risks of anesthesia or sedation outside the operating room: the role of the anesthesia care provider. Curr Opin Anaesthesiol. 2010;23(4):523–31.

43. MacRae MG. Closed claims studies in anesthesia: a literature review and implications for practice. AANA J. 2007;75(4):267–75.
44. Goudra B, Nuzat A, Singh PM, Borle A, Carlin A, Gouda G. Association between type of sedation and the adverse events associated with gastrointestinal endoscopy: an analysis of 5 years' data from a Tertiary Center in the USA. Clin Endosc. 2016;50(2):161–9.
45. Goudra BG, Singh PM, Sinha AC. Anesthesia for ERCP: impact of anesthesiologist's experience on outcome and cost. Anesthesiol Res Pract [Internet]. 2013 May 28 [cited 2013 Jun 7];2013. http://www.hindawi.com/journals/arp/2013/570518/abs/.
46. Tringali A, Mutignani M, Milano A, Perri V, Costamagna G. No difference between supine and prone position for ERCP in conscious sedated patients: a prospective randomized study. Endoscopy. 2008;40(2):93–7.
47. Vuyk J. Pharmacokinetic and pharmacodynamic interactions between opioids and propofol. J Clin Anesth. 1997;9(6 Suppl):23S–6S.
48. Vuyk J. TCI: supplementation and drug interactions. Anaesthesia. 1998;53(Suppl 1):35–41.
49. Goudra B, Singh PM, Gouda G, Borle A, Carlin A, Yadwad A. Propofol and non-propofol based sedation for outpatient colonoscopy-prospective comparison of depth of sedation using an EEG based SEDLine monitor. J Clin Monit Comput. 2015;30(5):551–7.
50. Standards for Basic Anesthetic Monitoring. Committee of origin: standards and practice parameters (approved by the ASA House of Delegates on October 21, 1986, last amended on October 20, 2010, and last affirmed on October 28, 2015).
51. Weaver J. The latest ASA mandate: $CO_2$ monitoring for moderate and deep sedation. Anesth Prog. 2011;58(3):111–2.
52. Statement on Nonoperating Room Anesthetizing Locations. Committee of origin: standards and practice parameters (approved by the ASA House of Delegates on October 19, and last amended on October 16, 2013).
53. Goudra BG, Singh PM, Penugonda LC, Speck RM, Sinha AC. Significantly reduced hypoxemic events in morbidly obese patients undergoing gastrointestinal endoscopy: predictors and practice effect. J Anaesthesiol Clin Pharmacol. 2014;30(1):71–7.
54. Goudra B, Alvarez A, Singh PM. Practical considerations in the development of a nonoperating room anesthesia practice. Curr Opin Anaesthesiol. 2016;30(1):71–7.
55. Perbtani YB, Summerlee RJ, Yang D, An Q, Suarez A, Williamson JB, et al. Impact of endotracheal intubation on interventional endoscopy unit efficiency metrics at a tertiary Academic Medical Center. Am J Gastroenterol. 2016 Jun;111(6):800–7.
56. Goudra B, Singh P, Sinha A. Outpatient endoscopic retrograde cholangiopancreatography: safety and efficacy of anesthetic management with a natural airway in 653 consecutive procedures. Saudi J Anaesth. 2013;7(3):259–65.
57. Akhondzadeh R, Ghomeishi A, Nesioonpour S, Nourizade S. A comparison between the effects of propofol-fentanyl with propofol-ketamine for sedation in patients undergoing endoscopic retrograde cholangiopancreatography outside the operating room. Biomed J. 2016;39(2):145–9.
58. Goyal R, Hasnain S, Mittal S, Shreevastava S. A randomized, controlled trial to compare the efficacy and safety profile of a dexmedetomidine-ketamine combination with a propofol-fentanyl combination for ERCP. Gastrointest Endosc. 2016;83(5):928–33.
59. Srikanth MS, Kahlstrom R, Oh KH, Fox SR, Fox ER, Fox KM. Topical benzocaine (Hurricaine) induced methemoglobinemia during endoscopic procedures in gastric bypass patients. Obes Surg. 2005;15(4):584–90.
60. Baron TH, Kozarek RA, Carr-Locke DL. ERCP. Philadelphia: Elsevier Health Sciences; 2012.
61. Schmitz A, Schmidt AR, Buehler PK, Schraner T, Frühauf M, Weiss M, et al. Gastric ultrasound as a preoperative bedside test for residual gastric contents volume in children. Paediatr Anaesth. 2016;26(12):1157–64.
62. Bouvet L, Chassard D. [Contribution of ultrasonography for the preoperative assessment of gastric contents]. Ann Fr Anesth Reanim. 2014;33(4):240–7.
63. Amer S, Horsley-Silva JL, Menias CO, Pannala R. Endoscopic retrograde cholangiopancreatography in patients with surgically altered gastrointestinal anatomy. Abdom Imaging. 2015;40(8):2921–31.

# Anesthesia for Colonoscopy

George A. Dumas

## Anesthesia Involvement

Colonoscopies are some of the most commonly performed outside of the operating room procedures. This procedure can be quite uncomfortable for the patient. Complex patients and advanced procedures require anesthetic assistance. Examples of these types of colonoscopies include: interventional colonoscopies, retrograde balloon-assisted deep enteroscopies, and other colonoscopies requiring deep levels of sedation. Patients with multiple comorbidities, pediatric patients, mentally impaired patients, uncooperative patients, patients with histories of substance use or abuse, patients on multiple or high-doses of pain medications or benzodiazepine therapy, patients with a history of difficult sedations, and patients with difficult airways are best served by an anesthesiologist. The best anesthetic technique will be determined by procedural and patient factors.

## Depth of Sedation Continuum

Many uncomplicated patients have been managed with a combination of opiates and benzodiazepines for colonoscopies. Due to the common use of propofol sedation for colonoscopies, it has

G. A. Dumas, M.D.
Department of Anesthesiology and Perioperative Medicine, University of Alabama at Birmingham, Birmingham, AL, USA
e-mail: gadumas@uabmc.edu

become essential for anesthesia providers to understand depth of sedation. Providers must have a thorough understanding of the physiological and anatomical changes occurring at different depths of sedation.

The American Society of Anesthesiologists has defined and described the depth of sedation continuum [1]. Minimal sedation is described as having normal response to verbal stimulation. The airway, spontaneous ventilation, and cardiovascular function are not affected in minimal sedation. Moderate sedation is described as purposeful response to tactile or verbal stimulation. It should be noted that reflex withdrawal to pain is not purposeful. No intervention is required for airway maintenance. Spontaneous ventilation is adequate and cardiovascular function is usually maintained. Deep sedation is described as purposeful response after repeated or painful stimulation. Reflex withdrawal to pain is not purposeful. An intervention to maintain the airway may be needed. Spontaneous ventilation may be inadequate and cardiovascular function is usually maintained.

General anesthesia is described as the patient being unarousable, even with painful stimulus. An airway intervention is often needed. Spontaneous ventilation is frequently inadequate and cardiovascular function may be impaired.

Conscious sedation refers to moderate sedation and analgesia. Colonoscopies are often performed with "conscious sedation." Since it is not always easy to predict how a patient may respond to various agents given for sedation and analgesia, anesthesia providers must be able to rescue patients from very deep levels of sedation [1]. More specifically, propofol use should be limited to those providers who are trained in the use of general anesthesia and are not involved in performing the procedure for which propofol administration is required [2].

## Preoperative Assessment

## Aspiration

Colonoscopy patients have an increased risk of aspiration and subsequent aspiration pneumonia. This risk is higher when deep sedation is used [3]. Upper airway protective reflexes are diminished with deeper levels of anesthesia. This places patients at greater risk of aspiration. In a study by Agostoni et al., aspiration occurred in 0.16% of colonoscopies [4]. Propofol sedation was used in most of the patients in this study. Swallowing impairment, a risk factor for aspiration, also occurs with deeper levels of sedation. At common infusion targets used during deep propofol sedation, aspiration due to swallowing impairment may occur [5]. Elderly patients and patients with an elevated BMI are at additional risk for swallowing impairment when propofol sedation is used [5]. About 15 min after return of consciousness from propofol sedation, reflexive swallowing completely returns [6]. When midazolam is used for colonoscopy, the swallowing reflex is depressed for 2 h after return of consciousness [7].

Active or passive regurgitation of gastric contents may occur. The patient's history will reveal predisposing conditions which may cause gastric aspiration. These conditions include: (1) increased gastric contents (delayed emptying, gastric hypersecretion, lack of adherence to fasting guidelines, overfeeding), (2) increased regurgitation risk (achalasia, Zenker's diverticulum, esophageal strictures and cancers, reduced lower esophageal sphincter tone, gastro-esophageal reflux disease, extremes of age), (3) diminished laryngeal function (stroke, multiple sclerosis, Parkinson's disease, Guillain-Barre, muscular dystrophy, cerebral palsy, head injury, trauma, burns) [8]. Aspiration management, in a deeply sedated or completely anesthetized patient, should begin with aggressive suctioning in the head down position and possible tracheal intubation with tracheal suctioning prior to initiation of ventilation [8]. Following fasting guidelines and consideration of pharmacotherapy with H-2 blockers, proton pump inhibitors, antacids, and/or prokinetic agents is essential in patients with risk factors. Consideration of tracheal intubation for airway protection in patients with elevated risk is also warranted.

## Bowel Preparation

The colon should be completely empty for a successful colonoscopy. Special consideration should be made when evaluating fluid restricted elderly patients who have had a bowel preparation. They are very susceptible to dehydration and can easily develop orthostatic hypotension. Polyethylene glycol preparations are very common. However, they have been associated with acute renal failure, particularly in geriatric patients [9]. Sodium phosphate can result in hyperphosphatemia, hypokalemia, and hypernatremia [10]. In elderly patients with renal insufficiency, heart failure, and volume overload, sodium phosphate preparations are contraindicated.

Split-dose bowel preparation solutions are often administered prior to colonoscopy. Improved bowel preparation is often obtained with split-dose regimens. However, the improved bowel prep only exists as long as the "runaway time" or time since the second and last dose of oral bowel preparation solution was administered does not exceed 5 h [11]. It should be noted that patients receiving split-dose bowel preparation solutions compared to single dose solutions given the evening before examination have similar residual gastric volumes [12]. Usually, a 2 h fasting period is sufficient after the second dose of bowel preparation solution.

## Cardiovascular Evaluation

Colonoscopy is considered a low risk procedure. In asymptomatic patients, preoperative cardiac testing is unnecessary. In patients with known cardiovascular disease, a routine 12-lead EKG is not indicated. Some patients may present with recent coronary interventions including bare-metal or drug-eluting cardiac stents. Consultation between anesthesiologist, endoscopist, and cardiologist may be required. Benefits of therapeutic or cancer staging procedures may outweigh other risks.

Implanted cardiac devices should be evaluated. During snare polyp resection, hot biopsy forceps application, or argon plasma coagulation, monopolar electrosurgical current may be used [13]. Because of this, precautions regarding function of pacemakers and implanted cardiac defibrillators should be undertaken. If electromagnetic interference is anticipated, recommendations should be obtained regarding device setting, magnet use, and device interrogation.

Obscure gastrointestinal bleeding and other disorders of the small bowel may be identified in a retrograde fashion. These retrograde balloon-assisted deep enteroscopies are often performed in elderly patients. Heyde's syndrome is an angiodysplastic bleeding syndrome due to acquired type-2A von Willebrand factor and is a result of aortic stenosis. It is therefore prudent to evaluate for signs and symptoms of aortic stenosis in elderly patients being evaluated for obscure gastrointestinal bleeding via retrograde balloon-assisted deep enteroscopy. It is important not to overlook this association as deep levels of sedation are typically required for completion of deep enteroscopy.

## Mask Ventilation Concerns

The likelihood of needing airway and ventilatory intervention increases in parallel with increased sedation depth. It is important to screen patients for potentially difficult mask ventilation. Difficult mask ventilation predictors include: age over 55 years, BMI >26 kg/m$^2$, presence of beard, history of sleep apnea or snoring, Mallampati III or IV, limited mandibular protrusion, male sex, lack of teeth, airway tumor or mass, neck irradiation, and neck circumference >40 cm [14–16]. Any of these predictors should raise the level of concern for a difficult mask ventilation, but greater than one predictor should increase concern much more [14]. The most significant predictor of impossible mask ventilation is neck irradiation [16]. In pediatric patients, difficult mask ventilation is especially concerning. This is due to the limited time to rescue the patient [15]. It should also be noted that in patients with a difficult mask ventilation, difficult intubation risk may be four times higher [14].

## Sedation Expectations

Patients often expect to be completely unconscious during colonoscopy. Patients that are the most concerned about awareness include: those who have never had the procedure and those who have not been counseled prior to their colonoscopy [17]. Chatman et al., surveyed patients before colonoscopy and found that anxiety about awareness during the procedure was high. Concerns of awareness trumped concerns related to incomplete colonic examination, respiratory complications, vomiting, and post-procedural drowsiness [17]. Patient expectations and satisfaction improved when a discussion about awareness during colonoscopy was undertaken prior to the colonoscopy.

## Intraoperative Concerns

### Prophylactic Antibiotics

Antibiotics are typically not required or indicated for colonoscopies. In patients with high risk cardiac conditions, it may be reasonable to give antibiotics [18]. This would apply to high risk patients with established gastrointestinal tract infections with enterococci. Antibiotic coverage, for prevention of infective endocarditis, with an antibiotic targeting enterococci may be reasonable.

## Monitoring

The standards for basic anesthetic monitoring apply during colonoscopy. Continuous pulse oximetry and exposure of the patient are used to evaluate and assess oxygenation. Continuous end-tidal carbon dioxide analysis and other clinical signs including auscultation of breath sounds and chest excursion are used to assess ventilation. Continuous display of the electrocardiogram, continuous heart rate monitoring, and blood pressure monitoring least every 5 min are used to evaluate circulation. Monitors including the EEG based BIS monitor or SEDLine monitor may be helpful for determining depth of sedation. These monitors are optional; however, use of these monitors may be beneficial in decreasing complications associated with deeper levels of sedation. Placement of monitors is straightforward. The patient is usually in the lateral decubitus position. Airway access is not compromised by the colonoscope. The head of the patient may be turned to the opposite side of the room from the anesthesia provider due to room setup.

## Sedation Depth

The anesthesia provider will need to consider multiple factors when determining the depth of sedation needed for colonoscopy. Factors which should be considered include: recall, patient movement, hypotension, airway events, aspiration, difficult colonoscopy, and cognitive recovery.

A recent study by Allen et al., looked at depth of sedation during colonoscopy with propofol and fentanyl [19]. "Light" sedation was defined as a bispectral index (BIS) of 70–80. "Deep" sedation was defined as a BIS of <60. Colonoscopy patients that required deep sedation had reduced movement, lower levels of recall, more hypotension, and increased airway obstruction. Despite a higher incidence of recall (12% versus 1%), the patients with less or light sedation were mostly satisfied. Light sedation leads to a more rapid recovery. Despite this, cognitive impairment was similar in both groups at hospital discharge [19].

It has been shown that propofol based sedation is associated with deeper levels of sedation than non-propofol based sedation [20]. Increased depth of sedation, as defined by propofol administration, has been associated with a higher risk of aspiration, colon perforation, and splenic injury [3]. Propofol titration to EEG based readings (SEDLine or BIS monitor) can help reduce the period of time patients are under deeper levels of anesthesia during colonoscopies. Risks associated with deeper levels of sedation (aspiration, hypotension, respiratory depression, etc.), can be reduced in this manner [20].

## Benzodiazepines and Opiates

Traditionally an opiate combined with a benzodiazepine has been used for sedation and analgesia during colonoscopy. Midazolam is usually the benzodiazepine of choice due to its rapid onset and short duration of action. Midazolam provides anxiolysis, amnesia, and sedation. Midazolam is also a respiratory depressant and has a reversal agent, flumazenil. Synergistic effects result when benzodiazepines are combined with opiates. This results in deeper levels of sedation, respiratory depression, and hemodynamic effects. Fentanyl, a rapid onset, short-acting opiate, has sedative and analgesic properties. Opiates can cause nausea and respiratory depression along with other side effects. Naloxone is the reversal agent for fentanyl and other opiates. Opiates including morphine and meperidine have also been used for sedation and analgesia during colonoscopy. However, they have a slower onset and longer duration of effect compared to fentanyl. Therefore, fentanyl may be a better choice for colonoscopy.

## Propofol

The popularity of propofol use during sedation for colonoscopy has increased dramatically due to its many favorable properties. Of these favorable properties, its rapid onset and rapid offset rank highly. Sedative and amnestic qualities of propofol are utilized. However, minimal analgesia is provided. Rapid cognitive function return, antiemetic properties, and short recovery times are all beneficial. Typically, onset of propofol sedation is 30–60 s and plasma half-life is 1–4 min [21]. A reversal agent for propofol does not exist. Also, consciousness levels can change rapidly during propofol anesthesia. Unintentional deep sedation or general anesthesia may occur during propofol administration. This can result in depression in respiratory, cardiovascular, and neurologic function. Rapidly changing levels of consciousness are associated with these physiologic alterations. Thus, the availability of a qualified anesthesia provider is essential. Recovery and discharge times are shorter with propofol compared to traditional sedative and analgesic agents (benzodiazepines and narcotics). Also, propofol based anesthesia results in higher patient satisfaction and side effects are not increased compared to traditional agents during colonoscopy [22, 23].

Better operating conditions and shorter procedure times are obtained when midazolam and or fentanyl are judiciously used to supplement propofol during colonoscopy [24]. If small amounts of midazolam are given, 2 mg or less, recovery time, patient satisfaction, and recall are similar to patients that only received propofol. When used to supplement propofol based sedation during colonoscopy, more than 2 mg of midazolam may be predictive of impaired cognitive function at discharge [24].

## Ketamine

Ketamine, which has analgesic and anesthetic properties, is a useful adjunct during sedation for colonoscopy. Minimal cardiovascular effects and maintenance of airway patency and respiratory drive at low doses make ketamine a good choice. Low-dose ketamine (0.3 mg/kg) supplementation to midazolam-fentanyl-propofol sedation improves multiple parameters [25]. Reduced propofol use and improvement of hemodynamic parameters were shown. Also, patients had fewer adverse sedation effects which included fewer airway support maneuvers. This study was performed on colonoscopy patients.

## Dexmedetomidine

Dexmedetomidine is an anxiolytic with sedative and analgesic properties. It is an alpha-2 agonist. Dexmedetomidine use does not result in significant respiratory depression. However, sympatholysis associated with its use has been associated with hypotension and bradycardia [26]. Hemodynamic instability, cost, and need for complex infusion are negatives associated with dexmedetomidine use during colonoscopy [27]. However, the positive benefits of dexmedetomidine has resulted in others supporting its use during colonoscopy [28].

## Remifentanil

Remifentanil, an ultra-short acting opioid agonist, is metabolized by nonspecific esterases. It has a context-sensitive half-time of 4 min regardless of infusion duration [29]. Compared to usual midazolam-meperidine sedation regimens, remifentanil alone anesthetics resulted in better communication between endoscopist and patient, enhanced patient satisfaction, and quicker recovery during colonoscopy [30, 31]. Cardiac and respiratory side effects may be reduced with lower doses of remifentanil (0.4 µg/kg loading dose and 0.04 µg/kg/min infusion dose) [31]. Additional sedation may be optional as patients are almost completely alert.

## Sevoflurane

In the ambulatory setting, sevoflurane has been studied for colonoscopy. Rapid patient psychomotor recovery and rapid discharge criteria readiness were shown [32]. In geriatric patients, fewer airway complications occurred with a sevoflurane anesthetic compared to a propofol anesthetic

[33]. Procedural conditions were the same for both groups. For administration of sevoflurane, a nasal airway connected to a semi-closed circuit may be considered. Proper scavenging should be utilized.

## Nitrous Oxide

Analgesia, short half-life, and minimal cardiorespiratory depression are some of the properties of nitrous oxide that make it appealing for use during colonoscopy. In systematic reviews of nitrous oxide use during colonoscopy, nitrous oxide with oxygen is shown to control discomfort and pain to an equal degree as conventional sedation [34, 35]. Use of nitrous oxide did not affect quality, difficulty, or duration of the procedures. Shorter hospital stays and faster patient recovery were shown when nitrous oxide was compared to traditional agents [34, 35]. Patient throughput may be improved by return of psychomotor function and fast recovery. This improved recovery profile may even allow some patients to drive themselves home after their procedure [36].

## Difficult Colonoscopy

Defining the difficult colonoscopy may be done a couple of different ways including: failure to reach the cecum, procedural time, patient discomfort, and physical exertion required by the endoscopist. Risk factors for difficult colonoscopy include: colon loops and angulations, poor bowel preparation, diverticular disease, extreme body habitus, female sex, prior surgery, young patients, and men with a history of constipation or laxative use [37–41].

Loops and angulations in the colon are a usual source of difficulty. These angulations and loops are common in the sigmoid colon. Control of the endoscope is difficult and patients can become uncomfortable. Often, increased sedation is needed. Successful intubation of the cecum is often proportional to level of sedation [41].

The colon may become more spastic due to diverticular disease. This can cause problems with bowel insufflation and bowel preparation [39, 41]. Visualization is difficult with poor bowel preparation. Obesity may make it challenging to apply abdominal counter-pressure. Ordinarily, this counter-pressure helps minimize looping. On the other extreme, lower body mass and reduced abdominal cavity size with reduced visceral fat makes it challenging to fold the colon [38]. Technical difficulty is also increased with a history of prior surgery, particularly abdominal hysterectomy [37]. The female colon can present difficulties. It is longer and more angulated as it crosses into the pelvis [41]. In men, constipation or laxative use may result in redundant colon. This redundancy makes reaching the cecum difficult [40]. Young patients exhibit discomfort with mesocolon stretching. Often the mesocolon is tight [39].

Scope advancement can be aided by changing the position of the patient. Patients may be turned to supine and subsequently to right lateral decubitus or prone to assist. It helps for the patient to not be overly sedated when positional changes are needed. Application of abdominal counter pressure is also useful. If the patient can hold a deep breath, this will lower the diaphragm. Lowering the diaphragm can help the scope pass the colonic flexure [41]. Scopes that are variable-stiffness also help.

Propofol sedation can aid in completing the colonoscopy. Deep propofol sedation increases axial and radial forces during scope advancement and withdrawal. Loops and angulations in the colon are able to be pushed through with deep propofol sedation. Examination time is reduced [42].

## Complications During Colonoscopy

Serious complications from colonoscopy are uncommon, but 33% of patients report minor, transient symptoms [43]. Death attributed to colonoscopy has been estimated to be 0.03% [43]. Therapeutic colonoscopies will increase complications.

## Cardiopulmonary Complications

Hypoxia, hypoventilation, arrhythmias, hemodynamic compromise, abdominal discomfort, and vasovagal reactions can result from sedation, mesenteric stretching and colonic distention. A study by Sharma et al. [44] revealed that cardiopulmonary complications occurred in 0.9% of procedures and were responsible for 67% of unplanned events in endoscopic studies where sedation was used. Transient hypoxemia and hypotension were the most common cardiopulmonary events. A much lower incidence of prolonged hypoxemia (0.78/100,000) during colonoscopy was revealed. Cardiopulmonary events are also more prevalent in patients with advanced age [45].

## Perforation and Splenic Injury

Deep levels of sedation may allow the endoscopist to complete the colonoscopy. However, deep sedation can lead to complications. These complications are in addition to aspiration and aspiration pneumonia and are thought to be increased by the inability of the patient to show discomfort when the colonoscope is advanced against resistance [46]. Perforation of the colon may occur from 0.6/1000 to 0.9/1000 colonoscopies [47, 48]. Persistent abdominal pain and abdominal distention are early symptoms. Peritonitis may develop later and an abdominal CT or plain film should be considered [49].

Splenic injury is more common in deeply sedated patients. This is due to increased patient toleration to loops in the colonoscope. The excessive force stresses colonic to splenic attachments and can cause injury [3].

## Hemorrhage

Although hemorrhage may occur during diagnostic colonoscopy, it is more common with polypectomy. Acute hemorrhage after polypectomy is apparent and can be treated endoscopically [49].

## Abdominal Pain or Discomfort

These are minor complications of colonoscopy. The reported incidence of bloating is 25% and reported incidence of abdominal pain or discomfort is 5–11% [50]. When carbon dioxide is used instead of standard air insufflation, there is less pain post-procedure [51].

## Gas Explosion

This is a very rare event. However, gas explosion may occur when the following are simultaneously present: hydrogen and methane gas in the colonic lumen, oxygen, and electrosurgical energy [49]. Electrocautery or argon plasma coagulation are examples of electrosurgical energy which may be used.

## Conclusion and Sedation Strategy

Reducing the period of time that the patient is in deep sedation during colonoscopy should help reduce risks related to deep sedation. These risks include: aspiration, endoscopic trauma, and respiratory compromise. It is always valuable to obtain a good history and physical exam and also describe what will be involved with the sedation. This will include a discussion about awareness. Propofol sedation offers several advantages. The ability to rapidly titrate sedation level is one of its best advantages. This will allow the provider to provide deep sedation to facilitate difficult portions of the exam but to lighten the anesthetic for other portions. Supplementation of propofol with small amounts of midazolam and fentanyl can be used. In difficult to sedate patients and patients with elevated anesthetic requirement, ketamine is a helpful adjunct. Ideally, ketamine should be used at lower doses. Sedation methods which require complex administration of inhaled or intravenous agents are best left for very unusual circumstances. Table 20.1 provides a summary of anesthesia considerations in patients undergoing colonoscopy.

**Table 20.1** Brief review of anesthesia for colonoscopy

| Plan/preparation/adverse events | Reasoning/management |
|---|---|
| For sedation cases, always have equipment available to provide positive pressure ventilation | Hypoxia is a common complication of sedation and sometimes positive pressure is required, particularly for patients that may be in a deeper plane od sedation than was intended |
| It is important to have emergency drugs available and intubation tools ready | If an emergency occurs, valuable time cannot be lost looking for supplies. Nasal trumpets and oral airways should be available |
| Pre-procedural evaluation | |
|   Aspiration risk | A major cause of morbidity and mortality is aspiration. Plan and use prophylaxis accordingly |
|   Bowel preparation | Elderly patients may be dehydrated |
|   Cardiovascular | Implanted cardiac devices should be evaluated particularly if electrosurgical current is used |
|   Difficult mask ventilation | Risk factors must be determined and airway devices must be available |
|   Patient expectations | Patients must be counseled about awareness |
| Position—left lateral decubitus | Ease of advancing the colonoscope. Positioning may be changed during the procedure |
| IV access—right hand (left hand OK if poor options) | Easy accessibility as this is the patient's top hand |
| Sedation | |
|   Propofol | Basis for most sedation plans due to its properties |
|   +/− Fentanyl | Helpful adjunct if used judiciously |
|   +/− Midazolam | Helpful adjunct if used judiciously |
|   +/− Ketamine | Useful in difficult to sedate patients (0.3 mg/kg) |
| Procedural adverse events<br>  Hypoxia<br>  Hypotension<br>  Arrhythmia<br>  Aspiration<br>  Perforation<br>  Hemorrhage<br>  Gas explosion | Aggressive treatment is required for hypoxia and airway related events. Otherwise, as indicated |
| Postoperative and post-discharge considerations<br>  Abdominal discomfort<br>  Perforation<br>  Hypoxia<br>  Hypotension | As indicated |

# References

1. American Society of Anesthesiologists; Quality Management and Departmental Administration. Continuum of depth of sedation: definition of general anesthesia and levels of sedation/analgesia [Internet]. 2014 [updated 2014 Oct 15; cited 2017 Mar 1]. http://www.asahq.org/~/media/Sites/ASAHQ/Files/Public/Resources/standards-guidelines/continuum-of-depth-of-sedation-definition-of-general-anesthesia-and-levels-of-sedation-analgesia.pdf.
2. American Society of Anesthesiologists; Quality Management and Departmental Administration. Statement on Safe Use of Propofol [Internet]. [updated 2014 Oct 15; cited 2017 Mar 1].http://www.asahq.org/~/media/Sites/ASAHQ/Files/Public/Resources/standards-guidelines/statement-on-safe-use-of-propofol.pdf.
3. Cooper GS, Kou TD, Rex DK. Complications following colonoscopy with anesthesia assistance: a population-based analysis. JAMA Intern Med. 2013;173(7):551–6. https://doi.org/10.1001/jamainternmed.2013.2908.
4. Agostoni M, Fanti L, Gemma M, Pasculli N, Beretta L, Testoni PA. Adverse events during monitored anesthesia care for GI endoscopy: an 8-year experience. Gastrointest Endosc. 2011;74(2):266–75. https://doi.org/10.1016/j.gie.2011.04.028.
5. Marco G, Laura P, Alessandro O, Massimo A, Francesca P, Barbara R, et al. Swallowing impairment during propofol target-controlled infusion. Anesth Analg. 2016;122(1):48–54. https://doi.org/10.1213/ane.0000000000000796.
6. Rimaniol JM, D'Honneur G, Duvaldestin P. Recovery of the swallowing reflex after propofol anesthesia. Anesth Analg. 1994;79(5):856–9.
7. D'Honneur G, Rimaniol JM, el Sayed A, Lambert Y, Duvaldestin P. Midazolam/propofol but not propofol

alone reversibly depress the swallowing reflex. Acta Anaesthesiol Scand. 1994;38(3):244–7.
8. Engelhardt T, Webster NR. Pulmonary aspiration of gastric contents in anaesthesia. Br J Anaesth. 1999;83(3):453–60.
9. Choi NK, Lee J, Chang Y, Jung SY, Kim YJ, Lee SM, et al. Polyethylene glycol bowel preparation does not eliminate the risk of acute renal failure: a population-based case-crossover study. Endoscopy. 2013;45(3):208–13. https://doi.org/10.1055/s-0032-1326031.
10. Qureshi WA, Zuckerman MJ, Adler DG, Davila RE, Egan JV, Gan SI, et al. ASGE guideline: modifications in endoscopic practice for the elderly. Gastrointest Endosc. 2006;63(4):566–9. https://doi.org/10.1016/j.gie.2006.02.001.
11. Bucci C, Rotondano G, Hassan C, Rea M, Bianco MA, Cipolletta L, et al. Optimal bowel cleansing for colonoscopy: split the dose! A series of meta-analyses of controlled studies. Gastrointest Endosc. 2014;80(4):566–76.e2. https://doi.org/10.1016/j.gie.2014.05.320.
12. Huffman M, Unger RZ, Thatikonda C, Amstutz S, Rex DK. Split-dose bowel preparation for colonoscopy and residual gastric fluid volume: an observational study. Gastrointest Endosc. 2010;72(3):516–22. https://doi.org/10.1016/j.gie.2010.03.1125.
13. Slivka A, Bosco JJ, Barkun AN, Isenberg GA, Nguyen CC, Petersen BT, et al. Electrosurgical generators: MAY 2003. Gastrointest Endosc. 2003;58(5):656–60.
14. Langeron O, Masso E, Huraux C, Guggiari M, Bianchi A, Coriat P, et al. Prediction of difficult mask ventilation. Anesthesiology. 2000;92(5):1229–36.
15. El-Orbany M, Woehlck HJ. Difficult mask ventilation. Anesth Analg. 2009;109(6):1870–80. https://doi.org/10.1213/ANE.0b013e3181b5881c.
16. Kheterpal S, Martin L, Shanks AM, Tremper KK. Prediction and outcomes of impossible mask ventilation: a review of 50,000 anesthetics. Anesthesiology. 2009;110(4):891–7. https://doi.org/10.1097/ALN.0b013e31819b5b87.
17. Chatman N, Sutherland JR, van der Zwan R, Abraham N. A survey of patient understanding and expectations of sedation/anaesthesia for colonoscopy. Anaesth Intensive Care. 2013;41(3):369–73.
18. Wilson W, Taubert KA, Gewitz M, Lockhart PB, Baddour LM, Levison M, et al. Prevention of infective endocarditis: guidelines from the American Heart Association: a guideline from the American Heart Association Rheumatic Fever, Endocarditis, and Kawasaki Disease Committee, Council on Cardiovascular Disease in the Young, and the Council on Clinical Cardiology, Council on Cardiovascular Surgery and Anesthesia, and the Quality of Care and Outcomes Research Interdisciplinary Working Group. Circulation. 2007;116(15):1736–54. https://doi.org/10.1161/circulationaha.106.183095.
19. Allen M, Leslie K, Hebbard G, Jones I, Mettho T, Maruff P. A randomized controlled trial of light versus deep propofol sedation for elective outpatient colonoscopy: recall, procedural conditions, and recovery.

Can J Anaesth. 2015;62(11):1169–78. https://doi.org/10.1007/s12630-015-0463-3.
20. Goudra B, Singh PM, Gouda G, Borle A, Carlin A, Yadwad A. Propofol and non-propofol based sedation for outpatient colonoscopy-prospective comparison of depth of sedation using an EEG based SEDLine monitor. J Clin Monit Comput. 2016;30(5):551–7. https://doi.org/10.1007/s10877-015-9769-5.
21. Training Committee. American Society for Gastrointestinal Endoscopy. Training guideline for use of propofol in gastrointestinal endoscopy. Gastrointest Endosc. 2004;60(2):167–72.
22. McQuaid KR, Laine L. A systematic review and meta-analysis of randomized, controlled trials of moderate sedation for routine endoscopic procedures. Gastrointest Endosc. 2008;67(6):910–23. https://doi.org/10.1016/j.gie.2007.12.046.
23. Singh H, Poluha W, Cheung M, Choptain N, Baron KI, Taback SP. Propofol for sedation during colonoscopy. Cochrane Database Syst Rev. 2008;8(4):CD006268. https://doi.org/10.1002/14651858.CD006268.pub2.
24. Padmanabhan U, Leslie K, Eer AS, Maruff P, Silbert BS. Early cognitive impairment after sedation for colonoscopy: the effect of adding midazolam and/or fentanyl to propofol. Anesth Analg. 2009;109(5):1448–55. https://doi.org/10.1213/ane.0b013e3181a6ad31.
25. Tuncali B, Pekcan YO, Celebi A, Zeyneloglu P. Addition of low-dose ketamine to midazolam-fentanyl-propofol-based sedation for colonoscopy: a randomized, double-blind, controlled trial. J Clin Anesth. 2015;27(4):301–6. https://doi.org/10.1016/j.jclinane.2015.03.017.
26. Bloor BC, Ward DS, Belleville JP, Maze M. Effects of intravenous dexmedetomidine in humans. II. Hemodynamic changes. Anesthesiology. 1992;77(6):1134–42.
27. Jalowiecki P, Rudner R, Gonciarz M, Kawecki P, Petelenz M, Dziurdzik P. Sole use of dexmedetomidine has limited utility for conscious sedation during outpatient colonoscopy. Anesthesiology. 2005;103(2):269–73.
28. Dere K, Sucullu I, Budak ET, Yeyen S, Filiz AI, Ozkan S, et al. A comparison of dexmedetomidine versus midazolam for sedation, pain and hemodynamic control, during colonoscopy under conscious sedation. Eur J Anaesthesiol. 2010;27(7):648–52. https://doi.org/10.1097/EJA.0b013e3283347bfe.
29. Westmoreland CL, Hoke JF, Sebel PS, Hug CC Jr, Muir KT. Pharmacokinetics of remifentanil (GI87084B) and its major metabolite (GI90291) in patients undergoing elective inpatient surgery. Anesthesiology. 1993;79(5):893–903.
30. Manolaraki MM, Theodoropoulou A, Stroumpos C, Vardas E, Oustamanolakis P, Gritzali A, et al. Remifentanil compared with midazolam and pethidine sedation during colonoscopy: a prospective, randomized study. Dig Dis Sci. 2008;53(1):34–40. https://doi.org/10.1007/s10620-007-9818-0.
31. Hong MJ, Sung IK, Lee SP, Cheon BK, Kang H, Kim TY. Randomized comparison of recovery time

after use of remifentanil alone versus midazolam and meperidine for colonoscopy anesthesia. Dig Endosc. 2015;27(1):113–20. https://doi.org/10.1111/den.12383.
32. Theodorou T, Hales P, Gillespie P, Robertson B. Total intravenous versus inhalational anaesthesia for colonoscopy: a prospective study of clinical recovery and psychomotor function. Anaesth Intensive Care. 2001;29(2):124–36.
33. Syaed El Ahl MI. Modified sevoflurane-based sedation technique versus propofol sedation technique: a randomized-controlled study. Saudi J Anaesth. 2015; 9(1):19–22. https://doi.org/10.4103/1658-354x.146265.
34. Welchman S, Cochrane S, Minto G, Lewis S. Systematic review: the use of nitrous oxide gas for lower gastrointestinal endoscopy. Aliment Pharmacol Ther. 2010;32(3):324–33. https://doi.org/10.1111/j.1365-2036.2010.04359.x.
35. Aboumarzouk OM, Agarwal T, Syed Nong Chek SA, Milewski PJ, Nelson RL. Nitrous oxide for colonoscopy. Cochrane Database Syst Rev. 2011; (8): CD008506. https://doi.org/10.1002/14651858. CD008506.pub2.
36. Martin JP, Sexton BF, Saunders BP, Atkin WS. Inhaled patient-administered nitrous oxide/oxygen mixture does not impair driving ability when used as analgesia during screening flexible sigmoidoscopy. Gastrointest Endosc. 2000;51(6):701–3.
37. Cirocco WC, Rusin LC. Factors that predict incomplete colonoscopy. Dis Colon Rectum. 1995;38(9): 964–8.
38. Anderson JC, Gonzalez JD, Messina CR, Pollack BJ. Factors that predict incomplete colonoscopy: thinner is not always better. Am J Gastroenterol. 2000;95(10):2784–7. https://doi.org/10.1111/j.1572-0241.2000.03186.x.
39. Waye JD. Completing colonoscopy. Am J Gastroenterol. 2000;95(10):2681–2. https://doi.org/10.1111/j.1572-0241.2000.03172.x.
40. Anderson JC, Messina CR, Cohn W, Gottfried E, Ingber S, Bernstein G, et al. Factors predictive of difficult colonoscopy. Gastrointest Endosc. 2001;54(5):558–62.
41. Witte TN, Enns R. The difficult colonoscopy. Can J Gastroenterol. 2007;21(8):487–90.
42. Korman LY, Haddad NG, Metz DC, Brandt LJ, Benjamin SB, Lazerow SK, et al. Effect of propofol anesthesia on force application during colonoscopy. Gastrointest Endosc. 2014;79(4):657–62. https://doi.org/10.1016/j.gie.2013.12.002.
43. Ko CW, Dominitz JA. Complications of colonoscopy: magnitude and management. Gastrointest Endosc Clin N Am. 2010;20(4):659–71. https://doi.org/10.1016/j.giec.2010.07.005.
44. Sharma VK, Nguyen CC, Crowell MD, Lieberman DA, de Garmo P, Fleischer DE. A national study of cardiopulmonary unplanned events after GI endoscopy. Gastrointest Endosc. 2007;66(1):27–34. https://doi.org/10.1016/j.gie.2006.12.040.
45. Warren JL, Klabunde CN, Mariotto AB, Meekins A, Topor M, Brown ML, et al. Adverse events after outpatient colonoscopy in the Medicare population. Ann Intern Med. 2009;150(12):849–57, w152
46. Adeyemo A, Bannazadeh M, Riggs T, Shellnut J, Barkel D, Wasvary H. Does sedation type affect colonoscopy perforation rates? Dis Colon Rectum. 2014;57(1):110–4. https://doi.org/10.1097/dcr.0000000000000002.
47. Levin TR, Zhao W, Conell C, Seeff LC, Manninen DL, Shapiro JA, et al. Complications of colonoscopy in an integrated health care delivery system. Ann Intern Med. 2006;145(12):880–6.
48. Ko CW, Riffle S, Michaels L, Morris C, Holub J, Shapiro JA, et al. Serious complications within 30 days of screening and surveillance colonoscopy are uncommon. Clin Gastroenterol Hepatol. 2010;8(2):166–73. https://doi.org/10.1016/j.cgh.2009.10.007.
49. Fisher DA, Maple JT, Ben-Menachem T, Cash BD, Decker GA, Early DS, et al. Complications of colonoscopy. Gastrointest Endosc. 2011;74(4):745–52. https://doi.org/10.1016/j.gie.2011.07.025.
50. Ko CW, Riffle S, Shapiro JA, Saunders MD, Lee SD, Tung BY, et al. Incidence of minor complications and time lost from normal activities after screening or surveillance colonoscopy. Gastrointest Endosc. 2007;65(4):648–56. https://doi.org/10.1016/j.gie.2006.06.020.
51. Wong JC, Yau KK, Cheung HY, Wong DC, Chung CC, Li MK. Towards painless colonoscopy: a randomized controlled trial on carbon dioxide-insufflating colonoscopy. ANZ J Surg. 2008;78(10):871–4. https://doi.org/10.1111/j.1445-2197.2008.04683.x.

# Anesthesia for Bronchoscopic Procedures

## 21

Mona Sarkiss

## Introduction and Historical Perspective

In the early 1800s, death related to foreign body aspiration was a recurrent theme. Dr. Gustav Killian, an ear nose and throat surgeon at that time, was inspired to invent a device that allows him to look inside the airway and retrieve the deadly foreign bodies. Soon after the invention of the first rigid laryngoscope in 1865, it was realized that overcoming airway reflexes and patient anxiety while inspecting the airway was the next plausible task. Initially the surgeon would practice on corpse or paid volunteers in order to be able to perform the procedure as fast as possible when a real patient is in need. During the actual procedure, an assistant would hold the patient's head in place while the surgeon introduces the rigid bronchoscope in the airway and retrieves the foreign body [1]. Attempts to desensitize the airway reflexes using available chemicals, such as belladonna, potassium bromide and ammonia were not successful, until cocaine was discovered and used to anesthetize the airway. Cocaine blunted the airway reflexes and altered the patient level of consciousness resembling a state of general anesthesia. A decade later, Ikeda invented the flexible bronchoscope in 1968. The need for the deep state of anesthesia created by cocaine was no longer necessary because of the small size and flexibility of the flexible bronchoscope. Conversely, the ease of use of the flexible bronchoscope has also led to the emergence of new procedures such as diagnostic airway exams; broncheo-alveolar lavage, endobronchial and transbronchial biopsies as well as some therapeutic procedures to debulk airway tumors, cauterize bleeder and insert airway stents [1]. The availability of newer local anesthetics such as lidocaine facilitated the performance of these procedures. However, the matter of patient anxiety, hypertension and tachycardia associated with the introduction of the flexible bronchoscope in the airway remained a concern and a hindered the completion of the procedure in some patients. The addition of different combinations of various anxiolytics and opioid analgesics to the local anesthesia during airway procedures was a natural progression as longer and more complicated airway procedure in a larger number of patients became common practice. Since the 1970s, the concept of conscious sedation with anxiolytics with or without opioids in addition to local anesthetics became and remained the mainstay for anesthesia for flexible bronchoscopic procedures.

M. Sarkiss, M.D., Ph.D.
Department of Anesthesiology and Perioperative Medicine, The University of Texas MD Anderson Cancer Center, Houston, TX, USA

Department of Pulmonary Medicine, The University of Texas MD Anderson Cancer Center, Houston, TX, USA
e-mail: msarkiss@mdanderson.org

In the early 1970, the field of interventional bronchoscopy emerged as a separate discipline. New procedures and devices were invented to manage benign and malignant critical airway obstruction, and debulk central airway tumors. Most of the interventional pulmonary procedures are best performed through a rigid bronchoscope where large specializes instruments can be introduced and stents can be easily deployed. The need for complimentary general anesthesia during rigid bronchoscopic procedures became a natural consequence. Needless to say, as anesthesia services became available to interventional pulmonologists for rigid bronchoscopic procedures, additional airway procedures that needed prolonged sedation, such as endobronchial ultrasound guided fine needle aspiration (EBUS-FNA) of mediastinal lymph nodes or pulmonary peripheral nodules and pleuroscopy, are currently being performed with anesthesia support in some centers [2].

The current guidelines left the choice of anesthesia technique to be used in various interventional pulmonary procedure to the bronchoscopist [2]. It is common practice that simple diagnostic and interventional procedures, of short duration in patients with uncompromising airway pathology, are performed under conscious sedation. Based on the availability of anesthesia support at different interventional pulmonary centers, more complex cases with significant central airway narrowing, expected long duration and/or patients with severe comorbidities are commonly performed under general anesthesia or are referred to tertiary center where anesthesia services are available to the interventional pulmonologists.

This chapter will give a brief description of the current interventional pulmonary procedures, pre-procedure evaluation, types of anesthesia, airway devices and mode of ventilation needed, possible complications and their management, post procedure care and how to set up anesthesia services in an out of the operating room bronchoscopy suite.

# Bronchoscopic Procedures

## Airway Exam

All bronchoscopic procedures begin with a thorough airway exam that begins at the vocal cords and ends at the second or third bronchial bifurcation where the flexible bronchoscope cannot reach any further. The goal of the airway exam is to clear the airway lumen of any secretions in order to detect any luminal or mucosal pathology such as, foreign body, tumor, or infections as well as narrowing of the central airway by external compression, all of which might necessitate an intervention. The central airway is richly supplied by sympathetic nerve ending that are stimulated once the airway is entered by the bronchoscopic. As a result, a sympathetic discharge in the form of tachycardia, hypertension as well as a coughing reflex are common occurrence during airway exam with the flexible bronchoscope. Topicalization of airway in a spray as you go manner through the bronchoscope with 1, 2 or 4% lidocaine is generally equally effective and adequate in calming both the hemodynamic changes and the cough reflex. Additionally, spraying lidocaine on the vocal cords before entering the airway is crucial to prevent laryngospasm during the procedure.

Once the airway exam is completed the indicated airway procedure is performed. Airway procedures are classified into diagnostic and therapeutic procedures.

## Diagnostic Procedure

### Broncheoalveolar Lavage (BAL)
BAL is a procedure to retrieve pulmonary secretions lining the alveoli and distal airway that might contain pathogens or inflammatory cells. The bronchoscope is introduced in the airway and wedged in the most distal accessible bronchus that leads the affected lung segment as seen on a radiologic test. Aliquots of normal saline with a total volume

between 100 and 300 mL is sequentially installed through the bronchoscope, immediately suctioned and sent for pathologic analysis. As BAL is considered a safe procedure that can be performed in a short time frame of 5–10 min, with no anticipated side effects, it is commonly performed under conscious sedation. However, patients who refuse conscious sedation due to anxiety or are considered high risk for conscious sedation can undergo the procedure under general anesthesia.

**Trans-Bronchial Aspiration (TBNA)**

TBNA through the flexible bronchoscope was first described in 1981. It is a procedure where a long needle is inserted in the flexible bronchoscope working channel through the tracheal or bronchial wall into mediastinal lymph nodes or a lesion in the lung parenchyma. The needle is then lunged several times into the lesion of interest while aspiration is applied at the proximal end of the needle in order to lodge cells or core tissue into the lumen of the needle. The aspirated material is then processed and sent for pathology analysis. The procedure can be performed blindly where the needle is inserted where the target lesion location is extrapolated from a radiologic image or it can be performed with ultrasound (EBUS-TBNA) or electromagnetic navigation guidance (EMN-TBNA) as described below.

Compared to open lung biopsy or mediastinoscopy for mediastinal lymph node biopsy, TBNA is considered a safer minimally invasive procedure. Conventional TBNA is commonly performed under conscious sedation while EBUS-TBNA and EMN-TBNA can be performed under conscious sedation or general anesthesia based on the case complexity, patient comorbidities and availability of anesthesia support.

**Endobronchial Ultrasound/ Transbronchial Lymph Node Biopsy (EBUS-FNA)**

EBUS is performed with a modified bronchoscope where an ultrasound transducer is built in at the tip of the bronchoscope. This causes the tip of the bronchoscope to have a diameter of 6.9–6.2 mm that is larger than a conventional flexible bronchoscope. The larger tip of the bronchoscope is more difficult to insert through the nose and is less tolerated when inserted through the mouth. Additionally, EBUS-FNA is performed for diagnosis of mediastinal lymph node or lung nodule pathology and/or staging of lung cancer. Consequently, some of the procedures can be lengthy and rather uncomfortable and unsafe when performed under conscious sedation. Therefore, practitioners may choose to perform all EBUS procedures or only the lengthy staging EBUS procedures under general anesthesia. Great controversy exists over performing EBUS under moderate sedation or general anesthesia. Recent study showed that more lymph nodes per patient and smaller lymph nodes were sampled more often when EBUS was performed under deep sedation or general anesthesia. In addition on-site cytology evaluation was used more frequently when general anesthesia was used [3]. However, several reports indicated no difference in patient satisfaction, yield, sensitivity or specificity of the EBUS procedure when performed under moderate sedation versus general anesthesia [4, 5].

**Electromagnetic Navigation Guided Lung Biopsy (EMN)**

EMN uses global positioning system to allow the bronchoscopist to reach distal peripheral lung lesion that cannot be reached with a conventional bronchoscope. The bronchoscopist uses a specialized long catheter to navigate the airway under electromagnetic guidance to reach the lesion of interest. Once the lesion is reached biopsies can be obtained by fine needle aspiration or therapy can be delivered by brachytherapy, microwave therapy or high frequency ablation [6].

**Pleuroscopy**

Medical pleuroscopy is performed to obtain biopsy of the parietal pleural in patients with persistent pleural effusion of unknown etiology. The procedure can also be used to install talc powder into the pleural space to obtain pleurodesis in patients with chronic pleural effusions. Different types of anesthesia has been described for patients undergoing pleuroscopy these include, general anesthesia, thoracic epidural, intercostal nerve blocks, local anesthesia, and conscious sedation.

## Therapeutic Procedures

Therapeutic interventional pulmonary procedures of short duration can be performed through the flexible bronchoscope under conscious sedation. Meanwhile, complex lengthy therapeutic airway procedures with compromised central airway are safely performed through the rigid bronchoscope. Despite few reports of rigid bronchoscopy performed under local anesthesia [7] or general anesthesia with spontaneous ventilation [8], the most common practice is to perform rigid bronchoscopy under general anesthesia with muscle relaxation [9]. Complex therapeutic procedure are commonly associated with frequent episodes of hypoxemia and hypercapnia that can be prevented and adequately managed with positive pressure or jet ventilation [8]. Alternatively, spontaneous or assisted ventilation can be used during rigid bronchoscopy based on the airway pathology [10].

## Pre-procedural Evaluation

### Airway Assessment

The ability of the patient to maintain a patent airway during moderate or deep sedation, difficulty of intubation in case of airway compromise or if rigid bronchoscopy is planned, and the ease of insertion of the laryngeal mask airway should be determined. Signs that can predict difficulty of intubation are: high Mallampati grade, decreased extension of the atlanto-occipital joint by more than two-third, decreased mouth opening below the normal range of 50–60 cm, thyromental distance measured in an extended neck from the mentum to the notch of the thyroid cartilage ≤6 cm in adults, short muscular neck, and receding mandible or history of obstructive sleep apnea.

Additionally, signs of airway changes secondary to radiotherapy treatment should be sought. For example, upper airway edema, neck scarring, poor laryngeal mobility with loss of the laryngeal click, limited mouth opening and/or known upper airway tumor.

### Dental Assessment

Examination of the teeth is necessary to identify the presence of loose teeth, dental prosthesis, chipped, missing teeth, bridges, crowns or denture. The presence of prominent or protruding maxillary incisors may alert the bronchoscopist to the possibility of difficult intubation and/or damage to the teeth during direct laryngoscopy or rigid bronchoscopy.

### Respiratory System Assessment

Special attention should be paid to Patients with high $FiO_2$ requirement and baseline use of supplemental oxygen, those with reactive, obstructive or restrictive airway disease. These can manifest as audible respiratory noises such as, stridor and wheezing, or visible signs of airway obstruction such as, the use of accessory muscles, nasal flaring and grunting, baseline saturation and the need for supplemental oxygen.

Reviewing computed tomography (CT) images, pulmonary function testing and flow volume loops are necessary to determine the location and ventilatory effects of the airway pathology at hand. For example; Upper airway pathology e.g. edema and/ or space occupying lesions, upper and mid tracheal pathology, tumors with ball valve effect, tumors and/or infections known to cause airway bleeding. All these finding are essential to guide the anesthesiologist in choosing the most suitable type of anesthesia, airway device and mode of ventilation during a particular airway procedure e.g.

## Cardiovascular System Assessment

Cardiac and circulatory co-morbidities related or unrelated to the pulmonary pathology need to be evaluated. For example, lung and/or mediastinal tumors can cause secondary hypoxemia and hypercarbia that may alter the patient's hemodynamics. Additionally, patients with known restrictive and obstructive pulmonary disease are known to have secondary pulmonary hypertension and core pulmonale as well as cardiac arrhythmias such as, atrial fibrillation, premature atrial beats, premature ventricular beats, supraventricular tachycardia and malignant ventricular tachycardia. Compressive and obstructive effect of the mediastinal pathology on the inflow and outflow of the cardiac chambers e.g., SVC syndrome, pulmonary veins occlusion, pulmonary artery thrombi and emboli, pericardial effusion, and pericardial tamponade can be detrimental under general anesthesia and need special care.

Appropriate choice of anesthesia technique, monitoring devices, and medications to support the circulatory system during the procedure is essential.

## Laboratory Testing

Common alterations in baseline laboratory test should be sought.

### CBC
Elevated white cell count can be secondary to an underlying pulmonary infection or the concurrent intake of steroids for the management of COPD or autoimmune pulmonary diseases. Acute anemia is commonly found in patients with massive hemoptysis. Alternatively, when thrombocytopenia is detected, especially in the setting of hemoptysis and/ or lung biopsies, the anesthesiologist should be alerted to order a type and screen and have packed RBCs and/or platelet available for transfusion in case of emergency bleeding during a bronchoscopic procedure.

### Electrolyte
Electrolyte abnormalities can also be encountered in patients with pulmonary pathology. For example, hyponatremia as a manifestation of paramalignant syndrome in patients with lung cancer, and/or elevated bicarbonate levels in patients with chronic carbon dioxide retention secondary to sleep apnea or other airway obstructive disease.

### Coagulation Studies
Simple bronchoscopic procedures such as airway exam and bronchoalveolar lavage can be safely performed in patients with coagulopathy. However, biopsy of airway pathology, mediastinal lymphadenopathy and/or lung parenchymal or rigid bronchoscopy for management of central airway tumor and hemoptysis might necessitate a normal baseline coagulation studies or correction of the coagulopathy before the procedure in order to perform the procedure safely.

### Renal and Hepatic Function
Baseline renal and liver function testing can be beneficial in the selection of anesthesia medications based on the drug metabolism and clearance.

### Type and Screen
Massive bleeding is rarely encountered in patients undergoing bronchoscopic procedures. However, a type and screen is considered judicious in patients undergoing rigid bronchoscopy for central airway tumor debulking and/or hemoptysis management.

**Nothing per os (NPO)** before the procedure for a period of 2 h for clear liquids, and 6–8 h for solids according to the current ASA guidelines. Patients with high risk of aspiration such as those with history of uncontrolled or untreated acid reflux; post esophagectomy or gastroparesis should be instructed to take the anti-reflux medication on the day of the procedure and can benefit from airway protection by endotracheal intubation.

**Consent** should be obtained from the patient after detailed explanation of the risks, benefits and possible alternatives of the procedure and sedation or anesthesia.

## Anesthesia Techniques

### Topical Anesthesia

The first synthetic local anesthetic, procaine, was introduced by Einhorn in 1905. Consequently, lidocaine was synthesized in 1943 by Löfgren. Synthetic local anesthetics have a lipophilic benzine ring linked via an amide or an ester bond to a hydrocarbon chain that is attached to a hydrophilic tertiary amine structure. Local anesthetics are classified according to the linking bond to either ester or amide local anesthetics. Ester and amide local anesthetics have different metabolism and potential to produce an allergic reaction. Amide local anesthetics, which are commonly used in bronchoscopy are metabolized by the liver microsomal enzymes and are also extracted through the lungs. The addition of epinephrine at 1:200,0000 (5 μg/mL) concentration or 0.25% phenylephrine causes local vasoconstriction, which slows down the absorption of the local anesthetic, prolongs its duration of action, and decreases its systemic toxicity.

## Side Effects of Local Anesthetics

Systemic toxicity of local anesthetics can be encountered when a large amounts of local anesthetics is absorbed from the application site or directly injected into a blood vessel. It is important to note that lidocaine plasma level of (5 μg/mL) or greater than 8.2 mg/kg of lidocaine instilled in the airway can result in systemic toxicity [2]. The toxic dose of benzocaine is 100 mg and the toxic dose of tetracaine is 100 mg (but toxicity has been reported at 40 mg).

Central nervous system (CNS) toxicity causes CNS excitation that manifests by restlessness, vertigo, tinnitus and slurred speech. The symptoms may progress to tonic–clonic seizure followed coma and death. Seizures can be immediately controlled with small doses of a benzodiazepine such as diazepam or midazolam, or intravenous thiopental or propofol. Supplemental oxygen should be provided if hypoxemia is noted. Additionally, hyperventilation and respiratory alkalosis causes hyperpolarization of the nerve membrane and increases the threshold for seizure as well as the amount of local anesthetic that is bound to protein and cannot cross the blood brain barrier. The airway should be intubated and protected in the event that the seizure activity cannot be controlled despite treatment.

Cardiovascular toxicity occur when the cardiac sodium channels are blocked by the binding of the local anesthetic. This can result in hypotension, long PR interval and widening of the QRS complex, cardiac arrhythmias, atrioventricular heart block and eventually cardiac arrest.

Methemoglobinemia is a rare side effect of local anesthetic that occurs when the hemoglobin iron molecule is oxidized into a ferric state. Methemoglobin cannot release bound oxygen to tissue causing tissue hypoxemia and cyanosis followed by stupor, coma and death. Methemoglobinemia is easily treated by the administration of 1–2 mg/kg of methylene blue intravenously.

Allergic reactions to local anesthetics are rare but are more common with ester local anesthetic metabolite para-aminobenzoic acid (PAPA). In addition, the preservatives used with either ester or amide local anesthetics (e.g., methylparaben) can be a source of allergic reaction. It is noteworthy that cross-sensitivity does not exist between ester and amide local anesthetics.

## Anesthesia of the Nasal Mucosa and Nasopharynx

Sensation to the nasal mucosa is provided by the middle division (V2) of the trigeminal nerve (CN V), the sphenopalatine ganglion and the ethmoid nerve. The nasal mucosa and the nasopharynx can be topicalized with a cotton-tipped applicators or pledgets dipped in a 1, 2 or 4% lidocaine solution with or without a vasoconstricting agent. The applicators are inserted inside the nose up to the inferior turbinate, the middle turbinate and the superior turbinate and left in place for 5 min each in order to achieve adequate topicalization.

## Anesthesia of the Mouth and Oropharynx

Sensory supply of the mouth and oropharynx is provided by branches of the glossopharyngeal, vagus and facial nerves. The lingual branch of the glossopharyngeal nerve provides sensation to the posterior third of the tongue, the vallecula, and the anterior surface of the epiglottis. The pharyngeal branch provides sensation to the posterior and lateral walls of the pharynx, and the tonsillar branch supplies the tonsillar pillars. Adequate anesthesia to the mouth and oropharynx can be provided by combination of the following methods:

- Application of a tongue blade coated with lidocaine gel directly on the tongue for several minutes.
- Inhalation of nebulized 4% Lidocaine or 0.5% Tetracaine.
- Spraying the posterior pharyngeal wall with Cetacaine atomizer spray (tetracaine and benzocaine combination).
- Gargling with 2–4 mL of viscous lidocaine for 30 s.

### Superior Laryngeal Nerve Block

The superior laryngeal nerve (SLN) is a branch of the vagus nerve that divides into internal and external branches at a point lateral to the cornu of the hyoid bone. The internal branch passes under the greater cornu of the hyoid bone, pierces the thyrohyoid membrane and enters the pyriform recess where it provides sensation to the base of the tongue, the superior epiglottis, the aryepiglottic folds, the arytenoids and the laryngeal mucosa above the vocal cords. The external branch provides motor innervation to the cricothyroid muscle.

SLN block the patient can be performed with the patient in a supine position with the head slightly extended. The landmark for the block is the greater horn of the hyoid bone that can be palpated above the thyroid cartilage. The needle (size 22 or 23 gauge) is insert towards the greater horn of the hyoid bone and directed caudally until a pop is felt as the thyroid ligament is pierced at a depth of about 1–2 cm. Negative aspiration is performed to avoid intravascular injection before 2–3 mL of 2% lidocaine with epinephrine is injected. Bilateral blocks should be performed.

### Recurrent Laryngeal Nerve Block (RLN)

The recurrent laryngeal provides motor and sensory innervation to the vocal cords as well as sensory innervation to the trachea. In a supine patient with hyperextended neck lidocaine 1–2% is injected into the skin over the cricothyroid membrane with a 22-gauge needle. A 22-gauge IV catheter is then inserted through the cricothyroid membrane into the tracheal lumen at an angle of 45° caudally. Air should be aspirated to confirm intra-tracheal position. The needle is removed leaving the catheter in the tracheal lumen. the patient is then asked to take a deep breath followed by forced exhalation while 3–4 cc of 1–2 or 4% lidocaine is injected into the tracheal lumen. This techniques causes coughing and spread of the local anesthetic over the vocal cords and the trachea.

## Conscious Sedation

Guidelines of the American college of chest physicians indicated in the 2011 consensus statement that "all physicians performing bronchoscopy should consider using topical anesthesia, analgesic and sedative agents, when feasible" [11]. Conscious sedation is needed to reduce patient's anxiety and pain. Additionally, conscious sedation in association with topical anesthesia reduces airway reflexes such as cough and gag, and sensation of difficulty breathing when the bronchoscope is inserted in the airway. It has been shown that patient satisfaction and willingness to undergo another bronchoscopic procedure increases when conscious sedation is used for bronchoscopic procedures. In addition, the ability of the bronchoscopist to complete an advanced diagnostic and therapeutic procedures of shorter duration improves with sedation.

Different drug regimens have been used, and they vary depending on the bronchoscopist' preference and experience. The most commonly used classes of drugs are benzodiazepines for anxiolysis and amnesia and opioids for suppression of cough and pain. The combination of narcotics and benzodiazepines has an additive effect on the suppression of the respiratory drive and cardiovascular hemodynamics thus increasing the likelihood of apnea, desaturation and hypotension. Therefore, these drugs should be titrated gradually to achieve the desired effect and avoid undesired side effects. Noteworthy is that the combination of an opioids and a benzodiazepine is associated with better patient's tolerance of bronchoscopy when compared to each agent alone [12].

## Monitored Anesthesia Care

Describes a situation where anesthesia services has been consulted to participate in the care of a patient undergoing a diagnostic or therapeutic procedure. It is important to note that MAC does not describe the depth of sedation. Under MAC, the anesthesiologist provides sedation or general anesthesia as needed and the post procedure recovery care. Situations where MAC is valuable are: when variable levels of sedation are needed to meets changes in the patient and the bronchoscopist needs during a procedure. Patients predisposed to respiratory failure or hemodynamic complications and resuscitation due to their sensitivity to sedating agents. Patients who need alternating periods of general anesthesia and lighter levels of sedation. Therefore, the drugs of choice for MAC should be the ultra-short-acting anesthetics that are easily titrated to match the patient tolerance to the procedure with rapid return to baseline status at the end of the procedure e.g. remifentanil, alfentanil, propofol, dexmedetomidine and fospropofol. In addition, midazolam, fentanyl, and morphine can also be an acceptable choices [13].

## General Anesthesia

The choice of general anesthesia for an interventional bronchoscopic procedure should be based on an open discussion between the anesthesiologist and the bronchoscopist. Factors to be considered are; procedure duration, location (e.g., trachea vs. Bronchi), degree of airway obstruction (e.g., complete vs. partial obstruction), depth of anesthesia needed, airway device options e.g., (none, endotracheal tube, laryngeal mask airway, or rigid bronchoscope), and the most suitable mode of ventilation (e.g., spontaneous ventilation, non-invasive positive pressure, assisted ventilation, mechanical ventilation or jet ventilation). In addition, the anesthesiologist should be remain open to altering the type of anesthesia provided as well as airway device used as the condition of airway is change throughout the procedure and particularly when complications occur.

**Total intravenous anesthesia (TIVA)** is the anesthetic technique of choice for interventional bronchoscopic procedures [5]. Inhalational anesthetics have multiple disadvantages when used during interventional bronchoscopic procedures, including the variable levels of anesthetic gas delivered when frequent suctioning occur during the procedure, and the contamination of the procedure room air by inhalation agents. However, it is important to emphasize that if bronchospasm is encountered during an airway procedure, inhalation agents are a better choice due to their potent bronchodilator effect. Propofol, Remifentanil, ketamine, Dexmedetomidine are the most commonly used anesthetics during interventional bronchoscopic procedures [13].

**Muscle relaxants** use during general anesthesia for interventional bronchoscopic procedure cannot be underestimated. Muscle paralysis is essential to prevent laryngospasm and coughing associated airway irritation when the bronchoscope is inserted in the airway. During therapeutic bronchoscopic procedures, muscle relaxation has many advantages. These include: facilitating the insertion of airway devices (e.g., LMA, endotracheal tube, and the rigid bronchoscope); better lung compliance during positive pressure ventilation or jet ventilation; providing the bronchoscopist with a still field when precise targeting of lesions adjacent to major vessels and the heart is needed; and maintaining the glottis aperture open during multiple insertion and removal of the bronchoscope and other instruments thus minimizing trauma to the vocal cord.

On the other hand, indiscriminate use of muscle relaxant in interventional bronchoscopy can be associated with severe complications. For example, there are several reports of loss of the airway patency after muscle relaxant was given in patients with large anterior mediastinal mass. Pneumothorax and/or pneumomediastinum can develop in patients with tracheo-esophageal fistulas, bronco-esophageal fistulas, or airway tears when muscle relaxant is given and positive pressure ventilation is used. In addition, prolonged unwanted muscle relaxation has been reported in patients with lung cancer associated with paraneoplastic Lambert–Eaton myasthenic syndrome.

In the event that muscle relaxation is deemed unsuitable, instillation of lidocaine on the vocal cord and the proximal airway is a better alternative to the use of muscle relaxation prior to insertion of the rigid bronchoscope or other airway devices.

**Fraction Inspired Oxygen (FiO$_2$)** of 100% is commonly needed to maintain the patient's oxygen saturation >90% during interventional bronchoscopic procedure. This is particularly true in patients with advanced lung pathology, poor baseline oxygen saturation, and/or the use supplemental oxygen. In addition, maintaining the FiO$_2$ around 100% becomes valuable when periods apnea or of complete airway occlusion occur e.g., during deployment or extraction of stents, balloon dilation of the airway, removal of a tumor mass where positive pressure ventilation can force the excised tumor down the airway causing acute obstruction, or during exchange of one rigid bronchoscope to a different type or size rigid bronchoscope.

Alternatively, low FiO$_2$ of less than 40% is required during electrocautery, laser, and argon plasma coagulation (APC) in order to avoid airway fire.

## Monitoring the Depth of Anesthesia

The use of processed electroencephalograms to monitor the depth of anesthesia has been shown to add a significant advantage when total intravenous anesthesia is used. In combination with the patient's clinical signs Monitoring the depth of anesthesia can guide the titration of intravenous anesthetics to achieve adequate depth of anesthesia while avoiding side effects of deep anesthesia such as respiratory failure or cardiovascular instability [14, 15].

## Airway Devices

The current guidelines recommend the use of supplemental oxygen during flexible bronchoscopic procedure with a goal to maintain oxygen saturation above 90%. should be monitored by pulse [2].

Nasal cannula, simple face mask, POM mask with special opening to introduce the bronchoscope can all be used in patients undergoing an airway procedure with conscious sedation. When general anesthesia is required a specialized airway device that does not interfere with the procedure or the airway pathology must be chosen.

## Laryngeal Mask Airway (LMA)

The LMA has many features that makes an ideal airway device for the introduction of the flexible bronchoscope into the airway and performing advanced bronchoscopic procedures. Compared to an endotracheal tube, the LMA is positioned above the larynx, allowing the bronchoscopist to inspect the entire length of the airway from the vocal cords to the distal bronchi. The large diameter of the lumen of the LMA allows for the insertion of the large therapeutic bronchoscopes, commonly used in therapeutic procedures, without compromise to the ventilation. Additionally, the LMA allows free mobility of the bronchoscope within the airway. Some of the LMA models such as the I-Gel has a built-in bite block that protects the bronchoscope from damage. Alternatively, it is important to understand the shortcomings of the LMA as an airway device. These shortcomings include the lack of protection against aspiration especially in patients with full stomach or at an increased risk of aspiration secondary to and underlying pathology. It is important to note that positive pressure ventilation with peak airway pressure above 20 cm H$_2$O can overcome the tone of the lower esophageal sphincter and insufflate the stomach with oxygen resulting in aspiration [16, 17].

Additionally, in patients with oral, pharyngeal, or laryngeal deformity secondary to airway pathology or radiotherapy, it is difficult to obtain adequate seal during positive pressure ventilation through the LMA.

## Endotracheal Tube (ETT)

The ETT is the most definitive and reliable airway devices in patients undergoing general anesthesia. However, it is important to note the limitations of the ETT when used as the main airway device during an interventional bronchoscopic procedure. Performing a bronchoscopic procedure in a patient with an ETT in place, can add challenges and limitation to the ability of the bronchoscopist to perform the procedure. The ETT limits the bronchoscopist ability to examine the vocal cords and the upper part of the trachea for pathology. The length of the ETT projecting from the patient's mouth limits the length of the flexible bronchoscope available for insertion into the airway. As a result, the proximal end of the ETT is commonly cut off after insertion in order to be able to advance the bronchoscope further in the airway. The insertion of the ETT in a patient with central airway narrowing or tumor undergoing a therapeutic bronchoscopic procedure can be harmful as the ETT can cause trauma and bleeding when it comes in contact with the airway pathology. Insertion of an ETT in a patient with pre-existing tracheal or bronchial stents also carries a risk of dislodging or deforming the stents, which can potentially result in airway compromise [18].

Additionally, the ETT can hinder the anesthesiologist ability to provide adequate ventilation to the patient when the therapeutic flexible bronchoscope with a large external diameter is used during the procedure. ETT with an internal diameter of 8.5 or 9 mm is needed in order to deliver adequate ventilation when therapeutic bronchoscope is used.

## Rigid Bronchoscope

The rigid bronchoscope is an ideal airway device in complicated interventional bronchoscopic procedures where multiple instruments and stents are used. Instruments can be introduced in the barrel of the rigid bronchoscope, while ventilation is delivered through a short stainless steel connector attached to the proximal end of the rigid bronchoscope. The side connector has multiple side ports to accommodate a jet ventilator, and the anesthesia circuit. The proximal end of the rigid bronchoscope can remain open to air to allow for insertion of instruments and the flexible bronchoscope, or it can be caped. If the proximal end is open, jet ventilation or spontaneous ventilation are the only possible modes of ventilation. Alternatively, when a cap is placed to seal the proximal end of the rigid bronchoscope, positive pressure ventilation delivered from the anesthesia ventilator or hand-bag ventilation can be used. Leak around the barrel of the rigid bronchoscope at the level of the vocal cords can be overcome by inserting a throat pack in the mouth and applying Vaseline gauze to occlude the nostrils [19].

The rigid bronchoscope has many advantages over the flexible bronchoscope. These include the ability to provide positive pressure ventilation during lengthy airway procedures and the ability to insert instruments with a large diameter into the airway such as the microdebrider, large suction catheter, and the deployment device for silicone stents. The rigid bronchoscope can also be used as a coring device to debulk airway tumors, dilate stenotic areas, stent the airway open in the case of external compression by mediastinal masses, and tamponade airway bleeding by applying direct pressure on the bleeder [20].

## Modes of Ventilation

### Spontaneous Ventilation

Spontaneous ventilation or negative pressure ventilation is invaluable in certain case scenarios. For example, patient with compromised integrity of the airway, such as tracheo-esophageal fistulas, broncho-esophageal fistulas, bronchopleural fistulas, and iatrogenic tears of the central airway. In such instances, positive pressure ventilation can result in pneumomediastinum, pneumothorax and possibly pneumoperitoneum with subsequent hemodynamic compromise. Conversion to spontaneous ventilation in a mechanically ventilated patient when an iatrogenic airway tear occurs during an airway procedure can be lifesaving. Central airway obstruction by an anterior mediastinum mass is another instance where spontaneous ventilation is considered a safer mode of ventilation. Spontaneous ventilation in patients with anterior mediastinal mass was adopted due to multiple reports of worsening of the central airway obstruction by the mediastinal mass after a muscle relaxant was given. Spontaneous ventilation is also essential when pleuroscopy is performed under deep sedation. The lung on the side of the procedure collapses once the chest wall is opened and has to remain collapsed for the duration of the procedure in order to achieve adequate visualization of the pleural space. Spontaneous ventilation maintains the lung collapse during pleuroscopy in the absence of double lumen tube or a bronchial blocker. In the event that intubation of the airway is needed in patient where muscle relaxation is contraindicated, the upper airway should be adequately topicalized with lidocaine after the induction of general anesthesia with Inhalation anesthetics or intravenous anesthetics. Alternatively, a small dose of succinylcholine can be administered to facilitate the intubation with subsequent rapid return to spontaneous ventilation.

## Assisted Ventilation

Spontaneous ventilation under general anesthesia can be inadequate causing hypoxia and/or hypercapnia. In a patient with an ETT or LMA in place, ventilation can be assisted by different modalities, such as intermittent hand-bag ventilation with a large tidal volume, pressure support, or synchronized intermittent mandatory ventilation. These ventilatory support techniques can help overcome atelectasis and improve ventilation and oxygenation during bronchoscopic procedures.

## Non-invasive Positive Pressure Ventilation (NIV)

NIV can be used in patients with sleep apnea or hypoxemic patients undergoing bronchoscopy under moderate or deep sedation. The use of NIV ventilation was shown to improve oxygenation and reduce the risk of acute respiratory failure after bronchoscopy in patients with impaired baseline oxygenation, such as chronic obstructive pulmonary disease (COPD) patients with pneumonia or immunocompromised patients [21, 22]. Nasal or full-face CPAP masks can be fitted out with a special adaptor that allows for the insertion of the bronchoscope. NIV should be considered when endotracheal intubation and mechanical ventilation carry an increased risk to the patient undergoing bronchoscopy.

## Positive Pressure/Controlled Mechanical Ventilation

Controlled positive pressure ventilation is needed in patients undergoing interventional bronchoscopic procedure that require muscle relaxation. Muscle paralysis can facilitate interventional bronchoscopic procedures by eliminating the cough reflex and ensuring a still field. This is particularly important when small lymph nodes are targeted during the EBUS procedure or when central airway tumors are vaporized with laser, Argon Plasma Coagulation (APC), or electrocautery. Positive pressure ventilation can be delivered through the LMA, ETT or rigid bronchoscope. When the LMA is used, care should be taken to maintain the peak airway pressure below 20 cm $H_2O$ to avoid inflating the stomach. Alternatively, when the rigid bronchoscope is used, capping of the rigid bronchoscope proximal end, packing of the mouth and occlusion of the nostril with Vaseline gauze, while using high oxygen flow rates is necessary to achieve adequate tidal volumes.

## Jet Ventilation

**Handheld Jet ventilation** can deliver 100% oxygen into a port at the proximal end of the rigid bronchoscope. However, air is entrained at the open proximal end of the rigid bronchoscope when oxygen is injected decreasing the delivered $FiO_2$ to less than 100%.

The pressure of the injected oxygen can be adjusted with a dial to achieve adequate chest rise without compromising the blood pressure by overinflating the chest. The frequency of ventilation is left to the operator to select and frequently ranges from 8 to 20 breaths per minute. Jet ventilation should be performed only when the proximal end of the rigid bronchoscope is open to air, to avoid barotrauma [23].

**High frequency mechanical jet ventilation** (Acutronic Medical Systems, Hirzel, Switzerland) has many advantages over the simple handheld jet ventilators [24]. These advantages include: ventilation frequency between 4 and 1600 breath per minute and high driving pressure up to 40 psi. The higher frequencies are particularly needed for patients with ARDS and tracheoesophageal fistulas. The high driving pressure produces high flow rate that ensures adequate ventilation, oxygenation with minimal atelectasis. Low intrapulmonary pressure with minimal chest wall movement can be achieved with high frequency jet ventilation as along as the proximal end of the rigid bronchoscope is open to air. The low intrapulmonary pressure produces an apnea like still field for the brochoscopist and makes the jet ventilator safe to use in patients with tracheoesophageal fistulas. The mechanical jet ventilator is also equipped with air-oxygen blender that allows for variation of the delivered $FiO_2$. Some models have a laser setting where immediate reduction of the $FiO_2$ to <40% can be achieved when laser is used in the airway. Barotrauma is prevented during the use of the mechanical jet ventilator by two alarm systems that will discontinue ventilation if the set maximum airway pressure limit is reached. These are the pause pressure monitoring and the airway pressure monitoring. Some models of the mechanical jet ventilator have special setting that allow for monitoring of $etCO_2$. One major advantage of the mechanical jet ventilator over the handheld jet ventilator is its ability to humidify the inspired oxygen up to 100%, enabling jet ventilation for longer procedures without the risks of airway mucosal dryness or damage to the ciliary function [24].

## Complication Associated with Interventional Pulmonary Procedures

### Airway Reactivity

Airway reactivity or bronchospasm can be encountered in patients with history of bronchial asthma or reactive airway disease, respiratory infections, COPD exacerbation. Additionally, irritation of the airway during the procedure by manipulation, instillation of normal saline or bleeding cause induce bronchospasm. Airway reactivity can be easily managed by Intra-procedural nebulization or inhalation of β-agonists e.g., Albuterol and the utilization of inhalation agents e.g., Sevoflurane.

### Bleeding

The source of bleeding can be a preexisting central or distal airway tumor, infection or bronchiectasis or Iatrogenic. Procedures that can be associated with central airway bleeding are, biopsy of central airway lesions, blind transbronchial lung biopsy (TBBx), biopsy of mediastinal lymph nodes, and debulking of central airway tumors during rigid bronchoscopy. Airway bleeding should be managed promptly and its management is based on the location and the severity of the bleeding. Superficial or mild to moderate bleeding can be managed with topical instillation of cold saline, diluted epinephrine, tranexamic acid or thrombin in the airway. Larger volume of bleeding threating to cause flooding of the airway and hypoxemia is best managed with the rigid bronchoscopy inserted in the airway. The rigid bronchoscope can exert direct compression and tamponade by the bleeder or Argon Plasma Coagulation (APC), LASER or electrocautery can be used to stop the bleeding. Additionally, tools for lung isolation such as bronchial blockers and double lumen tubes should be readily available and appropriately utilized as a temporizing measure while surgical management is arranged.

## Hypoxemia

Hypoxemia is an infrequent encounter during bronchoscopy and is defined as oxygen saturation <90% for more than 1 min. Hypoxemia can be due to oxygen independence, frequent suctioning, low $FiO_2$ used during laser and cautery, bleeding, bronchospasm, and airway obstruction by tumor, bleeding or instruments used for the procedure. The best management is to identify the cause. Meanwhile, increasing the oxygen flow and $FiO_2$ can be a temporizing measure while the etiology is sought and managed. Persistent hypoxemia unresponsive to increasing oxygen flow and $FiO_2$ warrants intubation with LMA or ETT and possible escalation of care.

## Hypercapnia

Hypercarbia and Hypercapnia during bronchoscopic procedure can be due to an underlying pulmonary pathology, respiratory depression due to deep sedation, inadequate ventilation, or airway obstruction by the bronchoscope or other instruments. Hypercapnia causes tachycardia and hypertension as well as difficulty waking from anesthesia due to somnolence. Pre-procedure bronchodilator therapy and or steroids can improve baseline reactive airway disease. Adequate reversal of muscle paralysis at the end of the procedure as well as utilizing of ultra-short acting anesthetics and sedative with no residual respiratory depression is essential to prevent hypercapnia during recovery. Reversal of the sedatives agents and/or insertion of an airway device such as LMA or ETT is necessary if procedures is performed under deep sedation.

## Airway Obstruction

Airway obstruction can occur before, during or after the bronchoscopic procedure. It can be due to external compression by benign or malignant space occupying lesions e.g., anterior mediastinal mass or Internal growth in the central airway, blood clots, mucous plugs, fungal infection. Airway obstruction should be managed by the interventional bronchoscopists while imposing several challenges to the anesthesiologists. Large obstructing lesions of the trachea and main bronchi pose a risk of air trapping behind the mass causing a ball-valve effect. If the air trapping went unnoticed, an increase in intrathoracic pressure ensue with impediment of the venous return and subsequent hemodynamic instability. Increasing the I:E ratio in these patients managed with positive pressure ventilation can reduce the risk of air trapping as it allows longer time for the passive exhalation. Additionally, applying suction with the flexible bronchoscope distal the ball-valve can decrease the hyperinflation and normalize the hemodynamics.

## Post-procedure Care

A standard designated recovery area with well-trained nursing staff is essential for safe recovery of patients who underwent an interventional bronchoscopic procedure. In the recovery room supplemental oxygen should be continued via a facemask or a nasal cannula and weaned off gradually. Meanwhile, vital signs should be monitored until discharge criteria are met usually within 30–45 min. Crash carts and emergency intubation equipment should be readily available in the post bronchoscopy recovery areas as post procedure respiratory failures and other complications that may require re-intubation, unplanned hospital stay, and/or ICU admission.

## Interventional Bronchoscopy Suite

Simple bronchoscopic procedures are commonly performed in an interventional bronchoscopy suite. Conscious sedation is provided by a trained bronchoscopy nurse under the supervision of the bronchoscopist. Meanwhile, rigid bronchoscopy or procedures that require general anesthesia are commonly performed in the operating room [25]. In most centers, the choice of the location of the procedure depends on the available anesthesia resources and the level of comfort of the anesthesia team to provide services for such complicated airway procedures outside the operating room. In recent years, interventional bronchoscopy departments that perform a large number of procedures on a daily basis have collaborated with the anesthesia department at their place of practice to design a specialized bronchoscopy suite with integrated anesthesia equipment. These specialized bronchoscopy suites are designed to be a replica of an operating room allowing the bronchoscopists to perform more procedures with anesthesia support under MAC or general anesthesia in the bronchoscopy suites. Interventional bronchoscopy suites have been operational for several years with great success in several centers in the United States and Europe [26].

# References

1. Becker HD. Bronchoscopy: the past, the present, and the future. Clin Chest Med. 2010;31(1):1–18, Table of Contents.
2. British Thoracic Society guidelines on diagnostic flexible bronchoscopy. Thorax. 2001;56(Suppl 1):i1–21.
3. Ost DE, Ernst A, Lei X, Feller-Kopman D, Eapen GA, Kovitz KL, Herth FJ, Simoff M. Diagnostic yield of endobronchial ultrasound-guided transbronchial needle aspiration: results of the AQuIRE Bronchoscopy Registry. Chest. 2011;140(6):1557–66.
4. Herth FJ, Eberhardt R, Krasnik M, Ernst A. Endobronchial ultrasound-guided transbronchial needle aspiration of lymph nodes in the radiologically and positron emission tomography-normal mediastinum in patients with lung cancer. Chest. 2008;133(4):887–91.
5. Sarkiss M, Kennedy M, Riedel B, Norman P, Morice R, Jimenez C, Eapen G. Anesthesia technique for endobronchial ultrasound-guided fine needle aspiration of mediastinal lymph node. J Cardiothorac Vasc Anesth. 2007;21(6):892–6.
6. Khan KA, Nardelli P, Jaeger A, O'Shea C, Cantillon-Murphy P, Kennedy MP. Navigational bronchoscopy for early lung cancer: a road to therapy. Adv Ther. 2016;33(4):580–96.
7. Conacher ID, Curran E. Local anaesthesia and sedation for rigid bronchoscopy for emergency relief of central airway obstruction. Anaesthesia. 2004;59(3):290–2.
8. Perrin G, Colt HG, Martin C, Mak MA, Dumon JF, Gouin F. Safety of interventional rigid bronchoscopy using intravenous anesthesia and spontaneous assisted ventilation. A prospective study. Chest. 1992;102(5):1526–30.
9. Ernst A, Silvestri GA, Johnstone D. Interventional pulmonary procedures: guidelines from the American College of Chest Physicians. Chest. 2003;123(5):1693–717.
10. Ausseur A, Chalons N. [Anesthesia in interventional bronchoscopy]. Rev Mal Respir. 1999;16(4 Pt 2):679–83.
11. Wahidi MM, Jain P, Jantz M, Lee P, Mackensen GB, Barbour SY, Lamb C, Silvestri GA. American College of Chest Physicians consensus statement on the use of topical anesthesia, analgesia, and sedation during flexible bronchoscopy in adult patients. Chest. 2011;140(5):1342–50.
12. Fox BD, Krylov Y, Leon P, Ben-Zvi I, Peled N, Shitrit D, Kramer MR. Benzodiazepine and opioid sedation attenuate the sympathetic response to fiberoptic bronchoscopy. Prophylactic labetalol gave no additional benefit. Results of a randomized double-blind placebo-controlled study. Respir Med. 2008;102(7):978–83.
13. Abdelmalak B, Makary L, Hoban J, Doyle DJ. Dexmedetomidine as sole sedative for awake intubation in management of the critical airway. J Clin Anesth. 2007;19(5):370–3.
14. Clark G, Licker M, Younossian AB, Soccal PM, Frey JG, Rochat T, Diaper J, Bridevaux PO, Tschopp JM. Titrated sedation with propofol or midazolam for flexible bronchoscopy: a randomised trial. Eur Respir J. 2009;34(6):1277–83.
15. Bruhn J, Myles PS, Sneyd R, Struys MM. Depth of anaesthesia monitoring: what's available, what's validated and what's next? Br J Anaesth. 2006;97(1):85–94.
16. Abdelmalak B, Ryckman JV, AlHaddad S, Sprung J. Respiratory arrest after successful neodymium:yttrium-aluminum-garnet laser treatment of subglottic tracheal stenosis. Anesth Analg. 2002;95(2):485–6, table of contents.
17. Hung WT, Liao SM, Su JM. Laryngeal mask airway in patients with tracheal stents who are undergoing non-airway related interventions: report of three cases. J Clin Anesth. 2004;16(3):214–6.
18. Kirsner KM, Sarkiss M, Brydges GJ. Treatment of tracheal and bronchial tumors and tracheal and bronchial stent placement. AANA J. 2010;78(5):413–9.
19. Ayers ML, Beamis JF Jr. Rigid bronchoscopy in the twenty-first century. Clin Chest Med. 2001;22(2):355–64.
20. Wahidi MM, Herth FJ, Ernst A. State of the art: interventional pulmonology. Chest. 2007;131(1):261–74.
21. Clouzeau B, Bui HN, Guilhon E, Grenouillet-Delacre M, Leger MS, Saghi T, Pillot J, Filloux B, Coz S, Boyer A, et al. Fiberoptic bronchoscopy under non-invasive ventilation and propofol target-controlled

infusion in hypoxemic patients. Intensive Care Med. 2011;37:1969–75.
22. Ambrosino N, Guarracino F. Unusual applications of noninvasive ventilation. European Respiratory Journal. 2011;38(2):440–9.
23. Fernandez-Bustamante A, Ibanez V, Alfaro JJ, de Miguel E, German MJ, Mayo A, Jimeno A, Perez-Cerda F, Escribano PM. High-frequency jet ventilation in interventional bronchoscopy: factors with predictive value on high-frequency jet ventilation complications. J Clin Anesth. 2006;18(5):349–56.
24. Kraincuk P, Kepka A, Ihra G, Schabernig C, Aloy A. A new prototype of an electronic jet-ventilator and its humidification system. Crit Care. 1999;3(4):101–10.
25. Vaitkeviciute IEJ. Con: Bronchial stenting and laser airway surgery should not take place outside the operating room. J Cardiothorac Vasc Anesth. 2005;19:121–2.
26. Amat B, Günther R, Carlos A, Antoni X, Antoni T. What is an interventional pulmonology unit in Europe? Clinical Pulmonary Medicine. 2010;17(1):42–6.

# Anesthesia for Cardioversion

## Michele L. Sumler and McKenzie Hollon

## Introduction

Cardioversion is a brief but painful procedure utilizing electrical current for the treatment of cardiac dysrhythmias. Direct current cardioversion can be used to normalize abnormal cardiac rhythms, stable or unstable, except ventricular fibrillation. Indications for electrical cardioversion include supraventricular tachycardias, atrial fibrillation, atrial flutter, ventricular tachycardia with pulse and any reentrant tachycardia with narrow or wide QRS which is unstable. Cardioversion is most commonly used to treat atrial fibrillation [1].

The circumstances for the procedure can vary widely, from an elective, off site anesthetic to an emergent procedure in a hemodynamically tenuous patient. In most cases, it is an outpatient procedure very rarely requiring an overnight hospital stay [2]. Beyond typical anesthetic considerations, the essential components of anesthetic management include understanding of the physiologic consequences of the underlying arrhythmia and the cardioversion. Familiarity with the defibrillation equipment and procedure, as well as knowledge of potential complications associated with cardioversions, are essential components of anesthetic management unique to this procedure.

Direct current cardioversion is preformed by sensing the intrinsic activity of the heart to synchronize the delivery of an electrical shock with the R wave of the QRS complex. The goal of synchronization is to ensure the electrical stimulation does not coincide with a vulnerable period of ventricular function. Synchronizing with the early portion of the QRS avoids the delivery of the shock during the terminal portion of the refractory state when adjacent myocardial fibers are in differing states of repolarization. Success of the cardioversion depends on multiple factors, including the patient's underlying disease as well as the effective delivery of electrical current to the atrial myocardium. Current may be delivered transcutaneously through chest electrodes, or more rarely through internal cardiac electrodes. Density of current delivered is influenced by the defibrillator's capacitor voltage, the output waveform, the size and position of the electrodes, and the impedance to flow between electrodes and the target myocardium [3]. The output waveform influences the energy delivery, and there are two types, monophasic and biphasic (Table 22.1).

Biphasic shocks have been shown to require the use of less energy than monophasic delivery and to have higher success rates of cardioversion. Currently biphasic shocks represent the present standard for cardioversion of atrial fibrillation [4]. Other independent factors predicting successful cardioversion are thoracic impedance and duration of dysrhythmia [5]. The American Heart Association provides guidelines on the

M. L. Sumler, M.D. (✉) · M. Hollon, M.D.
Department of Anesthesiology, Emory University Hospital, Atlanta, GA, USA
e-mail: msumler@emory.edu; mmayo2@emory.edu

Table 22.1 Comparison of monophasic and biphasic waveforms

| | Monophasic | Biphasic |
|---|---|---|
| Current direction | Unidirectional | Bidirectional |
| Waveform | Positive sinusoidal | Rectilinear |
| Typical energy level (J) | 200–300 | 100–200 |
| Median successful energy for cardioversion of AF (J) | 200 | 100 |

energy requirements based on which arrhythmia is being treated, with 120–200 J being the current initial requirement for biphasic cardioversion of atrial fibrillation [6]. To avoid myocardial damage, some have suggested that the interval between consecutive shocks should be at least 1 min [7].

Cardioversion is contraindicated in dysrhythmias due to enhanced automaticity, such as digitalis toxicity and catecholamine-induced arrhythmias. Not only is cardioversion ineffective in these enhanced automaticity states, it is also associated with a higher incidence of post shock ventricular tachycardia and fibrillation. Additionally, cardioversion is contraindicated in multifocal atrial tachycardia as it does not address the underlying cause of dysrhythmia.

## Focused History and Physical Findings in Patients Presenting for Elective Cardioversion

Patient assessment should begin with traditional pre-operative anesthetic evaluation, with particular attention paid to the cardiovascular system. The patient's history should be carefully reviewed for the presence of syncope, near-syncope, dizziness, chest pain, palpitations, and history of known bradycardias or tachycardias. Evaluation should include assessment of the electrocardiogram (EKG) to characterize the patient's current rhythm as well history of any known dysrhythmia triggers. It is important to be aware of prior pharmacologic and non-pharmacologic treatments of arrhythmias, as well as the details of any prior attempts at electrical conversion.

In the case of atrial fibrillation, the duration since onset may be unknown depending on the absence or presence of symptoms, and particular attention must be paid to the guidelines for evaluation of thrombus and appropriateness of anticoagulation. Further, the presence of implantable rhythm devices, pacemakers, ICDs, or dual devices, should be investigated. Improperly performed cardioversion in patients with these devices can damage the device or lead system and lead to malfunction or loss of capture. To ensure appropriate function, the device should be interrogated before and after cardioversion [8].

## Is the Patient in an Optimum State to Proceed with Anesthesia

Preoperative management of known cardiac conditions, including arrhythmias, congestive heart failure, ischemia, and hypertension should be assessed. Review of the medication history should pay particular attention to use of beta blockers, antihypertensives, antiarrythmics, and statins. If the patient is on digoxin, a level should be checked and the patient should be assessed for signs of toxicity, however it is not necessary to routinely discontinue it prior to the cardioversion. Many patients undergoing cardioversion are on anticoagulation to prevent systemic embolization of thrombus, it is important to ensure that anticoagulation is adequate prior to proceeding with the procedure. An electrolyte panel is necessary for all patients undergoing cardioversion. Evaluation of labs and familiarity with patient's history is essential as DC cardioversion is contraindicated in patients with digitalis toxicity or with hypokalemia [1].

Further testing, including echocardiogram for evaluation of the presence of thrombus, catheterization, and stress testing may be indicated based on the patient's presentation in accordance with current guidelines. In all elective cases, NPO guidelines should be followed. In the event that cardioverion is being performed emergently, full stomach measures should be taken. These measures include preoxygenation and tracheal intubation. Succinylcholine is not contraindicated in this setting but bradyarrythmias may be precipitated and hyperkalemia may be worsened with its use. Occasionally, pregnant patients may present for cardioversion. Cardioversion has been found to be safe in this patient population, although it has been associated with fetal arrhythmias [9]. In cases when the fetus is viable, it is prudent to monitor the fetal heart rate throughout the procedure.

## Preparation and Commonly Used Anesthetic Technique

It is common for these procedures to be done in off-site, or non-OR locations. Off site anesthetic challenges include unfamiliar equipment, personnel unfamiliar with anesthetic aspects of care and remoteness from additional anesthetic support. Preparing for an off-site anesthetic it is essential to ensure immediate availability of emergency drugs and airway equipment. American Society of Anesthesiologists (ASA) guidelines for standard monitors apply, and the minimum for cardioversion should include continuous EKG, pulse oximetry, BP monitoring, and likely continuous capnography [10]. An oxygen source, suction capability and a means to provide positive pressure ventilation should also be readily available.

A variety of anesthetics have been used successfully for cardioversion. Though external cardioversion is brief, the electrical stimulus can equal the intensity to that of surgical incision. An ideal anesthetic would provide analgesia, sedation, minimal hemodynamic compromise, and rapid recovery. The level of sedation required may depend on the setting and the patient, with adequate sedation allowing avoidance of recall of an unpleasant experience. Preventing or attenuating the effects of a catecholamine mediated stress response which could precipitate myocardial ischemia in this high risk population is paramount. The minimum appropriate anesthetic depth for elective cardioversion is likely deep sedation and often general anesthesia is required [1].

Volatile anesthetics are not often used for multiple reasons, including setting of the procedure often being offsite and very rarely requiring an endotracheal tube. There is no perfect IV drug however there are several small studies which have compared the efficacy of various IV agents including etomidate, propofol, fentanyl and benzodiazepines. Benzodiazepines have been shown to have a longer duration of effect and greater patient variability [11]. Propofol is associated with hypotension and a higher incidence of apnea than other IV anesthetics, but in comparison recovery time is more rapid. Etomidate produces myoclonus and pain on injection, however it's use is associated with less decrease in arterial blood pressure which may make it a better choice in patients with significant cardiac disease [12]. Comparison has been made between the combinations of etomidate and fentanyl, and propofol and fentanyl, with the etomidate and fentanyl combination having a shorter induction time and greater degree of hemodynamic stability [13]. A 2015 Cochrane database review looked at all the available literature and concluded that the evidence did not support superiority of any agent nor argue for the efficacy of additional analgesic medication to improve any metrics [14]. No matter which agent is most appropriate for the individual patient, careful titration to avoid hemodynamic compromise in a high risk population is prudent.

There are instances in which a transesophageal echocardiogram (TEE) is performed immediately prior to cardioversion to rule out the presence of thrombus. In these cases, the procedure may take up to 30 min. A nasal cannula will usually suffice, however further airway management may be required to keep a patient comfortable during the procedure. A study found that deep sedation with intravenous propofol and the use of a laryngeal mask airway (LMA), provided excellent conditions without the need to remove the TEE probe [15]. This provides a reasonable option in patients in which appropriate procedural sedation and airway maintenance become problematic.

## Anticipated Adverse Events

As with all procedures, the possibility of adverse events is always present. Prevention and management of adverse events should begin with preoperative planning, including obtaining adequate IV access for resuscitation, the use of monitors for early detection of adverse events, and the development of a plan for most likely adverse events.

Depending on the depth of anesthetic required, airway may become a particular concern in cases where deep sedation without a secured airway is employed. Airway management should include proper monitors, including $ETCO_2$, and preparation of plan of action for intervention in the case of airway compromise. It may be appropriate to bag valve mask ventilate the patient for such a brief procedure if there is no underlying pulmonary disease, the patient has been appropriately NPO, and there are no concerning findings on the airway exam. In patients with hemodynamic disturbances or concern for aspiration it may be wise to intubate the trachea for airway control.

The most common complications are arrhythmias, such as atrial, ventricular, and junctional premature beats. Other arrhythmias can also been seen transiently, including bradycardia and short periods of sinus arrest, and these commonly subside spontaneously [14] . Animal experiments have demonstrated a wide margin of safety between the energy required for cardioversion of atrial fibrillation and that associated with myocardial depression. Even without apparent myocardial damage, transient ST-segment elevation may appear on the EKG after cardioversion, and the anesthesia team should be aware of this potentially normal variant [16]. Rarely, high energy shocks can lead to myocardial necrosis which should manifest as immediate ST segment elevation which lasts for 1–2 min. EKG changes which last longer than 2 min typically indicate myocardial injury unrelated to the shock. However, more serious dysrhythmias, including ventricular fibrillation can result in cases of severe heart disease, improper synchronization, high amounts of electrical energy conduction, electrolyte abnormalities or digitalis toxicity. In some patients with longstanding atrial fibrillation, there may be underlying sinus node dysfunction or intrinsic conduction defects which are unmasked by cardioversion. These patients should be evaluated thoroughly by cardiology prior to cardioversion so that a transvenous or transcutaneous pacemaker can be used prophylactically if deemed appropriate [17].

Hemodynamic disturbances often occur and can lead to myocardial dysfunction. The population undergoing cardioversion is typically high risk, often with underlying cardiac disease and the absence of coronary perfusion during even a brief arrest may result in ischemia. Patients may experience a phenomenon called myocardial stunning which is myocardial dysfunction which is reversible within the first 24–48 h. To avoid inaccurate assessments, evaluation of cardiac function should be delayed until at least 48 h after the cardioversion [18]. Rarely, in patients with valvular heart disease or poor left ventricular systolic function, transient pulmonary edema may be seen.

Embolic and ischemic stroke are possible complications, and make this procedure contraindicated in patients with a known presence of thrombus. Thromboembolization is not uncommon, and has been associated with cardioversion in 1–7% of patients not give prophylactic anticoagulation before cardioversion of atrial fibrillation [19]. For this reason, evaluation of coagulopathy and assurance of adequate anticoagulation must be completed prior to the procedure. For elective cardioversions, patients who have been in atrial fibrillation for greater than 48 h, an echocardiogram should be performed to rule out the presence of an intracardiac thrombus. American College of Cardiology and American Heart Association guidelines recommend anticoagulation for 3–4 weeks before and after cardioversion. After completion of cardioversion, a neurologic exam for focal deficits should be assessed [1].

Painful skin burns can occur after cardioversion, and are most likely due to improper placement of the electrodes. Skin burns are less common with biphasic defibrillators and with the use of gel based pads. Some advocate prophylactic use of steroid cream and or topical ibuprofen to reduce pain and inflammation.

# References

1. American College of Cardiology/American Heart Association Task Force on Practice Guidelines; European Society of Cardiology Committee for Practice Guidelines (Writing Committee to Revise the 2001 Guidelines for Management of Patients With Atrial Fibrillation); European Heart Rhythm Association; Heart Rhythm Society. Circulation. 2006;114:e257–354.
2. Lesser MF. Safety and efficacy of in-office cardioversion for treatment of supraventricular arrhythmias. Am J Cardiol. 1990;66:1267–8.
3. Ewy GA. The optimal technique for electrical cardioversion of atrial fibrillation. Clin Cardiol. 1994;17:79–84.
4. Page RL, Kerber RE, Russell JK, et al. Biphasic versus monophasic shock waveform for conversion of atrial fibrillation: the results of an international randomized, double-blind multicenter trial. J Am Coll Cardiol. 2002;39:1956–63.
5. Mittal S, Ayati S, Stein KM, et al. Transthoracic cardioversion of atrial fibrillation: comparison of rectilinear biphasic versus damped sine wave monophasic shocks. Circulation. 2000;101:1282–7.
6. Atkins DL, Passman RS, Halperin HR, Samson RA, White RD, et al. Part 6: electrical therapies: automated external defibrillators, defibrillation, cardioversion, and pacing: 2010 American Heart Association Guidelines for Cardiopulmonary Resuscitation and Emergency Cardiovascular Care. Circulation. 2010;122(18 Suppl 3):S706–19.
7. Dahl CF, Ewy GA, Warner ED, et al. Myocardial necrosis from direct current countershock. Effect of paddle electrode size and time interval between discharges. Circulation. 1974;50:956–61.
8. Gould L, Patel S, Gomes GI, Chokshi AB. Pacemaker failure following external defibrillation. Pacing Clin Electrophysiol. 1981;4(5):575–7.
9. Schroeder JS, Harrison DC. Repeated cardioversion during pregnancy. Am J Cardiol. 1971;27:445–6.
10. Statement on Nonoperating Room Anesthetizing Locations Committee of Origin: standards and practice parameters (Approved by the ASA House of Delegates on October 19, 1994, and last amended on October 16, 2013).
11. Canessa R. Anesthesia for elective cardioversion: a comparison of four anesthetic agents. J Cardiothorac Vasc Anesth. 1991;5(6):566–8.
12. Desai PM, Kane D, Sarkar MS. Cardioversion: what to choose? Etomidate or propofol. Ann Card Anaesth. 2015;18(3):306–11.
13. Kalogridaki M. Anaesthesia for cardioversion: a prospective randomised comparison of propofol and etomidate combined with fentanyl. Hellenic J Cardiol. 2011;52(6):483–8.
14. Rabbino MD, Likoff W, Dreifus LS. Complications and limitations of direct current countershock. JAMA. 1964;190:417–20.
15. Ferson D, Thakar D, Swafford J, Sinha A, Sapire K, Arens J. Use of deep intravenous sedation with propofol and the laryngeal mask airway during transesophageal echocardiography. J Cardiovasc Vasc Anesth. 2003;17:443–6.
16. Lewis SR, Nicholson A, Reed SS, Kenth JJ, Alderson P, Smith AF. Anaesthetic and sedative agents used for electrical cardioversion. Cochrane Database Syst Rev. 2015;(3):CD010824.
17. Mancini GB, Goldberger AL. Cardioversion of atrial fibrillation: consideration of embolization, anticoagulation, prophylactic pacemaker, and long-term success. Am Heart J. 1982;104:617–21.
18. Kern KB, Hilwig RW, Rhee KH, Berg RA. Myocardial dysfunction after resuscitation from cardiac arrest: an example of global myocardial stunning. J Am Coll Cardiol. 1996;28(1):232–40.
19. Bjerkelund CJ, Orning OM. The efficacy of anticoagulant therapy in preventing embolism related to D.C. electrical conversion of atrial fibrillation. Am J Cardiol. 1969;23:208–16.

# Anesthesia for Dental Procedures

Carolyn Barbieri and Meghan Whitley

## Introduction

The Centers for Disease Control and Prevention (CDC) reports that dental caries and periodontal disease is the most common preventable chronic disease in the United States, despite all of the advances in modern medicine. Dental caries, the formation of cavities in teeth by bacteria, are four times more common than asthma in children. Dental disease significantly affects adults; 90% of people over the age of 20 have some degree of tooth or root decay [1]. Periodontal disease, inflammation and infections of the gums or bone, affects 47.2% of adults aged 30 years or older and 70.1% of adults 65 years or older [2].

## Human Dentition

### Dental Anatomy

A human tooth is broken down into three major parts; the crown, the neck, and the root. The crown of the tooth is the part of the tooth that is visible in the mouth and is responsible for slicing, ripping and grinding food (incisors, canines, and molars respectively). The neck of the tooth is the slightly constricted part of the tooth adjacent to the gingiva, residing between the crown and the root. The neck of the tooth is also referred to as the cementoenamel junction. The root portion yields strength and stability for the tooth and surrounding structures. The anterior teeth, incisors, and canines, are single rooted teeth and have a conical shape. The posterior teeth (premolars and molars) are multi rooted teeth and provide stability by the number of roots and direction of root implantation.

Every human tooth is composed of four different tissue types that serve various functions, enamel, dentin, pulp cavity, and the cementum. The enamel is the outmost layer of the crown, which provides the hard protective outer surface for the crown of the tooth. Just below the enamel lies the dentin which makes up the majority of the inner surface of the tooth. The dentin is a hard calcareous tissue, similar to but denser than bone. Dentin can only be seen on X-rays. Under the dentin, resides the pulp cavity. The pulp cavity is the central area of the tooth that contains the nerves and blood vessels for the tooth. The pulp cavity exists in both the crown and extends down into the root of the tooth. Lastly, the cementum makes up the outer surface of the dental root, which is much softer than the enamel and dentin.

C. Barbieri, M.D. (✉) • M. Whitley, D.O.
Department of Anesthesiology and Perioperative Medicine, Penn State Milton S. Hershey Medical Center, Hershey, PA, USA
e-mail: cbarbieri@pennstatehealth.psu.edu; mwhitley@pennstatehealth.psu.edu

The purpose of the cementum is to serve as a medium by which the periodontal ligaments can attach for tooth stability [3].

The periodontium is the supporting structures surrounding the root of the tooth. The periodontium is composed of the gingival and alveolar mucosa, the periodontal ligaments, and the alveolar bone. The gingival and alveolar mucosa (commonly referred to as gums) comprises the soft tissue covering all of the periodontal structures. The periodontal ligament attaches the external surface of the root (cementum) to the alveolar bone, acting as an anchor and shock absorber during mastication. The alveolar bone is a thickened ridge of bone that contains the tooth sockets. The alveolar bone can easily remodel, thus allowing orthodontic tooth movement. The alveolar bone abuts the deep supporting basal or skeletal bone of the mandible and maxilla. When teeth are lost or removed, the alveolar bone degenerates and the basal bone is evident in edentulous patients; forming the skeletal support for full or partial dentures.

## Dental Identification

There are two accepted dental identification systems commonly used today, the Universal Numbering System and the Palmer Notation System. In both systems the primary teeth (commonly referred to as baby teeth) are designated by letters and the permanent teeth are designated by numbers.

## Universal Numbering System

The most widely used system in United States is the Universal Numbering system. The Universal Numbering system starts identification at the farthest back upper right tooth moving right to left across the maxilla to the last upper left tooth, then moving to the farthest back lower left tooth moving left to right across the mandible to the last lower right tooth. Identification of primary dentition uses uppercase letters A through T, representing the twenty primary teeth, starting at the upper right second molar and ending at the lower right second molar, illustrated in Table 23.1. Identification of permanent dentition uses number 1 through 32, starting in the upper right third molar and continuing through to the lower right third molar, illustrated in Table 23.2 [4].

## Palmer Notation System

The Palmer Notation system is widely used in the United Kingdom and is the primary means of dental identification by orthodontists. The Palmer Notation system splits the dental arch into four quadrants, starting with the central incisor following distally and posteriorly, with all four quadrants designated by a symbol (⌐ ¬ ⌐ ¬). The primary dentition is assigned letters to the teeth from A to E in all four quadrants starting with the central incisor and moving distally, as shown in Table 23.3. The permanent dentition is assigned numbers from 1 to 8 in all four quadrants starting

**Table 23.1** Primary dentition: Universal Numbering system

| Upper right | | | | | Upper left | | | | |
|---|---|---|---|---|---|---|---|---|---|
| A | B | C | D | E | F | G | H | I | J |
| T | S | R | Q | P | O | N | M | L | K |
| Lower right | | | | | Lower left | | | | |

**Table 23.2** Permanent dentition: Universal Numbering system

| Upper right | | | | | | | | Upper left | | | | | | | |
|---|---|---|---|---|---|---|---|---|---|---|---|---|---|---|---|
| 1 | 2 | 3 | 4 | 5 | 6 | 7 | 8 | 9 | 10 | 11 | 12 | 13 | 14 | 15 | 16 |
| 32 | 31 | 30 | 29 | 28 | 27 | 26 | 25 | 24 | 23 | 22 | 21 | 20 | 19 | 18 | 17 |
| Lower right | | | | | | | | Lower left | | | | | | | |

**Table 23.3** Primary dentition: palmer notation system

| Upper right | | | | | Upper left | | | | |
|---|---|---|---|---|---|---|---|---|---|
| E⌋ | D⌋ | C⌋ | B⌋ | A⌋ | ⌊A | ⌊B | ⌊C | ⌊D | ⌊E |
| E⌉ | D⌉ | C⌉ | B⌉ | A⌉ | ⌈A | ⌈B | ⌈C | ⌈D | ⌈E |
| Lower right | | | | | Lower left | | | | |

**Table 23.4** Permanent dentition: palmer notation system

| Upper right | | | | | | | | Upper left | | | | | | | |
|---|---|---|---|---|---|---|---|---|---|---|---|---|---|---|---|
| 8⌋ | 7⌋ | 6⌋ | 5⌋ | 4⌋ | 3⌋ | 2⌋ | 1⌋ | ⌊1 | ⌊2 | ⌊3 | ⌊4 | ⌊5 | ⌊6 | ⌊7 | ⌊8 |
| 8⌉ | 7⌉ | 6⌉ | 5⌉ | 4⌉ | 3⌉ | 2⌉ | 1⌉ | ⌈1 | ⌈2 | ⌈3 | ⌈4 | ⌈5 | ⌈6 | ⌈7 | ⌈8 |
| Lower right | | | | | | | | Lower left | | | | | | | |

**Table 23.5** Continuum of Depth of Sedation: Definition of General Anesthesia and Levels of Sedation/Analgesia

| | Minimal sedation | Moderate sedation | Deep sedation | General anesthesia |
|---|---|---|---|---|
| Cognitive function | Normal response to verbal stimuli | Purposeful response to tactile stimuli | Purposeful response after repeated stimuli | Unarousable to painful stimuli |
| Ventilatory function | Unaffected | Unaffected | May be inadequate | Frequently Impaired; may require support |
| Cardiovascular function | Unaffected | Usually maintained | Usually maintained | May be impaired |
| Monitoring | Observation only | HR, O$_2$Sat, BP, RR | HR, O$_2$Sat, BP, RR | Standard ASA monitors |

with the central incisor and moving distally, as shown in Table 23.4 [5].

# Dental Procedures

The majority of dental procedures are performed in the outpatient dental office. For most dental procedures, local anesthesia with or without sedation is sufficient. However there are many patient medical conditions and procedural needs that may require additional monitoring and deeper levels of sedation than can be completed in the outpatient office. Consultation with an anesthesiologist is suggested, but are not limited to, the following medical conditions: pulmonary impairment with or with oxygen requirement, cardiovascular disease, neurologic compromise, morbid obesity, bleeding disorders, craniofacial abnormalities, orofacial trauma, or an increased risk of malignant hyperthermia [6–8].

# Levels of Sedation and Analgesia

Sedation and analgesia for procedures is defined as a continuum ranging from consciousness to unconsciousness. Sedation and analgesia can range from minimal sedation (anxiolysis), moderate sedation (conscious sedation), deep sedation (analgesia), to general anesthesia. The American Society of Anesthesiologists (ASA) has set forth guidelines for sedation and analgesia by non-anesthesiologists, as shown in Table 23.5 [9].

Minimal sedation, also known as anxiolysis, is a drug induced state where a patient responds normally to verbal commands, but cognitive function and coordination may be impaired. The patient's pulmonary and cardiovascular function remains unaffected by minimal sedation. Since pulmonary and cardiovascular function is maintained, it is not necessary to monitor or document vital signs, only visual observation of the patient is necessary. Sedation must be provided by a second qualified provider who is certified in Basic Life Support (BLS); sedation cannot be administered by the proceduralist themselves.

Moderate sedation, also known as conscious sedation, is a drug induced depression of consciousness where a patient responds purposefully to verbal commands. The patient's cognitive function is mildly impaired, but they should remain conscious throughout the procedure. The patient's pulmonary and cardiovascular function is maintained, but it is essential to monitor the patient's vital signs, including heart rate, oxygen saturation, blood pressure and respiratory rate. Sedation must be provided by a second qualified provider who is certified in BLS and ACLS, with all necessary emergency and resuscitative equipment.

Deep sedation, also known as analgesia, is the drug induced depression of consciousness where a patient cannot be easily aroused, but is arousable after repeated verbal or painful stimuli. The patient may have impaired spontaneous ventilation with or without partial or complete loss of airway and/or gag reflexes, thus respiratory support may be necessary. The patient's cardiovascular function is typically maintained during deep sedation, but vital signs must be monitored including heart rate, oxygen saturation, blood pressure and respiratory rate. Sedation must be provided by a second qualified provider who is certified in BLS and ACLS, with all necessary emergency and resuscitative equipment.

General anesthesia is a drug induced loss of consciousness where a patient is not arousable and no cognitive function is present. The patient's spontaneous ventilation is frequently inadequate and may require assistance. The patient may have partial or complete loss of airway and/or gag reflexes, thus respiratory support must be immediately available. The patient's cardiovascular function is impaired and standard ASA monitors are required. General anesthesia must be provided by an anesthesiologist, anesthesia resident or nurse anesthetist, with all necessary emergency and resuscitative equipment (see below).

## Monitoring and Emergency Equipment

All patients receiving Moderate Sedation, Deep Sedation and/or General Anesthesia must be in accordance with the current ASA guidelines; pulse oximetry, non-invasive blood pressure monitoring, and continuous electrocardiogram (EKG) (in additional to temperature and capnography for general anesthesia). Oxygen delivery devices most commonly used for dental procedures are nasal cannulas and many devices have been modified to allow for capnography.

When providing sedation for dental procedures, there may be impaired ventilation requiring assistance and possible endotracheal intubation and general anesthesia. As a result, all procedural rooms must have access to the following emergency equipment: emergency resuscitative medications, sedation medications, IV supplies, airway resuscitation equipment (including bag valve mask, nasal and oropharyngeal airways, endotracheal tubes, laryngoscopes, etc.), difficult airway equipment, and a dedicated anesthesia machine.

## Pharmacology of Dental Anesthesia

A number of medications are utilized by clinicians to assist with anxiolysis and maintenance of sedation and analgesia for dental procedures. These various medications are available through different routes of administration which can be tailored based on the cooperation of the patient, desired effect, and duration of action required. We will highlight some of the common agents which will be encountered in office-based dental suites.

Midazolam can be administered through a variety of routes tailored to the clinical situation. These include oral (PO), sublingual, intravenous (IV), intramuscular (IM) or rectal (PR). The onset and duration of action depend on the route used, but can range from 15 to 30 min and 60 to 90 min, respectively, for oral administration. The oral dosage is 0.25–0.5 mg/kg PO with a maximum cumulative dose of 15–20 mg orally. The intravenous dosage of midazolam is 0.05–0.1 mg/kg IV with a maximum cumulative dose of 10 mg IV. The intramuscular doasge of midazolam is 0.1–0.15 mg/kg IM with a maximum cumulative dose of 10 mg IM. The intranasal route can be used, but is irritating to the nasal mucosa. The retrograde amnesia which occurs with midazolam may improve compliance with further dental procedures if used during the initial procedure. As with all medications, clinicians should be aware of the risks associated with midazolam administration. There is a potential for airway obstruction and respiratory depression when combined with opioids. Therefore, it is recommended to reduce the dose by at least 25%, when used in combination [10, 11]. Flumazenil may be administered for benzodiazepine reversal, but may require redosing due to its short half-life when compared to that of benzodiazepines.

Another medication utilized for less stimulating procedures in neonates through children less than 3 years old is chloral hydrate [11]. Oral or rectal administration can be utilized, but there is a risk of incomplete absorption with the PR route. The onset is 30–60 min with a duration of action lasting 60–120 min. The suggested dose is 50–100 mg/kg with maximum dose of 2 g.

Chloral hydrate may also cause airway obstruction and respiratory depression at higher doses (75–100 mg/kg). Of note, there are significant differences in half life based on age. This ranges from 10 h in toddlers to as long as 40 h in preterm infants and therefore, may require prolonged recovery time and therefore may be poorly suited for outpatient offices [10, 11].

Demerol can be administered through multiple routes including PO, IV, subcutaneous or IM. The oral onset of action is 30–60 min with a duration of 2–4 h. The recommended dose is 1–2 mg/kg with a maximum dose of 50 mg. Demerol also has a risk of respiratory depression. Demerol has an active metabolite, normeperidine, that can cause seizures [11].

Ketamine can be administered through IV, IM, or PO routes. The dose is 3–10 mg/kg when used alone, but should be decreased by 50% when combined with midazolam given the additive effects [12]. There is a limited risk of respiratory depression with ketamine use.

A first generation H1 antagonist, hydroxyzine, can also be used for its sedation side effect. It can be administered through the PO or IM routes. The recommended dose is 1–2 mg/kg, and the maximum dose is 100 mg. The onset of action of hydroxyzine is within 15–30 min, and it has a duration of action lasting 2–4 h. There is a risk of QT prolongation, and this drug should be used with caution in susceptible patients [13].

Nitrous Oxide has an onset of action of less than 5 min with a rapid return to baseline. It ranges from minimal to moderate sedation depending on the concentration used. It is considered moderate sedation when administered in a greater than 50:50 ratio with or without the administration of sedatives or analgesics. The risk of hypoxia increases significantly with supplemental PO or IV agents and can occur with as minimal as 30% nitrous when chloral hydrate is also administered [12]. Nitrous oxide also requires specialized equipment for delivery, including a nasal mask, monitoring including $FiO_2$ sensing, and a scavenging system [11]. With respect to environmental risk, studies have shown an increased risk of spontaneous abortion and decreased conception rates in personnel routinely exposed to nitrous without scavenging equipment; however, this risk was not shown when this equipment was used [14].

## Local Anesthetics for Dental Anesthesia

Local anesthetics in the form of nerve blocks are typically used as the main source of analgesia for dental procedures. Local anesthetic selection is based on the patient's medical history, mental status, expected procedure duration, and planned administration of other adjunct medications. The local anesthetics typically available for dental procedures are contained below in Table 23.6 with maximum doses and anticipated duration of action [15, 16].

## General Anesthesia for Dental Procedures

General anesthesia can be induced for dental procedures or can unintentionally occur on the continuum of sedation. In patients who lack the ability to cooperate, have anticipated difficult airways, or need for significant dental work requiring a long procedure time, general anesthesia may be necessary.

General anesthesia techniques utilized include volatile anesthetics or total intravenous anesthesia (TIVA). Propofol can be utilized by itself, or the with the supplementation of opioids or other analgesics. Utilizing a TIVA technique does not require a scavenger system [17]. This can be beneficial in the outpatient setting where this equipment can be less common. With respect to post-operative nau-

**Table 23.6** Maximum Recommednded Dosage and Duration of Action of Local Anesthetic Medications

| Local anesthetic | Maximum dose (mg/kg) with epinephrine | Maximum dose (mg/kg) without epinephrine | Duration (min) |
|---|---|---|---|
| Atricaine | – | 7 | 60–230 |
| Bupivicaine | 2 | 3 | 240–480 |
| Lidocaine | 5 | 7 | 60–240 |
| Mepivicaine | 5 | 7 | 60–240 |
| Prilocaine | 7 | 10 | 60–120 |

sea and vomiting, Konig et al described no difference in emergence delirium or post-operative pain with propofol versus sevoflurane for anesthetic maintenance [12, 18]; therefore, this should not determine the anesthetic technique utilized. An important cause of post-operative nausea and vomiting following dental procedures is gastric blood. As a result, it is important to evacuate blood prior to the emergence of anesthesia, or prevent the initial occurrence with a throat pack.

## Intubation Techniques

If general endotracheal anesthesia is necessary, the authors' preferred technique is nasal endotracheal intubation. Nasal intubation is preferred over oral intubation due to the concern for potential obstruction due to dental equipment, and tube migration resulting in endobronchial intubation or unintentional extubation with head manipulation during the procedure. A thorough history must be elicited prior to all anesthetics, but with particular attention paid to a history of epistaxis or recent nasal or head trauma, which would preclude nasal tracheal intubation. The patient's risk of aspiration should also be assessed, as this may make an oral endotracheal intubation the preferred method when proceeding with a rapid sequence intubation.

The patient should be consented regarding the potential of epistaxis or mucosal damage, infection or creating a false passage with nasal intubation. In order to decrease the risk of epistaxis and mucosal damage, vasoconstrictors such as oxymetazoline (Afrin) can be administered. The recommended dose in children ages 2–5 is 2–3 drops of 0.025% solution [12]. Serial nare dilation can be utilized prior to attempted intubation to accommodate a nasotracheal tube. Bleeding can also be minimized by decreasing tube size by 0.5–1 mm I.D., warming the endotracheal tube (ETT) and covering the ETT tip on initial entry into the nare [12]. Endotracheal intubation can be assisted with Magill forceps or fiberoptic visualization. Special care should also be taken to pad and secure the nasal ETT in order to prevent Alar damage secondary to pressure during lengthy procedures.

## Complications of Dental Procedures

Anesthetic complications are no different than those that may occur in any form of moderate sedation to general anesthesia. However, there are specific complications that are more common while providing sedation or anesthesia for dental procedures. These include aspiration, hypoxia, airway obstruction, hemorrhage, intravascular injection of local anesthetic, spontaneous bacterial endocarditis, and cardiac arrhythmias.

## Subacute Bacterial Endocarditis (SBE)

Transient bacteremia (not present within 15 min) is noted in up to 65% of dental extractions and 16% of dental restorations and nasotracheal intubations. The two most common organisms responsible for SBE are Streptococcus viridans and Staphylococcus aureus [19]. While there is a risk with general dental maintenance such as flossing, the risk is greater with mucosal/gingival tissue perforation, or procedures involving the periapical region of the tooth [20]. While antibiotic administration for procedures used to be more common, the American Heart Association (AHA) 2007 guidelines limited SBE prophylaxis only to those at greatest risk of adverse complications from endocarditis [21].

Patients requiring SBE Prophylaxis [22]:

- History of prior infective endocarditis
- Prosthetic cardiac valves or prosthetic material used in valve repair
- Cyanotic congenital heart disease (CHD) with shunts or conduits
- Acyanotic (repaired) CHD within the first 6 months of repair with prosthetic material due to inadequate time for endothelialization
- Acyanotic (repaired) CHD with residual defects present near prosthetic material which presumably impedes endothelialization
- History of heart transplant with valvulopathy

## SBE Prophylaxis Dosing and Administration

For SBE prophylaxis, antibiotics should ideally be given 30–60 min prior to surgery; however, they can be given up to 2 h after the procedure, if needed [20, 21]. The standard antibiotic used for SBE prophylaxis is PO amoxicillin (50 mg/kg up to 2 g). However, the AHA offers alternatives for patients unable to tolerate PO or with penicillin allergies, including appropriate dosages [22]. In the event a patient requiring SBE prophylaxis is already on another antibiotic, the American Dental Association recommends a different class of antibiotics be administered for SBE prophylaxis [20]. Of note, there is no increased risk of prosthetic joint infections with dental procedures and SBE prophylaxis should not be administered to these patients unless there is another indication previously listed [23].

## Arrhythmias Associated with Dental Procedures

A number of case reports have described arrhythmias occurring in patients undergoing dental procedures. Some of the implicating factors described include intravascular epinephrine administration associated with local anesthetic use, as well as pain and anxiety since catecholamine levels can increase 40 fold with stress [24]. Other confounding factors include arrhythmias associated with hypoxia, hypercapnia and volatile anesthetic administration. Another potential cause of arrhythmias is attributed to trigeminal nerve stimulation. This can be alleviated or decreased by local infiltration to cranial nerve V or removing the surgical stimulus [19].

## Summary

This chapter has provided an overview of human dental anatomy, dental notation, levels of sedation, common anxiolytics and anesthetic practices, guidelines for the management of dental anesthesia, and potntial adverse events. Please refer to Table 23.7 as a summary of anesthetic considerations in patients undergoing dental anesthesia.

**Table 23.7** Summary of anesthesia considerations in patients undergoing dental procedures

| Plan/preparation/adverse events | Reasoning/management |
|---|---|
| Selection of appropriate sedation level<br>   Patient expectation/anxiety<br>   Medical comorbidities<br>   Airway abnormalities<br>   Potential risk of malignant hyperthermia | If any doubt exists regarding the ability to either maintain spontaneous ventilation one should intubate<br>Main causes of anesthesia related morbidity and mortality are related to hypoxemia, aspiration, and hypotension |
| Monitoring and supplies<br>   Standard ASA monitors + capnography<br>   Available supplies to convert to GETA<br>   Ability to give positive pressure ventilation | Pulse oximetry, arterial blood pressure, continuous ECG, temperature<br>Emergency drugs, sedative medications<br>Nasal and oropharyngeal airways, bag valve mask, endotracheal tubes, laryngoscopes, IV supplies, syringes, needles, oxygen nasal cannula with capnography, face masks<br>IV fluids and tubing<br>Difficult airway supplies (Video laryngoscope, LMA)<br>Dedicated anesthesia machine |
| Position—supine and bed turned 90 degrees | Maximizing space for the proceduralist |
| Most common complications<br>   Aspiration<br>   Airway obstruction<br>   Hypoxia<br>   Hypotension<br>   Hemorrhage | Risk factors for complications<br>Delayed gastric emptying (DM, Chronic Opioids), Achalasia, obesity<br>OSA, obesity, snoring<br>OSA, obesity, tobacco use, SOB, asthma, COPD, Home oxygen use, recent URI<br>Depressed cardiac function, hypovolemia<br>Coagulopathy, anticoagulation therapy |
| Procedure specific complications<br>   Intravascular injection of local anesthetic<br>   Spontaneous bacterial endocarditis<br>   Cardiac arrhythmias<br>   Hemorrhage | As indicated |

## References

1. Dye BA, Tan S, Smith V, Lewis BG, Barker LK, Thornton-Evans G, et al. Vital and health statistics series, series 11. 2007;248:1–92.
2. Eke PI, Dye B, Wei L, Thornton-Evans G, Genco R. Prevalence of periodontitis in adults in the United States: 2009 and 2010. J Dent Res. 2012;91(10):1–7.
3. Wright JT. Normal formation and development of defects of the human dentition. Pediatr Clin North Am. 2000;47(5):975–1000.
4. Oral Health Topics A-Z "Tooth Numbering Systems" [document on the internet]. American Dental Association; 2014 [cited 2015 Dec 20]. Available from: https://web.archive.org/web/20061102074427/http://www.ada.org/public/topics/tooth_number.asp.
5. Ferguson J. The Palmer notation system and its used with personal computer applications. Br Dent J. 2005;198:551–3.
6. Dougherty N, Romer M, Lee RS. Trends in special care training in pediatric dental residencies. ASDC J Dent Child. 2001;68(5–6):384–7, 303.
7. Shenkin JD, Davis MJ, Corbin SB. The oral health of special needs children: dentistry's challenge to provide care. ASDC J Dent Child. 2001;68(3):2001–5.
8. Waldman HB, Perlman SP. Children with both mental retardation and mental illness live in our communities and need dental care. ASDC J Dent Child. 2001;68(5-6):360–5.
9. Practice guidelines for sedation and analgesia by non-anesthesiologists: an updated report by the American Society of Anesthesiologists task force on sedation and analgesia by non-anesthesiologists [document on the Internet]. American Society of Anesthesiologists. Anesthesiology. 2002;96:1004–17 [cited 2015 Dec 20]. Available from: http://anesthesiology.pubs.asahq.org/article.aspx?articleid=1944958.
10. Anderson B, Lerman J, CotĐ C. Pharmacokinetics and pharmacology of drugs used in children. In: CotĐ C, Lerman J, Anderson B, editors. CotĐ and Lermans' practice of anesthesia for infants and children. 5th ed. Philadelphia: Elsevier; 2013.
11. Kaplan R, Cravero J, Yaster M, CotĐ C. Sedation for diagnostic and therapeutic procedures outside the operating room. In: CotĐ C, Lerman J, Anderson B, editors. CotĐ and Lermans' practice of anesthesia for infants and children. 5th ed. Philadelphia: Elsevier; 2013.
12. Herlich A, Martin B, Vecchione CF. Anesthesia for pediatric dentistry. In: Davis P, Cladis F, Motoyama E, editors. Smith's anesthesia for infants and children. 8th ed. Philadelphia: Elsevier; 2011.
13. Sakaguchi T, Itoh H, Ding W, Tsiju K, Nagaoka I, Oka Y, et al. Hydroxyzine, a first generation H(1)-receptor antagonist, inhibits human ether-a-go-go-related gene (HERG) current and causes syncope in a patient with the HERG mutation. J Pharmacol Sci. 2008;108(4):462–71.
14. Katz J, Holzman R. Occulational health. In: Barash P, Cullen B, Stoelting R, Cahalan M, Stock M, Ortega R, editors. Clinical anesthesia. 7th ed. Philadelphia: Lippincott Williams & Wilkins; 2013.
15. Guideline on use of local anesthesia for pediatric dental patients [document on the Internet]. American Academy of Pediatric Dentisty: Clinical Guidelines; 2005 [updated 2015; cited 2015 Dec 20]. Available from: http://www.aapd.org/media/policies_guidelines/g_localanesthesia.pdf.
16. Lin Y, Liu S. Local anesthetics. In: Barash P, Cullen B, Stoelting R, Cahalan M, Stock M, Ortega R, editors. Clinical anesthesia. 7th ed. Philadelphia: Lippincott Williams & Wilkins; 2013.
17. Hausman L, Rosenblatt M. Office-based anesthesia. In: Barash P, Cullen B, Stoelting R, Cahalan M, Stock M, Ortega R, editors. Clinical anesthesia. 7th ed. Philadelphia: Lippincott Williams & Wilkins; 2013.
18. Konig M, Varughese A, Brennen K, Barclay S, Shackleford T, Samuels P, et al. Quality of recovery from teo types of general anesthesia for ambulatory dental surgery in children: a double-blind, randomized trial. Paediatr Anaesth. 2009;19(8):748–55.
19. Olutoye O, Watcha M. Eyes, ears, nose and throat surgery. In: Gregory G, Andropoulos D, editors. Gregory's pediatric anesthesia. 5th ed. Oxford: Wiley-Blackwell; 2012. p. 777–809.
20. Guideline on antibiotic prophylaxis for dental patients at risk of infection [document on the Intenet]. American Academy of Pediatric Dentisty: Clinical Guidelines; 1990 [updated 2014; cited 2015 Dec 20]. Available from: http://www.aapd.org/media/policies_guidelines/g_antibioticprophylaxis.pdf.
21. Gertler R, Miller-Hance W. Essentials of cardiology. In: CotĐ C, Lerman J, Anderson B, editors. CotĐ and Lermans' practice of anesthesia for infants and children. 5th ed. Philadelphia: Elsevier; 2013.
22. Wilson W, Taubert K, Gewitz M, Lockhart P, Baddour L, Levinson M, et al. Prevention of infective endocarditis: guidelines from the American Heart Association. J Am Dent Assoc. 2008;139(Suppl 1):S3–9, S11–24.
23. Sollecito T, Abt E, Lockhart P, Truelove E, Paumier T, Tracy S, et al. The use of prophylactic antibiotics prior to dental procedures in patients with prosthetic joints. J Am Dent Assoc. 2015;146(1):11–6.
24. Manani G, Facco E, Casiglia E, Cancian M, Zanette G. Isolated atrial fibrillation (IAF) after local anaesthesia with epinephrine in an anxious dental patient. Br Dent J. 2008;205(10):539–41.

# Anesthesia for Electroconvulsive Therapy

## 24

Paul Su and Jonathan Z. Pan

## Introduction

Electroconvulsive therapy (ECT) is a procedure that can be used to treat psychiatric disorders when patients are unresponsive to other forms of therapy or as an emergent procedure in gravely debilitated patient populations [1]. Cerletti and Bini first reported the use of ECT for humans in Rome in 1938 after extensive studies of electrical induction of seizures in dogs [2, 3]. Since then, it is estimated that approximately one million patients receive ECT worldwide annually [4]. ECT has been studied and indicated for primarily unipolar and bipolar depression, mania, but also schizophrenia, schizoaffective disorders, mixed affective disorders, and catatonia [5, 6]. Further applications include depression secondary to neurological disorders such as multiple sclerosis and obsessive-compulsive disorder, although the efficacy of ECT in these contexts remains to be determined. Now, ECT is considered a low-risk, procedure routinely performed under general anesthesia with a mortality rate estimated to be between 0.01 and 0.1% and with a complication rate of 0.3% [1].

## Proposed Mechanism of Action

ECT involves applying an electrical shock to one or both cerebral hemispheres to induce a generalized seizure. The most important factor for success is the duration of seizures. An optimal duration of seizure is between 20 and 60 s. Clinical benefits become apparent after a cumulative 400–700 s of seizure activity; this typically translates into 2–3 weeks of treatment with 2–3 sessions per week [7]. The goal of the psychiatrist and anesthesiologist is therefore to determine a regimen of anesthetic agents, electrode placement, and stimulus intensities that produces seizures of optimum duration while minimizing side effects [8, 9]. Seizure monitoring is accomplished by electroencephalography and motor activity. A seizure longer than 120 s is prolonged and should be terminated via pharmacologic agents. Short-term amnesia is common after ECT and more rare but serious cognitive dysfunction has been described in the literature [1, 10]. Despite the clinical benefits, the exact mechanism of action behind ECT has yet to be elucidated. The prevailing hypotheses implicate the following processes: release of neurotransmitters (dopamine, serotonin, and GABA) during the induced seizure, or re-setting of neu-

---

Each part of the chapter is summarized in Table 24.1

P. Su, M.D., Ph.D. (✉)
Department of Anesthesia and Perioperative Care,
University of California, San Francisco, CA, USA
e-mail: Paul.Su@ucsf.edu

J.Z. Pan, M.D., Ph.D.
Department of Anesthesia and Perioperative Care,
Brain and Spinal Injury Center (BASIC),
University of California, San Francisco, CA, USA
e-mail: Jonathan.Pan@ucsf.edu

**Table 24.1** Summary of perioperative anesthesia considerations and plans for electroconvulsive therapy (ECT)

| Preparation/plan/adverse events | Reasoning/management |
|---|---|
| *Preoperative evaluation and considerations* | |
| ECT is typically performed in NORA procedural locations | Familiarize yourself with the NORA environment, location of emergency equipment (resuscitation, airway) and back up personnel |
| Strong relative contraindications:<br>– Pheochromocytoma<br>– Recent myocardial infarction (<3 months)<br>– Stroke (<1 month) | Consider and document the benefits of ECT weighted against the increased risk of complications associated with the contraindicated conditions |
| Preprocedural evaluation<br>Aspiration risk<br>Airway (OSA, Sleep apnea)<br>Cardiovascular comorbidities<br>Neurologic comorbidities<br>Home medication<br>Drug-drug interactions | ECTs are typically done without need for securing the airway, the induction agents and neuromuscular agents used are typically short acting. Airway equipment must always be ready and available including devices such as oral pharyngeal airway, supraglottic devices. High-risk airway patients may require intubation prior to ECT procedure<br>Patients with comorbidities should be medically optimized to minimize unnecessary risk and may require closer monitoring and intervention for this procedure |
| Position—supine | Patients are usually on transport gurney |
| IV access—small gauge IV will suffice | Required to administer intravenous medications. Volume resuscitation is rarely required |
| Monitors | |
| – EKG | For monitoring of heart rate, rhythm as well as ST segments which can vary significant with biphasic parasympathetic and sympathetic discharge |
| – Blood pressure | Would recommend cycling every minute during procedure given significant changes in blood pressure can be seen after application of electrical stimulus. Consider invasive arterial blood pressure monitoring for high risk patients |
| – Pulse oximeter | Provides oxygenation status as well as additional information regarding heart rate |
| – Seizure Monitoring: EEG, tourniquet method | EEG usually monitored by proceduralist. Blood pressure cuff applied on extremity (ipsilateral to electrode if unilateral) and inflated above systemic pressure prior to administration of neuromuscular blocker to monitor for seizure activity |
| *Procedural anesthetic plan* | |
| Anesthetic plan for ECT: | |
| – Induction Agent: typically with methohexital (0.5–1.5 mg/kg). Doses are adjusted after each ECT to optimize seizure duration and to minimize stimulus amplitude and side effects | Goal is to achieve seizure of >30 s<br>Methohexital: Preferred agent as it blunts hemodynamic response without changes in seizure duration, short activity<br>Propofol and thiopental can be used as it also blunts the hemodynamic response but can shorten seizure duration<br>Etomidate can prolong seizures, but requires longer recovery time than methohexital and often causes myoclonus, nausea and vomiting. Ketamine and sevoflurane can also increase seizure duration |
| – Neuromuscular blockade: typically with succinylcholine (0.5 mg/kg) | Short acting agent desirable so patient will recover airway reflexes immediately after seizure. Complete paralysis is not required Rocuronium (0.6 mg/kg) with rapid reversal with sugammadex (16 mg/kg) is comparable to succinylcholine. Make sure tourniquet is inflated prior to administration of neuromuscular blocker to be able to monitor seizure distal to tourniquet |
| – Hypocarbia | Hyperventilation to end tidal $CO_2$ of 30–35 mmHg helps to lengthen the duration of seizure |

**Table 24.1** (continued)

| Preparation/plan/adverse events | Reasoning/management |
|---|---|
| – Adjunctive agents<br>  Hemodynamic modulation | Consider short acting beta-blockers (esmolol), calcium channel blockers (clevidipine), and vasodilators (nitroglycerin) for patients at risks for myocardial ischemic or cerebrovascular injury<br>Glycopyrolate can reduce incidence of bradycardia and has anti-sialogogue effects |
| Analgesia | Short acting opioids (remifentanil, alfentanil, fentanyl) can decrease dose of induction agent<br>NISAIDs can be helpful in reducing headaches and myalgia |
| *Adverse events and post-procedure considerations* | |
| Procedural adverse events | |
| Bradycardia | Initial parasympathetic surge from electrical stimulus. May warrant pre-medication with glycopyrolate |
| Tachycardia/hypertension | Sympathetic surge after initial parasympathetic discharge. May warrant treatment with short acting beta-blockers, calcium channel blockers, or vasodilators if hypertension is not well tolerated |
| Dysrhythmias | Most often bradycardia and tachycardia from parasympathetic and sympathetic discharge. However, can sometimes see PVCs. ST segments and T wave abnormalities can be seen in cardiac patients with mismatch of myocardial oxygen supply and demand |
| Protracted seizures | Seizures greater than 120 s must be terminated with agents such as propofol or benzodiazepines |
| Aspiration | Minimize this risk with appropriate fasting periods. Suction equipment should be ready |
| Incontinence | From parasympathetic discharge. Recommend patients use the restrooms prior to procedure |
| Dental/oral trauma | Cautious placement of bite block and adequate neuromuscular blockade prior to delivering electrical shock |
| Post-procedure and discharge considerations | |
| Transient cognitive changes/memory impairment/post-ictal states | Common. Reassurance, support and reorientation. Consider dexmedetomidine for emergence agitation. Benzodiazepines may also be considered |
| Hyper/hypo glycemia | From sympathetic discharge, treat as indicated |
| Myalgia, pain and discomfort | Consider acetaminophen, NSAIDs. Typically, does not require opioid medications. Consider avoiding succinylcholine for future treatments |
| Nausea/vomiting | Consider typical anti-emetics |

rotransmitter levels after seizure activities, altered cerebral glucose metabolism and blood flow, modulation of the hypothalamic-pituitary-adrenal axis, changes in synaptic transmission and plasticity, and cell proliferation [11].

## Pathophysiological Responses

### Cardiovascular Effects

Seizures can be associated with marked cardiovascular swings. Initially, a tonic phase lasting 10–15 s is seen with an associated activation of the parasympathetic nervous system: bradycardia (and rarely asystole), premature atrial and ventricular contractions, hypotension, and salivation. Subsequently a more prominent myoclonic phase lasting 30–60 s follows with an associated activation of the sympathetic autonomic system: tachycardia (heart rate >130 beats per minute), hypertension (systolic blood pressure increases of 30–70 mmHg and diastolic blood pressure increase of 10–50 mmHg), premature ventricular contractions, and rarely ventricular tachycardia and changes in electrocardiogram (including ST segment changes, and T-wave inversion). These cardiovascular fluctuations are transient and resolves within minutes but occasional can continue into emergence and post-procedural period. ECT induced cardiovascular mortality has been reported as 0.03% and are most common in patients with known or suspected cardiovascular comorbidities [12, 13].

## Cerebral Effects

Electrical stimulation produces large increases in cerebral blood flow and thus intracranial pressure (ICP) [14]. It has been reported that after electrically induced seizures, CBF increases ~300% and cerebral metabolism increases ~200%. Additionally, there is evidence of a temporary increase in the vascular permeability of the blood brain barrier. The aforementioned physiologic effects must be considered in all patients with neurologic comorbidities such as those with cerebral aneurysms, arteriovenous malformations (AVMs), intracranial lesions/tumors, and those with increased intracranial pressure of unknown etiology. The cerebral effects can produce intracerebral hemorrhages, cortical blindness, and transient neurologic ischemic deficits [15, 16].

## Other Effects

Generalized convulsions have resulted in fractures, dislocations and muscle aches [17, 18]. Intraocular pressure can increase as a result of ECT and also secondary to the administration of succinylcholine [19]. Care should be taken in those with increased intraocular pressures and patients at high-risk for retinal detachment. Hyperglycemia can be seen post-ECT as a result of the stress response. It is recommended patient holds oral hypoglycemic and insulin in the morning of the procedure and reduces long acting insulin agents to reflect fasting states in preparation for anesthesia and the procedure [20].

## Patient Considerations

All patients should receive a careful pre-operative evaluation including a focused history and physical examination before receiving anesthetic care. Attention to cardiovascular, neurologic and pulmonary comorbidities is prudent given the significant physiologic stress ECT places on those organ systems. Pre-operative evaluation may require consultation with cardiologists, neurologists, and other specialists to medically optimize a patient prior to this elective procedure and to ascertain whether the potential benefits of treatment outweigh the risks. A 12-lead ECG should be done on all patients above the age of 60 [12].

According to the APA Task Force Report, there are no absolute contraindications to ECT. However, strong relative contraindications include pheochromocytoma, recent myocardial infarction (<3 months) or stroke (<1 month), and increased intracerebral pressure of any cause. Other relative contraindications include angina, poorly controlled heart failure, severe valvular disease; aortic and cerebral aneurysms or other vascular malformations subject to rupture with increased blood pressure; bone fractures, severe osteoporosis; high risk pregnancy (for which an obstetric service consult and fetal monitoring would be recommended); intraocular processes including glaucoma, and retinal detachment; and significant pulmonary disease including asthma/COPD. For higher risk patients, ECT may be safer performed in the operating room setting where the anesthesiologist has access to more emergency equipment, medications, and resources in the event of life-threatening complications [1].

## Special Patient Populations

*Patients with pacemakers/AICD:* The location of electrical stimulation for ECT is sufficiently distant from typical locations of pacemakers and AICDs that the presence of pacemakers or AICDs carries no procedural implication. One retrospective study of 146 ECT treatments in patients with pacemakers reported no pacemaker malfunctions or anesthesia related events. A magnet should be accessible to disable AICD function and/or to override a pacemaker to a fixed rate if necessary—especially if the patient experiences arrhythmias as a result of the cardiovascular responses to electrical stimulation. Patients with severe heart disease should be medically optimized prior to initiation of ECT. Electrolyte abnormalities should be corrected, and hypertension well-controlled [21]. For those at risk of an imbalance between myocardial oxygen supply and demand, invasive hemodynamic monitoring (arterial line) can be helpful in guiding the use of pharmacologic agents such as β blockers, calcium channel blockers, and vasodilators to blunt the sympathetic response.

*Pregnant patients:* The APA supports ECT as an appropriate treatment modality in the pregnant patient in the context of the negative impact of neglected psychiatric illness on the fetus by affecting development, gestation, and birth weight [22]. The most prudent way to optimize the chance of a safe anesthetic in obstetric patients is vigilance and close monitoring of both the mother and fetus before, during, and after ECT. ECT is safe and effective for pregnant patients and some would argue that it is safer than pharmacologic agents [23]. Most anesthetic agents and all induction agents are US FDA category B or C; methohexital, thiopental, etomidate, propofol, ketamine and sevoflurane can all be utilized in the pregnant woman. Only benzodiazepines have been categorized as category D (with positive evidence of risk to fetus, however potential benefits may outweigh potential risk), and cocaine is the only category X (contraindicated) anesthetic agent. Ideally, ECT should occur during the second and third trimesters as rapid organogenesis is occurring in the fetus during the first trimester. An obstetrical exam should occur prior to the initiation of ECT with documentation of fetal heart rate. Physiologic changes of pregnancy must be recognized and taken in consideration in providing anesthesia for the pregnant patient. First, with the expanding gravid uterus, the diaphragm is displaced upwards decreasing a pregnant patient's functional residual capacity (FRC). Taken together with increased oxygen demand and cardiac output, adequate pre-oxygenation is essential as she will be at risk of desaturation when compared to her non-pregnant peers. A semi-sitting position can help offset the change in FRC. The gravid uterus also can cause aortocaval compression, thus a right hip wedge or left tilt of the procedure bed to obtain left uterine displacement to relieve inferior vena cava compression should be performed after 20 weeks gestation. The pregnant woman is always regarded as having a full stomach and at increased risk of aspiration as early as the 12th week. Therefore the administration of a non-particulate antacid (Bicitra/sodium citrate 30 mL) and/or histamine-2 receptor blockers (ranitidine 50 mg IV 30–60 min prior to the procedure) should be considered. After 24 weeks gestational age, the patient should be intubated for airway protection by a rapid-sequence induction with cricoid pressure and maintenance via sevoflurane which can reduce the risk of uterine contractions. Non-invasive fetal heart monitoring is advised after ECT performed in the second and third trimester. Complications include premature labor due to increased levels of oxytocin produced after ECT and spontaneous abortion, and thus prophylactic tocolytic therapy may be useful in women with a history of premature labor who need ECT. Other complications include uterine contractions, vaginal bleeding, fetal arrhythmias specifically fetal bradycardia, and placental abruption. Depending on the gestational age and discussion with the psychiatrist, obstetrician and anesthesiologist, it may be best to perform ECT on pregnancy patients in facilities with immediate access to obstetrical care in the event of an emergency caesarian section. Certainly ECT is not without risk, and should be reserved for those with grave disability and psychiatric disorders recalcitrant to pharmacotherapy.

*Anticoagulated patients:* One small retrospective study of 35 patients receiving over 300 ECT treatments found no adverse effects attributed to ECT performed in patients on long-term warfarin therapy [24]. However, there is a single case report of hematuria in an anticoagulated patient status post ECT [25]; the presumed mechanism was induced hypertension in the presence of a preexisting vascular malformation.

*Children & adolescents:* ECT in the pediatric population is reserved only for rare circumstances such as adolescent depression or catatonic schizophrenia unresponsive to antidepressants or antipsychotic medications. There is a lack of ECT studies in the pediatric population due to ethics and other potential problems associated with this procedure on the developing brain. A recent literature review states that other forms of noninvasive brain stimulation (transcranial magnetic stimulation for example) in children and adolescents is safe with mainly mild transient side effects and relatively few serious adverse events, however these studies excluded ECT [26].

*Patients with cerebral aneurysms and intracranial masses:* The sympathetic surge after an induced seizure can place additional wall and sheer stress on an aneurysm increasing the probability of enlargement or rupture. Invasive hemodynamic monitoring may be beneficial in these patients. In addition, short acting pharmacologic agents can blunt the change in blood pressure such as nitroprusside, esmolol, clevidipine, etc. Increased intracranial pressure has long been considered an absolute contraindication to ECT, notably due to case reports of clinical deterioration of patients after ECT. However, early reported cases of adverse events were subsequently discovered to have underlying pre-existing intracranial processes. Nevertheless, proceeding with ECT in patients with increased intracranial pressure without mass effect can be concerning given the changes in cerebral blood flow. Patients could be optimized with pre-ECT steroids like dexamethasone to decrease surrounding vasogenic edema, diuretics such as furosemide, and hyperventilation if necessary [27].

## Procedure Considerations

Considerations for ECT start prior to the application of the electrical stimulus. Patients should continue their regular medications unless the medications are known to interfere with seizure generation or duration (for example, benzodiazepines, or theophyllines should be held or discontinued if possible) [28]. Certain drug-drug interactions should be considered: indirect sympathomimetic such as ephedrine can lead to hypertensive crisis in patients taking concurrent monoamine oxidase inhibitors; lithium can prolong the action of succinylcholine. Patients should be encouraged to empty their bladders before the procedure, as incontinence is common. Lastly, some patients may warrant administration of glycopyrolate or other anticholinergic agents to decrease salivation, and to blunt the initial parasympathetic activation.

The procedural framework of ECT is as follows: After the appropriate period of fasting per anesthesia society guidelines, standard monitors (EKG, blood pressure cuff, pulse oximetry) are applied to the patient. Following adequate preoxygenation, general anesthesia is induced typically with an intravenous agent such as methohexital. Prior to the administration of muscle relaxant, a blood pressure cuff is applied to one of the extremities and inflated above systolic blood pressure functioning as a tourniquet to prevent the circulation of the neuromuscular blocker distal to the cuff. Full relaxation is not required [29]. Stimulus electrodes are placed either bifrontotemporally (bilateral) or with one electrode placed frontotemporally and the second electrode placed on the ipsilateral side (unilateral). In unilateral ECT, the BP cuff should be on the same side as the electrodes to ensure that a bilateral seizure occurs [12]. Positive pressure mask hyperventilation with 100% oxygen serves to further preoxygenate the patient as well as induce mild hypocapnia (EtCO$_2$ 30–35 mmHg), which lengthens the seizure duration [30]. A bite block is placed to minimize oral trauma. Electrical stimulus is applied to induce a seizure. Seizure threshold varies greatly among patients and the lowest amount of electrical stimulus to induce a seizure of adequate duration should be used. Seizure monitoring is necessary and may be accomplished by an EEG and by the "BP cuff" technique, which allows motor activity to be visualized in the limb with the blood pressure cuff acting as a proxy. Bag mask ventilation can be resumed after the stimulus is applied, and the patient's airway supported until the patient wakes [1, 12].

## Pharmacologic Considerations

### Induction Agent

The desired seizure duration in ECT is one lasting more than 30 s. Induction agents can all affect seizure threshold and duration to some degree [29, 31]. Thoughtful preparation is warranted for a successful treatment—one with a minimal amplitude stimulus applied, minimal number of shocks needed to achieve a clinically acceptable seizure, and minimization of untoward side effects. According to Miller's Anesthesia, methohexital (0.5–1.5 mg/kg) is believed to be the gold standard agent to use for induction prior to ECT, as it blunts the hemodynamic response to ECT without a change in seizure duration [32]. Methohexital has minimal anticonvulsive properties on its own, and when compared to thiopental, propofol and etomidate, is viewed to be a superior agent [33, 34]. Propofol (0.75–2.5 mg/kg) and thiopental (1–2.5 mg/kg) both similarly blunt the hemodynamic response, but also minimally decrease seizure duration [35]. Of note, shortened seizure durations were observed with propofol doses of greater than 1.0 mg/kg; nevertheless, propofol can still be utilized with good effect. Etomidate (0.15–0.3 mg/kg) results in seizures of a longer duration compared to propofol and thiopental, however, regular use of etomidate is thwarted by myoclonus, nausea, vomiting, and a longer time to consciousness than methohexital. Furthermore, etomidate is not as effectively in blunting the hypertension and tachycardia associated with the sympathetic discharge with ECT. Interestingly, both ketamine (0.7–3 mg/kg) and volatile anesthetics (sevoflurane 6–8% for induction, followed by 1–2 MAC) can increase seizure duration, presumably because less induction agent is needed [36]. Similarly, sevoflurane is most advantageous in the pregnant patient but intravenous agents are most frequently utilized first. Initial dose is calculated using patient weight but subsequent doses are typically guided by previous response to ECT. All agents can be utilized and the variability in emergence and recovery should not be the sole factor in selection of induction agents.

## Neuromuscular Blockade

Prior to the participation of anesthesiologists in ECT in the 1950s the most common associated injuries included vertebral body compression fractures, broken limbs and dental damage secondary to tonic-clonic seizures. The use of neuromuscular blocking agents has prevented many of the aforementioned injuries. Paralysis need not be complete (as intubation is rarely required)—and often 0.5 mg/kg of the depolarizing agent succinycholine provides sufficient neuromuscular blockade for this short procedure [29]. Rarely is larger doses needed (up to 1.5 mg/kg; severe osteoporosis or pre-existing skeletal injury).

With the introduction of sugammadex, the use of rocuronium is emerging as an acceptable alternative, especially in settings where succinylcholine is contraindicated or less desirable. Studies comparing the recovery of neuromuscular blockade from succinylcholine (dosed at 1 mg/kg) was not significantly different from using rocuronium (0.6 mg/kg) followed by 16 mg/kg sugammadex immediately following seizure cessation [37]. When sugammadex was dosed at 4 mg/kg, the recovery was significantly slower than the succinylcholine group (absolute difference of about 100 s [38]. The use of sugammadex and rocuronium may have the added benefit of decreased myalgia and headache post ECT [39].

Other alternative neuromuscular blockers to consider include mivacurium (0.15–0.2 mg/kg) or atracurium (0.3–0.5 mg/kg) as short-acting non-depolarizing agents. It is important to be prepared for additional airway management and supportive measures for anticipated paralysis when using neuromuscular blockers. Mivacurium can result in clinically significant hypotension due to histamine release and is metabolized by pseudocholinesterase, thus patients with pseudocholinesterase deficiency are at risk for prolonged paralysis. If atracurium is utilized, reversal of neuromuscular blockade with atropine and edrophonium is required.

## Hemodynamic Modulation

β blockers can be administrated to blunt the sympathetic effects of ECT [40]. Atenolol is often administered pre-procedurally, whereas labetalol (0.05–0.4 mg/kg) and esmolol (1–2 mg/kg) are utilized during ECT. It is worthwhile to note some evidences suggest that labetalol and esmolol may reduce seizure duration [40]. Alternatively, calcium channel blockers such as nifedipine (0.1 mg/kg IV, 10 mg SL) and nicardipine (2.5–5 mg; 40 µg/kg) have been used without effects on seizure generation or duration, although nicardipine is traditionally favored due to its shorter duration of action [41, 42]. However, more recently, clevidipine, an even more rapid and short-acting late generation dihydropyridine calcium channel antagonist rapidly metabolized by plasma esterases, has been used to treat hypertension in many perioperative setting with great success [43]. Diltiazem may reduce seizure duration. Nitroglycerin, nitroprusside, and clonidine (0.05–0.3 mg, 60–90 min prior to induction) can blunt the hemodynamic response associated with ECT and may be warranted in the patient with high risk of myocardial ischemia or cerebrovascular injury. Of note, the α2 adrenergic receptor agonist dexmedetomidine administered pre-ECT increases sedation but does not blunt hemodynamic changes associated with the sympathetic surge [44]. When using sodium nitroprusside or nitroglycerin continuous blood pressure monitoring via an arterial line is recommended.

### Adjuvants

Anticholinergics are used primarily in blunting the initial parasympathetic response after electrical stimulation [45]. Glycopyrrolate or atropine can be administered to reduce the incidence of bradycardia and decrease oral secretions. Glycopyrrolate is thought to be superior given its anti-sialagogue effects, that it is not centrally acting, and its use results in less post-ECT tachycardia compared to atropine. Routine administration of atropine is not recommended.

### Analgesics (Opioids and NSAIDs)

Opioids as adjuncts can help decrease the dose of induction agent required and allow for a faster wake up. In this context, opioids such as remifentanil (1 µg/kg over 30–60 s), alfentanil (10–25 µg/kg), and fentanyl (1.5 µg/kg) with agents other than etomidate can lead to longer seizures using this dose-sparing effect [46]. NSAIDs can be useful to help reduce the incidence and severity of post-ECT headaches and myalgia [47].

## Medications and Techniques to Decrease the Seizure Threshold

Hyperventilation (hypocarbia) lengthens seizure duration and thus the effectiveness of ECT [30]. Intravenous caffeine, theophylline, and aminophyllines (xanthines) have been demonstrated to be an effective method of increasing seizure length, but the clinical efficacy has not been elucidated [48]. All methods of seizure enhancement run the risk of producing unacceptably long seizures and/or status epilepticus. A well-trained anesthesiologist should attempt to break a prolonged seizure using benzodiazepines or propofol.

## Complications/Adverse Events

Transient cognitive changes, memory impairment, and post-ictal confusions are the most commonly reported side effect after ECT. These symptoms can last from minutes to hours. Non-pharmacologic delirium interventions such as reassurance, support, and reorientation is all that is needed during this phase, however sometimes short-acting benzodiazepines such as midazolam can be used in some cases of emergence agitation but may delay discharge from PACU. Memory impairment is frequently reported and patients may note retrograde amnesia (difficulty in recalling information known/learned prior to ECT), anterograde amnesia (difficulty in retaining new information), or both. Typically, both retrograde and anterograde amnesia disappear after a period of days to weeks, although some patients have reported that memory did not return to their previous baseline after ECT. ECT has not been shown to be associated with permanent brain injury [49]. General somatic complaints (headaches, nausea, muscle soreness) are also common. Other adverse events include reactions to anesthetic and neuromuscular blocking agents, and dental and/or oral trauma despite the use of a bite block. Dexmedetomidine has been utilized for management of post-ictal/emergence delirium [50, 51]. While the goal is to elicit seizures of adequate duration, one should always be ready to terminate protracted seizures—for example, with propofol.

Management of the unprotected airway carries a plethora of different risks. Anesthesia providers must be familiar with difficult ventilation and difficult intubation algorithms during these rapid turnover procedures. Suction devices should always be ready and functional in events of vomiting, or increased oral secretions.

## Conclusion

ECT is an effective avenue of treatment for severe psychiatric illnesses. This relatively low risk procedure is typically performed in non-operating room anesthesia locations; but it can be associated with varied physiologic effects. Anesthesia providers should understand the physiology of ECT, the potential risks as it relates to each patient's medical history in order to provide safe care and to guard against any events.

## References

1. Rasmussen K. The practice of electroconvulsive therapy: recommendations for treatment, training, and privileging (second edition). J ECT. 2002;18(1):58–9.
2. Endler NS. The origins of electroconvulsive therapy (ECT). Convuls Ther. 1988;4(1):5–23.
3. Khan A, et al. Electroconvulsive therapy. Psychiatr Clin North Am. 1993;16(3):497–513.
4. Prudic J, Olfson M, Sackeim HA. Electro-convulsive therapy practices in the community. Psychol Med. 2001;31(5):929–34.
5. Lisanby SH. Electroconvulsive therapy for depression. N Engl J Med. 2007;357(19):1939–45.
6. Agarkar S, et al. ECT use in unipolar and bipolar depression. J ECT. 2012;28(3):e39–40.
7. Segman RH, et al. Onset and time course of antidepressant action: psychopharmacological implications of a controlled trial of electroconvulsive therapy. Psychopharmacology (Berl). 1995;119(4):440–8.
8. Loo C, Simpson B, MacPherson R. Augmentation strategies in electroconvulsive therapy. J ECT. 2010;26(3):202–7.
9. Sackeim HA, et al. Effects of electrode placement on the efficacy of titrated, low-dose ECT. Am J Psychiatry. 1987;144(11):1449–55.
10. Zachrisson OC, et al. No evident neuronal damage after electroconvulsive therapy. Psychiatry Res. 2000;96(2):157–65.
11. Rosenquist PB, Miller B, Pillai A. The antipsychotic effects of ECT: a review of possible mechanisms. J ECT. 2014;30(2):125–31.
12. Ding Z, White PF. Anesthesia for electroconvulsive therapy. Anesth Analg. 2002;94(5):1351–64.
13. Swartz CM. Physiological response to ECT stimulus dose. Psychiatry Res. 2000;97(2-3):229–35.
14. Saito S, et al. Regional cerebral oxygen saturation during electroconvulsive therapy: monitoring by near-infrared spectrophotometry. Anesth Analg. 1996;83(4):726–30.
15. Weisberg LA, Elliott D, Mielke D. Intracerebral hemorrhage following electroconvulsive therapy. Neurology. 1991;41(11):1849.
16. Rikher KV, Johnson R, Kamal M. Cortical blindness after electroconvulsive therapy. J Am Board Fam Pract. 1997;10(2):141–3.
17. Sarpel Y, et al. Central acetabular fracture-dislocation following electroconvulsive therapy: report of two similar cases. J Trauma. 1996;41(2):342–4.
18. Herriot PM, Cowain T, McLeod D. Use of vecuronium to prevent suxamethonium-induced myalgia after ECT. Br J Psychiatry. 1996;168(5):653–4.
19. Edwards RM, et al. Intraocular pressure changes in nonglaucomatous patients undergoing electroconvulsive therapy. Convuls Ther. 1990;6(3):209–13.
20. Ghanizadeh A, et al. The effect of electroconvulsive therapy on blood glucose, creatinine levels, and lipid profile and its association with the type of psychiatric disorders. Neurochem Int. 2012;61(7):1007–10.
21. MacPherson RD, Loo CK, Barrett N. Electroconvulsive therapy in patients with cardiac pacemakers. Anaesth Intensive Care. 2006;34(4):470–4.
22. Mander AJ, Norton B, Hoare P. The effect of maternal psychotic illness on a child. Br J Psychiatry. 1987;151:848–50.
23. Spodniakova B, Halmo M, Nosalova P. Electro convulsive therapy in pregnancy – a review. J Obstet Gynaecol. 2015;35(7):659–62.
24. Mehta V, et al. Safety of electroconvulsive therapy in patients receiving long-term warfarin therapy. Mayo Clin Proc. 2004;79(11):1396–401.
25. Blevins S, Greene G. Hematuria with electroconvulsive therapy: a case report. J ECT. 2009;25(4):287.
26. Krishnan C, et al. Safety of noninvasive brain stimulation in children and adolescents. Brain Stimul. 2015;8(1):76–87.
27. Patkar AA, et al. ECT in the presence of brain tumor and increased intracranial pressure: evaluation and reduction of risk. J ECT. 2000;16(2):189–97.
28. Rasmussen KG, Zorumski CF. Electroconvulsive therapy in patients taking theophylline. J Clin Psychiatry. 1993;54(11):427–31.

29. Wagner KJ, et al. Guide to anaesthetic selection for electroconvulsive therapy. CNS Drugs. 2005;19(9):745–58.
30. Sawayama E, et al. Moderate hyperventilation prolongs electroencephalogram seizure duration of the first electroconvulsive therapy. J ECT. 2008;24(3):195–8.
31. Lihua P, et al. Different regimens of intravenous sedatives or hypnotics for electroconvulsive therapy (ECT) in adult patients with depression. Cochrane Database Syst Rev. 2014;(4):CD009763.
32. Miller RD. Miller's anesthesia. 7th ed. Philadelphia: Churchill Livingstone/Elsevier; 2010.
33. Avramov MN, Husain MM, White PF. The comparative effects of methohexital, propofol, and etomidate for electroconvulsive therapy. Anesth Analg. 1995;81(3):596–602.
34. Singh PM, et al. Evaluation of etomidate for seizure duration in electroconvulsive therapy: a systematic review and meta-analysis. J ECT. 2015;31(4):213–25.
35. Rasmussen KG. Propofol for ECT anesthesia a review of the literature. J ECT. 2014;30(3):210–5.
36. Rasmussen KG, Jarvis MR, Zorumski CF. Ketamine anesthesia in electroconvulsive therapy. Convuls Ther. 1996;12(4):217–23.
37. Hoshi H, et al. Use of rocuronium-sugammadex, an alternative to succinylcholine, as a muscle relaxant during electroconvulsive therapy. J Anesth. 2011;25(2):286–90.
38. Kadoi Y, et al. Comparison of recovery times from rocuronium-induced muscle relaxation after reversal with three different doses of sugammadex and succinylcholine during electroconvulsive therapy. J Anesth. 2011;25(6):855–9.
39. Saricicek V, et al. Does rocuronium-sugammadex reduce myalgia and headache after electroconvulsive therapy in patients with major depression? J ECT. 2014;30(1):30–4.
40. Castelli I, et al. Comparative effects of esmolol and labetalol to attenuate hyperdynamic states after electroconvulsive therapy. Anesth Analg. 1995;80(3):557–61.
41. Avramov MN, et al. Effects of nicardipine and labetalol on the acute hemodynamic response to electroconvulsive therapy. J Clin Anesth. 1998;10(5):394–400.
42. Zhang Y, et al. The use of nicardipine for electroconvulsive therapy: a dose-ranging study. Anesth Analg. 2005;100(2):378–81.
43. Espinosa A, et al. Perioperative use of clevidipine: a systematic review and meta-analysis. PLoS One. 2016;11(3):e0150625.
44. Fu W, White PF. Dexmedetomidine failed to block the acute hyperdynamic response to electroconvulsive therapy. Anesthesiology. 1999;90(2):422–4.
45. Kramer BA. Anticholinergics and ECT. Convuls Ther. 1993;9(4):293–300.
46. Recart A, et al. The effect of remifentanil on seizure duration and acute hemodynamic responses to electroconvulsive therapy. Anesth Analg. 2003;96(4):1047–50, table of contents.
47. Leung M, Hollander Y, Brown GR. Pretreatment with ibuprofen to prevent electroconvulsive therapy-induced headache. J Clin Psychiatry. 2003;64(5):551–3.
48. Stern L, et al. Aminophylline increases seizure length during electroconvulsive therapy. J ECT. 1999;15(4):252–7.
49. Mander AJ, et al. Cerebral and brain stem changes after ECT revealed by nuclear magnetic resonance imaging. Br J Psychiatry. 1987;151:69–71.
50. Cohen MB, Stewart JT. Treatment of post-electroconvulsive therapy agitation with dexmedetomidine. J ECT. 2013;29(2):e23–4.
51. O'Brien EM, et al. Dexmedetomidine and the successful management of electroconvulsive therapy postictal agitation: a case report. J ECT. 2010;26(2):131–3.

# Anesthesia for MRI and CT

Gregory E. R. Weller

## Introduction

Magnetic resonance imaging (MRI) and computed tomography (CT) are advanced imaging technologies that offer unique diagnostic and therapeutic capabilities for our patients. MRI and CT imaging suites are usually far removed from main operating room complexes, and are generally not designed with optimal anesthetic care as a primary consideration. As clinical demand for MRI and CT studies continues to rise, there has been a concurrent increased demand for anesthesia services in these areas. As such, anesthesiologists must understand the unique hazards and challenges inherent in these non-operating room sites (Table 25.1).

This chapter first examines anesthesia in the MRI suite, detailing the key complexities and hazards unique to this environment, including strong magnetic fields, the ferromagnetic missile effect, radiofrequency thermal burns, cryogens, challenges with remote patient monitoring, and risks of magnetic contrast agents. The potential hazards of the MRI machine require extreme vigilance for patient safety. Anesthesiologists must work closely with MRI nurses and technologists to minimize MRI hazards, while still ensuring maximal anesthetic safety as usual.

G. E. R. Weller, M.D., Ph.D.
Penn State Hershey Medical Center,
Hershey, PA, USA
e-mail: gweller@pennstatehealth.psu.edu

Second, this chapter examines anesthesia in the CT suite, detailing hazards including ionizing radiation, challenging ergonomics, and radiocontrast agents. The CT suite introduces the additional challenge of occupational safety. Caring for an anesthetized patient in the CT scanner while trying to minimize occupational exposure to ionizing radiation requires careful planning and vigilance.

For both MRI and CT, various anesthetic strategies and their rationales are presented, offering an array of options for the provision of safe and effective anesthetic patient care. Patient indications for anesthesia, anesthesia equipment, imaging contrast agents, anesthetic techniques, and plans for emergency situations are discussed.

## Non-OR Anesthesia

Anesthesia outside of the usual operating room environment can be hazardous, with additional and unpredictable challenges that increase patient risk. Offsite locations generally are not designed to optimize anesthesia care, having limited space and non-ergonomic layouts. Personnel from other departments (e.g. Radiology) are unlikely to be familiar with the intricacies of safe anesthesia care, and may be less adroit and reliable in emergency situations. Case rhythms often deviate significantly from our usual OR routines, and are highly variable depending on procedure and location. Distractions and add-on cases are numerous, and communication is less predict-

**Table 25.1** Summary of anesthesia considerations in patients undergoing MRI and CT imaging

| Plan/preparation/adverse events | Reasoning/management |
|---|---|
| Careful planning and preparation, screening of patients and staff, and vigilance for the unique hazards of MR scanners | Hazards in MRI:<br>• Ferromagnetic missile effect<br>• Acoustic noise<br>• Burns<br>• Implanted medical device malfunction<br>• Patient far away |
| Careful planning and preparation, ionizing radiation protection for patient and staff, and vigilance for the unique hazards of CT scanners | Hazards in CT:<br>• Ionizing radiation<br>• Anesthesiologist may be physically remote from patient |
| Pre-procedural evaluation:<br>• Airway (OSA, Difficult airway)<br>• Aspiration risk<br>• Positioning issues<br>• Implanted medical devices<br>• Need for breath holds?<br>• Need for contrast?<br>• Renal function if contrast needed | • If any doubts exist regarding the ability to maintain safe spontaneous ventilation, an LMA or ETT should be used<br>• Implanted medical devices must be discussed with Radiology physicians and technologists<br>• Reactions to iodine-based radiocontrast agents are not unusual, and can be severe<br>• Reactions to gadolinium contrast are rare |
| If spontaneous ventilation is planned, have backup device for positive pressure ventilation immediately available | Desaturation and cardiorespiratory compromise as a result of inadequate spontaneous ventilation can present very quickly |
| Position: typically supine | Tomographic imaging around supine patient. |
| IV access: Required for all cases except non-contrast CT | Additional IV catheters may be required for contrast injectors |
| Anesthetic options:<br>(1) GA/TIVA with propofol & nasal cannula<br>(2) GA/LMA<br>(3) GA/ETT | (1) Nasal cannula offers increased efficiency; Avoids airway manipulation<br>(2) Choose LMA when spontaneous ventilation is unlikely to succeed (e.g. severe OSA)<br>(3) Choose ETT when secure airway is required |
| Adverse events:<br>• Failure of spontaneous ventilation<br>• Hypoxemia<br>• IV infiltration<br>• Contrast reaction<br>• Burns<br>• Implanted medical device malfunction | • Potential adverse events related to anesthetic technique (e.g. TIVA, spontaneous ventilation) or site (MRI)<br>• Prepare plans for adverse events, calling for assistance when needed, and emergencies<br>• For emergencies/codes in MRI → immediately remove patient from scanner room |
| Postoperative considerations:<br>• Monitor for contrast reactions<br>• Same PACU care as OR patients<br>• Neonates & infants may need prolonged PACU stays | Ideally, Radiology has dedicated PACU facilities<br>If not, transfer patient to central OR PACU |

able. Many offsite locations prioritize "the schedule" above anesthesiologists' requirements for patient safety.

It is important to understand that all out-of-the-OR anesthetics involve risk. Based on a closed claims analysis, events of inadequate oxygenation or ventilation occur seven times more frequently in the non-OR setting than in the OR [1]. Furthermore, adverse events in non-OR areas are four times more likely to be judged as being preventable by improved monitoring [1].

Optimizing anesthesia care in non-OR locations such as MRI and CT requires excellent communication within the anesthesia team, and with nurses, technologists, requesting physicians, radiologists, and patients and their families. Careful coordination between these different groups is essential. Efforts must be made to help anesthesia teams understand the unusual circumstances of each particular procedure or imaging site, and to help the local personnel understand anesthesia issues and our commitment to optimal patient safety.

## MRI: Basics

Providing safe and efficient anesthesia in the MRI suite can be a tall order. In addition to the standard challenges inherent in all out-of-the-OR sites, the MR machine creates unique safety hazards for the patient and unique difficulties for the anesthesiologist.

Familiarity with the underlying physics of magnetic resonance scanners, the physical layout of the MRI suite, potential effects on patients, safety terminology and rules allows anesthesiologists caring for adult or pediatric patients in the MRI suite to deliver optimal care. Anesthesia equipment issues in the magnetic environment must be addressed, and appropriate emergency plans developed. Anesthetic plans that account for the unique MRI hazards must be carefully developed pre-operatively, and effective communication with all care team members ensured.

## MRI: Physics

Atoms can be described by their intrinsic mass, electrical charge, and magnetic moment (spin). Atomic isotopes with an odd number of neutrons and protons display a magnetic moment (nonzero spin) and act like tiny magnets. Hydrogen protons, for example, are positively charged and spin around their axis like spinning tops. When such atomic nuclei are exposed to magnetic fields, they absorb and emit electromagnetic radiation, via a process called **nuclear magnetic resonance**.

The hydrogen atom is the most relevant nucleus for clinical MR systems, because hydrogen is highly abundant in water of biologic tissues. In a static (constant) magnetic field, a small excess fraction of hydrogen protons will align themselves with the magnetic field, producing an electromagnetic signal that is detectable by the MR scanner. Furthermore, external radiofrequency (RF) pulses applied to these atomic nuclei will induce disturbances in their spin axes. The rate at which each proton changes its spin orientation ("precession") is its resonance frequency. As the protons change their spin to align with the transient magnetic field, then revert to their orientation upon removal of the RF energy, the energy released is detectable by the MR detectors. The resonant frequency of a particular substance is proportional to the strength of the magnetic field. In a non-uniform (varying) magnetic field, the resonance frequencies of a sample are dependent upon the nuclei's locations, allowing for the extraction of spatial information from the detected signals, which is then translated into an image.

MRI scanners utilize three interacting electromagnetic fields: the static, gradient, and radiofrequency fields. The main (static) field is generated by a large electric current flowing through loops of bundled superconducting wires. This is the strongest of the three fields, and is constant over time. Modern clinical scanners employ enormously strong static magnetic fields, most commonly 1.5 or 3 Tesla (T). One Tesla equals 10,000 gauss, or approximately 10,000–30,000 times the strength of the Earth's natural magnetic field. MRI scanners typically have a cylindrical bore magnet, with the main static magnetic field oriented parallel to the bore. Three Tesla scanners have superior resolution and sensitivity. Caution is required, because ferromagnetic objects exposed to strong magnetic fields will be attracted to the source, becoming high-velocity projectiles that can harm or even kill patients and medical personnel.

The gradient magnetic field is time-varying, and much weaker than the main static field. It is rapidly turned on and off, inducing electrical currents in conductive material. This field is responsible for the high noise level in MRI scanners. Caution is required, because induced currents can disrupt medical equipment such as implantable cardiac devices.

The third and weakest field is the radiofrequency field. Radiofrequency energy is absorbed and released by tissues to produce signals detected by the receiver coils. Caution is required, because RF energy can heat biologic tissues, leading to burns.

MR scanners measure three properties of tissue: T1 relaxation (the time for the magnetization vector to re-align (relax) with the vertical/longitudinal axis of the static magnetic field), T2 decay (the time required for decay of transverse out-of-phase magnetization), and proton density.

MRI signals encode complex spatial information, and thus any patient movement can significantly diminish image quality. This is the most important reason that anesthesia is often required for MRI scans. It is at best challenging, and at worst impossible, for many patients to remain perfectly still for the necessary duration of 30–90 min. This is particularly true for pediatric patients.

To optimize electrical efficiency of the scanner, the wire bundles are cooled to superconducting temperature by submersion in cryogens, usually 1000–2000 L of liquid helium, maintained near absolute zero. The magnetic field can be emergently terminated by "quenching": rapidly releasing the cryogenic fluid in gaseous form. Since helium expands dramatically as it boils into gas, it must be vented to the outside through special escape valves and ventilation system. Quenching is considered hazardous, because if the ventilation system malfunctions or becomes obstructed, the expanding helium gas may escape into the scanner room, displacing the available air and leading to hypoxia or asphyxiation, ruptured eardrums, and frostbite. Thus, quenching is utilized only in emergencies to remove patients or equipment from the scanner.

In addition to standard MR anatomical imaging, additional techniques have been developed to study more complex tissue features. For example, MR angiography (MRA) and MR venography (MRV) evaluate blood vessels and vascular flow, and are used to assess vascular stenoses and aneurysms.

## MRI: Physical Layout

The centerpiece of the MRI suite is the scanner and its extremely powerful magnetic fields. The suite design should accommodate the needs of the radiologists, MRI technologists, anesthesiologists, outpatients, and inpatients. Standards for MRI suite design, and safe and responsible practices in the MR environment, are established by the American College of Radiology (ACR) [2].

Access to the scanner room and its dangerous magnetic fields must be restricted via card access or other barrier strategies. Of critical importance for cases requiring anesthesia, the suite should also be designed to facilitate anesthesia induction, maintenance of anesthesia in the scanner, emergence, and recovery.

To isolate the scanner from external electromagnetic interference, the walls of the MRI scanner room are sheathed with copper or aluminum, creating a Faraday cage to shield the scanner. Windows between the scanner room and the control room allow viewing of the patient; fine metal mesh embedded in the windows maintains Faraday cage continuity. Small access tubes ("wave guides") in the wall between the scanner room and the control room allow for passage of fiberoptic cables, IV tubing, anesthesia circuits, and other necessary components.

The ACR divides the MRI suite floorplan into four Zones [2], to facilitate safe practices (Table 25.2). Zone I includes all areas outside of the MRI facility, freely accessible to public. The

**Table 25.2** Conceptual division of MRI suites into four Zones, to ensure that access is carefully controlled and to optimize MR safety

| Zone | Areas | Details |
|---|---|---|
| I | • Locations outside of MRI complex | • No restrictions<br>• Fully accessible by everyone |
| II | • Initial portions of MRI complex<br>• Waiting room<br>• Nursing station<br>• Exam area | • Patient interviews & exams<br>• Supervised by Radiology staff<br>• Anesthesia induction area<br>• Recovery area |
| III | • MR Control room<br>• Corridor leading to scanner room | • Access strictly regulated<br>• Only screened patients and staff |
| IV | • MR Scanner room | • Extreme magnetic hazard<br>• Access strictly regulated<br>• Only screened patients and staff<br>• No ferromagnetic items allowed |

Based on the 2013 ACR Guidance Document on MR Safe Practices [2]

entire healthcare facility outside of the MRI department is part of Zone I. Zone II includes the MRI reception area, interview and exam area, and nursing station. Initial MRI screening will occur here, and patients will generally be supervised by Radiology personnel while in Zone II. This is the ideal location for anesthesia inductions and recovery. Zone III includes the MRI control room and adjoining spaces or hallways. Access to Zone III is strictly controlled due to hazards of ferromagnetic objects in strong magnetic fields. Only screened patients and personnel are allowed in Zone III, and physical barriers are required between Zones II and III, such as locked doors with card access. Finally, Zone IV is the MR scanner room itself. This room must be marked as "hazardous", and locked when not in use. MRI technologists must have direct visual control over Zone IV. Only trained personnel and properly screened patients may be allowed into Zones III and IV.

Anesthesiologists provide care in all four Zones, and must become familiar with the relevant safety and access regulations. Anesthesia induction and emergence should occur in a designated "induction area" within Zone II. This area should include all of the usual anesthesia equipment and supplies, including an anesthesia machine, suction, airway equipment, wall gas supplies, medications, intravenous access supplies, and access to a code cart with monitor/defibrillator. Having a fully-capable anesthesia induction suite in Zone II allows for the safest patient care, minimizing the impact of the magnetic field dangers in Zones III & IV.

The MR scanner room itself should contain built-in wall gas lines for oxygen, air, and nitrous oxide, as well as vacuum lines. The anesthesiologist's workstation in the control room should offer a reasonable view of the patient in the scanner, as well as any anesthesia machines, monitors, or other equipment being utilized.

## MRI: Safety

A significant factor contributing to the dangers associated with MR scanners is that they do not inherently "look" dangerous. Regardless of their benign appearance, they in fact have caused numerous incidents resulting in minor injuries, serious injuries, and death. Magnetic fields are invisible, MR scanner machines are always on, and hazard labeling and access restrictions in the past has been suboptimal, although this is improving.

A 2008 Sentinel Event Alert regarding MRI safety [3] cited 398 adverse MRI-related events in the prior decade, including nine fatalities. This report helped stimulate widespread efforts to improve patient safety in MRI suites. In 2013, the ACR published their updated Guidance Document on Safe MR Practices [2], including safe MR practice guidelines, MRI Zone definitions, patient flow recommendations, and equipment labeling policies.

An under-appreciated feature of MRI scanners is that the magnet <u>always stays on</u>. Even when the MRI scanner is not actively acquiring images, the large static magnetic field remains active, and thus ferromagnetic objects <u>always</u> present a hazard to patients and personnel in the MR environment. Precautions to restrict ferromagnetic items from the scanner room must be maintained at all times.

Why do adverse events occur in the MR suite? The most common causes include a lack of adequate training, the failure to follow proper procedures, e.g. screening of all patients and personnel for each entry into the scanner room, the use of inappropriate equipment, and inadequate labeling. Each institution utilizing MR scanners should develop and maintain robust systems for the reporting, investigation, and remediation of adverse events.

The 2013 American Society for Testing and Materials (ASTM) standards [4] require that all items used in MR environments be labeled with appropriate MR safety designations. Current MR safety terminology includes "MR Unsafe", "MR Conditional", and "MR Safe" (see Table 25.3). Labels may be displayed permanently on the item itself, or in the accompanying documentation. Color-coded, easily identifiable MR safety icons have been developed to enhance clarity and safety in MR suites. However, at this time many medical items still exhibit no MR safety informa-

**Table 25.3** MRI safety labels

| | | |
|---|---|---|
| MR Unsafe | Poses hazards in MR environments, and **must not** be allowed into MR scanner rooms | |
| MR Conditional | No known hazards in **specified** MR environments under **specified** conditions of use (e.g. specific static field strengths, scanning sequences, and RF/gradient coils) | |
| MR Safe | No known hazards, in all MR environments | |

Based on ASTM F2503-13: Standard Practice for Marking Medical Devices and Other Items for Safety in the Magnetic Resonance Environment [4]

tion. The lack of an MR safety label does not indicate compatibility with MRI. It is safest to assume that an unmarked item is MR-Unsafe, until reviewed in detail with the MR technologist.

## Effects on Patients

Over 30 years of experience with clinical MRI scanners has revealed no known significant physiological impacts on patients. This is in stark contrast to X-rays and CT, which utilize harmful ionizing radiation. There are reports that MRI can rarely cause transient vertigo and nausea, likely due to interference with the vestibular system. One study also showed transiently increased hemodynamic fluctuations in neonates undergoing MRI [5]. Overall, however, there is little evidence from either *in vitro* or *in vivo* studies that there is any adverse impact to biologic tissues from clinically-relevant MR exposure [6, 7]. Additionally, MRI is generally considered to be painless, with the exception of the requirement to lie in a single position (most commonly supine) for an extended duration, which may cause discomfort or pain in some patients.

However, this does not prove that MRI is entirely benign. MRI can present risks to our patients from the following sources: ferromagnetic devices or objects being drawn into the magnetic fields, acoustic hazard from loud MRI scanners, risk from MRI contrast agents, discomfort or pain from positioning, and the usual risks of anesthesia. These are discussed below.

## Temperature and Burns

MRI scanner rooms are maintained at cool temperatures (68–70 °F) to facilitate image quality. Infants and neonates are at risk for hypothermia, due to poorly developed thermal regulation and a large body surface area-to-volume ratio. For deep sedation or general anesthesia cases, the scanner's patient cooling fan should be turned off, and warm blankets used as needed. For neonates and infants, the patient's temperature should be checked prior to scanning, and the case postponed if already cool (<36.5 °C) [8].

MRI scans can also increase a patient's temperature or induce burns [3, 9]. Burns are the most common MRI injury, comprising 70% of the adverse events reported in the 2008 Sentinel Event Alert [3]. RF and gradient fields induce electric currents in any conductive material, especially if arranged in loops. Any metal wires or cables, even in MR-safe or MR-conditional equipment, may prove a burn risk for patients. Care must be taken to prevent monitoring cables or wires from kinking or looping near the patient.

Ideally, all patients in MRI should have their temperature monitored. Practically, this is difficult, because standard thermistors used in operating rooms are ferromagnetic and thus incompatible with the MRI environment. Recently, fiberoptic temperature probes have been developed for use in MRI. Consider employing an approved temperature probe in any patient at risk for significant temperature variations (e.g. neonates), or for longer-duration scans.

## Projectiles/Missile Effect

The most potentially devastating risk in the MR scanner is injury from high-velocity projectiles. In powerful magnetic fields, objects containing ferromagnetic material will be strongly attracted to the field source, becoming hazardous high-velocity projectiles. This is particularly true with clinical MR scanners, which have enormously powerful static fields. Any ferromagnetic object approaching the scanner will be pulled towards the bore. For example, in a 2001 tragedy, a 6 year-old child was killed in the MR scanner when an MR-Unsafe oxygen cylinder was accidentally brought near the scanner, becoming a high-velocity missile that caused fatal cranial trauma [10]. Objects susceptible to the MR missile effect include: phones, pagers, scissors, ID badges, jewelry, keys, watches, laryngoscopes, stethoscopes, monitors, IV poles, chairs, medical gas cylinders, stretchers, wheelchairs, and ventilators.

To minimize the risk from ferromagnetic projectiles, protocols for screening all patients and personnel entering the scanner area must be carefully designed and rigorously enforced. The MRI medical director or technologist is responsible for screening and access to the scanner. The anesthesiologist must collaborate with radiology personnel to ensure that all anesthesiology staff and patients are adequately checked. Screening must be in-person and methodical, with vigilance for all ferromagnetic metal objects and all medical devices or implants. Handheld detectors are useful adjuncts, as are walk-through detectors mounted on the MR scanner room doorway.

## Emergencies

Emergency situations requiring special consideration in the MRI scanner include codes, intentional or unintentional quenching, and fires. MR suites should have formal documented plans for each of these emergencies. Codes must **not** be conducted in Zone IV (the MR scanner room). Instead, the patient must be emergently transferred back to Zone II. This is because necessary equipment (code cart, monitor, defibrillator) is generally MR-unsafe, and may malfunction or cause serious harm near the scanner. There are currently no MR-safe or MR-conditional external defibrillators available.

## Implanted Medical Devices

Implanted medical devices present an additional hazard in MRI. In magnetic fields, implanted devices can heat and cause burns, become dislodged, or malfunction transiently or permanently. Radiology technologists consult online or print manuals detailing the MR safety status of thousands of studied medical devices [11]. Since new devices are being introduced constantly, and MR protocols are modified over time, not all devices have been tested under all scanning conditions. Due to the immense variety of medical devices encountered, the anesthesiologist must never make assumptions regarding the safety profile of a patient's device.

Examples of medical devices of concern in MRI include: programmable VP shunts (should be re-programmed post-scan), spinal cord stimulators, epidural catheters (some have steel wire coils), intracranial aneurysm clips (most currently available are non-ferrous), cochlear implants, ossicular prostheses, orthodontics, tracheostomy tubes (most Bivona tubes contain metallic fibers; switch to Shiley tubes for MR scan), tissue expanders for plastic surgery, prosthetic heart valves, cardiac stents (most are OK), prosthetic joints, shrapnel, and tattoos with metallic dyes.

## Cardiovascular Implantable Electronic Devices (CIEDs)

CIEDs such as pacemakers and automated implantable cardioverters-defibrillators (AICDs) pose a risk in MRI [12]. Strong magnetic fields can make them heat or malfunction, or become dislodged. Previous recommendations stated that patients with CIEDs should avoid MRI, but new MR-conditional devices are being developed [13]. In most cases, such MR-conditional devices require the weaker 1.5 T scanners.

Patients with CIEDs must have their devices carefully screened prior to MRI, consulting institutional guidelines and available literature. Prior to MRI, pacemakers should be re-programmed to non-sensing (e.g. VOO) safe mode, and AICDs disabled. After the scan, devices should again be interrogated and re-programmed as necessary.

## Acoustic Noise

Functioning MR scanners are extremely loud (3 T scanners ~100 decibels), and there are reports of patient hearing loss after MRI. Loud sounds in the scanner may also increase patient anxiety. Every patient must utilize hearing protection such as earmuffs and/or earplugs, whether awake, sedated, or anesthetized.

## Pregnancy

There are no published reports of fetal damage from MRI, and research indicates that MRI is probably safe for the fetus, patient, and radiology personnel. However, the ACR discourages pregnant women from getting MR scans unless considered necessary, and only after carefully assessing the risks of waiting until the end of the pregnancy. Gadolinium-based contrast should be avoided during pregnancy unless absolutely necessary, as these agents can cross the placenta into the fetal circulation.

## Occupational Safety

There is scant evidence regarding occupational safety in the MR environment, but in general the electromagnetic fields appear to be much less concerning than ionizing radiation. There are some reports that MRI can rarely cause transient vertigo and nausea, likely due to interference with the vestibular system [14]. Overall, however, there is little evidence from either clinical or laboratory studies that there is any detrimental biological impact from exposure to clinically-relevant static 1.5 T or 3 T magnetic fields [6, 7].

## MRI: Contrast Enhancement

Enhancement of MRI images is often performed with gadolinium-based contrast agents. Free gadolinium is toxic, so for clinical use, gadolinium is chelated to organic compounds to promote renal excretion and minimize toxic free ion release into the patient's tissues. Current U.S. Food and Drug Administration (FDA)-approved gadolinium-based MRI contrast agents include Ablavar (gadofosveset), Dotarem (gadoterate), Eovist (gadoxetate), Gadavist (gadobutrol), Magnevist (gadopentetate), MultiHance (gadobenate), Omniscan (gadodiamide), OptiMARK (gadoversetamide), and ProHance (gadoteridol). Gadolinium-based contrast agents do not create an osmotic load, unlike iodinated radiocontrast used for CT. Clearance of these contrast agents is renal, so is reduced in neonates and infants and those with renal impairment.

Gadolinium-based contrast agents are considered safe in patients with healthy kidneys [15], but in patients with renal impairment, these agents can cause **nephrogenic systemic fibrosis** (NSF) [16]. While clinical features vary significantly, NSF features often include: skin thickening and rash, most often affecting the extremities, neuropathic pain, muscle weakness, conjunctivitis, and gastroenteritis. There are treatments, but no complete cure, and NSF can be fatal. Patients with a glomerular filtration rate (GFR) <30 mL/

min/1.73 m² should not receive gadolinium-based contrast agents. Since gadolinium agents are dialyzable, consider dialyzing patients with significant renal dysfunction immediately after contrast-enhanced MR scans.

Other reactions to gadolinium agents include rashes, hives, nausea, vomiting, and headache. There is a risk for profound anaphylaxis, although gadolinium is considered less allergenic than X-ray contrast. Often, contrast agents are injected quickly ("power injection"); maintain vigilance for intravenous catheter infiltration/extravasation.

Oral contrast enhancement is sometimes utilized for MR abdominal imaging to enhance the gastrointestinal tract. Consider rapid sequence induction (RSI) after oral contrast administration, or consider administering contrast via an orogastric tube after anesthesia induction and tracheal intubation.

## MRI: Anesthesia Equipment

A full array of routine (usually MR-unsafe) anesthesia equipment should be available in Zone II, including an anesthesia machine, airway equipment, vascular access supplies, monitoring equipment, medications, and convenient access to a fully-stocked code cart including monitor/defibrillator. Appropriate MR-conditional or MR-safe anesthesia equipment should also be available for use within the scanner room. Of particular concern is the ability to monitor the patient in the scanner, deliver medications with IV pumps, and deliver ventilation and volatile agents with anesthesia machines.

Patient monitoring in MRI requires specialized equipment that minimizes risk of burns and malfunction. MRI **ECG** systems are shielded to minimize RF interference, utilize non-ferrous carbon graphite electrodes, and may be wireless. Electromagnetic interference from the scanner often causes transient ECG artifacts, hindering detection of morphologic ECG changes. MR-safe **pulse oximeters** are fiber-optic and often wireless. Conventional pneumatic oscillometric **blood pressure** monitoring works fine in MRI, and systems without ferrous components are available for this environment. Invasive blood pressure monitoring is challenging but possible using conventional disposable transducers, utilizing high pressure, low compliance extension tubing to allow the transducer to remain far away from the scanner. Alternatively, there are completely non-ferrous transducers available that are MR-safe. Fiberoptic **temperature** probes are available. There are currently no pulmonary artery catheters approved for MRI.

Total intravenous anesthesia (TIVA) is often employed in MRI, but most commonly-used **intravenous infusions systems** are MR-unsafe. A few MR-conditional infusion pumps are available, or MR-unsafe pumps can be used by restricting them to Zone III and using extended intravenous tubing fed through a wave guide into the scanner room.

Regular laryngoscopes are MR-unsafe, but MR-conditional plastic laryngoscopes are available for emergency airway management in the scanner. Endotracheal tubes (ETTs) are safe in MR. Most laryngeal mask airways (LMAs) present no problems in the scanner, although some have a metal spring in the inflation valve that can mildly distort MR images. If used during a head or neck scan, tape the inflation valve as far away from the patient as possible. Bags of intravenous fluids, and intravenous fluid lines are safe. MR-safe medical gas cylinders are available, made of aluminum and clearly marked as MR-safe. Be aware, there are many reported incidents of damage and injuries (including death) caused by MR-unsafe gas cylinders mistakenly brought near the scanner. Other miscellaneous anesthesia equipment needs to be evaluated on a case-by-case basis before being used in Zone IV.

The development of MR-conditional anesthesia machines has simplified controlled ventilation and inhalational techniques for MRI. These machines contain only minimal amounts of ferromagnetic materials, being constructed mostly of plastic, aluminum, stainless steel, and brass. Both Dräger and GE/Datex-Ohmeda offer advanced MR-conditional anesthesia machines. Due to missile hazards, all servicing of MR anesthesia machines must be performed outside of the scanner room. This includes vaporizer changes, gas cylinder changes, and repairs. Open MR scanners produce different magnetic field geometries, so anesthesia machines that are approved for use with standard cylindrical MR scanners have not been approved for open MR scanners, even though the overall static field strengths are lower (0.35–1.2 T).

If an MR-conditional machine is not available, a standard MR-unsafe anesthesia machine can be employed, but must be restricted to the Zone III control room. In a setup that is somewhat cumbersome but functional, an elongated ventilation circuit is extended through a wave guide into the scanner room. Be aware that elongated circuits may have very high compliance, distorting the anesthesia machine's interpretation of ventilator pressures and volumes. Vigilance for adequate chest rise is required; don't rely on the anesthesia machine's report of tidal volumes. One advantage of this setup is that it allows for breath holds while the operator remains in Zone III.

## MRI: Indications

Common indications for MRI include: seizures (new, follow-up, or evaluation for epilepsy surgery), hydrocephalus, developmental delay, hypotonia, failure to thrive, hearing loss, nonaccidental injury, spinal cord compression, meningomyelocele, tethered cord, nerve lesions, tumors and staging, skeletal abnormalities, ENT abnormalities, vascular anomalies (aneurysms, hemangiomas, etc.), osteomyelitis, and cardiac or aortic disease.

Adult indications that may require anesthesia for an MRI include: claustrophobia, pain, anxiety, movement disorders, developmental delay, poorly controlled GERD, recent vomiting, inability to lie flat due to respiratory disease, or unstable airways. Additionally, most children under 8–10 years require anesthesia due to the inability to remain motionless for the long scan duration.

## MRI: Anesthesia Techniques

In MRI, anesthesiologists should demand the same level of safety, equipment, and monitoring as in the main operating rooms, as specified by the ASA Statement on Nonoperating Room Anesthetizing Locations [17]. One of the key oddities and risks of MRI is that the anesthesiologist will be physically separated from patient, with the patient poorly accessible in the scanner bore, and the anesthesiologist in the control room. Due to this limited access, excellent preparation and vigilance are warranted. Depending on the body parts imaged, MRI scans can requires 30 min to 3 h or more. The **goals** of anesthesia for MRI are patient safety, patient comfort, anxiolysis, facilitating proper positioning, and minimizing patient movement.

Prior to anesthesia induction, a time-out (aka procedural pause for safety/safety checklist) should be performed, including the usual patient identifiers, allergies, and verification of consent, but should also include the specific type of imaging being performed, site (body part), and results of metal and device screening. Patients for MRI require full ASA monitors [18]. For pre-procedure anxiolysis, consider midazolam IV or PO. For children, consider parental presence at induction for appropriately selected patients and caregivers.

Induction of anesthesia must occur in Zone II, where MR-unsafe equipment can safely be employed. Once safely anesthetized, the patient is transferred into the scanner room, positioned and padded carefully, ventilation tubing and intravenous tubing attached as necessary, ear protection applied, and monitors adjusted. As anesthetic issues arise during the scan, the anesthesiologist must determine whether each issue is urgent or minor. Urgent issues such as airway loss, IV infiltration, or cardiorespiratory compromise require immediate re-entry into the scanner room. Non-urgent minor tasks such as adjusting ventilator parameters or re-positioning a nasal cannula can usually wait a few minutes until the next available pause in imaging sequences.

Post-operatively, recovery care must conform to the same standards as in the ORs [13]. Ex-premature and young infants may require extended post-op stays due to an increased risk of apnea [19]. Ideally the Radiology suites have a dedicated recovery area, but transport to the operating room PACU is also acceptable.

In terms of anesthetic strategy, the first question is whether to employ sedation or general anesthesia. While this author prefers general anesthesia for most cases, opinions and practice vary widely between institutions. Malviya et al. examined sedation and anesthesia in children for MRI and CT [20], reporting that procedural failure, excessive motion, and hypoxemia occurred more frequently in children receiving sedation compared with general anesthesia. Other studies also show potential adverse events with moderate sedation or light anesthesia, including respiratory depression, oxygen desaturations, airway obstruction, agitation, and vomiting [21].

In terms of specific anesthesia technique, there remains little convincing data demonstrating the superiority of any specific anesthesia techniques over others in MRI. Many techniques have been used successfully [22, 23], and strategies vary tremendously based on the institution, the anesthesiologist, and the patient.

## Monitored Anesthesia Care/Sedation

Intravenous agents are preferred, because oral and intramuscular methods generally offer less predictable onset and depth of anesthesia, and possibly prolonged recovery time compared with IV medications. Specific agents to consider include: benzodiazepines, narcotics, dexmedetomidine, ketamine, and low-dose propofol. While chloral hydrate has been heavily used in the past, it currently is considered inferior to other agents due to adverse consequences such as airway obstruction, procedural failure, and prolonged sedation. Regardless of the agents utilized, vigilance for airway and respiratory complications must be maintained. It may be difficult to identify airway or respiratory issues due to the obstructed view of patient's head and chest, and it may take longer to remedy airway or respiratory issues due to the extra time required to unlock and enter the scanner room.

## General Anesthesia

For general anesthesia for MRI, the most common options are TIVA with propofol infusion and nasal cannula oxygen, or general anesthesia with an LMA or ETT. Considerations should include co-morbidities (especially airway risk) and duration of imaging procedure, since longer scans may require more airway protection due to patient fatigue, secretions, and airway obstruction.

Airway options include nasal cannula (with spontaneous ventilation), LMA (with spontaneous, assisted, or controlled ventilation), or an ETT (with assisted or controlled ventilation). If the scan requires breath holds (some cardiac, thoracic, and abdominal scans), then the best options are an LMA or ETT. If the scan requires oral contrast, then appropriate options include either a rapid sequence induction following contrast administration, or a standard induction followed by intubation and placement of an orogastric tube to allow contrast administration after securing the airway. All patients with increased suspicion for airway compromise should receive an LMA or ETT.

Agents for general anesthesia in MRI include most standard intravenous and volatile agents. For TIVA, the most commonly employed agent is **propofol** (50–150 µg/kg/min for adults, 100–300 µg/kg/min for children) [24]. With its rapid onset and recovery, easy titration, and reliable loss of consciousness, propofol can provide an effective, safe TIVA with spontaneous ventilation, especially in children. In adults, it may be more challenging to find an appropriate therapeutic window allowing both adequate anesthesia and spontaneous ventilation. **Dexmedetomidine** preserves respiratory drive, but can cause moderate cardiovascular fluctuations, and may not be quite as reliable as propofol. Ketamine is cardio-stable and preserves respiratory drive, but can cause hallucinations or nightmares. **Narcotics** are used only rarely in MRI, for pre-existing pain. Use caution in patients with native airways and nasal cannulas, as narcotics can cause significant respiratory depression. If an LMA or ETT is employed, then **volatile agents** may be used. Sevoflurane is the most common agent, due to its minimal airway stimulation. Desflurane is not available on MR-compatible machines due to its extra wiring.

For **children** with uncomplicated airways, our most common strategy is TIVA with propofol and nasal cannula. After induction, the airway and respiratory drive are re-assessed. Mild airway obstruction can often be mitigated by a shoulder roll, head re-positioning, or placement of an oral airway. If spontaneous ventilation appears unlikely to succeed, an LMA or ETT is placed. If an advanced airway is used, anesthesia maintenance can be achieved with TIVA, mixed volatile and IV agents, or volatiles alone. For children with potentially complicated airways (young neonates, severe OSA, airway anomalies), the primary strategy is LMA or ETT.

For **adults**, our most common strategy is an LMA, due to the high rate of airway obstruction under anesthesia in adults. Due to limited access to the patient's airway during the scan, obstruction cannot be relieved via simple manual jaw thrust (as would often be utilized during other nasal cannula cases such as colonoscopy). Thin, healthy adult patients may succeed with nasal cannula airway, but we find that the majority merit LMAs.

## Infant Immobilizers

In many cases, young infants can be swaddled to achieve a natural sleep and consequent lack of movement [25]. Vacuum papoose systems offer a great mechanism for achieving high-quality scan images without requiring sedation or general anesthesia [26]. A special airtight bean bag is swaddled around the infant patient and secured, effectively locking the infant in position, but doing so comfortably, akin to traditional swaddling. This concept works best on babies 3 months old or younger, and is most successful if used approximately 30–45 min after feeding, which encourages the infant to sleep naturally.

## Cardiovascular MRI

Cardiovascular MRI is used to image the heart and great vessels. Cardiac MRA is used to study pressure gradients, flows, and volumes. These techniques often require ECG gating, in which the image sequencing is synchronized to the patient's cardiac cycle. Breath holds may also be required, to minimize image artifacts from pulmonary excursion, necessitating LMA or ETT placement. Consider muscle relaxation to minimize patient movements and optimize image gating. Extra vigilance for screening is required, due to a higher incidence of implanted devices in cardiac patients.

## MRI: Intraoperative MRI

A relatively new twist on MR imaging is intraoperative MRI. This venue must be treated with extra caution like all MRI facilities. Essentially, this is an OR suite, with a built-in MR scanner housed in an adjacent room. The MR scanner is utilized intermittently during neurosurgical procedures, to verify adequacy of tissue excision, or identify landmarks intraoperatively. Either the magnet is moved towards the patient, or the patient is transported to the adjacent scanner. Vigilant screening of all personnel & patients prior to entry is required. This special OR must be "MR-equipped" with no ferromagnetic devices. Only MR-safe and MR-conditional equipment is acceptable during scans. Ideally, this special suite is physically separated from the main ORs, to facilitate screening.

## CT: Basics

Like MRI, the CT suite presents some unique challenges that must be recognized and overcome to allow for safe anesthesia care. Anesthesiologists caring for adult or pediatric patients in the CT suite must be familiar with the underlying physics of CT scanners and the effects of ionizing radiation on their patients and themselves. Safety issues and techniques for sedation and general anesthesia are presented.

## CT: Physics and Radiation

CT scanners employ an X-ray tube that rotates axially around the patient, taking a series of X-ray images from numerous different angles. A computer then uses this data to calculate tomographic cross-sectional images. CT measures tissue electron density (X-ray attenuation) to differentiate between high-density tissues (bone, calcium, bone, iron, and contrast-enhanced areas) and lower-density tissues (water, muscle, fat, and air).

X-rays are high-frequency electromagnetic radiation that carry energy that displaces electrons from their atoms in a process called ionization. Biologically, ionizing radiation can directly or indirectly damage DNA. Undifferentiated or highly mitotic cells are most susceptible to ionizing radiation, placing at risk tissue such as the epidermis, eye lens, bone marrow, thymus, and gonads. This causes cell damage or death, leading to a wide range of problems including radiation burns, teratogenesis, cataracts, and sterility. Damaged DNA can also eventually lead to cancer.

The danger from CT scanners is invisible and painless, and thus difficult to acutely appreciate. The radiation dose from one CT scan is 100–1000 millirem, equivalent to 10–100 chest X-rays. These high radiation exposures are of particular concern in pediatric patients, as CT scans have been shown to increase the risk of leukemia and brain tumors [27]. In 2011, the Joint Commission released a Sentinel Event Alert regarding the radiation risks of diagnostic imaging [28], declaring that physicians should ensure the "right test" (consider non-ionizing radiation if possible, e.g. ultrasound or MRI) and "right dose" (minimize radiation dose), and promote a culture of safety. Anesthesiologists should work closely with radiologists and CT technologists to ensure that ionizing radiation doses are "as low as reasonably achievable", to minimize risk to both the patient and staff.

Unlike MRI, the CT environment does not place constraints on equipment. Rather, it requires radiation protection for the anesthesiologist. Ionizing radiation exposure is inversely proportional to the square of the distance from the source (inverse-square law). Radiation sources include: direct radiation from scanner beams, scatter radiation from patient, and leaked radiation from scanner.

## CT: Safety

Use lead shielding for patients as feasible, especially around reproductive organs. If possible, anesthesiologists should remain outside the scanner room, in the control room, watching anesthetized patients and monitors through the control window. If the anesthesiologist must stay in the scanner room, they should don a wraparound lead apron, lead jacket, thyroid shield, and leaded eyeglasses, and remain as far from the scanner bore as feasible. Consider mobile radiation barriers, made of transparent leaded acrylic, placed between the anesthesiologist and the scanner. The anesthesiologist should wear a radiation badge (dosimeter) to monitor dose accrual over time.

## CT: Physical Layout

To restrict the spread of ionizing radiation, CT scanner rooms are lined with lead, and the control room has large lead-infused windows to allow for direct visualization of patients from the safety of the control room. If anesthesia is to be performed, the CT scanner room should have built-in wall gas lines, vacuum suction, and available electric outlets. CT scanners are smaller than MR scanners, with shorter bores that only mildly inhibit access to the patient.

## CT: Contrast Enhancement

Enhancement of CT images is often performed with radiopaque contrast agents, to improve visualization of vascular structures and tissue differentiation. These iodine-based agents have a high rate of adverse events, up to 5%, including anaphylaxis, hypersensitivity/anaphylactoid reactions, thyroid dysfunction, and kidney injury [29, 30], with serious morbidity in approximately 1 per 1000 patients. The highest rate of adverse reactions are with older, high-osmolar contrast agents. Recently approved low-osmolar and iso-osmolar agents offer considerably improved safety profiles. Patients with a history of previous anaphylactoid reaction may benefit from pre-treatment with steroids and histamine blockers 1 h prior to contrast. If an anaphylactic reaction is suspected, call for assistance, ensure adequate monitoring, and administer oxygen, fluids, antihistamines, steroids, bronchodilators, and epinephrine as needed.

Radiocontrast agents can be nephrotoxic, causing acute kidney injury, aka contrast-induced nephropathy (iatrogenic acute renal failure). This effect is dose-dependent, so anesthesiologists should consult with radiologists to minimize the dose. Rates of contrast-induced nephropathy are much higher in patients with pre-existing renal disease (GFR <30 mL/min/1.73 $m^2$) [30]. Anesthesiologists should check renal function preoperatively. Radiocontrast agents are hypertonic relative to plasma, thus may cause transient hypertension, followed by a hyperosmotic diuresis.

Gastrointestinal imaging studies may employ oral contrast enhancement with diatrizoate agents such as Gastrografin. This water-soluble agent at full strength is quite hypertonic (3%), and pulmonary aspiration of this highly osmotic fluid may be dangerous. It is preferable to use diluted agent (1.5%, isotonic), which has a lower risk of aspiration sequelae. Typically, the CT scan is performed 1 h after ingestion of the oral contrast agent. Even though Gastrografin likely qualifies as a clear fluid, this still violates standard NPO guidelines, so consider a rapid sequence induction, or consider administering contrast via orogastric tube after anesthesia induction and tracheal intubation.

## CT: Anesthesia Equipment

A full array of anesthesia equipment should be available in the CT scanner room, including an anesthesia machine, airway equipment, vascular access supplies, monitoring equipment, medications, and convenient access to a fully-stocked code cart including monitor/defibrillator. Many CT anesthetics utilize TIVA, so an infusion pump may be useful. Standard monitors, anesthesia machines, infusion pumps, gas cylinders, laryngoscopes, and other equipment can be safely used in the CT suite without risk of electromagnetic interference or injury. Both the anesthesiologist (if remaining in the CT room during scanning) and the patient (as applicable) should wear lead shielding.

## CT: Indications

Indications for CT scan include intracranial hemorrhage, mental status changes, encephalopathy, cranial trauma, seizures, focal neurologic abnormalities, airway abnormalities, headache, visual defects, hydrocephalus, tumors and staging, bone lesions, soft tissue lesions, abscesses and cysts, mediastinal mass, and foreign bodies.

Most adults and children will not require anesthesia for CT scan, due to the quick duration of the imaging procedure, usually only a few minutes. However, anesthesia may still be needed for patients with young age (<3–5 years), significant anxiety or claustrophobia, positional pain, movement disorders, developmental delay, neurologic impairment, complex or fragile cardiorespiratory problems, or if breath holds are requested (e.g. for chest CT).

## CT: Anesthesia Techniques

Anesthesia for CT follows most of the same principles as for MRI (see above). However, CT scans are much shorter than MRI, usually lasting 2–10 min depending on body parts imaged and the need for contrast. Just like for MRI, patients for CT require full ASA monitors, and should receive the same fully-resourced care as in the operating suites. Inhibition of patient movement is particularly important during contrast-enhanced scans, because these images cannot be easily repeated, due to maximum contrast dose restrictions.

As with MRI, this author recommends general anesthesia over sedation for most CT cases. For children, our most common technique is mask induction, followed by intravenous catheter placement. TIVA is initiated with propofol and nasal cannula, the patient positioned and secured to the scanner gantry, and the anesthesiologist retreats to the control room for the brief duration of the scan. Patients with OSA may require an oral airway. Alternatively, sevoflurane can be used; the patient can be mildly hyperventilated via mask immediately prior to the scan. After verifying that the recorded images are satisfactory, the patient is emerged and taken to recovery.

Cases requiring breath holds are facilitated via LMA placement, to allow manual control of ventilation during the scan (while wearing full protective gear). A few patients, such as those with unstable airways or vomiting, may require endotracheal intubation.

Specific agents are similar to those recommended for MRI (see above). Propofol and dexmedetomidine are excellent intravenous agents, and sevoflurane is useful for mask induction and maintenance. Narcotics are only rarely needed.

Many invasive procedures are performed under CT guidance, such as biopsies, drain placements, and ablations. For these procedures, the anesthesiologist generally needs to remain in the scanner room, and should wear appropriate lead protection. CT-guided procedures take much longer than simple CT scans, lasting 30–120 min. Positioning is potentially cumbersome, lateral or prone positioning may be required, and the CT gantry table is narrow and hard. While many such cases can be performed safely with nasal cannula, most will require LMA or ETT placement to better secure the airway.

Special concern is required for patients with known or suspected mediastinal mass. The mass may acutely compromise thoracic vascular and pulmonary structures, with potentially catastrophic consequences for the patient. The best plan is to maintain spontaneous ventilation and cardiorespiratory status quo.

While regional anesthesia is not useful for standard CT imaging, it may be appropriate for invasive CT image-guided procedures. For example, peripheral nerve blocks for procedures on the extremities, or intercostal blocks for lung biopsies or biliary stent placements.

## References

1. Metzner J, Posner KL, Domino KB, et al. The risk and safety of anesthesia at remote locations: the US closed claim analysis. Curr Opin Anaesthesiol. 2009;22:502–8.
2. Expert Panel on MR Safety, Kanal E, Barkovich AJ, Bell C, et al. ACR guidance document on MR safe practices: 2013. J Magn Reson Imaging. 2013;37:501–30.
3. The Joint Commission. Preventing accidents and injuries in the MRI suite. Sentinel Event Alert, Issue 38; 14 Feb 2008. http://www.jointcommission.org/assets/1/18/SEA_38.pdf. Accessed 24 March 2017.
4. ASTM International. Standard practice for marking medical devices and other items for safety in the magnetic resonance environment. Designation: F2503-13. West Conshohocken; 2013.
5. Philbin MK, Taber KH, Hayman LA. Preliminary report: changes in vital signs of term newborns during MR. AJNR Am J Neuroradiol. 1996;17:1033–6.
6. International Commission on Non-Ionizing Radiation Protection, Vecchia P, Hietanen M, Ahlbom A, et al. Guidelines on limits of exposure to static magnetic fields. Health Phys. 2009;96:504–14.
7. Hartwig V, Giovannetti G, Vanello N, et al. Biological effects and safety in magnetic resonance imaging: a review. Int J Environ Res Public Health. 2009;6:1778–98.
8. Dalal PG, Porath J, Parekh U, et al. A quality improvement project to reduce hypothermia in infants undergoing MRI scanning. Pediatr Radiol. 2016;46:1187–98.
9. Brown TR, Goldstein B, Little J. Severe burns resulting from magnetic resonance imaging with cardiopulmonary monitoring: risks and relevant safety precautions. Am J Phys Med Rehabil. 1993;72:166–7.
10. Martinez J, Ferraro S, Siemaszko C. Freak MRI accident kills W'Chester boy. New York Daily News; 31 July 2001.
11. Shellock FG. Reference manual for magnetic resonance safety, implants and devices: 2015 edition. Los Angeles: Biomedical Research Publishing Group; 2015.
12. Levine GN, Gomes AS, Arai AE, et al. Safety of magnetic resonance imaging in patients with cardiovascular devices: an American Heart Association scientific statement from the Committee on Diagnostic and Interventional Cardiac Catheterization, Council on Clinical Cardiology, and the Council on Cardiovascular Radiology and Intervention. Circulation. 2007;116:2878–91.
13. Practice advisory on anesthetic care for magnetic resonance imaging: an updated report by the American Society of Anesthesiologists Task Force on

Anesthetic Care for Magnetic Resonance Imaging. Anesthesiology. 2015;122:495–520.
14. Roberts DC, Marcelli V, Gillen JS, et al. MRI magnetic field stimulates rotational sensors of the brain. Curr Biol. 2011;21:1635–40.
15. Prince MR, Arnoldus C, Frisoli JK. Nephrotoxicity of high-dose gadolinium compared with iodinated contrast. J Magn Reson Imaging. 1996;6:162–6.
16. Marckmann P, Skov L. Nephrogenic systemic fibrosis: clinical picture and treatment. Radiol Clin North Am. 2009;47:833–40.
17. ASA Statement on nonoperating room anesthetizing locations. Approved by the ASA House of Delegates on October 19, 1994, and last amended on October 16, 2013. Schaumburg: American Society of Anesthesiologists.
18. ASA Standards on basic anesthetic monitoring. Approved by the ASA House of Delegates on October 21, 1986, last amended on October 20, 2010, and last affirmed on October 28, 2015. Schaumburg: American Society of Anesthesiologists.
19. Coté CJ, Zaslavsky A, Downes JJ, et al. Postoperative apnea in former preterm infants and inguinal herniorrhaphy: a combined analysis. Anesthesiology. 1995;82:809–22.
20. Malviya S, Voepel-Lewis T, Eldevik OP, et al. Sedation and general anaesthesia in children undergoing MRI and CT: adverse events and outcomes. Br J Anaesth. 2000;84:743–8.
21. Sanborn PA, Michna E, Zurakowski D, et al. Adverse cardiovascular and respiratory events during sedation of pediatric patients for imaging examinations. Radiology. 2005;237:288–94.
22. De Sanctis Briggs V. Magnetic resonance imaging under sedation in newborns and infants: a study of 640 cases using sevoflurane. Pediatr Anesth. 2005;15:9–15.
23. Heard C, Harutunians M, Houck J, et al. Propofol anesthesia for children undergoing magnetic resonance imaging: a comparison with isoflurane, nitrous oxide, and a laryngeal mask airway. Anesth Analg. 2015;120:157–64.
24. Wu J, Mahmoud M, Schmitt M, et al. Comparison of propofol and dexmedetomedine techniques in children undergoing magnetic resonance imaging. Pediatr Anesth. 2014;24(8):813.
25. Antonov NK, Ruzal-Shapiro CB, Morel KD, et al. Feed and wrap MRI technique in infants. Clin Pediatr. 2016. https://doi.org/10.1177/0009922816677806.
26. Golan A, Marco R, Raz H, et al. Imaging in the newborn: infant immobilizer obviates the need for anesthesia. Isr Med Assoc J. 2011;13:663–5.
27. Pearce MS, Salotti JA, Little MP, et al. Radiation exposure from CT scans in childhood and subsequent risk of leukaemia and brain tumours: a retrospective cohort study. Lancet. 2012;380:499–505.
28. The Joint Commission. Radiation risks of diagnostic imaging. Sentinel Event Alert, Issue 47; 24 Aug 2011. http://www.jointcommission.org/assets/1/18/SEA_47.pdf. Accessed 24 March 1973.
29. Andreucci M, Solomon R, Tasanarong A. Side effects of radiographic contrast media: pathogenesis, risk factors, and prevention. Biomed Res Int. 2014;2014:741018.
30. Davenport MS, Cohan RH, Ellis JH. Contrast media controversies in 2015: imaging patients with renal impairment or risk of contrast reaction. AJR Am J Roentgenol. 2015;204:1174–81.

# Radiotherapy and Anesthesia

Bharathi Gourkanti, David Mulvihill, Jill Kalariya, and Yue Li

## Introduction

Radiation oncologists use externally or internally directed photons or charged particles (e.g. protons) to target tumor cells for a variety of cancers in pediatric and adult populations [1–3]. The need for immobility in order to avoid damage to healthy tissues is paramount, and may be difficult to achieve without sedation or anesthesia in children, patients with anxiety, or patients with disease-specific conditions that may make immobility difficult (e.g. high respiratory rate, pain with prolonged immobility) [4]. Furthermore, insertion of internal radiation seeds, or brachytherapy, can be painful and would require analgesia and sedation or anesthesia [3, 5].

Anesthesia for radiation therapy becomes a unique challenge to the anesthesiologist in a number of ways. In order to optimize healing of healthy cells, the total radiation therapy is fractionated into several therapy sessions, requiring multiple anesthetics. The anesthesiologist is required to safely plan each session carefully in order to minimize or avoid harm. The anesthesiologist is also challenged by the location of radiation suites. Radiation suites can be far from operating theaters, and in the case of proton therapy, a stand-alone building. Furthermore, anesthesiologists are far from the patient during treatment as healthcare providers are required to be out of the radiation suite.

This chapter starts with an introduction to radiation oncology relevant to the anesthesiologist. Then, anesthetic goals and management are detailed, focusing on external beam radiation, brachytherapy .and intraoperative radiation therapy. Finally, complications of radiation therapy affecting future anesthetics will be described.

## Radiation Therapy

### Overview

An estimated 1/3 of patients including children diagnosed with cancer will require radiation therapy at some point during their lifetime, alone or in combination with chemotherapy and surgery. While survival from childhood cancers increased significantly and the use of therapeutic radiation for pediatric malignancies decreased in recent decades, radiation therapy is still utilized in treatment of many pediatric solid tumors [6–8]. Utilizing radiation in the management of childhood cancer presents unique challenges.

B. Gourkanti, M.D. (✉) · J. Kalariya, M.D.
Y. Li, M.D.
Department of Anesthesiology, Cooper University Hospital, Camden, NJ, USA
e-mail: gourkanti-bharathi@cooperhealth.edu; kalariya-jill@cooperhealth.edu; li-yue@cooperhealth.edu

D. Mulvihill, M.D.
Department of Radiation Oncology, Cooper University Hospital, Camden, NJ, USA
e-mail: mulvihill-david@cooperhealth.edu

Radiation therapy must be delivered with high accuracy and precision to a clearly defined target to avoid irradiating normal tissues and structures which often lie in proximity to the tumor. Achieving this level of accuracy and precision in a pediatric patient necessitates extra time, effort and resources beyond that which is required for a compliant adult patient [9].

## Therapeutic Radiation

Radiation can be classified as ionizing or nonionizing. Ionizing radiation can disrupt the atomic architecture of a cell and cellular DNA. In the therapeutic setting, radiation is delivered either by particle (electrons, protons, neutrons) or photon (X-rays, gamma rays). Radiation dose (Table 26.1) is based on factors including therapeutic intent (palliative versus curative), radiosensitivity or resistance of a tumor, and radiation tolerance of surrounding normal tissues and structures. The total dose to a tumor is frequently broken up into smaller daily doses. Fractionation allows for dose to be delivered within a therapeutic window so that normal tissues and cells are able to repair the damage from ionizing radiation.

**Table 26.1** Radiation for pediatric tumors

| Tumor | Dose (Gy) | Number of treatments |
|---|---|---|
| CNS | | |
| Craniopharyngioma | 54 | 30 sessions |
| Ependymoma | 54–60 | 30–33 sessions |
| Germinoma | 45–50 | 25–27 sessions |
| Low grade glioma | 45–54 | 25–30 sessions |
| Medulloblastoma | 54 | 30 sessions |
| Retinoblastoma | 42–45 | 21–25 |
| Extremity/thoracic | | |
| Rhabdomyosarcoma (high risk) | 36–50.4 | 20–28 sessions |
| Osteosarcoma (inoperable) | 60–75 | 30–37 sessions |
| Ewing sarcoma (definitive) | 55.8 | 31 |

Some examples of childhood solid tumors and the associated radiation dose and number of treatment sessions required to treat

## Treatment Planning and Delivery

Radiation therapy is typically delivered in an outpatient setting, although it can be delivered to an inpatient while in an emergent situation such as spinal cord compression, SVC syndrome, or as palliation for intractable pain from metastatic disease. The radiation oncologist will determine the clinical need and appropriateness for therapy. The next step involves patient simulation in the treatment position. During simulation, patient is placed in the treatment planning position and immobilized, which is reproduced during subsequent treatment sessions, so as to minimize motion of the target volumes and normal structures to ensure the accuracy and precision of treatment. The imaging scan is reviewed by the radiation oncologist and the tumor volume is identified and contoured, and a treatment plan is devised [10]. Features of a plan include radiation modality (particle or photon), beam angles, treatment time, tumor dose, and dose to normal structures. The patient then undergoes daily treatments, utilizing the same setup and immobilization as employed in the simulation.

## Immobilization

Patient immobilization is critical in ensuring the accuracy, precision, and reproducibility of radiation treatments (Fig. 26.1). A compliant adult patient is typically able to tolerate immobilization devices, and able to cooperate with instructions to remain still. However, in the pediatric setting, not all patients are able to comprehend or cooperate with instruction, and immobilization becomes much more of a challenge. Underscoring the need for patient immobilization is a host of potential treatment-related side effects from radiation therapy. Toxicities from treatment in the pediatric patient may include endocrinologic consequences such as growth-hormone deficiency, hypothyroidism, diabetes, and gonadal disorders including infertility [11, 12]. Additionally, pediatric patients are perhaps even more susceptible to risk of secondary malignancy owing to the fact that their organ systems are still

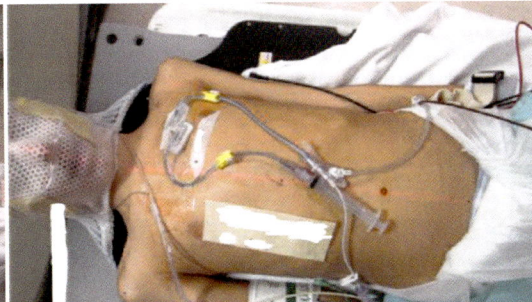
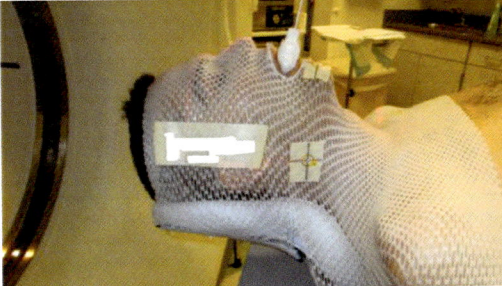
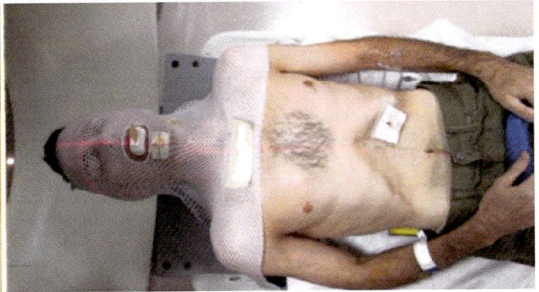

**Fig. 26.1** A patient undergoing radiotherapy with the head immobilized in a personalized device

undergoing development and therefore more vulnerable to damage [13]. In a review of pediatric patients treated at Indiana University Health Proton Therapy Center, it was found that 100% of patients aged 3 and under required anesthesia/sedation for radiation therapy. While this number decreased with increasing patient age, pediatric patients aged 13 and older still required anesthesia/sedation in 10% of the cases [14]. Another study estimated that 57% of children aged 3–12 years and 62.3% of children aged 5–8 years required daily anesthesia for radiation therapy [15]. Duration of anesthesia/sedation will depend on duration of treatment. Treatment for Ewing sarcoma could be as long as 31 fractions delivered over greater than 6 weeks, whereas preventative cranial irradiation for pediatric leukemia may be as short as ten fractions delivered over 2 weeks [16]. Certain treatment modalities, such as proton therapy, require elaborate setup and thereby consume more time. One report estimated the median time under anesthesia to be 49.7 min, with a range of 30–90 min [17]. Despite the complexities associated with pediatric anesthesia/sedation in the delivery of therapeutic radiation, the largest reported series of repetitive anesthesia/sedation in this population reported only a 0.0074% occurrence of medical events in a series of patients treated over 4 years [17].

"Pediatric patient undergoing CT simulation for radiation therapy planning. An aquaplast head mask is used for immobilization of the cranium and neck. Wrist restraints are used to prevent upper extremity motion, while a leg rest and foot block are utilized to maintain lower body immobilization and position. Vital signs are continuously monitored while the patient is under anesthesia, and IV access and oxygen administration are likewise maintained."

## Anesthetic Goals

Anesthetic goals for radiotherapy include adequate anxiolysis, sedation, analgesia, and immobility. Anxiolysis should be provided for patients because they are in an unfamiliar environment and will be kept alone in the treatment area due to occupational hazards of radiation to the providers. Due to discomfort during positioning, immobilization devices, especially those applied to the face and head, claustrophobia, and altered mental status or preexisting developmental delay. There have also been reports of unusual odor during radiotherapy of the brain [18–20]. Implantation or removal of radioactive material during brachytherapy can be painful and therefore patients should be given analgesia [18]. There is a need for accurate positioning and immobility of patients to direct external beam radiation precisely to destroy the targeted tissue while avoiding damage to healthy tissues surrounding the area. Another reason for immobility is during brachytherapy when an applicator for administration of radioactive substance is implanted [18, 19].

## Anesthetic Management for External Beam Radiotherapy

External beam radiotherapy is painless, so adults can tolerate it without any anesthesia. Anesthesia is usually required for children, especially younger children, and adults with developmental delays, altered mental status, and other comorbidities that preclude immobility.

### Pre-procedure

Evaluation of the patient begins with a thorough identification of comorbidities and complications from the cancer and cancer treatments. For example, intracranial space occupying lesions for radiotherapy should focus on identifying signs and symptoms of raised intracranial pressure like nausea, vomiting, and altered sensorium. This should alert the anesthesiologist to prepare for ICP monitoring if clinically indicated and methods to reduce ICP preoperatively [20].

Children with raised intra-abdominal pressure (e.g. Wilms tumor) and patients with concomitant chemotherapy induced nausea and vomiting [19] should be give aspiration prophylaxis in the preoperative period. These patients would benefit from rapid sequence induction for general anesthesia. Evaluation by consultants should be sought if side effects of cytotoxic or immunosuppressive chemotherapy is suggested [20]. Cardiopulmonary toxicity and sepsis may present unique challenges during anesthesia. Children undergoing repeated radiation sessions may need permanent central venous access [19].

Pediatric patients may be fearful of the treatment area and staff members. Special attention may be required to adequately prepare them for the simulation and treatment sessions. Some centers take older children to the Proton Beam Therapy (PBT) facility to help alleviate anxiety and improve familiarity. A child friendly environment recognizes, encourages and supports the emotional and physiologic needs of children. Environmental modification by the use of cartoon painted mask, bedding and body fixtures can have a great impact on the patient experience [21].

### Intra-procedure

A unique challenge to the anesthesiologist is the radiotherapy room. The room is sealed with a large leaded door, and the patient is isolated limiting access and monitoring. For appropriate monitoring, a video camera should focus on the patient and additional camera on the monitor [19]. An interfaced system of closed-circuit television and telemetric microphones is used along with standard ASA monitoring [22]. In the event of a problem, shutdown of the radiation beam and immediate access to the patient (within 20–30 s) is crucial [20].

The radiation suite itself has unique equipment and machinery that can be a physical barrier, limiting the access to the patient. Immobilization devices that are applied to the face and head cause limited access to the airway [20]. It is useful to have a checklist like the one in Table 26.2.

The anesthetic technique has to be individualized to each patient with modifications determined by the procedure and comorbidities. Additional considerations include the ability to access and secure the airway during the procedure; risk of aspiration; ability to remain supine and motionless for extended periods of time; and conditions such as obstructive sleep apnea, COPD, and congestive heart failure. Clear communication is essential between the

**Table 26.2** Procedural checklist for anesthesia management [23]

| |
|---|
| **Pre-procedure:** Anesthesia consultation, cardiology/pulmonary consultation if required and Informed consent |
| **Personnel:** Anesthesiologist, Radiation oncologist, Radiation therapists, Nurse, Family member |
| **Establish:** Proper anesthetic plan, Ease of intravenous access, Risk of aspiration, Location and adequacy of recovery room, Back-up plan for transfer or admission to hospital |
| **Monitoring of the patient:** ECG, Pulse oximetry, NIBP, $EtCO_2$, Temperature, Two Closed circuit cameras—one for patient and one for monitor |
| **Airway:** Oxygen supply, tubing, A self-refilling Bag-valve mask, Oral and nasal airways, Tongue blade, Laryngeal mask, Intubation equipment, Suction |
| **Intravenous management:** All necessary drugs for anesthesia and resuscitation, Intravenous supplies (tubing, normal saline, pole, syringes etc.), Automated syringe pump (e.g. for controlled continuous infusion of intravenous anesthetic agent) |
| **Standby:** Anesthetic drug cart, Difficult airway cart, Cardiac arrest cart, Anesthesia machine |
| **Miscellaneous:** Safety belt, Sliding board, Stretcher, Blankets |

Modified from Clinical Oncology (2001) 13:416–421
*ECG* electrocardiography, *NIBP* non invasive blood pressure, $EtCO_2$ end tidal $CO_2$

anesthesiologist and the radiation therapist regarding the anticipated length of procedure, level of procedural stimulation and pain, patient positioning, need for patient cooperation, and recovery [24].

There is currently no anesthetic technique that is clearly superior, and the same procedure may be performed under light sedation, or a general anesthetic, depending on patient characteristics or procedural concerns.

Sedation with Dexmedetomidine in radiotherapy is not common. This is most likely due to a 10-min loading dose and relatively frequent need for repeated boluses [25]. Single-dose IV ketamine 0.5–0.8 mg/kg provides effective sedation, but with a greater half-life and more adverse effects (e.g., vomiting) than propofol [26]. In cases like retinoblastoma, deep sedation with propofol or general anesthesia is needed to keep the eye immobile, ensuring appropriate radiating conditions. Ketamine, with its side effect of lateral nystagmus, is not appropriate in these cases [26]. General Anesthesia (GA) may be provided as Inhalational anesthesia or Total Intravenous Anesthesia (TIVA).

## Monitoring

All anesthetics should comply with the ASA Standards for Basic Anesthetic Monitoring [27]. Monitoring of exhaled carbon dioxide should be considered for all patients receiving sedation because of the difficulty of monitoring adequacy of ventilation in patients once the imaging equipment and drapes have been positioned [28]. Patient access and visual monitoring can be challenging because of the significant distance from the patient and the obstruction by the imaging equipment. The anesthesia machine must be far enough away to not interfere with the movement of equipment, so extensions on the intravenous tubing, oxygen supply, and ventilator tubing are commonly required. Backup equipment, especially adjunct airway devices, oxygen, and other resources, should be readily available in the event of an unexpected difficult airway [24].

## Post-procedure

The recovery of patients undergoing conscious sedation and general anesthesia should be consistent with the standards of postanesthesia care set forth by the ASA [29]. A discussion between the anesthesia provider and the radiologist about the patient's recovery needs should take place before the procedure so appropriate arrangements can be in place [24]. There should be adequate staffing and monitoring for the patient when being transported to PACU with supplemental oxygen and monitors until complete recovery [19]. Patients are discharged according to the standard discharge criteria of the hospital.

## Anesthesia for Brachytherapy

Brachytherapy is administered by inserting a radiation source inside a specific cancer site. Both the insertion and removal of the implant requires some form of anesthesia. Local anesthetics are often used when administering brachytherapy, although this can be painful for the patient and lead to suboptimal placement due to patient movement. Sedation can be administered without the anesthesia staff, but this should be done with caution as the inherent side effects of medications such as respiratory depression should be monitored closely for patient safety. Sedation has the benefit of providing the patient with more analgesia [18, 30, 31].

Regional anesthesia techniques, including spinal, epidural, combined spinal epidural (CSE), and caudal can be used when targeting the inferior half of the body. Advantages of these techniques when compared to local anesthesia and sedation include complete analgesia when using spinal or epidural, immobility under spinal anesthesia, increased patient satisfaction, and safe transport of patients [18]. The onset of spinal anesthesia is rapid and termination of effect can be reasonably predicted [30]. Once in place, an epidural catheter offers the benefit of being used later when the applicator is being removed [30]. A CSE combines the advantages of using the spinal component while the epidural can be used for extended analgesia [18]. Caudal epidural blocks have been used for gynecological brachytherapy, though it has been shown to provide an inferior level of analgesia compared to other regional anesthetics and be difficult in placement especially in the obese population. Contraindications to neuraxial anesthesia including patient refusal, infection in the area, bleeding diathesis and anticoagulation should be followed.

General anesthesia (GA) can be used in populations where indicated. This includes when regional is contraindicated, location of brachytherapy is in the upper body, or those unable to tolerate sedation or a local anesthetic. GA can be an option for all brachytherapy cases. GA requires the necessary equipment, including ventilator, airway devices, and appropriate monitoring. Transport of patient to MRI while under general anesthesia may be necessary, and MRI-compatible equipment should be available.

## Anesthesia for Radiation Beam Therapy

Beam radiation can be performed on the patient daily for weeks. An important component is precise positioning; radiation should target the exact same area on the skin, which is marked using tattoos. Molds masks and immobilizers are used to minimize damage to surrounding tissues. Moderate or deep sedation can be adequate in both adults and children provided a patent airway can be established. It is ideal to monitor vital signs more frequently (every 2 min) during the induction of moderate to deep sedation. The anesthesia provider must keep in mind that face mask immobilizers may limit access to the airway. General anesthesia can be performed when moderate or deep sedation is inadequate due to patient positioning, airway protection, muscle paralysis requirement (such as in retinoblastoma), or other indications. When GA is provided, care must be taken to make sure anesthesia equipment including ventilator do not interfere with the X-ray beam and that all extensions are long enough.

## Anesthesia for Intraoperative Radiation Therapy (IORT)

IORT is commonly used in breast-conserving surgery for the treatment of breast carcinoma. Formerly, anesthetized patients were transported from operating room to the location of linear accelerator. Nowadays, mobile accelerators are transported to the OR to deliver radiation, thereby eliminating the need to transport the patient. The benefit of IORT is the ability to irradiate tumor margins immediately after surgically removing the tumor while the patient is under general anesthesia, thus eliminating the need for delayed treatment in adjuvant settings and shortened course of treatment (min vs.

# 26 Radiotherapy and Anesthesia

**Table 26.3** Advantages and disadvantages of anesthetic techniques

| Type of anesthesia | Advantages | Disadvantages |
|---|---|---|
| Local | May be done by the radiotherapist if anesthesia staff unavailable | Analgesia may be inadequate<br>Patient immobility may be inadequate |
| Sedation | May be done by the radiotherapist if anesthesia staff unavailable | Analgesia may be inadequate |
| | Sedation may be useful for applicator removal | If performed by a radiotherapist, may need assistance if the patient has respiratory depression |
| Regional | Useful for procedures of lower body | Patient must be an appropriate candidate (e.g. no coagulopathy) for spinal/epidural |
| | In a functioning epidural or spinal block, provides adequate analgesia | Lengthy procedures may outlast a spinal or single shot epidural block |
| | Easy to safely transport especially if the anesthesia provider needs to bring the patient immobilized to a scanner or treatment room | |
| | Few complications | |
| | Epidural catheters left in place allow for use during applicator removal | |
| General | Immobility and analgesia requirements easily met | Requires full anesthesia equipment/ventilator, which may be unavailable if scans in other areas of the hospital must be performed |
| | Must be done for certain cases such as upper body | |
| | Fewer complications | |

With permission from Out of Operating Room Anesthesia, Springer Nature

weeks). The anesthetic technique of choice is general endotracheal anesthesia with/without muscle relaxation [32].

Unique issues here are described below:

1. Moving the mobile accelerator into the OR and appropriately aligning the accelerator with the surgical field requires communication, planning and coordinated actions of members of all the teams.
2. Because of radiation hazard to the OR personnel, all personnel must exit the OR prior to delivery of the dose.
3. Monitoring the patient from outside the OR may be done by turning patient monitor toward hallway or displaying vital signs on the monitors outside OR [32].

## Repeated Sedation

Tachyphylaxis is a phenomenon which describes an acute rapid decrease in responses to a drug which is known to occur with repeated IV anesthetic administration. Patients require increased doses to achieve the same effect. Repeated general anesthesia carries risks of airway complications such as trauma to vocal cords and trachea (which can result in tracheal stenosis). Other complications include oral/dental injuries, corneal damage (exposure keratitis), and positioning-related neuropathies. Children requiring daily anesthesia for radiation therapy also have the risk of nutritional deficits due to NPO status until time of procedure; this paired with effects of radiation, malignancy itself, and chemotherapy can cause malnutrition, anorexia, and malaise.

The advantages and disadvantages of anesthetic techniques are summarized on Table 26.3.

## Radiation Safety

### Safety of Healthcare Providers from Radiotherapy (Radiation)

When patients receive radiation therapy, the safety of healthcare workers is a priority. Today, almost all facilities that offer radiation therapy have established guidelines to prevent unnecessary radiation exposure to their workers. Regular monitoring of the healthcare worker and the facility is now the norm whenever radiation therapy is offered to the patients. Overall, people who work in the radiation therapy department are exposed to low levels of radiation. In practice, any amount of radiation exposure is considered harmful, but at very low exposure, the estimated increase in risk is minimal.

Unfortunately, medical experts cannot seem to agree on how much chronic radiation is safe. The health effects of radiation may occur after months or years of chronic exposure. In every country, there is a regulatory board that sets the amount of radiation that health care workers can receive. Most countries follow the US guidelines established by the OSHA (Occupational Safety and Health Administration). The amount that healthcare workers can be exposed to per calendar quarter in Rem (a unit of effective absorbed dose of ionizing radiation in human tissue, equivalent to one roentgen of X-rays) is as follows:

1. Whole body—1¼
2. Hands, forearms, feet and ankles—18¾
3. Skin of the entire body—7½

During any calendar quarter, the radiation dose to the workers shall not exceed 3 Rems [33].

A more practical radiation exposure limited is defined by the NCRP (National Council on Radiation Protection and Measurements) #91/116. This whole body exposure limit is defined as 50 mSv/year. Individual organs such as the lens (150 mSv/year) and the hands (500 mSv/year) can tolerate slightly higher doses of radiation. In reality, however, most radiation workers are exposed to approximately 2 mSv/year. A Sievert is a unit of measurement designed to measure the health effects of low levels of ionizing radiation. It is expressed in Joules/kg.

Some healthcare providers go by rules set as ALARA (as low as reasonably achievable) [34]. This agency states that no amount of radiation is safe and that every possible precaution should be taken to prevent radiation exposure in healthcare workers.

Healthcare workers take extreme precautions to prevent unnecessary radiation exposure. In most hospitals, the following protective measures are recommended to limit radiation exposure:

1. Wearing lead gloves and aprons
2. Installing lead plated glass that acts as a barrier wall. This allows the doctor to see the patient while at the same time minimizing exposure to radiation
3. Addition of lead strips during the radiation procedure
4. Standing at a safe distance from the radiation source
5. Performing the radiation treatment in room with protective walls
6. Wearing radiation badges that can calculate the amount of radiation dose one has been exposed to

It is important to understand that despite these precautions, some amount of radiation exposure will pass through. That is why healthcare facilities now make sure that all healthcare workers should wear radiation badges (Dosimeter) during the workday. This badge collects and records the amount of radiation exposure received by the healthcare worker. After every 3 months, the badge is analyzed and if the total amount of radiation exposure is more than the recommended dose, then the healthcare worker is pulled off the radiation department for a few months [34, 35].

## Complications

There are two types of complications. Radiation related and anesthesia related as shown in the table [36]. Sepsis may be caused by catheter (central line) related bloodstream infection in immunocompromised patients or due to chemo-radiation induced leukopenia. Respiratory complications include airway obstruction, laryngospasm, apnea, and desaturation. Hemodynamic complications include tachycardia and hypotension. Tachyphylaxis

**Table 26.4** Complications of radiation therapy

| Anesthesia related | Radiation related |
|---|---|
| Respiratory | General |
| Cough, Wheeze, Desaturation, Airway obstruction, Laryngospasm, Bronchospasm, Apnea, Aspiration pneumonitis, Trauma/Tracheal stenosis from repeated intubations | Fever, Sepsis, Malaise, Hair loss, Skin itching, dryness, blistering, Secondary malignancies |
| Cardiac | Site-specific |
| Hypotension, Hypertension, Bradycardia, Tachycardia, Arrhythmias | Head & neck: Dry mouth, gum sores, trismus, dysphagia |
| Drug related: Anaphylaxis, Tachyphylaxis | Chest: Dyspnea, dysphagia, radiation pneumonitis, radiation fibrosis |
| Positioning related: Peripheral nerve damage | Abdomen: anorexia, nausea, vomiting, diarrhea |
| Postoperative nausea vomiting | Pelvis: rectal bleed, incontinence, bladder irritation |

due to repeated administration of IV anesthetics such as propofol and ketamine (vs. volatile agents do not) [29]. Damage from repeated intubations has a potential for tracheal stenosis over time (can be avoided with MAC or LMA).

Study conducted by Anghelescu et al. showed that significant risk factors for anesthesia related complications are duration of procedure, total propofol dose, the use of adjunct agents with propofol (opioids, benzodiazepines and/or ketamine) and simulation (vs. radiation therapy). Simulations require a greater total dose of propofol and longer anesthesia time than radiation therapy sessions [1]. Study conducted by Vivek Verma et al. showed that rates of anesthetic complications during radiation therapy are similar to anesthetic complications during controlled operating room setting, referring that anesthesia for pediatric radiation therapy is safe. Lowest anesthetic complications happened during propofol infusion and oxygen delivery via nasal cannula [4]. The complications of radiation therapy are summarized in Table 26.4.

## Summary

Anesthesia for radiation therapy presents with a unique set of challenges to the anesthesiologist. Hazards of ionizing radiation, limited access to the patient and airway, and remote locations are among the many concerns. Anesthesiologists are often called to provide care for children and adult patients with claustrophobia, altered mental status and mental retardation. Good communication with the radiation therapist and advanced individualized planning are imperative to provide safe anesthesia in a demanding environment.

## References

1. Anghelescu DL, Burgoyne LL, Liu W, et al. Safe anesthesia for radiotherapy in pediatric oncology: St. Jude Children's Research Hospital Experience, 2004–2006. Int J Radiat Oncol Biol Phys. 2008;71(2): 491–7.
2. Mahmoud M, Mason KP. Anesthesia and sedation for pediatric procedures outside the operating room. In: Davis PJ, Cladis FP, editors. Smith's anesthesia for infants and children 9th ed. Philadelphia: Elsevier; 2017. p. 1035–1054.e5.
3. Barnett KM, Lu AC, Tollinche LE. Anesthesia and radiotherapy suite. In Goudra BG, Singh PM (eds). Out of operating room anesthesia: A comprehensive review. 1st ed. New York: Springer; 2017. p. 347–55.
4. Verma V, Beethe AB, Leriger M, et al. Anesthesia complications of pediatric radiation therapy. Pract Radiat Oncol. 2016;6(3):143–54.
5. Smith MD, Todd JG, Symonds RP. Analgesia for pelvic brachytherapy. Br J Anaesth. 2002;88(2):270–6.
6. Latham GJ. Anesthesia for the child with cancer. Anesthesiol Clin. 2014;32(1):185–213.
7. Hess CB, et al. Exposure risks among children undergoing radiation therapy: considerations in the era of image guided radiation therapy. Int J Radiat Oncol Biol Phys. 2016;94(5):978–92.
8. Gibbs IC, Tuamokumo N, Yock TI. Role of radiation therapy in pediatric cancer. Hematol Oncol Clin North Am. 2006;20(2):455–70.

9. McMullen KP, Kerstiens J, Johnstone PA. Practical aspects of pediatric proton radiation therapy. Cancer J. 2014;20(6):393–6.
10. Spiotto MT, Connell PP. Strategies to overcome late complications from radiotherapy for childhood head and neck cancers. Oral Maxillofac Surg Clin North Am. 2016;28(1):115–26.
11. Coura CF, Modesto PC. Impact of late radiation effects on cancer survivor children: an integrative review. Einstein (Sao Paulo). 2016;14(1):71–6.
12. Bereket A. Endocrinologic consequences of pediatric posterior fossa tumours. J Clin Res Pediatr Endocrinol. 2015;7(4):253–9.
13. Kamran SC, et al. Therapeutic radiation and the potential risk of second malignancies. Cancer. 2016;122(12):1809–21.
14. McMullen KP, et al. Parameters of anesthesia/sedation in children receiving radiotherapy. Radiat Oncol. 2015;10:65.
15. Scott MT, et al. Reducing anesthesia and health care cost through utilization of child life specialists in pediatric radiation oncology. Int J Radiat Oncol Biol Phys. 2016;96(2):401–5.
16. Halperin EC. Pediatric radiation oncology. New York: Raven Press; 1989. p. xii, 434p.
17. Buchsbaum JC, et al. Repetitive pediatric anesthesia in a non-hospital setting. Int J Radiat Oncol Biol Phys. 2013;85(5):1296–300.
18. Barnett KM, Lu AC, Tollinche LE. Anesthesia and radiotherapy suite. In: Goudra BG, Singh PM, editors. Out of operating room anesthesia: a comprehensive review. Cham: Springer; 2017. p. 347–55.
19. Diaz CD, Luther RC. Pediatric anesthesia in the radiology suite. In: Weiss MS, Fleisher LA, editors. Nonoperating room anesthesia. Philadelphia: Elsevier Saunders; 2015. p. 161–70.
20. Souter KJ, Pittaway AJ. Nonoperating room anesthesia (NORA). In Barash PG, Cullen BF, Cahalan RK, et al. (eds). Clinical Anesthesia. 7th edition. Philadelphia: Lippincott Williams and Wilkins; 2013. p. 885–6.
21. Mizumoto M, Oshiro Y, Ayuzawa K, et al. Preparation of pediatric patients for treatment with proton beam therapy. Radiother Oncol. 2015;114:245–8.
22. McFadyen GJ, Pelly N, Orr RJ. Sedation and anesthesia for the pediatric patient undergoing radiotherapy. Curr Opin Anaesthesiol. 2011;24:433–8.
23. Tsang RW, Solow HL, Ananthanarayan C, et al. Daily general anaesthesia for radiotherapy in uncooperative patients: ingredients for successful management. Clin Oncol. 2001;13:416–21.
24. Rubin D. Anesthesia for ambulatory diagnostic and therapeutic radiology procedures. Anesthesiol Clin. 2014;32:371–80.
25. Shukry M, Ramadhyani U. Dexmedetomidine as the primary sedative agent for brain radiation therapy in a 21-month old child. Paediatr Anaesth. 2005;15:241–2.
26. Pradhan DG, Sandridge AL, Mullaney P, et al. Radiation therapy for retinoblastoma: a retrospective review of 120 patients. Int J Radiat Oncol Biol Phys. 1997;39:3–13.
27. American Society of Anesthesiologists. Standards for basic anesthetic monitoring. Last amended 20 Oct 2010. Available at http://www.asahq.org/For-Members/Standards-Guidelines-and-Statements.aspx.
28. Lightdale JR, Goldmann DA, Feldman HA, et al. Microstream capnography improves patient monitoring during moderate sedation: a randomized, controlled trial. Pediatrics. 2006;117:e1170–8.
29. American Society of Anesthesiologists. Standards for postanesthesia care. Last amended 1 Oct 2009. Available at http://www.asahq.org/For-Members/Standards-Guidelines-and-Statements.aspx.
30. Roessler B, Lucia S, Gustorff B. Anaesthesia for brachytherapy. Curr Opin Anaesthesiol. 2008;21(4):514–8.
31. Lim KH, Lu JJ, Wynne CJ, et al. A study of complications arising from different methods of anesthesia used in high-dose-rate BT for cervical cancer. Am J Clin Oncol. 2004;27:449–51.
32. Kathryn M, Glynn MD, Adam I, Riker MD. Anesthetic considerations for intraoperative radiation therapy. Ochsner J. 2015;15(4):438–40.
33. United States Department of Labor. Occupational safety and health standards/toxic and hazardous substances. Washington, DC: Occupational Safety and Health Administration (OSHA); Regulations (Standards - 29 e-CFR - 1910.1096).
34. Agency for Toxic Substances and Disease Registry (ATSDR). Public health statement for ionizing radiation. Atlanta: U.S. Department of Health and Human Services, Public Health Service; 1999.
35. Association of Surgical Technologists. AST standards of practice for ionizing radiation exposure in the perioperative setting, Littleton; 2010.
36. Seiler G, Vol ED, Khafaga Y, et al. Evaluation of the safety and efficacy of repeated sedations for the radiotherapy of young children with cancer: a prospective study of 1033 consecutive sedations. Int J Radiat Oncol Biol Phys. 2001;49(3):771–83.

# Anesthesia for Office Based Cosmetic Procedures

## Sally S. Dawood and Michael Stuart Green

## Introduction

Office based anesthesia (OBA) is defined as the administration anesthesia services in an out of hospital setting which is not an accredited ambulatory surgical center. OBA differs from non-operating room anesthesia (NORA) in that NORA typically takes place outside of the operating room but still within a hospital facility.

The trend towards OBA for cosmetic procedures has been growing steadily in the past decade. The American Society of Aesthetic Plastic Surgery reported that outpatient cosmetic procedures increased over 400% in the period between 19970 and 2007 [1]. In the USA, $15 billion were spent on aesthetic cosmetic procedures in 2016, with surgical procedures accounting for 56% of the total expenditures [2].

## Patient Selection

The selection of patients who are appropriate for OBA can be controversial topic. Ideally, patients who are ASA physical status 1 or 2 are the best candidates. These patients still require preoperative evaluation, consent and any laboratory evaluation prior to procedure as deemed necessary by anesthesia staff [3]. The real dilemma is created by ASA 3 and 4 patients with complex medical history and multiple comorbidities. The anesthesiologist should have a preoperative evaluation including history and physical examination within a 30 day period, necessary laboratory work, medical consultation and clearance along with the feasibility to reach out to the patient for any perioperative optimization for the patient's condition [4].

Patients that are generally not recommended for OBA include patients experiencing severe respiratory symptoms, history of adverse reactions to local anesthetics, history of substance abuse, potentially difficult airway, significant drug allergies, and patients with aspiration risk, morbid obesity [5], obstructive sleep apnea and susceptibility to malignant hyperthermia [6]. Anesthesiologists performing OBA still need case-by-case selection and exclusion of certain patients according to the availability of trained personnel and equipment within the office-based setting.

## Office Facilities

As anesthesiologists are keen patient advocates, the anesthesia team should be certain that the extent of the procedure, the training credentials of the surgeon and the presence of trained

S. S. Dawood, M.D.
M. S. Green, D.O., M.B.A.
Department of Anesthesiology and Perioperative Medicine, Drexel University College of Medicine, Philadelphia, PA, USA
e-mail: Michael.Green@Drexelmed.edu

**Table 27.1** Types of office based procedures performed in the USA

| Surgical procedures | | Nonsurgical procedures | |
|---|---|---|---|
| Liposuction | 414,335 | Botulinum toxin | 4,597,886 |
| Breast augmentation | 310,444 | Hyaluronic acid | 2,494,814 |
| Tummy Tuck | 181,540 | Hair removal | 1,035,783 |
| Eyelid surgery | 173,883 | Photorejuventation | 657,172 |
| Breast lift | 161,412 | Chemical peel | 616,225 |

personnel available for immediate help in case of emergencies are readily available. The surgeon or practitioner must have enough training or board certification for the performed procedures, and must be eligible to perform the same procedures in accredited hospitals.

Safe administration of anesthesia in an office setting is no different than anywhere else in terms of preparation, equipment stocking and maintenance. ASA monitors should be readily available at all times including temperature, capnography, non-invasive blood pressure cuffs of different sizes, heart rate and pulse oximetry. A variety of airway devices should be accessible and office staff should be trained to support. The office setting should have a variety of nasal cannulas, oral and nasal airways, self-inflating masks, different sizes and types of laryngoscopes and endotracheal tubes, different sizes of LMA, suction, emergency airway kits. A variety of medications including anesthetics medications, ACLS medications and a malignant hyperthermia kit may need to be present if triggering agents are to be utilized.

## Procedures

From a simple facial filler to liposuction, cosmetic office-based procedures are increasing in popularity for patients, surgeons and anesthesiologists due to their convenience, easier scheduling, improved patient care and privacy, and significantly contained expenses along with the newer less invasive cosmetic procedures and safer anesthetic techniques [7, 8]. This all contributes to an increase in complexity of the procedures performed and an increase in the number of patients with more complex comorbidities undergoing anesthesia in an office-based setting rather than in a hospital-based setting.

Examples of cosmetic procedures performed in the office setting include abdomen reduction, circumferential body lift, liposuction, breast augmentation, reduction and lift, Botox injections, dermabrasion, wrinkle treatment, facial contouring, laser hair removal, blepharoplasty and rhinoplasty.

The top five procedures performed in 2016 as stated by the American Society for Aesthetic Plastic Surgery (Table 27.1) [2].

## Anesthetic Management and Techniques

With increased complexity of procedures, the choice of anesthetic technique has progressed from sedation to general and regional anesthesia. The ASA has mandated the use of end tidal capnography for moderate and deep sedation cases and encouraged for lighter levels of sedation. The choice between sedation and general anesthesia can sometimes be controversial, and different studies have alternatingly favored one over the other. Sedation and general anesthesia have low complication rates and favorable safety profiles with experienced providers [9, 10]. Although general anesthesia can require more preparation and training, it is still considered the optimum airway management technique.

The choice of intravenous anesthetics is variable and based largely on user discretion. Propofol, fentanyl, ketamine, benzodiazepines and others have been used widely alone or in combinations in OBA. Although occasionally they have been implicated with abuse and morbidity and mortality, care should be exercised for side effects and safety profile.

An increasing number of anesthesia providers are utilizing the combination of ketamine and propofol, under the name ketofol. No standard dose exists but the combination has been most studied at a 1:1 ratio. Ketamine provides a more stabile hemodynamic profile, while the propofol offsets the sympathomimetic effects of ketamine. Ketofol provides adequate sedation and analgesia with the added benefit of the non-emetogenic properties of propofol [11, 12].

The combination of benzodiazepines and ketamine is another popular combination. This combination is short acting, has minimal cardiac and respiratory depression and reduced PONV. The benefit is especially significant when given as an adjunct with propofol and no added opiates [13, 14]. One study used intravenous diazepam and low dose ketamine to provide dissociative anesthesia allowing for local anesthetic injection found very favorable results regarding analgesia and PONV [15].

The use of local anesthetics in regional anesthesia provides outstanding postoperative pain management with minimal airway manipulation in combination with sedation and is considered as an excellent choice for OBA [7]. The choice can be tailored for each procedure with multiple options. Local infiltration at the surgical site for rhinoplasty, anterior intercostal nerve blocks for breast surgery, or posterior intercostal blocks done bilaterally for abdominoplasty [16] are all reasonable options. Although intercostal nerve blocks have been avoided due to complications such as pneumothorax and local anesthetic toxicity, it has been shown that the abovementioned complication rate is minimal once the technique is mastered [16]. These techniques are mostly combined with sedation and occasionally with general anesthesia, to minimize the need for parenteral opioids.

Tumescent anesthesia is another common anesthetic technique than can be administered in an office setting. Its use has expanded form abdominal liposuction to other procedures such as breast surgery and segmental liposuction. Tumescent anesthesia involves the injection of a very diluted local anesthetic, such as lidocaine (0.05–0.1%), usually mixed with epinephrine (1:100,000) with a dose ranging between 35 and 40 mg/kg of lidocaine [17, 18]. The injected fluid is around 3–4 mL per expected aspirated fat volume. The regional anesthesia achieved with the tumescent technique accompanied with IV sedation or to a lesser extent general anesthesia provides excellent anesthesia without the added risk of IV narcotics [18]. Local anesthetic toxicity and volume overload are still significant concerns regarding the tumescent technique, but a high margin of safety without added risk of hypervolemia or rate of local anesthetic toxicity has been proven [5, 17]. The range of bleeding in tumescent anesthesia is less than 1% of the aspirated volume [19].

Liposuction is the most commonly performed surgical procedure in the office setting. Deposits of fats underneath the skin are removed via cannulas inserted through small incisions with the assistance of a powerful vacuum. There are different types of liposuction; dry, wet, super wet and the most common type tumescent liposuction. When liposuction is performed and a small volume is removed related adverse events are rare, however aspiration of a large volume, mostly more than 4 L, can be associated with more adverse effects [19]. During tumescent anesthesia hemodynamic changes associated with the large volume liposuction include an increased heart rate, mean pulmonary arterial pressure, stroke volume index and cardiac index. These increases are associated with a decrease in mean arterial blood pressure and systemic vascular resistance with no significant change in central venous pressure [20]. The raised cardiac index is contributed to epinephrine levels and hemodilution. Hypothermia is another major concern and has been associated with liposuction of large volumes and longer surgical duration.

During longer procedures and high volume liposuction accounting for the infiltrated and aspirated tumescent fluid is crucial. In managing intraoperative fluids occasionally invasive monitoring such as central venous pressure monitoring and invasive arterial pressure monitoring may be needed if large fluid shifts are expected. Intraoperative fluid volume ratio, defined as the infiltrated plus intravenous fluids divided by aspirated fluid, should be calculated and kept at a ratio around 1.2 for large volume liposuction more than 5 L to prevent dehydration or fluid overload [21]. Liposuction has been associated with several complications including hypervolemia, hypothermia, pulmonary edema, fat embolus, abdominal viscera perforation and local anesthetic toxicity. Patient positioning can vary according to the areas being liposuctioned, so the anesthesiologist must be vigilant with protection of pressure points, nerves prone to injury, and eyes, ears, and nose as they must be properly protected and padded [19].

Airway management and maintaining oxygenation in rhinoplasty and rhytidectomy can be challenging especially with electrocautery. An interesting technique was developed using a 16 Fr. Levin stomach tube that is threaded through a No. 7 NPA or a Berman OPA and then attached to a universal adaptor with oxygen source. The patient's oxygenation and saturation can be controlled through oxygen flow and can be interrupted whenever needed [16].

Facial cosmetic surgery can range from surgical procedures on the eyelid, nose surgery, fat transfer to the face and face lift to non-surgical procedures such as photorejuvenation, chemical peel and injectables like Botulinum toxin or hyaluronic acid. Facial cosmetic surgery occasionally entails providing anesthesia without direct constant access to the patient's airway, which can make response to respiratory complications challenging for the anesthesiologists. Moderate controlled hypotension and local anesthetics with epinephrine infiltration to the surgical field can be used to ensure a clear surgical field, which is crucial for facial surgeries due to the high vascularity of these regions as even a tiny amount of bleeding can hinder the surgical exposure [22].

Choice of anesthetic management for facial cosmetic procedures varies from sedation with local anesthetic infiltration to general anesthesia using endotracheal tube or laryngeal mask airway. Although occasionally deeper levels of sedation can be needed to ensure patient immobility and optimal surgical conditions. Emergence from anesthesia after facial cosmetic procedures should be smooth to prevent patient staining and to prevent hematoma formation [23]. Topical anesthetics like EMLA cream have been used effectively for providing analgesia in non-surgical facial cosmetic procedures examples being chemical peeling or photorejuvenation [24].

## Special Considerations

Morbidly obese patients are a growing population that seeks cosmetic procedures in the office setting. This population poses a different set of physiological and pathological challenges. These patients have obesity related comorbidities such as hypertension, hyperlipidemia, diabetes mellitus, obstructive sleep apnea, venous stasis and gastroesophegeal reflux disease which place them at an elevated risk [25]. Extreme care and vigilance with positioning of the patient should be performed with all equipment ready for anticipated difficult intubation along with adequate prophylaxis for venous thromboembolism [5].

Obstructive sleep apnea (OSA) poses a challenge to the anesthesiologist in the office-based setting. The mainstay of diagnosis of OSA is overnight polysomnography and measuring the hypopnea index. This is defined by measuring the number episodes of apnea and hypopnea lasting more than 10 s/h. Since OSA is often under diagnosed, a survey questionnaire to screen for patients at risk for OSA should be used. The STOP BANG questionnaire is one of the most commonly utilized. The STOP BANG questionnaire looks for symptoms such as snoring, tiredness, observed apnea by others and high blood pressure along with patient criteria like body mass index >35 kg/m$^2$, age more than 50 years old, neck circumference more than 15 in. and male gender [26].

OSA patients carry perioperative risks like upper airway obstruction that may lead to hypercapnia and hypoxia, respiratory depression, arrhythmias, hypertensive episodes, pulmonary hypertension, myocardial infarction, stroke and increase sensitivity to opioids [26]. Multimodal use of different analgesics to minimize the use of opioids is generally recommended for OSA patients [27]. The most conventional treatment of OSA is continuous positive airway pressure (CPAP), which can improve the associated respiratory and cardiovascular adverse effects. CPAP can be applied intraoperatively but studies have shown that approximately 30% of OSA patients are intolerant to CPAP [28]. Anesthesiologist should be zealously cautious on selecting patients suffering from OSA for anesthesia in an office based setting. It is generally recommended that patients suffering from severe OSA are not appropriate for OBA.

Elderly patients are an increasing population due to the relative longevity and because of the safer anesthesia techniques. More are presenting for OBA for cosmetic surgeries [5]. One should bear in mind that although the procedure may be considered minimal and noninvasive, the complex physiology of the elderly population could be challenging and lead to added morbidity.

Pulmonary embolism and deep vein thrombosis prophylaxis are known complications. The use of sequential compression devices, early ambulation, avoidance of hypervolemia, with identification of risk factors of coagulopathy, such as oral contraceptives, should all be employed [3].

Postoperative nausea and vomiting (PONV) is a major concern in the office settings as it causes patient discomfort, delay in discharge and increases the overall cost of the procedure. PONV is usually an underestimated complication following office based procedures. Risk assessment for PONV prophylaxis and treatment, as stated by Apfel et al., should never be overlooked for patients scheduled for elective emetogenic surgery such as cosmetic procedures lasting more than 2 h [29]. Studies have shown that PONV rate is related to the duration of anesthesia, particularly if more than 4 h [30]. Risk factors for PONV include female gender, history of motion sickness or PONV, non smoking, use of nitrous oxide or desflurane and use of opioids [31].

As PONV etiology is multifactorial, ranging between the patient's demographics, medical condition, and type and length of surgery, the prophylaxis must be always multimodal. Prophylactic agents vary between the traditional mainstays of PONV prophylaxis like serotonin receptor antagonists, dexamethasone, anticholenergics, droperidol and metoclopramide along with the non-traditional antiemetics like clonidine, propofol and supplemental oxygen [32]. Aprepitant, a newer antiemetic, is a selective high affinity antagonist to substance P and neurokinin-1 receptors. Aprepitant has been studied for PONV prophylaxis and showed reduction in the rate of immediate PONV when administered 1 h preoperatively [33]. Most studies have shown that the rate of PONV is decreased if risk factors are avoided and the appropriate prophylaxis is utilized [32].

## Patient Safety

OBA is a vastly expanding anesthetic subspecialty taking place in a setting that is very different from where most anesthesiology training occurs. Hence, the anesthesiologists recently joining OBA practice can face some difficulties when they become the sole anesthesiologist in an office setting. Safety precautions and setting are often different than training provided. Currently, only 2% of anesthesia residency training programs provides adequate OBA training [7, 16].

While OBA throughout the past decade has proven its higher safety margin, studies have shown that OBA safety profile is comparable to an accredited surgical center or hospital [34, 35]. The American Association for Accreditation of Ambulatory Surgery Facilities conducted a study with over 400,000 procedures, of which 63% were cosmetic surgeries, over 5-year period. The overall anesthesia related mortality was five cases. The causes of death were cardiac arrest, tension pneumothorax, cerebral hypoxia, stroke and one case of unexplained death [34]. Worth noting, the studies conducted only surveyed accredited surgical offices. Adverse events in those offices may not have been completely documented. Currently, only 27 states have regulations for OBA by one of the major organizations responsible for accrediting a surgical office including, the accreditation Association for Ambulatory Health Care, the American Association for Ambulatory Surgical Facilities and the Joint Commission for Accreditation of Healthcare Organizations (JCAHO) [36].

# References

1. Shapiro FE. Anesthesia for outpatient cosmetic surgery. Curr Opin Anaesthesiol. 2008;21(6):704–10.
2. Surgery TASfAP. Cosmetic surgery national data bank statistics 2016. Available from: https://www.surgery.org/sites/default/files/ASAPS-Stats2016.pdf.
3. Hunstad JP, Walk PH. Office-based anesthesia. Semin Plast Surg. 2007;21(2):103–7.
4. Weaver JM. The safety of both fixed and transportable office-based anesthesia for dentistry. Anesth Prog. 1999;46(1):1–2.
5. Ellsworth WA, Basu CB, Iverson RE. Perioperative considerations for patient safety during cosmetic surgery – preventing complications. Can J Plast Surg. 2009;17(1):9–16.
6. Shapiro FE, Punwani N, Rosenberg NM, Valedon A, Twersky R, Urman RD. Office-based anesthesia: safety and outcomes. Anesth Analg. 2014;119(2):276–85.
7. Hausman LM, Frost EA. Office-based surgery: expanding the role of the anesthesiologist. Middle East J Anaesthesiol. 2007;19(2):291–310.
8. Spring MA, Stoker DA, Holloway J, Weintraub M, Stevens WG. Office-based plastic surgery with general anesthesia: efficiency of cost and time. Semin Plast Surg. 2007;21(2):99–101.
9. Bitar G, Mullis W, Jacobs W, Matthews D, Beasley M, Smith K, et al. Safety and efficacy of office-based surgery with monitored anesthesia care/sedation in 4778 consecutive plastic surgery procedures. Plast Reconstr Surg. 2003;111(1):150–6; discussion 157–8.
10. Johnson PJ. General anesthesia in an office-based plastic surgical facility: a report on more than 23,000 consecutive office-based procedures under general anesthesia with no significant anesthetic complications. Arch Facial Plast Surg. 2001;3(4):287.
11. Friedberg BL. Propofol in office-based plastic surgery. Semin Plast Surg. 2007;21(2):129–32.
12. Friedberg BL. Propofol ketamine anesthesia for cosmetic surgery in the office suite. Int Anesthesiol Clin. 2003;41(2):39–50.
13. Vinnik CA. Dissociative anesthesia in an office-based plastic surgery practice. Semin Plast Surg. 2007;21(2):109–14.
14. Friedberg BL. Propofol-ketamine technique. Aesthetic Plast Surg. 1993;17(4):297–300.
15. Quttainah A, Carlsen L, Voice S, Taylor J. Ketamine-diazepam protocol for intravenous sedation: the cosmetic surgery hospital experience. Can J Plast Surg. 2004;12(3):141–3.
16. Blake DR. Office-based anesthesia: dispelling common myths. Aesthet Surg J. 2008;28(5):564–70; discussion 571–2.
17. Wang G, Cao WG, Li SL, Liu LN, Jiang ZH. Safe extensive tumescent liposuction with segmental infiltration of lower concentration lidocaine under monitored anesthesia care. Ann Plast Surg. 2015;74(1):6–11.
18. Klein JA. Tumescent technique for regional anesthesia permits lidocaine doses of 35 mg/kg for liposuction. J Dermatol Surg Oncol. 1990;16(3):248–63.
19. Sood J, Jayaraman L, Sethi N. Liposuction: anaesthesia challenges. Indian J Anaesth. 2011;55(3):220–7.
20. Kenkel JM, Lipschitz AH, Luby M, Kallmeyer I, Sorokin E, Appelt E, et al. Hemodynamic physiology and thermoregulation in liposuction. Plast Reconstr Surg. 2004;114(2):503–13; discussion 514–5.
21. Rohrich RJ, Leedy JE, Swamy R, Brown SA, Coleman J. Fluid resuscitation in liposuction: a retrospective review of 89 consecutive patients. Plast Reconstr Surg. 2006;117(2):431–5.
22. Nekhendzy V, Ramaiah VK. Prevention of perioperative and anesthesia-related complications in facial cosmetic surgery. Facial Plast Surg Clin North Am. 2013;21(4):559–77.
23. Beer GM, Goldscheider E, Weber A, Lehmann K. Prevention of acute hematoma after face-lifts. Aesthetic Plast Surg. 2010;34(4):502–7.
24. Iannitti T, Capone S, Palmieri B. Short review on face rejuvenation procedures: focus on preoperative antiseptic and anesthetic delivery by JetPeel-3 (a high pressure oxygen delivery device). Minerva Chir. 2011;66(3 Suppl 1):1–8.
25. Byrne TK. Complications of surgery for obesity. Surg Clin North Am. 2001;81(5):1181–93; vii–viii.
26. Ganzberg S. Obstructive sleep apnea and office-based surgery. Anesth Prog. 2016;63(2):53–4.
27. Joshi GP, Ankichetty SP, Gan TJ, Chung F. Society for Ambulatory Anesthesia consensus statement on preoperative selection of adult patients with obstructive sleep apnea scheduled for ambulatory surgery. Anesth Analg. 2012;115(5):1060–8.
28. Tan KB, Toh ST, Guilleminault C, Holty JE. A cost-effectiveness analysis of surgery for middle-aged men with severe obstructive sleep apnea intolerant of CPAP. J Clin Sleep Med. 2015;11(5):525–35.
29. Apfel CC, Korttila K, Abdalla M, Kerger H, Turan A, Vedder I, et al. A factorial trial of six interventions for the prevention of postoperative nausea and vomiting. N Engl J Med. 2004;350(24):2441–51.
30. Phillips BT, Wang ED, Rodman AJ, Watterson PA, Smith KL, Finical SJ, et al. Anesthesia duration as a marker for surgical complications in office-based plastic surgery. Ann Plast Surg. 2012;69(4):408–11.
31. Yi MS, Kang H, Kim MK, Choi GJ, Park YH, Baek CW, Jung YH, Woo YC. Relationship between the incidence and risk factors of postoperative nausea and vomiting in patients with intravenous patient-controlled analgesia. Asian J Surg. 2017. https://doi.org/10.1016/j.asjsur.2017.01.005. pii: S1015-9584(16)30464-X. PMID 28372932.
32. Fujii Y. Prophylaxis of postoperative nausea and vomiting in patients scheduled for breast surgery. Clin Drug Investig. 2006;26(8):427–37.

33. Trimas SJ, Trimas MD. Use of aprepitant and factors associated with incidence of postoperative nausea and vomiting in patients undergoing facial plastic surgery. JAMA Facial Plast Surg. 2015;17(4):251–5.
34. Morello DC, Colon GA, Fredricks S, Iverson RE, Singer R. Patient safety in accredited office surgical facilities. Plast Reconstr Surg. 1997;99(6):1496–500.
35. Keyes GR, Singer R, Iverson RE, McGuire M, Yates J, Gold A, et al. Mortality in outpatient surgery. Plast Reconstr Surg. 2008;122(1):245–50; discussion 251–3.
36. Urman RD, Punwani N, Shapiro FE. Office-based surgical and medical procedures: educational gaps. Ochsner J. 2012;12(4):383–8.

# Anesthesia for Upper GI Endoscopy Including Advanced Endoscopic Procedures

## 28

Mary Elizabeth McAlevy and John Levenick

## Introduction

Anesthesia providers are increasingly consulted to provide sedation for newer, more complex endoscopic procedures. The basic principles and guidelines for evaluating and preparing a patient for a screening upper endoscopy are applicable to the anesthetic management of these advanced endoscopic procedures. In addition, the anesthesia provider must be knowledgeable of the indication, technique, complexity and length of these new procedures. Understanding the risks, complications and patient comorbidities is crucial to providing safe sedation.

The Endoscopy suite where the authors practice is managed by a University Hospital and is located in an outpatient clinic building adjacent to the main hospital. At the time of publication all mentioned procedures are performed in this Endoscopy Suite with the exception of POEM, which is performed in the operating room setting. Upper endoscopic procedures are done for either diagnostic, prognostic, and/or therapeutic purposes. The interventions discussed in this chapter include: standard endoscopy (EGD), endoscopic ultrasound (EUS), endoscopic cystenterostomy, pancreatic necrosectomy and per-oral endoscopic myotomy (POEM).

## Procedure Description and Technical Considerations

### EGD

A flexible forward viewing endoscope is passed through a mouth piece, over the tongue with visual access to the esophagus, stomach, and duodenum. Through a working channel, instruments can be passed through the scope to perform biopsies, treat bleeding, or deploy instruments including luminal stents. Common indications for EGDs include: Evaluation of reflux disease and its sequelae, evaluation and possible treatment of dysphagia/odynophagia, dyspepsia and peptic ulcer disease, iron deficiency anemia, assessment for celiac disease or other proximal small bowel mucosal pathology, screening for and/or treat esophageal varices, and diagnosis and possible palliation of luminal foregut tumors.

### EUS (Endoscopic Ultrasound)

Similar to an EGD, a flexible forward viewing endoscope is passed through a mouth piece, over the tongue with visual access to the esophagus,

M. E. McAlevy, M.D. (✉)
Department of Anesthesiology and Perioperative Medicine, Hershey, PA, USA
e-mail: mmcalevy@pennstatehealth.psu.edu

J. Levenick, M.D.
Department of Gastroenterology, Hershey, PA, USA
e-mail: jlevenick@pennstatehealth.psu.edu

stomach, and duodenum. However this type of endoscope utilizes an oblique angled luminal camera making visualization of the lumen difficult. There are two different types of echoendoscopes. The first classified as Radial; gives 360° ultrasound images perpendicular to the scope tip. This is used for evaluation of esophageal cancer and subepithelial masses. This scope does not have the capability for biopsy. The second is classified as Linear; which gives a focused ~170° image along the access of the probe used to guide fine needle aspiration under direct visualization. This type of echoendsocope is used primarily to locally stage foregut tumors as well as diagnose non-luminal foregut tumors (pancreas, liver, abdominal and mediastinal lymph nodes) and pancreatic cysts using fine needle aspiration [2]. Of note it has the highest sensitivity for diagnosis of choledocholithiasis and small pancreatic masses of any imaging modality.

## Endoscopic Cystenterostomy (Cystgastrostomy)

Cystenterostomy is usually performed using a linear EUS followed by needle aspiration of the cyst cavity. After needle aspiration a wire is coiled in the cyst under fluoroscopy, and then the tract is sequentially dilated up 10–20 mm in size. Trans-luminal stent(s) are then placed to allow ongoing drainage and formation of an enterocystic fistula [2]. Creation of a trans-luminal ostomy between the lumen and a cyst is usually either symptomatic walled off pancreatic necrosis or pseudocyst and facilitates drainage and possible access for debridement (necrosectomy).

## Endoscopic Necrosectomy

After creation or revision of a cystenterostomy, an endoscope is driven through the enteric lumen into the cyst cavity to perform direct necrosectomy of necrotic solid material. This material is gently pulled free from the cavity walls and deposited usually in the stomach or duodenum, but a large piece may be removed per os [3]. These procedures are frequently lengthy, lasting >90–120 min.

## POEM (Per Oral Endoscopic Myotomy)

This procedure is becoming the treatment of choice for achalasia. It utilizes a standard upper endoscope and advanced per oral cavity as in normal EGD. An incision is made through the mucosa into the submucosa of the esophagus ~10–15 cm proximal to the gastroesophageal junction, and using endoscopic dissection, a tunnel is made distally extending 2–3 cm into the stomach [4] The esophageal muscles, preferentially the circular muscles, are incised. The incision is about 2 cm into the stomach and 7 cm proximal into the esophagus [4]. The incision site into the tunnel is then closed with multiple clips or sutures.

## Preoperative Evaluation and Optimization for Patients Undergoing Upper GI Endoscopy

The same principles used for pre-anesthetic evaluation of surgical cases should be applied to pre-evaluation of GI endoscopy procedures including but not limited to a review of medical, anesthetic and medication history and completion of a focused physical examination with review of any pertinent diagnostic studies [5]. Preoperative evaluation for endoscopy requires a well-defined process in order to prevent the presentation of patients with inadequate work up on the day of the procedure. The majority of endoscopy centers perform a phone history and triage patients prior to the procedure date. Any concerning findings are flagged and reviewed by a physician to determine if further workup is indicated. In of consideration of these new advanced endoscopic procedures, it is imperative to determine during the preanesthetic evaluation the most appropriate location for performing the procedure (Endoscopy suite versus Operating Room). The anesthesia provider must take into account patient comorbidities and complication risk of procedure to ensure the availability of specialized monitoring, airway equipment and additional personnel in the event of serious complications.

Obtain a prior anesthetic history to determine if patient has had adverse anesthetic reactions, difficult airway or family history of malignant hyperthermia. Keep in mind that many of the indications for performing upper GI endoscopy are signs and symptoms worrisome for increased risk of aspiration including: severe gastroesophageal reflux disease, delayed gastric emptying (diabetes, chronic opioid use, pregnancy), dysphagia, achalasia, increased intraabdominal pressure (ascites, obesity) [6]. Determination of aspiration risk will dictate need for protection of airway with endotracheal intubation. Past medical history to determine risk of airway obstruction, hypoxia and increased risk of bleeding is crucial in formulating anesthetic plan for endoscopy. Patient history that is concerning for increased risk of airway obstruction includes, snoring, obstructive sleep apnea (OSA), excessive daytime sleepiness. History concerning for increased incidence of hypoxia during sedation includes, OSA, obesity, tobacco use, shortness of breath, asthma, COPD, home oxygen use, reactive airway disease or recent upper respiratory infection [7]. These patients may exhibit increased volume of secretions which could predispose to coughing, bronchospasm and laryngospasm during procedure. Risk of bleeding is increased with history of liver disease, esophageal varices, prior GI bleeding, anticoagulation, known coagulopathies (e.g. Hemophilia).

A focused physical exam on day of the procedure should evaluate for factors increasing the risk of obstruction/hypoxia, aspiration and cardiopulmonary depression. The physical exam should include an airway exam noting the Mallampati score, neck circumference, thyromental distance, presence of craniofacial anomalies, and neck range of motion. Pulmonary auscultation with documentation baseline breath sounds should be performed. Visual inspection and palpation of abdomen for ascites in patients with history of liver disease as a paracentesis may be required pre procedure if there is respiratory compromise. Cardiac auscultation should be performed with documentation of new murmurs or other abnormal findings. Dental examination for any loose teeth that may become dislodged due to bite block, endoscope or instrumentation of the airway should be completed and documented. Check lab values for hemoglobin levels in patients with history of GI bleed and anemia, or are undergoing advanced endoscopy procedures with an increased risk of bleeding.

As with any preoperative evaluation, the goal is to determine whether the patient's medical problems are optimized prior to delivery of an anesthetic. These same principles apply to anesthesia out of the operating room for endoscopic procedures. The severity of the patient's comorbidities is weighed against the procedure risk. EGD is considered a minimally invasive low risk procedure. EUS, Pancreatic Cystgastrostomy, Necrosectomy, and POEM are considered higher risk procedures. Emergent or urgent procedures may not allow time for complete patient optimization and as a result are considered to be higher risk. Cardiac optimization should follow 2014 ACC/AHA guidelines on perioperative cardiovascular evaluation and management of patients undergoing noncardiac surgery. Patients with Cardiac Implantable Electronic Device (Pacemaker and AICD) should be optimized per consensus guidelines published in July 2011 as a joint project involving the Heart Rhythm Society, American Society of Anesthesiologists, American Heart Association and the Society of Thoracic Surgeons. Respiratory symptoms should be at baseline without recent increase in oxygen requirements, dyspnea, and hospitalizations or emergency room visits for pulmonary disease exacerbations. Anticoagulant management and recommendations should be determined by the most recent guidelines from the ASGE. These are formulated by determination of the risk of bleeding versus the risk of thromboembolic event. Patients presenting with achalasia for POEM procedure should be given strict guidelines for clear liquid diet 2 days prior to procedure to reduce aspiration risk [4].

## Anesthetic Considerations

### Selection of Appropriate Sedation Level

Sedation requirements for upper endoscopic interventions are dependent on patient demographics and the exact procedure to be performed. Sedation may range from light/moderate sedation to general anesthesia [8]. General anesthesia may be provided with or without endotracheal intubation. Determination of appropriate sedation technique must take into account medical history, sedation history, patient preference, and level of discomfort anticipated by procedure. EGDs are short in duration and less invasive; typically, general anesthesia is not required. Conversely, EUS is more complex and uncomfortable. The EUS scope is larger in caliber, needle aspiration is performed to obtain biopsies and duration of procedure is longer. All of these factors necessitate deep sedation/general anesthesia for patient comfort and optimal operating conditions for the endoscopist. Pancreatic Cystgastrostomy and Necrosectomy require general anesthesia with or without endotracheal intubation. These procedures are the longest and most complex. They carry a higher risk of aspiration and complication rate compared to EGD. POEM procedures require general anesthesia with endotracheal intubation. The population with achalasia is at high risk of aspiration. General anesthesia with endotracheal intubation is favored as it allows a still patient and a controlled airway in case of pneumothorax, pneumomediastinum or pneumoperitoneum.

Moderate sedation for EGD is achieved by combination of opioid and benzodiazepine administration. This level of sedation may be conducted by any physician licensed to administer moderate sedation that may or may not be a trained anesthesia professional. Anesthesia providers may choose to provide moderate sedation based on criteria above or may be consulted based on complex patient medical history. General anesthesia for EGD may be indicated due to factors which include but are not limited to failed moderate sedation, patient preference, procedure requirement, and need for endotracheal intubation for airway protection. Patients with higher risk of aspiration as detailed above in preprocedure evaluation will require airway protection with endotracheal tube placement. Induction of general anesthesia by rapid sequence induction must be considered to further prevent aspiration. Medications used for induction are chosen based on the patient's medical history. Due to the short duration of most endoscopy procedures, a short acting neuromuscular blocking agent may be preferred to facilitate endotracheal intubation. Maintenance of general anesthesia is achieved with inhalational agents or intravenous infusion. Fortunately, in the majority of cases for upper endoscopy endotracheal intubation is not required and general anesthesia is safely administered via intravenous infusion and supplemental oxygen.

### Monitoring and Supplies

All patients require continuous monitoring according to the current ASA guidelines: pulse oximetry, arterial blood pressure monitoring, continuous ECG, temperature, and capnography. Many devices for supplemental oxygen delivery have been modified to also allow for carbon dioxide sensing. Oxygen delivery devices most commonly used for upper endoscopy procedures are nasal cannulas or a bite block with an oxygen delivery system incorporated. In addition, facemasks have been developed that provide oxygen delivery/carbon dioxide sampling modified with a port to allow endoscope passage.

When providing sedation for any upper endoscopy, there may be a need for unanticipated endotracheal intubation and endotracheal anesthesia. This need is increased for EUS and mandatory for necrosectomy and POEM. As a result, the procedure rooms should be equipped accordingly. A typical anesthesia cart used in the nonoperating room anesthesia endoscopy suite should contain emergency drugs, sedative medications, nasal and oropharyngeal airways, bag valve mask, endotracheal tubes, laryngoscopes, IV supplies, syringes, needles, oxygen nasal cannulas, face masks, intravenous fluids and tubing. In addition, access to difficult airway supplies such as a Video Laryngoscope, Intubating LMA, and fiberoptic bronchoscope may be necessary. Consider having at least one of these types of backups available in case of unanticipated difficult airway. A dedicated anesthesia machine is not mandatory for standard EGD, however is recommended for advanced endoscopy procedures where administration of general endotracheal anesthesia is more common.

## Patient Positioning

Patients are positioned in left lateral decubitus for all EGD and EUS procedures. This may aid in prevention of airway obstruction and aspiration. Positioning for Cystgastrostomy and Necrosectomy varies from left lateral decubitus to supine depending upon preference, patient anatomy and need for fluoroscopy. POEM procedures are always performed in supine position.

## Sedative Medications

Most commonly used medications for moderate sedation include midazolam and fentanyl. Another opioid to consider for sedation includes Meperidine, but has become less popular over the last decade. Alfentanil may also be considered in place of fentanyl. Benefits of alfentanil include faster onset and shorter duration of action when administered in small bolus doses. The most popular agent and technique used to achieve general anesthesia for endoscopy is via Propofol infusion [9]. Propofol may be administered alone or in combination with a benzodiazepine or opioid depending upon patient sedation requirements. Propofol may be administered either as an intermittent bolus to achieve desired effect for procedures of short duration or as an infusion for longer procedures. Benefits of providing general anesthesia using propofol include, faster onset of desired level of sedation, quicker recovery time, and improved quality of examination. Propofol has been shown to facilitate the performance of higher volume of procedures compared with moderate sedation [9]. Other intravenous agents that have been studied and used to provide sedation for endoscopy include; dexmetatomidine, ketamine, and remifentanil. Dexmetatomidine infusion will provide sedation with less risk of respiratory depression. There has been conflicting data published on its use for endoscopy. Sedation quality, patient and endoscopist satisfaction are comparable to midazolam and fentanyl [10]. Potential concerns include delayed onset to achieve level of sedation, hypotension, bradycardia and longer recovery time. Ketamine has been investigated for use as a sole agent or for use in conjunction with other sedatives. The majority of studies have been with pediatric patients. Benefits include the ability to administer intramuscularly if have a combative patient or patient in which cannot obtain intravenous access while unsedated. Ketamine does not cause respiratory depression and has minimal effect on hemodynamics. An antisialagogue should be coadministered to prevent excess secretions. Increased secretions during upper endoscopy will require frequent suctioning to prevent excess cough and laryngospasm. Remifentanil provides profound analgesia and sedation with a very short recovery time. However in studies looking at its use for endoscopy at doses to achieve optimal sedation there was frequent apnea necessitating positive pressure ventilation [11]. Topicalization with local anesthetic of the posterior oropharynx may be used as an adjunct to sedation. Topicalization may improve endoscope passage by depressing gag reflex and decrease patient coughing and straining [12]. Benzocaine and lidocaine are local agents most commonly used. Caution with Benzocaine sprays as it has risk of causing methemoglobinemia. Metered single dose benzocaine sprays are available to aid in preventing overdose and side effect of methemoglobinemia. Lidocaine is available in various preparations for topicalization including, liquid, viscous and ointment. Lidocaine topicalization is applied with use of atomizers or by direct application [13].

## Prevention and Management of Adverse Events

Knowledge and awareness of the common adverse events during upper endoscopy allows the anesthesia provider to better prepare and manage these potential complications. The principles for management of these complications do not differ from management in the operating room, but anesthesia providers must appreciate that the resources available to handle these problems may not be as readily accessible in the endo suite. This includes not only equipment but also experienced personnel comfortable in managing patient with acute cardiopulmonary depression.

Airway obstruction is one of the primary complications encountered during upper endoscopy and if not managed appropriately can ultimately lead to a serious cardiopulmonary event. Management of upper airway obstruction is achieved by first providing neck extension and jaw thrust maneuvers. If the airway remains obstructed a nasal trumpet may be inserted. Placement of nasal airway must be done cautiously as to not cause trauma or epistaxis. Failure of these attempts to relieve obstruction with ensuing signs of hypoxia will necessitate communication with endoscopist to abort procedure to allow definitive airway management. The patient may require placement of oral airway, face mask, supraglottic airway or ETT for positive pressure ventilation.

Another common complication during the procedure is hypoxia. It may occur even in the absence of airway obstruction. Hypoxia may be attributed to one or many of multiple physiologic factors that occur during sedation including but not limited to change in tidal volume, functional residual capacity, minute ventilation, ventilation perfusion mismatch, and apnea during sedation. The initial management is to increase amount of supplemental oxygen provided and rule out other causes e.g. obstruction and aspiration. Endotracheal intubation with positive pressure ventilation may be required if hypoxia does not improve with these maneuvers.

Aspiration is a serious complication leading to hypoxia and potential unplanned admission. Prevention of aspiration can be achieved by adherence to American Society of Anesthesiology NPO guidelines. Patient positioning on left side not only lessens risk of obstruction but also aspiration. In addition may consider placing bed in reverse Trendelenburg. If gastric contents are observed after placement of endoscope there are two management options. (1) Suctioned under direct visualization through the endoscope if are thin and low volume. (2) Removal of endoscope and placement of endotracheal tube via rapid sequence induction if gastric contents are thick and increased volume. General anesthesia with endotracheal intubation via rapid sequence induction should be performed from the start in patients with known history of gastroparesis, achalasia and food impaction.

Air embolism is a rare complication of upper endoscopic procedure but possesses the potential to be severe and fatal. The use of carbon dioxide for insufflation decreases the risk of air embolism as it is easily absorbed. Patient's at higher risk for air embolism include history of previous interventions or surgeries of the bile duct system, TIPS, inflammation of the digestive system, post-surgical gastrointestinal fistula, gastrointestinal tumors and certain interventional techniques [14]. Air embolism should be part of the differential diagnosis in patients with sudden cardiopulmonary instability and neurologic changes especially during EUS, pancreatic necrosectomy and cystgastrostomy. Simple maneuvers to perform to decrease impact of air embolism while definitive diagnosis is established include: stopping procedure, administer high flow 100% oxygen, initiate high volume normal saline infusion, place patient in Trendelenburg and left lateral decubitus position to minimize air migration to brain and force air from the RVOT. Definitive diagnosis is via bedside echocardiogram [14].

Hemorrhage is possible during any upper endoscopy procedure. GI bleeding is a common indication for endoscopy and in these instances endoscopy is intended to treat and stop hemorrhage. Patients are managed expectantly with appropriate volume resuscitation. However in some cases hemorrhage can be a complication of the procedure itself. This is most commonly seen with endoscopic necrosectomy. It will typically occur during access to the collection, particularly if a vessel is punctured during dilation of the transmural tract or during the direct debridement of the necrotic cavity [15]. Hemorrhage may also occur from retroperitoneal vessels such as the portal vein during the direct debridement of the necrotic material, representing a sometimes drastic complication that may require emergent angiography or even surgery. It is important to verify in each patient the coagulation status and ensure that anticoagulation medications appropriately discontinued. Plan to obtain adequate IV access and consider type and screen for possible administration blood products.

## Preferred Technique

The author's preferred technique and recommendations for providing sedation and anesthesia for upper endoscopic procedures takes into consideration all of the above referenced material, preoperative evaluation/optimization, knowledge of anesthetic risks, and known procedural complications. This is then applied to each patient encounter and anesthetic plan is determined based on three main factors: (1) Procedure type, (2) Aspiration Risk, and (3) Individual patient comorbidities. An EGD/EUS performed on patients with a low aspiration risk and no other major medical comorbidities may be performed safely in an Endoscopy suite with MAC IV sedation or IV general anesthesia. This author's preferred method for this patient population is to provide general anesthesia with intravenous infusion of Propofol as it will provide optimal conditions for endoscopy procedure with more rapid recovery compared to IV sedation with opioids and benzodiazepines. Deep sedation is especially important during EUS, as these procedures are lengthier and require the patient to be motionless during needle biopsies. In addition, the specialized ultrasound endoscope is larger than a standard endoscope, and insertion may cause more patient discomfort requiring deeper levels of sedation or general anesthesia.

In preparation for providing sedation for upper endoscopy, always ensure that there are adequate supplies and medications available in case of need for urgent conversion to general endotracheal anesthesia for airway protection or in the event of cardiopulmonary collapse. After appropriate preoperative evaluation the patient is brought to the endoscopy procedure room. Standard monitors are placed and supplemental oxygen is provided by a carbon dioxide sensing nasal cannula. A single metered dose spray of cetacaine spray is applied to posterior oropharynx. This will aid in blunting gag reflex which is especially helpful during EUS. Another adjunct to consider is the administration of 0.2 mg IV glycopyrrolate preprocedure. This author finds it beneficial to aid in decreasing amount of oral secretions that may interfere leading to excessive cough, obstruction and laryngospasm. The patient is positioned in left lateral decubitus position to comfort with the head elevated and bed in slight reverse Trendelenburg. This positioning helps to further decrease aspiration risk. The protective bite block is placed carefully prior to administration of sedative medications as to not cause any dental injury. Propofol is administered via infusion or incremental bolus to achieve desired level of sedation in order to allow easy passage of the endoscope from posterior oropharynx into esophagus. Depending upon individual patient sedation requirements may also consider administration of other medications as adjuncts to propofol. This includes but is not limited to midazolam, fentanyl, ketamine, dexmetatomidine. Continuous monitoring for obstruction and apnea and suctioning of secretions is frequent.

EGD/EUS performed on patients with a low aspiration risk and severe medical comorbidities requires early determination of appropriate location. Patient safety is improved by providing anesthesia care in an operating room or endoscopy suite within the hospital as opposed to a free standing facility. Patients with known difficult airways will require the availability of various airway adjuncts and personnel comfortable with aiding anesthesia providers in case of emergency. Serious medical issues especially those putting patient's at high risk for cardiopulmonary complications also mandate a higher level of monitoring during and after the procedure that may not be able to be safely provided in an outpatient endoscopy suite. The anesthesia provider must make this determination based on the available resources provided in their facility.

EGD/EUS performed on patients with high aspiration risk and have no other major medical comorbidities requires general anesthesia with placement of endotracheal tube for airway protection. A rapid sequence induction should be considered. Procedure may be performed in any location as long as appropriate equipment and personnel for management and recovery of GETA are available.

EGD/EUS in patients with both high aspiration risk and major medical problems must be performed in a location with immediate access to invasive monitoring supplies, personnel trained to aid anesthesia providers in management of severe cardiopulmonary complications and difficult airway management. General endotracheal anesthesia for airway protection is necessary. Endoscopy suite location and access to before mentioned supplies may affect the decision to move location of procedure to operating room complex for safety.

Primary cystenterostomy and necrosectomy carry the highest complication risk of any upper endoscopy procedure. As a result this author recommends general endotracheal anesthesia. Airway protection is crucial as cyst fluid and necrotic debris from the pancreas will be drained into the stomach and may be snared by endoscope and removed via oral cavity. Depending on patient's medical comorbidities and complexity of procedure consider performing in an OR versus outpatient endoscopy suite. There must be resources available to manage acute blood loss and supplies to provide rapid blood transfusion. Hemorrhage risk is elevated especially during primary necrosectomy when the tract is being established with the endoscope for the first time therefore it is important to obtain a type and screen and ensure adequate IV access. In addition, confirm that antiplatelet and other anticoagulation medications have been held preprocedure. There is also an elevated risk of inducing bacteremia during access of infected necrotic pancreatic fluid and tissue. The anesthesia provider must be aware to monitor for hypotension, tachycardia and fever. Post procedure the patient will likely require admission for observation if not already an inpatient. Patients for repeat necrosectomy still require ETT for airway protection. Bleeding is less likely than compared to primary necrosectomy however must still be considered.

The author's preferred anesthetic technique for POEM requires a rapid sequence induction for GETA to provide airway protection from aspiration due to achalasia. Intubation allows for controlled ventilation, and close monitoring of end tidal carbon dioxide during dissection and insufflation. To date there have been no studies suggesting clinical importance of anesthetic agent use during POEM procedures [16]. Use of Propofol or Sevoflurane is acceptable. The patient is positioned supine and draped to allow access to abdomen and chest for urgent needle decompression of pneumoperitoneum and pneumothorax. Positive pressure ventilation will minimize the risk for pneumomediastinum. Observation of sudden increase in end tidal carbon dioxide tension may be a sign of subcutaneous emphysema while a sudden increase in peak inspiratory pressures may point to capnothorax. The majority of cases of subcutaneous emphysema resolve with conservative treatment. This author currently recommends performing these procedures in an operating room to allow for rapid surgical management of these serious procedural complications.

## Adverse Events and Post Procedure Complications

Anesthetic complications for endoscopy are no different from those that may occur in the operating room. Risks of moderate sedation and general anesthesia apply to all patients regardless of procedure type and location. However, there are specific complications that are more common while providing anesthesia for upper endoscopic procedure. Providers much have awareness of these events which include: aspiration, obstruction, apnea, hypoxia, and laryngospasm. Sedation and general anesthesia provided without placement of a definitive airway puts patients at risk for aspiration, upper airway obstruction, laryngospasm and apnea. Many of the indications for performing EGD include patients with signs and symptoms worrisome for aspiration including but not limited to GERD, dysphagia, achalasia, and gastroparesis. Medications administered to achieve appropriate levels of sedation lead to relaxation and collapse of tissue in the oropharynx promoting obstruction of upper airway. Laryngospasm may be caused by direct stimulation by secretions or the endoscope. This is most common if the patient has not reached an adequate level of sedation or presence of inadequate topicalization. Apnea is caused by upper airway obstruction, laryngospasm or as a side effect of excess administration of sedative medications. Dental injury is increased during EGD, even in the absence of direct laryngoscopy and ETT placement. In order to prevent damage to endoscope an oral plastic bite block is placed between the patient's teeth and fastened around the back of the neck with an elastic band. During the procedure the patient may bite down with excessive force or manipulation of the endoscope may cause the bite block to cause dental dislodgement or chipping. Injury and swelling of the lips has also been described. The lip may be entrapped between teeth and bite block leading to ischemic or mechanical trauma.

In addition, it is important to also be knowledgeable of the common complications that may occur as a direct result of the procedure itself. Procedural complications of a standard EGD include aspiration, perforation (1/5–10,000), bleeding and missed lesion [17]. Procedural complications for EUS are the same as with standard EGD with the additional slight increased perforation risk with a more rigid scope tip and oblique view, especially in the oropharynx or duodenal sweep [2]. If FNA of pancreas is performed during EUS there is a 1% chance of developing pancreatitis requiring hospital admission.

Cystenterostomy/necrosectomy complications include those for a standard EGD with the additional risk of Air/$CO_2$ embolus (up to 2%), perforation (at the cyst-enteric fistula) or cyst wall dehiscence (5%) and massive bleeding [3]. Perforation may not be diagnosed until patient is in the recovery room. Perforation during upper endoscopy most commonly occurs with dilation of esophageal strictures or achalasia, removal of foreign bodies or application of esophageal endoprostheses [18]. Perforation causes leaking of gastrointestinal contents into mediastinum or peritoneum resulting in mediastinitis and severe sepsis. Patients most commonly complain of pain in the recovery area. Subcutaneous emphysema may also be palpated. Fever, sepsis and pneumothorax are later findings. Any patient with worsening pain after instrumentation and interventional procedures during upper endoscopy should be evaluated for perforation. The gastroenterologist should be notified and patient should be sent for barium swallow study and chest X-ray.

POEM procedural complications include capnomediastinum, capnothorax, capnoperitoneum (small ones are common). There is a 1–2% chance of bleeding and <1% chance of mediastinitis [19]. Post procedure the patient is admitted and maintained NPO for 24 h and a water-soluble contrast study of the esophagus is obtained to rule out a leak and assure passage into the stomach. Under ideal circumstances patients may be discharged home the day after the procedure.

Anesthetic planning key point overview for upper endoscopy procedures

| | |
|---|---|
| Selection of appropriate sedation level<br>  Patient expectation<br>  Medical history<br>  Procedure type | Procedure type recommended sedation<br>  EGD-Moderate or Deep Sedation, GETA<br>  EUS-Deep Sedation, GETA<br>  Necrosectomy/Cystgastrostomy-GETA<br>  POEM-GETA |
| Most common complications | Risk factors for complications |
|   Aspiration | Delayed gastric emptying (DM, Chronic Opioids), Dysphagia, Achalasia, Ascites, Obesity |
|   Airway obstruction | OSA, Obesity, Snoring |
|   Hypoxia | OSA, Obesity, Tobacco use, SOB, Asthma, COPD, Home oxygen use, Recent URI |
|   Hemorrhage | Varices, History of GI Bleed, Coagulopathy, Anticoagulation therapy, Procedure type |
| Procedure specific complications | EGD-Aspiration, Perforation, Hemorrhage<br>EUS-Higher risk Perforation, Pancreatitis<br>Necrosectomy-Air embolism, Higher risk of perforation and hemorrhage<br>POEM-Capnomediastinum, Capnothorax, Capnothorax, Mediastinitis, Hemorrhage |
| Monitoring and supplies<br>  Standard ASA monitors + Capnography<br>  Available supplies to convert to GETA<br>  Ability to give positive pressure ventilation | Pulse oximetry, arterial blood pressure, continuous ECG, temperature<br>Emergency drugs, sedative medications, nasal and oropharyngeal airways, bag valve mask, endotracheal tubes, laryngoscopes, IV supplies, syringes, needles, oxygen nasal cannulae with capnography sensing ability, face masks, IV fluids and tubing<br>Difficult airway supplies (Video laryngoscope, LMA)<br>Dedicated anesthesia machine for advanced Endoscopy procedures |
| Patient positioning | EGD/EUS-Left lateral decubitis<br>Necrosectomy-supine or Left lateral<br>POEM-Supine |
| Focused exam | Airway<br>Pulmonary<br>Cardiac<br>Abdominal (hx Ascites)<br>Dental exam for loose teeth<br>Check hemoglobin (anemia)<br>Type and Screen if needed |

# References

1. Goulson DT, Fragneto RY. Anesthesia for gatrointestinal endoscopic procedures. Anesthesiol Clin. 2009;27:71–85.
2. Wiersema MJ, Vilmann P, Giovannini M, et al. Endosonography-guided fine-needle aspiration biopsy: diagnostic accuracy and complication assessment. Gastroenterology. 1997;112:1087.
3. Gardner TB, et al. Direct endoscopic necrosectomy for the treatment of walled-off pancreatic necrosis: results from a multicenter U.S. series. Gastrointest Endosc. 2011;73:718–26.
4. Ponsky JL, Marks JM, Pauli EM. How I do it: per-oral endoscopic myotomy (POEM). J Gastrointest Surg. 2012;16:1251–5.
5. Practice Advisory for Preanesthesia Evaluation an updated report by the American Society of Anesthesiologists Task Force on Preanesthesia Evaluation. Anesthesiology. 2012;116:1–17.
6. Engelhardt T, Webster NR. Review article pulmonary aspiration of gastric contents in anaesthesia. Br J Anaesth. 1999;83:453–60.
7. Smetana GW. Preoperative pulmonary evaluation: identifying and reducing risks for pulmonary complications. Cleve Clin J Med. 2006;73:3646.
8. Cohen LB, Wecsler JS, Gaetano JN, et al. Endoscopic sedation in the United States: results from a nationwide survey. Am J Gastroenterol. 2006;101:967–74.
9. Trummel J. Sedation for gastrointestinal endoscopy: the changing landscape. Curr Opin Anaesthesiol. 2007;20:359–64.

10. Demirarany Y, Korkut E, Tamer A, et al. The comparison of dexmedetomidine and midazolam used for sedation of patients during upper endoscopy: a prospective, randomized study. Can J Gastroenterol. 2007;21:25–9.
11. Litman RS. Conscious sedation with remifentanil during painful medical procedures. J Pain Symptom Manage. 2000;19:468–71.
12. Evans LT, Saberi S, Kim HM, et al. Pharyngeal anesthesia during sedated EGDs: is "the spray" beneficial? A meta-analysis and systematic review. Gastrointest Endosc. 2006;63:761–6.
13. Ayoub C, Skoury A, Abdul-Baki H, et al. Lidocaine lollipop as single-agent anesthesia in upper GI endoscopy. Gastrointest Endosc. 2007;66:786–93.
14. Donepudi S, Chavalitdhamrong D, Pu L, Draganov P. Air embolisim complicating gastrointestinal endoscopy: a systematic review. World J Gastrointest Endosc. 2013;5(8):359–65.
15. Giovannini M, Binmoeller K, Seifert H. Endoscopic ultrasound-guided cystogastrostomy. Endoscopy. 2003;35:239–45.
16. Tanaka E, Murata H, Minami H, Sumikawa K. Anesthetic management of peroral endoscopic myotomy for esophageal achalasia: a retrospective case series. J Anesth. 2014;28:456–9.
17. Chirica M, Champault A, Dray X, et al. Esophageal perforations. J Visc Surg. 2010;147:e117.
18. Cotton PB. Outcomes of endoscopy procedures: struggling towards definitions. Gastrointest Endosc. 1994;40:514.
19. Inoue H, Tianle KM, Ikeda H, Hosoya T, Onimaru M, Yoshida A, Minami H, Kudo SE. Peroral endoscopic myotomy for esophageal achalasia: technique, indication, and outcomes. Thorac Surg Clin. 2011;21:519–25.

# Part III

# Pediatric Anesthesia

# Anesthesia for Fetal Intervention and Surgery

## 29

Jagroop Mavi

## Maternal Anesthetic Considerations

There are specific physiologic changes that occur with pregnancy that have an impact on the anesthetic management of the mother. To ensure maternal and fetal safety, the anesthesiologist must understand how these physiologic changes affect anesthetic management and must take an active role in perioperative management of both parties [1]. Left uterine displacement to prevent aortocaval compression and resulting compromised uteroplacental perfusion should be employed beginning as early as 13–16 weeks of gestation [1]. In terms of the respiratory system, there is decreased functional residual capacity and increased minute ventilation, which leads to faster oxygen desaturation with apnea. Decreases in capillary oncotic pressure and increases in capillary permeability increase the risk of pulmonary edema especially when magnesium sulfate is used for tocolysis. Upper airway edema and mucosal congestion leads to potentially difficult mask ventilation and intubation. Adequate precautions should be taken to prevent aspiration, as there is a reduced lower esophageal sphincter tone due to elevated progesterone and estrogen levels along with increased intra-abdominal pressure from the gravid uterus. Intravenous metoclopramide and oral sodium citrate are administered preoperatively to reduce gastric secretion and increase gastric pH. There is a pregnancy-induced decrease in MAC leading to an increased sensitivity to anesthetics, and in addition an engorged epidural venous plexus results in increased sensitivity to neuraxial local anesthetics. The thrombophilic state of pregnancy combined with a prolonged surgical procedure places the mother at risk for venous thromboembolic events, thus pneumatic compression boots are indicated until the patient is fully ambulatory [2]. The parturient is also at risk for amniotic fluid embolism during labor or intra-abdominal surgery.

There are preoperative and intraoperative factors that can compromise uteroplacental circulation. Causes of impaired uteroplacental blood flow or oxygenation include reduced maternal oxygenation or hemoglobin concentration, maternal hemorrhage, aortocaval compression, drugs reducing uterine blood flow, uterine contractions, and maternal catecholamine production increasing uteroplacental vascular resistance [1].

## Fetal Anesthetic Considerations

Risks to the fetus, which include renal failure, fetal demise, CNS injuries, postoperative amniotic fluid leaks, membrane separation, preterm rupture of membranes, preterm labor, and preterm delivery are relatively high [1]. There are preoperative and

J. Mavi, M.D.
Department of Anesthesiology and Pain Management, Cincinnati Children's Hospital Medical Center, Cincinnati, OH, USA
e-mail: Jagroop.Mavi@cchmc.org

**Table 29.1** Anesthetic management for fetal interventions

|  | Minimally invasive procedures | Midgestation open procedures | EXIT procedures |
|---|---|---|---|
| Maternal anesthesia | Local or neuraxial anesthesia ± intravenous sedation | General endotracheal anesthesia with postoperative epidural analgesia | General endotracheal anesthesia with postoperative epidural analgesia OR regional anesthesia (epidural, combined spinal epidural) |
| Fetal anesthesia | ±IM medications | Transplacental and IM | Transplacental and IM/IV |

intraoperative factors that can compromise fetoplacental circulation. Causes of impaired umbilical blood flow or fetal circulatory redistribution include umbilical vessel spasm, reduced fetal cardiac output, fetal hemorrhage, impaired uteroplacental blood flow, fetal hypothermia, umbilical cord kinking, and increased fetal catecholamine production [1]. Fetal heart rate (FHR) is the most important determinant of cardiac output. Fetal bradycardia (heart rate <100 bpm) is a strong indicator of fetal distress, which may include hypoxia, hypothermia or noxious stimuli. Changes in fetal heart or cardiac contractility may be tolerated for only a brief period and appropriate interventions should be performed immediately to prevent end organ damage. Noxious stimuli can elicit neuroendocrine and hemodynamic responses by 18–20 weeks gestation, which leads to the requirement for fetal analgesia in open midgestation cases and select EXIT procedures [3]. Long-term positive and negative effects of such anesthesia and analgesia on fetal neurodevelopment are still unclear. Both neurogenesis and neuronal migration accelerate and reach a peak during and after the second trimester. These processes are extremely sensitive to environmental and pharmacological influences. Synaptogenesis begins as early as the third trimester and extends to the first few years of life. Although data on the fetal brain are limited, most animal studies indicate that the developing fetal brain is at risk from maternal anesthesia especially during the second trimester [4].

During surgery, maintenance of normothermia is hampered by exposure of the fetus, whose thin skin is susceptible to evaporative fluid and heat loss. This evaporative heat loss is minimized by only partial fetal delivery and through amnioinfusion with warm saline. In a preterm fetus, the effects and duration of anesthetic agents are increased owing to immature organ function, incomplete myelination, and delayed elimination. Altered coagulation factors and immature liver function predispose the fetus to bleeding. In addition, the small blood volume of the fetus contributes to a low threshold for blood transfusion. Table 29.1 lists the anesthetic considerations in the management for fetal interventions.

## Preoperative Evaluation

Preoperative anesthetic evaluation should include a detailed maternal history of medical problems, allergies, complications with previous anesthetics, and obstetric history. A focused physical exam of the heart, lungs, airway, and spine must be performed during the preanesthetic assessment. Preoperative fetal ultrasound, echocardiography, and/or MRI to document baseline cardiac function in addition to physiologic and anatomic defects in the fetus are required. Imaging studies are also helpful as they provide information on placental location and anatomy that may alter the surgical approach, patient positioning, and necessitate modification of the anesthetic plan. Maternal type and screen is adequate for minimally invasive procedures but type and crossmatch should be ordered for midgestation open fetal cases and EXIT procedures. Leukocyte reduced, irradiated, CMV-negative, O-negative blood should be readily available to the fetus in every case.

## Intraoperative Anesthetic Management

### Minimally Invasive Procedure

Minimally invasive procedures are the most common fetal interventions performed and include both needle-based ultrasound guided procedures and fetoscopic interventions (laser photocoagulation for twin-twin transfusion, ablation of posterior urethral valves, amniotic band release, tracheal occlusion). These interventions are performed in early or midgestation with local or neuraxial anesthesia. If the procedure involves multiple needle punctures at various locations, large instruments, or a mini laparotomy, neuraxial anesthesia provides superior pain control for maternal comfort [1]. The mother is monitored with standard ASA monitors and maternal blood pressure is maintained to within 20% of baseline. The wellbeing of the fetus is assessed at the beginning and end of the procedure using ultrasound. Supplemental analgesia (opioids), anxiolysis (midazolam) and propofol infusion (starting at 25–50 μg/kg/min) for sedation administered to the mother may provide minimal fetal immobility and some analgesia from placental transfer. Intravenous fluids are restricted during these procedures to prevent pulmonary edema postoperatively with the addition of tocolytics to halt preterm labor. A plan should be in place for treatment of fetal distress and should include having fetal weight-based doses of emergency drugs for fetal resuscitation (atropine, epinephrine) immediately available. Persistent fetal bradycardia or fetal compromise may require an emergency cesarean section if the gestational age is compatible with extrauterine viability. The anesthesiologist should therefore be prepared to deliver general anesthesia in emergency situations. Table 29.2 lists various indications for minimally invasive fetoscopic surgery.

## Open Midgestation Procedure

Table 29.3 lists various indications for open midgestation fetal surgery. In addition to anesthetic considerations for minimally invasive fetal procedures, open fetal procedures have some unique issues. There is need for profound uterine relaxation, intraoperative fetal monitoring, fetal analgesia, postoperative maternal analgesia, and the potential for maternal or fetal fluid shifts and blood loss. In midgestation open procedures the fetal part is exteriorized for surgery and after completion the fetus is placed back into the uterus and continues to grow for the rest for the gestation [5]. Currently the most common indication for a midgestation case is myelomeningocele (MMC) repair, but other interventions such as congenital cystic adenomatoid malformation (CCAM) resection and sacrococcygeal teratoma (SCT) resections are also performed. Open procedures are typically performed under general endotracheal anesthesia. A preoperative epidural (T12–L1) catheter is inserted for postoperative pain control but not bolused until the end of surgery due to anticipated intraoperative hemodynamic instability [3].

The mother is positioned supine with left uterine displacement and standard ASA monitors are applied. An arterial line is placed for close blood pressure monitoring due to the elevated levels of volatile anesthetics used and potential for significant blood loss. Desflurane is the volatile anesthetic of choice for these cases as it is easily titratable. Desflurane is administered at normal anesthetic concentrations before and after hysterotomy but increased to 2–3 MAC during uterine manipulation for relaxation and surgical exposure. This technique is associated with maternal

**Table 29.2** Indications for minimally invasive fetoscopic surgery

| Disease | Procedure |
|---|---|
| Twin-twin transfusion syndrome | Laser photocoagulation of placental vessels |
| Twin reversed arterial perfusion | Radiofrequency ablation |
| Amniotic band syndrome | Division of amniotic bands |
| Obstructive uropathy | Shunt insertion and valve ablation |
| Cyanotic heart disease | Atrial septostomy |

**Table 29.3** Indications for open midgestation fetal surgery

| Disease | Procedure |
|---|---|
| Myelomeningocele | Repair of neural canal defect |
| Sacrococcygeal teratoma | Resection or debulking of teratoma |
| Intrathoracic masses | Resection of mass |
| Congenital diaphragmatic hernia with low lung-to-head ratio | Tracheal occlusion |

hypotension and significant fetal cardiac dysfunction [3]. An alternative technique utilizes intravenous anesthesia prior to and after uterine manipulation with addition of desflurane during hysterotomy to achieve uterine relaxation. This supplemental IV anesthesia technique is associated with more stable maternal hemodynamics, improved uterine blood flow and better fetal acid-base status than exposure to high dose desflurane for the entirety of the case [6].

Intermittent intravenous doses of nitroglycerin (50–200 μg IV) may be used as a supplement for optimizing uterine relaxation [1]. Arterial blood pressure is maintained with IV phenylephrine or ephedrine as needed to maintain mean arterial blood pressure >65 mmHg. A phenylephrine infusion may be required. An intramuscular cocktail of fentanyl (20 μg/kg), vecuronium (0.2 mg/kg), atropine (20 μg/kg) is administered to the fetus by the surgeon to ensure complete blockade of the fetal stress response in addition to immobilizing the fetus to optimize surgical conditions. When the procedure is completed the hysterotomy is closed and aggressive tocolysis and pain control are maintained postoperatively.

## EXIT Procedure

Table 29.4 lists various indications for ex utero intrapartum therapy (EXIT). The EXIT procedure is usually deferred until as late in gestation as possible, based on both the maternal and fetal condition. The particular intervention performed in an EXIT procedure varies by indication and may involve securing an airway, resecting an intrathoracic mass, resecting a neck mass in a controlled setting, special circumstances with thoracoomphalopagus conjoined twins, or inserting cannulas for extracorporeal membrane oxygenation (ECMO). EXIT allows extended uteroplacental support while the airway is secured by direct laryngoscopy, rigid or fiberoptic bronchoscopy, and possible insertion of an ECMO cannula if required. With emphasis on techniques aimed to maximize uterine relaxation and maintain uteroplacental blood flow, it is now possible to maintain placental support for up to 180 min before delivery and separation from placental circulation [11].

A preoperative decision between the surgery and anesthesia team is made as to whether the EXIT procedure is suitable to be performed solely under lumbar (L4–5) epidural anesthesia, in which case the epidural is dosed with local anesthetic and a T4–T6 level is confirmed prior to incision. EXIT procedures often require general anesthesia for both the mother and fetus, as time is needed to perform a fetal intervention while on placental circulation prior to delivery. The anesthesia plan in this case is similar to open midgestation cases. After adequate preoxygenation, a rapid-sequence induction is performed, and the airway is secured with a cuffed endotracheal tube. Emergency airway equipment should always be immediately available. Following intubation, additional intravenous access is obtained, and intra-arterial and foley catheters are inserted. Ultrasonography is used just before surgical preparation to verify fetal wellbeing and identify the location of the placenta. Before uterine incision, complete uterine relaxation is induced using at least two MAC of volatile anesthetic, supplemented by incremental doses of nitroglycerin followed by an infusion to 0.5–1 μg/kg/min, if needed [7].

High doses of volatile anesthetics invariably decrease maternal systemic vascular resistance and cardiac output. Thus, ephedrine and phenyl-

**Table 29.4** Indications for ex utero intrapartum therapy (EXIT)

| Disease | Procedure |
|---|---|
| Severe aortic stenosis or left lung hypoplasia | ECMO cannulation |
| Congenital diaphragmatic hernia | Removal of tracheal clip or balloon that was placed in utero |
| | ECMO cannulation |
| Congenital high upper airway obstruction syndrome | Tracheostomy |
| Giant cervical neck mass | Resection of mass |
| Severe pulmonary hypoplasia from intrathoracic mass (congenital pulmonary airway malformation or CPAM) | Resection of mass |
| | ECMO cannulation |
| Anticipated difficult intubation | Obtain surgical airway |

ephrine are titrated to maintain maternal systolic blood pressure within 20% of baseline. As drug passage is dependent upon maternal drug concentration and uteroplacental perfusion, the fetal response to these maternally administered drugs must be closely evaluated. Fetal bradycardia is a reliable indicator of fetal distress and must be immediately addressed.

Once the surgical site is confirmed, to minimize maternal bleeding, a stapled hysterotomy is performed using a hemostatic uterine stapling device. The placenta is localized by ultrasound and a 5 cm margin from placental edge to hysterotomy incision is ensured to reduce the risk of placental abruption [7]. Warm uterine irrigation is performed to prevent fetal hypothermia and to maintain uterine volume. Adequate uteroplacental blood flow is ensured by attention to complete uterine relaxation, maintenance of maternal blood pressure and oxygenation, and avoidance of kinking or compression of the umbilical cord. After delivery of the placenta IV oxytocin 20 units/1 L of fluids is administered to restore uterine tone. Intramuscular methylergonovine 0.2 mg and/or intramuscular carboprost tromethamine 250 μg may be required for refractory uterine atony.

To monitor the fetus, a sterile pulse oximeter probe is placed on an extremity and covered with foil to deflect ambient light. Supplemental fetal anesthesia is administered as an intramuscular cocktail as in open midgestation cases. Intermittently, sterile fetal echocardiography can monitor cardiac function, ductal patency, and volume status.

## Postoperative Management

Postoperative maternal management after fetal surgery includes close monitoring of fetal heart rate and uterine activity during the immediate postoperative period after minimally invasive procedures and for the first 24–48 h after open fetal surgery. Adequate maternal analgesia is provided using a multimodal regimen with acetaminophen, opioids (oral, parenteral, or neuraxial), neuraxial and local anesthetics, non-pharmacologic modalities, or a combination of these. There should be consideration of venous thromboprophylaxis, especially in those patients with limited mobility. Postoperative tocolytic administration is crucial as part of a regimen designed to prevent preterm labor in minimally invasive and open midgestation cases [8].

## References

1. Rollins M, Rosen M. Anesthesia for fetal intervention and surgery. In: Part 3 practice of pediatric anesthesia. Gregory's pediatric anesthesia, John Wiley and Sons. Chap. 19. 5th ed. 2012. p. 444–74.
2. Moldenhauer JS. Ex utero intrapartum therapy. Semin Pediatr Surg. 2013;22:44–9. (p10).
3. Hoagland M, Chatterjee D. Anesthesia for fetal surgery. Pediatr Anesth. 2017;27:346–57.
4. Palanisamy A. Maternal anesthesia and fetal neurodevelopment. Int J Obstet Anesth. 2012;21:152–62.
5. Saxena K. Anaesthesia for fetal surgeries. Indian J Anaesth. 2009;53(5):554–9.
6. Ngamprasertwong P, et al. Anesthetic techniques for fetal surgery: effects of maternal anesthesia on intraoperative fetal outcomes in a sheep model. Anesthesiology. 2013;118:796–808.
7. Oluyinka O, Olutoye O. EXIT procedure for fetal neck masses. Curr Opin Pediatr. 2012;24:386–93. (p13).
8. Sviggum H, Kodali B. Maternal anesthesia for fetal surgery. Clin Perinatol. 2013;40:413–27.
9. Moaddab A, et al. Ethical issues in fetal therapy. Best Pract Res Clin Obstet Gynecol. 2017. https://doi.org/10.1016/j.bpobgyn.2017.02.005.
10. Van de Valde M, De Buck F. Fetal and maternal analgesia/anesthesia for fetal procedures. Fetal Diagn Ther. 2012;31:201–9.
11. Mavi J, Previte J. Anesthetic complications of fetal surgery: EXIT procedures. Fleisher/Rosenbaum. Complications in anesthesia 3e. Elsevier, Chapter 149; Elsevier-Health Sciences Division. 3rd ed. 2017.

# Anesthesia for Neurosurgical Procedures

## 30

Jaya L. Varadarajan

Neurosurgical conditions in the pediatric population have unique management considerations with distinct manifestations, making them different from those of adults. There are age related differences in the incidence, anatomy, and pathology of surgical lesions. Children demonstrate differences in the physiological responses to surgery and anesthesia from adults; in addition, variation among age groups is what sets children apart and makes management decisions often different from the norm of adult neuro-anesthetic practice. Over the last decade or more, there have been numerous technological advances in neurosurgery; this coupled with sub-specialization, and a better understanding of postoperative needs of pediatric patients has dramatically improved outcomes in infants and children with neurosurgical lesions [1].

## Neuroanatomy, Neurophysiology and Developmental Considerations

The infant cranial vault is unique in that the intracranial space is compliant owing to open fontanelles and sutures, allowing for a slow expansion of intracranial volume. The posterior fontanelle is the first to close around 2–3 months of age; sphenoid and mastoid fontanelles follow with the anterior fontanelle being the last to close around 2–3 years of age. Infants thus demonstrate an exception to the Munro-Kellie hypothesis, as the infant skull is pliable up until 2 years of age [2]. The mass effect of a slow growing tumor or hemorrhage is often masked by compensatory distension of the fontanelle and widening of the cranial sutures. Acute increases in volume due to massive hemorrhage or an obstructed ventricular system cannot be attenuated by this expansion, and can result in life-threatening increases in intracranial pressure (ICP) or herniation [3] (Fig. 30.1).

Intracranial compliance is the change in ICP relative to the intracranial volume. Once the fontanelles and sutures have closed, children have a smaller cranial volume and lower intracranial compliance than adults, putting them at a higher risk for herniation (Fig. 30.2) [4]. The infant brain triples its weight in the first year after birth. Eighty percent of the intracranial volume consists of brain and interstitial fluid, with blood and cerebrospinal fluid (CSF) making up the remainder. CSF volume is larger in infants and neonates (4 mL/kg) compared to adults (2 mL/kg).

There are unique differences in cerebrovascular physiology that distinguish children from adults. Cerebral metabolic rate for oxygen ($CMRO_2$) is higher in children at ~5.8 mL/100 g/min compared to adult levels of 3.5 mL/100 g/min. CBF in healthy children is believed to be ~100 mL/100 g/min compared to adults at

J. L. Varadarajan, M.D.
Department of Anesthesiology, Section of Pediatric Anesthesiology, Medical College of Wisconsin, Children's Hospital of Wisconsin, PO Box 1997, MS 735, 9000 W.Wisconsin Avenue, Milwaukee, 53201-3022 WI, USA

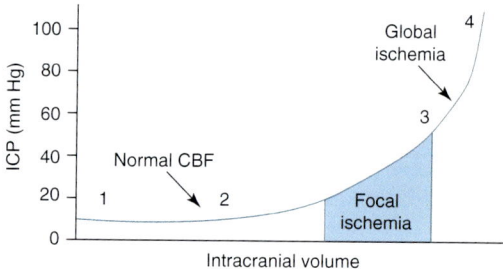

**Fig. 30.2** Intracranial compliance curve. At normal intracranial volumes (1), ICP is low but compliance is high and remains so despite small increases in volume. As intracranial volume acutely rises (2), the ability to compensate is rapidly overwhelmed, even when the ICP is still within normal limits, but the compliance is low. At higher ICP (3), a threshold is quickly reached where further volume expansion leads to rapid and higher increase in ICP. (4) Reflects maximal intracranial volume and high ICP. *Adapted from Smith's Anesthesia for Infants and Children. 8th Edition*

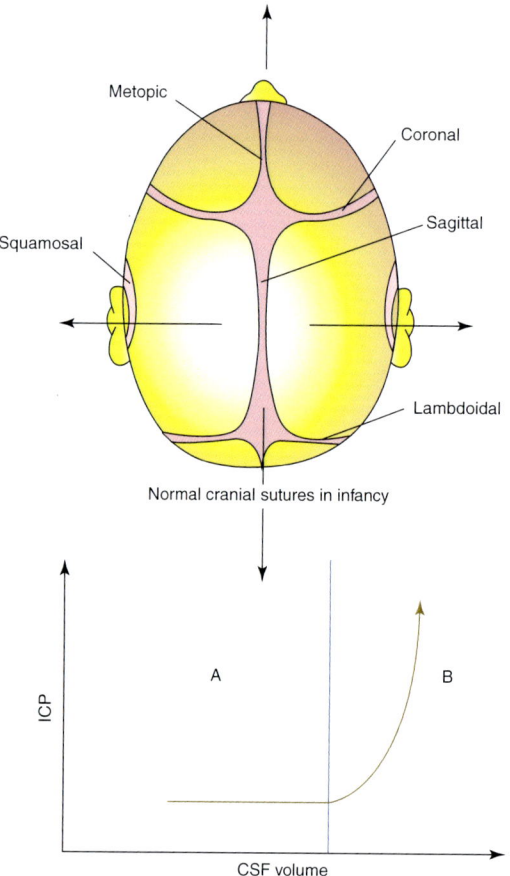

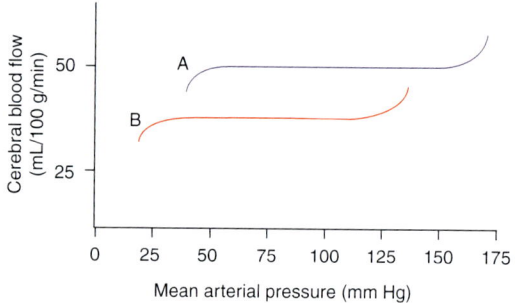

**Fig. 30.1** Cranial sutures and fontanelle in neonates and infants. Initially the compliant skull of the neonate minimizes insidious increases in intracranial volume. However, acute increases in intracranial volume will lead to rapid rises in intracranial pressure. *Adapted from Smith's Anesthesia for Infants and Children. 8th Edition*

**Fig. 30.3** Autoregulation of cerebral circulation—Neonates (Curve B) & Adults (Curve A). *Adapted from Smith's Anesthesia for Infants and Children. 8th Edition*

50 mL/100 g/min. Cerebral blood flow (CBF) is tightly coupled to cerebral metabolism and $CMRO_2$ at global and regional levels. Both CBF and metabolic demand increase immediately after birth, the changes mirroring neuroanatomical and psychomotor growth, which in turn reflect cognitive growth. CBF is 10–20% of the cardiac output in the first 6 months of life, peaking at 55% between ages 2–4, settling into adult levels of 15% by 7–8 years [5]. In adults, cerebral autoregulation ensures that CBF remains relatively constant within a mean arterial pressure (MAP) range of 50–150 mmHg, outside of which CBF becomes pressure dependent. This autoregulation occurs at undefined lower absolute values in infants and children (Fig. 30.3). There is data that children as young as 6 months of age autoregulate CBF as well as older children, but none on the lower limit of autoregulation (LLA) in healthy neonates. It was believed that neonates are especially vulnerable to cerebral ischemia and intraventricular hemorrhage due to a narrow autoregulatory range. Previously held beliefs that the LLA is lower in infants than older children, has been challenged [6]. Since blood pressure increases with age, infants are likely at increased risk for cerebral ischemia due to lower blood pressure reserve (mean arterial pressure—LLA). Analysis of cerebral perfusion in infants and

children undergoing cardiopulmonary bypass surgery reveals a wide range in the lower limits of autoregulation, suggesting individual variability and highlights the limitations of currently available monitors to measure and optimize cerebral perfusion [7]. It has been suggested that diastolic blood pressure is a better indicator of cerebral perfusion pressure (CPP) than systolic arterial pressure in this population [8]. Cerebral ischemia occurs at CBF values of ~25–40 mL/100 g/min and is heralded by EEG slowing, followed by neuronal damage that is initially reversible. Rapid cell death occurs at a CBF <6 mL/100 g/min. The lower the CBF at ischemic levels, the shorter the duration allowable before irreversible neuronal damage. Tight blood pressure control is therefore essential in the management of neonates to minimize both cerebral ischemia during hypotension and intraventricular hemorrhage with hypertension. A clinically accepted "Rule of Thumb" is that acceptable MAP for a neonate approximates the gestational age.

The vasoreactivity to $CO_2$ is also believed to be higher in children than adults. In comparison, the influence of $PaO_2$ is of much less clinical significance. There are minimal changes in cerebral blood flow (CBF) with changes in $PaO_2$ above 50 mmHg. Below a $PaO_2$ of 50 mmHg, CBF increases to maintain adequate cerebral oxygen delivery [9]. This lower threshold of $PaO_2$ is lower in neonates. The influence of hyperoxia is controversial, but it is believed to decrease CBF.

Despite these observations, the mechanisms of normal cerebral autoregulation in healthy children, and adaptations in acute disease are not completely understood. To complicate things further, both anatomic and physiologic maturation might play a role in the development of a fully developed autoregulatory response as the child grows. There may also be an increased latency in the autoregulatory response in young children, that is age dependent.

## Preoperative Evaluation

Many pediatric neurosurgical conditions are of an emergent nature. Despite this, a thorough preoperative evaluation and organ system review is essential to identify coexisting conditions, and anticipate potential physiologic derangements, that might increase the likelihood of perioperative complications. In the setting of emergent surgery, children with a preexisting upper or lower respiratory infection, a full stomach, gastrointestinal reflux, or ongoing emesis are at higher risk and appropriate precautions should be taken to prevent complications. Children whose presenting symptoms include repeated emesis, and those who have had prolonged fasting periods are at risk for hypovolemia and hypoglycemia, both of which can cause hemodynamic and metabolic perturbations under anesthesia. Many neurosurgical patients have comorbidities that are part of a syndrome, and return to the operating room for repeat procedures. It is useful to enquire about prior anesthetic experiences and issues in the postoperative period.

Premature infants are prone to postoperative apneic spells at baseline; this could be amplified by the neurological condition. Intraoperative management, and postoperative disposition should take this into account. Some craniofacial anomalies may make airway management a challenge; this should be anticipated, with special equipment and techniques utilized as necessary. Congenital heart disease might complicate the perioperative course, especially in the newborn. A thorough evaluation with input from a pediatric cardiologist might be warranted to optimize cardiac function when the acuity of the condition allows. Workup might include an echocardiogram. Children with suprasellar masses might need an Endocrinology evaluation. There are certain neurological conditions that warrant special considerations in the preoperative period, as outlined in Table 30.1.

Preoperative physical examination in all neurosurgical patients should document the level of consciousness, motor and sensory function, cranial nerves, pupillary reflexes, and signs and symptoms of raised ICP. This will serve as a baseline for postoperative assessment. The signs of raised ICP vary based on the age of the child, as outlined in Table 30.2. Brainstem lesions can present with cranial nerve dysfunction such as impaired gag reflex and swallow, respiratory

**Table 30.1** Anesthetic concerns in neurosurgery

| | |
|---|---|
| Denervation injuries | Hyperkalemia after succinylcholine—use NDPMR |
| | Resistance to non-depolarizing muscle relaxants |
| Chronic exposure to anti-seizure medications | Hepatic dysfunction |
| | Hematologic abnormalities |
| | Increased metabolism of anesthetic agents |
| | Require increased doses and frequent redosing |
| Arteriovenous malformations | Potential for congestive heart failure |
| Moyamoya disease | Risk of perioperative ischemia |
| Neuromuscular disease | Malignant hyperthermia |
| | Respiratory failure |
| | Sudden cardiac death |
| Arnold Chiari malformation | Postoperative apnea |
| | Aspiration pneumonia |
| | Postoperative stridor |
| Hypothalamic and pituitary lesions | Adrenal insufficiency/excess |
| | Thyroid abnormalities |
| | Diabetes insipidus/SIADH |
| Craniofacial abnormalities | Difficult airway |
| | Significant blood loss |
| Neural tube defects (myelomeningocele) | Latex sensitivity, allergy and risk of anaphylaxis |

**Table 30.2** Signs of intracranial hypertension in infants and children

| Infants | Children | Infants and children |
|---|---|---|
| Irritability | Headache | Decreased consciousness |
| Full Fontanelle | Diplopia | Cranial Nerve (III & IV) palsies |
| Widely separated sutures | Papilledema | Loss of upward gaze (setting sun sign) |
| Cranial enlargement | Vomiting | Signs of herniation, Cushing's triad, pupillary changes |

Adapted from Smith's Anesthesia for Infants and Children, 8th Edition

distress, diplopia, and aspiration. Visual field changes are a clue to suprasellar masses. A clinical assessment of volume status is imperative. Preoperative laboratory tests are tailored to the neurological condition, surgery being performed, anticipated blood loss, and general health of the child. Liver function tests and hematologic profile may be necessary in children who are on chronic anticonvulsants. Type and cross-matched blood should be available for surgeries with large volumes of predicted blood loss, such as resection of large tumors, and craniofacial reconstructions. Unanticipated blood loss is a risk with interventional procedures for vascular malformations in the Radiology suite. As blood-draws can be challenging in infants, it is reasonable to draw a hematocrit, PT and PTT soon after induction in the operating room to minimize trauma to the child.

Premedication should be utilized judiciously in the pediatric patient requiring neurosurgery. In infants and younger children, it is best to administer this in the preoperative area, to ease separation from parents [10, 11]. Premedication is especially necessary in certain conditions such as moyamoya disease to avoid agitation and crying, or in the case of an arteriovenous malformation that has recently bled. Oral Midazolam is usually the drug of choice; it may be administered parenterally if an intravenous catheter is present, and titrated to effect under the direct supervision of a medical provider. The decision to premedicate should be weighed against the risk of oversedation in a neurologically impaired patient, in whom hypoventilation might increase the risk of intracranial hypertension.

## Intraoperative and Postoperative Management

The general principles of intraoperative management need to be modified for specific disease states in neurosurgical cases. Induction technique and choice of induction agent is based on the preoperative status of the patient, a rapid sequence induction being mandatory in the somnolent child with signs of raised intracranial pressure owing to the risk of aspiration. The goal during induction is minimizing further increases in ICP. In general, most intravenous drugs minimize CBF, metabolism and ICP. In neurologically stable patients, a mask induction with sevoflurane and nitrous oxide can be performed. Manual hyperventilation can be utilized during this time if necessary to decrease ICP.

Positioning requirements vary among neurosurgical cases. Special attention should be paid during positioning to optimize access for both surgeon and anesthesiologist, while ensuring safety of the patient. Many neurosurgical procedures require prone positioning with the head of the bed turned 90–180° away from the anesthesiologist. The head is secured in cranial fixation pins, or a Mayfield frame with the neck flexed or extended to facilitate surgical exposure. Extreme rotation of the head can impede venous return or compromise cerebral perfusion, extreme flexion can cause migration of the endotracheal tube into a mainstem bronchus, and cause brainstem compression in posterior fossa lesions, while extreme extension can lead to unplanned extubation. Sometimes it is required that the head be higher than the torso to facilitate venous and CSF drainage from the surgical site, increasing the risk of venous air embolism (VAE) [12]. In infants VAE can occur even in the lateral, prone, or supine position, as the larger head rests above the heart [13, 14]. The risk is increased in children with intracardiac shunts. Precordial Doppler is the most sensitive monitor to detect VAE but prone positioning may preclude its use on the chest. In infants weighing <6 kg the Doppler could be placed on the posterior thorax between the scapulae. In addition to the characteristic changes in Doppler sounds, a sudden decrease in end-tidal $CO_2$, dysrhythmias, and ischemic changes in the EKG should alert one to the occurrence of VAE.

Two large peripheral venous catheters and an arterial line are sufficient for most procedures. Central venous catheters are not routinely used, as the narrow-gauge catheters used in children are often unsuccessful in aspirating air in the event of a VAE. Currently, EEG is considered the most reliable intraoperative monitor for focal cerebral ischemia. Near Infrared Spectroscopy (NIRS) is increasingly proving useful for early detection of global cerebral ischemia. It provides a non-invasive assessment of venous oxy-Hgb saturation and has been reported to correlate with jugular bulb saturation. EMG is useful in identification and dissection of functional nerve roots in tethered spinal cord syndrome. In surgeries involving the spine, SSEP is utilized to assess the dorsal sensory pathways of the spinal cord and MEP to monitor the integrity of the corticospinal tracts that transmit motor impulses. Electrocorticography (ECoG) is used for cortical stimulation in seizure surgery. Preoperative planning should include a discussion of the type and extent of neurophysiologic monitoring to be used, as many anesthetic agents have a depressant effect on some monitors.

Maintenance of anesthesia is achieved with an opioid-based balanced technique, that includes low dose volatile agent, and a muscle relaxant. Muscle relaxation should be avoided in cases where intraoperative EMG, MEP, or muscle stimulation is utilized. Nitrous oxide is avoided after the initial mask induction until the dura is opened, as intracranial air can persist for up to 3 weeks after a craniotomy and the rapid expansion of air cavities can cause a tension pneumocephalus. Meticulous fluid management is essential and although there is no absolute formula, maintenance of normovolemia is key in most situations. Normal saline or Plasmalyte are commonly used as maintenance fluids. The use of colloids in the setting of a disrupted blood brain barrier is controversial. The decision to transfuse blood is based on the type and duration of surgery, underlying condition of the child and potential for ongoing blood loss. Brain swelling and raised ICP is managed with a combination of judicious hyperventilation, and hyperosmolar therapy that may include mannitol and hypertonic saline, along with Furosemide [15]. Hypertonic saline may be associated with natriuresis, central pontine myelinolysis and rebound increase in ICP. The decision to extubate after surgery is based on numerous factors. Airway edema is a concern in prolonged prone cases with significant blood loss requiring large volume replacement. The risk of postoperative apnea and vocal cord paralysis should be considered in surgeries involving the brainstem. If extubation is planned, drugs should be titrated to facilitate neurological assessment at emergence. Postoperative care for the large majority of neurosurgical cases is optimally provided in the Intensive Care Unit for 2–3 days after surgery, where close monitoring of neurologic status can be achieved. One should be alert to the occurrence of postoperative seizures; although the incidence is low, the effects can be devastating. The routine use of prophylactic anticonvulsants is debatable [16].

## Considerations for Specific Disease States and Surgeries

### Congenital Anomalies

Spinal dysraphism is a midline defect that can be minor involving only superficial bone and membranous structures or may include malformed neural tissue; it can involve the head (encephalocele) or spine. Spina bifida refers to a spectrum of spine defects, a defect containing CSF is a meningocele; a meningomyelocele also includes neural tissue. These are often associated with hydrocephalus and Arnold Chiari malformations. Primary closure is often undertaken on the first 1–2 days of life. This is a field where in-utero closure is increasingly being undertaken as the defect is identified on prenatal ultrasound. Special attention is paid at induction to positioning, with a "donut" ring being used to avoid pressure on the defect if intubation is attempted in the supine position. In the case of large defects, intubation in the lateral position may be necessary. These patients are at high risk for developing latex sensitivity and anaphylaxis, as they are subject to repeated exposure to latex products, both in surgery for coexisting orthopedic and urologic problems, and in routine care as in repeated bladder catheterizations. These children may develop a tethered spinal cord as they grow, that can cause nerve root distortion, progressive neurologic deficits and chronic pain. As mentioned, EMG monitoring intraoperatively can help identify functional nerve roots and avoid inadvertent injury that can lead to fecal or urinary incontinence. Selective Dorsal Rhizotomy is a procedure performed for severe spasticity associated with cerebral palsy. This involves surgical division of dorsal rootlets to decrease afferent input to motor neurons in the spinal cord. The rootlets are identified by direct stimulation and noting the corresponding muscle action potential with EMG. These patients have severe somatic pain postoperatively, along with dysesthesia, hyperesthesia and muscle spasms. A multimodal postoperative pain management strategy is imperative [17].

### Arnold Chiari Malformations

These consist of four grades of abnormalities of the posterior fossa, leading to varying ranges of caudad displacement of the cerebellar vermis through the foramen magnum. Children with Type I have milder symptoms, Type II often have coexisting hydrocephalus, Type III have the most severe symptoms with long term disability, and Type IV is characterized by cerebellar hypoplasia or aplasia. Care should be taken in these patients to avoid extreme head flexion during intubation as it can cause brainstem compression. Abnormal responses to hypoxia and hypercarbia should be anticipated as they have cranial nerve and brainstem dysfunction.

### Tumors

Brain tumors are the second most common childhood malignancy, next to leukemias. The majority are infratentorial and include medulloblastomas, cerebellar astrocytomas, brainstem gliomas, and ependymomas of the fourth ventricle. Supratentorial tumors account for 25–40% of brain tumors in children and include astrocytomas, oligodendrogliomas, ependymomas, and glioblastomas. Infratentorial tumors can obstruct CSF flow, thereby leading to intracranial hypertension and hydrocephalus. Surgery for resection is accompanied by anesthetic challenges at every stage. Positioning is usually prone with the head fixed in pins, and turned 90–180° away from the anesthesiologist based on surgeon preference. Skull fractures, intracranial hematomas and dural tears are risks during pinning. Sinus tears, VAE and massive blood loss are risks during raising of the bone flap, and require constant vigilance. Elevated ICP is managed by altering ventilation techniques, mannitol, or by the insertion of a ventricular or lumbar catheter by the surgeon. Arrhythmias and hemodynamic perturbations are not uncommon during brainstem manipulation. Postoperative concerns include apnea and airway obstruction from damage to the respiratory centers and cranial nerves.

Other tumors seen in children include craniopharyngiomas, pituitary adenomas, optic nerve gliomas, hypothalamic tumors, and papillomas of the choroid plexus. Precocious puberty is often the presentation in hypothalamic tumors. Of the perisellar tumors, craniopharyngiomas are the most common and can be accompanied by endocrine derangements; steroids are often necessary as the hypothalamic-pituitary-adrenal axis is affected. Diabetes insipidus commonly occurs both pre, intra, and postoperatively. Urine output should be closely monitored along with serum electrolytes, and osmolality. The transsphenoidal approach is sometimes used in older children; one should however be prepared to convert to an open craniotomy in the event of massive bleeding.

## Hydrocephalus

Hydrocephalus is a condition where there is an increase in CSF volume as the result of a mismatch of CSF production and absorption, leading to increased intracranial pressure. It is the most common neurosurgical condition in pediatrics. It can result from the obstruction of CSF flow, or an inability to absorb CSF. In neonates, especially premies, intraventricular or subarachnoid hemorrhage is a common cause, as is congenital aqueductal stenosis. Other causes include trauma, infection and tumors. Hydrocephalus may be non-obstructive (communicating) or obstructive (non-communicating) based on whether there is unimpeded flow of CSF around the spinal cord. The acuity of presentation depends on the rapidity of development of hydrocephalus and the intracranial compliance. In the infant, the cerebral vault gradually expands to accommodate the increased CSF volume, if hydrocephalus develops over time. In older children whose sutures are fused, the risk of herniation is higher as the skull cannot expand and compensate. These children present to the ER with increasing lethargy, vomiting, rapidly develop cranial nerve dysfunction and bradycardia, and are definite aspiration risks. Following a rapid sequence induction, hyperventilation is instituted to control the ICP. Definitive treatment is correction of the cause, but immediate treatment involves placement of a ventricular drain or ventriculoperitoneal shunt with the goal of controlling the ICP by rapidly relieving the obstruction. VP shunts divert CSF from the ventricles to the peritoneal cavity. When absorption through the peritoneum is compromised, as in peritonitis, the distal end of the shunt is placed in the right atrium or pleural cavity. Shunts often need to be replaced as the child grows or the pathophysiology changes, requiring repeat trips to the operating room. Shunts with programmable valves help minimize this to some extent. Acute obstruction of a shunt needs to be treated urgently as it can have lethal consequences. Shunt infection is not uncommon in this population; in this situation, the entire shunt system is removed and an external ventricular drain (EVD) established temporarily. A new shunt is placed after treatment of the infection. Transportation and moving of patients with EVDs requires special attention to avoid sudden drainage of CSF or dislodgement of the tubing. Excess drainage of CSF can lead to slit ventricle syndrome [18]. Fluid overload should be avoided in these patients to minimize brain swelling. Endoscopic third ventriculostomy is a procedure that creates an alternative route from one area of CSF to another, thus bypassing an area of obstruction. Common locations for a ventriculostomy are through the septum pellucidum allowing the lateral ventricles to communicate, or through the floor of the third ventricle into the CSF cisterns. Cauterization of the choroid plexus in addition, helps to reduce excessive CSF production. Damage to the basilar artery and its branches, or neural injuries are a concern with these procedures.

## Seizures

Seizures are a common neurological disorder, and can be a component of various epilepsy syndromes. Vagal nerve stimulators inhibit seizures at the brainstem/cortical levels. Surgical resection of the seizure focus is the last recourse when a child has intractable epilepsy, and involves serial craniotomies. The first is for insertion of intracranial grid-and-strip electrodes on the exposed cortex of the brain. The patient is then monitored for seizures in the electrophysiology unit to map the location of the seizure foci, which then serves to guide the neurosurgeon for resection. It is important to avoid agents that may suppress seizures during and after the surgery, i.e. benzodiazepines. It may take several days but typically the patient returns to the operating room in 2–3 days. Surgical risk and anesthetic concerns are dependent on the location of the seizure focus, its proximity to vital structures, and the age of the patient. Intraoperative neurophysiologic monitoring is used to guide the resection; this might include cortical stimulation to identify the motor strip, EEG, and EMG. Advances in neurophysiologic monitoring have made these procedures safer and more accurate. The anesthetic technique is tailored to the patient's specific requirements with the goal of not compromising the monitoring, especially when the seizure foci involve functional areas of the brain [19]. A narcotic based general anesthetic with low levels of volatile agent is optimal. Muscle relaxation is avoided if cortical stimulation of motor cortex or EMG is being used.

Upregulation of the hepatic P450 enzymes from chronic use of anticonvulsants can result in rapid metabolism and clearance of neuromuscular blockers and opioids in these patients [20]. Awake craniotomies are rarely undertaken in children but may be considered in older and cooperative teenagers when ongoing assessment of neural function is imperative. Anesthesia for an awake craniotomy can range from no sedation with local anesthesia alone, to alternating "asleep-awake-asleep" techniques in which general anesthesia is limited to the period before and after functional testing [21]. Following induction of general anesthesia, the airway is secured with either an endotracheal tube or a laryngeal mask airway, and the patient is kept asleep during the craniotomy. The anesthetic is discontinued and the patient extubated during the period of functional neurological testing, during which time a psychologist is also present in the operating room. Once testing is completed, general anesthesia is reinstituted. With this technique, the patient is completely anesthetized for the painful parts of the surgery. A disadvantage is the unpredictability of the patient's emergence and reactions under surgical drapes. Deep sedation with a natural airway, using propofol and dexmedetomidine, combined with an opioid is an alternative. Not all older children are good candidates for an awake craniotomy; patient selection should take into consideration their maturity, psychological preparedness, and ability to cooperate in an unfamiliar environment.

## Craniosynostosis

Premature closure of one or more cranial sutures occurs in about 1 in 2000 births; it may be associated with a variety of syndromes, some of which are harbingers of a difficult airway. Uncorrected craniosynostosis can result in increased ICP and brain compression, with neurologic sequelae. Correction is usually undertaken in the first 3–6 months of life, as brain growth is rapid during this period and the skull bones more malleable. The procedure may be a single strip craniectomy or a complete craniofacial reconstruction.

These procedures fall into the purview of Plastic Surgery, but more extensive cranial exposures involve neurosurgeons. Although extradural, blood loss from the scalp and cranium can be significant, and VAE is a significant risk. Adequate venous access and invasive monitoring are imperative. The use of antifibrinolytics is controversial, but may have some utility. Less invasive neuroendoscopic techniques aim for smaller incisions, minimal dissection and blood loss, and fewer complications, allowing for less aggressive fluid replacement, less invasive hemodynamic monitoring, and possibly less mortality [22, 23].

## Vascular Malformations

Vascular anomalies in children are rare, and most are congenital lesions. Large arteriovenous malformations (AVMs), such as those of the Vein of Galen in neonates are associated with high output congestive heart failure. Initial treatment often consists of serial embolizations in the interventional radiology suite, during which they require inotropic support, or antihypertensive treatment with vasodilators [24]. Intracranial AVMs may be associated with vascular or lymphatic malformations in the spinal cord, or face.

Moyamoya disease is a rare condition characterized by chronic progressive steno-occlusion of the arteries of the Circle of Willis, usually the intracranial portion of the internal carotid arteries, with collateral vessel formation at the base of the brain [25]. The syndrome can be associated with neurofibromatosis, tuberous sclerosis, Marfan's syndrome, Noonan Syndrome, homocystinuria, thalassemia, sickle cell disease, congenital heart disease optic nerve gliomas, basal brain tumors, and chromosomal disorders such as Down's, William's and Turner's syndromes. These children present with frequent transient ischemic attacks or recurrent strokes. Surgical treatment aims to increase collateral flow by direct or indirect revascularization procedures, using the external carotid circulation as the donor supply. Perioperative ischemia is a significant risk; it is imperative to maintain normocapnia, normotension, normovolemia, and normothermia,

concepts that are contrary to what is practiced for other neurosurgical cases, and continue them into the perioperative period [26]. Both hypercapnia and hypocapnia can be detrimental, a cerebral steal phenomenon diverting blood flow away from the compromised ischemic area of the brain. Indirect procedures are now commonly used in children. In pial synangiosis, an intact superficial temporal artery is fixed to the pial surface with the creation of a wide opening of dura and arachnoid; over time, there is ingrowth of new vessels through the opening to the poorly perfused area of the brain. Anesthetic technique should not interfere with EEG monitoring.

## Neuroimaging

Neurosurgical patients go through several imaging studies as part of their workup, which may include CT, MRI, Nuclear Medicine scans etc., for which younger children require sedation or general anesthesia. Stereotactic procedures can start out in the Radiology suite where the patient is often anesthetized, prior to application of the frame and the anesthetized patient is then transported to the operating room. The need for intraoperative MRI for procedures such as laser thermoablation has led to the construction of hybrid suites where imaging and surgery can be performed in a sterile environment. Access to the patient is a challenge in this situation, as is the need for MRI compatible or MRI conditional equipment.

## Neurotrauma

Traumatic brain injury (TBI) is the leading cause of death and disability in children over 1 year of age in the USA. Spinal cord injury is often concurrent. In children, cervical spine fractures can occur without neurological deficit, and deficits can occur without a radiologic fracture. Decreased perfusion to the brain and cerebral ischemia occur in the first 6–12 h after a TBI, followed by hyperemia and raised ICP. Children with a GCS score <9 should be intubated for airway protection and management of raised ICP. Cerebral autoregulation may be impaired and the CPP threshold required to prevent cerebral hypoperfusion is not well understood. Current recommendation is to avoid CPP <40 mmHg, however the threshold to prevent ischemia is likely age-dependent with older children requiring a higher CPP [27]. A systolic BP higher than normal, may be needed to maintain CPP. The goal of surgery in TBI is to optimize viable brain recovery by removal of massive hemorrhages or lesions. There is a high risk of VAE and massive blood loss in craniotomies for evacuation of epidural or subdural hematomas. Anesthetic goals include mild hyperventilation to prevent brainstem herniation and intracranial hypertension. Head cooling and mild hypothermia may be protective; although this may be controversial, hyperthermia should be avoided. When a child presents with a conglomeration of chronic and acute subdural hematomas, subarachnoid hemorrhage, skull fractures in various stages of healing, with or without other injuries out of proportion to the history, non-accidental or inflicted trauma should be suspected. Outcomes are usually poor.

## Summary

The management of pediatric neurosurgical patients presents challenges to both surgeon and anesthesiologist. Understanding the age-related differences in this population is vital and goes a long way in being prepared for complex cases, thus avoiding complications. Formulating a thoughtful plan well in advance, being aware of the riskier portions of the surgery, and maintaining open dialogue with the surgeon through the procedure, is essential to minimizing perioperative morbidity and mortality.

## References

1. Chumas P, Kenny T, Stiller C. Subspecialisation in neurosurgery-does size matter? Acta Neurochir. 2011;153(6):1231–6.
2. Mokri B. The Monro-Kellie hypothesis: applications in CSF volume depletion. Neurology. 2001;56(12):1746–8.
3. Shapiro K, Marmarou A, Shulman K. Characterization of clinical CSF dynamics and neural axis compliance using the pressure-volume index: I. The normal pressure-volume index. Ann Neurol. 1980;7(6):508–14.
4. Vavilala M, Soriano S, Krane E. Anesthesia for neurosurgery. In: Davis P, Cladis FP, editors. Smith's anesthesia for infants and children. 8th ed. Philadelphia: Elsevier; 2017. p. 744–5.
5. Wintermark M, Lepori D, Cotting J, Roulet E, van Melle G, Meuli R, et al. Brain perfusion in children: evolution with age assessed by quantitative perfusion computed tomography. Pediatrics. 2004;113(6):1642–52.
6. Vavilala MS, Lee LA, Lam AM. The lower limit of cerebral autoregulation in children during sevoflurane anesthesia. J Neurosurg Anesthesiol. 2003;15(4):307–12.
7. Brady KM, Mytar JO, Lee JK, Cameron DE, Vricella LA, Thompson WR, et al. Monitoring cerebral blood flow pressure autoregulation in pediatric patients during cardiac surgery. Stroke. 2010;41(9):1957–62.
8. Rhee CJ, Fraser CD, Kibler K, Easley RB, Andropoulos DB, Czosnyka M, et al. The ontogeny of cerebrovascular pressure autoregulation in premature infants. J Perinatol. 2014;34(12):926–31.
9. Ellingsen I, Hauge A, Nicolaysen G, Thoresen M, Walloe L. Changes in human cerebral blood flow due to step changes in PAO2 and PACO2. Acta Physiol Scand. 1987;129(2):157–63.
10. McCann ME, Kain ZN. The management of preoperative anxiety in children: an update. Anesth Analg. 2001;93(1):98–105.
11. Kain ZN, Caldwell-Andrews AA, Krivutza DM, Weinberg ME, Wang SM, Gaal D. Trends in the practice of parental presence during induction of anesthesia and the use of preoperative sedative premedication in the United States, 1995-2002: results of a follow-up national survey. Anesth Analg. 2004;98(5):1252–9, table of contents.
12. Grady MS, Bedford RF, Park TS. Changes in superior sagittal sinus pressure in children with head elevation, jugular venous compression, and PEEP. J Neurosurg. 1986;65(2):199–202.
13. Harris MM, Yemen TA, Davidson A, Strafford MA, Rowe RW, Sanders SP, et al. Venous embolism during craniectomy in supine infants. Anesthesiology. 1987;67(5):816–9.
14. Faberowski LW, Black S, Mickle JP. Incidence of venous air embolism during craniectomy for craniosynostosis repair. Anesthesiology. 2000;92(1):20–3.
15. Piper BJ, Harrigan PW. Hypertonic saline in paediatric traumatic brain injury: a review of nine years' experience with 23.4% hypertonic saline as standard hyperosmolar therapy. Anaesth Intensive Care. 2015;43(2):204–10.

16. Hardesty DA, Sanborn MR, Parker WE, Storm PB. Perioperative seizure incidence and risk factors in 223 pediatric brain tumor patients without prior seizures. J Neurosurg Pediatr. 2011;7(6):609–15.
17. Geiduschek JM, Haberkern CM, McLaughlin JF. Pain management for children following selective dorsal rhizotomy. Can J Anaesth. 1997;41:492–6.
18. Elredge EA, Rockoff MA, Medlock MA, Scott RM, Millis MB. Postoperative cerebral edema occurring in children with slit ventricles. Pediatrics. 1997;99:625–30.
19. Eldredge A, Soriano SG, Rockoff MA. Neuroanesthesia. Neurosurg Clin N Am. 1995;6:505–20.
20. Soriano SG, Martyn JA. Antiepileptic-induced resistance to neuromuscular blockers: mechanisms and clinical significance. Clin Pharmacokinet. 2004;43(2):71–81.
21. Sarang A, Dinsmore J. Anaesthesia for awake craniotomy--evolution of a technique that facilitates awake neurological testing. Br J Anaesth. 2003;90(2):161–5.
22. Jimenez DF, Barone CM. Endoscopic craniectomy for early surgical correction of sagittal craniosynostosis. J Neurosurg. 1998;88(1):77–81.
23. Jimenez DF, Barone CM, Cartwright CC, Baker L. Early management of craniosynostosis using endoscopic-assisted strip craniectomies and cranial orthotic molding therapy. Pediatrics. 2002;110(1 Pt 1):97–104.
24. Burrows PE, Robertson RL. Neonatal central nervous system vascular disorders. Neurosurg Clin N Am. 1998;9(1):155–80.
25. Baykan N, Ozgen S, Ustalar ZS, Dagcinar A, Ozek MM. Moyamoya disease and anesthesia. Paediatr Anaesth. 2005;15(12):1111–5.
26. Parray T, Martin TW, Siddiqui S. Moyamoya disease: a review of the disease and anesthetic management. J Neurosurg Anesthesiol. 2011;23(2):100–9.
27. Vavilala MS, Kernic MA, Wang J. Acute care clinical indictors associated with discharge outcomes in children with severe traumatic brain injury. Pediatric Guideline Adherence and Outcomes Study. Crit Care Med. 2014;42(10):2258–66.

# Anesthesia for Thoracic Surgery

## David S. Beebe and Kumar G. Belani

## Introduction

Pediatric Anesthesiologists often have to provide care for babies and children who have to undergo thoracic procedures. While management of older children and teenagers is often similar to management of adults undergoing thoracic and video-assisted thoracoscopic procedures, the physiology of babies and small children undergoing thoracotomies can be quite different than adults. Both the response to lateral positioning and, if necessary, one lung ventilation is different and can be more difficult to manage in infants and small children than older children or adults. There now is equipment for lung isolation specifically designed for pediatric patients, but may not always be safe or effective to use in every patient.

In this chapter we will we will review the preoperative evaluation and perioperative anesthetic care of babies and children undergoing thoracic surgery. In addition, we will: (1) Review the response to lateral positioning and ventilation in small children and contrast that with adults or older children. (2) Review the techniques and management of lung isolation and one-lung ventilation as well as the use of $CO_2$ insufflation. (3) Discuss the techniques used for post-operative analgesia.

## Preoperative Evaluation

In the preoperative evaluation attention should be paid to the underlying reason the patient is scheduled for thoracic surgery. Conditions such as an anterior mediastinal mass are more common in children and can make anesthetic induction hazardous. Symptoms can be deceiving. Children can lose a large amount of functioning lung tissue and be asymptomatic. The development of dyspnea or exercise intolerance indicates severe disease progression. The children should be examined for the presence of wheezing, decreased breath sounds or asymmetric breathing patterns. Chest X ray, CT scans and MRI studies should be examined to determine if airway or vascular compromise is present or likely to occur with induction of general anesthesia. Most patients should receive a hemoglobin determination, and blood should be type and screened for all major thoracic operations. However preoperative arterial blood gases are usually not necessary. Measurement of oxygen saturation by pulse oximetry and evaluation of venous $HCO_3$, elevated in children with chronic $CO_2$ retention, are usually sufficient. Standard pulmonary function tests are also difficult to interpret in children who are often uncooperative [1].

D. S. Beebe, M.D. (✉)
K. G. Belani, M.B.B.S., M.S.
Department of Anesthesiology, University of Minnesota Medical School, Masonic Childrens' Hospital, Minneapolis, MN, USA
e-mail: beebe001@umn.edu

## Induction and Management of Anesthesia for Thoracic Surgery and Perioperative Monitoring

For standard thoracic procedures in children where lesions are not likely to result in hemodynamic compromise, either an inhaled induction of general anesthesia with sevoflurane or an intravenous induction with propofol is usually well tolerated. In patients with significant loss of lung tissue or who are chronically hypoxic, 100% oxygen should be used without Nitrous Oxide during either an inhaled or intravenous induction of general anesthesia to prevent hypoxia. Skeletal muscle relaxation is usually administered to aid tracheal intubation and provide relaxation for surgery. Sevoflurane and low-dose narcotics such as fentanyl are most commonly used for maintenance of anesthesia. Total intravenous anesthesia with propofol can also be used and has the advantage of diminished postoperative nausea and vomiting and may improve oxygenation because of improved matching of ventilation with perfusion in the lateral position. Nitrous Oxide is not often used for thoracic procedures, however, because it can diffuse into blebs and closed air spaces that may develop in a thoracic procedures and cause a pneumothorax. Nitrous Oxide also prevents the administration of 100% oxygen which is often necessary in thoracic operations. In most cases following tracheal intubation patients are ventilated using a tidal volume of 7 mL/kg, a low level of PEEP to prevent atelectasis (5 cm $H_2O$), and a respiratory rate adjusted to maintain an end-tidal $CO_2$ between 30 and 40 mmHg. An air-oxygen mixture is often used initially at an $FiO_2$ adequate to maintain oxygenation. However, if one-lung ventilation is required, 100% oxygen is usually necessary [1].

In addition to the standard monitoring used in all patients undergoing anesthesia (ECG, blood pressure, end-tidal gas analysis, pulse oximetry), patients undergoing major thoracic procedures often benefit from an arterial catheter to allow blood gas analysis. In more minor procedures, such as most thoracoscopic operations, arterial catheters are not necessary. In all thoracic operations the anesthesia provider team must be aware of the airway pressures and delivered tidal volumes measured by the ventilator because they can be affected during the operation and require adjustment to ensure adequate ventilation [1].

One condition occasionally seen in children that can make administration of anesthesia hazardous is an anterior mediastinal mass. Anesthetic induction with loss of spontaneous ventilation can cause compression of the anterior mediastinal structures by the mass. Not only can the trachea be compressed causing airway obstruction, but the pulmonary artery and the superior vena cava can also become compressed, resulting in cardiac arrest. If possible, local anesthesia alone should be utilized if a biopsy of the mass is required. If general anesthesia is necessary, careful induction with spontaneous ventilation or awake tracheal intubation may be used. A large bore peripheral venous catheter should be placed in the lower extremity. Spontaneous ventilation should be maintained. A surgeon who can do rigid bronchoscopy should be present to open the airway if tracheal collapse occurs. There also are a few reports of cardiopulmonary bypass being used as a last resort, and perhaps should be considered in high risk patients [1, 2].

## Physiology of Positioning and Ventilation for Thoracotomy in Infants Compared to Older Children and Adults

Most, although not all, thoracic procedures are performed in the lateral position. The operative side, which is usually the side with the pathology, is in the non-dependent position. Due to the low pressures generated by the right heart in the pulmonary circulation and the compliant nature of the pulmonary vasculature, this results normally in more of the blood flow being delivered to the dependent lung in older children or adults. This is beneficial because more blood is delivered to healthy, non-operative lung where it can absorb oxygen. Therefore, most older children and adults can tolerate thoracic surgery in the lateral position even if the operative, non-dependent lung is not ventilated [1].

In contrast in babies or infants the hydrostatic pressure gradient between the dependent and non-dependent lungs is not as high and the blood flow is more uniform between the two lungs. Also the chest wall of infants and babies under 1 year of age is significantly more compliant than that of older children or adults. When infants are placed in the lateral position the chest wall partially collapses due to gravity and impedes ventilation to the dependent lung more than in older children or adults. Also Infants normally consume 6–8 mL/kg/min of $O_2$ compared with a normal $O_2$ consumption in adults of 2–3 mL/kg/min. For these reasons, infants are at increased risk of significant oxygen desaturation during surgery in the lateral decubitus position than older children or adults even if 100% oxygen is utilized [1].

## Techniques and Management of One-Lung Ventilation and $CO_2$ Insufflation

Often pediatric surgeons request that the operative lung be collapsed during the operation to facilitate exposure, minimize trauma to the lung during dissection and occasionally to protect the non-operative lung from spillage or infection from the lung having surgery. There are several techniques and devices that have been developed over the years. All will work well in older children or teenagers. Infants and babies are more problematic.

1. Endobronchial intubation. This is the oldest technique but still can be useful, particularly in an emergency situation. For example, the normal lung can be isolated from hemorrhage from an injured lung in the emergency room by intubating the bronchus to the good lung. Verification can be confirmed by bronchoscopy. Patients can be managed during surgery with this technique as well, but better devices are available to be used electively for most patients. One advantage to this technique, however, is that it can be used in patients of all sizes. Successful one lung ventilation in infants less than 10-kg has been described using selective bronchial intubation [3].

2. Bronchial blockers. Balloon tipped, Fogarty catheters were originally used to occlude the bronchus of lung that is to be collapsed in infants or small children. The catheter is advanced into the bronchus under bronchoscopic guidance and the balloon inflated. The trachea then can be intubated alongside the catheter. The air is absorbed from the blocked lung and it eventually collapses. This technique can be used in patients of all sizes. However, the balloon is a high-pressure, low volume device not designed for use in the airway and potentially can cause mucosal injury. It also is not possible to suction the blocked lung using this device, or apply oxygen or CPAP to the dependent lung. A bronchial blocking device has been developed with a lower pressure balloon that can be placed through the endotracheal tube (Arndt Endobronchial Blocker)—the latter tube has been designed to allow easier placement using bronchoscopic guidance. The bronchoscope is placed through an adaptor following intubation that allows ventilation through the endotracheal tube while the blocker is manipulated into position. The adapter fixes the blocker in position. The blocker has a small lumen which allows suctioning of the blocked lung. In small infants <10 kg where the blocker would occlude the lumen of the tracheal tube it has been placed extraluminally and successfully used for one lung ventilation. Another device, the Univent™ tube, has a bronchial blocker built into the side of the tube. A bronchoscope is utilized following intubation with the tracheal tube to guide the blocked into the bronchus. It also has a small lumen in the blocker to allow suctioning, and the fixation device is built into the tube. Both devices have a small lumen in the center of the blocker which allow more rapid deflation of the blocked lung as well as suctioning of the collapsed lung and the application of CPAP. The bronchial balloon is of a high pressure, low volume type which may cause mucosal injury [1, 3].

3. Double lumen endotracheal tubes. Double lumen endotracheal tubes are usually placed in the left bronchus and allows ventilation to each lung independently. The left sided double lumen tubes are usually used for surgery on either lung because right sided tubes are more difficult to properly place because of the high takeoff of the right upper lobe. Due to the fact there are two lumens they are quite wide and were never utilized in children for many years for fear of injuring the bronchus. Currently there is a 28 F endotracheal tube designed to be used in children as young as 8 years of age. Placement is the same as in adults i.e. the tube is rotated to the left as the trachea is intubated and advanced into the left main stem bronchus. Tube and proper cuff placement is confirmed by bronchoscopy. The cuffs of the double lumen tubes are also low-pressure and high volume to minimize mucosal injury. Double-lumen tubes allow easy suctioning and CPAP application to the non-ventilated lung, and are very stable after taping in place. Therefore, double-tubes are handy to use in children or teenagers large enough to accommodate their size. One disadvantage to using a double-lumen tube compared to a bronchial blocker is that the double lumen tube must be changed to a single lumen tube if the patient is to remain tracheally intubated after surgery. In contrast, if a bronchial blocker is used only the device must be removed and the tracheal tube can stay in place [1].

When placing a bronchial blocker or double-lumen tracheal tube it is important to ventilate the patient with 100% oxygen. This allows for more rapid absorption of air from the non-ventilated lung and a more rapid collapse of the lung tissue. Collapse can be hastened by applying suction to the non-ventilated lung. In most cases 100% oxygen is utilized both to maximize oxygen delivery to the ventilated lung and to act as a pulmonary vasodilator. This causes more blood to flow from the hypoxic, non-ventilated lung to the ventilated lung where oxygen can be taken up. Patients are ventilated at a tidal volume of 7 mL/kg with the rate adjusted maintain a constant end-tidal carbon dioxide concentration, with a low level of PEEP (5 cm of $H_2O$) to prevent atelectasis. The airway pressures must be monitored and the tidal volumes and ventilatory rates adjusted to prevent barotrauma. Ventilation of both lungs is then established at the completion of surgery [1].

Often surgeons will have insufflated carbon dioxide into the pleural space at low pressures (5–15 mmHg) similar to laparoscopy, either to hasten the lung collapse or to partially collapse the lung for the operation without requiring one lung ventilation. This has been common for short, thoracoscopic procedures and avoids the need for the placement of bronchial blockers or double lumen tracheal tubes. Carbon dioxide insufflation is usually well tolerated [1]. However, there have been cases reported where the insufflation of carbon dioxide caused hypotension, bradycardia and cardiovascular collapse. The mechanism for this

**Table 31.1** Evaluation and correction of hypoxemia during one-lung ventilation

| Steps | Action |
|---|---|
| 1 | Place the patient on 100% oxygen if not on it already |
| 2 | Resume two-lung ventilation if hypoxemia severe |
| 3 | Evaluate tube and cuff positions with bronchoscopy and auscultation |
| 4 | Suction the tracheal tube lumen(s) to be sure there is no obstruction from secretions |
| 5 | Apply CPAP (5–10 cm $H_2O$) to the non-ventilated lung |
| 6 | Apply a low-level of PEEP (5 cm of $H_2O$) to the ventilated lung. Avoid high levels of PEEP because it may divert blood to the non-ventilated lung |
| 7 | Ventilate the non-dependent lung with a recruitment maneuver intermittently |
| 8 | Change from an inhalational to intravenous anesthesia ± phenylephrine infusion to improve hypoxic pulmonary vasoconstriction and therefore matching of ventilation to perfusion |
| 9 | If these maneuvers fail, complete the surgery using two-lung ventilation |

is unknown, but may be related to the insufflation being performed too rapidly [4].

With the use of 100% oxygen most patients tolerate one lung ventilation. Adjustments often have to be made, however (Table 31.1). If difficulty in oxygenation or ventilation occurs, position of the cuffs on the double lumen tube may have to be checked using the bronchoscope to be sure displacement or herniation has not occurred. CPAP (5 cm $H_2O$) applied to the non-ventilated lung may improve oxygenation by forcing more blood to the ventilated lung where oxygenation can occur. However, some patients, especially infants and small children, may not tolerate one lung ventilation not matter what is done and it may have to be abandoned [5].

## Postoperative Analgesia

Postoperative analgesia is a serious problem for infants and children who have had thoracic surgery. Prior to surgery a plan for analgesia should be discussed with the parents and children themselves if they are mature enough because some of the analgesic techniques necessary may be invasive. If the patients are already receiving pain medications the management may be even more difficult. All children should have a plan for non-narcotic oral analgesics postoperatively such as scheduled acetaminophen, ibuprofen, and gabapentin. Intraoperative and perioperative administration of dexmedetomodine and ketamine may help diminish postoperative pain as well. There are four basic approaches that are commonly used, some concurrently, for analgesia in the perioperative period. All of them have limitations and potential complications.

1. Thoracic Epidural Analgesia. Classically thoracic epidural analgesia has been used for pain relief after thoracotomies or painful thoracoscopic procedures (i.e. pectus excavatum repair). It is usually placed at the T5–T7 levels. In older children or teenagers, it can be placed preoperatively. In younger children or infants they can be placed following induction of general anesthesia. Dilute infusions of local anesthetics (i.e. Ropivacaine 0.1%) often combined with clonidine or fentanyl are administered by an infusion pump at rates from 0.3 to 0.5 mg/kg/h. Although this technique is technically familiar to anesthesiologists and is generally effective, complications such as hypotension and itching can occur. Serious spinal cord injuries have also occurred and caused several institutions to abandoned this technique for analgesia for pectus excavatum repair [6].

2. Paravertebral blocks. Paravertebral analgesia has become popular for analgesia post thoracotomy. It has the advantage of being able to provide analgesia to only the operative side. Bilateral paravertebral catheters can be used for thoracic procedures such as pectus excavatum repairs, and can receive local anesthetic infusions similar to epidural analgesia. The degree of analgesia is usually similar to epidural analgesia without the hypotension or weakness seen with the epidural technique. Patients may ambulate after receiving paravertebral analgesia and have been sent home with continuous infusions. Placement of paravertebral catheters is currently easier to do with the use of ultrasound; they generally take longer to place than an epidural catheter. Complications such as pneumothorax or inadvertent epidural or intrathecal catheter placement resulting in spinal block may still occur [6, 7].

3. Chest Wall Infusion. Catheters placed along the chest wall spanning the incision can be infused with local anesthetic to block the nerves along the incision site. This technique is easy to do. It was associated with less nausea and vomiting but comparable pain scores similar to thoracic epidural analgesia for pectus excavatum repair [8].

4. Intravenous Patient Controlled Analgesia. Patient controlled analgesia is often required to supplement the other techniques if the analgesia they provide is inadequate. Patient controlled analgesia used alone also compared favorably to thoracic epidural analgesia in in a recent small study of pediatric cancer patients undergoing thoracotomy. Pain scores, time to

ambulation and voiding as well as discharge to home were similar among the groups but hospital costs were lower if patient controlled analgesia alone was utilized [9].

## Summary

Anesthesia for thoracic anesthesia in children can be performed safely and effectively as in adults. However the equipment and techniques for both perioperative management and postoperative analgesia must be modified for their smaller size, different response to positioning and distinctive physiology.

## References

1. Goliana B, Hammer GB. Pediatric thoracic anesthesia. Curr Opin Anaesthesiol. 2005;18:5–11.
2. Blank RS, de Souza DC. Anesthetic management of patients with an anterior mediastinal mass: continuing professional development. Can J Anesth. 2011;58:853–67.
3. Sutton CJ, Naguib A, Puri S, Sprenker CJ, Camporesi EM. One-lung ventilation in infants and small children: blood gas values. J Anesth. 2012;26:670–4.
4. Harris RJD, Benveniste G, Pfitzner J. Cardiovascular collapse caused by carbon dioxide insufflation during one-lung anesthesia for thoracoscopic dorsal sympathectomy. Anaesth Intensive Care. 2001;30:86–9.
5. Fitzgerald J, Evans F. Techniques for single lung ventilation in infants and children. Anaesthesia Tutorial of the Week 2015. http://www.wfsahq.org. Accessed 23 Oct 2015.
6. Hall Burton DM, Boretsky KR. A comparison of paravertebral nerve block catheters for postoperative analgesia following the Nuss procedure for pectus excavatum repair. Paediatr Anaesth. 2014;24:516–20.
7. Hutchins J, Castro C, Wang Q, Chinnakotla S. Postoperative pain control with paravertebral catheters after pediatric total pancreatectomy and islet autotransplantation: a retrospective study. Paediatr Anaesth. 2016;26:315–20.
8. Choudry DK, Brenn R, Sacks K, Reichard K. Continuous chest wall infusion for analgesia in children undergoing the Nuss procedure: a comparison with thoracic epidural. Paediatr Anaesth. 2016;26:582–9.
9. Gonzalez KW, Dalton BG, Millspaugh DL, Thomas PG, St. Peter SW. Epidural versus patient-controlled analgesia after pediatric thoracotomy of malignancy: a preliminary review. Eur J Pediatr Surg. 2016;26:340–3.

# Anesthesia for Specific Cardiac Lesions: Right-to Left Shunts

## 32

J. R. Paquin, J. E. Lam, and E. P. Lin

## Introduction

Congenital heart disease is reported in approximately 9 per 1000 live births worldwide and continues to increase [1–3]. Cyanotic heart disease, wherein deoxygenated blood bypasses the lungs and shunts across a defect into the systemic circulation, accounts for approximately 15% of all CHD [4]. These lesions can be further classified as right-sided obstructive lesions or intracardiac mixing lesions. The clinical significance of a right-to-left shunt will vary with the degree of obstruction and mixing, leading to pressure overload, volume overload and varying degrees of hypoxemia. The presence of these shunts requires appropriate attention from the anesthesia provider to optimize pulmonary blood flow and oxygenation while maintaining cardiac function.

## Pathophysiology

Shunts can be due to either intracardiac connections between chambers or extracardiac connections between a systemic and pulmonary artery. The direction of blood flow through intracardiac communications is determined by the pressure gradient across the defect. Primary determinants include the size of the defect, whether it is restrictive or not, and the degree of anatomic and dynamic obstruction. For extracardiac communications, the relative resistance on either side, specifically the systemic vascular resistance (SVR) and pulmonary vascular resistance (PVR), play a significant role. Systemic vascular resistance is a measure of vasomotor tone that reflects ventricular afterload, while PVR is a measure of the vascular tone within the pulmonary vasculature [5]. The balance between SVR and PVR is a dynamic process that can be quantified as a ratio of measured pulmonary blood flow (Qp) to measured systemic blood flow (Qs). A normal Qp:Qs should be close to 1, whereas right-to-left shunting results in a Qp:Qs less than 1. Pulmonary vascular resistance is affected by mechanical ventilation, arterial partial pressure of carbon dioxide ($PaCO_2$), and the arterial partial pressure of oxygen ($PaO_2$). Systemic vascular resistance is decreased by many anesthetic agents and increased by alpha-agonists and increased intravascular volume [6]. Other factors that affect PVR and SVR are listed in Table 32.1. When caring for a patient with a right-to-left shunt, the aim is to preserve or even improve the systemic and pulmonary blood flow balance. Under anesthesia this is accomplished by adjusting ventilator parameters including inspired oxygen concentration to address the $PaCO_2$ and the $PaO_2$ [7]. In addition, the balance between systemic and pulmonic blood flow can be accomplished with judicious use of fluids and inotropic support [7].

J. R. Paquin (✉) · J. E. Lam · E. P. Lin
Anesthesia and Pediatrics, Cincinnati Children's Hospital Medical Center, Cincinnati, OH, USA
e-mail: joanna.rosing@cchmc.org; jennifer.lam@cchmc.org; erica.lin@cchmc.org

**Table 32.1** Factors effecting changes in SVR and PVR

| Increased SVR | Decreased SVR |
|---|---|
| – Increased intravascular volume<br>– Medications: alpha-agonists (phenylephrine, dopamine, norepinephrine, ephedrine, epinephrine) | – Hypovolemia<br>– Acidosis<br>– Hypoxia<br>– Vasodilation<br>– Medications: anesthetic agents (Sevoflurane, Isoflurane, Desflurane, propofol), diuretics, ACEI |
| Increased PVR | Decreased PVR |
| – Hypoxia<br>– Acidosis<br>– Increased $PaCO_2$<br>– Decreased $PaO_2$<br>– Lung volumes<br>  – Above FRC<br>  – At RV (hypoxic pulmonary vasoconstriction)<br>– Infundibular spasm<br>– Hypothermia | – Oxygen<br>– Increased $PaO_2$<br>– Decreased $PaCO_2$<br>– Vasodilation: inhaled nitric oxide, prostacyclins, endothelin receptor antagonists, phosphodiesterase inhibitors |

The most common extracardiac shunt in the neonatal period is the ductus arteriosus. Patients with critical obstruction are dependent on blood flow through a patent ductus arteriosus to maintain adequate mixing. For these ductal-dependent patients, the balance between SVR and PVR is important to maintain to ensure adequate pulmonary blood flow and cardiac output. In this situation, prostaglandin E1 ($PGE_1$) is used to maintain patency postnatally until a palliative or corrective procedure can be performed.

Cardiac defects due to right-sided obstructive lesions typically occur in the presence of a right ventricular outflow tract obstruction (RVOTO). Over time, RVOTO causes the right ventricular wall to thicken in response to the pressure overload, but the hypertrophy can further increase the dynamic obstruction of the outflow tract [8]. As ventricular compliance deteriorates, the increase in end-diastolic pressure promotes more right-to-left blood flow through intracardiac communications. These communications can be restrictive or nonrestrictive. A restrictive communication limits the degree of shunting, while a nonrestrictive communication has the potential for extensive blood flow between the right and left sides of the heart. Thus, a nonrestrictive communication is more likely to be clinically significant, as it can further decrease pulmonary blood flow, thereby worsening the degree of hypoxemia.

Complex mixing lesions, such as TGA and TA, differ from right-sided obstructive lesions in that they can have normal or even increased pulmonary blood flow. Instead, the cyanosis results from the mixture of pulmonary and systemic circulation, with an $SpO_2$ of 75–80% indicative of a fairly balanced Qp:Qs. During the first few days and weeks of life, the fall in pulmonary vascular resistance allows for an increase in pulmonary blood flow, which in mixing patients can result in a higher saturation. Unfortunately, this pulmonary overcirculation imposes a volume load and can lead to chamber dilation. Clinically, patients develop congestive heart failure. Furthermore, exposure of the pulmonary arteries to increased circulation can accelerate the development of pulmonary vascular disease.

Conditions that result from right-to-left shunts are important to acknowledge because they contribute to increased morbidity and mortality under anesthesia. Sequelae from cyanotic CHD are the result of the body's compensatory response to chronic hypoxemia, volume overload and pressure overload. Hypoxemia produces long term effects on most organ systems including the hematopoietic system and the liver, which can lead to polycythemia and coagulation disorders. Chronic hypoxemia alters the coagulation profile by stimulating the production of erythropoietin, known as secondary erythrocytosis [9]. This process increases the body's red blood cell mass to increase the oxygen carrying capacity. These patients are at risk for thrombosis due to the resulting hyperviscosity; however, they are also at risk of thrombocytopenia. Thrombocytopenia results from decreased production and increased activation of platelets from the shear stress of blood hyperviscosity [10, 11]. Additional studies suggest impaired fibrinogen function and clot strength contribute to bleeding disorders in cyanotic CHD [9]. Deficiencies of vitamin K-dependent factors also result from poor cardiac output and chronic venous congestion in the liver. Thus, bleeding is also of concern in the presence of secondary erythrocytosis.

In addition to erythrocytosis, other compensatory mechanisms of cyanosis exist to balance the effects of right-to-left shunts. An increase in cardiac output facilitates oxygen delivery. Increased nitric oxide production from the endothelium of the coronary arteries promotes vasodilation, and increased levels of 2,3-diphosphoglycerate shift the oxygen dissociation curve rightward encouraging tissue unloading of oxygen [12, 13].

In defects associated with right-to-left shunts, cardiac failure can result from sustained increases in both pressure and volume load [8]. Volume overload typically occurs with pulmonary overcirculation or with valve regurgitation that leads to chamber dilation. Pressure overload occurs in the face of obstruction, leading to hypertrophy. The heart is left at a mechanical disadvantage, and function progressively deteriorates. Cardiac failure in infants can present as poor feeding, failure to thrive, tachypnea, tachycardia, and other signs of poor perfusion.

Patients with CHD are more vulnerable to the consequences of abnormal heart rhythms. They are also more susceptible to arrhythmias due to strain on the conduction system and the presence of necrosis or fibrosis extending into the conduction system [5]. Strain on the conduction system results from heart chamber dilation in response to persistently increased pressure and/or volume load [8]. For instance, patients with Ebstein's anomaly have significant tricuspid valve pathology that causes right atrial dilation, putting them at risk of atrial tachycardia. Patients who have undergone surgical repair can have fibrotic scar tissue extending into the conduction system. Due to incisional scars and surgical patches in the RVOT region, repaired TOF patients are particularly susceptible to ventricular tachyarrhythmias.

Pulmonary hypertension is a documented perioperative risk factor in children with CHD, and results from an increase in PVR, ventricular dysfunction, and hypoperfusion of the coronary arteries [14]. A pulmonary hypertensive crisis can develop rapidly, and in the presence of an intracardiac communication will either increase right-to-left shunting or reverse left-to-right shunting. The treatment of an acute crisis is aimed at lowering PVR while supporting right ventricular function. Modalities to improve PVR include supplemental oxygen, inhaled nitric oxide, and the correction of acidosis, while inotropic support can be used to augment ventricular function.

In summary, cyanotic CHD leads to compromised organ systems because of chronic hypoxemia, volume overload, and pressure overload. Overtime these patients are unable to compensate for their disease, leading to life-threatening sequela, such as cardiac failure, arrhythmias, and/or pulmonary hypertension. These significant comorbidities place a patient with cyanotic CHD at higher risk in the perioperative setting [15]. Therefore, it is imperative that the anesthesia provider understand CHD pathophysiology to formulate an appropriate plan to deliver the safest anesthetic possible [16].

## Specific Lesions

Right-to-left shunts are the result of abnormal intracardiac or vascular connections allowing deoxygenated blood to move systemically. The most common cyanotic CHD lesions include Tetralogy of Fallot, TGA, TA, TAPVR, and tricuspid valve abnormalities.

## Tetralogy of Fallot

Tetralogy of Fallot is widely recognized as the most common cyanotic CHD. The four anatomic hallmarks are: right ventricular outflow tract obstruction, a nonrestrictive ventricular septal defect (VSD), an overriding aorta, and right ventricular hypertrophy. The degree of RVOTO determines the degree of right-to-left shunting through the VSD due to elevated right ventricular pressures. Patients with Tetralogy of Fallot can suffer from acute hypercyanotic episodes, termed 'tet spells'. During these spells, an increase in right-to-left shunting occurs in response to worsening obstruction due to RVOT infundibular spasm, combined with a decrease in SVR. The resulting severe hypoxia and acidosis can lead to complete cardiovascular collapse if not treated expeditiously. Management goals focus on decreasing PVR, increasing SVR, and augmenting pulmonary blood flow. Treatment includes oxygen, fluids, phenylephrine, propranolol, and bicarbonate.

## Transposition of the Great Arteries

Transposition of the great arteries is a condition with discordant ventricular-arterial connections that result in two parallel circulations. In dextro-TGA (d-TGA) configuration, the aorta arises from the right ventricle and the pulmonary artery arises from the left ventricle. A point of mixing that allows oxygenated blood into the systemic circulation is necessary for survival. In the newborn infant, it is likely to be the ductus arteriosus. After the ductus closes, an ASD or VSD must be present. The adequacy of the mixing influences the degree of cyanosis. After birth as the pulmonary resistance falls, there is an increase in pulmonary blood flow that can lead to significant pulmonary overcirculation. These patients are at risk for the rapid development of irreversible pulmonary vascular disease if left untreated.

## Truncus Arteriosus

In truncus arteriosus, the combined ventricular output is directed through a single great artery that arises from the base of the heart to supply the coronary, pulmonary, and systemic circulations. The resistances in the pulmonary and systemic vascular beds dictate the flow. Infants with TA are susceptible to pulmonary overcirculation at the expense of systemic circulation. Therefore, measures must be taken to avoid decreases in PVR which could result in congestive heart failure, fluid overload and low cardiac output. Truncus arteriosus is associated with DiGeorge and velocardiofacial syndromes which may have additional implications for safe anesthetic management. These patients are also at risk for accelerated development of pulmonary vascular disease.

## Total Anomalous Pulmonary Venous Return

Total anomalous pulmonary venous return is a condition where all four pulmonary veins attach either directly or indirectly to the right side of the heart instead of the left atrium. There are four different types of TAPVR based on the location of anomalous vessels: supracardiac, cardiac, infracardiac, or mixed connections. Total anomalous pulmonary venous return results in left-to-right shunting at the level of pulmonary vein insertion. However, right-to-left shunting occurs at the atrial level due to the presence of an ASD/PFO, and is necessary to introduce oxygenated blood into the left side of the heart and maintain cardiac output. Prostaglandins may be indicated to allow right-to-left shunting through a PDA in newborns; although, the resulting decrease in PBF may worsen cyanosis [17]. When these connections are obstructive, usually in infracardiac connections, the patient develops life-threatening cyanosis requiring emergent surgical repair.

## Tricuspid Valve Abnormalities

Ebstein's anomaly, the most common tricuspid valve abnormality, is a relatively rare defect that constitutes <1% of CHD. It consists of downward displacement of the septal and posterior tricuspid valve leaflets at the inlet of the right ventricle leading to an 'atrialized' portion of the right ventricle and a malformed right ventricular chamber [18]. The dysplastic tricuspid valve usually causes significant regurgitation, resulting in increased right atrial pressure and decreased pulmonary blood flow. The elevated right atrial pressure prevents the PFO from closing at birth, allowing for right-to-left shunting. Additional pathology associated with Ebstein's anomaly includes atrial tachycardia due to right atrial dilation.

## Other Lesions

Other anomalies which are likely to have a right-to-left shunting component include but are not limited to pulmonary atresia/pulmonary stenosis, single ventricle pathology, Eisenmenger Syndrome, heterotaxy syndromes and non-cardiac sources such as liver disease with pulmonary fistulas.

## Perioperative Anesthetic Considerations

These are detailed in Table 32.2.

## Preoperative Assessment

Children with CHD commonly present for elective and non-elective procedures as they are just as likely to be afflicted with childhood disorders as children without CHD; however, their perioperative morbidity and mortality are higher [19–23]. The Pediatric Perioperative Cardiac Arrest (POCA) registry reported that most arrests occurred during non-cardiac surgery [22, 24]. Therefore, a thorough anesthetic preoperative assessment is imperative. A preoperative evaluation should include a detailed history and physical with focus on the patient's functional status, cardiac anatomy and function, long-term physiologic sequela, and a detailed review of cardiac imaging. Specific attention should be paid to the following:

*Neurological status*: Children with CHD may present with a history of neurological insult (i.e. stroke, transient ischemic attack) after prior cardiothoracic surgical repairs or after low cardiac output states [2]. It is recommended to assess for residual symptoms.

**Table 32.2** Perioperative anesthetic considerations for children with right-to-left shunts undergoing surgery

| Plan/preparation/adverse events | Reasoning management |
|---|---|
| Preprocedural evaluation<br>  – Anesthetic history<br>  – Airway (hypoventilation, hypercapnia, PHTN crisis)<br>  – Cardiovascular status (baseline oxygen saturations, cardiac function, surgical history, arrhythmias, pacemaker dependence)<br>  – Review of imaging<br>  – Review of medications<br>  – Review of laboratory data | Children with cyanotic CHD have a higher risk of morbidity and mortality perioperatively than children without CHD. Therefore, it is imperative to perform a thorough preprocedural evaluation to identify risks and to plan a safe anesthetic |
| Position—Will depend on the surgical procedure for which the patient presents. Evaluate if the position of the procedure is likely to impede preload, cardiac function, and/or ventilation | Patient positioning that effects preload, cardiac function, and ventilation is likely to increase a right-to-left shunt and worsen cyanosis. Prone, lateral decubitus, trendelenburg, and laparoscopic techniques are more likely to have deleterious effects on shunting |
| IV access—Appropriate access will depend on the surgical procedure and the patient's clinical status<br>  – Reliable peripheral iv<br>  – Arterial line<br>  – Central line | Complex patients with congenital heart disease may prove to be difficult to obtain iv access. This may be the result of multiple previous access points, prior procedures, and/or abnormal vasculature. Consider arterial and central access if indicated by the patient's clinical status and surgical procedure |

(continued)

**Table 32.2** (continued)

| Plan/preparation/adverse events | Reasoning management |
|---|---|
| Deep Sedation<br>General Anesthesia—induction technique<br>– Inhalational induction<br>– Intravenous induction<br>– Endotracheal tube | While deep sedation may be possible in this patient population. Concern for increased $PaCO_2$ with hypoventilation and acidosis will increase right-to-left shunts<br>Inhalational induction is appropriate in some patients with cyanotic CHD. However, inhalational induction may cause vasodilation decreasing the SVR and increasing right-to-left shunts. In addition, inhalational induction will be slower when right-to-left shunts are present<br>Intravenous induction provides more hemodynamic stability and more rapid onset. However, there is an increased risk of a paradoxical air embolism through an intracardiac connection<br>Controlled ventilation maintains a balance of SVR and PVR by preventing hypoventilation |
| Procedural adverse events:<br>  Hypotension<br>  Cyanosis<br>  PHTN crisis<br>  Arrhythmias<br>  Cardiac collapse | It is important that the anesthesia providers work to optimize pulmonary blood flow, oxygenation, and cardiac function. Procedural adverse events can occur; therefore, preparation to treat adverse events expeditiously is imperative |
| Postoperative and Post-discharge Considerations<br>– Cardiac stability<br>– Baseline cardiac function<br>– Cardiology consult/intensivist/patient's cardiologist<br>– Postoperative monitoring for hypoxia<br>– Respiratory difficulties | Postoperatively patients with CHD will benefit from optimizing oxygen delivery and maintaining end organ function as cardiac output may be decreased due to the lingering effects of anesthesia and/or surgical stress. These patients also have increased metabolic demands with maladaptive responses to stress |

*Cardiovascular status:* Evaluation of the patient's current functional status, surgical history, presence of arrhythmias and/or pacemaker/defibrillator-dependence, and baseline oxygen saturation delineates the patient's baseline health. It is vital to recognize if the patient's oxygen saturations correspond with the cardiac lesion. Oxygen saturations higher or lower than expected may indicate an altered physiology from baseline. The direction of blood flow across intracardiac and vascular shunts provides valuable information on pressure gradients. Clinical symptoms that must be ascertained include fatiguability, dyspnea, poor feeding, cyanotic episodes, diaphoresis, failure to gain weight, and vomiting. A review of available imaging is crucial. Close attention to these many factors will assist in identifying and understanding each patients' anatomy, physiology, and current cardiovascular function.

*Respiratory:* Respiratory infections can result in increased pulmonary vascular resistance and lead to increased hypoxemia in a child with cyanotic CHD [16]. Appropriate communication with the patient's cardiologist and surgeon regarding procedure urgency is advised when a recent respiratory infection has been detected. It is also useful to identify prior history of prolonged intubation, vocal cord paralysis, lung compliance, and operations with resulting nerve damage (i.e. phrenic and/or vagus injury) to plan efficient ventilation strategies. Depending on the surgery, a preoperative chest radiograph may be indicated.

*Medications*: Cardiac medications such as angiotensin converting enzyme inhibitors (ACEI) are historically linked to instability on induction of anesthesia due to excessive venodilation. Thus, many recommend withholding ACEIs on the day of surgery. In addition, the use of diuretics may further exacerbate venodilation due to dehydration [25]. Anticoagulation medications should also be evaluated to assess the risks of thrombosis versus perioperative bleeding. High risk patients may need to continue anticoagulation. The risks and benefits should be communicated with all team members. Interactions with other common cardiac medications such as digoxin with dexmedetomidine are important to identify to avoid significant bradycardia. Typically, all other cardiac medications are continued; however, it is recommended to carefully examine a patient's medication list for potential interactions or complications.

*Laboratory studies:* Hematologic and chemical profiles as well as coagulation studies may be indicated in the face of renal and hepatic dysfunction or anticoagulation therapy.

*Imaging:* Echocardiograms, cardiac catheterization results, cardiac MRI, and CT results should be reviewed.

*Physical exam:* Each patient should be examined for cardiac-specific findings. Common signs include clubbing, cyanosis, mottled skin, delayed capillary refill, lethargy, failure to thrive, murmurs, hepatomegaly, tachypnea, pre- and post-ductal oxygen saturation discrepancies and decreased pulses.

*Intravenous access*: Intravenous access may be difficult in patients with CHD. This may be the result of scarring from multiple access points during prior procedures or hospitalizations, clotted vessels from central lines and/or abnormal vasculature. Radiographs may be reviewed to confirm location of indwelling lines such as PICC and umbilical catheters.

*Spontaneous Bacterial Endocarditis Prophylaxis:* Tables 32.3 and 32.4 emphasize when prophylactic antibiotics are indicated per recent guidelines [26, 27].

**Table 32.3** Endocarditis prophylaxis

| |
|---|
| Cardiac conditions associated with the highest risk of adverse outcome from endocarditis for which prophylaxis with dental procedures is reasonable |
| Prosthetic cardiac valve or prosthetic material used for cardiac valve repair |
| Previous endocarditis |
| Congenital Heart Disease (CHD)[a] <br> – Unrepaired cyanotic CHD, including palliative shunts and conduits <br> – Completely repaired CHD with prosthetic material or device, whether placed by surgery or catheter intervention, during the first 6 months after the procedure[b] <br> – Repaired CHD with residual defects in the site or adjacent to a site of a prosthetic patch or prosthetic device (which inhibit endothelialization) |
| Cardiac transplantation recipients who develop cardiac valulopathy |

Circulation. 2007; 116: 1736–54
[a]Except for conditions listed above, antibiotic prophylaxis is no longer recommended for any other form of CHD
[b]Prophylaxis is reasonable because endothelialization of prosthetic material occurs within first 6 months

**Table 32.4** Antibiotic regimen for endocarditis prophylaxis

| Regimens for dental procedures, respiratory tract procedures (incision or biopsy of mucosa), infected skin, skin structure, or musculoskeletal tissue (single dose 30–60 min before procedure) | | | |
|---|---|---|---|
| | Agent | Adults | Children[a] |
| Standard | Amoxicillin | 2 g PO | 50 mg/kg PO |
| Unable to take oral medications | Ampicillin or <br> Cefazolin or Ceftriaxone | 2 g IM/IV <br> 1 g IM/IV | 50 mg/kg IM/IV <br> 50 mg/kg IM/IV |
| Allergic to penicillin or ampicillin | Cephalexin or <br> Clindamycin or <br> Azithromycin or <br> Clarithromycin | 2 g PO <br> 600 mg PO <br> 500 mg PO | 50 mg/kg PO <br> 20 mg/kg PO <br> 15 mg/kg PO |
| Allergic to penicillin or ampicillin and unable to take oral medication | Cefazolin or <br> Ceftriaxone or <br> Clindamycin | 1 g IM/IV <br> 600 mg IM/IV | 50 mg/kg IM/IV <br> 20 mg/kg IM/IV |

Circulation. 2007; 116: 1736–54
[a]Total pediatric dose should not exceed adult dose

*Premedication:* It is beneficial to minimize stress in this patient population as increased anxiety can result in increased PVR and subsequent right-to-left shunting. The most common premedication used is midazolam (oral, intravenous, intranasal). Intranasal dexmedetomidine has also proven helpful for anxiolysis. However, caution is advised as patients presenting with heart block from previous surgeries, significant pulmonary hypertension or taking AV nodal blocking agents should not be considered candidates for dexmedetomidine [28].

*Available resources:* Communication among the different patient care teams is imperative. It is recommended to involve the patient's cardiologist or cardiology consult services on site, intensive care services, cardiothoracic surgeon, adjunct medical services (i.e. otolaryngology, pulmonology), and ECMO support team when appropriate [19, 25].

*Cardiac anesthesia specialized care:* There is no consensus that anesthesiologists who care for children with CHD require formal congenital cardiac training; however, it is recommended that the anesthesia provider be familiar with CHD anatomy and physiology [19].

## Intraoperative Management

### Monitoring

Patient monitoring should include all standard ASA monitors in addition to those indicated by the patient's cardiac disease and functional status. The level of monitoring should be tailored for the procedure that will take place. Arterial blood pressure monitoring should be considered when hemodynamic values are likely to be significantly affected during the procedure, and/or the ventilation may be altered. In addition, central line placement is necessary when peripheral venous access is problematic, and monitoring central venous pressure provides valuable information on the cardiac filling pressure. Central access also allows for the administration of potent vasoactive agents. Both arterial and central access allow frequent blood sample monitoring. In severely ill children, there may also be utility for a transesophageal echocardiogram (TEE). However, TEE is contraindicated in patients with TAPVR, as it can cause occlusion of pulmonary veins.

### Induction

Induction of anesthesia will vary based on the individual patient's cardiac defect and functional status. Considerations should be made for the presence of shunts, myocardial contractility, ventricular dilation or hypertrophy, outflow tract obstructions, dysrhythmias, and pulmonary hypertension when formulating an anesthetic plan [6, 29]. In patients with right-to-left shunts, the goal during induction is to optimize Qp:Qs. In most patients, this involves minimizing decreases in SVR and increases in PVR. However, in some neonates with pulmonary overcirculation, it is prudent to maintain PVR by limiting $FiO_2$ and allowing judicious hypoventilation to promote systemic outflow. Other goals during induction include the maintenance of ventricular function and normal sinus rhythm [29].

Some patients may be appropriate for an inhalational induction; however, induction speed will be decreased. Inhaled anesthetic concentrations are decreased in the presence of right-to-left shunts as blood moves to the systemic circulation without circulation through the lungs to absorb the anesthetic agent. Therefore, the arterial concentration of inhaled agents is diluted in the presence of right-to-left shunts given that the partial pressure ratio in the lungs: brain is never achieved [30]. The most common inhalational agent used is sevoflurane, which can reduce myocardial contractility and decrease SVR by vasodilation. Nevertheless, because heart rate increases with sevoflurane, the cardiac output is generally not affected. It has been shown to result in less hypotension and less negative inotropy when compared to halothane [29].

Nitrous oxide, often used during induction of anesthesia for its second gas effect, allows for use of less sevoflurane, thereby ameliorating the decrease in SVR and hypotension during induction [6, 31]. Nitrous oxide is also known to expand an air embolism which is a significant risk in patients with right-to-left shunts. While nitrous oxide has a utility in inhalational induction of anesthesia in cyanotic CHD, the risk of air embolism makes it a poor choice for maintenance of anesthesia.

In an intravenous induction when a right-to-left shunt is present, medications pass directly to the left ventricle, bypassing the pulmonary vascular system. The result is a more rapid onset. Varying agents are available for use in intravenous induction, including fentanyl, propofol, ketamine, and etomidate.

Fentanyl, a synthetic opioid, is known to blunt the surgical stress response with minimal effect on cardiac function, though it can lower the heart rate, especially in higher doses. Caution should be made in heart failure patients whose cardiac output may be dependent on the heart rate. Fentanyl can also be used as a maintenance agent with intermittent bolus doses or as an infusion.

Propofol is a sedative-hypnotic that causes a dose-dependent reduction in mean arterial pressure (MAP) due to decreased preload and afterload from venous and arterial dilation. These effects may lead to an increase in right-to-left shunting with a subsequent decrease in oxygen saturation [19, 32]. Changes in heart rate, pulmonary artery pressure, or PVR have not been noted with propofol. While propofol may be appropriate in some patients with cyanotic CHD, careful titration is recommended and in certain patients it may be preferable to use in conjunction with ketamine.

Ketamine is a popular induction agent in children with CHD due to its stimulation of the sympathetic nervous system, resulting in a release of endogenous catecholamines. It is generally associated with an increase in heart rate, MAP and cardiac output with minimal changes in SVR. However, caution must be taken in those who may be catecholamine depleted, as ketamine's direct myocardial depressant effects will be unmasked in these patients. Ketamine is typically well tolerated in the setting of pulmonary hypertension and may be preferred over propofol due to its effects on SVR.

Etomidate exerts its hemodynamic effects through GABA receptors. It has no effect on systemic or pulmonary hemodynamics and therefore has minimal hemodynamic effects on shunt lesions [19, 33]. However, there is concern for adrenal suppression in as little as one dose [15, 19].

In patients with right-to-left shunting and systemic desaturation, it is most important to maintain oxygenation and ventilation. Airway management and efficient ventilation are essential [6]. For all intravenous medication administrations, caution for air bubbles is imperative as these patients are at risk for paradoxical embolism through the shunt. A multimodal, slowly titrated, patient-specific approach is recommended to maintain cardiac function and hemodynamic balance during induction of anesthesia.

## Maintenance

The goal during maintenance of anesthesia is to minimize physiologic changes that upset the delicate balance of pulmonary blood flow and systemic circulation. The specifics must be tailored to the patient. For instance, maintaining and even increasing PVR can be beneficial in patients with pulmonary overcirculation. In other patients with inadequate pulmonary blood flow, it is necessary to decrease PVR and maintain SVR to avoid worsening of right-to-left shunting. Under anesthesia this is accomplished by adjusting ventilator parameters, managing fluid status, providing adequate analgesia, and careful attention to patient positioning. Volatile anesthetic gases, fentanyl, propofol in judicious doses, and ketamine can be safely used for maintenance with minimal to no effect on shunting [25].

Inspired oxygen has profound effects on PVR. Higher concentrations can vasodilate the pulmonary vascular bed, and is an effective therapy in the treatment of pulmonary hypertension due to high PVR.

Paralytic agents may be required to maintain adequate surgical conditions. Succinylcholine, a depolarizing muscle relaxant, is known for its rapid onset. Patients with CHD may be more prone to the bradycardic effects of succinylcholine administration. These effects may be diminished with the pretreatment of atropine. Nondepolarizing neuromuscular blockers, such as vecuronium, rocuronium, and cisatracurium, generally lack cardiovascular effects and are appropriate choices for neuromuscular blockade in CHD.

The decision on controlled ventilation versus spontaneous ventilation in patients with CHD should be made based on the nature of the surgical procedure as well as the patient's physiology. Controlled ventilation may be preferred in these patients out of concern for hypoventilation which could lead to an increase in PVR. Hypoventilation will increase the $PaCO_2$ causing acidosis, increasing the PVR and worsening right-to-left shunts. Mechanical ventilation at functional residual capacity will maintain a normal $PaCO_2$, avoid hypoxemia, and optimize the pH [7, 34].

Regional and neuraxial anesthesia may be considered in select patients with CHD. Epidural or caudal analgesia may facilitate a balanced general anesthetic, minimize administration of myocardial depressant anesthetic medications, and allow for early extubation. Potential adverse effects, such as decreased preload, are a major concern [23, 35]. High blocks are not likely to be well tolerated in children with CHD due to excessive vasodilation and blockade of cardiac accelerators. If neuraxial anesthesia is considered, an epidural may be preferable over a spinal blockade because it is titratable, thereby avoiding a rapid sympathetic block. Furthermore, an epidural can be used in the post-operative period to provide narcotic-sparing pain control. Unfortunately, baseline coagulapathies and perioperative anticoagulation therapies may prohibit the use of regional and neuraxial anesthesia.

Fluid strategies intraoperatively may be challenging in patients with CHD. Ensuring adequate intravascular volume is important to maintain SVR and preload and lessen right-to-left shunting. However, it must be recognized that children with cyanotic CHD often require a higher hematocrit for increased oxygen-carrying capacity. Heavy use of lactated ringers or normal saline may result in significant hemodilution, leading to increased hypoxemia. Additionally, fluid overload may not be well-tolerated in patients in heart failure. Therefore, careful attention must be paid to hematocrit with fluid administration, and blood products may be required.

Considerations should be made for surgical positioning of patients with cyanotic CHD. Specifically, the prone and lateral decubitus positions, in addition to laparoscopic procedures with increased intraabdominal pressures, can have a deleterious effect on right-to-left shunting. These positions may impede the patient's physiology by affecting preload, afterload, or impeding ventilation.

Adverse events can occur precipitously, so immediate availability of cardiac medications and therapies such as epinephrine, phenylephrine, milrinone, and inhaled nitric oxide can be life-saving. Knowledge about personnel resources, especially during off-hours or when practicing in a remote location, is also helpful during crisis management.

## Postoperative Management

Postoperatively, patients with CHD will benefit from optimizing oxygen delivery and maintaining end-organ function as cardiac output may be decreased from lingering anesthesia and/or surgical stress [36]. These patients may have increased metabolic demands with maladaptive responses to stress [36]. Appropriate postoperative analgesia is beneficial to achieving these goals. A multimodal approach is preferred, as hypoventilation from opioid-induced narcosis can result in hypercarbia, increased PVR, and worsening a right-to-left shunt.

Postoperative recovery location should be based on the patient's cyanotic CHD, complexity of surgical procedure, and postoperative risk factors. Regardless, the patient should be monitored for respiratory difficulties, hemodynamic instability, desaturations, and arrhythmias [5]. Preoperative discussion with the patient's cardiologist, intensivist, and surgeon will help facilitate postoperative patient disposition especially if postoperative intensive care is necessary. However, outpatient surgery may be reasonable with appropriately selected patients for certain surgeries.

## Conclusion

The complexity and variation of CHD does not allow for a universal anesthetic plan. The plan of care must be individualized to each patient and their disease. Understanding the anatomy and physiology will allow the provider to safely care for the patient.

## References

1. Khoshnood B, Lelong N, Houyel L, Thieulin AC, Jouannic JM, Magnier S, et al. Prevalence, timing of diagnosis and mortality of newborns with congenital heart defects: a population-based study. Heart. 2012;98:1667.
2. Marino BS, Lipkin PH, Newburger JW, Peacock G, Gerdes M, Gaynor JW, et al. Neurodevelopmental outcomes in children with congenital heart disease: evaluation and management: a scientific statement from the American Heart Association. Circulation. 2012;126:1143–72.
3. Botto LD, Correa A, Erickson JD. Racial and temporal variations in the prevalence of heart defects. Pediatrics. 2001;107:E32.
4. Reller MD, Strickland MJ, Riehle-Colarusso T, Mahle WT, Correa A. Prevalence of congenital heart defects in metropolitan Atlanta, 1998–2005. J Pediatr. 2008;153:807.
5. Andropoulos DB, Stayer S, Mossad EB, Miller-Hance WC. Anesthesia for congenital heart disease. 3rd ed. Hoboken: Wiley; 2015.
6. Chiu CL, Wang CY. Sevoflurane for dental extraction in children with Tetralogy of Fallot. Paediatr Anaesth. 1999;9:268–70.
7. Walker A, Stokes M, Moriarty A. Anesthesia for major general surgery in neonates with complex cardiac defects. Paediatr Anaesth. 2009;19:119–25.
8. Kwiatkowski DM, Hanley FL, Krawczeski CD. Right ventricular outflow tract obstruction: pulmonary atresia with intact ventricular septum, pulmonary stenosis, and Ebstein's malformation. Pediatr Crit Care Med. 2016;17(8):S323–9.
9. Zabala LM, Guzzetta NA. Cyanotic congenital heart disease: focus on hypoxemia, secondary erythrocytosis, and coagulation alterations. Pediatr Anesth. 2015;25:981–9.
10. Horigone H, Hiramatsu Y, Shigeta O, Nagasawa T, Matsui A. Overproduction of platelet microparticles in cyanotic congenital heart disease with polycythemia. J Am Coll Cardiol. 2002;39:1072–7.
11. Lill MC, Perloff JK, Child JS. Pathogenesis of thrombocytopenia in cyanotic congenital heart disease. Am J Cardiol. 2006;98:254–8.
12. Broberg C, Jayaweera AR, Diller GP, Prasad SK, Thein SL, Bax BE, et al. Seeking optimal relation between oxygen saturation and hemoglobin concentration in adults with cyanosis from congenital heart disease. Am J Cardiol. 2001;107:595–9.
13. Rudolph AM, Nadas AA, Borges WH. Hematologic adjustments to cyanotic congenital heart disease. Pediatrics. 1953;11:454–65.
14. Friesen RH, Williams GD. Anesthetic management of children with pulmonary arterial hypertension. Pediatr Anesth. 2008;18:208–16.
15. Wijesingha S, White M. Anaesthetic implications of congenital heart disease for children undergoing non-cardiac surgery. Anaesth Intensive Care Med. 2015;16(8):395–400.
16. Cabalka AK. Physiologic risk factors for respiratory viral infections and immunoprophylaxis for respiratory syncytial virus in young children with congenital heart disease. Pediatr Infect Dis J. 2004;23(1):S41–5.
17. Patregnani J. Total anomalous pulmonary venous return. In: Jones MB, Klugman D, Fitzgerald RK, Kohr LM, Berger JT, Costello JM, et al., editors. Pediatric cardiac intensive care handbook. Washington, DC: Pediatric Cardiac Intensive Care Books; 2015. p. 121–3.
18. Driscoll DJ, Dearani JA. Ebstein anomaly of the tricuspid valve. In: Moeller JH, JIE H, editors. Pediatric cardiovascular medicine. 2nd ed. Oxford, UK: Wiley-Blackwell/Wiley; 2012. p. 509–17.
19. White MC. Approach to managing children with heart disease for noncardiac surgery. Paediatr Anaesth. 2001;21:522–9.
20. Hennein HA, Mendeloff EN, Cilley RE, et al. Predictors of postoperative outcome after general surgical procedures in patients with congenital heart disease. J Pediatr Surg. 1994;29:866–70.
21. Baum VC, Barton DM, Gutgesell HP. Influence of congenital heart disease on mortality after noncardiac surgery in hospitalized children. Pediatrics. 2000;105:332–5.
22. Ramamoorthy C, Haberkern CM, Bhananker SM, Domino KB, Posner KL, Campos JS, et al. Anesthesia-related cardiac arrests in children with heart disease: data from the Pediatric Perioperative Cardiac Arrest (POCA) Registry. Anesth Analg. 2010;110:1376–82.
23. Kachko L, Birk E, Simhi E, Tzeitlin E, Freud E, Katz J. Spinal anesthesia for noncardiac surgery in infants with congenital heart disease. Pediatr Anesth. 2012;22:647–53.
24. Morray JP, Geiduschek JM, Ramamoorthy C, Haberkern CM, Hackel A, Caplan RA, et al. Anesthesia-related cardiac arrest in children: initial findings of the Pediatric Perioperative Cardiac Arrest (POCA) Registry. Anesthesiology. 2000;93:6–14.
25. Rosenthal DN, Hammer GB. Cardiomyopathy and heart failure in children: anesthetic implications. Pediatr Anesth. 2011;21:577–84.
26. Wilson W, Taubert KA, Gewitz M, Lockhart PB, Baddour LM, Levison M, et al. Prevention of infective endocarditis: guidelines from the American Heart Association: a guideline from the American Heart Association Rheumatic Fever, Endocarditis, and Kawasaki Disease Committee, Council on

Cardiovascular Disease in the Young, and the Council on Clinical Cardiology, Council on Cardiovascular Surgery and Anesthesia, and the Quality of Care and Outcomes Research Interdisciplinary Working Group. Circulation. 2007;116:1736–54.
27. National Institute for Health and Clinical Excellence. Prophylaxis against infective endocarditis. www.nice.org.uk/CG064. Accessed March 2017.
28. Pasin L, Febres D, Testa V, Frati E, Borghi G, Landoni G, et al. Dexmedetomidine vs midazolam as preanesthetic medication in children: a meta-analysis of randomized controlled trials. Paediatr Anaeth. 2015;25(5):468–76. https://doi.org/10.1111/pan.12587.
29. Rivenes SM, Lewin MB, Stayer SA, Bent ST, Schoenig HM, McKenzie ED. Cardiovascular effects of sevoflurane, isoflurane, halothane, and fentanyl-midazolam in children with congenital heart disease: an echocardiographic study of myocardial contractility and hemodynamics. Anesthesiology. 2001;94(2):223–9.
30. Huntington JH, Malviya S, Voepel-Lewis T, Lloyd TR, Massey KD. The effect of a right-to-left intracardiac shunt on the rate of rise of arterial and end-tidal halothane in children. Anesth Analg. 1999;88:759–62.
31. Chin C. ABCs of neonatal cardiac anesthesia. Artif Organs. 2013;37(1):100–2.
32. Williams GD, Jones TK, Hanson KA, Morray JP. The hemodynamic effects of propofol in children with congenital heart disease. Anesth Analg. 1999;89:1411–6.
33. Dhawan N, Chauhan S, Kothari SS, Kiran U, Das S, Makhija N. Hemodynamic responses to etomidate in pediatric patients with congenital cardiac shunt lesions. J Cardiothorac Vasc Anesth. 2010;24(5):802–7.
34. Fletcher R. Gas exchange during anaesthesia and controlled ventilation in children with congenital heart disease. Paediatr Anaesth. 1993;3:5–17.
35. Holzman RS, Nargozian CD, Marnach R, McMillan CO. Epidural anesthesia in patients with palliated cyanotic congenital heart disease. J Cardiothorac Vasc Anesth. 1992;6(3):340–3.
36. Tweddell JS, Hoffman GM. Postoperative management in patients with complex congenital heart disease. Semin Thorac Cardiovasc Surg Pediatr Card Surg Annu. 2002;5:187–205.

# Aortic Stenosis: Anesthesia Considerations

## Benjamin Kloesel and Kumar Belani

## Introduction

Aortic stenosis in children is a very different disease entity compared to its adult counterpart. In adults, aortic stenosis can be hereditary or acquired. The most frequent hereditary presentation is a bicuspid aortic valve. Acquired valve disease results from progressive calcification with subsequent restriction of leaflet mobility and obstruction of outflow. In developing countries, acquired aortic valve stenosis is frequently seen in the setting of rheumatic heart disease.

While stenosis at the valvular level is the most commonly encountered left ventricular outflow tract obstruction, supravalvular and subvalvular aortic stenosis can occur. Each of those groups has different pathomechanisms and treatment approaches. In addition, pediatric aortic stenosis can often be associated with a myriad of syndromes that may have other manifestations of congenital heart disease or organ involvement leading to specific implications on anesthetic management.

This chapter will review the different left ventricular outflow tract subtypes and provide an insight into pathophysiology and management strategies for pediatric patients undergoing diagnostic and surgical procedures.

## Subtypes of Left Ventricular Outflow Tract Obstruction

### Supravalvular Aortic Stenosis

Supravalvular aortic stenosis, the least common form of left ventricular outflow tract obstruction, describes a narrowing above the aortic valve at either the sinotubular junction or proximal ascending aorta. The underlying etiology is a genetic mutation causing a defect in elastin production. Three distinct forms have been defined: a sporadic mutation; a mutation as part of Williams syndrome (also known as Williams-Beuren syndrome); and a familial autosomal dominant form [1].

### Subvalvular Aortic stenosis

Subvalvular aortic stenosis accounts for about 8–20% of all forms of left ventricular outflow tract obstruction [2]. It is characterized by the presence of a space-occupying lesion below the aortic valve. Examples include thin membranes consisting of endocardial folds and fibrous tissue, fibromuscular ridges formed by a thickened membrane; diffuse tunnel-like fibromuscular

B. Kloesel, M.D., M.S.B.S. (✉)
K. Belani, MBBS, MS, FACA, FAAP
Department of Anesthesiology, University of Minnesota, Masonic Children's Hospital, Minneapolis, MN, USA
e-mail: bkloesel@umn.edu

obstructions or duplications of the anterior mitral valve leaflet. An association with other congenital cardiac anomalies is described in 50–60% of cases and most cases present before the age of 10 years [3].

## Valvular Aortic stenosis

Aortic valve stenosis accounts for 60–75% of pediatric left ventricular outflow tract obstructive lesions and is associated with other congenital heart anomalies in 15–20% of patients [4]. It can present at any age, from the neonatal period to adulthood. The majority of valvular aortic stenosis in children is congenital and related to abnormalities of the aortic valve leaflets, which may be unicuspid, bicuspid, tricuspid and rarely quadricuspid.

Severe and critical aortic stenosis in the neonate is frequently associated with a unicuspid valve and may present with the patient in cardiogenic shock. Systemic blood flow through the stenosed orifice is severely compromised; survival is initially dependent on a right-to-left shunt via a patent ductus arteriosus. Neonatal aortic stenosis is frequently associated with hypoplasia of left-sided structures.

## Pathophysiology

Stenosis at any of the previously mentioned levels leads to left ventricular outflow tract obstruction, which places a pressure burden on the left ventricle. This increase in afterload elicits remodeling processes in the left ventricle that include myocardial hypertrophy and fibrosis. Concentric hypertrophy in response to increased wall stress initially aids in maintaining contractility, but proves to be detrimental in the long-term [5]. In adult patients, increases in ventricular myocardium size are not accompanied by increases in the number of supplying arteries. The hypertrophic ventricle becomes subject to demand-supply mismatch, creating a state that predisposes to ischemia and systolic as well as diastolic dysfunction [5, 6].

In contrast, the myocardium in children has some regenerative capabilities and is able to increase its vascular supply; hence, the development of cardiac dysfunction and failure is delayed. Still, coronary artery flow is compromised due to a combination of the following factors: (a) development of some degree of subendocardial fibrosis; (b) alterations in aortic reflected waves which typically augment diastolic pressure, but with increased aortic stiffness loose this benefit; (c) prolonged time spent in systole due to left ventricular outflow tract obstruction at the expense of time spent in diastole and (d) decreased ventricular compliance results in an increase in left ventricular end-diastolic pressure [6]. Ultimately, changes precipitated from left ventricular outflow tract obstruction may lead to the long-term complication of congestive heart failure; in the immediate perioperative periods, those patients are predisposed to development of myocardial ischemia, which can progress to acute heart failure and even cardiac arrest.

## Treatment

When left ventricular outflow tract obstruction reaches a specific point, the only treatment alternative is to relieve the obstruction; this can be accomplished either surgically (resection of obstructing tissue, outflow tract reconstruction, valvulotomy, valve repair/replacement) or by interventional approaches (balloon dilation, stent placement).

## Anesthetic Considerations: Neonatal Critical Aortic Stenosis

The neonate with critical aortic stenosis represents a unique and challenging patient population that requires special anesthetic considerations.

Frequently, a neonate with critical aortic stenosis presents with cardiogenic shock. The initial resuscitative steps include maintenance of blood flow through the ductus arteriosus by using a prostaglandin infusion to avoid ductal closure.

This will provide systemic blood flow via a right-to-left shunt. These babies require endotracheal intubation and mechanical ventilation to optimize oxygenation, control ventilation and reduce oxygen consumption. It is not uncommon for these babies to additionally require inotropic support with dopamine or epinephrine. When systemic perfusion is dependent on a right-to-left shunt via the patent ductus arteriosus, there may be very little antegrade flow through the valve. As a consequence, the coronary arteries are perfused in a retrograde fashion by systemic venous blood from the right-to-left shunt that can exacerbate myocardial ischemia. There is debate about the optimal approach to neonatal critical aortic stenosis: some proponents advocate early surgical valvotomy while others consider aortic balloon dilation as the best treatment modality (see Fig. 33.1). The decision is influenced by factors including patient size, comorbidities and valve anatomy [7, 8].

Anesthetic considerations for the management during surgical valvotomy are beyond the scope of this chapter and interested readers are referred to pediatric cardiac anesthesiology textbooks. For balloon valvotomies in the cardiac catheterization lab, the patient should be kept intubated, anesthetized and relaxed with neuromuscular blockers to allow the best imaging and access conditions. Infusions including prostaglandins and inotropes should be continued without interruption, ideally via a central venous line or peripherally inserted central catheter. Blood products should be readily available and defibrillator pads along with 5-lead ECG monitoring should be placed before draping. Adequate intravenous access lines need to be established before the procedure. Invasive arterial blood pressure monitoring may be available in form of an umbilical artery catheter but could also be obtained from the arterial access site placed by the cardiologist. Anesthesia can be maintained with a low-dose volatile agent supplemented by opioids. At time of balloon inflation, hypotension and arrhythmias may occur and need to be immediately treated to prevent cardiac arrest. A potential complication of aortic balloon valvotomy is aortic insufficiency that, if severe, may require urgent surgical intervention. The same applies for perforation of the cardiac wall or large blood vessels.

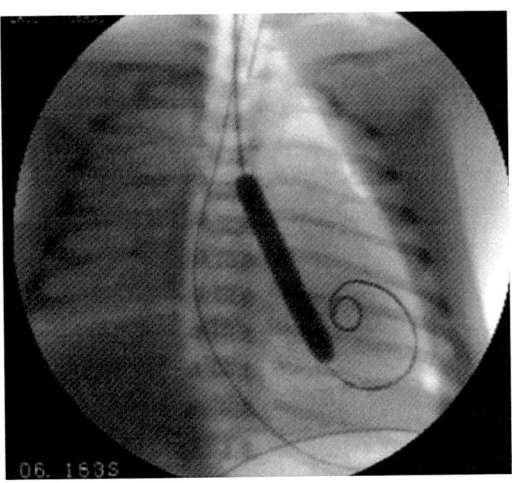

**Fig. 33.1** Fluoroscopic radiograph of a baby undergoing percutaneous transluminal aortic valvuloplasty for critical aortic stenosis. (From: Hirofumi Saki and Hideaki Senzaki. Congenital Aortic Stenosis in Children. In *Medicine: Cardiology and Cardiovascular Medicine: Calcific Aortic Valve Disease. Chapter 18 (open access).* Elena Aikawa (Editor). ISBN: 978-953-51-1150-4)

## Anesthetic Considerations: Hemodynamic Management

### Heart Rate

Tachycardia negatively affects patients with left ventricular outflow tract obstruction in two ways: (1) as heart rate increases, the time spent in diastole decreases more than the time spent in systole. Perfusion of the left ventricular myocardium occurs in diastole and is therefore decreased. (2) Tachycardia imposes a higher workload on the ventricular myocardium and increases oxygen demand. Consequently, care should be taken to maintain a normal heart rate and avoid tachycardia while preventing the occurrence of bradycardia. This is in contrast to adult practice, where beta-blockers are frequently used to even induce slight bradycardia. Neonates and young infants are dependent on their heart rate to maintain and modify cardiac output. As such, heart rate modification may compromise cardiac output and should be considered with caution. In the setting of heart rate changes, the ECG can aid in detection of developing ischemia.

## Contractility

Contractility should be maintained. Negative inotropic agents can compromise cardiac output and should be avoided. Positive inotropic agents tend to create problems in hypertrophic obstructive cardiomyopathy but should also be used cautiously if a component of dynamic left ventricular outflow tract obstruction has been identified.

## Preload

Maintaining adequate preload with even a tendency to increased preload is important in hypertrophic obstructive cardiomyopathy to counteract the dynamic outflow tract obstruction. In aortic stenosis, hypovolemia can, by means of preload reduction, further compromise cardiac output through a left ventricular outflow tract obstruction and should be avoided. A slight increase in preload may be beneficial if left ventricular hypertrophy is present—a stiff ventricle with decreased compliance requires slightly higher filling pressures to function optimally, although fluid overload should be avoided.

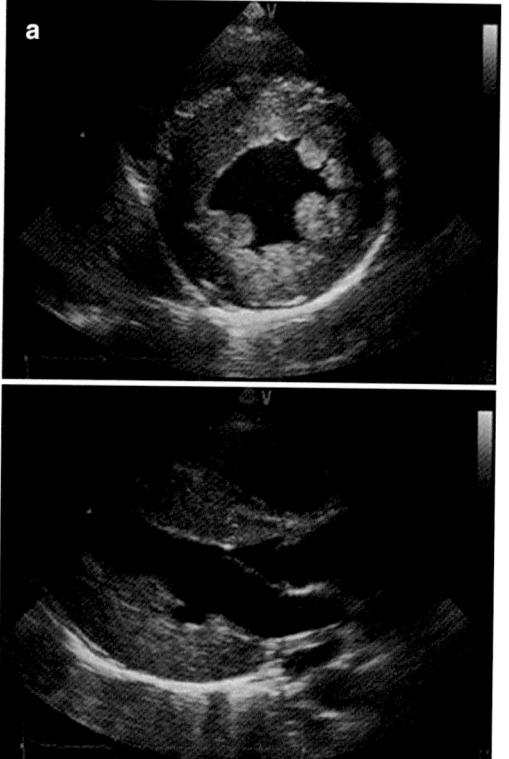

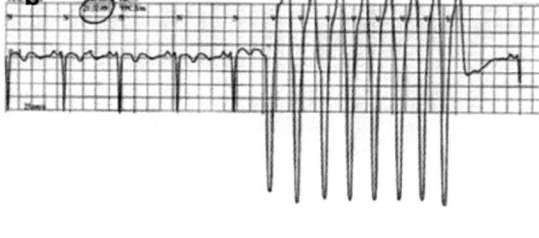

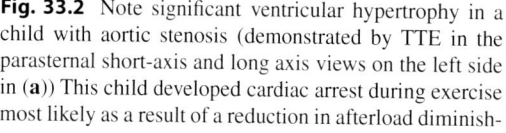

**Fig. 33.2** Note significant ventricular hypertrophy in a child with aortic stenosis (demonstrated by TTE in the parasternal short-axis and long axis views on the left side in (**a**)) This child developed cardiac arrest during exercise most likely as a result of a reduction in afterload diminishing coronary perfusion and creating ventricular ischemia. Two weeks after resuscitation this child demonstrated the occurrence of episodes of ventricular tachycardia as seen in (**b**). From: [13]

## Afterload

Coronary artery perfusion is dependent on diastolic blood pressure; a significant drop in afterload, combined with a fixed left ventricular outflow tract obstruction, can have detrimental effects on coronary perfusion pressure and may precipitate ischemia. If the left ventricular outflow tract obstruction has been present for some time and resulted in left ventricular hypertrophy, the induced ischemia is worse due to a more marked supply-demand mismatch. A further reduction in cardiac function occurs that may result in a vicious circle (see Fig. 33.2).

## Heart Rhythm

Maintenance of sinus rhythm is important for patients with left ventricular outflow tract obstruction as the coordinated atrial and ventricular systole allows maintenance of preload and cardiac output. Tachycardias (supraventricular, ventricular, junctional) and bradycardias should be treated expeditiously.

## Anesthetic Considerations: Supravalvular Aortic Stenosis Associated with Williams Syndrome

Williams's syndrome is an autosomal dominant genetic disorder due to deletions on chromosome 7. Manifestations of this condition include "Elfin" facies, supravalvular aortic stenosis, elastin arteriopathy of medium and large arteries with involvement of the coronary arteries, intellectual disability, short stature and distinctive personality and behavioral traits ("cocktail party personality"). It is well documented in the literature that Williams-Beuren patients are at higher risk for sudden cardiac death, especially when undergoing diagnostic or surgical procedures [9, 10]. The predisposition arises from a combination of factors: impairment of coronary artery blood flow from ostial and diffuse right and left coronary artery stenosis, mechanical impairment of coronary artery blood flow at the aortic leaflet level, subendocardial ischemia from right and left ventricular hypertrophy and left outflow tract obstruction [11]. Another defining factor is the low likelihood of successful resuscitation after witnessed cardiac arrest. Published literature on anesthetic care of these patients emphasizes careful planning and patient monitoring, adequate back-up mechanisms (including intensive care and ECMO capabilities), preservation of sinus rhythm, maintenance of preload, contractility and afterload as well as avoidance of anesthetic drugs that may precipitate or worsen myocardial ischemia [12].

Table 33.1 summarizes the essentials of anesthetic management in newborns, children and adolescents with left ventricular outflow tract obstruction.

Table 33.1 Essential points summarizing care of newborns, children and adolescents with left ventricular outflow tract obstruction

| Plan/preparation/adverse events | Reasoning/management |
|---|---|
| Ensure adequate monitoring prior to induction of anesthesia | • Standard ASA monitors (blood pressure cuff, ECG, pulse oximetry, temperature)<br>• Use 5-lead ECG monitoring with V5 to increase sensitivity to detect ischemia<br>• Cycle blood pressure cuff every minute during induction<br>• Consider placement of invasive arterial blood pressure monitoring (if appropriate for planned procedure)<br>• For severe left ventricular outflow tract obstruction, consider placement of defibrillator pads |

| Plan/preparation/adverse events | Reasoning/management |
|---|---|
| Employ gentle induction technique that avoids tachycardia and severe decreases in afterload and contractility | Depending on severity of left ventricular outflow tract obstruction (LVOTO) and left ventricular systolic function, consider<br>• Adequate premedication<br>• Etomidate (severe LVOTO)<br>• Midazolam/Fentanyl (severe LVOTO)<br>• Gentle mask induction (mild-moderate LVOTO) |
| General goals for intraoperative management of left ventricular outflow tract obstruction | • Heart rate: slightly bradycardic to normofrequent, avoid tachycardia and severe bradycardia<br>• Heart rhythm: maintain sinus rhythm<br>• Preload: maintain euvolemia, consider careful volume expansion to induce mild hypervolemia<br>• Afterload: maintain, avoid decreases in systemic vascular resistance<br>• Contractility: maintain, avoid agents with negative inotropy |

## Conclusions

Newborns, infants and children with aortic stenosis can present with distinct clinical features all of which relate to left ventricular outflow obstruction. When critical obstruction is present, these pediatric patients are at high risk for sudden death. A thorough preoperative evaluation including a cardiac work up is essential before anesthesia induction. The goals of anesthesia care include the avoidance of arrhythmias, assuring a stable heart rate along with an undisturbed pre and afterload and strong inotropy.

## References

1. Mitchell MB, Goldberg SP. Supravalvar aortic stenosis in infancy. Semin Thorac Cardiovasc Surg Pediatr Card Surg Annu. 2011;14(1):85–91.
2. Darcin OT, Yagdi T, Atay Y, Engin C, Levent E, Buket S, et al. Discrete subaortic stenosis: surgical outcomes and follow-up results. Tex Heart Inst J. 2003;30(4):286–92.
3. Etnel JR, Takkenberg JJ, Spaans LG, Bogers AJ, Helbing WA. Paediatric subvalvular aortic stenosis: a systematic review and meta-analysis of natural history and surgical outcome. Eur J Cardiothorac Surg. 2015;48(2):212–20.
4. Singh GK. Aortic stenosis. Indian J Pediatr. 2002;69(4):351–8.
5. Carabello BA. Aortic stenosis: from pressure overload to heart failure. Heart Fail Clin. 2006;2(4):435–42.
6. Jashari H, Rydberg A, Ibrahimi P, Bajraktari G, Henein MY. Left ventricular response to pressure afterload in children: aortic stenosis and coarctation: a systematic review of the current evidence. Int J Cardiol. 2015;178:203–9.
7. Benson L. Neonatal aortic stenosis is a surgical disease: an interventional cardiologist view. Semin Thorac Cardiovasc Surg Pediatr Card Surg Annu. 2016;19(1):6–9.
8. Hraska V. Neonatal aortic stenosis is a surgical disease. Semin Thorac Cardiovasc Surg Pediatr Card Surg Annu. 2016;19(1):2–5.
9. Bird LM, Billman GF, Lacro RV, Spicer RL, Jariwala LK, Hoyme HE, et al. Sudden death in Williams syndrome: report of ten cases. J Pediatr. 1996;129(6):926–31.
10. Horowitz PE, Akhtar S, Wulff JA, Al Fadley F, Al Halees Z. Coronary artery disease and anesthesia-related death in children with Williams syndrome. J Cardiothorac Vasc Anesth. 2002;16(6):739–41.
11. Burch TM, McGowan FX Jr, Kussman BD, Powell AJ, DiNardo JA. Congenital supravalvular aortic stenosis and sudden death associated with anesthesia: what's the mystery? Anesth Analg. 2008;107(6):1848–54.
12. Matisoff AJ, Olivieri L, Schwartz JM, Deutsch N. Risk assessment and anesthetic management of patients with Williams syndrome: a comprehensive review. Paediatr Anaesth. 2015;25(12):1207–15.
13. Saiki H, Sugimoto M, Senzaki H. Exercise-induced cardiopulmonary arrest in a child with aortic stenosis. Cardiol Young. 2016;26(5):1013–6.

# Anesthesia for Spinal Surgery in Children

**34**

Ali Kandil, Deepika S. Rao, and Mohamed Mahmoud

## Introduction

According to the American Association of Neurologic Surgeons, the incidence of adolescent idiopathic scoliosis is approximately 2–3% of the general population. An estimated six to nine million adolescents in the United States between the ages of 10 and 18 have some degree of spinal deformity. Consequently, every year, these patients make more than 600,000 visits to private physician offices; 30,000 are fitted with a brace, and 38,000 patients undergo spinal fusion surgery. As such, most pediatric anesthesia providers will care for some percentage of these children, and a firm understanding of their unique anesthetic considerations is crucial to their perioperative success.

In addition to scoliosis, spinal dysraphism (myelomeningocele and tethered cord) are pathologies that commonly necessitate pediatric spine surgery. Myelomeningocele (MMC) results from failure of neural tube fusion during the first 4 weeks of gestation, leading to herniation of the meninges with neural elements, and can occur at any level of the spinal cord. Most commonly, MMC occurs at the level of the lumbar spinal cord. Usually associated with Arnold Chiari II malformation, this pathology requires some level of surgical intervention both during the neonatal period and as the child ages [1]. The spinal cord below the defect is often tethered, which over time can result in neuromuscular scoliosis.

This chapter will focus on the clinical pathophysiology and perioperative management of scoliosis, myelomeningocele, and tethered cord and discuss the anesthetic considerations thereof. The role of intraoperative neurophysiological monitoring will be discussed as well as anesthetic considerations for optimization of this monitoring in pediatric patients.

## Scoliosis

### Preoperative Assessment

As with most complex surgical treatments, the key to successful perioperative management of children undergoing spinal deformity surgery is a multidisciplinary approach. The role of effective communication cannot be understated and patients and families should have realistic expectations regarding perioperative course. A thorough preoperative evaluation must be performed highlighting cardiac and pulmonary status. Additionally, patients must be evaluated and optimized hematologically, nutritionally, and psychologically.

A. Kandil, D.O., M.P.H. (✉) · D. S. Rao, M.D.
M. Mahmoud, M.D.
Cincinnati Children's Hospital Medical Center, Cincinnati, OH, USA
e-mail: ali.kandil@cchmc.org; Deepika.Rao@cchmc.org; Mohamed.Mahmoud@cchmc.org

## Pulmonary Status

Preoperative evaluation and optimization of pulmonary status is paramount in preparation for spinal surgery. Kyphoscoliosis can alter the anatomy and physiology of the lungs by restricting ventilation. As the curve increases in these patients, the restrictive lung disease worsens. Specifically, there is a decrease in vital capacity (VC) and forced expiratory volume in 1 s (FEV1). The effects of this restrictive physiology can range from clinically insignificant to debilitating. Hypoventilation, hypoxia, and ventilation-perfusion mismatch (V-Q mismatch) can lead to pulmonary hypertension and ultimately cor pulmonale [2]. The degree of curvature is measured by the Cobb angle, and a Cobb angle greater than 100° can cause severe respiratory compromise decreasing VC to 45% or less or forced vital capacity (FVC) to 30% less than predicted. Such decrements can portend the need for postoperative mechanical ventilation [3, 4]. As standard practice, certain patients require further pulmonary function testing prior to spinal deformity surgery. These include patients with severe deformity (Cobb angle > 80°), neuromuscular scoliosis, patients with baseline reactive airway disease, and patients with decreased functional status. Proper vetting of patients can improve patient outcomes.

## Cardiac Status

Cardiac function is typically preserved in adolescent idiopathic scoliosis. However, the presence of severe restrictive lung disease can lead to pulmonary hypertension and cor pulmonale. The incidence of cardiac dysfunction in patients with neuromuscular scoliosis (i.e. scoliosis associated with neuromuscular disease) is higher. Mitral valve prolapse and coarctation of the aorta are the two most common cardiac pathologies associated with scoliosis [2]. In addition, children with muscular dystrophy and spinal muscular atrophy (SMA) can present with cardiomyopathies and suffer arrhythmias that pose challenges to the anesthesia provider [5]. Patients with neuromuscular scoliosis and patients with severe spinal deformity (Cobb angle > 100°) should have preoperative cardiac testing which includes an electrocardiogram (EKG) and an echocardiogram [6].

## Hematologic Status

The extent of bleeding varies from one patient to the next, but it is clear that spinal deformity surgery may encounter major blood loss totaling more than half the child's blood volume with higher blood loss expected with ponte osteotomies and vertebral column resection. Accordingly, a complete blood count (CBC) and coagulation profile should be obtained prior to surgery. Thrombocytopenia and coagulopathy can be at least partially corrected prior to surgery, potentially preventing intraoperative transfusion. A blood type and crossmatch should be done prior to scoliosis surgery. Children with neuromuscular scoliosis are at nearly seven-times greater risk for massive blood loss, and thus for transfusion of blood products perioperatively, than are patients with idiopathic scoliosis [7]. The onus is on the perioperative team to plan for this eventuality and be prepared for transfusion of blood products. Further, the use of antifibrinolytic agents like tranexamic acid (TXA) and aminocaproic acid (ACA) can be administered intraoperatively to decrease blood loss. The hematologic literature supports the use of antifibrinolytic drugs to reduce perioperative blood loss and the amount of blood transfused in children undergoing surgical correction of scoliosis [8]. Autologous blood donation, use of cell-saver and preoperative erythropoietin have also been used to minimize need for allogenic blood transfusion.

## Nutritional Status

Nutritional status in children undergoing spinal deformity plays a profound role in the perioperative course, especially in patients with neuromuscular scoliosis [9]. The nutritional effects on the clotting cascade are significant and preoperative blood work is necessary. A basic metabolic profile, assays for iron, albumin, and even vitamin K can help identify deficiencies that can play a role intraoperatively. These deficiencies can frequently be corrected prior to surgery, decreasing the risk of intraoperative transfusion.

## Intraoperative Management

### Induction of Anesthesia

Induction of anesthesia in a pediatric patient is dependent on the age and level of cooperation of the patient. In older patients who are able to cooperate, an intravenous induction is ideal. In addition, airway management in children with neuromuscular scoliosis can be challenging, and pre-induction intravenous catheter placement should be considered. For younger children or patients who cannot cooperate, an inhalation induction can be performed. The use of nitrous oxide as a proxy for premedication can facilitate ease of induction, when used prior to introducing sevoflurane. Further, nitrous oxide can allow for smoother induction with sevoflurane. Sevoflurane is the most commonly used volatile agent for induction, not only because of its safety profile but also because it is less pungent and irritating than other volatile agents. Intravenous induction agents include propofol, ketamine, etomidate, and midazolam. Given the frequent use of total intravenous anesthesia (TIVA) in patients undergoing spinal deformity surgery, propofol is the most commonly used intravenous induction agent. Neuromuscular blockade may improve intubating conditions, but because intraoperative neuromonitoring is standard of care for these procedures, its use should be limited to patients who do not require pre-positioning baseline somatosensory and transcranial motor evoked potentials (SSEPs and TcMEPs). In patients with adolescent idiopathic scoliosis (AIS), pre-positioning baseline SSEPs and TcMEPs are not necessary, and thus a single dose of non-depolarizing neuromuscular blocking agents can be used. Succinylcholine, a depolarizing neuromuscular blocking drug may be a suitable alternative, as it is rapidly metabolized and typically does not have lasting effects on TcMEPs. Certain conditions preclude the use of succinylcholine; for instance, patients with muscular dystrophies, certain myopathies, and some neuromuscular diseases may be at risk for severe hyperkalemia and malignant hyperthermia. As such, prior to administration of this drug, a thorough review of medical history should be performed.

### Airway Management

Both during and after appropriate induction of anesthesia, airway management is a critical consideration in the perioperative course. The ability to mask ventilate a patient is the most important step, and the use of an oropharyngeal or nasopharyngeal airway to alleviate upper airway obstruction can facilitate ventilation. Children with AIS rarely pose challenges in airway management, whereas children with neuromuscular scoliosis oftentimes require additional airway intervention. Patients with spinal muscular atrophy syndrome, Duchenne's muscular dystrophy, Klippel-Feil syndrome, any of the mucopolysaccharidoses, and other complex congenital syndromes may be associated with particularly difficult airway anatomy necessitating special equipment such as fiberoptic bronchoscopy or video laryngoscopy.

Spinal deformity surgery typically requires prone positioning for extended periods of time, so maintenance of endotracheal tube patency is critical. The use of reinforced or armored tubes can prevent occlusion of the tube after positioning. Proper securement of the endotracheal tube is also critical, as the prone position will preclude adjustment of the tube intraoperatively. Moreover, use of dental guards and protective soft bite-blocks will be necessary to present tongue trauma in the prone position due to neuromonitoring.

### Maintenance of Anesthesia

At an institutional level, the importance of streamlining the anesthetic regimen is important to optimize the perioperative course, as different anesthetic agents affect intraoperative neuromonitoring potentials and hemodynamics differently. By creating a protocol for maintenance of anesthesia, the effect of the anesthetic on these important variables can be relatively controlled. The use of total intravenous anesthesia (TIVA) has been advocated in both the adult and pediatric population to limit the deleterious effects anesthetics have on SSEPs and TcMEPs. Inhalational agents cause a dose-dependent decrement in the amplitude of the TcMEPs and to a lesser extent the SSEPs. As such, the use of continuous infusions of propofol and an opioid like remifentanil

**Table 34.1** Ability to obtain reliable neurophysiologic monitoring in children [10]

| | Exhibit monitorable SSEPs (%) | Exhibit monitorable TcMEPs (%) |
|---|---|---|
| Children under 24 months of age | 57 | 86 |
| Children 2–4 years old | 83 | 100 |
| Children 4–6 years old | 93 | 97 |
| Children 0–6 years old | 76 | 94 |

Adapted from: McIntyre IW, Francis L, McAuliffe JJ. Transcranial motor-evoked potentials are more readily acquired than somatosensory-evoked potenitals in children younger than 6 years. Anesth Analg 2016;122:212–18

or sufentanil are suggested for these types of surgeries. Especially in children, where obtaining robust responses may be more challenging, limiting anesthetic effects can be the difference between a response that can be monitored and one that cannot. In fact, in children under 2 years old, obtaining reliable SSEPs occurs only a little more than half the time. Additionally, if a TIVA technique is used, obtaining reliable TcMEPs occurs about 86% of the time in children under 2 years old [10] (Table 34.1). Accordingly, the anesthetic technique plays a large role in the ability to obtain robust potentials in these young patients who already pose difficulty because of the relative immaturity of their motor tracts [11].

## Hemodynamic Monitoring

The duration of surgery in spinal deformity correction is surgeon and institution-dependent, but universally are considered major surgeries in children. Monitoring modalities should include continuous electrocardiography, pulse oximetry, capnography, invasive and non-invasive blood pressure monitoring, temperature monitoring, and urine output. Monitoring central venous pressure (CVP) should be performed in patients with significant cardiopulmonary disease and in cases where major blood loss is anticipated. Invasive blood pressure monitoring with an intra-arterial line is critical not only because of potential for significant hemodynamic changes, but also because it allows for frequent lab draws to evaluate acid-base status, blood counts, and electrolytes. Body temperature is an important variable in surgical outcomes, and rectal or nasal probes are most effective at monitoring core temperature and are preferred to skin temperature monitoring. Hypothermia has been implicated in increased infection rate and increased bleeding, and thus warming modalities should be widely used. Warming, convection blankets, warm air mattresses, and fluid warmers are all devices that can facilitate maintenance of body temperature [12].

## Intraoperative Neurophysiologic Monitoring

Intraoperative neurophysiologic monitoring is an essential component of spinal deformity surgery and most spine surgeries in children and adults. Somatosensory evoked potentials (SSEPs) in concert with transcranial motor evoked potentials (TcMEPs) provide the most effective monitoring schema for children undergoing surgical correction of scloliosis (Fig. 34.1). During exposure, hardware placement, correction and distraction, these modalities provide a critical layer of protection for the patient. Accordingly, it is incumbent upon the anesthesia provider to have a working knowledge of how their anesthetic agents affect the neurophysiologic responses, so that changes in these potentials are not a result of the anesthetic. Most anesthetics exert their effects on SSEPs and TcMEPs by altering neuronal excitability at the level of the synapse [13].

SSEPs give a neurophysiologic depiction of the integrity of the ascending dorsal column pathway. In order to elicit these responses, patients are stimulated peripherally and a response is generated centrally. These responses are less sensitive to volatile anesthetics than other modalities, but are still affected by volatile anesthetics in a dose-dependent fashion, resulting in increased latency and decreased amplitude of the cortical responses. A change is considered significant if there is a 10% increase in latency or a 50% decrease in amplitude [14–16]. Nitrous oxide typically only decreases cortical response

**Fig. 34.1** Normal TcMEP (right sided) (**a**) and normal SSEP (lower extremity) (**b**)

amplitudes less than 50% and does not affect other components of the SSEPs [17, 18].

TcMEPs give neurophysiologic depiction of the integrity of the corticospinal tracts. In order to elicit these responses, the patient is stimulated transcranially (centrally) and a response is recorded peripherally. These potentials are quite sensitive to the effects of volatile anesthetics in children, and the use of all volatile anesthetics, including nitrous oxide, for anesthesia maintenance is virtually prohibitive for TcMEPs [19]. Further, these responses cannot be elicited if neuromuscular blocking agents like succinylcholine or cisatracurium are in use. Thus the utilization of this modality requires communication between the neuromonitoring team and the anesthesia team in order to administer an anesthetic that can optimize these responses. Again, propofol infusion with a opioid infusion has been advocated [20–22]. Bolus administration of most intravenous anesthetics cause transient amplitude and latency effects, and thus infusions of short-acting, easily-titratable drugs like remifentanil and propofol seem to be the most effective strategy for maintenance of anesthesia. Dexmedetomidine, a relatively new alpha-agonist sedative, can be used as an anesthetic adjunct at target plasma concentrations of up to 0.6 ng/mL, since it does not alter SSEPs and TcMEPs during complex spine surgery by any clinically significant amount [23]. The use of intraoperative neurophysiologic monitoring is the gold-standard for surgical correction of scoliosis and for most spine surgeries in children.

## Postoperative Management

Most patients undergoing surgical correction of AIS are safely extubated at the conclusion of surgery, as long as blood loss is acceptable, changes in neurophysiologic monitoring are not prohibitive, and patient's respiratory status has been stable throughout the case. Patients with neuromuscular scoliosis oftentimes require a higher level of care postoperatively, which may include monitoring in an intensive care setting, postoperative mechanical ventilation, and postoperative transfusion of blood products. In general, at the heart of postoperative care in these patients is sufficient postoperative analgesia. At our institution, the acute pain service is consulted on each scoliosis patient to formulate a plan, which typically is multimodal in approach. It begins with patient-controlled analgesia (PCA) with morphine, hydromorphone, or fentanyl. Adjunctive medications such as gabapentin, methadone, acetaminophen, diazepam, methocarbamol, and ketorolac are also important components of a good post-surgical pain plan. Such a plan provides for efficient discharge of these patients and optimizes their perioperative experience.

## Myelomeningocele (MMC)

### Introduction

Myelomeningocele (MMC) is the most common congenital primary neural defect, with an incidence of 1–2/1000 live births. Overall rates of neural tube defects have decreased since the benefits of folate supplementation during pregnancy have become widely known, but MMC is still a frequent finding with many systemic and long-term effects [24, 25]. MMC is a highly morbid condition, in which the meninges and neural tissue are exposed to and damaged by the intrauterine environment. The abnormal fusion of the embryologic neural tube during the first month of gestation results in a range of congenital presentations known as spina bifida. The milder defects in neural tube closure may result in a meningocele, a sac-like herniation of the dura and arachnoid membranes. More severe defects may result in a myelo-meningocele (MMC), in which neural elements are present with the meninges within the hernia sac. These neural elements include nerve tissue and cerebrospinal fluid. Most commonly, the failure of the neural tube closure occurs in the middle or caudal neural groove, which results in a thoracic or lumbosacral meningomyelocele [26].

As a general principle, higher or more cephalad defects result in more severely affected clinical presentations [11, 27]. However, MMC at any spinal level can result in severe permanent disabilities, including paraplegia, bowel and bladder dysfunction, sexual dysfunction, skeletal deformations, mental impairment, and cranial nerve dysfunction [28]. Other associated conditions include the development of scoliosis, which, depending on the severity of curvature, may result in chronic pain and progressive restrictive lung disease [29, 30]. Tethered cord is also associated with neural tube defects, and will be discussed separately [31]. Additionally, syringomyelia may develop as a sequelae of MMC. This condition is characterized by the development of a fluid-filled cavity or cyst within the spinal cord, and may lead to progressive neurologic symptoms including motor, sensory, and autonomic dysfunction [30]. Almost all infants born with MMC have supraspinal neurologic anomalies, with 80–90% affected by obstructive hydrocephalus [32]. Arnold–Chiari II malformation is present in 20–35% of patients, and is characterized by a small posterior fossa, leading to the herniation of the cerebellar vermis through the foramen Magnum. This downward displacement of the medulla, cerebellum, and fourth ventricle into the spinal canal results in obstructive hydrocephalus [33, 34]. Ventriculoperitoneal shunting is required in 80–90% of these children, and may precede or may follow MMC repair [34]. Despite shunting, some children will suffer permanent developmental deficits. These issues include central hypoventilation and apnea, bradycardia, vocal cord dysfunction and stridor, and abnormal swallow and gag leading to frequent aspiration [35]. Thus, children with MMC associated with Chiari malformation will require careful assessment and management during the perioperative period.

### Etiology/Pathogenesis

Idiopathic or non-syndromic MMC may result from intrauterine exposures that predispose to abnormal neural tube fusion. MMC is commonly associated with maternal folic acid deficiency. It may also be associated with intra-uterine exposure to the anti-epileptic medications valproate and carbamazepine. Maternal obesity and diabetes during gestation may play a role as well [24, 36]. Chromosomal abnormalities including trisomy 13, trisomy 18, and triploidy have all been associated with higher rates of MMC development [24, 25]. MMC may also be present as part of a constellation of systemic congenital anomalies associated with VACTERL (vertebral anomalies, anal anomalies, cardiac defects, tracheo-esophageal fistula, renal/genitourinary anomalies, limb malformations).

The primary failure in neurulation that produces the spinal defect directly causes myelodysplasia. Myelodysplasia, or the abnormal development of neural tissue, directly leads to neuronal dysfunction [24, 25]. Fetal surgery to repair MMC before the 26th week of gestation may interrupt progression of neurologic damage and preserve neurologic function. Fetal surgery may also decrease the chances of requiring a postnatal ventriculoperitoneal shunt by 50% [34]. Early closure to minimize both direct traumatic damage as well as bacterial contamination is recommended, because the defective neural tissue is in open communication with the environment [37, 38]. Studies have shown that MMC repair within the first 24–48 h of life significantly decreases the risk of irreversible neurologic damage and infection rates [39], and improves long-term urologic/bladder function [40].

## Preop Considerations

Preanesthetic preparation should begin with an assessment of the patient's overall physical condition and co-morbidities. Even the stable neonatal patient is likely to present challenges with vascular access, thermal regulation, glucose monitoring, fluid management, and positioning. Premature, small-for-gestational-age, or syndromic neonates are more likely to require assessment of systemic comorbidities such as cardiac disease, or respiratory distress syndrome [41, 42].

Infants with Chiari malformations and hydrocephalus may also present with neurologic symptoms. The severity of tonsillar herniation should be assessed with imaging, and severely affected patients must be monitored for the possible development of brainstem herniation. Cranial nerve or brainstem dysfunction must be evaluated for the increased risk of central apnea. Abnormal swallow and gag reflexes may increase the risk of aspiration. There may also be an increased risk of vocal cord dysfunction, stridor, or bradycardia. Neck extension should be limited due to the risk of brainstem compression in these patients [28, 32, 33, 41].

Imaging of the spine and brain should be reviewed. Cardiac evaluation with electrocardiogram and echocardiogram is recommended due to the high rate of comorbid congenital heart disease [43]. Pulmonary disease may prompt further imaging, including possible chest x-ray.

Laboratory evaluation should include a complete blood count to assess starting hemoglobin and hematocrit. The patient should be typed and crossmatched for possible intraoperative blood transfusion. Baseline blood chemistries should be established, including glucose levels [1, 41]. Preoperative care of the neonate with MMC should center around protection of the exposed neural tissue. The prevention of trauma is paramount. A soaked gauze or silo should cover the exposed MMC, both to protect and to decrease insensible fluid losses. Possible continuous CSF leakage should be countered by an infusion of a balanced salt solution. Caution should be taken to prevent hypothermia. Latex precautions are nearly always pre-emptively instituted for the MMC patient, due to the high likelihood of requiring multiple surgeries [1].

## Intraoperative Considerations

Appropriate positioning for induction and intubation to avoid physical trauma to the hernia sac presents a challenge. Supine positioning provides the best conditions for ventilation and intubation, but the MMC sac must be cushioned in a foam or gel "doughnut" ring that puts no pressure on the lesion. However, the doughnut will disproportionately elevate one part of the body; the rest of the patient should be supported with padding or rolled towels to remain on a level. Lateral positioning for induction will prevent trauma to the MMC defect, but will lead to difficulty with ventilation and intubation. Prone positioning should be avoided during induction, but will be required for surgery [1]. Inhalational or IV induction may be used. Consider premedication with 20 mcg/kg atropine for neonates at risk for bradycardia. Note that succinylcholine is not associated with excessive hyperkalemia in these patients. Endotracheal intubation is required; an armored tube may be of benefit in appropriately-sized patients [41, 42].

After induction, the patient is placed in a prone position for the actual surgery. Rolls of foam, soft towels, or gel bolsters must be carefully positioned under the shoulders and the pelvis to allow free thoraco-abdominal excursion during ventilation. The extremities must be padded, and the face supported on a foam or gel pillow that puts no pressure on the eyes. Kinks in the endotracheal tube must be avoided [1].

Consider arterial and central venous access depending on the size of the lesion, the risk of blood loss, and the presence of complicating comorbidities. Invasive monitoring may not be required for the healthy patient. Intraoperative monitoring should include measurement of urine output. Blood loss is usually small, but may increase if it becomes necessary to undermine a large area of tissue to achieve primary closure. Core temperature should be closely monitored. Conservation of body heat is important, since autonomic control below the defect is often impaired. Appropriate strategies include underbody or overbody warmers, radiant warming devices, and increasing the room temperature. Maintenance of anesthesia is most frequently done with an inhalational agent in an air-oxygen mixture. Prolonged use of nitrous oxide should be avoided due to the small risk of pneumocephalus and venous air embolism. Muscle relaxants may be used if nerve stimulation or neuromonitoring is not planned. Pain control is typically achieved with narcotics and/or adjunctive medications such as acetaminophen. Sensory levels are difficult to ascertain in the neonatal period, so analgesic requirements will vary [1, 41, 42].

## Postoperative Considerations

Extubation may be possible after an uncomplicated surgery in the otherwise healthy patient. However, consider keeping patients with significant cardiopulmonary disease or other comorbidities intubated and ventilated. Surgeries complicated by significant fluid shifts and prolonged prone positioning may increase the risk of glottic edema and post-operative respiratory distress [1]. Chiari II patients without shunts to relieve hydrocephalus require close monitoring in the postoperative period as well. They can demonstrate an abnormal ventilatory response to hypoxia, and are at increased risk of postoperative apnea or even respiratory arrest. Impingement on the brainstem can lead to higher risk for vocal cord dysfunction and postoperative stridor. For these reasons, careful consideration is required before extubating these patients, and careful postoperative monitoring is required [1, 35]. These patients usually require a multidisciplinary approach to their long term postoperative care. Surgical and medical teams must work in conjunction with physical therapists and social workers to improve functionality and quality of life for these children. Additionally, these patients frequently require repeated surgical interventions most commonly for tethered cord syndrome and ventriculoperitoneal shunt revisions, urologic procedures to improve bladder function, and orthopedic procedures to mitigate scoliosis, contractures, and hip dislocations [39, 44, 45].

## Tethered Cord Syndrome (TCS)

### Introduction

Tethered cord (TC) refers to a spinal cord that is fixed and held taut at some point in the spinal canal. Normally, the spinal cord is loose and able to move within the spinal canal. But the abnormal tethering of the spinal cord limits its movement, and stretch-related damage results. In the pediatric population, this stretch commonly occurs as children grow; this leads to progressive spinal cord damage and progressive neurologic symptoms. Due to the variation of the growth rate among children, both symptom progression and age of presentation are highly variable. Tethered cord syndrome (TCS) refers to the range of symptoms, neurological and otherwise, that are caused by this type of progressive spinal cord damage. A diagnosis of TCS is based on the presence of both neurologic symptoms and an abnormally tethered spinal cord [46].

### Causes

The primary cause of TCS is an inelastic or thickened filum terminale. The filum terminale is a strand of delicate fibrous tissue that connects the apex of the conus medullaris to the coccyx, and normally has a high viscoelasticity to permit movement of the spinal cord. Normally, the spinal cord begins to ascend within the spinal canal as the spinal column starts to grow in the ninth week of gestation. By 3 months of age, the tip of the spinal cord has ascended to between the T12 and L2 vertebrae, facilitated by the elastic filum terminale. However, the loss of elasticity caused to the deposition of abnormal fibrous material will abnormally anchor the spinal cord, and result in the forcible elongation of the lumbosacral spinal cord. Types of spina bifida associated with tethered cord syndrome include tight filum terminale, dermal sinus tracts that connect intraspinal connective tissue to the skin, diastematomyelia or split spinal cord syndrome, myelomeningocele and lipomyelomeningocele. Note that spina bifida patients may have neurologic symptoms similar to TCS, but may or may not actually have a spinal cord that is abnormally tethered. In these patients, true TCS may also develop from scar tissue formed during surgical correction of spina bifida [31].

**Signs and Symptoms**

Tethered cord syndrome presents with a range of symptoms, and the severity and progression of disease vary from patient to patient. In most cases, individuals experience symptoms during infancy or childhood. Others may not develop any symptoms until reaching adulthood. Physical exam findings that may indicate the presence of tethered cord are also consistent with other forms of neural tube defects. These signs are typically located in the sacral area of the spinal column, and usually overlie the area of defect. Signs may include tufts of hair, dimples, benign lipomatous tumors or skin tags, aberrant skin pigmentation, or hemangiomas. These findings may be the only evidence for tethered cord in infants, as many lower extremity motor and sensory abnormalities are difficult to assess [24, 46]. Neurologic symptoms typically involve a combination of the motor, sensory, and autonomic systems. One common presenting motor symptom in the pediatric population the development of toe walking, which may progress to more severe gait disturbance over time. Both upper and lower motor neuron findings may be present in the same limb, such as hyperreflexia, pathologic plantar response, and muscle atrophy. Associated musculoskeletal abnormalities may also present in the spinal column as scoliosis or exaggerated lumbar lordosis. Sensory changes may be limited to areas of decreased sensation, or may be profound and involve the loss of pain, temperature, and proprioception. Bowel and bladder dysfunction, both incontinence and retention, is present in more than 50% of patients. The most significant sign of TCS in teenagers and adults is back pain that is aggravated by flexion or strain of the lumbosacral spine; this motion elongates the lumbosacral spinal canal and stretches the lower spinal cord [46, 47].

Identifying the presence of a tethered spinal cord is typically achieved via imaging. Ultrasound is often the first diagnostic tool in utero, and is useful in infants under 2 months of age. In some instances, ultrasound images may still be useful in toddlers or small children. While CT imaging can provide supportive evidence, diagnosis via MRI imaging remains the gold standard. A thickened filum terminale or "low conus medullaris" is evidence for tethered cord. The conus medullaris normally terminates at or above the L1-2 disk space. After 3 months of age, a conus that ends below the L1-2 vertebral level may indicate a tethered cord; a conus that ends below L3-4 is highly likely to be tethered. The tethered cord syndrome, however, is a clinical diagnosis based on neurological and musculoskeletal findings in combination with a tethered spinal cord. Abnormal sacral anatomy in the neonate—including dimples, hairy patches, draining pits, or masses—should always prompt an immediate evaluation for spina bifida and tethered cord. Abnormal bowel or bladder function is often one of the earliest presenting symptoms and must also be fully investigated for spinal dysfunction [31, 46].

## Preoperative Considerations

Surgery to de-tether the spinal cord is performed in a effort to improve or prevent the progression of neurologic symptoms. The surgical approach will depend on the etiology of TCS, such as an inelastic filum, myelomeningocele, or dermal sinus tract [47]. Imaging of the spine and brain should be reviewed. The degree of neurologic involvement must be assessed; the patients will require personalized approaches to positioning, pain management, and bowel/bladder management. Children with concomitant myelomeningocele require thorough evaluation and preparation, as discussed previously [1]. Complex or re-do surgeries may require intraoperative blood transfusion, and those patients should be typed and crossmatched in advance. Laboratory evaluation should include a complete blood count to assess starting hemoglobin and hematocrit.

## Intraoperative Considerations

For the typical TCS patient, an inhalational or intravenous induction in the supine position is appropriate. The patient is then placed in a prone position. Rolls of foam, soft towels, or gel bolsters must be carefully positioned under the shoulders and the pelvis to allow free thoracoabdominal excursion during ventilation. Arterial lines, central venous access, and blood transfusion is rarely necessary, unless surgical repair of a more complex spinal defect is planned or unless the patient has significant comorbidities. Maintenance of anesthesia can be done via an intravenous or inhalational technique. Neuromuscular blockade should be avoided if nerve stimulation or neuromonitoring is planned. Analgesia is usually achieved with a combination of narcotics, adjunctive drugs such as acetaminophen, and infiltration of local anesthetics. Extubation is usually possible after an uncomplicated surgery.

## Postop Considerations

Around 80% of patients who presented with back pain experience relief after an de-tethering surgery. Around 50% experience improvement with bladder function and muscle weakness. De-tethering surgery that is necessary at a younger age is associated with a worse neurologic outcome. After repair, the spinal cord may become "re-tethered" due to development of adhesions and scar tissue, and additional surgery may be required. However, patients who have undergone multiple TCS operations in the past usually experience less symptom relief and increased morbidity with subsequent procedures [47, 48].

## Conclusion

The preoperative, intraoperative, and postoperative management of spinal deformity and spinal cord surgery in children requires meticulous attention to detail and a thorough understanding of the anesthetic implications in these disease processes. It is very important to have an anesthesia consult for these patients in order to have adequate preparation. The acuity of patients with scoliosis, myelomeningocele, and tethered cord is variable and with if the anesthesia and perioperative team is prepared, surgical correction of these conditions can be done safely. At our institution, there are protocols in place for intraoperative neurophysiological monitoring, infection prevention, and postoperative pain management. Having such protocols in place can streamline care of these complex patients and prevent gaps in perioperative management.

## References

1. Singh D, Rath GP, Dash HH, Bithal PK. Anesthetic concerns and perioperative complications in repair of myelomeningocele: a retrospective review of 135 cases. J Neurosurg Anesthesiol. 2010;22:11–5.

2. Barois A. Respiratory problems in severe scoliosis. Bull Acad Natl Med. 1999;183(4):721–30.
3. Salem MR, Klowden AJ. Anesthesia for orthopedic surgery. In: Gregory GA, editor. Pediatric anesthesia. New York: Churchill Livingstone; 2002. p. 617–61.
4. Yuan N, Skaggs DL, Dorey F, Keens TG. Preoperative predictors of prolonged postoperative mechanical ventilation in children following scoliosis repair. Pediatr Pulmonol. 2005;40(5):414–9.
5. Raw DA, Beattie JK, Hunter JM. Anaesthesia for spinal surgery in adults. Br J Anaesth. 2003;91:886–904.
6. DiCindio S, Arai L, McCulloch M, Sadacharam K, Shah SA, Gabos P, Dabney K, Theroux MC. Clinical relevance of echocardiogram in patients with cerebral palsy undergoing posterior spinal fusion. Paediatr Anaesth. 2015;25(8):840–5.
7. Edler A, Murray DJ, Forbes RB. Blood loss during posterior spinal fusion surgery in patients with neuromuscular disease: is there an increased risk? Paediatr Anaesth. 2003;13:818–22.
8. Florentino-Pineda I, Thompson GH, Poe-Kochert C, Huang RP, Haber LL, Blakemore LC. The effect of amicar on perioperative blood loss in idiopathic scoliosis: the results of a prospective, randomized double-blind study. Spine (Phila Pa 1976). 2004;29:233–8.
9. Jevsevar DS, Karlin LI. The relationship between preoperative nutritional status and complications after an operation for scoliosis in patients who have cerebral palsy. J Bone Joint Surg Am. 1993;75:880–4.
10. McIntyre IW, Francis L, McAuliffe JJ. Transcranial motor-evoked potentials are more readily acquired than somatosensory-evoked potenitals in children younger than 6 years. Anesth Analg. 2016;122:212–8.
11. Szelényi A, Bueno de Camargo A, Deletis V. Neurophysiological evaluation of the corticospinal tract by D-wave recordings in young children. Childs Nerv Syst. 2003;19:30–4. Cracco JB, Cracco RQ. Spinal somatosensory evoked potentials: maturational and clinical studies. Ann N Y Acad Sci. 1982;388:526–37.
12. Kurz A, Sessler DI, Lenhardt R. Study of Wound Infection and Temperature Group. Perioperative normothermia to reduce the incidence of surgical-wound infection and shorten hospitalization. N Engl J Med. 1996;334:1209–15.
13. Sloan TB. Anesthetics and the brain. Anesthesiol Clin North Am. 2002;20:265–92.
14. Samra SK, Vanderzant CW, Domer PA, Sackellares JC. Differential effects of isoflurane on human median nerve somatosensory evoked potentials. Anesthesiology. 1987;66:29–35.
15. Peterson DO, Drummond JC, Todd MM. Effects of halothane, enflurane, isoflurane, and nitrous oxide on somatosensory evoked potentials in humans. Anesthesiology. 1986;65:35–40.
16. McPherson RW, Mahla M, Johnson R, Traystman RJ. Effects of enflurane, isoflurane, and nitrous oxide on somatosensory evoked potentials during fentanyl anesthesia. Anesthesiology. 1985;62:626–33.
17. Schindler E, Müller M, Zickmann B, Osmer C, Wozniak G, Hempelmann G. Modulation of somatosensory evoked potentials under various concentrations of desflurane with and without nitrous oxide. J Neurosurg Anesthesiol. 1998;10:218–23.
18. Wolfe DE, Drummond JC. Differential effects of isoflurane/nitrous oxide on posterior tibial somatosensory evoked responses of cortical and subcortical origin. Anesth Analg. 1988;67:852–9.
19. Thees C, Scheufler KM, Nadstawek J, et al. Influence of fentanyl, alfentanil, and sufentanil on motor evoked potentials. J Neurosurg Anesthesiol. 1999;11:112–8.
20. Ubags LH, Kalkman CJ, Been HD, Drummond JC. Differential effects of nitrous oxide and propofol on myogenic transcranial motor evoked responses during sufentanil anaesthesia. Br J Anaesth. 1997;79:590–4.
21. Lo YL, Dan YF, Tan YE, et al. Intraoperative motor-evoked potential monitoring in scoliosis surgery: comparison of desflurane/nitrous oxide with propofol total intravenous anesthetic regimens. J Neurosurg Anesthesiol. 2006;18:211–4.
22. Lotto ML, Banoub M, Schubert A. Effects of anesthetic agents and physiologic changes on intraoperative motor evoked potentials. J Neurosurg Anesthesiol. 2004;16:32–42.
23. Bala E, Sessler DI, Nair DR, McLain R, Dalton JE, Farag E. Motor and somatosensory evoked potentials are well maintained in patients given dexmedetomidine during spine surgery. Anesthesiology. 2008;109:417–25.
24. Au KS, Northrup H, Allison-Koch A. Epidemiology and genetic aspects of spina bifida and other neural tube defects. Dev Disabil Res Rev. 2010;16:6–15.
25. Milunsky A, Jick H, Jick SS, Bruell CL, MacLaughlin DS, Rothman KJ, Willett W. Multivitamin/folic acid supplementation in early pregnancy reduces the prevalence of neural tube defects. JAMA 1989;262(20):2847–52.
26. McLone DG, Knepper PA. The cause of Chiari II malformations: a unified theory. Pediatr Neurosci. 1989;15:1–12.
27. Fletcher JM, Copeland K, Frederick JA, Blaser SE, Kramer LA, Northrup H, Hannay HJ, Brandt ME, Francis DJ, Villarreal G, Drake JM, Laurent JP, Townsend I, Inwood S, Boudousquie A, Dennis M. Spinal lesion level in spina bifida: a source of neural and cognitive heterogeneity. J Neurosurg. 2005;102(3 Suppl):268–79.
28. Dennis M, Salman MS, Juranek J, Fletcher JM. Cerebellar motor function in spina bifida meningomyelocele. Cerebellum. 2010;9(4):484–98.
29. Dias MS. Neurosurgical causes of scoliosis in patients with myelomeningocele: an evidence-based literature review. J Neurosurg. 2005;103(1 Suppl):24–35.

30. Samuelsson L, Eklöf O. Scoliosis in myelomeningocele. Acta Orthop Scand. 1988;59:122–7.
31. Hudgins RJ, Gilreath CL. Tethered spinal cord following repair of myelomeningocele. Neurosurg Focus. 2004;16(2):E7.
32. Tamburrini G, Frassanito P, Iakovaki K, Pignotti F, Rendeli C, Murolo D, Di Rocco C. Myelomeningocele: the management of the associated hydrocephalus. Childs Nerv Syst. 2013;29(9):1569–79.
33. Messing-Jünger M, Röhrig A. Primary and secondary management of the Chiari II malformation in children with myelomeningocele. Childs Nerv Syst. 2013;29(9):1553–62.
34. Rintoul NE, Sutton LN, Hubbard AM, Cohen B, Melchionni J, Pasquariello PS, Adzick NS. A new look at myelomeningoceles: functional level, vertebral level, shunting, and the implications for fetal intervention. Pediatrics. 2002;109(3):409–13.
35. Oren J, Kelly DH, Todres ID. Respiratory complications in patients with myelodysplasia and Arnold-Chiari malformation. Am J Dis Child. 1986;140:221–4.
36. Wu YW, Croen LA, Henning L, Najjar DV, Schembri M, Croughan MS. Potential association between infertility and spinal neural tube defects in offspring. Birth Defects Res A Clin Mol Teratol. 2006;76(10):718–22.
37. Dias MS. Neurosurgical management of myelomeningocele (Spina Bifida). Pediatr Rev. 2005;26(2):50–9.
38. Pollack IF, Kinnunen D, Albright AL. The effect of early craniocervical decompression on functional outcome in neonates and young infants with myelodysplasia and symptomatic Chiari II malformations: results from a prospective series. Neurosurgery. 1996;38(4):703–10.
39. Attenello FJ, Tuchman A, Christian EA, Wen T, Chang KE, Nallapa S, Cen SY, Mack WJ, Krieger MD, McComb JG. Infection rate correlated with time to repair of open neural tube defects (myelomeningoceles): an institutional and national study. Childs Nerv Syst. 2016;32(9):1675–81.
40. Tarcan T, Onol FF, Ilker Y, Alpay H, Simşek F, Ozek M. The timing of primary neurosurgical repair significantly affects neurogenic bladder prognosis in children with myelomeningocele. J Urol. 2006;176(3):1161–5.
41. Conran AM, Kahana M. Anesthetic considerations in neonatal neurosurgical patients. Neurosurg Clin N Am. 1998;9(1):181–5.
42. Mellor DJ, Lerman J. Anesthesia for neonatal surgical emergencies. Semin Perinatol. 1998;22(5):363–79.
43. Ritter S, Tani LY, Shaddy RE, Minich LL. Are screening echocardiograms warranted for neonates with meningomyelocele? Arch Pediatr Adolesc Med. 1999;153:1264–6.
44. Bowman RM, Mclone DG, Grant JA, Tomita T. Spina bifida outcome: a 25-year prospective. Pediatr Neurosurg. 2001;34(3):114–20.
45. Talamonti G, D'Aliberti G, Colice M. Myelomeningocele: long-term neurosurgical treatment and follow-up in 202 patients. J Neurosurg. 2007;107(5 Suppl):368–86.
46. Lew SM, Kothbauer KF. Tethered cord syndrome: an updated review. Pediatr Neurosurg. 2007;43(3):236–48.
47. Al-Holou WN, Muraszko KM, Garton HJ, Buchman SR, Maher CO. The outcome of tethered cord release in secondary and multiple repeat tethered cord syndrome. J Neurosurg Pediatr. 2009;4(1):28–36.
48. Maher CO, Goumnerova L, Madsen JR, Proctor M, Scott RM. Outcome following multiple repeated spinal cord untethering operations. J Neurosurg. 2007;106(6 Suppl):434–8.

# Anesthesia for Pediatric Plastic and Craniofacial Surgery

Shelley Joseph George and Michael Stuart Green

## Common Pediatric Plastic Surgery Procedures

### Otoplasty

Otoplasty is the surgical correction of protruding ears. This surgery may be done under general anesthesia or a local anesthetic [1, 2]. A common complication of general anesthesia is severe nausea and vomiting that may last 2 days postoperatively. Airway devices can include laryngeal mask airways or the Ring-Adair-Elwyn (RAE) tube, to provide optimal positioning. If local anesthetic is not used, a total intravenous anesthetic technique may be beneficial to minimize vomiting. Non-narcotic analgesics, such as acetaminophen and ibuprofen, may be used for postoperative pain relief.

### Syndactyly

Syndactyly may be a singular malformation or part of a syndrome. It is highly associated with prolonged QT syndrome, so patients having surgical correction should have an electrocardiogram preoperatively [3]. Regional anesthesia provides excellent surgical and postoperative pain relief.

### Trauma

Considerations for patients undergoing trauma surgery are to elucidate all injuries, despite diagnosing obvious conditions, obtain a thorough medical history, minimize aspiration risks, and promote the use of local or regional techniques where possible.

### Orbital Hypertelorism

Surgery is performed to decrease the interpupillary distance. This is seen with various congenital anomalies [4]. Anesthetic considerations for this procedure include a thorough preoperative assessment for concomitant congenital abnormalities. General anesthesia with an endotracheal tube is used as the surgery involves a frontal craniectomy. The provider must be cautious as the oculocardiac reflex may be prompted during surgery [3]. If an obvious difficult airway is excluded the patient may undergo an inhalational induction. Blood loss may be significant and may require transfusion. The patient must be monitored for respiratory distress post operatively.

S. J. George, M.D. · M. S. Green, D.O., M.B.A. (✉)
Department of Anesthesiology and Perioperative Medicine, Drexel University College of Medicine, Philadelphia, PA, USA
e-mail: sjg62@drexel.edu; Michael.Green@Drexelmed.edu

## Midface Procedures

Midface surgery is used to improve maxillary hypoplasia and can be seen in patients that suffer other facial abnormalities. The Lefort I osteotomy is the most common osteotomy. Children who have midface and mandibular hypoplasia include Pierre Robin, Apert, Treacher Collins, Saethre-Chotzen, CHARGE, Stickler, Nager, Godenhar, and Pfeiffer syndromes [5]. Specific anesthetic concerns include protecting the cornea, ocular dislocation, difficult mask ventilation and difficult intubation [6]. There must be a discussion regarding the need for the exchange of tracheal tubes during the surgery [3]. If the surgeon requests that the oral tube be changed to a nasotracheal tube after completing the midfacial osteotomies, this must be done with sterile technique and is often complicated by blood and an edematous airway. A tube exchanger should be passed through the nare and lined up with the oral endotracheal tube. As the nasal endotracheal is passed over the tube exchanger through the vocal cords, the oral endotracheal tube is removed. Before extubation an air leak must be confirmed and wire cutters must be in close proximity.

## Orthognathic Procedures

Orthognathic surgery is done to correct maxillary or mandibular hypoplasia. Nasal fiberoptic intubation is useful as many patients are difficult airways and have atlanotaxial instability [7]. This operation is unique to many pediatric craniofacial surgeries as it often employs controlled hypotension to minimize intraoperative blood loss [8]. In order to be done safely an arterial catheter is placed. Steroids and the close placement of wire cutters are necessary as airway edema is a possible postoperative complication.

## Hemifacial Microsomia

These disorders include orbital distortion, mandibular hypoplasia, ear anomaly, nerve involvement, and soft tissue deficiency. Treacher Collins and Goldenhaar syndromes are in the category [9]. If the defect is bilateral, the chance for difficult intubation increases. Maintaining spontaneous ventilation until the airway is secured is recommended.

## Cleft Lip and Palate

Difficult intubation decreases with age. Because cleft palate surgery reduces the pharyngeal space the patient is at an increased risk for obstruction, and should only be extubated after airway reflexes have returned. To facilitate respiration postoperatively the surgeon can place a nasopharyngeal tube, which is especially helpful when using opioids for postoperative pain management [3].

## Craniosynostosis

Craniosynosis occurs in 1 in every 3000 live births and leads to abnormal skull growth that can lead to a myriad of complications, as the child's head and brain continues to grow [10]. Craniosynostosis is caused by the premature closure of one or more suture lines. The cranial vault is comprised of the temporal, parietal, frontal, and occipital bones (Fig. 35.1). Various mechanisms may cause craniosynostosis (Table 35.1). It can be due to a mechanical issue such as intrauterine constraint, a genetic defect, or metabolic and hematologic abnormalities [10]. It often presents as a single finding, but 20% of the time it can present as a syndrome (Table 35.2). If syndromic often it is associated with a genetic mutation. Mutations

**Fig. 35.1** Suture lines of the cranium

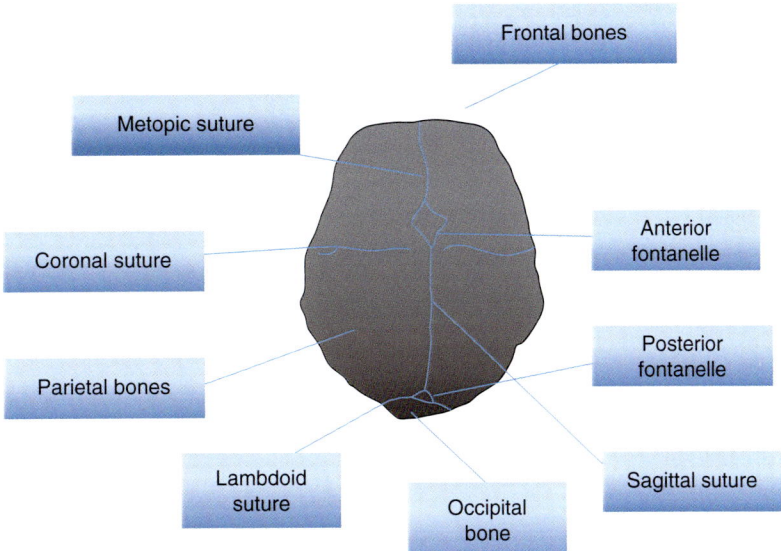

**Table 35.1** Types of craniosynostosis and the affected sutures

| Types of craniosynostosis | Suture affected |
|---|---|
| Scaphocephaly | Sagittal |
| Triogonocephaly | Metopic |
| Plagiocephaly | Unilateral coronal |
| Brachiocephaly | Bicoronal |
| Acrocephaly, turricephaly, oxycephaly | Multiple sutures |

in the gene coding for fibroblastic growth factor receptors (FGF) is most often implicated as the cause for syndromic craniosynostosis. Often this is an autosomal dominant mutation [11]. The sequeale of the premature closure of the skull may lead to multiple medical issues including increased ICP from hydrocephalus, airway obstruction or craniocerebral disproportion that then may lead to seizures, developmental delay, blindness and death. As a result of the complications, craniofacial surgery is indicated for improving neurological function, ocular, nasal, dental and auditory deformities, cosmetic appearance and psychological function.

## Considerations for the Timing of Surgery

The timing of the surgery is dependent upon on the urgency of related issues. Examples of urgent issues include if the patient needs to immediately protect their airway or eyes, or if the ICP is raised, then surgery must take place as soon as possible [10].

Other considerations include:

The pliability of the cranial bone is optimal at 3–6 months. After 1 year of age the skull may not ossify small defects and bone grafting may be necessary.

Blood loss has a greater effect in earlier infancy. Six to eight months of age is when the hematocrit stabilizes. At this age bony structures are also slightly firmer and easier to remodel [12].

Table 35.2 Common craniosynostosis syndromes along with associated features and anesthetic concerns

| Common craniosynostosis syndromes | Associated features | Anesthetic concerns |
|---|---|---|
| Apert | Bicoronal synostosis, brachycephaly, cleft palate, midface hypoplasia → OSA, proptosis, symmetrical syndactyly<br>Midface hypoplasia and proptosis<br>Fused cervical vertebrae<br>Hydrocephalus | Limited neck mobility<br>Smaller ETT than anticipated<br>Risk of bronchospasm<br>Difficult mask ventilation |
| Crouzon | Bicoronal sutures affected<br>Maxillary hypoplasia | Limited neck mobility<br>Smaller ETT than anticipated |
| Pfeieffer | Thumbs and great toes deviate<br>Maxillary hypoplasia, mandibular prognathism | Limited neck mobility<br>Smaller ETT than anticipated |
| Muenke | Most common, facial features are mildly affected, sensorineural hearing loss | |
| Saethre-chotzen | Bicoronal abnormalities<br>Beaked nose ptosis | |

## Types of Surgeries for Synostosis

### Surgeries for Sagittal Synostosis

Strip craniectomy originally described in the late 1890s, is a procedure where the fused sagittal suture is excised [13]. This technique has limited success, as there is a high restenosis rate and new techniques that have built on this have shown improved outcomes [14, 15].

### Spring-Assisted Cranioplasty

The Spring assisted cranioplasty includes a strip craniectomy followed by the placement of calibrated springs inserted between the edges of the cut bone, thus allowing for cranial expansion and normalization of skull shape. The springs are removed 6 months later under general anesthesia [16]. The main disadvantage of this surgery is the need for a second surgery.

Similarly there is an endoscopic technique that uses parietal barrel-stave osteotomies through two small incisions and then postoperatively, the child is placed in cranial molding orthotics for 6 months [17]. The main disadvantage of the surgery is the need for a helmet after.

These surgeries are done around 6 months of age, usually do not require blood transfusions, and often allow the patient to be discharged postoperative day 1 [14].

### Cranial Vault Deformities

Repair for Non sagittal synostosis, sagittal synostosis found late, and syndromic craniosynostosis [14].

Total Calvarial Reconstruction is the mainstay of corrective surgery. This surgery allows for all deformities of the skull to be addressed not just the fused suture [18]. The procedure is a very complex and has several complications that must be monitored. Complications include massive hemorrhage, venous air embolization especially when there is an elevated head position; venous outflow obstruction and upper airway edema and bleeding are attributed to the sphinx position.

The Fronto-Orbital advancement and reconstruction is used to release the synostosed suture and decompress the cranial vault, reshape the vault, advance the frontal bone, and advance the supraorbital bar [19]. The procedure is done in the supine position as a wide coronal incision and frontal craniotomy are made. Epinephrine in the scalp, scalp sutures, and scalp clips helps promote hemostasis. A zig-zag incision helps hide the scar after hair grows back. When the surgeon is operating near the orbits, the oculocardiac reflex may be stimulated. If symptomatic, the surgeon must release pressure and medicate where necessary.

Posterior Cranial Vault Reconstruction is primarily for infants with late presentation of sagittal synostosis or residual deformity from initial sagittal synostosis surgery, or syndromic patients. The procedure is done in the prone position with bicoronal incision. These patients typically do not have airway management issues and the child can be induced with inhaled anesthetic [14].

## Anesthetic Concerns

A very distinctive concern for this subset of patients and families is their emotional state. The child may already have decreased cognitive function, behavioral problems, poor self-esteem and anxiety as they approach a surgery that will change their appearance and may develop a loss in identity. This particularly affects older children.

## Airway Evaluation

The airway can present as a specific concern in many patients who present for craniofacial surgery. Although a difficult airway is not common in single suture craniosynostis, the possibility for difficult intubation or mask ventilation increases if the patient has been diagnosed with a known syndrome. Consider difficult mask ventilation with patients who are known to have airway obstructions such as choanal atresia, stenosis, macroglossia, and micrognathia. Look for signs of obstruction like mouth breathing or snoring. Fifty percent of patents with Apert, Crouzon, or Pfeifer syndrome develop OSA. Nasopharyngeal airways may be required in the operating room and CPAP may be necessary postoperatively. Alternatively, some centers schedule a tracheostomy prior to craniofacial surgery. A preoperative sleep study may be particularly helpful if unsure about patient's status. Examine the patient for cervical anomalies and neck motion.

## Neurologic Evaluation

Assess the need for ICP monitoring, as patients may have already been diagnosed with increased ICP via headaches on physical exam, ophthalmological exam or head computerized tomography.

## Cardiac and Pulmonary Evaluation

Status should be evaluated as children with diagnosed congenital syndromes often present with multiorgan disease. Tests that may be beneficial include arterial blood gas evaluation, chest x-ray, pulmonary function testing, electrocardiograms, electrolyte evaluation.

## Communication

Communication is imperative in the perioperative setting as the surgery may include multiple operators, difficult patient airway and positioning, and several potential severe complications.

## Intraoperative Management

Preoperative medications may still be required after proper psychological preparation has been allowed for. Sedation should not be given in patients with increased ICP or possible airway obstruction. Benzodiazepines may be given transrectally, Fentanyl can be administered transmucosaly, local anesthetic cream can be placed at the IV insertion site when needed. If an antisalogogue is warranted, the side effects of dry mouth and fever should be monitored for and considered.

ICP lowering techniques should be maintained throughout this time even if the ICP is normal because patients do not always present with signs and symptoms. There is also the possibility for regional increased intracranial pressure and certain areas of the cranial vault may not be able to accommodate the brain.

## Induction

Often two or more anesthesiologists are present in the operating suite, as one may focus on the airway and one can work on access and invasive lines. Intravenous or inhalational inductions are both possibilities that need to be assessed after determining the possibility for difficult airway and IV access. Syndromic patients may have a higher chance for difficult airway but also have more difficult IV securement due to the fat on the dorsum of the hand. The practitioner should have multiple plans and varied equipment ready to attack the airway [20]. Spontaneous ventilation is preferred if possible until controlled ventilation is established. Facemask fit may be improved by building up the face with gauze, applying a large mask and using high gas flows. Techniques to assist with mask ventilation include maintaining sniffing position, opening the mouth, jaw thrust, and the use of nasopharyngeal or oral airways. Intubation by direct laryngoscopy is often impossible because of anatomy. The use of LMA as bridge to fiberoptic intubation is often used. LMA's can be placed in awake infants with topical anesthesia. Video assisted endoscopes and rigid bronchoscopes can assist. Tracheostomy, if reintubation will be necessary or difficult securement of airway, should be considered [12]. The endotracheal tube must be secured such that despite changing the patient's positioning there is not a possibility for inadvertent extubation or endobronchial intubation.

## Positioning

The length of surgery can last anywhere from 4 to 12 h therefore proper positioning is key. The child may be placed in the supine, prone or modified prone position (sphinx). In the sphinx position the patient is placed in the prone position and the neck and head are extended to rest the chin on a support. Hyperextension of the neck may lead to spinal cord injury [21]. Postoperative airway complications could result from macroglossia caused by compromised venous and lymphatic draining with neck flexion. Neutral positioning without tilt down or up helps to decrease the chance for venous air embolism and bleeding. Corneal injury can be minimized by using a topical lubricant. If the patient is in the prone position the head can be lifted 3–4 times in an hour to allow for venous and lymphatic drainage.

## Temperature Regulation

Temperature regulation is key as large tissue exposure, high perfusion, anesthetic effects and resuscitation with fluids may lead to hypothermia and coagulopathy. It is recommended to drape as quickly as possible, warm the room to 23–24 °C, use heat lamps, warming blankets, warm fluids, heat and humidify gasses, and bathe the skull in warm irrigant.

## Monitoring

Along with standard ASA monitors, an arterial line and central venous catheter are recommended as there is always the possibility for dynamic cardiovascular changes and rapid blood loss. In addition, a central venous catheter may also be used to aspirate air in event of venous air embolization.

## Neuromonitoring

Medications that cause an increase in intracranial volume should not be used. The patient may be mildly hyperventilated to a paCO2 of 30–35 mmHg. If possible, keeping the head elevated at 20°–30° and the use of diuretics help in the management of intracranial pressure and maintaining cerebral perfusion pressure. The determination of the need for a CSF drain should be made with the surgeon. Venous air embolism is a known and significant complication of surgical procedures for craniosynostosis. The incidence may be has high as 83% for open procedures, but the majority are not clinically significant [22].

## Hemorrhage

The absolute percentage of blood volume lost increases in smaller and younger children due to the relatively large head creating an increased surface area [23]. Prolonged surgery, greater than 5 h, has been associated with increased blood loss [24]. It is also noted that perioperative teams with greater experience have lower levels of blood loss [12]. As there is a possibility that the patient can lose up to 400% of blood volume vigilance is key [23]. Often total blood loss cannot be explained by what is found in the suction canister, as the drapes and surgical field must be examined. Because it is often difficult to get a true sense of the actual blood loss serial hemoglobin levels should be ordered and a cutoff value to manage vitals is often determined. Major bleeding from osseous venous plexus, arterial bleeds, or accidental puncture of the dural sinus is not uncommon. It is also imperative for the anesthesiologist to be aware that during the scalp incision and while raising the periosteum rapid blood loss is known to occur. The administration of albumin increases the incidence of postoperative coagulation [23].

To reduce the need for homologous blood transfusion, techniques to optimize the patient's hemoglobin prior to surgery are used. Currently strategies to minimize blood transfusion rates intraoperatively are being debated as none have been shown to be without complication. Scarring and adhesions on repeat operations increase bleeding. Older children can initially be treated with IVF and blood products. If a 1:1 PRBC: FFP is not used and there is massive transfusion the likelihood of coagulopathy increases. Metabolic derangements are usually secondary to blood transfusion and resuscitation. Severe hyperkalemia can be seen with blood products that have a prolonged shelf time or were irradiated. Deliberate hypotension is more appropriate for extracranial surgery as there may already be compromise to perfusion in intracranial surgery. It is encouraged to have standardization of transfusion policies with in the institution.

## Pain Management

Currently the mainstay of therapy is an intraoperative opiate-based approach, which is continued along with acetaminophen in the postoperative period. An audit of 26 patients on a morphine nurse controlled analgesia regimen showed promising pain control with minimal sedation [24].

## Nausea and Vomiting

Both ondansetron and dexamethasone in the perioperative period have been shown effective to decrease the incidence of vomiting in this population and high-risk population subset [25, 26].

## Postoperative

Extubation of the patient depends on the patient's own risk factors and operative risks such as increased volume given for resuscitation [27]. Patients should be transferred to the intensive care unit. Careful monitoring for blood loss and hyponatremia is necessary at this time.

## References

1. Karapurkar SA, Garasia MB, Deval DB. Anaesthesia and craniofacial surgery. J Postgrad Med. 1994;40:3–6.
2. Laberge LC. Local anesthesia for otoplasty in children. Clin Plast Surg. 2013;40(4):671–86.
3. Engelhardt T, Crawford MW, Lerman J. Plastic and reconstructive surgery. In: Coté CJ, Lerman J, David Todres I, editors. A practice of anesthesia in infants and children. Philadelphia: Saunders Elsevier; 2009. p. 701–13.

4. Sharma RK. Hypertelorism. Indian J Plast Surg. 2014;47(3):284–92. https://doi.org/10.4103/0970-0358.146572.
5. Perkins JA, Sie KC, Milczuk H, Richardson MA. Airway management in children with craniofacial anomalies. Cleft Palate Craniofac J. 1997;34(2):135–40.
6. Raj D, Luginbuehl I. Managing the difficult airway in the syndromic child. Contin Educ Anaesth Crit Care Pain. 2015;15(1):7–13. https://doi.org/10.1093/bjaceaccp/mku004.
7. Kellman RM, Losquadro WD. Comprehensive airway management of patients with maxillofacial trauma. Craniomaxillofac Trauma Reconstr. 2008;1(1):39–47. https://doi.org/10.1055/s-0028-1098962.
8. Barak M, Yoav L, Abu el-Naaj I. Hypotensive anesthesia versus normotensive anesthesia during major maxillofacial surgery: a review of the literature. Sci World J. 2015;2015:480728. https://doi.org/10.1155/2015/480728.
9. Sinkueakunkit A, Chowchuen B, Kantanabat C, Sriraj W, Wongswadiwat M, Bunsangjaroen P, Chantawong S, Wittayapairoj A. Outcome of anesthetic management for children with craniofacial deformities. Pediatr Int. 2013;55:360–5. https://doi.org/10.1111/ped.12080.
10. Thomas K, Hughes C, Johnson D, Das S. Anesthesia for surgery related to craniosynostosis: a review. Part 1. Paediatr Anaesth. 2012;22(11):1022–41.
11. Johnson D, Wilkie AOM. Craniosynostosis. Eur J Hum Genet. 2011;19(4):369–76. https://doi.org/10.1038/ejhg.2010.235.
12. Schindler E, Martini M, Messin-Junger M. Anesthesia for plastic and craniofacial surgery. In: Gregory GA, Andropoulos DB, editors. Pediatric anesthesia. Hoboken: Blackwell Publishing Ltd; 2012. p. 810–44.
13. Bir SC, Ambekar S, Notarianni C, Nanda A. Odilon Marc Lannelongue (1840-1911) and strip craniectomy for craniosynostosis. Neurosurg Focus. 2014;36(4):E16.
14. Stricker PA, Fiadjoe JE. Anesthesia for craniofacial surgery in infancy. Anesthesiol Clin. 2013;32:215–35.
15. Proctor MR. Endoscopic craniosynostosis repair. Transl Pediatr. 2014;3(3):247–58. https://doi.org/10.3978/j.issn.2224-4336.2014.07.03.
16. Rodgers W, Glass GE, Schievano S, Borghi A, Rodriguez-Florez N, Tahim A, Angullia F, Breakey W, Knoops P, Tenhagen M, O'Hara J, Ponniah A, James G, Dunaway DJ, Jeelani N. Spring assisted cranioplasty for the correction of non-syndromic scaphocephaly: a quantitative analysis of 100 consecutive cases. Plast Reconstr Surg. 2017;140(1):125–34.
17. Jimenez DF, Barone CM. Endoscopic craniectomy for early surgical correction of sagittal craniosynostosis. J Neurosurg. 1998;88(1):77–81.
18. Chen EH, Gilardino MS, Whitaker LA, Bartlett SP. Evaluation of the safety of posterior cranial vault reconstruction. Plast Reconstr Surg. 2009;123(3):995–1001.
19. Mendonca D, Gejje S, Kaladagi N. Fronto-orbital advancement: revisited. J Cleft Lip Palate Craniofac Anomal. 2015;2:20–6.
20. Fiadjoe J, Stricker P. Pediatric difficult airway management: current devices and techniques. Anesthesiol Clin. 2009;27(2):185–95. https://doi.org/10.1016/j.anclin.2009.06.002.
21. Francel P, Bell A, Jane J. Operative positioning for patients undergoing repair of craniosynostosis. Neurosurgery. 1994;35:304–6.
22. Faberowski L, Black S, Mickle J. Incidence of venous air embolism during craniectomy for craniosynostosis repair. Anesthesiology. 2000;92:20–3.
23. Stricker P, Shaw T, Desouza DE. Blood loss, replacement and associated morbidity in infants and children undergoing craniofacial surgery. Pediatr Anesth. 2010;20:150–9.
24. Hughes C, Thomas K, Johnson D, Das S. Anesthesia for surgery related to craniosynostosis: a review. Part 2. Pediatr Anesth. 2012;23:22–7.
25. Gurler T, Celik N, Total S. Prophylactic use of ondansetron for emesis after craniofacial operations in children. J Craniofac Surg. 1999;10:45–8.
26. The Association of Paediatric Anaesthetists of Great Britain and Ireland. Guidelines on the prevention of post operative vomiting in children; 2009.
27. Hasan R, Nikolis A, Dutta S. Clinical outcome of perioperative airway and ventilatory management in children undergoing craniofacial surgery. J Craniofac Surg. 2004;15:655–61.

# Anesthesia for Ears, Nose, and Throat Surgery

**36**

Edward Cooper, Tobias Everett, James Koziol, and Rajeev Subramanyam

## Ear Surgery

### Pressure Equalization Tube Insertion (PET)

PE Tubes or pressure equalizer tube insertion is perhaps the most common pediatric surgery done in the United States. PE tubes are also known as tympanostomy tubes or ventilation tubes, and are inserted to help prevent ear infections. The insertion procedure is generally undertaken on an outpatient basis and in patients between 1 and 3 years of age. Following inhalational induction, the airway is generally maintained with assisted bag-mask ventilation. Intravenous (IV) access is not routinely obtained. Analgesia can be provided with intranasal fentanyl (1 mcg/kg) and rectal acetaminophen (30 mg/kg). Alternatively, pre- or post-operative oral acetaminophen and/or ibuprofen may be used. The combination of fentanyl and intramuscular ketorolac has been found to be associated with superior analgesia, reduced rescue analgesic requirements, while not prolonging recovery times or increasing risk of post-operative emesis [1].

Although this is a relatively safe and non-invasive procedure, vigilance is required due to the potential for upper airway obstruction, laryngospasm, cardiac dysrhythmia and other adverse events. Many children may present with a recent or concurrent upper respiratory infection with increased airway reactivity. Recent or concurrent respiratory illness is the most significant predictor for perioperative adverse events during PE tube placement [2].

### Cochlear Implantation

#### General Considerations

Cochlear implantation is the placement of an electronic device that directly stimulates auditory nerves in response to sound waves received by microphone. As a result, this electronic signal bypasses the cochlear apparatus and provides functional hearing for many conditions associated with sensorineural hearing loss. Much pediatric

---

E. Cooper, M.D.
Department of Anesthesia, Cincinnati Children's Hospital Medical Center, University of Cincinnati School of Medicine, Cincinnati, OH, USA
e-mail: edward.cooper@cchmc.org

T. Everett, M.B.Ch.B., F.R.C.A.
Department of Anesthesia, The Hospital for Sick Children, University of Toronto,
Toronto, ON, Canada
e-mail: tobias.everett@sickkids.ca

J. Koziol, F.A.N.Z.C.A.
Department of Anaesthesia and Pain Medicine,
Royal Children's Hospital, Parkville, VIC, Australia

R. Subramanyam, M.D., M.S. (✉)
Department of Anesthesia, Cincinnati Children's Hospital Medical Center, University of Cincinnati School of Medicine, Cincinnati, OH, USA

Children's Hospital of Philadelphia,
Philadelphia, PA, USA
e-mail: subramanyr@email.chop.edu

hearing loss can be attributed to perinatal TORCH infections [3]. Other common etiologies of pediatric hearing loss are congenital syndromes resulting in bony abnormalities and consequent conductive hearing loss. Common stigmata of these syndromes include facial abnormalities, difficult airway concerns (e.g. Treacher-Collins, Klippel-Feil), or systemic disease (e.g. Alport's syndrome and renal failure, Jarvell syndrome and cardiac conduction abnormalities) that may contribute to perioperative morbidity.

Hearing correction is frequently attempted prior to 2.5 years of age secondary to the potential for improved expressive and receptive language developmental outcomes. Some clinicians advocate for surgery as young as 1 year of age. When possible, children at high-risk of hearing loss should receive brainstem auditory testing to screen for deficits within the first year of life [4].

Modern cochlear devices contain both an internal (electrode stimulator) and external component (microphone apparatus). Internal electrodes are placed via a mastoidotomy into the mastoid antrum and directly stimulate the cochlear nerve. The electrodes have multiple channels to better process auditory signals. Due to the proximity of the overlying facial nerve, care must be taken not to dissect the nerve inadvertently. Neuromonitoring techniques are often employed for this surveillance. Once implanted, the electrodes and accompanying generator must be calibrated using electrically evoked audio responses. The two main measures to be ascertained are the Elicited Stapedius Reflex Threshold (ESRT) and the Elicited Compound Action Potential (ECAP). ECAP corresponds to the "noise floor"—the point at which any less stimulation will not be interpreted as sound. ESRT determines the maximum stimulus before sound is associated with pain.

## Anesthetic Considerations

Standard preoperative evaluation should be completed prior to the procedure with particular attention to potential syndromic co-morbidities. Evaluation and communication with these patients may be challenging in the context of profound hearing loss. Deferral of premedication may be advantageous when patient-provider interaction may already be challenging at baseline.

Wide-latitude can be given regarding method of induction, but intraoperative maintenance of anesthesia is of critical importance. Because of limited airway accessibility during the procedure is limited and operative time often usually exceeds 3 hours, placement of an endotracheal tube is required. Direct arterial monitoring is not required and would only be used for patient-specific indications. The cautious avoidance of hypertension facilitates maintaining a bloodless field and aids surgical dissection. Muscle relaxation is avoided, aside from facilitation of intubation, so that the facial nerve may be monitored during the case.

Volatile anesthetics result in a dose dependent increase in the measurement of ESRT, this may result in an implant that is "too loud" on first testing. The use of propofol and nitrous oxide are recommended instead because they do not demonstrate this effect [5]. ECAP is relatively unaffected by anesthetic technique. Adjunctive use of a remifentanil infusion at 0.2–0.3 mcg/kg/min may also help to limit movement and provide additional hemodynamic stability. Despite this phenomenon the use of volatile agents is not an absolute contraindication, and may provide a more reliable depth of anesthesia than a traditional total intravenous anesthetic (TIVA) technique. A secondary benefit of TIVA is a decreased incidence of postoperative nausea and emesis in the post-operative period.

At conclusion of the case, extubation should be as smooth as possible to prevent coughing and trauma to the surgical site. This may be facilitated by deep extubation after the resumption of spontaneous ventilation or by a low-dose maintenance infusion of remifentanil (0.05–0.1 mcg/kg/min) until emergence. Post-operative analgesia requirements are modest, but a titrated opioid infusion or patient controlled analgesia (PCA) may be required as part of a multimodal analgesia technique. Complications are rare, but if present are generally perisurgical infection, CSF leak, meningitis, device migration or failure [6]. Once implanted, the receiver device is at risk of magnet displacement and magnetic resonance imaging (MRI) as well as evoked potentials for neuromonitoring are contraindicated. Despite these precautions even exposures to relatively weak magnetic fields, such as those in children's toys, have been identified to result in magnet displacement. A displaced magnet requires a second exposure to general anesthesia to correct.

## Nasal Surgery

### Functional Endoscopic Sinus Surgery

#### General Considerations

There exists a high disease burden of both adult and pediatric chronic rhinosinusitis and nasal obstruction. Pathology may arise from hypertrophy of turbinate tissue leading to anterior nasal blockage or from deviations of the bony or cartilaginous septum due to trauma. Disease also arises from inflammation of sinuses within the facial bones, usually in the maxillary and ethmoid sinuses, and more rarely in the sphenoid and frontal sinuses. Chronic rhinosinusitis with post-nasal drip has also been implicated as a factor that exacerbates asthma symptoms [7].

Surgical intervention is normally reserved for those patients refractory to medical therapies including intranasal vasoconstrictors (e.g. phenylephrine) and topical corticosteroids (e.g. fluticasone) [8]. Systemic corticosteroid therapy may be used for short periods of time and is typically administered prior to surgery to reduce inflammatory burden and improve operating conditions. Nasal surgery to relieve obstruction is planned after preoperative imaging of the sinuses with computed tomography and/or direct examination of the nasal passages with fiberoptic endoscopy [9].

Turbinectomy or turbinoplasty is planned when obstruction is due to enlarged or collapsing turbinates that obstruct anterior nasal passages. Septoplasty is performed to correct congenital or acquired deviations of the nasal septum when it contributes to blockage of either nostril. Functional endoscopic sinus surgery (FESS) is performed to relieve obstructions by widening the ostia of affected sinuses. Of note because of the close proximity of the sinus ostia to the orbit, possible penetration of the endoscope through the inflamed and compromised sinus tissue into the sterile orbit or skull base is of surgical concern [10]. The above surgeries are often performed together to facilitate access to the sinuses.

#### Anesthetic Considerations

The majority of patients undergoing nasal surgery are otherwise well. It is unusual to consider surgery beyond simple turbinoplasty in children under the age of 10 years, as facial bones and nasal cartilages are expected to continue to grow and shift with age [11]. Chronic sinus infections, including fungal infections, are more commonly observed in children who are immunosuppressed, including those with poorly controlled diabetes.

The choice of anesthetic technique varies amongst the authors, but invariably includes general anesthesia. Regarding choice of airway, many would advocate for placement of a secure oral endotracheal tube due to lack of access to the patient's head during the procedure. There is invariably post nasal drip of blood, debris, and mucus related to the surgery, which should be kept clear of the airway and also from the esophagus and stomach where blood can be highly emetogenic. Placement of a throat pack in association with an endotracheal tube is mandatory, along with associated safety precautions to ensure its removal at the end of surgery. An alternative anesthetic strategy is to use a reinforced laryngeal mask airway as its greater bulk may be beneficial in limiting further passage of blood into the stomach [12]. Positive pressure ventilation with the laryngeal mask airway may be limited and may also result in air leak reaching the nasal passages, interfering with operating conditions. This complication may be mitigated with placement of a throat pack to provide additional support to closing the soft palate against the posterior pharyngeal wall.

Intranasal vasoconstrictors are usually applied prior to commencement of surgery. Possible solutions include phenylephrine, oxymetazoline, and cocaine. Cocaine has the dual benefit of being both an avid vasoconstrictor and a local anesthetic. Surgeons may also request hemodynamic parameters to be kept at relatively low normal physiologic ranges to improve operating conditions. The authors believe that it is reasonable to avoid hypertension and tachycardia, but do not advocate for the use of permissive hypotension without deliberate consideration of end-organ perfusion. The use of titrated propofol and remifentanil infusions may also be advantageous, as post-operative pain following nasal surgery is relatively unusual and this technique decreases surgical site vasodilatation with the additional benefit of diminished incidence of post-operative nausea and emesis when compared with volatile anesthesia [13].

Post-operative pain relief requirements are mild due to the concomitant use of topical anesthesia, acetaminophen with a low dose opioid available for breakthrough pain is all that is typically required. Post-operative nausea and vomiting (PONV) is common, and should be treated prophylactically. Intraoperative dexamethasone is indicated to reduce nasal swelling and decrease PONV. Post-operative bleeding complications are not uncommon and may be related to hypertension and/or tachycardia. This complication is addressed with surgical packing of the nasal passages to provide pressure hemostasis. The packing may be dissolvable (e.g. gelatin based sponges), but may lead to nasal obstruction post-operatively [14]. Post-operative administration of antihypertensives may be of benefit (e.g. clonidine). Anterior and posterior-nasal drip is to be expected and it is critical to keep the airway protected until airway reflexes are intact after emergence. Return to the operating room for bleeding is unusual, but if bleeding is significant, an overwhelming amount of blood in the stomach must also be assumed and addressed accordingly on repeat induction. Recovery is enhanced through the utilization of intra-nasal saline washes, which also aid in dissolving surgical packing [15]. Topical corticosteroids are often prescribed to reduce the risk of adhesion of healing tissue that may form a new obstruction.

## Throat Surgery

## Airway Endoscopy

### General Considerations
Continued advances in medical optic technology and persistent miniaturization of existing equipment continue to broaden the range of applications, procedures, and patient populations that could potentially benefit from an endoscopic airway techniques. We will discuss the nature of some of these procedures and additional considerations specific to the pediatric anesthesiologist that one should be aware of prior to facilitating such cases.

With the utilization of flexible fiberoptic bronchoscopy a proceduralist can ascertain significant dynamic and static diagnostic information regarding the functional anatomy of the patient's airway from the level of the nare to the distal bronchial tree [16]. Conversely with the implementation of rigid bronchoscopy, the scale of anatomic structures able to be visualized safely may be limited relative to flexible bronchoscopy, but the range of possible therapeutic interventions expands dramatically. Because of the complementary functions of both of these instruments, it is not uncommon for both endoscopes to be used within the same anesthetic encounter. Consequently the sequence of procedures and goals of each intervention should be communicated clearly and understood by all medical providers in order to optimize conditions for a successful procedure and anesthetic.

Common indications for the use of flexible fiberoptic laryngoscopy or bronchoscopy include the diagnostic evaluation of stridor, chronic wheeze, aspiration, persistent pneumonia or distal airway disease, tracheostomy surveillance, and hemoptysis. The therapeutic utility of the flexible scope includes evaluation and intubation of the difficult airway, clearance of pulmonary secretions, and an evolving role in interventional techniques such as tracheal stent placement [17]. The use of rigid bronchoscopy not only provides critical information in the diagnosis and management of conditions listed above, but can also be applied in the evaluation and removal of airway foreign bodies, blunt dissection and evaluation of laryngeal anatomy, and management of airway masses [18, 19].

### Anesthetic Considerations
Because of the inherent nature of airway endoscopic procedures, "sharing the airway" with the surgeon demands critical communication and anticipation of both planned and unplanned events by all providers. The anesthesiologist should be focused in particular about maintaining

airway patency, oxygenation, ventilation, and minimizing complications such as aspiration and airway fires throughout instrumentation and perioperative recovery. These objectives should all be met while maintaining an adequate plane of anesthesia as required by the goals of the intervention and optimizing the surgical field for the surgeon through the absence of independent patient movement or external manipulation of the airway, suppression of airway reflexes, and minimization of secretions. If possible, conditions should be optimized to allow for extended periods of unassisted ventilatory stability without significant patient decompensation in order to diminish interruptions of the procedure. These aims, even with exceptional communication and intraprovider familiarity, can be difficult to successfully accomplish at all times and even more challenging when the anesthesiologist and proceduralist are simultaneously working in the same anatomic field with an unsecured airway.

Prior to beginning bronchoscopy, patients should receive a comprehensive pre-anesthetic evaluation with thorough documentation of existing co-morbidities. A large fraction of the patients requiring airway endoscopy have secondary medical conditions such as congenital cardiac defects, alveolar lung disease, and difficult airway concerns that may dramatically influence the anesthetic plan. In addition, the goals of the procedure should be clearly delineated. For instance, if evaluating for etiologies of stridor or wheeze, dynamic function and potential airway collapse during the respiratory cycle should be observed. This assessment is ideally accomplished with the absence of neuromuscular blockade, a relatively light plane of anesthesia, and a spontaneously breathing patient.

Standard American Society of Anesthesiologists (ASA) monitors should be used and universal *nil per os* (NPO) guidelines followed. If no intravenous access is present and the patient is deemed safe for an inhalational induction the anesthetic can be initiated via spontaneous breathing of a volatile agent and intravenous access subsequently obtained [20]. Alternatively, if IV access is available prior to induction, induction of anesthesia can be accomplished via judicious titration of amnestic and analgesic medications by means of bolus and/or infusion technique. Given the difficultly in scavenging the anesthetic agent in an open airway case, the variability of consistent delivery of volatile anesthetics during the procedure, loss of reliable end-tidal and anesthetic gas monitoring, and potentially superimposed ventilation-perfusion (V/Q) mismatch secondary to intermittent hypoventilation and underlying lung disease, maintenance of anesthesia is best preserved via the intravenous route. It is our practice to use a propofol infusion (usually between 150 and 300 mcg/kg/min) paired with short-acting opioids, such as fentanyl or remifentanil via bolus or infusion delivery [21–23]. Other intravenous drug combinations utilizing these medications, or others such as dexmedetomidine or ketamine have comparable efficacy. These medications are then titrated to the desired clinical effect of a spontaneous but unconscious patient that tolerates the procedure well. Prior to instrumentation of the airway, atomized lidocaine (up to 5 mg/kg) is directly applied to the vocal cords, minimizing the risk of potential laryngospasm and reducing the need for systemic anesthetic agents. Additional adjunctive intravenous medications such as glycopyrrolate or atropine may prove beneficial in minimizing secretions, and the use of topical oxymetazoline may mitigate traumatic bleeding and edema of the mucosa. If adequate oxygenation becomes challenging during the flexible bronchoscopy, the patient may benefit from supplemental oxygen delivery above the level of the carina either via the bronchoscope, if available, or supraglottic oxygen via an endotracheal tube placed in the oropharynx. Alternatively, if oxygenation and ventilation become prohibitive in completing the procedure safely consider utilizing the fiberoptic bronchoscope through an adequately sized endotracheal tube in order to provide more reliable tidal volumes and oxygen delivery.

After completion of the dynamic airway evaluation via flexible fiberoptic bronchoscopy and supraglottic evaluation via rigid bronchoscopy, the persistence of a spontaneous respiratory pattern becomes less imperative. This circumstance, coupled with the increased noxious stimulation generated via rigid bronchoscopy and heightened risk of complications with patient movement is an indication for deepening of the plane of anesthesia and potential dosing of neuromuscular blockade medications depending on the nature of the procedure to follow. Inspired oxygen fraction should be reduced to appropriate levels to mitigate airway fires if electric cauterization is planned. Satisfactory oxygenation and ventilation can usually be maintained using the ventilating side-arm of the bronchoscope and the anesthesia circuit.

Following completion of the procedure, infusions and volatile agents can be discontinued, reversal agents given if germane, and the patient delivered assisted respirations until emergence from anesthesia. Glucocorticoid administration may prove beneficial in minimizing airway edema and clinical signs of stridor or increased work of breathing.

## Airway Foreign Body Aspiration

### General Considerations

The removal of an airway foreign body is a relatively common procedure in the toddler demographic. Airway foreign bodies have a predilection to be localized to the right mainstem bronchus secondary to its' wider diameter and less acute angle of separation from the trachea relative to the left. Though plain radiographs may be strongly suggestive of a foreign body located in the airway, clinicians should be prepared if necessary to follow the procedure with esophagoscopy if the foreign body is unable to be directly visualized and/or to assess for additional masses and trauma [24].

### Anesthetic Considerations

Focus on physical exam and degree of respiratory distress is paramount in helping to determine timing and anesthetic plan. Coughing, unilateral wheezing, dyspnea, and decreased transmission of breath sounds are often appreciated. Atelectasis, air trapping, or superimposed pneumonia may be present on radiographs. Both posterior-anterior and lateral radiographs may be beneficial to better characterized the size, location, and nature of the foreign body. We recommend that standard NPO guidelines should be followed. If the patient is exhibiting signs of respiratory distress or the mass appears to be in a tenuous position, NPO guideline violation is acceptable in favor of removal of the foreign body [25, 26].

Induction of anesthesia can be commenced via the inhalational or intravenous route. If access was not present at time of induction, it is subsequently obtained. It is our practice to recommend preservation of spontaneous respiratory effort and direct topicalization of the airway with lidocaine (up to 5 mg/kg). If the foreign body can be easily observed in the laryngeal inlet upon the attempted administration of local anesthetics, efforts can be made to remove the object with forceps. Adequate depth of anesthesia is maintained via a continuous intravenous infusion of propofol augmented with a short-acting opioid. Using a total intravenous anesthetic technique provides a more reliable and consistent delivery of anesthetic agent throughout the procedure, minimizing the risk of cough, dislodgement, object migration, and additional airway trauma with the surgical instruments or the foreign body [27, 28]. Some providers advocate for early muscle relaxation upon induction and subsequent positive-pressure ventilation to eliminate risk of patient reactivity and subsequent trauma that may occur when having a spontaneously breathing patient with potential for variable depth of anesthesia. Use of this positive pressure ventilation dependent technique may increase the risk of distal migration of the foreign body. There is currently a paucity of data definitively supporting one strategy over the other.

Subsequent to intubation of the glottis with the bronchoscope, assisted ventilation may be provided via the side-port. Ventilation may become more challenging during the course of the procedure with instruments obstructing the working channel of the rigid bronchoscope and repeated attempts at removal eliciting progressive worsening of airway trauma and inflammation. Periodic suctioning and ventilation without instrumentation may be necessary to bring physiologic parameters into acceptable physiologic range. Acute awareness and diminution of the possibility for foreign body migration, either by surgical manipulation or patient responsiveness, that can result in the complete inability to maintain ventilation is crucial. Subsequent to removal of the object, patients should be intubated, anesthetic discontinued, patient recovered, and administered glucocorticoids to decrease airway edema. Though rare, procedural complications such as laryngospasm, bronchospasm, hypoxia, and pneumothorax can be observed [29].

## Obstructive Sleep Apnea and Sleep Disordered Breathing

### General Considerations

Obstructive sleep apnea (OSA) represents the most severe form of sleep disordered breathing. The prevalence of OSA is 2–4% in the pediatric population and can be as high as 50% in obese children. Evaluation for OSA begins with a detailed history of snoring, related sleep disturbances, and physical examination. The prevalence of primary snoring is only 10% and history alone does not help to distinguish snoring from an OSA diagnosis. The gold standard to diagnose pediatric OSA is an overnight polysomnography test. Polysomnography determines the severity of OSA based on measuring rates of apnea, hypopnea, and obstructive events. Obstructive hypoventilation resulting in $CO_2$ levels above 50 mmHg for at least 25% of the total sleep time is diagnostic [30]. Screening questionnaires available for pediatric patients include a 22-point validated questionnaire validated for children aged 2–18 years [31], the American Society of Anesthesiologists screening tool [32], and the Snoring, Troubled breathing, Unrefreshed (STBUR) questionnaire [33]. Other diagnostic modalities for OSA evaluation include direct examination by an otolaryngologist, home testing, overnight oximetry, ambulatory polysomnography, MRI, and drug induced sleep endoscopy (DISE). Although the use of MRI and DISE are not clearly linked to outcomes, both of these procedures involve anesthesia or sedation in order to obtain diagnostic results [34, 35].

The medical management of pediatric OSA is directed towards weight loss, continuous positive airway pressure therapy (CPAP), use of anti-inflammatory medications (montelukast, intranasal corticosteroids), oral appliances, orthodontic treatment, and ultimately surgery. The primary surgical therapy for pediatric OSA in children older than 2 years of age is adenotonsillectomy. Other surgical options include nasal surgery, uvulopalatopharyngoplasty, lingual tonsillectomy, base of tongue surgery, supraglottoplasty, and craniofacial procedures [30].

### Anesthetic Considerations

There are several crucial anesthetic plan implications for children diagnosed with OSA. These considerations are dependent on the nature of the procedure to be completed and the severity of the patient's disordered breathing. Close communication between the surgical team and the anesthesiologist is required to help ensure a safe outcome for these high-risk patients. Children with long-standing severe OSA should have a cardiac assessment prior to procedure, including documentation of symptomatic history, and consideration of electrocardiogram and echocardiogram testing. In contrast to adult OSA patients, because CPAP therapy is often poorly tolerated in the pediatric patient, CPAP is an option in only a small minority of children with persistent post-tonsillectomy OSA or those who are deemed to be poor surgical candidates [30].

Children with OSA are at an increased risk of perioperative complications [36, 37]. Chronic hypoventilation is associated with increased analgesic sensitivity to opioids [38]. Standard opioid doses should be empirically reduced by 30–50% when compared to a similar patient without OSA. A comprehensive plan for perioperative management and thoughtful and safe postoperative disposition plan should be established a-priori. A multimodal pain treatment regime should be followed with the utilization of short acting narcotics coupled with acetaminophen, NSAIDs, ketamine, and/or dexmedetomidine if not otherwise contraindicated

[39]. Secondary to variably inherited metabolism, codeine should *not* be administered to any patient with OSA. Several deaths have been reported in patients who are ultra-rapid metabolizers of codeine due to life severe respiratory depression and profound hypoxia. Other opioids metabolized through CYP2D6 pathway may also be accompanied by higher risk of respiratory arrest in patients with OSA [40].

Inpatient postoperative monitoring should be continued overnight in patients with severe OSA with continuous pulse oximetry and capnography. Planned postoperative admission to the intensive care unit should be considered in morbidly obese children with severe OSA.

## Drug Induced Sleep Endoscopy (DISE)

DISE is a diagnostic procedure performed to identify dynamic airway collapse and anatomic localization of obstruction in patients with OSA [41]. DISE is commonly indicated in order to assess persistent airway obstruction in patients with OSA after tonsillectomy or pharyngoplasty. The procedure can be challenging since the diagnostic goals of inducing airway collapse while mimicking natural REM sleep is diametrically opposed to the clinical goal of maintaining a safe patent airway in order to minimize adverse respiratory events.

DISE in pediatric patients' can be performed both inside and outside the operating room depending on specific institutional resource availability. Patients are usually induced with a volatile anesthetic, intravenous access is obtained and the patient is then transitioned to an intravenous technique utilizing one of many various anesthetic regimens in combination or monotherapy with agents such as propofol, ketamine, remifentanil and/or dexmedetomidine [42]. Our experience has demonstrated that the use of a dexmedetomidine infusion coupled with ketamine promotes stable hemodynamics and successful clinical conditions to query the native airway with minimal adverse events [43, 44]. A bolus dose of 1–2 mcg/kg dexmedetomidine is administered along with 1–2 mg/kg ketamine. This induction regimen is then followed by a high dose infusion of dexmedetomidine [43].

## Airway Magnetic Resonance Imaging (MRI)

Cine MRI is a dynamic imaging examination of the airway used to help identify sites of anatomical upper airway obstruction. When completed in optimal conditions, MRI identifies obstruction in majority of patients with the added advantage of no radiation exposure [34]. Unfortunately, the use of this diagnostic modality is significantly limited by complexity of managing these patients under anesthesia for an extended time course and often with an exaggerated distance between clinician and patient.

Propofol and dexmedetomidine infusions are the most commonly used anesthetics to achieve motion control for sleep MRI. Dexmedetomidine monotherapy has been observed to provide higher diagnostically useful studies with the need for less artificial airway support when compared to propofol [45]. The high dexmedetomidine dose required to improve diagnostic yield carries a hemodynamic instability risk of bradycardia and hypotension. Our practice is not to administer prophylactic anticholinergics, but to have such agents readily available in the case of a crisis [46]. Fluid loading with 10 mL/kg of normal saline prior to dexmedetomidine administration is recommended to reduce the incidence of hypotension [47]. The anesthetic management is comparable to DISE, with the exception that the use of ketamine is rarely needed. The use of airway adjuncts is not preferred as this will undermine the diagnostic utility of the examination. A risk-benefit discussion with the otolaryngologist, sleep physician and the radiologist is recommended to safely balance the diagnostic value of the test with the safety of the patient when airway management becomes predictably challenging.

## Tonsillectomy

### General Considerations

Tonsillectomy is one of the most common surgeries performed in the pediatric patient population. The primary indication for the majority of pediatric tonsillectomies is sleep disordered breathing, with the second most prevalent indication being a history of recurrent pharyngeal infections. A randomized controlled trial comparing adenotonsillectomy versus watchful waiting in 464 children aged 5–9 years concluded that surgical treatment reduced symptoms and improved outcomes related to behavior, quality of life, and polysomnographic findings [48]. Another meta-analysis has shown that tonsillectomy can produce short-term improvement in sleep outcomes when compared with no surgery in children with OSA [49]. Although tonsillectomy is a routine and ubiquitously performed procedure it still carries the risk of significant postoperative complications, morbidities, mortalities, and malpractice claims [50].

## Anesthetic Considerations

The majority of patients are induced with a volatile agent and then an IV access is obtained. The intraoperative fractional inspiration of oxygen is reduced to less than 30% to reduce the risk of airway fire. Nitrous oxide has combustible properties and should not be used to reduce the inspired oxygen concentration. The airway is secured using an endotracheal tube Intraoperative management consists of IV fentanyl or IV morphine or a combination of both drugs, IV dexamethasone 0.5 mg/kg up to a maximum of 16 mg [51], and an IV $5HT_3$ receptor antagonist [39]. IV opioid doses are reduced in patients with OSA as noted above in the OSA section. Acetaminophen IV is often used at the following doses: <4 weeks of age 7.5 mg/kg, >4 weeks to 2 years 10 mg/kg, and >2 years 15 mg/kg [52]. Routine antibiotic use is presently not recommended.

The post anesthesia care time is brief unless other significant co-morbidities are present. While complications are rare, when they occur they are most often respiratory in nature. Additional morbidities include re-bleeding, inconsolable pain, nausea, emesis, and dehydration. Postoperative management of tonsillectomy consists of oral acetaminophen, ibuprofen and dexamethasone (Table 36.1). Postoperative opioids should be used with caution and are generally prescribed only for patients of school age or older [39].

## Laryngeal Cleft Repair and Supraglottoplasty

### General Considerations

Benjamin and Inglis classified degrees of laryngeal cleft defects into four grades [53]. The extent of the continuity between the laryngeal and tracheal lumens dictates the grade of cleft and will influence the surgical management, operative duration and the complexity of the anesthetic technique. Low-grade clefts may present late in life or not at all. These relatively benign clefts can be repaired endoscopically. In contrast, the more complex type four clefts usually present early in life with florid symptomatology such as persistent cough, repeated aspiration, and profound respiratory distress. Surgical repair may require extensive open exposure including both the neck and thoracic cavity. Specific circumstances may necessitate extracorporeal membrane oxygenation or cardiopulmonary bypass particularly if a congenital cardiac lesion will be addressed during the same surgical encounter.

Laryngomalacia is a laxity of the arytenoid, aryepiglottic and epiglottic structures that collapse inwards with negative pressure inspiration. Laryngomalacia often clinically presents with stridor, gastroesophageal reflux, and failure to thrive. Generally this lesion can be managed nonoperatively, but with more severe manifestations a supraglottoplasty may be indicated. Supraglottoplasty, also termed an aryepiglottic fold division, is an endoscopic technique. It has simplified the treatment for laryngomalacia which historically might have otherwise involved prolonged tube feeding and tracheostomy. The surgery may be accomplished with "cold instruments" or a carbon dioxide laser and is discussed below.

### Anesthetic Considerations

In preparation for providing anesthesia for laryngeal cleft repair the anesthesiologist should take care to exclude the multiple associated anomalies that can accompany this anatomic defect (e.g. Opitz-G, CHARGE or VACTERL syndromes). Preoperative chest plain films, echocardiogram and abdominal ultrasound scan may all prove informative.

**Table 36.1** Perioperative management of tonsillectomy

| | |
|---|---|
| Preoperative | History and physical examination<br>Screening for OSA/SDB<br>Review polysomnography<br>Cardio pulmonary comorbidities<br>Obesity<br>Failure to thrive<br>Syndromes |
| Postoperative disposition | *Overnight stay*<br>• <3 years of age<br>• Severe OSA/SDB<br>• Comorbidities<br>• Adverse events |
| | *? ICU stay*<br>• Morbid obesity (>99th percentile) with severe OSA/SDB |
| | *Same day discharge*<br>• Patients with none of the above perioperative factors mentioned under overnight stay and ICU stay are eligible for same day discharge. |
| Anesthesia | Premedication (30–50% of dose in OSA/SDB) vs. parental presence<br>Inhalational vs. intravenous induction<br>Reduce oxygen concentration to <30% (avoid Nitrous oxide)<br>Monitor airway pressure<br>Conservative opioid dosing in patients with OSA/SDB<br>Intravenous acetaminophen; Ibuprofen<br>Intravenous dexamethasone 0.5 mg/kg (max. 8–25 mg)<br>Intravenous antiemetic<br>Hydration up to 30–40 mL/kg lactated ringer's solution<br>No routine antibiotics<br>Deep vs. awake extubation |
| Postoperative | Routine PACU stay ~90 min<br>PACU fentanyl and morphine<br>Rescue antiemetics<br>Watch for perioperative respiratory adverse events<br>Opioid prescription to >6 years of age or elect to skip opioids<br>Oral acetaminophen<br>Oral dexamethasone for 3 days<br>Discharge instructions<br>Adverse events: bleeding, nausea/vomiting, dehydration, pain<br>Readmissions; redo surgery |

*ICU* intensive care unit, *OSA* obstructive sleep apnea, *PACU* post anesthesia care unit, *SDB* sleep disordered breathing

Complex microlaryngeal surgery can pose significant challenges to the anesthesiologist. Similar to other otolaryngological surgeries, profound general anesthesia, reflex suppression and akinesia is required, all without abolishing spontaneous respiration. Complicating this goal, is that those patients with complex lesions will often require prolonged, multiphase anesthetic exposures at a young age with significant pre-existing comorbidities. Like many other airway procedures these surgeries generally begin with suspension laryngoscopy and rigid bronchoscopy to evaluate the complete tracheobronchial tree. The anesthesia technique is similar for both surgeries, usually with a natural airway, though periodically supraglottoplasty procedures will be completed with the aid of a nasal endotracheal tube. With both procedures the target should be a consistent and stable plane of general anesthesia with spontaneous ventilation. This may be achieved with techniques involving a combination of both volatile and intravenous anesthetic agents. Though because of the variability in volatile anesthetic delivery and limitation of monitoring with a natural airway (*see bronchoscopy section above*), utilizing a TIVA technique may prove to be a more reliable anesthetic strategy. With TIVA, anesthetic delivery is independent of the operative site, procedural interruptions, airway obstruction, and patient respiratory effort.

TIVA techniques with combination therapy of dexmedetomidine and propofol infusions, with an adjunctive remifentanil infusion titrated to respiratory rate can provide deep plane of anesthesia while maintaining spontaneous respiration. A dedicated TIVA infusion line may prove helpful in preventing unintentional anesthetic medication boluses while delivering other medication and fluids during the procedure. Topicalization of the airway with local anesthetics is encouraged to minimize the hazard of patient movement and coughing that can occur with serious consequences. Oxygen is administered via the side port on the suspension laryngoscope or a nasopharyngeal oxygen insufflation catheter. Because end-tidal gas monitoring is frequently challenging, vigilant observation, auscultation, and palpation of the patient is imperative.

Postoperative intensive care is indicated for all but the simplest cleft repairs. Low grade repairs are ideally left spontaneously breathing without an endotracheal tube. High grade clefts may need extended sedation plans and consequently prolonged postoperative ventilation in order to minimize patient motion and potential trauma to the at-risk surgical site. In most cases an endotracheal tube is usually adequate, though with some patients an elective tracheostomy may be preferable. Postoperative disposition for supraglottoplasty procedures should be dictated by the usual patient factors but this specific surgery in and of itself does not inherently necessitate escalated post-procedural observation beyond those considerations that one would exercise for routine otolaryngological surgeries.

## LASER (Light Amplification by Stimulated Emission of Radiation)

LASERs are commonly used to treat airway papillomas, webs, and redundant subglottic tissue. The advantages are minimal tissue injury and rapid healing with minimal postoperative pain. Like many otorhinolaryngology procedures, anesthetic challenges include sharing of the airway with other providers, potential for airway fire, damage to other neighboring anatomic structures, hypoxemia, flume, and hazards to operating room personnel.

A tubeless, spontaneously breathing technique is often utilized for LASER procedures, though a nasal endotracheal tube can be used if not obstructing the surgeon's view or activity. Particular perioperative management safety concerns specific to LASER cases should be emphasized to ensure the well-being of both patient and provider. Meticulous consideration should be given to averting airway fires [54]. If a nasal endotracheal tube is used, a LASER-safe tube or tube covering should be selected. If an open airway technique is employed, then the fraction of inspired oxygen and nitrous oxide should be decreased in order to minimize combustibility. In addition, carbon dioxide LASERs commonly used in ENT procedures carry a risk of corneal damage upon direct exposure. LASER specific eye protection, coupled with clear warning signs posted outside the operating room, and close communication with the surgeon and LASER technician are prerequisites for the safe management of these cases.

## Epiglottitis

### General Considerations

Epiglottis is an airway emergency and results in the acute inflammation and swelling of the epiglottis, and may be associated with other stigmata of a systemic inflammatory process. Fortunately, the incidence of epiglottitis has decreased significantly with the advent and wide-spread use of the *Haemophilus Influenza* type B vaccination [55, 56]. Despite the near eradication of *H. Influenza* as the offending microbiologic pathogen, strains of beta-hemolytic streptococci, staphylococci, pneumococci, and other lesser known organisms in immunocompromised patients have been documented as specific etiologic agents for this condition [57]. Patients often present with fever, stridor, respiratory distress, dysphagia, and significant drooling. Classic "tripod" positioning may be exemplified in order to facilitate patency of the airway and assist respiratory effort.

**Anesthetic Considerations**

Expeditious treatment and immediate intubation of the airway is vital. Risk of progression to total laryngeal obstruction if untreated, is high. Plain neck radiographs, laboratory tests, and other investigation are not necessary, and often discouraged secondary to the time-sensitive nature of the condition and/or potential for laryngospasm with noxious stimulation. If radiographs have already been obtained, the "thumb-sign" indicative of a swollen and enlarged epiglottis may be present. In the pediatric patient, visualization of the epiglottis or maneuvers to establish or confirm the diagnosis should not be attempted prior to anesthesia as this may precipitate acute obstruction and subsequent hypoxemic arrest. If no intravenous access in present, intravenous access or intramuscular injection should not be attempted [58]. Calm awake inhalational induction should be attempted in the operating room with an experienced airway surgeon available at the bedside for emergent tracheostomy if needed [59]. After induction, early continuous positive airway pressure is often needed to maintain airway patency. Intravenous access can be attempted under general anesthesia with subsequent securement of the airway via direct laryngoscopy. A wide-selection of different sized endotracheal tubes should be available secondary to the high probability of glottic narrowing. The patient should receive appropriate wide-spectrum empiric antibiotics and remain intubated post-procedure in the intensive care unit for at least 24–48 h post-presentation. When appropriate, consider trial of extubation in the operating room environment.

**Acknowledgment** *Conflict of Interest*: None.

## References

1. Stricker PA, Muhly WT, Jantzen EC, Li Y, Jawad AF, Long AS, et al. Intramuscular fentanyl and ketorolac associated with superior pain control after pediatric bilateral myringotomy and tube placement surgery: a retrospective cohort study. Anesth Analg. 2017;124(1):245–53.
2. Hoffmann KK, Thompson GK, Burke BL, Derkay CS. Anesthetic complications of tympanostomy tube placement in children. Arch Otolaryngol Head Neck Surg. 2002;128(9):1040–3.
3. Bilavsky E, Shahar-Nissan K, Pardo J, Attias J, Amir J. Hearing outcome of infants with congenital cytomegalovirus and hearing impairment. Arch Dis Child. 2016;101(5):433–8.
4. Connor CM, Craig HK, Raudenbush SW, Heavner K, Zwolan TA. The age at which young deaf children receive cochlear implants and their vocabulary and speech-production growth: is there an added value for early implantation? Ear Hear. 2006;27(6):628–44.
5. Crawford MW, White MC, Propst EJ, Zaarour C, Cushing S, Pehora C, et al. Dose-dependent suppression of the electrically elicited stapedius reflex by general anesthetics in children undergoing cochlear implant surgery. Anesth Analg. 2009;108(5):1480–7.
6. Migirov L, Carmel E, Kronenberg J. Cochlear implantation in infants: special surgical and medical aspects. Laryngoscope. 2008;118(11):2024–7.
7. Vashishta R, Soler ZM, Nguyen SA, Schlosser RJ. A systematic review and meta-analysis of asthma outcomes following endoscopic sinus surgery for chronic rhinosinusitis. Int Forum Allergy Rhinol. 2013;3(10):788–94.
8. Fokkens WJ, Lund VJ, Mullol J, Bachert C, Alobid I, Baroody F, et al. European position paper on rhinosinusitis and nasal polyps 2012. Rhinol Suppl. 2012;(23):3 p preceding table of contents, 1–298.
9. Ramakrishnan Y, Zammit-Maempel I, Jones NS, Carrie S. Paranasal sinus computed tomography anatomy: a surgeon's perspective. J Laryngol Otol. 2011;125(11):1141–7.
10. Hosemann W, Draf C. Danger points, complications and medico-legal aspects in endoscopic sinus surgery. GMS Curr Top Otorhinolaryngol Head Neck Surg. 2013;12:Doc06.
11. Rizzi MD, Kazahaya K. Pediatric chronic rhinosinusitis: when should we operate? Curr Opin Otolaryngol Head Neck Surg. 2014;22(1):27–33.
12. Kaplan A, Crosby GJ, Bhattacharyya N. Airway protection and the laryngeal mask airway in sinus and nasal surgery. Laryngoscope. 2004;114(4):652–5.
13. Eberhart LH, Folz BJ, Wulf H, Geldner G. Intravenous anesthesia provides optimal surgical conditions during microscopic and endoscopic sinus surgery. Laryngoscope. 2003;113(8):1369–73.
14. Weber RK. Nasal packing and stenting. GMS Curr Top Otorhinolaryngol Head Neck Surg. 2009;8:Doc02.
15. Thomas WW 3rd, Harvey RJ, Rudmik L, Hwang PH, Schlosser RJ. Distribution of topical agents to the paranasal sinuses: an evidence-based review with recommendations. Int Forum Allergy Rhinol. 2013;3(9):691–703.
16. Tobias JD. Sedation and anesthesia for pediatric bronchoscopy. Curr Opin Pediatr. 1997;9(3):198–206.

17. Wood RE. Pediatric bronchoscopy. Chest Surg Clin N Am. 1996;6(2):237–51.
18. Todres ID. Pediatric airway control and ventilation. Ann Emerg Med. 1993;22(2 Pt 2):440–4.
19. Miller JI Jr. Rigid bronchoscopy. Chest Surg Clin N Am. 1996;6(2):161–7.
20. Hu S, Dong HL, Sun YY, Xiong DF, Zhang HP, Chen SY, et al. Anesthesia with sevoflurane and remifentanil under spontaneous respiration assisted with high-frequency jet ventilation for tracheobronchial foreign body removal in 586 children. Paediatr Anaesth. 2012;22(11):1100–4.
21. Cai Y, Li W, Chen K. Efficacy and safety of spontaneous ventilation technique using dexmedetomidine for rigid bronchoscopic airway foreign body removal in children. Paediatr Anaesth. 2013;23(11):1048–53.
22. Chai J, Wu XY, Han N, Wang LY, Chen WM. A retrospective study of anesthesia during rigid bronchoscopy for airway foreign body removal in children: propofol and sevoflurane with spontaneous ventilation. Paediatr Anaesth. 2014;24(10):1031–6.
23. Chen KZ, Ye M, Hu CB, Shen X. Dexmedetomidine vs remifentanil intravenous anaesthesia and spontaneous ventilation for airway foreign body removal in children. Br J Anaesth. 2014;112(5):892–7.
24. Farrell PT. Rigid bronchoscopy for foreign body removal: anaesthesia and ventilation. Paediatr Anaesth. 2004;14(1):84–9.
25. Fidkowski CW, Zheng H, Firth PG. The anesthetic considerations of tracheobronchial foreign bodies in children: a literature review of 12,979 cases. Anesth Analg. 2010;111(4):1016–25.
26. Malherbe S, Whyte S, Singh P, Amari E, King A, Ansermino JM. Total intravenous anesthesia and spontaneous respiration for airway endoscopy in children—a prospective evaluation. Paediatr Anaesth. 2010;20(5):434–8.
27. Shen X, Hu CB, Ye M, Chen YZ. Propofol-remifentanil intravenous anesthesia and spontaneous ventilation for airway foreign body removal in children with preoperative respiratory impairment. Paediatr Anaesth. 2012;22(12):1166–70.
28. Soodan A, Pawar D, Subramanium R. Anesthesia for removal of inhaled foreign bodies in children. Paediatr Anaesth. 2004;14(11):947–52.
29. Tomaske M, Gerber AC, Weiss M. Anesthesia and periinterventional morbidity of rigid bronchoscopy for tracheobronchial foreign body diagnosis and removal. Paediatr Anaesth. 2006;16(2):123–9.
30. Ehsan Z, Ishman SL. Pediatric obstructive sleep apnea. Otolaryngol Clin North Am. 2016;49(6):1449–64.
31. Chervin RD, Weatherly RA, Garetz SL, Ruzicka DL, Giordani BJ, Hodges EK, et al. Pediatric sleep questionnaire: prediction of sleep apnea and outcomes. Arch Otolaryngol Head Neck Surg. 2007;133(3):216–22.
32. American Society of Anesthesiologists Task Force on Perioperative Management of Patients with Obstructive Sleep Apnea. Practice guidelines for the perioperative management of patients with obstructive sleep apnea: an updated report by the American Society of Anesthesiologists Task Force on Perioperative Management of patients with obstructive sleep apnea. Anesthesiology. 2014;120(2):268–86.
33. Tait AR, Voepel-Lewis T, Christensen R, O'Brien LM. The STBUR questionnaire for predicting perioperative respiratory adverse events in children at risk for sleep-disordered breathing. Paediatr Anaesth. 2013;23(6):510–6.
34. Manickam PV, Shott SR, Boss EF, Cohen AP, Meinzen-Derr JK, Amin RS, et al. Systematic review of site of obstruction identification and non-CPAP treatment options for children with persistent pediatric obstructive sleep apnea. Laryngoscope. 2016;126(2):491–500.
35. Chatterjee D, Friedman N, Shott S, Mahmoud M. Anesthetic dilemmas for dynamic evaluation of the pediatric upper airway. Semin Cardiothorac Vasc Anesth. 2014;18(4):371–8.
36. Brown KA. Outcome, risk, and error and the child with obstructive sleep apnea. Paediatr Anaesth. 2011;21(7):771–80.
37. Cote CJ. Risk, error, outcome, and prevention in pediatric anesthesia: so many issues, lots of good solutions, but where do we find the resources? Paediatr Anaesth. 2011;21(7):713–5.
38. Brown KA, Laferriere A, Lakheeram I, Moss IR. Recurrent hypoxemia in children is associated with increased analgesic sensitivity to opiates. Anesthesiology. 2006;105(4):665–9.
39. Subramanyam R, Varughese A, Willging JP, Sadhasivam S. Future of pediatric tonsillectomy and perioperative outcomes. Int J Pediatr Otorhinolaryngol. 2013;77(2):194–9.
40. Crews KR, Gaedigk A, Dunnenberger HM, Leeder JS, Klein TE, Caudle KE, et al. Clinical Pharmacogenetics Implementation Consortium guidelines for cytochrome P450 2D6 genotype and codeine therapy: 2014 update. Clin Pharmacol Ther. 2014;95(4):376–82.
41. Friedman NR, Parikh SR, Ishman SL, Ruiz AG, El-Hakim H, Ulualp SO, et al. The current state of pediatric drug-induced sleep endoscopy. Laryngoscope. 2017;127(1):266–72.
42. Nguyen-Famulare N, Nassar M. Sleep endoscopy and anesthetic considerations in pediatric obstructive sleep apnea: a review. Int Anesthesiol Clin. 2017;55(1):33–41.
43. Kandil A, Subramanyam R, Hossain MM, Ishman S, Shott S, Tewari A, et al. Comparison of the combination of dexmedetomidine and ketamine to propofol or propofol/sevoflurane for drug-induced sleep endoscopy in children. Paediatr Anaesth. 2016;26(7):742–51.
44. Ehsan Z, Mahmoud M, Shott SR, Amin RS, Ishman SL. The effects of anesthesia and opioids on the upper airway: a systematic review. Laryngoscope. 2016;126(1):270–84.

45. Mahmoud M, Gunter J, Donnelly LF, Wang Y, Nick TG, Sadhasivam S. A comparison of dexmedetomidine with propofol for magnetic resonance imaging sleep studies in children. Anesth Analg. 2009;109(3):745–53.
46. Subramanyam R, Cudilo EM, Hossain MM, McAuliffe J, Wu J, Patino M, et al. To pretreat or not to pretreat: prophylactic anticholinergic administration before dexmedetomidine in pediatric imaging. Anesth Analg. 2015;121(2):479–85.
47. Mason KP, Turner DP, Houle TT, Fontaine PJ, Lerman J. Hemodynamic response to fluid management in children undergoing dexmedetomidine sedation for MRI. AJR Am J Roentgenol. 2014;202(6):W574–9.
48. Marcus CL, Moore RH, Rosen CL, Giordani B, Garetz SL, Taylor HG, et al. A randomized trial of adenotonsillectomy for childhood sleep apnea. N Engl J Med. 2013;368(25):2366–76.
49. Chinnadurai S, Jordan AK, Sathe NA, Fonnesbeck C, McPheeters ML, Francis DO. Tonsillectomy for obstructive sleep-disordered breathing: a meta-analysis. Pediatrics. 2017;139(2):e20163491.
50. Subramanyam R, Chidambaran V, Ding L, Myer CM 3rd, Sadhasivam S. Anesthesia- and opioids-related malpractice claims following tonsillectomy in USA: LexisNexis claims database 1984-2012. Paediatr Anaesth. 2014;24(4):412–20.
51. Baugh RF, Archer SM, Mitchell RB, Rosenfeld RM, Amin R, Burns JJ, et al. Clinical practice guideline: tonsillectomy in children. Otolaryngol Head Neck Surg. 2011;144(1 Suppl):S1–30.
52. Subramanyam R, Varughese A, Kurth CD, Eckman MH. Cost-effectiveness of intravenous acetaminophen for pediatric tonsillectomy. Paediatr Anaesth. 2014;24(5):467–75.
53. Benjamin B, Inglis A. Minor congenital laryngeal clefts: diagnosis and classification. Ann Otol Rhinol Laryngol. 1989;98(6):417–20.
54. Apfelbaum JL, Caplan RA, Barker SJ, Connis RT, Cowles C, Ehrenwerth J, et al. Practice advisory for the prevention and management of operating room fires: an updated report by the American Society of Anesthesiologists Task Force on Operating Room Fires. Anesthesiology. 2013;118(2):271–90.
55. Wurtele P. Acute epiglottitis in children and adults: a large-scale incidence study. Otolaryngol Head Neck Surg. 1990;103(6):902–8.
56. Reilly BK, Reddy SK, Verghese ST. Acute epiglottitis in the era of post-Haemophilus influenzae type B (HIB) vaccine. J Anesth. 2013;27(2):316–7.
57. Walker P, Crysdale WS. Croup, epiglottitis, retropharyngeal abscess, and bacterial tracheitis: evolving patterns of occurrence and care. Int Anesthesiol Clin. 1992;30(4):57–70.
58. Damm M, Eckel HE, Jungehulsing M, Roth B. Airway endoscopy in the interdisciplinary management of acute epiglottitis. Int J Pediatr Otorhinolaryngol. 1996;38(1):41–51.
59. Spalding MB, Ala-Kokko TI. The use of inhaled sevoflurane for endotracheal intubation in epiglottitis. Anesthesiology. 1998;89(4):1025–6.

# Anesthesia for Ophthalmological Procedures

## 37

Charlotte Walter

## Introduction

Ophthalmic cases are frequently encountered by pediatric anesthesiologists and present unique challenges for successful management. A good understanding of the anatomy and physiology of the eye is mandatory to understand the management of various pediatric ophthalmic conditions. Also, ophthalmic surgery is associated a unique subset of medications whose pharmacology must be appreciated. In addition, drugs commonly used during an anesthetic can cause unwanted side effects that are detrimental to the eye. Finally, there are several ophthalmic conditions that are seen when taking care of a pediatric population. A good understanding of these conditions and their management is necessary.

## Anatomy and Physiology of the Eye

### Anatomy

The eye itself is protected by the orbit; the orbits are conical structures made up of six different bones [1]. A child's orbit is rounder than an adult but the width increases with age [2]. There are several accessory visual structures which include the eyelids, extraocular muscles, mucous membranes lining the eyelids and the lacrimal apparatus [3]. The eyeball is outpouching of the brain [2]. The eyeball is divided into three layers and two chambers [4]. The layers are the outer fibrous layer, a middle layer called the vascular coat and an inner layer consisting of the retina [3]. The outer fibrous layer is made of the sclera, the white of eye, and the cornea, the transparent part of the fibrous layer covering the anterior portion of the eye [1]. The vascular layer consists of the choroid, the ciliary body and the iris. The iris contains muscles that allow for pupillary dilation by sympathetic stimulation and pupillary constriction by parasympathetic stimulation [3]. The iris also divides the anterior chamber of the eye filled with aqueous humor from the posterior chamber of the eye filled with vitreous humor [1]. The inner layer contains the retina which is made up of the pigment cell and neural layers that transmit visual signals via the optic nerve (cranial nerve II) [3]. The sensory innervation of the eye is provided by the ophthalmic branch of the trigeminal nerve [3].

The seven extraocular muscles of the orbit are responsible for moving the superior eyelids and the eyeball. There are four recti muscles that attach to the anterior surface of the eye forming a cone [1]. Three recti muscles are innervated by CN III as well as the inferior oblique muscle (the oculomotor nerve) while the lateral recti are innervated by CN VI (abducens nerve) [1]. The superior oblique muscle is innervated by CN IV (the trochlear nerve) [1].

C. Walter, M.D.
Department of Anesthesia, Cincinnati Children's Hospital Medical Center, University of Cincinnati, Cincinnati, OH, USA
e-mail: Charlotte.walter@cchmc.org

## Physiology

Understanding intraocular pressure (IOP) is key to understanding the physiology of the eye. Normal IOP ranges from 10 to 20 mmHg [5]. Pressures are somewhat lower at birth [6]. IOP is determined by many different factors including intraocular volume. Intraocular volume is determined by the volumes of the vitreous humor and the aqueous humor [6]. Vitreous humor volume is constant. Aqueous humor production and elimination play the biggest role in influencing IOP [6]. Outflow of the aqueous humor can fluctuate based on the dilation of the pupil. The sympathetic nervous system causes mydriasis or pupil constriction thereby decreasing outflow and increasing IOP [6]. Parasympathetic does the opposite; it causes miosis or widening of the iris allowing more outflow and a decrease in IOP [6]. Other factors such as sclera rigidity, blood volume, venous pressure and external pressure on the eye can also play a role [5].

## Anesthetic Implications

An acute rise in IOP can lead to serious complications. High IOP impairs blood flow to the retina; this can lead to loss of optic nerve function and blindness [5]. Also, an increase in IOP can be dangerous for patients with perforating eye injuries and glaucoma. Many different common and necessary anesthetic practices can cause an increase in IOP such as endotracheal intubation and laryngoscopy [5]. Other common occurrences under anesthesia such as vomiting and coughing also increase IOP [7]. Furthermore, blood volume of the eye and therefore IOP is sensitive to respiratory acidosis and alkalosis. Respiratory acidosis increases blood volume and IOP while respiratory alkalosis lowers blood volume and IOP [7].

## Oculocardiac Reflex

### Physiology

During ophthalmic surgery, the oculocardiac reflex is at risk for being triggered. The oculocardiac reflex is peripheral subtype of the trigeminal cardiac reflex [8]. It is defined as a sudden drop in heart rate of more than 20% of baseline from the stimuli of pressure on the globe, conjunctiva and orbital structures or traction of the extraocular muscles [9]. The bradycardia can also lead to other arrhythmias including junctional rhythm, AV block ventricular bigeminy and asystole. It can also lead to hypotension, apnea and gastric hypermotility [8]. A stimulus such as pressure on the globe triggers the afferent pathway of the V1 branch of the trigeminal nerve to send a signal to the Gasserian ganglion where the sensory nucleus of the trigeminal nerve is located [8]. In the Gasserian ganglion, the efferent limb of the reflex is triggered by cross connections to the motor nucleus of the vagus nerve [8]. The stimulation of the vagus nerve causes bradycardia through its parasympathetic motor function. The bradycardia may be profound leading to asystole and cardiac arrest. The response usually stops once the stimulation stops [10].

### Anesthetic Implications

There are many ways to reduce the risk of the oculocardiac reflex including avoiding hypercarbia and hypoxia, achieving an adequate depth of anesthesia, gentle surgical manipulation and prophylactic anticholinergic medications such as atropine or glycopyrrolate [10]. However, the prophylactic use of anticholinergics remains controversial secondary to their side effect profile. The treatment for the reflex is generally stopping the surgical manipulation. If the bradycardia persists, atropine should be administered [11].

## Pharmacology and Ophthalmic Surgery

### Ophthalmic Medications (Table 37.1)

Many different drugs are used to treat ophthalmic conditions and/or create optimal surgical conditions. These drugs have side effects that play an important role in the anesthetic. Eye drops can drain through the nasolacrimal system and be absorbed by nasal mucosa [12].

**Table 37.1** Common ophthalmic medications and their effect on Anesthesia

| Drug name | Mechanism of action | Effect on the eye | Anesthetic important side effects |
|---|---|---|---|
| Echothiophate | Irreversible cholinesterase inhibitor | Pupillary constriction that can be used to treat glaucoma | Prolongs the effects of succinylcholine even for weeks after discontinuation |
| Phenylephrine | Alpha agonist | Pupillary dilation to facilitate access to the posterior eye | Hypertension, bradycardia, pulmonary edema |
| Timolol | Beta-antagonist | Decreases IOP | Bradycardia, hypotension, bronchospasm, apnea in infants |

Echothiophate is a potent, irreversible cholinesterase that can be used to treat esotropia and glaucoma [13]. It is such a potent cholinesterase that it can prolong the effects of succinylcholine. In children who receive echothiophate ophthalmic drops daily, cholinesterase activity declines as soon as treatment is started and can last several weeks after the drop are discontinued [14].

Phenylephrine eye drops are used in ophthalmic surgery as a mydriatic agent to facilitate reaching the posterior eye. These drops can have systemic absorption leading to systemic effects. Hypertension, heart rate alterations and pulmonary edema can occur after administration [15]. Since phenylephrine drops are usually administered preoperatively, these cardiopulmonary effects can be seen by the anesthesiologist intraoperatively.

Timolol is a nonselective beta-antagonist that decrease IOP and can be used to treat glaucoma. Timolol can cause severe cardiac and pulmonary effects including bradycardia, hypotension and bronchospasm [12]. In neonates, timolol administration is associated with apnea and is contraindicated [16].

## Anesthetic Medications

Many drugs commonly used in anesthesia have impacts on the eye; sometimes these effects can have serious side effects. Drugs administered to patients during anesthesia can affect intraocular pressure by directly causing changes to the eye and its function and indirectly by causing changes to the cardiopulmonary systems [7].

Nitrous oxide can have serious complications if given during some ophthalmic surgeries. In retinal detachment surgeries, an expandable gas sulfur hexafluoride sometimes is injecting into the vitreous to cause internal tamponade of the retinal break [7]. Nitrous oxide is 117 times more soluble than sulfur hexafluoride; if nitrous oxide is used as part of the anesthetic when the sulfur hexafluoride gas bubble is inserted into the eye, it will diffuse into the bubble faster than the sulfur hexafluoride can diffuse out leading to a rapid threefold increase in the volume of the bubble [7]. This can cause an increase in intraocular pressure and retinal ischemia.

Succinylcholine has been shown to increase IOP by causing the extraocular muscle to contract and external pressure on the eye to increase [7]. Succinylcholine 1 mg/kg IV causes ocular muscle contraction for at least 15 min after administration [17]. Studies have shown that nondepolarizing muscle relaxants may cause a small decrease in IOP [18, 19].

Ketamine has been postulated to increase IOP by an increase in blood pressure, an increase in tone of extraocular muscles and a direct effect on the central homeostatic mechanism responsible for regulating IOP [20]. Several studies have shown that this increase in IOP associated with ketamine doses in children is small (1–2 mmHg) and transient [20, 21]. Ketamine is also associated with a nystagmus and blepharospasm that may be unwanted during certain ophthalmic procedures [7].

Volatile agents such as desflurane and sevoflurane have been shown to decrease intraocular pressure and are frequently utilized in pediatric ophthalmology cases [5].

## Anesthetic Considerations: Surgery and Condition Specific Strabismus

### Pathology

Strabismus is an abnormal alignment of the eyes. Strabismus has a high prevalence (3–5%) among pediatric patients making strabismus repair a common surgery for the pediatric anesthesiologist [22]. To repair strabismus, the extraocular muscles responsible for the abnormal alignment are either resected or recessed [6]. Strabismus can be either idiopathic or associated with a myriad of conditions including neuromuscular disorders or several congenital diseases such as Marfan syndrome, myotonic dystrophy, Stickler syndrome and Turner's syndrome [6].

## Anesthetic Considerations

Strabismus repair is considered a high risk for postoperative nausea and vomiting [23]. Hence, strabismus repair cases should receive double prophylaxis with two antiemetic medications given during general anesthesia [24]. Serotonin receptor antagonist such as ondansetron have been used successfully to reduce the risk of the PONV after strabismus surgery [25]. Other complications from strabismus repair include emergence delirium and activation of the oculocardiac reflex [26].

During strabismus repair, surgeons may conduct a forced duction test. A forced duction test is performed by grasping the sclera and moving the eye into each gaze field by traction and assesses the mechanical restriction to movement of the eye muscles [27]. The test differentiates between a paretic muscle and an ocular movement restriction and requires absent muscle tone [27]. Some surgeons may request neuromuscular blockade during strabismus repair for these reasons. However, succinylcholine can interfere with the forced duction test up to 20 min after administration [17]. Therefore, if muscle relaxants are requested to perform a forced duction test, nondepolarizing agents should be considered.

## Ruptured Globe

### Pathology

Ruptured globe is defined as a full thickness injury to the outer layer of the eye; ruptured globe has an incidence of 2–3.8/100,000 in the US with most pediatric cases occurring at home and from a penetrating sharp object [28]. When the outer layer of the eye is not intact, any increase an IOP may cause extrusion of aqueous and vitreous humor and permanent vison deficits [29].

## Anesthetic Considerations

Ruptured globe is a surgical emergency often mandating the need for rapid sequence intubation secondary to full stomach and aspiration risks. The child with the ruptured globe, as with any trauma, is at risk for being emotionally upset and crying which can cause an unwanted increase in IOP. As previously discussed, succinylcholine in isolation can also raise IOP [30]. However, there is controversy as to whether succinylcholine is contraindicated for an open globe surgery that needs a rapid sequence intubation [31]. Some studies have shown that the increase in IOP that occurs after succinylcholine administration is not related to an increased risk of extrusion of eye contents [32]. Also, adequate depth at induction with the addition of short acting opioids has been shown to minimize the increase in IOP associated with succinylcholine [32]. In spite of this, most anesthesiologists avoid succinylcholine for induction in these cases and choose a nondepolarizing muscle relaxant [32].

## Retinopathy of Prematurity

### Pathology

Retinopathy of prematurity (ROP) is common blinding disease in the developed world. The two main risks factors for ROP are exposure to oxygen and gestational age [6]. The retina develops it blood flow from the fourth month of gestation through right before birth [33]. Premature infants, therefore, are born with incomplete retinal vessel development. ROP occurs in two phases. The first phase is marked by vessel loss; the extrauterine environment is relatively hyperoxic to premature infant; this relatively hyperoxia spurs a period of regression of developed retinal vessels and avascular areas on the retina [34]. The avascular areas eventually lead to tissue hypoxia [34]. The second phase is marked by vessel proliferation; the previous avascular areas on the retina undergo neo-revascularization induced by tissue hypoxia [34]. This revascularization can occur up to 44 weeks post conception. This neo-vascularization results in a pathologic growth of vessels causing a scar formation [34]. This scar can retract and pull away the retina causing retinal detachment and blindness [34]. It has not been determined the best oxygen levels for reducing ROP [35].

## Anesthetic Considerations

Early treatment of ROP is often performed to help avoid the late devastating complications such as retinal detachment and blindness. Laser photocoagulation and cryotherapy are routine treatments for ROP [36]. These cases are performed both in the operating room suite with an anesthesiologist and in the neonatal intensive care unit with a neonatologists running the sedation. Various anesthesia modalities have been successfully used including topical eye drops, general anesthesia and intravenous sedation with mechanical ventilation [37, 38]. Difficulties in accessing a pediatric anesthesiologist, preference of the ophthalmologists and institutional practices of the neonatal intensive care unit all contribute to the decision of which modality to perform [37]. During transport and throughout anesthesia, the amount of oxygen must be carefully monitored and regulated for all neonatal patients to decrease the risk of ROP [39].

The late consequences of ROP include need for vitrectomy and other invasive procedures. These surgeries usually mandate a general anesthetic in the operating room [6].

## References

1. Presland A, Price J. Ocular anatomy and physiology relevant to anesthesia. Anaesth Intensive Care Med. 2010;11(10):438–43.
2. Turvey TA, Golden BA. Orbital anatomy for the surgeon. Oral Maxillofac Surg Clin North Am. 2012;24(4):525–36.
3. Moore KL, Dalley AF. Clinically oriented anatomy. 5th ed. Philadelphia: Lippincott; 2006.
4. Kels BD, Grzybowski A, Grant-Kels JM. Human ocular anatomy. Clin Dermatol. 2015;33:140–6.
5. Park JT, Lim HK, Jang KY, Um DJ. The effects of desflurane and sevoflurane on the intraocular pressure associated with endotracheal intubation in pediatric ophthalmic surgery. Koren J Anesthesiol. 2013;64(2):117–21.
6. Davis PJ, Cladis FP, Motomoya EK. Smith's anesthesia for infants and children. 8th ed. St. Louis: Elsevier Mosby; 2011.
7. Cunningham AJ, Barry P. Intraocular pressure-physiology and implications for anesthetic management. Can Anaesth Soc J. 1986;33(2):195–208.
8. Meuwly C, Golanov E, Chowdhury T, Erne P, Schaller B. Trigeminal cardiac reflex: new thinking model about the definition based on a literature review. Medicine. 2015;94(5):e484.
9. Song IA, Seo KS, Oh AY, Baik JS, Kim JH, Hwang JW, Jeon YT. Dexmedetomidine injection during strabismus surgery reduces emergence agitation without increasing oculocardiac reflex in children: a randomized controlled trial. PLoS One. 2016;11(9):e0162785.
10. Rodger A, Cox RG. Anesthetic management for pediatric strabismus surgery: continuing professional development. Can J Anesth. 2010;57:602–17.
11. Lubbers HT, Zweifel D, Gratz KW, Kruse A. Classification of potential risk factors for trigeminocardiac reflex in craniomaxillofacial surgery. J Oral Maxillofac Surg. 2010;68:1317–21.
12. Kiryazov K, Stefova M, Iotova V. Can ophthalmic drops cause central nervous system depression and cardiogenic shock in infants? Pediatr Emerg Care. 2013;29:1207–9.
13. Cavallaro RJ, Krumperman LW, Kugler F. Effect of ecthothiophate therapy on the metabolism of succinylcholine in man. Anesth Analg. 1968;47(5):570–4.
14. Ellis PP, Esterdahl M. Echothiophate iodide therapy in children: effect upon cholinesterase levels. Arch Ophthalmol. 1967;77(5):598–601.
15. Sbaraglia F, Mores N, Garra R, Giuratrabocchetta G, Lepore D, Molle F, Savino G, Piastra M, Pulitano S, Sammartino M. Phenylephrine eye drops in pediatric anesthesia patients undergoing ophthalmic surgery: incidence, presentation, and management of complications during general anesthesia. Pediatr Anesth. 2014;24:400–5.
16. Bailey PL. Timolol and postoperative apnea in neonates and young infants. Anesthesiology. 1984;61:622.
17. France NK, France TD, Woodburn JD, Burbank DP. Succinylcholine alteration of the forced duction test. Ophthalmology. 1980;87(12):1282–7.
18. Chiu CL, Wang CY. Effect of rocuronium compared with succinylcholine on intraocular pressure during rapid sequence induction of anaesthesia. BMJ. 1999;82(5):757–60.
19. Vinik HR. Intraocular pressure changes during rapid sequence induction and intubation: a comparison of

rocuronium, atracurium and succinylcholine. J Clin Anesth. 1999;11(2):95–100.
20. Nagdeve NG, Yaddanapudi S, Pandav SS. The effect of different doses of ketamine on intraocular pressure in anesthetized children. J Pediatr Ophthalmol Strabismus. 2006;43(4):219–23.
21. Wadia S, Bhola R, Lorenz D, Padmanabhan P, Gross J, Stevenson M. Ketamine and intraocular pressure in children. Ann Emerg Med. 2014;64(4):385–8.
22. Ying GS, Maguire MG, Cyert LA, Ciner E, Quinn GE, Kulp MT, Orel-Bixler D, Moore B. Prevalence of vision disorders by racial and ethnic group among children participating in Head Start. Ophthalmology. 2014;121(3):630–6.
23. Gan TJ, Diemunsch P, Habib AS, Kovac A, et al. Consensus guidelines for the management of postoperative nausea and vomiting. Anesth Analg. 2014;118(1):85–113.
24. Hohne C. Postoperative nausea and vomiting in pediatric anesthesia. Curr Opin Anaesthesiol. 2014;27(3):303–8.
25. Bowhay AR, May HA, Rudnicka AR, Booker PD. A randomized controlled trial of the antiemetic effect of three doses of ondansetron after strabismus surgery in children. Pediatr Anaesth. 2001;11:215–2.
26. Ibrahim AN, Shabana T. Sub-Tenon's injection versus paracetamol in pediatric strabismus surgery. Saudi J Anaesth. 2017;11(1):72–6.
27. Dell R, Williams B. Anaesthesia for strabismus surgery: a regional survey. Br J Anaesth. 1999;82(5):761–3.
28. Li X, Zarbin MA, Bhagat N. Pediatric open globe injury: a review of the literature. J Emerg Trauma Shock. 2015;8(4):216–23.
29. Mowafi HA, Aldossary N, Ismail SA, Algahtani J. Effect of dexmedetomidine premedication on the intraocular pressure changes after succinylcholine and intubation. Br J Anaesth. 2008;100(4):485–9.
30. Pandey K, Badola RP, Kumar S. Time course of intraocular hypertension produced by suxamethonium. Br J Anaesth. 1972;44(2):191–6.
31. Vachon CA, Warner DO, Bacon DR. Succinylcholine and the open globe. Tracing the teaching. Anesthesiology. 2003;99(1):220–3.
32. Seidel J, Dorman T. Anesthetic management of preschool children with penetrating eye injuries: postal surgery of pediatric anesthetists and review of the available evidence. Pediatr Anesth. 2006;16:769–76.
33. Quimson SK. Retinopathy of prematurity: pathogenesis and current treatment options. Neonatal Netw. 2015;34(5):284–7.
34. Chen J, Smith LEH. Retinopathy of prematurity. Angiogenesis. 2007;10:133–40.
35. Hartnett ME, Lane RH. Effects of oxygen on the development and severity of retinopathy of prematurity. J AAPOS. 2013;17(3):229–34.
36. Gorbe E, Vamos R, Joo GJ, Jeager J, et al. Perioperative analgesia of infants during the therapy for retinopathy of prematurity. Med Sci Monit. 2010;16(4):186–9.
37. Jian JB, Stauss R, Luo XQ, Nie C, et al. Anaesthesia modalities during laser photocoagulation for retinopathy of prematurity: a retrospective, longitudinal study. BMJ Open. 2017;7:e013344.
38. Sammartino M, Bocci MG, Ferro G, Mercurio G, et al. Efficacy and safety of continuous intravenous infusion of remifentanil in preterm infants undergoing laser therapy in retinopathy of prematurity: clinical experience. Pediatr Anaesth. 2003;13:596–602.
39. Kinochi K. Anaesthetic considerations for the management of very low and extremely low birth weight infants. Best Pract Res Clin Anaesthesiol. 2004;18(2):273–90.

# Anesthesia for Neonatal Emergencies: General Principles

## 38

Jakob Guenther and Kumar G. Belani

## Introduction

On a daily basis, pediatric anesthesiologists encounter challenges related to the size of their patients, "competition" for surface area to utilize monitoring equipment, as well as gaining access to the airway and blood vessels. All these challenges are further aggravated in premature infants and neonates, and yet again more aggravated in emergent situations.

Medical advances during the last few decades have resulted in improved survival of younger and smaller infants. At the same time this has created an increase of interventions in low/very low/ extremely low birth weight infants who present with significant physiologic and anatomic immaturity as well as significant morbidity. These babies are more vulnerable to suffer complications that may result in significant challenges in the perioperative period.

This chapter will focus on some basic recommendations regarding neonatal physiology (glucose management, fluid management, transfusion management, neonatal shock), and the challenges awaiting the anesthesiologist in the perioperative phase, as well as strategies to optimize monitoring and therapy. The anesthetic management of specific cardiac and anatomic conditions

J. Guenther, M.D. (✉) · K. G. Belani, M.B.B.S., M.S.
University of Minnesota Masonic Children's Hospital, Minneapolis, MN, USA
e-mail: jguenthe@umn.edu

(Examples: gastroschisis, TEF, CDH, Pyloric stenosis) are being covered in other chapters.

## Glucose and Fluid Management in Neonatal Emergencies

While most term neonates are able to tolerate several hours without active glucose administration, certain neonatal populations depend on parenteral glucose and nutrition administration during emergencies, especially very and extremely low birth weight premature infants, as well as children with diabetic mothers.

Both hypoglycemia and hyperglycemia (necrotizing enterocolitis, intraventricular hemorrhage) have been associated with higher morbidity [1–3], and while frequent blood glucose testing may be desirable, it may be difficult to achieve during surgery. Capillary blood sticks may be impossible due to inability to reach the child, while frequent blood draws from intravenous or arterial catheters may result in anemia, hemodilution, inadvertent bolus of continuous medications or loss of function of the access line.

During the first days of life, for fluid resuscitation in the neonate one typically avoids active administration of sodium due to prevalent excess of sodium in the neonate's extracellular space. Fluid replacement is typically done with hypotonic and glucose containing fluids. However, this changes when the patient is losing significant amounts of extracellular fluids due to either abnormal anatomy or physiology (Surgical access to abdominal or thoracic cavity, Gastroschisis, NEC, etc.). These losses include loss of electrolytes that require replacement with isotonic fluids, not hypotonic fluids [4].

Anticipating these requirements and making appropriate infusions available prior to surgery may result in better resuscitation and avoidance of overloading the immature kidneys of the neonate.

Even in not critically ill neonates the optimal maintenance therapy remains somewhat unclear. While fluid resuscitation of children older than 6 months should be done with isotonic fluids, data for neonates and younger infants is scarce [4].

The often applied "4-2-1 rule" based on physiology knowledge of the 1950s, and is an estimate based on both the caloric requirements of a child and the use hypotonic and glucose containing fluids. This rule is not meant to calculate deficits in the perioperative environment or in management of critically sick infants. The original authors updated their recommendations in 2004, discussing several caveats to the application of the "4-2-1" rule, which are reflected in the summary below [5, 6].

To summarize:

- Neonates and Infants may require significant amounts of fluid resuscitation during large surgeries, especially intra-abdominal and intrathoracic procedures. Perioperative fluid resuscitation should be done with **isotonic crystalloids, colloids or blood products**. Large boluses of hypotonic fluid can result in life threatening hyponatremia [4, 7]
- A simplified guideline for perioperative fluid resuscitation, in heart and kidney healthy children, and in the absence of major bleeding the following strategy is recommended:
  - 20–40 mL/kg of ISOTONIC fluids in perioperative phase (intra- and postop)
  - Up to 80 mL/kg possible, if severe dehydration suspected
  - Recovery: "2-1-0.5" rule (2 mL/kg for 1–10 kg, 1 mL/kg for next 10 kg, 0.5 mL/kg for every kg above 20 kg)
  - If patient remains NPO after surgery, switch back to hypotonic saline and "4-2-1"

- If the patient arrives on Glucose containing maintenance or Total Parenteral Nutrition, it can be continued, but the volume may need to be reduced in this setting, since the surgical stress can result in hyperglycemia. Concerns for hyponatremia also apply in this setting.
- Urine output as a measure of adequate fluid resuscitation may be difficult to assess in neonates. In the first 24–48 h a low urine output is physiologic. After this period, neonates will ideally produce at least 1–2 mL/kg/h. Premature and even term infants have a decreased ability to concentrate urine higher than a maximum osmolality of 700 mEq/L compared to 1400 mEq/L in adults. As a result, there is no "concentrated urine" to indicate improving or decreasing urine production. **Neonates either micturate — or they don't**. Diapers only allow post-surgical assessment of urine output (weighing), while the typically fairly large bore tubing of urine catheters may not show even "adequate" urine output for hours. On the other hand, if a neonate does not produce any urine in spite of prolonged aggressive fluid resuscitation, concerns for kidney failure or obstruction of the urogenital system should be raised.
- There is no easy way to predict fluid responsiveness to improve cardiac output in pediatric patients under general anesthesia. Typical monitors, such as blood pressure, pulse pressure variation, heart rate, plethysmography or central venous pressure and even filling status of the IVC via ultrasound do not reliably predict fluid responsiveness. The only predictive variable is doppler echocardiography of respiratory variation in aortic blood flow peak velocity. Further studies may be required, since there is no consensus on the degree of variation to predict fluid responsiveness [8, 9].
- Near Infrared Spectroscopy (NIRS) is sensitive, but not specific, to give a valuable estimate of perfusion trends, but has to be interpreted within the entire situation. It is an excellent monitor to give an early warning about worsening oxygen debt, but does not specify the underlying cause. The perfusion decrease may be a sign of cardiac failure, ane-

mia, regional ischemia (NEC) or actual hypovolemia. The value of NIRS as an additional monitor will be discussed later in this chapter.

## Temperature Regulation in Neonates

Hypothermia is a common, dangerous and preventable occurrence during neonatal surgery. It is associated with a higher risk of infection, poor wound healing, coagulation impediment (both platelet function and coagulation enzyme cascade), delayed emergence and increased oxygen consumption that may result in ischemia of organs.

Mechanism of heat loss in neonates and infants lose compared to adults include the following:

- Radiation (40%): A relatively large surface area including a large and mostly bald head contributes to the additional heat loss.
- Convection (35%): Less natural insulation (fat tissue) is prevalent compared to older children and adults. Brown fat (compared to later developing white fat) has less insulating but actually heat producing capacities via specialized mitochondria. Forcing the neonate to produce additional heat is a highly energy and oxygen demanding process that can worsen oxygen debt.
- Evaporation (25%): Water evaporation results in active cooling of the surrounding area, and can happen both on exposed surface areas (sweating, surgical field) and in the infant's airway due to a dry ventilation gas–mix.
- Conduction in a dressed and covered neonate on a warmed surface will play a minor role, but a cold gel mat on the OR table may cause significant heat conduction from the neonate into the underlying surface and this may progress to hypothermia.

Strategies to treat hypothermia include

- **Prevention is key**: If the surgery takes place in a temperature controlled environment (OR versus ICU), the anesthesia team should ensure a warm operating environment, availability of heat radiating devices, as well as starting to warm the OR table surface, when feasible.
- **Radiation:** Heat lamps and high room temperature can decrease the heat gradient between infant and environment. The less the heat gradient is, the less radiation loss occurs. These are excellent measures during times when the patient tends to be partially uncovered (Induction, line placement, emergence).
- **Convection:** Forced air warming devices and heated blankets are effective, but there are concerns of increased surgical infection rates with forced air which may result in delayed utilization until the child is completely draped. Only a partial cover is possible due to interference with the surgical field. Forced air mats "under" the infants technically do not actually flow under the child, since this would create a rather unstable surface, the forced warm air flows mostly to the sides.
- **Evaporation:** Avoidance of sweaty and wet skin or moisturized heated air in the breathing circuit can decrease evaporation. Keep in mind that passive air moisturizers (HME devices) increase dead space and unless pre-moisturized may require time to trap enough moisture to make a difference.
- **Conduction:** Gel mats and circulating heated fluid surfaces may require pre-warming, otherwise they can actually contribute to hypothermia. On the other hand, once they are warm, they may contribute to hyperthermia, since they take a prolonged time to cool down. A newer blanket called the "hot-dog" is now available that has electronic precise temperature control but needs to be evaluated in this age group.
- **Warm fluids** are only effective when given as a bolus. A slowly infusing "maintenance" drip in a neonate will be likely back to room temperature by the time it reaches the neonate, unless the heating happens immediately before entering the body.
- **Shivering** as a mode of heat generation is not an option because of lack of effective muscle mass and would therefore be less effective

## Transfusion Considerations in Neonatal Emergencies

While healthy neonates typically present with a high hemoglobin and hematocrit, the anesthesia team has to keep in mind that especially during the first weeks of life most of the hemoglobin (50–95%) consists of the fetal type (HbF). Fetal hemoglobin has a higher oxygen affinity compared to the adult type (left shifted on oxygen dissociation curve), which is a result of poor interaction with 2,3-DPG.

The higher oxygen affinity of HbF allows the fetus to better extract oxygen from placental maternal blood, which—due to placental anatomy—has a decreased oxygen saturation compared to maternal arterial blood.

This mechanism loses its benefits after birth, once more efficient lung oxygenation is available to the infant, assuming the lung is healthy. At this point the higher oxygen affinity of HbF (P50 = 19 mmHg $PO_2$) will release **less** Oxygen to the tissue than HbA (P50 = 27 mmHg $PO_2$) at the same $PO_2$.

As a result, infant tissues may build up more oxygen debt before HbF releases adequate amounts of oxygen. A physiologic higher hemoglobin makes up for this, but an anemic neonate may experience significant tissue oxygen debt, especially in the setting of a higher oxygen metabolism.

The tested red cell blood products in the USA on the other hand exclusively contain HbA which can improve tissue oxygenation. Unfortunately, 2,3-DPG within the PRBC is consumed within 1 week of storage, so the longer the PRBC is being stored, the higher the oxygen affinity of the stored blood HbA will be [10].

Apart from concerns of hemolysis and high potassium content, 2,3-DPG depletion should also be considered as a reason to use "fresh blood" whenever feasible. While the infant has the ability to produce 2,3-DPG, a single adult PRBC (300 mL, often derived from 500 mL donated blood) is a "quasi exchange transfusion" for an infant of 3 kg body weight, and it will take the infant some time to build up enough 2,3 DPG to fully benefit from the available HbA.

Overall, transfusion practice has shifted to a more restrictive approach (with certain exemptions), but exact recommendations for transfusion thresholds are hard to define, since the metabolism and physiology of a 24-week gestational age preemie versus a 36-week gestational age at birth baby may be vastly different. On the other hand, an intrauterine growth retarded 36-week gestational age baby may have significantly more issues than a fairly adequately developed 32-week gestational age preemie with sufficiently matured lungs. Cyanotic heart defects or ECMO requirements will yet again influence the need for blood oxygen content and may push the transfusion threshold to a hematocrit of 40% (12.5–13 g/dL of hemoglobin).

Recommendations derived from studies in this field are based on week of ex utero life (not gestational age) and the need for respiratory support (defined as $FiO_2$ > 0.25 or any mechanical support). In the first week of life for otherwise normal babies transfusion is recommend for a hemoglobin threshold of 10 g/dL (11.5 g/dL with respiratory support), 8.5 g/dL (10 g/dL with respiratory support) in the second week and 7.5 g/dL (8.5 g/dL with respiratory support) during and after the third week of life, respectively [11, 12].

## Perioperative Monitoring: Why Standard Monitors Are Not Sufficient in Neonates

The typical perioperative monitoring in adult and pediatric monitoring (Pulse Oximetry, invasive or noninvasive blood pressure, ECG, Temperature, End Tidal $CO_2$ and other ventilation parameters) have significant shortfalls in neonates and especially critically sick neonates.

Blood pressure poorly reflects tissue oxygenation in the neonatal and pediatric population and an increasing unrecognized oxygen debt can build up, while the neonate attempts to compensate the beginning shock by increasing vasoconstriction. Blood pressure — as an expression of the bodies SVR — was found to be essentially unrelated to Oxygen delivery ($DO_2$) in infants and neonates. In other words, "serious hemorrhage and organ hypoperfusion can occur without significant change in blood pressure, even in anesthetized patients" [13].

Cardiac output (CO) is described as a function of stroke volume (SV) and heart rate (CO = SV × HR). A different approach (Ohm's law) takes blood pressures and vascular resistance (SVR) into consideration with an inverse correlation between cardiac output and SVR (CO = BP/SVR). This formula essentially states that with a CONSTANT blood pressure and INCREASING vascular resistance, the Cardiac output DECREASES.

Applied to the clinical picture: Neonatal stress response caused by sepsis, heart failure, anemia or hypovolemia consists of sympathetic upregulation, which results in vasoconstriction (centralization) and a "normal" blood pressure reading. Due to the neonate's inability to improve inotropy (thin cardiac walls), the cardiac output actually decreases in this setting [13]. Hypoperfusion and ischemia can occur in tissues distal to the constricted arterial system.

Especially in non-sedated or non-anesthetized neonates the blood pressure can be preserved until acute decompensation of cardiac function (cardiac arrest) occurs. Anesthetized infants tend to have decreases in their blood pressure sooner, since sympathetic response may be blunted, but still may be in a critical oxygen debt by the time the blood pressure significantly drops.

Other perfusion monitors that could be used to assess perfusion status in adults may also fall short in neonates.

- Pulse oximetry is rather a description of the pulmonary function than a perfusion measurement. Arterial oxygenation contributes to arterial oxygen content ($CaO_2$), but alone does not give adequate information about $DO_2$. More advanced use of plethysmography (Perfusion Index) may allow assessment of peripheral blood flow, but only limited assessment of visceral blood flow or tissue oxygenation status.
- Heart rate does correlate to a certain degree with cardiac output, but is highly variable and is inversely related to stroke volume. In the setting of sympathetic stress response (surgery) or changing intra-abdominal pressures due to surgical stimulation—with effects on preload and afterload—heart rate readings or even trends are not very exact. Anesthesia itself may blunt adequate sympathetic response and cover up a trend towards tachycardia. By the time the neonate responds with a clear trend, a significant tissue oxygen debt may have built up. Overall, it has a poor predictive value.
- End tidal $CO_2$ ($ETCO_2$) correlates fairly well with cardiac output, but due to (relatively) large dead space within the circuit, higher respiratory rates as well as surgical manipulation or peritoneal insufflation of $CO_2$, a reliable exhaled $CO_2$ curve or $CO_2$ trend may not be available.
- ECG remains an essential monitor to assess arrhythmias and cardiac ischemia, but the incidence of arrhythmia other than hypoxia induced bradycardias is very low in otherwise heart healthy neonates and infants. Coronary events would likely only occur in congenital abnormalities or associated with significant hypoxemia. While ECG may show signs of cardiac ischemia during a severe hemodynamic failure, it does not predict shock.

## The Importance of Additional Monitors in Critically Sick Neonates and Infants

In the following, the relationship of oxygen delivery ($DO_2$), consumption ($VO_2$) and extraction is further explained to introduce the benefits of NIRS (Near-infrared spectroscopy), which in the neonatal and pediatric world can act as a reliable early warning system for worsening tissue oxygen debt.

The purpose of our cardiovascular and pulmonary system is the adequate delivery of substrate (i.e. oxygen and others) to the tissues that eventually utilize it (oxygen consumption). Standing alone, none of the monitored vital signs can give a comprehensive picture of the perfusion status of the patient. Even the combination of multiple different vital signs comes short in giving a clear picture and require interpretation based on the (simplified) physiologic understanding of our bodies.

Oxygen delivery ($DO_2$) is defined as the arterial oxygen content ($CaO_2$) that is delivered by cardiac output, expressed in the formula:

$$DO_2 = CaO_2 \times CO - \text{with } CaO_2 = 1.34 \times Hgb \times SaO_2 + 0.003 \times PaO_2.$$

Oxygen consumption ($VO_2$) is the amount of $O_2$ consumed by perfused tissues, expressed as the difference between arterial and venous oxygen content multiplied by cardiac output:

$$VO_2 = CO \times (CaO_2 - CvO_2)$$

Oxygen extraction ($O_2ER$) expresses oxygen consumption as a fraction between the delivered and consumed Oxygen as an **indicator of perfusion. A higher than normal oxygen extraction points to "Oxygen hunger" of the tissue.**

$$O_2ER = VO_2 / DO_2 = (CaO_2 - CvO_2) / CaO_2$$
When neglecting dissolved oxygen : $O_2ER = (SaO_2 - SvO_2)/SaO_2$.

$VO_2$ can remain stable even in the setting of decreasing $DO_2$, since the body is able to increase $O_2ER$ (inverse relationship between extraction and delivery). Unfortunately, the ability of the body to extract Oxygen from the blood is limited, so once $DO_2$ falls below a critical threshold, $VO_2$ will decrease, resulting in anaerobic metabolism and worsening oxygen debt [14].

There is no easy direct measurement of $VO_2$ available, but indirect measures such as increasing lactate in the setting of metabolic acidosis can be used to describe a trend. Unfortunately, lactate can be influenced by other factors and is a late indicator of perfusion deficit (when the damage is done). It also requires frequent blood draws to follow which can deplete urgently needed oxygen carriers in the blood stream.

Mixed venous blood gases can be used to assess venous saturation ($SvO_2$), which can be used as a measurement of $O_2ER$—when neglecting dissolved oxygen. An increasing difference between $SaO_2$ and $SvO_2$ may be an expression of the bodies increasing oxygen debt. Decreasing CO will result in decreased tissue perfusion resulting in higher extraction of $O_2$ by the organs.

In the neonate world, true mixed venous blood gas samples are rare, since the risk of placing pulmonary artery catheters clearly outweighs the benefits in this population. Even if a PA sample was drawn, it would only reflect total extraction, ignoring the fact that the body may perfuse certain tissue beds better than others (brain versus intestines). A near normal value may suggest adequate perfusion, while ongoing hypoperfusion of the intestines is causing ischemia and potential permanent damage such as necrotizing enterocolitis (NEC).

Most of the time only a measurement of superior or inferior caval vein blood, or — in absence of a central line — peripheral venous blood is possible with the same limitation as described above. SVC blood may give a more adequate picture of brain perfusion, while IVC blood reflects intestinal perfusion better.

The importance of venous saturation changes cannot be underestimated, since it reflects a beginning oxygen debt significantly earlier than blood pressure or heart rate in a slowly developing shock picture. It allows earlier diagnosis, prevention and treatment of an acute cardiovascular event [13].

The disadvantage of blood samples is their quality of being rather a "spot check", making it more difficult to describe trends. Too frequent sampling will yet again result in anemia and decreased oxygen carriers. Continuous invasive venous saturation ($ScvO_2$) monitoring may not be available in neonates and still has the disadvantage of only reflecting either SVC or IVC perfusion area changes.

## Noninvasive SvO₂ Monitoring (NIRS)

As previously discussed, when neglecting the dissolved $O_2$ (which becomes less relevant with higher hemoglobin), extraction can be expressed as the difference between $SaO_2$ and $SvO_2$. Near-infrared Spectroscopy (NIRS)—without getting into too much detail about the physics involved—is a technology not un-similar to pulse oximetry. It can be considered the "pulse-ox for tissues and the circulation" [13]. It uses a different spectrum of wavelengths to focus less on the pulsatile changes within a tissue, but more on the overall "color" of the hemoglobin within a tissue (saturated and desaturated blood).

Most tissues have a significantly higher amount of post-capillary (deoxygenated) blood. Based on this assumption, NIRS calculates a continuous (and regional) noninvasive estimate of the venous oxygen saturation. The oxygenation extraction as an indicator of perfusion can be calculated by applying the modified formula:

$$O_2ER = (SaO_2 - SvO_2) / SaO_2$$

It is important to understand that the gradient between arterial and venous saturation is more important than the actual venous saturation. Cardiac patients may present with a decreased $SaO_2$ at baseline, and the venous saturation will be decreased accordingly, often without significantly higher $O_2ER$. The importance of NIRS in cardiac and single ventricle pathophysiology could fill an entire chapter on its own and—unfortunately—cannot adequately be covered here.

Different tissues have a different $O_2ER$ at baseline and will be perfused depending on their vital priority in the setting of beginning shock. A multi-site NIRS approach (2–3 stickers) allows to assess the perfusion of several organ systems as well as an estimate of the overall perfusion. A significant decrease in only one area may reflect centralization of perfusion, or occlusion of vessels perfusing the organ. Changes in all measured area may be a sign of a general hypoperfusion and imminent shock.

The most typical locations of NIRS utilization with expected baseline values and tissue specific characteristics are described below:

- **Cerebral Oximetry:** Depending on head size and weight one or two forehead NIRS probes can describe cortex perfusion. Due to its high energy metabolism, the brain extracts more oxygen at baseline than other tissues. Considering a normal $SaO_2$ and $PaCO_2$ the venous saturation in the jugular vein bulb is expected to be around 60% ($O_2ER$ = 40%). Due to measurement of a mixed sample of blood flow in the cortex a normal cerebral oximetry typically ranges between 70 and 80%. Brain perfusion is dependent on $PaCO_2$, and both hyper- and hypoventilation may influence perfusion and — therefore — extraction. Auto-regulatory blood flow mechanisms will keep the brain perfusion fairly intact until a critical perfusion pressure has been reached (anaerobic threshold). Below this threshold a rapid decline of venous oxygenation can be observed. Regional mechanisms such as occlusion of vessels will result in cardiac output independent changes of perfusion and venous saturation.

- **Renal Oximetry:** Due to its mostly arterial blood flow as a "public organ" and minimal $O_2ER$, the venous saturation is expected to be high in a well perfused kidney. A NIRS reading of 90% ($O_2ER$ = 10%) is a normal reading in a healthy infant with normal $SaO_2$. Renal NIRS is sensitive to autonomic tone (centralization) and can be an early indicator of increasing tissue oxygen debt (kidneys are "shock-organs"). Typically values below 50% are considered a critical value and correlate with kidney injury if not corrected.

- **Intestinal/Splanchnic Oximetry:** Application of abdominal wall NIRS allows a sensitive picture of intestinal perfusion. A NIRS reading of 80% ($O_2ER$ = 20%) is considered normal with a normal $SaO_2$. Intestinal NIRS can be an important monitor in prevention, diagnosis and treatment of necrotizing enterocolitis (NEC). Intraoperative use of abdominal wall NIRS is somewhat limited since a significant part of neonatal surgery involves the abdominal compartment (competes with surgical field for surface area). It plays a bigger role in the ICU, but can be an excellent alternative location for

NIRS placement, if renal placement is not possible.
- **Somatic/Muscle Oximetry:** Placement of NIRS over muscle tissue can be a backup option, if placement over abdomen or kidneys is not feasible. A NIRS reading of 80% ($O_2ER = 20\%$) is considered normal with a normal $SaO_2$. The predictive value as a generalized perfusion monitor is less established compared to renal and splanchnic oximetry, but can be utilized to measure extremity perfusion during catheterization of arteries or can add value as a preductal/postductal monitor in cardiac patients.
- **MULTISITE NIRS:** Using at least two NIRS sites (cerebral and renal/abdominal) significantly increases the predictive value of NIRS. Decline in one versus both sites can give additional information about the location and severity of a perfusion deficit and can be an early indicator of shock [13].

As a general guideline, NIRS must be interpreted within the clinical situation and in reference to other measured vital signs (especially $SaO_2$ to assess the actual arteriovenous difference). Hypotension without changes in NIRS should **not** be ignored and appropriately assessed and treated. On the other hand, a declining NIRS in the setting of a "normal" blood pressure requires assessment and potentially treatment, and may be even more alarming [13].

Sources of error for NIRS include uncertainty about which tissue is actually being measured. While it seems reasonable to postulate that — in a skinny neonate — measurements over an organ may actually reflect perfusion of the underlying organ — due to short distances between skin and organ — increasing subcutaneous fat tissue or thicker muscle layers may not allow the same assumption in older patients.

Certain "colorful" substances can interfere with adequate measurements of NIRS. Bilirubin (neonates, liver disease) and meconium are known to result in false low readings. Newer NIRS monitors utilize up to five wavelengths that allow for measurements outside the absorption ranges of these substances to create more reliable numbers. Depending on the monitor available at a location, these substances can acutely falsify measurements (false low) and decrease the usability of NIRS.

NIRS algorithms assume a certain ratio of arterial and venous blood within a certain organ and weigh the measurement accordingly. Physiologic variability in the monitored area or placing the NIRS probe at an incorrect location (classic example: rib cage while actually trying to measure renal NIRS) may decrease accuracy of NIRS. Using the same algorithm for all tissues may also result in less reliable numbers. In response, manufacturers have begun to develop organ specific algorithms and the ability to "tell" the monitor which organ is monitored. This resulted in FDA certification to use the calculated saturation as absolutes and not only as a trend monitor for some manufacturers.

Schneider et al. did a side by side comparison of four different NIRS technologies resulting in significant differences in the measurements, and raised some concerns about the "absolute versus trend" issue. While it cannot be excluded that one of the system is highly accurate (but difficult to prove which one), the conclusion of this study was to only use NIRS as a trend monitor in the neonate population and not fully rely on the absolutes [15]. Dix et al. found similar issues in their comparison of different NIRS technologies [16].

## Preoperative Considerations

In the preoperative assessment of the sick neonate undergoing emergent surgery, time is of the essence. Neonates may be critically ill and on their way to build up tissue oxygen debt and shock, while clinically and para-clinically appear to be "stable" (see above).

A focused baseline exam including the airway — this may very likely be the first airway intervention in the baby's life — to prepare for potential difficulties, and a quick chart review regarding known cardiac or lung issues may be the only anesthesia intervention possible due to time constraints.

At the same time the parents or guardians of the newborn will need reassurance of the importance of handing the most precious being in their lives to complete strangers who will insert tubes, needles and knives into their child.

Nevertheless, a focused brief with the surgeon and the OR staff should not be avoided to clarify need of antibiotics, availability of blood products, and access requirements needed to be able to resuscitate the child. Improvising these issues become very challenging once the neonate is draped.

The surface area to apply monitors (ECG, blood pressures cuff, NIRS stickers) versus surgical needs (operative field, grounding pads) is very limited and establishing boundaries before applying the monitors not only saves time, but also costs, if single use monitor probes have to be discarded or replaced.

Gaining additional access must be taken into serious consideration. Even peripheral intravenous catheters can be a time consuming challenge, and central access as well as arterial access even more so. While additional or central access makes intraoperative optimization easier, the repercussion of adding an hour's worth of general anesthesia in a critically sick child may worsen the overall outcome.

## Intraoperative Considerations

From the time the patient arrives in the OR until the drapes are covering the patient, there is a time window for the anesthesia team to assure the adequate securement of airway, lines and all body parts of the neonate, including avoidance of pull on lines and airway. Once the drapes are up, things get significantly more challenging.

At the same time, adequate temperature control needs to be established. It is very easy to forget about hypothermia during a prolonged induction period with 2–3 people trying to gain additional access on each limb while the patient lies essentially uncovered on the OR table. Heat lamps and raised room temperature are essential here.

Neonates present with their own airway challenges, and going into too much detail would probably expand the volume of this chapter too much. Major considerations include:

- Neonates require PEEP to avoid atelectasis, especially after induction of anesthesia. The functional residual capacity of a newborn often overlaps with their closing capacity. Apnea or decreased respiratory drive quickly results in atelectasis and desaturation. Once desaturation has occurred, it may require high positive pressures to adequately inflate the lungs again.
- Positive pressure mask ventilation may result in epigastric air inflation, worsening the ability to ventilate the lungs due to increasing pressure on the thorax from below. A quick insertion of a suction catheter may be necessary to improve ventilation and decrease atelectasis. While cricoid pressure has a questionable benefit in avoidance of aspiration, it has been shown to reliably prevent inflation of the abdomen during mask ventilation, when applied correctly [17].
- High intrathoracic pressures may decrease preload and cardiac output thereby worsening perfusion and oxygen debt in spite of "adequate" arterial oxygenation.
- The trachea of neonates and especially preemies is very short and small changes of ETT position may result in extubation or main stem intubation with inability to adequately ventilate and oxygenate.
- The combination of drooling, being edentulous and possible reflux from the stomach makes it essential to secure the ETT thoroughly and with materials that are moisture resistant. Paper and silk tape can become unreliable quickly, if not covered and protected against moisture.
- It pays off to assess adequacy of ventilation with neck extension and flexion (if no contraindications exist) to assure the ETT remains in the trachea above the carina. Carinal stimulation by an ETT can cause severe vagal reactions in the neonatal and pediatric population. Inadvertent main stem intubation may cause significant desaturation in newborns, especially with prevalent respiratory failure and immature lungs.
- The airways of newborns are more cephalad and it can be difficult to pick up the often floppy epiglottis with a standard Miller blade.

Using a Miller blade purposefully as a MAC blade usually provides a decent view of the vocal cords allowing quick intubation and therefore apnea time. In short: if one thinks intubation is possible with the current view, one should intubate with the current view.
- Low and extremely low birth weight preemies may present with an uncuffed ETT due to the small size of their airways. In patients with expected high intra-abdominal pressures due to edema or planned capno-peritoneum, adequate ventilation may become difficult with an uncuffed ETT. The anesthesia team has to consider and potentially test for leak before the surgery starts to allow appropriate oxygenation and ventilation.

Establishing access is challenging on multiple levels. Not only can the placement of intravenous access be time consuming and difficult due to patient size and hemodynamic status, but also the eventual use of every line has to be considered before the patient is draped. During emergent surgeries with expected fluid shifts or blood loss, ideally at least two independent intravenous lines are required.

One has to allow continuous administration of fluids and glucose as required. This line may also function well as a carrier for continuous hemodynamically active, anesthetic or narcotic drug delivery, especially in the NICU setting.

Another independent line is often required to bolus medications, as well as fluids in form of crystalloids, colloids or blood products. Not dividing these lines may result in unwanted boluses of anesthetic or hemodynamically active drugs.

The smaller the patient, the greater the consideration in properly calculating large fluid boluses to deliver a medication. In a patient of less than 1000 g weight, every infused milliliter results in more than 1 mL/kg of fluid delivery. Flushing in medications can quickly become high volume fluid resuscitation and challenge the immature kidneys of these newborns.

Using Albumin or balanced crystalloids (instead of Normal Saline) as flush may be desirable. Neonatal ICUs often provide small volume flush-lines (less than 1 mL) of adequate length that reach outside the drapes. These lines—on the other hand—are not well equipped to give large fluid boluses or blood products.

High pressure delivery through a small-volume flush line may result in hemolysis of red blood cells or in rare cases damage to the actual line delivering the bolus, resulting in infiltration, damage to tissues and inability to deliver anesthetic and potentially life-saving medications.

An ideal flush line consists of two components that split very proximal to the access site of the patient—one component consisting of a small volume extension to deliver medications with minimal fluid addition to avoid fluid overload, and the other component consisting of a larger bore tubing to allow adequate fluid resuscitation. Keep in mind, that — unless this contraption is prepared and established before the patient is draped — it will be difficult to later connect to the patient.

## Surgery in the NICU

Neonatal emergent surgeries usually take place in two main locations — the operating room and the Neonatal ICU. Reasons to perform procedure in the ICU include respiratory or hemodynamic instability of the child. Respiratory failure in very small infants with premature lungs may result in the need for special ventilators or even High Frequency Oscillatory ventilation, that are typically not easy to transport and the chances for accidental extubation or inward movement to a main stem in these little babies can result in quick respiratory decompensation.

The baby may also not respond well hemodynamically to being moved and repositioned between ICU bed and OR table and even short environmental exposure can result in significant temperature dysregulation with detrimental effects.

Providing anesthesia in an ICU setting brings challenges of space utilization, unavailability of anesthesia equipment or the use of unknown equipment such as ICU ventilators. These ventilators — in contrast to many OR ventilators — are optimized to ventilate even the smallest patients, but are almost never equipped to deliver anesthesia gas. This turns every anesthetic in this setting into a TIVA, with all of its benefits and disadvantages.

The neonatal crib typically allows good access to the baby, but provides very limited space to position equipment and most of the surface area will be utilized by the surgeon. Once the patient is draped in this setting, it is near impossible to access the patient without disrupting the surgery.

The NICU staff can be an excellent resource to provide additional hands and to help utilizing the existing equipment. However, different philosophies about patient care and management — especially in critical situations — may result in communication challenges. Guidelines or a brief discussion about the expectations of both NICU and the anesthesia team may optimize patient care. Rule of thumb — only change what REALLY needs to be changed.

## Postoperative Considerations

Even before completion of the surgical procedure an increase of the room temperature is helpful to avoid postoperative hypothermia in the neonate. Removal of the drapes with exposure to room temperature, wiping off surgical antiseptic solution residue with saline, high flow ventilation to wash out volatile anesthetics may all contribute to rapid loss of heat, even if adequate body temperature was achieved during the procedure.

Depending on the preoperative status and intraoperative changes, it is worthwhile to consider extubation even after larger surgical procedures, if the initial problem has been "fixed". Contraindications include hemodynamic instability, concerns for respiratory failure due to pre-existing conditions, fluid overload, airway edema, over-sedation or insufficient reversal of neuromuscular blockade. In addition, preemies and neonates may present with apnea, especially in very small neonates or anemic patients. Extubation in some instances may be done in the NICU if the distance between the O.R. and NICU is considerable.

Potential advantages of early extubation include avoidance of additional sedation in the NICU with decreased risk of Ileus, quicker enteral feeding and even faster discharge.

The reversal of neuromuscular blockade can be more challenging in neonates. While the typical weight adjusted doses of neostigmine and glycopyrrolate typically produce the same results as in adults, a reliable measurement of "Train of four" as well as "First to Fourth twitch" ratio maybe difficult due to the size of the neonatal forearm. Both position of the stimulation electrode and strength of stimulus may easily result in direct stimulation of muscle rather than ulnar nerve.

Successful case reports of Sugammadex use (with a typical dose of 4 mg/kg) as a reliable and safe way to reverse Rocuronium and Vecuronium can be found in the literature [18]. Higher doses may be required with deep neuromuscular blockade, so even with the use of Sugammadex an assessment of neuromuscular blockade is recommended.

Transport complications may include airway issues due to incidental movement of the endotracheal tube, loss of IV access and — as always — hypothermia. Warm blankets, or heat producing gel mats are helpful to warm the infant on transport, since the warming function of the crib is typically disabled without active power supply.

Once the newborn is safely transported to the NICU a thorough report is given to the NICU staff to whom care is reassigned.

## References

1. Maayan-Metzger A, Itzchak A, Mazkereth R, Kuint J. Necrotizing enterocolitis in full-term infants: case–control study and review of the literature. J Perinatol. 2004;24(8):494–9.
2. Hall N, Peters M, Eaton S, Pierro A. Hyperglycemia is associated with increased morbidity and mortality rates in neonates with necrotizing enterocolitis. J Pediatr Surg. 2004;39:898–901.
3. Van der Lugt M. Short and long term outcome of neonatal hyperglycemia in very preterm infants: a retrospective follow-up study. BMC Pediatr. 2010;10:52.
4. Loennqvist P. Fluid management in association with neonatal surgery: even tiny guys need their salt. Br J Anaesth. 2014;112(3):404–6.

5. Holliday M, Friedman A, Segar W. Acute hospital-induced hyponatremia in children: a physiologic approach. J Pediatr. 2004;145:584–7.
6. Holliday M, Segar W, Friedman A. Reducing errors in fluid therapy management. Pediatrics. 2003;111:424–5.
7. Loennqvist P. Inappropriate perioperative fluid management in children: time for a solution. Paediatr Anaesth. 2007;17:203–5.
8. Gan H, Cannesson M, Chandler J, Ansermino J. Predicting fluid responsiveness in children: a systematic review. Anesth Analg. 2013;117(6):1380–92.
9. Desgranges F, Desebbe O, Pereira de Souza Neto E, Raphael D, Chassard D. Respiratory variation in aortic blood flow peak velocity to predict fluid responsiveness in mechanically ventilated children: a systematic review and meta-analysis. Paediatr Anaesth. 2016;26(1):37–47.
10. D'Alessandro A, Liumbruno G, Grazzini G, Zolla L. Red blood cell storage: the story so far. Blood Transfus. 2010;8:82–8.
11. Kirpalani H, Whyte R, Andersen C, Asztalos E, Heddle N, Blajchman M, Peliowski A, Rios A, LaCorte M, Connelly R, Barrington K, Roberts R. The Premature Infants in Need of Transfusion (PINT) study: a randomized, controlled trial of a restrictive (low) versus liberal (high) transfusion threshold for extremely low birth weight infants. J Pediatr. 2006;149(3):301–7.
12. Chen H, Tseng H, Lu C, Yang S, Fan H, Yang R. Effect of blood transfusions on the outcome of very low body weight preterm infants under two different transfusion criteria. Pediatr Neonatol. 2009;50(3):110–6.
13. Scott J, Hoffman G. Near-infrared spectroscopy: exposing the dark (venous) side of the circulation. Pediatr Anesth. 2014;24:74–88.
14. Vincent J. $D_{O_2}/V$. In: Functional hemodynamic monitoring. Berlin: Springer; 2005. p. 251–8.
15. Schneider A, Minnich B, Hofstaetter E, Weisser C, Hattinger-Juergenssen E, Wald M. Comparison of four near-infrared spectroscopy devices shows that they are only suitable for monitoring cerebral oxygenation trends in preterm infants. Acta Paediatr. 2014;103:934–8.
16. Dix L, Van Bel F, Baerts W, Lemmers P. Comparing near-infrared spectroscopy devices and their sensors for monitoring regional cerebral oxygen saturation in the neonate. Pediatr Res. 2013;74:557–63.
17. Moynihan R, Archer B-UJJ, Feld L, Kreitzman T. The effect of cricoid pressure on preventing gastric insufflation in infants and children. Anesthesiology. 1993;78(4):652–6.
18. Alonso A, de Boer H, Booij L. Reversal of rocuronium-induced neuromuscular block by sugammadex in neonates. Eur J Anaesthesiol. 2014;31:163.

# Anesthesia for Tracheoesophageal Fistula

## 39

Pornswan Ngamprasertwong

## Introduction

Tracheoesophageal fistula (TEF) with or without esophageal atresia (EA) is a rare congenital anomaly, with an incidence of 1:2500–3000 live births. The majority of cases are sporadic, but can be associated with VACTERL (vertebral defects, anal atresia, cardiac defects, tracheoesophageal fistula, renal anomalies, and limb abnormalities) [1]. There are two common classifications, by Gross and Vogt, using anatomical structure to classify this anomaly into five different types. The most common type is Gross type C (Vogt type IIIb), which is EA (blind upper pouch) with a distal fistula (TEF of the lower pouch). Typically, TEF with EA patients require surgical intervention in the very first few days of life. The TEF without EA patients (Gross type H) might be undetected during the neonatal period, but generally present later on with recurrent aspiration and pneumonia. For isolated EA (Gross type A), patients are managed by gastrostomy, follow by re-anastomosis in the next few months. Due to an intact tracheal lumen, the isolated EA poses less respiratory and anesthetic challenges. The summary of anesthetic plan with reasoning is demonstrated in (Table 39.1).

P. Ngamprasertwong, M.D., M.Sc
Department of Anesthesia and Pediatrics, Cincinnati Children's Hospital Medical Center,
Cincinnati, OH, USA
e-mail: pornswan.ngamprasertwong@cchmc.org

## Pathophysiology and Clinical Features

In contrast to many other congenital anomalies, TEF is frequently missed prenatally despite the many advances in prenatal diagnosis. Polyhydramnios and the absence of a stomach bubble in the prenatal ultrasound are nonspecific signs of EA with a positive predictive value of 56% [1]. In EA with TEF patients, air in the stomach may be present and the finding on the prenatal ultrasound is less specific. The diagnosis of EA with TEF is usually made shortly after birth based on clinical symptoms including: coughing, wheezing, excessive salivation, choking, cyanosis with feeding, and the inability to pass a nasogastric tube more than 10–15 cm. Definitive diagnosis is confirmed by coiling of a large caliber nasogastric tube (Replogle tube) in the upper esophageal pouch. Chest and abdominal X-ray demonstrate intestinal gas, which indicates the presence of a distal tracheoesophageal fistula. Surgical repair via right thoracotomy or thoracoscopy is typically performed in the first 24–72 h of life in otherwise healthy neonates [2].

Low birth weight and associated cardiac anomalies are independent predictors of mortality in infants undergoing EA/TEF repair [3]. The survival rate after EA/TEF repair in less than 2 kg neonates with major cardiac anomalies is only 27% as compared to a survival rate of 100% in greater than 2 kg neonates without heart disease [4]. Due to the high incidence of associated

Table 39.1 Summary of the plan of anesthesia with reasoning

| Plan | Reasoning |
| --- | --- |
| The patient should be stabilized in the neonatal intensive care unit in a 30° head up position with continuous suctioning of the upper esophageal pouch | To minimize the risk of aspiration and the development of pneumonia |
| Preoperative intravenous fluid and antibiotic prophylaxis should be administered | To prevent dehydration, hypoglycemia and to reduce the risk of respiratory tract infection |
| Preoperative echocardiogram is required | Due to the high incidence of associated cardiac anomalies and to identify the side of the aortic arch |
| The key to airway management for TEF is the placement of the endotracheal tube with the tip lying below the fistula but above the carina | To provide adequate ventilation while minimizing gastric distention |
| Avoid awake intubation | Awake intubation in a vigorous baby, especially a preterm baby, can result in intraventricular hemorrhage |
| Standard management includes induction of general anesthesia with muscle relaxation and endotracheal intubation | The majority of TEFs are small and appear to be low risk for difficult ventilation, even if they are located below the tip of the ETT |
| Rigid bronchoscopy is also routinely performed in the same anesthetic prior to the onset of surgical repair of the TEF in many centers | To identify the location and size of the fistula, to characterize airway anatomy and to place a Fogarty catheter to occlude a large TEF |
| The end-tidal carbon dioxide ($EtCO_2$) tracing needs to be carefully monitored, together with prompt availability of a flexible bronchoscope, intubation equipment and suction | The small size of the ETT and working around the tracheal area during TEF repair pose additional risks of ETT dislocation and kinking and plugging of the ETT with mucus or blood |
| An arterial line is indicated in patients with congenital heart disease, prematurity, poor pulmonary compliance, and a large fistula with preoperative ventilatory compromise | These high risk patients require continuous monitoring of mean arterial pressure, frequent blood sampling and following of blood gas analysis |
| An arterial line is also indicated in patients undergoing thoracoscopic repair | During one lung ventilation, the $ETCO_2$ is falsely low and arterial blood gas is a better monitor of ventilation |
| The patient can be extubated immediately postoperatively in select patients. However, the majority of patients remain intubated in the neonatal intensive care unit after surgery | Extubation can be complicated by poor pain control, tracheomalacia, and vocal cord paralysis. If the patient requires emergency reintubation, there may be more disadvantages due to a traumatic intubation, leakage at the anastomotic site, or accidental removal of the trans-anastomotic feeding tube |

cardiac anomalies (29%), preoperative echocardiogram is required in all patients undergoing TEF repair. Beside the heart structures, the position of the aortic arch also needs to be identified. In 2.5% of EA/TEF patients, the aortic arch is located on the right side. The left thoracotomy approach is much easier than the usual right thoracotomy incision in patients with a right sided aortic arch [1]. Preoperative lumbar ultrasound is beneficial in neonates with a sacral dimple due to the high incidence of vertebra anomalies if caudal catheter placement is planned for postoperative pain control.

Severe pneumonia or dependence on mechanical ventilations are no longer prognostic indicators of mortality in neonates with EA/TEF. The improvement in neonatal care including the use of maternal steroids and the availability of exogenous surfactant has significantly reduced the incidence of respiratory distress syndrome which complicated prematurity and aspiration pneumonia [5].

## Anesthetic Management

### Preoperative Preparation

The surgical repair of EA/TEF is urgent, but not emergent. Delay in surgical correction results in increased risk of aspiration and pneumonitis. The patient should be stabilized in the neonatal unit and maintained in a 30° head up position with continuous suction of the upper esophageal pouch. Preoperative intravenous fluids should be administered to prevent dehydration and hypoglycemia. Prophylactic antibiotics are required to reduce the risk of respiratory tract infection.

## Airway Management

The key to airway management for TEF is the placement of the endotracheal tube with the tip lying below the fistula but above the carina in order to provide adequate ventilation while minimizing gastric distension. A cuffed endotracheal tube (ETT) is preferable during the surgical repair. Not only does a cuffed ETT provide better tidal volumes with minimal leakage while facing increase in intrathoracic pressure during thoracotomy, the cuff can be used to occlude the TEF [6]. For the uncuffed ETT, use the ETT without a side hole and face the bevel of the ETT to the front of the trachea to minimize the chance of ventilation through the TEF in the back of the trachea [7].

Traditionally, the literature recommended awake intubation, the avoidance of positive pressure ventilation and the avoidance of muscle relaxant until the fistula was surgically controlled. There are many disadvantages of this approach. First, awake intubation in a vigorous baby, especially a preterm baby, can result in intraventricular hemorrhage. Second, adequate ventilation and good surgical conditions are difficult to achieve during open thoracotomy without muscle relaxant. Third, the majority of TEF are small and appear to be low risk for difficult ventilation, even if it is located below the tip of ETT [8]. Therefore, the current standard management is induction of general anesthesia with muscle relaxant and endotracheal intubation.

Rigid bronchoscopy is also routinely performed in the same anesthetic prior to surgical repair in many centers in order to locate and size the TEF. Rigid bronchoscopy can also identify other associated anomalies in the airway such as laryngomalacia, tracheomalacia, multiple fistulas, and external compression from a vascular ring [9]. When the fistula is large and lies just above the carina, maintaining proper position of the ETT is challenging. Adequate ventilation can be achieved by occlusion of this fistula using a Fogarty catheter with placement under rigid bronchoscopy visualization. With this approach, rigid bronchoscopy will be performed under general anesthesia while the patient is spontaneously ventilating. After identification of the location and structure of the fistula(s), the Fogarty catheter is placed via a rigid bronchoscope and inflated. Then, muscle relaxant can be given, followed by endotracheal intubation. The ETT is placed in the trachea, next to the Fogarty catheter. The proper placement of the ETT can also be checked using a flexible bronchoscope. After control of the TEF is obtained, the Fogarty balloon is deflated and removed while the ETT is still in place.

When a rigid bronchoscope or small fiber optic bronchoscope is not available, the conservative method is to place the ETT using direct laryngoscopy into the main stem bronchus. The ETT is then slowly pulled back until the breath sounds are heard bilaterally and the patient is well ventilated with minimal gastric distension. If conditions are not optimized, the patient may require one lung ventilation. The tip of the ETT must be on the opposite side of the surgical incision (lower lung in lateral decubitus position). The down side of bronchial intubation is bronchial edema resulting in prolong collapsed of the upper lobe [10]. After surgical repair, the ETT will be moved up into the trachea to achieve two lung ventilation.

## General Considerations

The patient typically arrives in the operating room with intravenous fluids replacement, a suction in the upper esophageal pouch, and in the head up position. Aggressive bag mask ventilation should be avoided, since it leads to excessive gastric distension. After inhalational induction, if there is no plan for bronchoscopy, many pediatric anesthesiologists routinely paralyze the patient after successful gentle bag mask ventilation before intubation. Good intubating conditions can be achieved with deep inhalational anesthesia, but thoracotomy without muscle relaxant is very challenging. With a small fistula, the tip of the ETT can be well above the fistula and still provide adequate ventilation. Either surgical ligation of the fistula or clamping of lower esophagus [11] will prevent further gastric insufflation. This approach avoids the need to re-tape and readjust the ETT position from a single lung to a tracheal intubation while the baby is under the drapes in the lateral decubitus position. Expansion of the lung may also be required to correct hypoxia during the procedure and at the end of the procedure to manage atelectasis.

## Anesthesia for Gastrostomy

Preoperative gastrostomy is rarely performed due to the loss of the ability to ventilate and leakage of air through the open gastrostomy. A small TEF rarely affects the ability to ventilate. Rigid bronchoscopy and placement of a Fogarty catheter allow for occlusion of a large TEF prior to a definitive repair. In very rare circumstances, when the patient presents with respiratory compromise and requires emergency gastrostomy prior to definitive repair, spontaneous breathing should be maintained. After inhalational induction, a small dose of intravenous fentanyl and topical lidocaine on the vocal cords can be used to facilitate intubation. In premature infants with a severely dilated stomach, a large angiocatheter may also be placed into the abdomen to rapidly achieve a gastrostomy without general anesthesia. It is important to note, however, that adequate ventilation may not be achieved after stomach decompression due to air leakage via the gastrostomy. Temporary occlusion of the gastrostomy or retrograde occlusion via the gastrostomy site may be required to improve ventilation until the fistula is surgically controlled.

The most common indications of gastrostomy placement are as a part of a staged repair for feeding and to improve nutrition in very low birth weight neonates [12] while waiting for delayed primary repair, or in patients with long gap esophageal atresia.

## Anesthesia for Open Thoracotomy Repair of TEF

It is essential to always obtain an echo cardiogram to identify the position and location of the aortic arch. Routinely, patients will undergo a right thoracotomy. If the patient has a right sided aortic arch, surgical approach will be much easier and safer via a left thoracotomy.

Besides routine care of a neonate undergoing general anesthesia (i.e. keeping the patient warm, placing standard ASA monitors, having two peripheral intravenous lines for fluid management), airway management and adequate ventilation are always challenging during TEF repair. The small size of the ETT and working around the trachea area pose the additional risks of ETT dislocation, or kinking and plugging of the ETT with mucus or blood. Ventilation during thoracotomy and surgical retraction is often inadequate. In addition to the standard ASA monitors, an arterial line is also required in high risk patients including those with congenital heart disease, prematurity, poor pulmonary compliance, and a large fistula with preoperative ventilatory compromise. An arterial line not only provides continuous monitoring of the mean arterial pressure, it also allows frequent blood sampling and following blood gas analysis. The end-tidal carbon dioxide ($EtCO_2$) tracing needs to be carefully monitored together with prompt availability of flexible bronchoscopy and intubation equipment as well as suction to interrogate the ETT if clogging or dislodgement is suspected.

After the TEF is ligated, the esophagus is then reanastomosed. The trans-anastomosis feeding tube is passed and becomes a critical tube. This feeding tube promotes nutrition by allowing enteral feeding and reducing the incidence of gastroesophageal reflux as compared to a gastrostomy tube [1]. A caudal catheter advanced to T6–T7 provides good postoperative analgesia and avoids narcotics there by promoting early extubation [2]. In selective populations, the patient can be extubated immediately postoperatively. This results in less trauma from rubbing of the ETT against tracheal mucosa. However, extubation can be complicated by poor pain control, tracheomalacia, and vocal cord paralysis [5]. If the patient requires emergency reintubation, there may be greater disadvantages due to trauma, leakage at the anastomosis site, or accidental remove of the trans-anastomosis feeding tube.

## Anesthesia for Thoracoscopic Repair of TEF

Surgeons are increasingly trying to repair TEFs via a thoracoscopic approach. The patients will be in the semi-prone position with 45° elevation of the right side with the right arm above the head. These patients receive the same intraoperative anesthesia management, however an arterial line is always required. Due to insufflation of carbon dioxide ($CO_2$) to collapse the right lung, ventilation during the thoracoscopic surgery is often compromised. In a case series by Krosnar et al. from Edinburg, all patients undergoing thoracoscopic repair desaturated to 84–91% and most of them required 100% oxygen during 5 mmHg of $CO_2$ insufflation [10]. During one lung ventilation, the $ETCO_2$ is falsely low and therefore serial arterial blood gas sampling is a better monitor of ventilation.

## Postoperative Complications and Considerations

Major postoperative complications include sepsis, pneumothorax, unilateral or bilateral vocal cord paralysis, tracheomalacia, renal insufficiency, anastomosis leakage, esophageal stricture, gastroesophageal reflux and recurrent tracheoesophageal fistula [3]. Recurrent TEF occurs in 3–20% of patients after TEF repair depending on the TEF type and surgical technique. Endoscopic repair of recurrent TEF using a ventilating rigid tracheoscope simultaneous with flexible esophagoscope to de-epithelize and seal the fistula with fibrin glue, results in lower morbidity but higher rate of recurrence compared to open approaches. Ideal candidates for this technique are patients with a long, thin and small fistula located proximally where the cuffed endotracheal tube can be placed beyond the fistula site [13].

Long gap esophageal atresia is a gap wider than 3 cm or two vertebral bodies. Patients with long gap esophageal atresia can be a surgical challenge. Since a primary anastomosis is not possible, this group of patients require G-tube placement and delayed repair. Traction suture of the upper and lower esophageal pouch can be placed when a primary anastomosis is not feasible. This traction results in esophageal elongation which facilitates delayed primary repair. Besides esophageal lengthening, esophageal replacement using colonic interposition or gastric tube interposition has been proven effective. However, the risks of esophageal stricture, leakage, recurrent TEF, and esophageal mucosal outpouching increase with a complicated repair [14]. There is a strong association between gastroesophageal reflux, anastomotic tension and leakage of the anastomosis with esophageal anastomotic stricture [1].

## References

1. Spitz L. Esophageal atresia. Lessons I have learned in a 40-year experience. J Pediatr Surg. 2006;41(10):1635–40.
2. Gayle JA, Gomez SL, Baluch A, Fox C, Lock S, Kaye A. Anesthetic considerations for the neonate with tracheoesophageal fistula. Middle East J Anaesthesiol. 2008;19(6):1241–54.
3. Diaz LK, Akpek EA, Dinavahi R, Andropoulos DB. Tracheoesophageal fistula and associated congenital heart disease: implications for anesthetic management and survival. Paediatr Anaesth. 2005;15(10):862–9.
4. Okamoto T, Takamizawa S, Arai H, Bitoh Y, Nakao M, Yokoi A, et al. Esophageal atresia: prognostic classification revisited. Surgery. 2009;145(6):675–81.
5. Broemling N, Campbell F. Anesthetic management of congenital tracheoesophageal fistula. Paediatr Anaesth. 2011;21(11):1092–9.
6. Greemberg L, Fisher A, Katz A. Novel use of neonatal cuffed tracheal tube to occlude tracheo-oesophageal fistula. Paediatr Anaesth. 1999;9(4):339–41.

7. Baraka A, Akel S, Haroun S, Yazigi A. One-lung ventilation of the newborn with tracheoesophageal fistula. Anesth Analg. 1988;67(2):189–91.
8. Andropoulos DB, Rowe RW, Betts JM. Anaesthetic and surgical airway management during tracheo-oesophageal fistula repair. Paediatr Anaesth. 1998;8(4):313–9.
9. Kane TD, Atri P, Potoka DA. Triple fistula: management of a double tracheoesophageal fistula with a third H-type proximal fistula. J Pediatr Surg. 2007;42(6):E1–3.
10. Krosnar S, Baxter A. Thoracoscopic repair of esophageal atresia with tracheoesophageal fistula: anesthetic and intensive care management of a series of eight neonates. Paediatr Anaesth. 2005;15(7):541–6.
11. Ni Y, Yao Y, Liang P. Simple strategy of anesthesia for the neonate with tracheoesophageal fistula: a case report. Int J Clin Exp Med. 2014;7(1):327–8.
12. Petrosyan M, Estrada J, Hunter C, Woo R, Stein J, Ford HR, et al. Esophageal atresia/tracheoesophageal fistula in very low-birth-weight neonates: improved outcomes with staged repair. J Pediatr Surg. 2009;44(12):2278–81.
13. Richter GT, Ryckman F, Brown RL, Rutter MJ. Endoscopic management of recurrent tracheoesophageal fistula. J Pediatr Surg. 2008;43(1):238–45.
14. Al-Shanafey S, Harvey J. Long gap esophageal atresia: an Australian experience. J Pediatr Surg. 2008;43(4):597–601.

# Anesthesia for Congenital Diaphragmatic Hernia

Bobby Das, Nathaniel Lata, and Ximena Soler

Congenital Diaphragmatic hernia is a defect in the diaphragm that occurs during fetal development, causing abdominal contents to herniate in the pleural space, leading to compromised lung function. Some of the earliest medical descriptions of CDH are from the 1600s [1]. Surgical interventions were well documented in the late 1800s by Dr. O'Dwyer [2]. Current treatment strategies are based of the work started by Donovan in 1945 emphasizing early repair and the need to decompress the bowel [1]. Congenital Diaphragmatic Hernia occurs in approximately 1 in 2000 live births. About 50–60% of patients have isolated CDH. The remaining have additional malformations like congenital heart defects (40–60%)—or chromosomal abnormalities 5–15% [3].

B. Das (✉)
Cincinnati Children's Hospital Medical Center, Cincinnati, OH, USA
e-mail: bobby.das@cchmc.org

N. Lata
University of Missouri, Kansas City, Kansas City, MO, USA

Children's Mercy Hospital, Kansas City, MO, USA
e-mail: Njlata@cmh.edu

X. Soler
Department of Anesthesiology, Cincinnati Children's Hospital, Cincinnati, OH, USA
e-mail: Ximena.soler@cchmc.org

## Embryology

The formation of the diaphragm starts during the first few weeks of gestation. On day 20 begins the formation of the U-shaped intraembryonic coelom with the approachment of the neural ectoderm. By the end of the fifth week the septum transversum and the pleuroperitoneal fold, migrate, and meet halfway to complete the diaphragmatic muscle. Between days 41 and 52, the posterior diaphragm appears to descend to the lower thoracic final position. This is a result of the rapid growth of the dorsal embryo compared to the ventral part. During weeks 9–12 the pleural cavities enlarge and cover the lateral walls. Body wall tissue splits off medially. Extension of the pleural cavities into the body walls form the costodiaphragmatic recesses.

If the pleuroperitoneal membrane is not fused to the septum transversus when the intestines return to the abdomen from the umbilical cord, usually in week 11; they may migrate into the thoracic cavity, along with other abdominal organs, depending on the size of the defect [4].

The diaphragmatic tissue fuses in weeks 7–10. Thus, a defect occurring during the pseudoglandular phase—when multiplication of proximal airway divisions and supporting pulmonary arterial vasculature take place-is likely to produce pulmonary hypoplasia and respiratory failure at birth. Lung hypoplasia is associated with decreased number of alveolar type II cells. The earlier the defect occurs the more severe the hypoplasia and resulting comorbidities. In 70–80% of the cases, the posterior diaphragm fails to close, forming a triangular defect known as the foramen of Bochdalek since the right pleuroperitoneal opening tends to close early. Hence, a bilateral defect implies an earlier and more serious one. Right sided hernias may manifest later in life and with milder signs. Approximately 9% are anterior or Morgagni. CDH occurs approximately 85% of the time on the left side, 10% on the right and less than 5% bilaterally [5].

## Genetics

Once the diagnosis of CDH has been established it is classified phenotypically as being isolated or complex. The genetic counselor will obtain a three-generation family history with attention to other congenital malformations or perinatal deaths. Infants identified prenatally have a 550 band chromosome analysis. Children with complex CDH are evaluated with aCGH, and arrays targeting typical "hotspots" such as 15q26 [6]. Most individuals with isolated CDH are the only affected member of the family. Based on data from consecutive series, the risk of recurrence of isolated Bochdalek hernias in a sibling is less than 2%. Counseling of individuals with complex CDH is problematic and should be addressed on a case by case basis. The estimated recurrence risk to siblings is "low" since most families have low recurrence. As survival continues to improve, an increasing number of infants with repaired CDH will be having children of their own. If dominant *de novo* variants are responsible for most of those cases, a survivor's risk of having a child with CDH would be as high as 50%—given complete penetrance. New studies will be needed to clarify this risk, as more children survive with more complex defects.

## Comorbidities

The principal problems encountered in children with CDH are related to pulmonary hypoplasia secondary to abdominal viscera in the thorax. Pulmonary hypertension is common and its management is paramount to patient outcome. About one-third have cardiovascular malformations. Smaller proportions have skeletal, neurologic, genitourinary, gastrointestinal, and other defects. In the neonatal period, persistence of fetal circulation is potential. Syndromes that can involve CDH include: Pallister-Killian, Fryns, Ghersoni-Baruch, WAGR, Denys-Drash, Brachman-De Lange, Donnai-Barrow, and Wolf-Hirschhorn. Chromosomal anomalies that are associated with CDH include: trisomy 13, trisomy 18, tetrasomy, and 12p mosaicism [5]. There has not been specific associations with any one chromosomal defect [7].

## Diagnosis and Testing

### Prenatal

With increasing utilization of ultrasound for anatomy screenings in industrialized nations, more than 70% of cases of congenital diaphragmatic hernia are identified antenatally [8]. Ultrasound, in conjunction with MRI, can also have prognostic utility. Pulmonary hypoplasia and pulmonary hypertension are the two main determinants of neonatal morbidity and mortality, and severe cases require proper evaluation of prognosis for fetal surgery [9].

Abdominal organs in the thoracic cavity are a classic identifier for CDH on ultrasound. In the more common (85–90%) left-sided CDH, the mediastinum is shifted to the right [10]. Herniated viscera may show peristalsis, while fetal lung is more echogenic. The liver is visible in the chest in right-sided CDH. This can be challenging to identify because the liver is echogenic like fetal lung, requiring Doppler studies of the umbilical vein and hepatic vessels or location of the gall bladder for landmarks [8]. Findings suggestive of CDH include polyhydramnios, intrathoracic gastric bubble and mediastinal shift.

Observed-to-expected lung-to-head ratio, liver position, and total lung volume have been shown to correlate with neonatal morbidity and mortality [11, 12]. Lung-to-head ratio(LHR) is measured by ultrasound and shows the ratio of the contralateral lung area, at the level of the four-chamber view of the heart, to the head circumference. Total fetal lung volume is the sum of both lung volumes measured by MRI. In a recent meta-analysis, LHR < 1 was predictive for ECMO use. LHR < 1 and liver herniation on ultrasound showed that odds of survival were 0.14 and 0.21 respectively [12].

For this high-risk group, fetal surgical techniques have been developed and attempted. Percutaneous Fetal Endoluminal Tracheal Occlusion (FETO) is performed between 25 and 28 weeks of gestation, usually under maternal epidural anesthesia. At the end of pregnancy, the balloon is released followed by Ex Utero Intrapartum Treatment Procedure (EXIT) to securement of the airway, or controlled delivery in a tertiary center. The idea behind this technique is to trap surfactant-rich fetal lung fluid in the lung that will help expand the tissue against the pressure of the herniated organs [12]. Even if no fetal surgery is planned, prenatal diagnosis of the defect will allow for the transfer of the mother to a tertiary center where proper care of the sick neonate can be offered.

After diagnosis, planned vaginal or cesarean section after a gestational age of 37 weeks in a designated tertiary center should be pursued. In case of preterm labor prior to 34 weeks of gestation, antenatal steroids should be given [13]. When diagnosis is made antenatally, amniocentesis and karyotyping are performed [8].

## Postnatal

Less commonly, CDH can present after delivery. Diagnosis is made based on symptoms and physical signs [10]. Typically, infants present with acute respiratory distress in the neonatal period [8]. Classically, a physical examination would reveal cyanosis, scaphoid abdomen, diminished breath sounds, distant heart sounds, and bowel sounds in the chest. Plan x-ray of the thorax and abdomen would show position of the herniated viscera. Blood gas can be useful to show efficiency of gas exchange. Echocardiography of the heart can rule out associated malformations, measuring right to left shunt, and estimating severity of pulmonary HTN [10]. Figure 40.1 is an MRI image that shows lung compression from abdominal contents invading pleural space.

Rarely, children can have late presentation, but prognosis for these cases is excellent. Age range and presentations can be variable. GI and respiratory symptoms are most frequent and diagnosis can be made with a variety of imaging studies including CT and GI contrast radiographs. Also, a nasogastric tube on radiographs can help establish diagnosis [14].

## Anesthetic Management

### Pre-operative

The patient with CDH can present to the anesthesiology team in a few different circumstances. Prenatally, severe cases can be intervened upon with fetal surgical techniques, previously open correction of the defect and now fetal endoluminal tracheal occlusion [15, 16]. In the intrapartum period, patients can present for EXIT procedure to deflate endoluminal tracheal occlusion balloon or, in severe cases, place the neonate directly on to extracorporeal membrane oxygenation

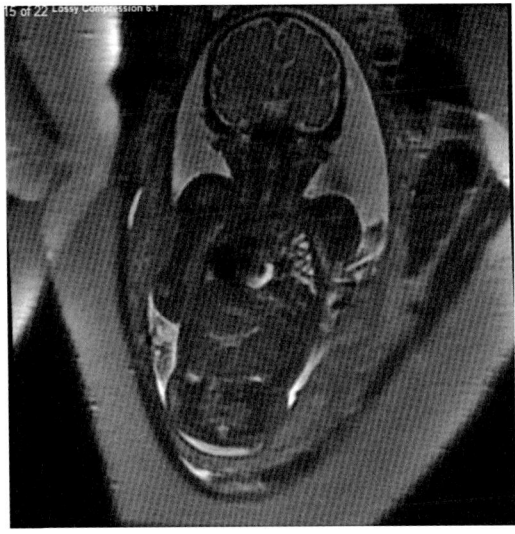

**Fig. 40.1** Coronal MRI image of fetal CDH showing lung compression from abdominal contents invading pleural space

(ECMO) [17]. Postnatally, CDH predominantly is repaired in the neonatal period. The timing of the procedure is variable, but optimization of the patient's ventilation and oxygenation prior to surgical intervention is recommended [13, 18].

Up until the early 1990s, CDH was treated like a surgical emergency and pulmonary hypertension was aggressively controlled with hyperventilation, frequently using high peak inspiratory pressures, oxygen concentrations, and ventilator rates [19]. This paradigm has shifted to optimization of the patient with a number of modalities (ECMO, inhaled nitric oxide (iNO), high frequency oscillator ventilation) prior to proceeding with surgery. In terms of ventilation, minimization of iatrogenic barotrauma has become a priority, characterized by permissive hypercapnia, preservation of spontaneous respiration, and avoidance of high ventilator pressures [19]. The delayed surgical repair of CDH after birth allows time for stabilization of the patient in the intensive care unit and for adequate assessment by the anesthesiologist.

For the postnatal patient, preoperative evaluation involves preparing for a neonatal anesthetic with special consideration for comorbidities seen with CDH. Birth history should be elicited from the family. Neonates born earlier have shorter time for lung development, and thus have poorer outcomes [20]. Management of ventilation and perfusion in the neonatal ICU should also be identified. It is recommended that patients with CDH be intubated immediately after birth to reduce the risk of pulmonary hypertension due to prolonged acidosis and hypoxia with delayed intubation [13]. Mode of ventilation (mechanical, HOFV, oscillation), peak pressures, and tidal volumes achieved, are important for continued management of ventilation in the operating room. Treatments are adapted to reach a preductal saturation between 85 and 95%, with target $PaCO_2$ range of 45–60 mmHg [13].

If ventilation and oxygenation strategies are inadequate, ECMO is an option for these children. It can act as a temporizing measure before surgery to allow the lungs to rest, during surgery to ensure adequate perfusion and oxygenation during repair, or after surgery if a patient decompensates after repair [21]. Criteria for ECMO include: inability to maintain preductal saturations >85% or postductal saturations >70%, Increased $PaCO_2$ and respiratory acidosis <7.15, peak inspiratory pressure > 28 $cmH_2O$ or mean airway pressure > 17 $cmH_2O$ required to maintain preductal saturation > 85%, inadequate oxygen delivery with metabolic acidosis as measured with elevated lactate >5 mmol/L, systemic hypotension, oxygenation index >40 [13]. The role of ECMO in patients with CDH remains unclear, but some studies have shown positive effects on outcome [13].

Echocardiography reveals concurrent congenital cardiac anomalies, persistence of fetal circulation, and degree of pulmonary hypertension. Cranial ultrasonography can diagnose intraventricular bleeding, a contraindication to heparinization for ECMO [22]. Optimization of systemic blood pressure with epinephrine, dopamine, and calcium infusions are used to maintain blood pressure at a normal level for gestational age [13]. Sedation is used to decrease neurohumoral stress and prevent increases in pulmonary vascular resistance. Inhaled nitric oxide can help with complicated, refractory pulmonary hypertension, but might not reduce the need for ECMO or decrease mortality [23]. Prostaglandin E1 and sildenafil may also be of use [13]. Use of surfactant is typically avoided for both term and preterm infants with CDH [13].

## Intraoperative

Most neonates will require respiratory support, so they frequently already have a definitive airway upon presentation to the anesthesia team [16]. Induction of anesthesia is variable depending on the severity of the cardiopulmonary comorbidities, but typically a rapid sequence intubation with propofol and relaxant is sufficient. Positive pressure via mask is avoided to prevent insufflation of the viscera in the thorax. Upon intubation, decompression of the stomach and intestines with a nasogastric tube helps prevent encroachment upon lung volumes by the herniated viscera. Ventilation strategies involve balancing optimal oxygenation and ventilation in the setting of elevated pulmonary vascular resistance, while minimizing peak airway pressures to avoid iatrogenic lung trauma. High-dose opioid techniques reduce the patient's response to surgical stimulation and avoid increases in pulmonary vascular resistance. If the patient is on ECMO, medication doses may need to be increased secondary to increased clearance of the drug in the circuit. Patient's with CDH may tolerate low dose volatile anesthetic, but this is dependent on cardiopulmonary function. Nitrous oxide should be avoided to due to the potential for expansion of herniated bowel in the thorax, causing mass effect on lung volumes [5, 17].

Monitors include two pulse oximeters (pre- and post-ductal), EKG, NIBP, temperature, and end-tidal $CO_2$. Vascular access for these cases include arterial, peripheral, and central lines. Pre-ductal arterial placement is recommended for systemic blood pressure monitoring and frequent blood gas sampling. Central access is useful to maintain potentially long-term vasoactive infusions. Ideally, venous access should be avoided in the lower extremities because repair of the hernia can result in inferior vena cava compression, limiting the effectiveness of delivered drugs and infusions. Heating blankets and plastic wrap on the neonate's head can be used to maintain euthermia [5, 17].

Analgesic techniques vary depending on the surgical approach and specific presentation for the patient. In the intubated neonate, long acting narcotics and sedatives are frequently used. Regional anesthesia via neuraxial analgesic techniques including epidural and caudal have been especially in patients who have late presentation. Patients on ECMO are systemically anticoagulated, contraindicating neuraxial techniques.

Fluid management involves delivery of dextrose-containing solution for maintenance and then replacement of insensible losses with isotonic crystalloid. In the first day of life, restrictive fluid management of 40 mL/kg/day is used, with increases of intake thereafter [13]. Glucose, lipids, and proteins are delivered parentally until the defect is repaired. Blood products should be available upon repair of the defect, especially if the patient is on ECMO.

Right to left shunting contributes to hypoxia in the presence of pulmonary hypertension. Occasionally prostaglandin $PGE_1$ is used to maintain a patent ductus arteriosus and reduce right ventricular afterload. Other techniques introduced in the acute neonatal treatment phase include nitric oxide (iNO), prostacycline, tolazoline, dipyridamole. Other authors recommend the use of surfactant and perflubron. If the patient is refractory to this management, as evidenced by $PaO_2 < 50$ mmHg with $FiO_2$ of 100%, extracorporeal Membrane Oxygenation should be started to avoid further lung injury.

## Post-operative

Patients that presented with challenging cardiopulmonary disease should remain intubated and mechanically ventilated postoperatively. Slow weaning of hemodynamic and ventilatory support occurs in the intensive care unit. Enteral feeding starts post-operatively. Nutritional morbidity and gastroesophageal reflux is commonly encountered in the first year of life [13].

Long-term complications for CDH survivors include: pulmonary morbidity including restrictive and obstructive defects secondary to altered lung structure and prolonged ventilatory support, persistent pulmonary hypertension, GERD, cardiovascular disease, neurocognitive defects, and musculoskeletal abnormalities [24] (Table 40.1).

**Table 40.1** Summary of the perioperative management for congenital diaphragmatic hernia

| Pre-operative: |
| --- |
| • Obtain birth history-prematurity etc. |
| • Check co-morbidities: Syndrome, pulmonary hypertension (HTN), etc. |
| • Obtain Echo to check cardiac function, evidence of pulmonary HTN |
| • Determine ECMO settings/type: V-V vs. V-A |
| • Check ventilator settings/ type of ventilator |
| • Labs: CBC, electrolytes, Coags, ABG, and Type and Screen |
| • Check medication and obtain necessary infusion: Pressors, iNO, sildenafil, etc. |
| Intra-operative: |
| • Secure airway with RSI |
| • Consider using NICU ventilator (piston based) or HOFV |
| • Vent setting to avoid barotrauma |
| • Judicious use of opiates to decrease PVR and for pain control |
| • ECMO |
| • Low dose volatile anesthetic depending upon cardiac function |
| • Access: 2 peripheral IV's, arterial line, and consider central line for pressors |
| • Standard ASA monitors: Consider preductal placement of arterial line, NIBP, or pulse oximetry |
| • Warming blanket and warm OR temperature |
| • Regional: Consider epidural or caudal with late presentation of CDH, unless on ECMO |
| • Use D10 containing isotonic crystalloid for glucose management |
| • Blood on hold |
| • Have pressors, iNO, ICU drips ready if needed |
| Post-operative: |
| • ICU transport |
| • Slow wean of ventilator settings prior to extubation |
| • Sedation infusions while intubated |
| • Nasogastric tube for enteral feeding |
| • Possible need for ECMO |
| Long-term morbidity: |
| • Pulmonary hypertension |
| • GERD |
| • Cardiovascular disease |
| • Neurocognitive deficits |
| • Musculoskeletal abnormalities |
| ECMO criteria: |
| • Inability to maintain preductal saturations >85% or post-ductal saturations >70% |
| • Increased $PaCO_2$ |
| • Respiratory acidosis <7.15 |
| • Peak inspiratory pressure >28 $cmH_2O$ or mean airway pressure > 17 $cmH_2O$ required to maintain preductal saturation >85% |
| • Inadequate oxygen delivery with metabolic acidosis as measured with elevated lactate >5 mmol/L |
| • Systemic hypotension |
| • Oxygenation index >40 |

# References

1. Golombek SG. The history of congenital diaphragmatic hernia from 1850s to the present. J Perinatol. 2002;22(3):242–6.
2. O'Dwyer J. Operation for relief of congenital diaphragmatic hernia. Arch Pediatr. 1889;9:130–2.
3. Pober BR, Russell MK, Ackerman KG. Congenital diaphragmatic hernia overview. GeneReviews. NCBI Bookshelf, National Library of Medicine. 2010;(3):1–29.
4. Dicovery.lifemapsc.com. LifeMap Discovery Medical embryology. Pansky B. In: Schoenwolf G, Bleyl S, Brauer P, et al., editors. Larsen's human embryology, 5th ed. Philadelphia, PA: Churchill Livingstone; 2014.
5. Bachiller PR, Chou JH, Romanelli TM, Roberts JD. Cote and Lerman's. A practice of anestheisa for infants and children. 5th edn. p 757–8.
6. Kantarce S, Casavant D, Russell M, Pober BR. Findings from aCGH in patients with CDH: a possible locums for Fryns syndrome. Am J Med Genet. 2006;140A(1):17–23.

7. Borys D, Taxy J. Congenital diaphragmatic hernia and chromosomal anomalies: autopsy study. Pediatr Dev Pathol. 2004;7(1):35–8.
8. Kotecha A, Barbato A, Bush A, Claus F, Davenport M, Midulla F. Congenital diaphragmatic hernia. Eur Respir J. 2012;39(4):820–9.
9. Benachi A, Cordier AG, Cannie M, Jani J. Advances in prenatal diagnosis of congenital diaphragmatic hernia. Semin Fetal Neonatal Med. 2014;19(6):331–7.
10. Leeuwen L, Fitzgerald D. Congenital diaphragmatic hernia. J Paediatr Child Health. 2014;50(9):667–73.
11. Oluyomi-Obi T, Kuret V, Puligandla P, Lodha A, Lee-Robertson H, Ryan G, et al. Antenatal predictors of outcome in prenatally diagnosed congenital diaphragmatic hernia (CDH). J Pediatr Surg. 2016;52(5):881–8.
12. Deprest J, Jam J, Van Schoubroeck D. Current consequences of prenatal diagnosis of CDH. J Pediatr Surg. 2006;41(2):423–30.
13. Snoek KG, Reiss IK, Greenough A, Capolupo I, Urlesberger B, Tibboel D, et al. Standardized postnatal management of infants with congenital diaphragmatic hernia in Europe: the CDH EURO consortium consensus—2015 update. Neonatology. 2016;110(1):66–74.
14. Ciqdem MK, Onen A, Otcu S, Okur H. Late presentation of Bochdalek-type congenital diaphragmatic hernia in children: a 23-year experience at a single center. Surg Today. 2007;37(8):642–5.
15. Tovar JA. Congenital diaphragmatic hernia. Orphanet J Rare Dis. 2012;7:1.
16. Bosenberg A, Brown RA. Management of congenital diaphragmatic hernia. Curr Opin Anaesthesiol. 2008;21(3):323–31.
17. Diu M, Mancuso T. Pediatric diseases; congenital diaphragmatic hernia. Stoelting's Anesthesia and Co-Existing Disease. 2012;6:594–6.
18. Hedrick H. Management of prenatally diagnosed congenital diaphragmatic hernia. Semin Pediatr Surg. 2013;22(1):37–43.
19. Boloker J, Bateman DA, Wung JT, Stolar CJ. Congenital diaphragmatic hernia in 120 infants treated consecutively with permissive hypercapnea/spontaneous respiration/elective repair. J Pediatr Surg. 2002;37(3):357–66.
20. Bouchghoul H, Senat MV, Storme L, de Lagausie P, Begue L, Benachi A. Congenital diaphragmatic hernia: does gestational age at diagnosis matter when evaluating morbidity and mortality? Am J Obstet Gynecol. 2015;213(4):535.e1–7.
21. Shieh HF, Wilson JM, Sheils CA, Smithers CJ, Kharasch VS, Buchmiller TL. Does the ex utero intrapartum treatment to extracorporeal membrane oxygenation procedure change morbidity outcomes for high-risk congenital diaphragmatic hernia survivors? J Pediatr Surg. 2017;52(10):22–5.
22. Chapman RL, Peterec SM, Bizzarro MJ, Mercurio MR. Patient selection for neonatal extracorporeal membrane oxygenation: beyond severity of illness. J Perinatol. 2009;29(9):606–11.
23. Finer F, Ehrenkranz R, et al. Inhaled nitric oxide and hypoxic respiratory failure in infants with congenital diaphragmatic hernia. The Neonatal Inhaled Nitric Oxide Study Group (NINOS). Pediatrics. 1997;99(6):838–45.
24. Peetsold MG, Heij HA, Kneepkens CM, Nagelkerke AF, Huisman J, Gemke RJ. The long-term follow-up of patients with a congenital diaphragmatic hernia: a broad spectrum of morbidity. Pediatr Surg Int. 2009;25(1):1–17.

# Omphalocele and Gastroschisis

## Wendy Nguyen and Kumar Belani

In this chapter, the differences between the two defects will be discussed. In addition, the preoperative management, anesthetic intraoperative monitoring, anesthetic goals, and postoperative outcomes will be outlined. Table 41.1 provides a summary of anesthesia considerations in patients undergoing surgery for Omphalocele and Gastroschisis.

## Introduction

An omphalocele is a central defect of the umbilical ring where the abdominal contents eviscerate into the intact umbilical sac. They are frequently accompanied with other anomalies and require detailed further work-up.

Gastroschisis is a full thickness abdominal wall defect with evisceration of bowel through the defect. The bowel contents are exposed, without a covering membrane. Gastroschises most frequently present as the only anomaly.

W. Nguyen, M.D. (✉)
Department of Anesthesiology, University of Minnesota School of Medicine,
Minneapolis, MN, USA

University of Minnesota, Masonic Children's Hospital, Minneapolis, MN, USA
e-mail: nguye747@umn.edu

K. Belani, M.B.B.S., M.S., F.A.C.A., F.A.A.P
University of Minnesota, Masonic Children's Hospital, Minneapolis, MN, USA

For the practicing anesthesiologist, omphaloceles and gastroschises are relatively common, but the size and complexity of the defect can present unique challenges. Its accompanying anomalies may be significant enough to play a larger role in outcomes. As such, patients with these abdominal wall defects may present repeatedly for complications related to abdominal wall defect closures and/or for other procedures related to their other anomalies (Fig. 41.1).

## Omphalocele

### Definition and Diagnosis

In omphaloceles, the umbilical cord inserts in the protruding sac, containing the internal peritoneal membrane, Wharton's jelly, and an external amniotic membrane. The sac frequently contains the stomach, loops of the small and large intestines, liver (up to 50% of the time), and sometimes gonads.

Omphaloceles occur due to a failure of bowel loops to return to the abdominal cavity following the physiological herniation of the umbilical cord between the 6th and 11th week of development. Small to medium omphaloceles are considered 2–4 cm in size. Although there is no consensus, most surgeons define giant omphaloceles (GOC) as 5 cm or larger [7]. In cases of GOC, the thoracic cavity may be abnormally shaped and

**Table 41.1** Summary of anesthesia considerations in patients undergoing surgery for omphalocele and gastroschisis

| Plan/preparation/adverse events | Reasoning/management |
|---|---|
| Pre-procedural evaluation<br>– Pre-operative work-up; related co-morbidities<br>– Airway<br>– Size and complexity of the defect | Management may change significantly if there are any other anomalies such as cardiac conditions.<br>Securing of the airway may be necessary if there is significant respiratory compromise from the defect and/or other anomalies.<br>The size and the complexity of the defect guides the route of the delivery, surgical and anesthetic management, and outcomes. |
| Access and monitoring<br>– PICC, PIV ± arterial line<br>– Orogastric or nasogastric tube | Central access is necessary for TPN. It is also helpful for the measurement of CVP to monitor for increased abdominal pressures. A larger PIV is helpful for transfusing and administering drugs quickly. An arterial line may be helpful for monitoring labs and blood pressure, but may not be necessary if the patient is otherwise stable.<br>An orogastric or nasogastric tube is necessary for abdominal decompression. |
| Intraoperative management<br>– Maintain normothermia<br>– Maintenance fluid and replacement of insensible loss<br>– Monitor for increased abdominal pressures<br>– Consider extubation for small abdominal wall defects. Neuraxial analgesia may help facilitate this | Maintaining normothermia can be challenging due to the amount of insensible losses from the exposed abdominal organs.<br>Similarly, insensible losses must be aggressively replaced to maintain intravascular volume.<br>Intravesical line is helpful for monitoring for intraabdominal pressures during closure. In lieu of an intravesical pressure monitoring, end tidal $CO_2$ and airway pressures can be tracked.<br>Although not widely adapted, use of neuraxial anesthesia would be helpful for post-operative pain control and facilitate extubation in the operating room. |
| Post-operative management and discharge considerations<br>– Monitor for signs of abdominal compartment syndrome<br>– Monitor for surgically-related complications<br>– Extubate when surgically and hemodynamically stable<br>– Manage co-existing anomalies<br>– May require prolonged TPN | Abdominal compartment syndrome is an emergency requiring expedient decompression to avoid ischemia and subsequent short gut syndrome.<br>Some will require multiple procedures to mitigate complications, such as adhesions and volvulus, from the initial procedure.<br>If there is significant pulmonary compromise prior to surgical closure, prolonged intubation is likely.<br>Patients with small abdominal wall defects tend to be fair better than those with large or complex defects.<br>Co-existing anomalies, if significant, such as cardiac or pulmonary hypoplasia, may play a more significant role in outcomes than the abdominal wall defect itself. |

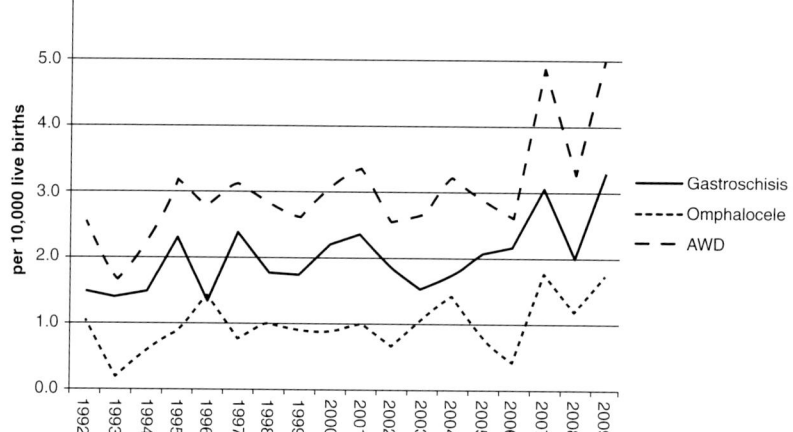

**Fig. 41.1** The incidences of both omphalocele and gastroschisis have been increasing as outlined in this study by Kong and associates [6]

reduced in size, which may lead to pulmonary hypoplasia.

Prenatal diagnosis is made by ultrasound screening during late first trimester to mid-second trimester. An elevated maternal alpha fetoprotein level may be present, but is not diagnostic. Antenatal echocardiography should be performed as up to 50% of fetuses will have cardiac defects. Most common cardiac lesions include muscular ventricular septal defect, atrial septal defect, and coarctation of the aorta [8].

A recent study using a large multi-center clinical database in North America found the incidence of at least one other anomaly with omphaloceles was 35% [9]. Interestingly, another recent large study examined births in Texas from 1999 to 2008 and found 80% of omphaloceles had other anomalies [10]. This is more in line with other studies that report multiple anomalies occurred in 67–88% of omphaloceles [11].

Omphaloceles have been known to be associated with complex syndromes including cloacal exstrophy, Donnai-Barrow syndrome, Beckwith-Wiedeman syndrome, and Pentalogy of Cantrell. Chromosomal defects (Trisomy 13, 18 or 21) are observed in up to 30–40% of babies with omphalocele [12–15].

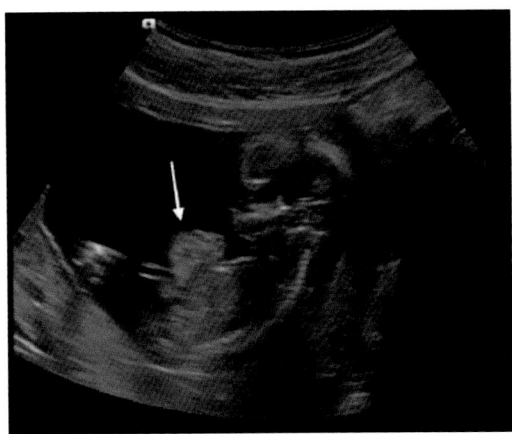

**Fig. 41.2** An antenatal ultrasound examination at 14 weeks of pregnancy. Note the presence of an abdominal wall defect as pointed by the arrow [22]

## Treatment

There is no benefit to delivering prior to 37 weeks unless there are complicating features, such as polyhydramnios [12]. However, the route of delivery is controversial. Retrospective studies reveal no differences in fetal outcome with a C-section delivery [16]. However, these studies did not stratify outcome by the severity of the omphalocele. As such, when the defect includes an extra-abdominal liver, C-section may be prudent to avoid hepatic injury [17].

Repair is not urgent. Once delivered, goals include stabilization, and characterization of abnormalities. All newborns with omphalocele must undergo an evaluation for other defects because even though an antenatal ultrasound and cardiac echocardiogram suggests an isolated anomaly, additional multiple defects are not uncommon [18, 19]. Thus, soon after birth, additional studies include transthoracic echocardiography, renal ultrasound, karyotyping, and additional genetic evaluation as indicated (Fig. 41.2).

Preoperative care may require securing the airway, use of oscillator ventilation, nitric oxide, and even extracorporeal membrane oxygenation (ECMO) because of significant ventilatory compromise related to pulmonary hypoplasia and other defects [15]. More than gastroschisis, babies with omphalocele carry a higher risk of having pulmonary hypertension [9].

Bowel decompression minimizes aspiration risk and worsening bowel distension. Antibiotics are required to prevent infection. Intravenous iso-osmotic fluids three to four times the usual maintenance rate may be needed to provide adequate hydration and to compensate for insensible losses secondary to peritonitis, edema, ischemia, and protein loss. Urine output goal should be approximately 1–2 mL/kg/h, and acid base-status and electrolytes should be frequently monitored.

A bowel bag over the sac has been useful to mitigate heat loss [20]. Gauze may be used as well. In the past, super moist gauze had been advocated, but the moisture will cool and can lead to hypothermia [15]. Great care needs to be taken to not rupture the sac as that increases infection risk. Central and arterial umbilical lines are avoided. Early placement of a peripherally inserted central catheter (PICC) is helpful, as these babies will need total parental nutrition.

The primary goal of omphalocele repair is to return of the viscera to the abdominal cavity. The secondary goal is to close the fascia and skin. Two to four centimeter omphalocele defects may be undergo a primary closure with a good surgical outcome.

On the other hand, larger omphaloceles will require a staged repair. This entails the use of a silo chimney or prosthesis [21]. The sac is removed and a silo mesh (usually Silastic™ or Teflon™) is sutured to fascia of the defect. Then, the extra-abdominal organs are gradually returned to the peritoneal cavity in approximately 3–10 days. After the herniated bowel is reduced, the prosthesis is removed, and the defect closed under anesthesia in the operating room. For complex omphaloceles, a conservative non-operative delayed closure is suggested. This procedure involves placement of a topical solution, such as silver sulfadiazine, directly to the sac to promote neoepithelialization and then eventual closure of the remaining ventral hernia (Fig. 41.3) [7, 22].

## Anesthetic Considerations

A thorough preoperative analysis is essential to define the extent of involvement and compromise due to associated defects. These babies may already be intubated at birth due to respiratory compromise from the lesion and/or pulmonary hypoplasia. Babies not intubated will require decompression of the stomach with a nasogastric or orogastric tube. Following this, a rapid-sequence induction of anesthesia is accomplished in babies with a normal upper airway. Cardiac status will dictate the choice of anesthetic agents. However, nitrous oxide is avoided to reduce bowel distension.

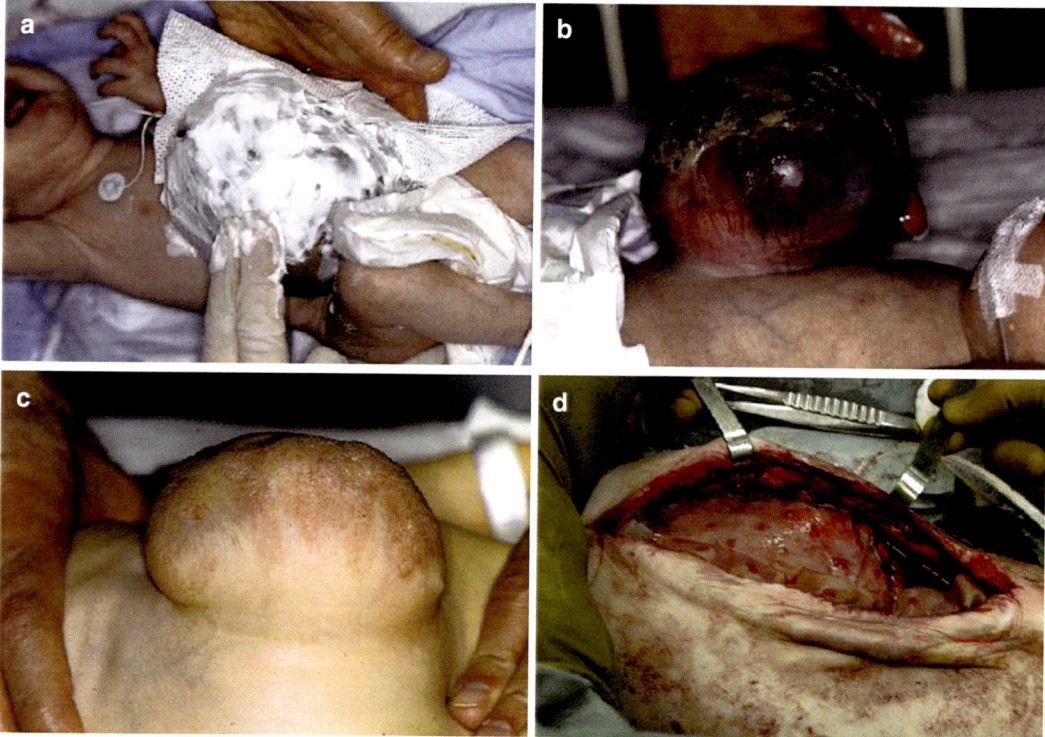

**Fig. 41.3** Complex large omphaloceles may be treated conservatively with escharotic treatment with the initial application of silversulfadiazine (**a**). This allows epithelialization and eschar formation (**b**, **c**). The baby then is taken to the operating room for repair of a ventral hernia after reducing contents of the omphalocele [11]

For intraoperative monitoring, an arterial line is helpful, but not necessary for closure. Placement of a central line is recommended to allow not only measuring central venous pressure but also for biochemical monitoring. Patients with Beckwith-Wiedemann syndrome require attentive management of glucose. Maintenance and/or total parenteral nutrition (TPN) may be infused through the central line. A peripheral intravenous (PIV) line is placed for administering drugs and fluids. It is important to keep up with insensible losses during the case with an iso-osmotic solution at a rate of 8–15 mL/kg/h. Maintaining normothermia is important and can be challenging with large abdominal defects.

Another challenge in babies with large omphaloceles is the increase in intraabdominal pressure during closure. With tight closures, there will be pressure on the inferior vena cava, aorta, and diaphragm. This can result in detrimental increases in intrathoracic pressure, intracranial pressure, and diminished perfusion of splanchnic organs. The severity of the ensuing changes can be gauged at the bedside by evaluating intragastric and intravesical pressure via an orogastric tube and urinary catheter [12], increase in end-tidal $CO_2$ and peak airway pressures, and reductions in $SPO_2$ (pulse oximetry) [11]. Intragastric pressure more than 20 mmHg and central venous pressure (CVP) less than 4 mmHg may be associated with decreased venous return and cardiac index requiring surgical decompression [11, 23]. Otherwise, abdominal compartment syndrome (ACS) can ensue causing diminished perfusion to abdominal organs and congestion in the brain due to increased intracranial pressure by way of increased intrathoracic pressure [11, 24].

Following closure of small omphaloceles and without other major significant anomalies, the babies can be extubated after surgery. For neonates undergoing a gradual reduction after an uncomplicated primary closure, mechanical ventilation is usually required for 24–48 h or longer. Thereafter, respiratory compliance usually improves dramatically [25]. Adjuncts to general anesthesia include a caudal catheter and chloroprocaine infusion to help facilitate extubation [26].

## Post-operative Care and Outcomes

Postoperatively, respiratory status, signs of infection, inferior vena cava compression (blue lower limbs, or bowel ischemia), abdominal pressures are monitored. TPN may need to be continued for weeks due to ileus [12]. Babies with complex omphaloceles or GOC may require unusual levels of PEEP, months or "even years of positive pressure support via a tracheostomy" [15].

Most patients with small omphaloceles recover well and do not present any long-term issues. However, only a small percentage have a truly isolated lesion [18]. Isolated lesions confer to a 95–97% survival [27, 28]. Larger lesions including GOC and those with liver involvement have worse outcomes [29, 30]. For GOC, nonoperative delayed closure may confer to reduced mortality compared to staged closure (21.8% versus 23.4%) [7].

Morbidity and mortality may also be related to the side effects of intravenous alimentation (e.g., liver failure or sepsis). Complications related to the initial surgical care such as bowel perforation, and presence of malrotation, adhesions, obstruction will require additional procedures. If malrotation is not treated in a timely manner, midgut volvulus could lead to short bowel syndrome [11].

In cases of omphaloceles with other anomalies, survival and morbidity is often dependent on the associated defects such as cardiac malfunction and intestinal atresia [12]. Compared to gastroschises, babies with omphaloceles have a higher mortality (18% compared to 4%) [9].

## Gastroschisis

## Definition and Diagnosis

Gastroschisis is usually 2–5 cm in diameter and almost always to the right of the umbilical cord. The eviscerated bowel is often small and large bowel. The liver is rarely present. The bowel contents are exposed, without a covering membrane. Cryptorchidism coexists when the testes exit along with the bowel.

Although some institutions recommend planned late preterm delivery to avoid ongoing in utero inflammation, the increased risks associated with preterm delivery must be weighed against the risk for intrauterine fetal demise [31]. No consensus has been reached and no concrete evidence supports induced early delivery [11]. Interestingly, spontaneous preterm delivery at approximately 36.5 weeks gestational age is more common in mothers whose babies have gastroschisises than the general population (28% versus 6%) [32]. This may be secondary to the inflammatory stimulus [12].

There are different theories regarding the pathogenesis of gastroschisis. Exposure to acetaminophen, aspirin, and pseudoephedrine in utero has been associated with an increased incidence [33, 34]. Smoking has also been implicated [12]. One theory suggests that gastroschisis is associated with an earlier embryologic event related to abnormal development to the right omphalomesenteric artery or right umbilical vein, causing ischemia to the right paraumbilical area [11]. Another theory postulates that they are caused by an imbalance between cell proliferation and planned cell death (apoptosis) during the critical embryonic development period [13]. Stevens et al., hypothesized that gastroschisis may be the result of failure of the yolk sac and vitelline structures to be included into the body stalk [35].

Similar to omphalocele, the prenatal diagnosis of gastroschisis is made towards the end of first trimester (Fig. 41.2), after the physiological closure of the abdominal wall around 10 weeks of gestation. The discerning factor is whether a membrane is present [12]. An elevated maternal alpha fetoprotein level may be seen and is more common in gastroschisis than omphalocele.

Babies with gastroschisis do not usually have any associated syndromes, nor do they have any genetic defects. Thus, fetal karyotyping is not routine [36]. Babies with complex gastroschisis usually have intestinal atresia (around 10% of cases), stenosis, necrosis or volvulus [37, 38]. However, cardiac, renal, musculoskeletal, and central nervous system anomalies can occur [39]. A recent study found that gastroschises had associated anomalies 32% of time compared to 80% of omphaloceles [10].

## Treatment

Swift protection of extruded bowel is mandatory at birth by means of sterile moist sponges and sterile covering, such as a plastic bag. Babies should be cared for in the right flank decubitus position to limit ischemic injury [12]. Similar to the treatment of omphaloceles, normothermia, antibiotics, bowel decompression, monitoring acid-base status, and obtaining reliable access are important. Since the protruding small and large intestines are without a covering membrane, patients with gastroschisis can require even more aggressive fluid management. Urine output needs to be closely monitored.

Definitive cover, either primary or staged, should be undertaken within the next 4–7 h [40, 41]. If the herniated loops are without matting and peel, it is possible to perform the reduction at the bedside [42], under mild sedation [40]. However, surgeons need to know when it is no longer safe to perform a bedside reduction and convert to a reduction in the operative room under general anesthesia. If the loops are edematous and covered by an inflammatory peel, primary reduction may still be feasible under general anesthesia [12]. On the other hand, if the herniated loops are very edematous, covered by a thick peel and/or tightly matted together, then a stage reduction is indicated. The process is similar to that of an omphalocele staged reduction. An extracorporeal bag is sutured around the enlarged defect, or inserted within the abdomen when using a preformed spring-loaded silo, and hung from the roof of the crib. The intestine is gradually returned to the abdomen via gentle pressure. It is not necessary to keep the infant intubated and/or sedated while the bag is in place and during manual reduction [12]. Similar to omphaloceles, it usually takes approximately 7–10 days for the loops to return the abdomen. Then, the patient is brought to the operating room to remove the bag and close the abdominal wall.

## Anesthetic Considerations

The anesthetic considerations for the closure of gastroschisis are similar to that of omphaloceles. As part of routine evaluation, these babies should also be evaluated for additional anomalies. Gastroschisis babies will require more fluid secondary to insensible losses. Monitoring for intraabdominal hypertension during closure via peak pressures, end tidal $CO_2$, CVP, $SPO_2$ and/or bladder catheter is important in preventing abdominal compartment syndrome.

Vane et al., described using a spinal anesthetic in selected patients with gastroschisis as an effective sole anesthetic [43]. Raghavan et al., described using neuraxial anesthesia as an adjunct technique with general anesthesia of 22 neonates and noted a decreased need for postoperative ventilation requirement (23% vs. 88% with general anesthesia only) [44].

## Post-operative Care and Outcome

The post-operative course depends on the severity of intestinal damage, co-existing stenosis, atretic segments of small intestines, and the occurrence of complications such as bowel perforation or volvulus [11, 27, 38]. With simple cases, the more common scenario, primary reduction occurs in 70% of cases with quicker start of gastric feeding and achievement of full feeds, lower complication rate, and shorter hospital stay. Survival is greater than 95% if patients are treated in pediatric centers [45]. In complex cases with atresias, stenosis, perforations, and/or volvulus, all parameters are worse, including mortality [27]. They often require multiple operations and prolonged parenteral nutrition [12]. In these situations, survival decreases to 70% [27, 46].

## References

1. Wilson RD, Johnson MP. Congenital abdominal wall defects: an update. Fetal Diagn Ther. 2004;19(5):385–98.
2. Zaccara A, Iacobelli B, Calzolari A, Turchetta A, Orazi C, Schingo P, et al. Cardiopulmonary perfomances in young children and adolescents born with large abdominal wall defects. J Pediatr Surg. 2003;38(3):478–81.
3. Jones KL, Benirschke K, Chambers CD. Gastroschisis: etiology and developmental pathogenesis. Clin Genet. 2009;74(4):322–5.
4. Goldbaum G, Daling J, Milham S. Risk factors for gastroschisis. Teratology. 1990;42(4):397–403.
5. Siega-Riz AM, Herring AH, Olshan AF, Smith J, Moore C. The joint effects of maternal prepregnancy body mass index and age on the risk of gastroschisis. Paediatr Perinat Epidemiol. 2009;23(1):51–7.
6. Kong JK, Yeo KT, Abdel-Latif ME, Bajuk B, Holland AJA, Adams S, et al. Outcomes of infants with abdominal wall defects over 18 years. J Pediatr Surg. 2016;51(10):1644–9.
7. Bauman B, Stephens D, Gershone H, Bongiorno C, Osterholm AB, et al. Management of giant omphaloceles: a systemic review of methods of staged surgical vs. nonoperative delayed closure. J Pediatr Surg. 2015;51:1725–30.
8. Gibbin C, Touch S, Broth RE, Berghella V. Abdominal wall defects and congenital heart disease. Ultrasound Obstet Gynecol. 2003;21(4):334–7.
9. Corey KM, Hornik CP, Laughon MM, McHutchison K, Clark RH, Smith PB. Frequency of anomalies and hospital outcomes in infants with gastroschisis and omphalocele. Early Hum Dev. 2014;90(80):421–4.
10. Benjamin B, Wilson GN. Anomalies associated with gastroschisis and omphalocele: analysis of 2825 cases from the Texas Birth Defects Registry. J Pediatr Surg. 2014;49(4):514–9.
11. Christison-Lagay ER, Kelleher CM, Langer JC. Neonatal abdominal wall defects. Semin Fetal Neonatal Med. 2011;16:164–72.
12. Gamba P, Midrio P. Abdominal wall defects: prenatal diagnosis, newborn management, and long-term outcomes. Semin Pediatr Surg. 2014;23:283–90.
13. Robinson JN, Abuhamad AZ. Abdominal wall and umbilical abnormalities. Clin Perinatol. 2000;4:947–78.
14. Weber TR, Au-Fliegner M, Downard CD, Fishman SJ. Abdominal wall defects. Curr Opin Pediatr. 2002;14(4):491–7.
15. Mann S, Blinman TA, Wilson RD. Prenatal and postnatal management of omphalocele. Prenat Diagn. 2008;28:626–32.
16. Anteby EY, Yagel S. Route of delivery of fetuses with structural anomalies. Eur J Obstet Gynecol Reprod Biol. 2003;106(1):5–9.
17. Island S. Advances in surgery for abdominal wall defects. Gastroschisis and omphalocele. Clin Perinatol. 2012;39:375–86.
18. Fratelli N, Papageoghiou AT, Bhide A, Sharma A, Okoye B, Thilaganathan B. Outcome of antenatally diagnosed abdominal wall defects. Ultrasound Obstet Gynecol. 2007;30:266–70.
19. Cohen-Overbeek TE, Tong WH, Hatzmann TR, Wilms JF, Govaerts LCP, Galjaard RJH, et al.

Omphalocele: comparison of outcome following prenatal or postnatal diagnosis. Ultrasound Obstet Gynecol. 2010;36(6):687–92.
20. Towne BH, Peters G, Chang JH. The problem of "giant" omphalocele. J Pediatr Surg. 1980;15:543–8.
21. Schuster SR. A new method for staged repair of large omphaloceles. Surg Gynecol Obstet. 1967;125(4):837–50.
22. Varghese AS, Vause S, Kamupira SR, Emmerson AJB. Congenital abdominal wall defects. Arch Dis Child Educ Pract Ed. 2017;102(1):19.
23. Yaster M, Buck JR, Dudgeon DL, Manolio TA, Simmons RS, Zeller P, et al. Hemodynamic effects of primary closure of Omphalocele/gastroschisis in human newborns. Anesthesiology. 1988;69:84–8.
24. Rosenthal RJ, Friedman RL, Chidambaram A, Khan AK, Martz J, Shi Q, et al. Effects of hyperventilation and hypoventilation on $PaCO_2$ and intracranial pressure during acute elevations of intraabdominal pressure with $CO_2$ pneumoperitoneum: large animal observations. J Am Coll Surg. 1998;187:32–8.
25. Nakayama DK, Mutich R, Motoyama EK. Pulmonary dysfunction after primary closure of an abdominal wall defect and its improvement with bronchodilators. Pediatr Pulmonol. 1992;12:174–80.
26. Tobias JD, Rasmussen GE, Holcomb GW III, Brock JW, Morgan WM. Continuous caudal anesthesia with chloroprocaine as an adjunct to general anaesthesia in neonates. Can J Anaesth. 1996;43:69–72.
27. Molik KA, Gingalewski CA, West KW, Rescorla FJ, Scherer LR III, Engum SA. Gastroschisis: a plea for categorization. J Pediatr Surg. 2001;36:51–5.
28. Henrich K, Huemmer HP, Reingruber B, Weber PG. Gastroschisis and omphalocele: treatments and long-term outcomes. Pediatr Surg Int. 2008;24:167–73.
29. Tsakayannis DE, Zurakowski D, Lillehei CW. Respiratory insufficiency at birth: a predictor of mortality for infants with omphalocele. J Pediatr Surg. 1996;31(8):1088–90.
30. Biard JM, Wilson RD, Johnson MP, Hedrick HL, Schwarz U, Flake AW. Prenatally diagnosed giant omphaloceles: short- and long-term outcomes. Prenat Diagn. 2004;24(6):434–9.
31. Carnaghan H, Pereira S, James CP, Charlesworth PB, Ghionzoli M, Mohamed E, et al. Is early delivery beneficial in gastroschisis? J Pediatr Surg. 2014;49:928–33.
32. Lausman AY, Langer JC, Tai M, Seaward PGR, Windrim RC, Kelly EN. Gastroschisis: what is the average gestational age of spontaneous delivery? J Pediatr Surg. 2007;42:1816–21.
33. Werler MM, Sheehan JE, Mitchell AA. Maternal medication use and risks of gastroschisis and small intestinal atresia. Am J Epidemiol. 2002;155:26–31.
34. Baerg J, Kaban G, Tonita J, Pahwa P, Reid D. Gastroschisis: a sixteen-year review. J Pediatr Surg. 2003;38:771–4.
35. Stevenson RE, Rogers RC, Chandler JC, Gauderer MWL, Hunger AGW. Escape of the yolk sac: a hypothesis to explain the embryogenesis of gastroschisis. Clin Genet. 2009;75:326–33.
36. Mastroiacovo P, Lisi A, Castilla EE, Martinez-Frias M, Bermejo E, Marengo L. Gastroschisis and associated defects: an international study. Am J Med Genet. 2007;143A:660–71.
37. Ghionzoli M, James CP, David AL, Dimple S, Tan AWC, Iskaros J, et al. Gastroschisis with intestinal atresia -predictive value of antenatal diagnosis and outcome of postnatal treatment. J Pediatr Surg. 2012;47:322–8.
38. Bergholz R, et al. Complex gastroschisis is a different entity to simple gastroschisis affecting morbidity and mortality—a systematic review and meta-analysis. J Pediatr Surg. 2014;49(10):1527–32.
39. Kunz LH, Gilbert WM, Tower DR. Increased incidence of cardiac anomalies in pregnancies complicated by gastroschisis. Am J Obstet Gynecol. 2005;193:1248–52.
40. Cauchi J, Parikh DH, Samuel M, Gornall P. Does gastroschisis reduction require general anesthesia? A comparative analysis. J Pediatr Surg. 2006;41:1294–7.
41. Singh SJ, Fraser A, Leditschke JF, Spence K, Kimble R, Dalby-Payne J, et al. Gastroschisis: determinants of neonatal outcome. Pediatr Surg Int. 2003;19(4):260–5.
42. Bianchi A, Dickson AP, Alizai NK. Elective delayed midgut reduction -no anaesthesia for gastroschisis: selection and conversion criteria. J Pediatr Surg. 2002;37:1334–6.
43. Vane DW, Abajian JC, Hong AR. Spinal anesthesia for primary repair of gastroschisis: a new and safe technique for selected patients. J Pediatr Surg. 1994;29(9):1234–5.
44. Raghavan M, Montgomerie J. Anesthetic management of gastrochisis—a review of our practice over the past 5 years. Pediatr Anesth. 2008;18:1055–9.
45. Long AM, Court J, Morabito A, Gillham JC. Antenatal diagnosis of bowel dilatation in gastroschisis is predictive of poor postnatal outcome. J Pediatr Surg. 2011;46:1070–5.
46. Arnold MA, Chang DC, Nabaweesi R, Colombani PM, Fischer AC, Lau HT. Development and validation of a risk stratification index to predict death in gastroschisis. J Pediatr Surg. 2007;42:950–6.

# Anesthesia for Hypertrophic Pyloric Stenosis

Trung Du

## Introduction

Pyloromyotomy for HPS is the most common surgical procedure performed in infancy with a reported incidence of 0.9–5.1:1000 live births [1].

The classic historical description is of an infant in the first weeks with progressively worse, non-bilious non-bloody, projectile vomiting. The child remains desperately hungry, but with progressive dehydration and fatigue, the desire to feed wanes. On physical examination, palpation of an "olive" in the right upper quadrant of the abdomen, the hypertrophied pyloric muscle, is pathognomonic for HPS [2]. Analysis of the blood chemistry presents the triad of hypochloremia, hypokalemia and metabolic alkalosis.

In reality, the situation can be a little more variable. Presentation typically occurs between 2 and 12 weeks, with a peak at 5 weeks of age, and is more common in first-born males [3]. It is reported that up to 4% of presenting infants may have bilious vomiting, and blood may be present where the effort of emesis damages the lining of the stomach [4]. As few as 13.6% (though some historical studies suggest greater than 50%) of infants who are eventually diagnosed with HPS have a palpable olive on presentation [5]. Finally, normal blood chemistry is an increasingly common finding: 60% of 505 patients identified with HPS in a study conducted from 2008 to 2014 having no electrolytic abnormality at presentation [6].

Ultrasound imaging rather than physical examination, has been increasingly relied on as the definitive method for diagnosis. Ultrasound has proven to have high accuracy when performed by an appropriately trained physician, surgeon or radiologist, with a sensitivity and specificity of up to 99.5% and 100%, respectively [7]. A pyloric muscle thickness of 3 mm and a pyloric canal length of >15 mm is considered diagnostic of HPS [8].

This shifting reliance on ultrasound to diagnose HPS is likely to be a major factor in the early detection, and the associated reduction in the biochemical derangement that is seen in the presenting population.

## Applied Anatomy and Pathophysiology

Described by Danish Pediatrician, Harald Hirschsprung in 1888, HPS results from the progressive hypertrophy of the muscular pyloric sphincter leading to gastric obstruction and impaired emptying [9]. Since that time, while the medical community has developed a greater understanding of how to diagnose, medically manage, and surgically treat HPS, the pathophysiological cause remains elusive.

T. Du
Lady Cilento Children's Hospital, South Brisbane, QLD, Australia
e-mail: Trung.Du@health.qld.gov.au

One theory offered suggests that HPS is caused by a relative deficiency of nitric oxide synthase (NOS) [10]. The subsequently deficiency of the nitric oxide and impaired ability to relax the pyloric sphincter leads to spasm and hypertrophy. This proposition is supported by studies in mice that have demonstrated hormonal NOS inhibition can cause muscular thickening at the pyloric sphincter with resultant HPS [11].

However, in human studies, only a slightly higher occurrence of genomic variation in neuronal NOS coding, and hence NOS pathway failure, has been observed in HPS patients [12].

While the true cause remains unknown, HPS has been associated with a mixture of genetic and environmental factors. There is a male predominance of 5 to 1, and a significantly lower incidence of HPS in African and Asian populations [5, 13]. It occurs in familial cluster, with increased concordance in monozygotic twins (>200-fold likelihood) [14]. Interestingly, as birth order increases the risk of HPS decreases [15].

Maternal factors associated with greater incidence are hyperthyroidism, smoking, young age, high pre-pregnancy BMI, exposure to macrolide antibiotic, and use of nasal decongestants [16]. Babies that are bottle fed are more likely to develop HPS compared to their breast-fed counterparts [17].

## Surgical Options

Pyloromyotomy was originally described by the German surgeon, Conrad Ramstedt in 1912 [18]. It involves longitudinal division of the pyloric muscle down to the level of the mucosa, with the incision extending from the limits of the circular fibers of the stomach to the vein of Mayo at the duodenum end. Resolution of the mechanical obstruction, and absence of leak from inadvertent perforation is tested by injecting air into the stomach and ensuring passage only into the duodenum.

Prior to this, pyloric dilation, pyloroplasty and gastroenterostomy to bypass the obstruction had been performed for HPS with poor surgical outcomes. With the advent and adoption of pyloromyotomy as a curative procedure, mortality from HPS is exceeding low (<0.3%) [19].

A supraumbilical surgical approach may be preferred by the surgeon for cosmetic purposes. However, this may be stymied by difficulty in delivering the pylorus into a more distant wound opening, with the attendant risks of serosal tears or need to extend the original incision [20].

Pyloromyotomy via laparoscopic surgery in the infant offers the advantage of smaller incisions (and hence a reduced likelihood for pain and scarring), and a shorter hospital stay, with a more rapid return to feeding, bowel function and normal activity when compared to the equivalent open technique [21]. Advancement in surgical techniques have led to the development of the microlaparoscopic pyloromyotomy, and single incision laparoscopic techniques with the view of further improving cosmetic outcomes and reducing complication rates.

Laparoscopic surgery in the infant attracts some important anesthetic considerations. On initiation of pneumoperitoneum or with the insertion of trochars, the higher vagal tone in the pediatric patient exposes them to a greater risk of bradycardia and asystole than adults. This risk can be reduced by a more gradual insufflation of gas [22].

Intraoperative inflation pressures as low as 6 cm $H_2O$ (though up to 12 cm $H_2O$ may be required) can facilitate successful surgery. Endeavoring to have the procedure complete at the lowest viable pressure reduces the potential for: cardiovascular instability from reduced cardiac output, impairment of ventilation from reduced thoracic compliance, and tube migration with endobronchial intubation upwards displacement of the diaphragm and lungs [22].

While carbon dioxide pneumoperitoneum for the duration of the procedure has been shown to cause a gradual increase in blood pressure and end tidal carbon dioxide, this is well tolerated by the infant without deleterious alteration of regional brain oxygenation [23].

There exists a slightly greater risk of incomplete myotomy (1.17% vs. 0.29%), and perforation (0.83% vs. 0.29%) when comparing the laparoscopic technique to open techniques [24, 25].

Regardless of which technique is chosen, pyloromyotomy has the least number complications where it is performed by a specialist pediatric surgeon at a tertiary level pediatric hospital [26]. Given its non-emergent nature, there is little reason to attempt it outside this setting.

## Non-surgical options

Atropine sulphate purportedly reduces pyloric spasm, and is an effective medical treatment option that has a reported success rate of 88%. However, this treatment option requires the child to be hospitalized for intravenous feeding until the resolution of the mechanical obstruction. A study of 19 infants found that an average of 13 days (with a range of 6–20 days) of intravenous atropine treatment was needed [27]. With oral atropine, 4–6 weeks of treatment are required to be effective [28]. In both studies there was a small (10% and 25%, respectively) but not insignificant rate of infants that failed medical treatment and required pyloromyotomy.

Taking into consideration the low rates of complication, and the high rate of success of surgery, and comparing that to the high resource and time cost of treatment with atropine, it would seem the latter would only be preferable where the infant state of health made anesthesia or surgery untenable.

## Pre-operative Evaluation

HPS does not constitute a surgical emergency and operative treatments should be delayed until the infant has been adequately resuscitated. While the patient population is young, the majority are born at term and HPS is not associated with other congenital abnormalities or organ dysfunction.

## Correction of Electrolytes

The primary focus is correction of the biochemical derangement and dehydration. The gastric outlet obstruction is at the level of the pylorus, therefore the vomitus is lacking the usual alkaline secretion from the small bowel. Hypochloremia, and hypokalemia results from loss of chloride, potassium, sodium and hydrogen ions from repeated episodes of vomiting.

The observed metabolic alkalosis is multifactorial. There are gastric losses of hydrogen ions in the vomitus. Renal homeostasis is perturbed, with bicarbonate reabsorbed in the setting of low chloride to maintain electroneutrality. Similarly, sodium is reabsorbed in exchange for hydrogen ions, with a paradoxical aciduria resulting [13].

Multiple regimes have been formulated to correct the dehydration and biochemical anomalies observed in HPS. A continuous infusion approach is preferred to the episodic boluses administered in some institutions. However, neither approach has been demonstrated to be superior, with most infants achieving adequate resuscitation and operative readiness within 24 h of presentation [29].

When gauging the adequacy of resuscitation, chloride or the bicarbonate levels is often used as the decisive value in determining the endpoint. The cut off values chosen are largely based on expert consensus rather than any clear evidence base [30].

Similarly, there is limited guidance in the literature as to the degree to which the metabolic alkalosis needs to be corrected to permit safe anesthesia. However, alkalemia (and concomitant alkalosis of the cerebral spinal fluid), may impair respiratory drive in the perioperative period, and reduce cerebral oxygenation under anesthesia [31].

More recently, Dalton conducted a regression analysis of 542 cases suggesting that chloride is a more sensitive and specific indicator of adequacy of resuscitation than bicarbonate [6]. The study defined a normal electrolyte profile as a chloride of >100 mmol/L, bicarbonate of <30 mmol/L and a potassium of <3.4 or >5.2 mmol/L, which is in keep with a prevailing expert opinion.

Dalton found that to achieve a normal chloride level, most infants with chloride less that 85 mmol/L on arrival required 3 × 20 mL/kg saline boluses, while those with chloride with less than 97 mmol/L required 2 × 20 mL/kg saline boluses. The fluid boluses were given at hourly intervals.

Where chloride was normal, a bicarbonate of ≥40 required 3 × 20 mL/kg saline bolus, and bicarbonate of ≥33 2 × 20 mL/kg saline boluses for correction. Milder derangements in chloride, bicarbonate and potassium were treated with a single saline bolus of 20 mL/kg. Confirmatory lab tests were only drawn after the prescribed fluid regime was completed.

This strategy not only predicted the volume required for resuscitation, and reduced the number of unnecessary lab draws, but also reduced the delays in clinical care that occur while waiting for labs values to become available to guide therapy.

Yanchar found that once acceptable blood chemistry has been achieved, it is unlikely to deviate from the acceptable range and further rechecking just prior to surgery is probably unnecessarily cautious [32].

## Anesthesia Considerations

Standard anesthesia monitoring should be instituted for induction, with particular care being paid to the temperature management of the child. A forced air warming blanket with temperature guided by rectal temperatures is a straightforward approach.

## Management of Aspiration Risk

With mechanical obstruction at the pylorus, the accumulation of gastric fluids poses an increased risk of aspiration on induction of anesthesia. The amount of accumulated gastric fluid is independent of the presence of a pre-operative nasogastric tube, or duration of fasting. Blind suctioning of the infant in supine and decubitus positions is recommended, but cannot be relied on to completely empty the stomach. Cook-Sather found infants had 1–1.8 mL/kg remaining in the stomach despite blind suctioning [33].

While administration of an atropine has been advocated to blunt the vagal response to suctioning, and pre-empt the possible bradycardias that may occur on intubation, safe practice has been demonstrated without its use [34].

Previously, awake endotracheal intubation was a common practice, however this technique may be complicated by bradycardia, laryngospasm, hypoxia, aspiration, and trauma to the airway. In a study comparing it to RSI, it was shown to expose the infant to a greater risk of prolonged or failed intubation. In the absence of any clear advantage, this technique should be avoided [35].

Classic rapid sequence induction (RSI), with pre-oxygenation, avoidance of apneic ventilation, administration of suxamethonium, and the application of cricoid pressure to compress the esophagus during intubation, also has attendant difficulties in the infant population.

With the infant's high oxygen consumption, and a high closing capacity relative to their functional residual capacity, rapid desaturation after induction but prior to muscle relaxation being adequate for intubation. This can happen despite attempts to pre-oxygenate the child.

When applied incorrectly, cricoid pressure can distort the anatomy, and increase difficulty in ventilation and intubation. The clinical value of cricoid pressure in reducing reflux of gastric contents continues to erode in the adult population, and should be also be reevaluated in the pediatric sphere [36].

Alternative RSI techniques have been described that offer a greater margin of safety for the induction of pediatric patients. Neuhaus advocates a controlled RSI, with bag-valve mask ventilation (<10 to 12 cm $H_2O$), avoidance of cricoid pressure, and the administration of a non-depolarizing muscle relaxant. In a retrospective review of 1001 pediatric patient (including 64 infants) undergoing intubation with this controlled RSI technique, a smaller incidence of desaturation, and bradycardia was observed compared to classic RSI. It was found to offered better intubating conditions and there was no greater aspiration risk seen [37].

Successful inhalation induction has been reported by Scimgeour. Across an 8 year period, 252 patients with HPS underwent inhalational induction with sevoflurane and nitrous [38]. There were no reports of aspiration, but the study was not designed nor powered to demonstrate increased safety compared to RSI. In addition, the need to perform an inhalation induction in a child who almost universally presents for anesthesia with intravenous access has been questioned [39]. The value of this technique may be limited to a small population of infants where securing intravenous (or intraosseous) access is as undesirable prior to induction of anesthesia.

## Drug Selection

Inadequate sedation and paralysis on induction, can lead to lead to laryngospasm, hypoxia, bradycardia and delayed or failed intubation [35].

In the absence of other risk factors, reports of complications to suxamethonium are rare, and it continues to offer the advantage of rapid onset and offset of muscle relaxation for RSI. Rocuronium at 1.2 mg/kg can offer good intubating, in a similar time frame, however, the overall duration of action may be undesirable. This consequence can be mitigated with the availability of the reversal agent, sugammadex. Indeed, Plaud demonstrated that sugammadex (2 mg/kg) produced more rapid reversal, 0.6 min for a train-of-four ratio of 0.9, in the infant population compared to the older groups, where 1.1–1.2 min were necessary [40].

Alternatively, a smaller dose of rocuronium (0.3–0.7 mg/kg) can be used on induction with the understanding that there will be will be a delay before complete muscle relaxation occurs, and some oxygenation and ventilation with the bag-valve-mask will be required. This may theoretically expose the infant to a greater risk of aspiration [41].

Whatever drug choice is made for muscle relaxation, it important to be aware that the neonatal and infant population exhibit a greater sensitivity to neuromuscular blocking agent [42]. Judicious dosing as well as routine administration of reversal agents at the end of the case are advised.

Propofol is the predominant hypnotic agent in use in the western world, and is thought to offer a more rapid recovery profile with fewer cardio-respiratory complications that its predecessor, thiopentone. Westrin found that a larger dose of propofol (3.0 ± 0.2 mL/kg) are needed to achieve loss of lid reflex in children aged 1–6 months, as compared to the 10–16 year old group (2.4 ± 0.1 mL/kg) [43]. Both thiopentone and propofol can cause hypotension, and this may be more marked in infant who has been inadequately resuscitated.

While less commonly used and studied, ketamine appears safe and effective in the neonatal and infant population [44]. It may offer greater hemodynamic stability with its sympathomimetic effects serving to maintain heart rate, and blood pressure.

Inhalational anesthesia is commonly used as maintenance for this procedure. While sevoflurane is the most common agent currently in use, emergence and extubation in this population is prolonged when compared to the use of desflurane at the same MAC. In that study, it was found that there was no difference in apnea risk between the two volatile agents [45].

Nitrous can cause expansion of bowel gas, and it's use in maintenance should be particularly avoided for infants with an obstructive pathology.

Intraoperative and post-operative analgesia with acetaminophen and the addition of non-steroidal anti-inflammatory agents (NSAIDs), if necessary, are usually sufficient to treat the limited surgical pain that is caused by pyloromotomy. There seems to be no advantage offered by intravenous (7.6 ± 1.8 mg/kg) as compared to rectal (30.2 + 5.5 mg/kg) administration of acetaminophen [30]. Some reluctance with NSAIDs usage persist given the risk of decreased renal perfusion, platelet dysfunction, and increased pulmonary pressures [46].

Systemic analgesics can be augmented by infiltration of long acting local anesthesia at the wound site, or as part of a regional anesthetic technique. Intraoperative opiates are best avoided in the perioperative period in this population to avoid increasing the risk of post-operative apneas.

## Regional Techniques

Regional techniques have been employed successfully as the sole anesthetic technique, as an adjuncts to general anesthesia and as component of the postoperative analgesia regime.

Both spinal and single shot epidural, as the sole anesthetic with or without endotracheal intubation, has been used to facilitate open and laparoscopic pyloromyotomy. This technique reportedly consumes less time in the operating room, with a more rapid delivery of infant to surgical readiness as well as a more rapid emergence and exit from the operation room [47–49].

Single-shot rectus sheath, para-vertebral, and end of case caudal blocks have been performed as adjuncts to general anesthesia and can reduce the need for the administration of muscle relaxants or opiates, and permit earlier extubation at the completion of surgery.

A potential benefit of a pure regional technique is avoidance of apnea, as well as the potential neurotoxic effects of general anesthesia on the developing brain. However, the GAS trial, concerned with inguinal hernia repair in a similarly aged population undergoing a procedure of similar length, reports that while early apnea (0–30 min) was less common (1% vs. 3%), the incidence of late apneas (up to 12 h post op) was the same [50].

When measured 2 years later, neurodevelopment outcomes for the cohort were unchanged compared to matched controls. This is consistent with the finding of the recent multicenter PANDA study investing cognitive outcomes after general anesthesia in infants [51].

**Table 42.1** Checklist of perioperative management of infants with pyloric stenosis presenting for pyloromyotomy

| Plan/preparation/adverse events | Reasoning/management |
|---|---|
| For optimal outcomes, where practicable, the infant should be transferred to have their surgery at a dedicated pediatric center by a specialist pediatric surgeon | Pyloromyotomy is not a surgical emergency<br>Resuscitation and correction of biochemical derangement is the priority |
| Preprocedural evaluation<br>  Biochemistry<br>  Adequacy of resuscitation<br>  Reduction of gastric volume<br>  Administration of atropine | Commonly accepted biochemical endpoints are, chloride of $\geq 100$ mmol/L, and bicarbonate of $\leq 30$ mmol/L<br>Preoperative suctioning of the infant's stomach immediately prior to induction reduces the volume of gastric contents that could reflux<br>Common practice to prevent bradycardia on laryngoscopy, with little supporting evidence |
| General anesthesia<br>  Rapid sequence induction (RSI)<br>  Gas induction<br>Regional<br>  Spinal, caudal, and thoracic epidural without endotracheal intubation<br>  Rectus sheath, paravertebral and end of case caudal | RSI with intravenous access remains the most common induction method. Gentle ventilation on induction can reduce the likelihood and severity of hypoxia. Succinylcholine may be preferred due to its rapid onset and limited duration of activity<br>Gas induction without complication has been reported, but is not been proven to be superior<br>Additional anesthesia interventions are reportedly required in 4–25% of intended sole spinal anesthesia<br>Regional can also be used as an adjunct for post-operative analgesia |
| Procedural adverse events<br>  Aspiration<br>  Hypotension (from poor resuscitation)<br>  Bradycardia | The risk of adverse events under laparoscopy can be reduced by minimizing pneumoperitoneum pressures. Aim for <12 mmHg |
| Postoperative and post-discharge considerations<br>  Post-operative apneas<br>  Post-operative analgesia | Post-operative apnea is more common in this age group. The risk may be more pronounced due to persisting metabolic alkalosis, the use of peri-operative opiate analgesia, or anemia (hemoglobin <10 g/dL)<br>Wound infiltration with local anesthesia and non-opiate analgesia is typically adequate |

## Conclusion

While the cause of HPS remains unknown, treatment with pyloromyotomy has made infant mortality from this pathological process an extremely rare occurrence. The use of ultrasound has led to earlier diagnosis and an associated reduction in the of biochemical anomalies found in infants on presentation. Fluid resuscitation and correction of chloride to >100 mmol/L, and bicarbonate to <30 is desirable prior to having surgery. Perioperative considerations are summarized in Table 42.1.

While there is no consensus for the optimal plan for management of the aspiration risk during induction for HPS infants, RSI with controlled ventilation seems like a reasonable compromise between the risk of desaturation on induction and the risk of aspiration. Awake intubation should be avoided, and inhalation induction seems reserved for very specialized circumstances.

HPS surgery is generally short in duration, and medication and dose selection for induction muscle relaxation needs careful consideration. For laparoscopic procedures cardiorespiratory embarrassment can be lessened by maintaining low abdominal insufflation pressures.

Regional anesthesia for HPS is a viable sole anesthetic or may be used as an adjunct to general anesthesia. In experienced hands it seems to offer greater operating room efficiencies than a general anesthetic technique.

Opiate usage in this population may increase the risk of apneas in the perioperative period, and acetaminophen and NSAIDS may be adequate analgesia in combination with local infiltration or regional block.

Current evidence suggests that brief anesthesia for infants to undergo pyloromyotomy does not cause any neurodevelopmental delay.

## References

1. MacMahon B. The continuing enigma of pyloricstenosis of infancy: a review. Epidemiology. 2006;17:195–201.
2. de Laffolie J, Turial S, Heckmann M, Zimmer KP, Schier F. Decline in infantile hypertrophic pyloric stenosis in Germany in 2000–2008. Pediatrics. 2012;129:e901–6.
3. Aboagye J, Goldstein SD, Salazar JH, et al. Age at presentation of common pediatric surgical conditions: re-examining dogma. J Pediatr Surg. 2014;49:995–9.
4. Piroutek MJ, Brown L, Thorp AW. Bilious vomiting does not rule out infantile hypertrophic pyloric stenosis. Clin Pediatr (Phila). 2012;51(3):214–8. https://doi.org/10.1177/0009922811431159. Epub 2011 Dec 12.
5. Glatsein M, Carbell G, Boddu SK. The changing clinical presentation of hypertrophic pyloric stenosis: the experience of a large, tertiary care pediatric hospital. Clin Pediatr. 2011;50:192–5.
6. Dalton BG, Gonzalez KW, Boda S, Thomas PG, Sherman AK, St Peter SD. Optimizing fluid resuscitation in hypertrophic pyloric stenosis. J Pediatr Surg. 2016;51(8):1279–82. https://doi.org/10.1016/j.jpedsurg.2016.01.013. Epub 2016 Feb 3.
7. White MC, Langer JC, Don S, et al. Sensitivity and cost minimization analysis of radiology versus palpation for the diagnosis of hypertrophic pyloric stenosis. J Pediatr Surg. 1998;33:913–7.
8. Hernanz-Schulman M. Pyloric stenosis: role of imaging. Pediatr Radiol. 2009;39:S134–9.
9. Hirschsprung H. Falle von angeborener pyloric stenose. Jahrb Kinderhik. 1888;27:61.
10. Kusafuka T, Puri P. Altered messenger RNA expression of the neuronal nitric oxide synthase gene in infantile hypertrophic pyloric stenosis. Pediatr Surg Int. 1997;12:576–9.
11. Boybeyi O, Soyer T, Atasoy P, Gunal YD, Aslan MK. Investigation of the effects of enteral hormones on the pyloric muscle in newborn rats. J Pediatr Surg. 2015;50:408–12.
12. Serra A, Schuchardt K, Genuneit J, Leriche C, Fitze G. Genomic variants in the coding region of neuronal nitric oxide synthase (NOS1) in infantile hypertrophic pyloric stenosis. J Pediatr Surg. 2011;46:1903–8.
13. Aspelund G, Langer JC. Current management of hypertrophic pyloric stenosis. Semin Pediatr Surg. 2007;16:27–33.
14. Krogh C, Fischer TK, Skotte L, Biggar RJ, Øyen N, Skytthe A, et al. Familial aggregation and heritability of pyloric stenosis. JAMA. 2010;303(23):2393.
15. Gladstein K, Spence MA. A statistical analysis of birth-order effects with application to data on pyloric stenosis. Ann Hum Genet. 1978;42:213–7.
16. Vermes GG, László D, Czeizel A, Acs N. Maternal factors in the origin of infantile hypertrophic pyloric stenosis—a population-based case-control study. Congenit Anom. 2016;56(2):65–72.
17. Krogh C, Biggar RJ, Fischer TK, Lindholm M, Wohlfahrt J, Melbye M. Bottle-feeding and the risk of pyloric stenosis. Pediatrics. 2012;130:e943–9.
18. Rammstedt C. Zur operation der angeborenen pylorus stenose. Med Klin. 1912;8:1702–5.
19. Perger L, Fuchs JR, Komidar L, Mooney DP. Impact of surgical approach on outcome in 622 consecutive

19. pyloromyotomies at a paediatric teaching institution. J Pediatr Surg. 2009;44:2119–25.
20. Eltayeb AA, Othman MH. Supraumbilical pyloromyotomy: a comparative study between intracavitary and extracavitary techniques. J Surg Educ. 2011;68:134–7.
21. Pelizzo G, Bernardi L, Carlini V, et al. Laparoscopy in children and its impact on brain oxygenation during routine inguinal hernia repair. J Minim Access Surg. 2017;13(1):51–6. https://doi.org/10.4103/0972-9941.181800.
22. Gupta R, Singh S. Challenges in paediatric laparoscopic surgeries. Indian J Anaesth. 2009;53(5):560–6.
23. Tytgat SH, Stolwijk LJ, Keunen K, Milstein DM, Lemmers PM, van der Zee DC. Brain oxygenation during laparoscopic correction of hypertrophicpyloric stenosis. J Laparoendosc Adv Surg Tech A. 2015;25:352–7.
24. Hall NJ, Van Der Zee J, Tan L, Pierro A. Meta-analysis of laparoscopic versus open pyloromyotomy. Ann Surg. 2004;240:774–8.
25. Hall NJ, Eaton S, Seims A, et al. Risk of incomplete pyloromyotomy and mucosal perforation in open and laparoscopic pyloromyotomy. J Pediatr Surg. 2014;49:1083–6.
26. Ednie AC, Amram O, Creaser JC, Schuurman N, Leclerc S, Yanchar N. Hypertrophic pyloric stenosis in the maritimes: examining the waves of change over time. Can J Surg. 2016;59(6):383–90. https://doi.org/10.1503/cjs.002816.
27. Kawahara H, Takama Y, Yoshida H, et al. Medical treatment of hypertrophic pyloric stenosis: should we always slice the olive? J Pediatr Surg. 2005;40:1848–51.
28. Lukac M, Antunovic SS, Vujovic D, et al. Is abandonment of nonoperative management of hypertrophic pyloric stenosis warranted? Eur J Pediatr Surg. 2013;23:80–4.
29. Peters B, Oomen MW, Bakx R, Benninga MA. Advances in infantile hypertrophic pyloric stenosis. Expert Rev Gastroenterol Hepatol. 2014;8:533–41.
30. Kamata M, Cartabuke RS, Tobias JD. Perioperative care of infants with pyloric stenosis. Paediatr Anaesth. 2015;25:1193–206. https://doi.org/10.1111/pan.12792.
31. Nissen M, Cernaianu G, Thranhardt R, Vahad M, Barenberg K, et al. Does metabolic alkalosis influence cerebral oxygenation in infantile hypertrophic pyloric stenosis. J Surg Res. 212:229–37.
32. Yanchar NL, Rangu S. Corrected to uncorrected? The metabolic conundrum of hypertrophic pyloric stenosis. J Pediatr Surg. 2017;52(5):734–8. https://doi.org/10.1016/j.jpedsurg.2017.01.024. Epub 2017 Jan 28.
33. Cook-Sather SD, Tulloch HV, Liacouras CA, et al. Gastric fluid volume in infants for pyloromyotomy. Can J Anaesth. 1997;44:278–83.
34. Fastle RK, Roback MG. Pediatric rapid sequence intubation: incidence of reflex bradycardia and effects of pretreatment with atropine. Pediatr Emerg Care. 2004;20(10):651–5.
35. Cook-Sather SD, Tulloch HV, Cnaan A, et al. A comparison of awake versus paralyzed tracheal intubation for infants with pyloric stenosis. Anesth Analg. 1998;86:945–51.
36. Algie CM, Mahar RK, Tan HB, et al. Effectiveness and risks of cricoid pressure during rapid sequence induction for endotracheal intubation. Cochrane Database Syst Rev. 2015;(11):CD011656. Published online 2015 Nov 18.
37. Neuhaus D, Schmitz A, Gerber A. Controlled rapid sequence induction and intubation—an analysis of 1001 children. Pediatr Anesth. 2013;23:734–40.
38. Scrimgeour GE, Leather NW, Perry RS, et al. Gas induction for pyloromyotomy. Pediatr Anesth. 2015;25:677–80.
39. Wang JT, Mancuso TJ. How to best induce anesthesia in infants with pyloric stenosis? Paediatr Anaesth. 2015;25(7):652–3. https://doi.org/10.1111/pan.12690.
40. Plaud B, Meretoja O, Hofmockel R, et al. Reversal of rocuronium-induced neuromuscular blockade with sugammadex in pediatric and adult surgical patients. Anesthesiology. 2009;110:284–94.
41. Bouvet L, Albert ML, Augris C, Boselli E, et al. Real-time detection of gastric insufflation related to facemask pressure–controlled ventilation using ultrasonography of the antrum and epigastric auscultation in nonparalyzed patients: a prospective, randomized, double-blind study. Anesthesiology. 2014;120(2):326–34.
42. Saldien V, Vermeyen KM, Wuyts FL. Target-controlled infusion of rocuronium in infants, children, and adults: a comparison of the pharmacokinetic and pharmacodynamic relationship. Anesth Analg. 2003;97:44–9.
43. Westrin P. The induction dose of propofol in infants 1-6 months of age and in children 10-16 years of age. Anesthesiology. 1991;74:455–8.
44. Pani N, Panda CK. Anaesthetic consideration for neonatal surgical emergencies. Indian J Anaesth. 2012;56(5):463–9. https://doi.org/10.4103/0019-5049.103962.
45. Sale SM, Read JA, Stoddart PA, et al. Prospective comparison of sevoflurane and desflurane in formerly premature infants undergoing inguinal herniotomy. Br J Anaesth. 2006;96:774–8.
46. Haidon JL, Cunliffe M. Analgesia for neonates. Contin Educ Anaesth Crit Care Pain. 2010;10(4):123–7. https://doi.org/10.1093/bjaceaccp/mkq016.
47. Willschke H, Machata AM, Rebhandl W, et al. Management of hypertrophic pylorus stenosis with ultrasound guided single shot epidural anaesthesia-a retrospective analysis of 20 cases. Pediatr Anesth. 2011;21:110–5.

48. Somri M, Gaitini LA, Vaida SJ, et al. The effectiveness and safety of spinal anaesthesia in the pyloromyotomy procedure. Paediatr Anaesth. 2003;13:32–7.
49. Islam S, Larson SD, Kays DW, et al. Feasibility of laparoscopic pyloromyotomy under spinal anesthesia. J Pediatr Surg. 2014;49:1485–7.
50. Davidson AJ, Morton NS, Arnup SJ, et al. Apnea after awake-regional and general anesthesia in infants: the general anesthesia compared to spinal anesthesia (GAS) study: comparing apnea and neurodevelopmental outcomes, a randomized controlled trial. Anesthesiology. 2015;123(1):38–54.
51. Sun LS, Li G, DiMaggio CJ, et al. Feasibility and Pilot Study of the Pediatric Anesthesia NeuroDevelopment Assessment (PANDA) Project. J Neurosurg Anesthesiol. 2012;24(4):382–8.

# Anesthesia for Intestinal Obstruction

## 43

Ilana Fromer and Kumar G. Belani

## Introduction

Acute intestinal obstruction is not uncommon in newborns, infants and children. In newborns, intestinal obstruction most often presents within the first few days of life—generally recognized as a failure to pass meconium—and is almost always a surgical emergency following optimization of electrolyte and fluid status. Most causes of intestinal obstruction in the newborn are congenital with the most common being imperforate anus, duodenal and jejunoileal atresias, Hirschsprung's disease, and malrotation with volvulus. Although less common than in the neonatal period, infants and older children may also present with signs and symptoms of intestinal obstruction necessitating surgical correction and anesthesia. Pyloric stenosis (which will be discussed in its own chapter) is a frequent reason for intestinal obstruction in the older infant followed by intussusception, malrotation, incarcerated hernias, and acute appendicitis.

Intestinal obstruction in the pediatric patient will often present itself as a surgical emergency, leaving the anesthesiologist with little time to prepare. Although there are many different etiologies of intestinal obstruction, the pathophysiology is comparable, requiring similar anesthetic considerations, goals, and principles of care (see figure) [1].

## Neonatal Intestinal Obstruction

Intestinal obstruction in the newborn is a common reason for admission to neonatal ICU's with an approximate incidence of 1/2000 [2]. Most often the obstruction is due to congenital rather than acquired causes and is usually recognized early in the postnatal period. However, a delay in diagnosis can be detrimental. Symptoms and signs of obstruction can range from mild vomiting and distention to intestinal perforation with infection, bowel necrosis, sepsis, and respiratory distress in the newborn. While a timely surgical intervention is crucial, optimization of the patient's metabolic status is of primary importance and should not be delayed until after surgery. Although there are several different underlying causes of bowel obstruction in the newborn—the most common of which will be discussed in this chapter—it is important to note perioperative and anesthetic care follows similar guidelines and principles.

Ano-rectal malformations are among the more common congenital malformations in the neonate. Etiology is unknown and most likely multifactorial. The incidence of these malformations is approximately 1:2000 to 1:5000 live

---

I. Fromer, M.D. (✉) · K. G. Belani, M.B.B.S., M.S.
Department of Anesthesiology, University of Minnesota, Masonic Children's Hospital, Minneapolis, MN, USA

births and ranges from complete anal atresia (otherwise referred to as an imperforate anus) to a mild stenosis [3]. If there is total bowel obstruction, as seen more commonly in male infants, surgical treatment is an emergency. If this occurs it is important to consider the presence of associated anomalies in the neonate. The incidence of associated anomalies ranges from 45 to 65%, with cardiac, renal, and skeletal anomalies (as part of the VACTERL association) the most common [3, 4]. Anesthetic management will vary depending on the severity of the lesion and complexity of the planned surgery that can range from a simple anoplasty to a diverting colostomy with or without an extensive intraabdominal repair. In most instances the surgeons prefer a staged procedure [3, 5].

Duodenal atresia occurs in 1/5000–1/10,000 live births [6] with an increased frequency in males vs. females. Although duodenal atresia can exist as a singular anomaly, more than half are associated with other significant anomalies. Down's Syndrome is present in roughly 30% of cases and congenital heart disease will be present in another 20–30% [6, 7]. Currently, duodenal atresia is usually diagnosed in utero via a fetal ultrasound as early as the late second or early third trimester, most commonly after the mother presents with polyhydramnios. When not diagnosed prenatally, the classic presentation is usually an otherwise stable newborn with bilious emesis and the characteristic "double bubble" sign on abdominal radiograph. Once diagnosis has been made, prompt treatment with gastric decompression and intravenous fluids should be achieved [2, 6]. Surgical intervention can either be done laparoscopically or by open duodenoduodenostomy. A delay in treatment and/or diagnosis may progress to dehydration and subsequently hypochloremic alkalosis.

Jejunoileal atresia (JIA) can cause obstruction and occurs in 1:5000 live births. Although the triggering factors are unknown it is thought to arise from intrauterine vascular events [2]. The clinical presentation can be variable and depends on the anatomic location of the obstruction, and may present similar to duodenal atresia if the lesion is more proximal. JIA is often diagnosed using ultrasonography showing distended bowel or abdominal radiographs showing dilated intestinal loops and air-fluid levels [8]. Maternal polyhydramnios has been reported in approximately 20% of babies with this congenital disorder with up to 50% being born prematurely [8, 9]. Unlike duodenal atresia, the presence of other anomalies or syndromes is not as common due to its occurrence in later fetal development. Despite this, gastrointestinal malformations (including gastroschisis and omphalocele) are noted in 25–35% of cases and 10–15% are associated with cystic fibrosis [8, 9]. JIA and stenosis are classified into four different types grouped by location and severity of the lesion, although more than one lesion may be found in up to 25% of babies [2]. Treatment should proceed with gastric decompression, IV fluids, and antibiotics to avoid metabolic disturbances. Surgery, although not always emergent, should be expeditious and will depend on the pathologic findings and circumstances of each case.

Meconium ileus (MI) is a distal luminal obstruction of the bowel caused by abnormally thickened meconium. It has an estimated incidence of 2–6 per 1000 live births a year [10] and accounts for 10–30% of neonatal intestinal obstructions [11], though it can also present later in life as well. Meconium ileus is almost always unique to patients with cystic fibrosis (CF), however, only 13–17% of CF patients will present with MI at birth [10]. Diagnosis is usually made after a newborn has failed to pass meconium in the first 1–2 days of life and frequently abdominal distention will be present along with "palpable doughy bowel loops" [11]. Unlike the earlier mentioned causes of neonatal intestinal obstruction, patients usually do not exhibit symptoms of abdominal tenderness or respiratory distress. Radiographs may indicate the typical "ground glass" appearance from swallowed air and dilated loops of bowel, but air-fluid levels are usually absent [2, 11]. Often the family history will be positive for CF. Once diagnosis has been made, treatment is initially begun non-operatively with a water-soluble contrast enema to loosen and soften the meconium in order to enable evacuation. Adequate IV hydration should be maintained in conjunction with this procedure [6]. If there is no progress after 2–3 attempts, a surgical intervention is indicated [2] usually involving irrigation of the meconium via an enterotomy until the bowel is cleared [2, 6]. Because meconium ileus usually manifests in the neonatal period, respiratory symptoms of cystic fibrosis are typically not present nor of clinical concern to the anesthesia care team at this time.

Congenital aganglionic megacolon, commonly known as Hirschsprung's disease (HD), is the most common congenital neurointestinal disease with an incidence estimated to be 1/5000 live births [12]. It results from the failure of the enteric neural crest cells to complete their migration leaving the distal end of the bowel (usually the rectum or sigmoid colon) devoid of motility and unable to relax causing a distal bowel obstruction [12]. Hirschsprung's disease is associated with other genetic abnormalities in roughly 20% of cases, and is most commonly associated with trisomy 21 found in 4–16% of all patients with HD [2]. Approximately 90% of children are diagnosed during the neonatal period because of failure to pass meconium in the first couple days of life. Diagnosis usually involves abdominal films revealing dilated loops of bowel and a contrast enema demonstrating a transition zone between the proximal dilated bowel and the aganglionic dilated rectum. However, a definitive diagnosis can only be made with a rectal biopsy (usually done at bedside without anesthesia) showing an absence of ganglionic cells. Surgical correction remains the mainstay of treatment, most commonly a transanal endorectal pull-through, often with laparoscopic assistance.

## Intestinal Obstruction in Infants

Malrotation is an early embryologic aberrancy resulting in an abnormal rotation of the bowel. It is often associated with areas of ischemia, atresia, and obstruction. Malrotation itself is not a surgical emergency, however, when associated with midgut volvulus—a twisting of the intestine causing an obstruction—it requires immediate surgical correction and if not recognized early can have catastrophic results [13, 14]. Malrotation is infrequently diagnosed prenatally with most cases discovered within the first month of life and nearly 90% by the first year of life [15]. Although the incidence is predicted to be around 1/6000 live births, autopsy studies suggest it may be as high as 1/200 births postulating that many patients enter adulthood undiagnosed [2, 15]. Malrotation is only weakly associated with other genetic or chromosomal abnormalities, however, it is present in the majority of children with heterotaxia syndromes [16] and is almost always present in conjunction with congenital diaphragmatic hernia, gastroschisis, and omphalocele [14] though volvulus is rare in these cases.

The classic presentation of a neonate with malrotation and volvulus is almost always bilious vomiting, many in the first 10 days of life [17], and a diagnostic workup should be done immediately so as not to delay treatment if clinical suspicion is strong. In infants and children clinical presentation of malrotation is often vague and maybe be either acute or chronic, usually including non-specific symptoms such as diarrhea, constipation, abdominal pain, and/or failure to thrive. In these cases, an upper gastrointestinal series is the preferred diagnostic study and surgical correction with either an open or a laparoscopic Ladd procedure involving a counterclockwise detorsion of the bowel and excision of the peritoneal "Ladd bands" is the preferred treatment [2, 18].

Intussusception occurs when a segment of proximal bowel telescopes into the adjacent segment of distal bowel often resulting in obstruction. It can occur in both the small and large intestine [19] and is the most common form of intestinal obstruction in infancy and early childhood (most often 4 months to 2 years) with peak incidence between 4 and 9 months and an almost 2:1 male preponderance [19–21]. Although earlier studies suggested incidence to be as high as 1/1000 live births, a world-wide literature review published in 2013 estimated incidence to be much lower, occurring in only 74 of 100,000 live births, although varying substantially by region [21]. The etiology of intussusception is almost always idiopathic with only 10% found to be associated with an anatomical pathology such as Meckel's diverticulum or an intestinal lymphadenopathy [19, 20]. Clinical presentation of intussusception has classically been described as a triad of abdominal pain, vomiting, and blood and mucus "currant jelly" in stool, however, in more than 2/3 of patients, presentation is often nebulous and non-specific making diagnosis difficult [19, 20, 22]. If left untreated, the bowel can become gangrenous resulting in perforation and sepsis. In 85–90% of cases this condition will resolve after reduction with either ultrasound or fluoroscopic guided fluoroscopic air or contrast enema [19, 23] done without the need for sedation or general anesthesia. If this is not successful or there is evidence of bowel necrosis, urgent laparoscopic or open surgical intervention will be necessary.

## Preoperative and Intraoperative Anesthetic Concerns for Intestinal Obstruction in Neonates and Infants

Prior to any planned elective or emergent procedure, it is important to understand the underlying type and cause of intestinal obstruction and its possible correlation to other syndromes and/or chromosomal abnormalities, as these may have a large influence on anesthetic care. If necessary, a cardiac workup including echocardiography should be done to rule-out any significant form of congenital heart disease prior to the induction of anesthesia.

Anesthetic management should focus on the patient's clinical status and the type of surgical intervention to be performed. If the child is septic or in shock, he or she should be optimized prior to induction of anesthesia. Correcting electrolyte and fluid deficits is one of the principal anesthesia concerns. Restoration of an adequate vascular fluid volume is critical to preserve cardiovascular stability, organ perfusion and tissue oxygenation.

Normotonic replacement fluid should be used along with crystalloid or colloid boluses—usually 10–20 mL/kg [24]. If surgery is to proceed with an open laparotomy, the exposed bowel will lead to insensible fluid losses and aggressive fluid resuscitation is critical. Third space losses are estimated to be around 15–20 mL/kg/h in open abdominal procedures and up to 50 mL/kg/h in premature infants with a septic bowel [24]. If blood loss is a risk for the planned surgery, blood should be ordered and ready in the operating room to avoid a delay in treatment. Blood losses should be replaced with either a 1:1 ratio of blood or colloid or 3:1 ratio for crystalloid [24]. Adequate access should also be obtained prior to initiation of surgery. Ideally two intravenous lines should be available, especially in the setting of hypovolemia. A central line and invasive arterial monitoring needs to be considered if warranted by patient's clinical status (Table 43.1).

Often these patients will be NPO due to the nature of their lesion and early diagnosis, however full stomach precautions should still be taken as there is still a significant risk for pulmonary aspiration during induction of anesthesia. Preoperative gastric decompression with an oral or nasal gastric tube is important prior to a rapid-sequence induction. If the neonate or premie is severely debilitated or there is a concern about the upper airway, awake intubation is a suitable option. Critically ill neonates will have an even higher rate of oxygen consumption. Coupled with abdominal distention and a decreased functional residual capacity, they will be prone to rapid desaturations in the setting of apnea. Timely and safely securing the airway is crucial and may be aided by use of an endotracheal tube with a preformed stylet and video laryngoscope if available.

If there is concern for hemodynamic instability, anesthesia should be induced with ketamine or etomidate, however it is important to bear in mind that there is controversy over the use of etomidate

**Table 43.1** A guide to the care of newborns, infants and children with intestinal obstruction

| Plan/preparation/adverse events | Reasoning/management |
|---|---|
| Preoperative evaluation<br>– Associated congenital abnormalities<br>– Airway compromise<br>– Ventilation difficulties<br>– Fluid status and electrolyte status<br>– Signs of sepsis and/or shock | Although most pediatric intestinal obstructions are surgical emergencies, they are first and foremost medical emergencies and a thorough preoperative evaluation must be done to ensure optimization of patients clinical status prior to induction of anesthesia |
| Intubation<br>– RSI<br>– Gastric decompression<br>– Stylleted tube<br>– Videolaryngoscope<br>– Extra personnel<br>– Backup tubes, blades, LMA available | Intestinal obstruction requires full stomach precautions. Many neonates and infants with intestinal obstruction will have increased oxygen demand and decreased FRC. Quick and careful intubation is critical and one must be prepared for any difficulties that may arise |
| Intraoperative management<br>– 2 intravenous lines<br>– Aggressive IV fluid hydration<br>– Electrolyte balance<br>– Temperature management<br>– Avoid nitrous oxide | Distended bowel will increase third-spacing and fluid deficits which can lead to hemodynamic compromise and electrolyte abnormalities<br>Expose distended bowel will increase risk of hypothermia<br>Nitrous oxide can worsen bowel distention |
| Postoperative management<br>– Extubation v. Postoperative mechanical ventilation<br>– Supportive therapy<br>– Pain control; regional anesthesia | Many patients will require ICU management and ventilator support post-operatively. Extubation criteria should be strictly adhered to<br>Neuraxial and regional anesthesia may decrease IV and inhaled anesthetic requirements both intraoperatively and postoperatively and promote earlier extubation and decreased hospital stay |

in septic patients related to its negative effect on adrenocorticoid synthesis [25]. Anesthesia can be maintained with either inhalational or intravenous anesthetics titrated to the baby's clinical picture and requirements. If extubation is planned, opioids should be used prudently. Nitrous oxide should be avoided as it may worsen bowel distention [26, 27]. A neuromuscular agent is often helpful in improving surgical conditions and ventilation. Additionally, adequate neuromuscular blockade will allow lower but required concentrations of inhaled anesthetics to be used.

Regional anesthesia combined with general anesthesia has also proven to be safe and beneficial during major abdominal surgeries in the neonate and infant. Both lumbar epidurals and caudal catheters have potential benefits of earlier tracheal extubation, blunting of the surgical stress response, and providing hemodynamic stability, limiting the need for parenteral opioids, and reducing use of intraoperative volatile anesthetics [28–30]. Although demonstrated to be safe in the neonate and infant, regional anesthesia procedures are not devoid of serious adverse effects, most commonly related to the placement of the needle or catheter and the physiologic effects of the infused medicines. While not encouraged in the adult population, the placement of regional anesthesia post-induction is common practice in pediatric patients. Although this is an acceptable standard of care, performing a neuraxial block in an anesthetized patient increases the risk of injury to the spinal cord and should only be practiced by an experienced provider.

Hypothermia is also an important consideration in neonatal surgery (and explained in detail in another chapter in this book), especially when a large surface of bowel will be exposed. Increasing the ambient temperature of the operating room, forced air warming, humidification of airway gases, and warming of intravenous fluids and blood is essential to compensate for the obligatory surgery related heat loss in these critically ill babies.

## Extubation and Postoperative Management

The preoperative presentation and effects of associated anomalies as well as the intraoperative course and surgical intervention will greatly influence postoperative management. Many patients will require continued postoperative ventilator support in the setting of respiratory compromise and hemodynamic instability. If this is the case, extubation will not be an option. For more minimally invasive or laparoscopic surgeries, extubation may be appropriate assuming no cardiovascular or respiratory instability. Postoperative pain can be challenging to evaluate in the neonate and infant, and treatment can be difficult to standardize given the diversity of patients and clinical situations. Currently pain is best managed with a multi-modal approach including opioids, acetaminophen and NSAIDs [30]. Just like in adults the use of regional and neuraxial blocks and infusions in the postoperative period are becoming increasingly common, however, careful administration of local anesthetic should be adhered to given the risk of local anesthetic toxicity in this patient population [30].

## Intestinal Obstruction in Children

Appendicitis is the most common cause of acute abdominal pain in children with a lifetime risk of nearly 8%. Up to 70,000 children are hospitalized annually for appendicitis in the United States alone [31], accounting for 88% of emergency surgical admissions [32]. Appendicitis is thought to result from an obstruction of the lumen of the appendix—usually by fecal matter—that leads to edema, inflammation, and infection. If left untreated, the affected appendix can rupture, ultimately leading to peritonitis (commonly referred to as complicated appendicitis) and sepsis. Classically children with appendicitis will present with fever, anorexia, nausea, vomiting, and abdominal pain—often periumbilical or localized to the right lower quadrant. Despite this common presentation, correctly diagnosing appendicitis can be challenging with missed diagnoses ranging from 20 to 40% and rates of negative appendectomy up to 34% [33] thus necessitating the need for radiographic confirmation. Although CT imaging is the gold standard of diagnosis, radiation exposure and long-term cancer risk is a major concern in the pediatric population, suggesting that ultrasound scanning should be the preferred diagnostic modality in children [33]. Once diagnosed, management is usually an open or laparoscopic appendectomy. If perforation has already occurred at the time of diagnosis, intravenous fluid resuscitation and broad spectrum antibiotics should be initiated.

If diagnosis of acute appendicitis is made prior to perforation, anesthetic management is typically uncomplicated. Fluid deficits should be assessed and managed preoperatively in the setting of vomiting, decreased oral intake, and fever. If a perforated appendix and peritonitis or sepsis is suspected, fluid resuscitation should be aggressive with adequate hydration initiated prior to induction of anesthesia. A large bore or second IV line and invasive arterial monitoring may be necessary depending on clinical assessment. Full stomach precautions should be followed despite NPO time as paralytic ileus can be a complication of acute appendicitis [34] and a rapid sequence induction and endotracheal intubation should be performed. Premedication with IV midazolam or pain medications should be used at the discretion of the anesthesia care team and based on the clinical presentation of each patient prior to induction of anesthesia.

Although post-operative pain control is usually straightforward, many children may be undertreated postoperatively. A recent U.S. study reported that up to 1/3 of pediatric patients who underwent a laparoscopic appendectomy demonstrated pain scores of >4 on a 1–10 scale over 60% of the time. Initiating the use of a multimodal postoperative pain regimen with local anesthetic infiltration, oral acetaminophen, NSAIDs, and opioid PCA reduced this rate significantly [35]. Open appendectomy is usually more painful than laparoscopic procedure and patients may benefit from the addition of an ultrasound-guided transverse abdominis plane (TAP) block in addition to other pain therapy [36].

Indirect inguinal hernias are one of the most common pediatric surgical conditions with incidence ranging from 1 to 5% [37, 38]. The overall risk of incarceration is up to 16% in children but may be as high as 31% in premature infants, usually occurring in their first year of life [37]. Most often, inguinal hernias are asymptomatic and found on a routine examination, however, they may also present more emergently when peritoneal contents are trapped in the hernia sac causing compromise to their vascular supply. Children with incarcerated inguinal hernias will often exhibit signs of acute bowel obstruction. They may have severe pain, be inconsolable, and have bloody stools and/or bilious emesis [39]. Non-operative reduction may be tried initially, but if not successful, the child should be taken for an emergent surgery which can be done either open or laparoscopically. Both general and regional anesthesia are safe for inguinal hernia repair and choice of anesthesia will vary based on the child's clinical appearance at the time of surgery. If a true bowel obstruction or strangulation is suspected, anesthetic requirements will be similar to those for the other pathologies of intestinal obstruction.

Figure 43.1 summarizes the general principles of care in children with intestinal obstruction.

## Outcomes and Conclusion

Pediatric intestinal obstruction is caused by a variety of intestinal pathologies with diverse clinical presentations. While advances in the diagnosis and treatment of the pediatric patient with intestinal obstruction has decreased patient morbidity and mortality, many of these patients are critically ill at the time of surgical intervention and anesthesia. A familiarity with the most common intestinal lesions, their pathophysiology and presentation, and means of surgical correction will be helpful in the anesthetic care and management of this patient population.

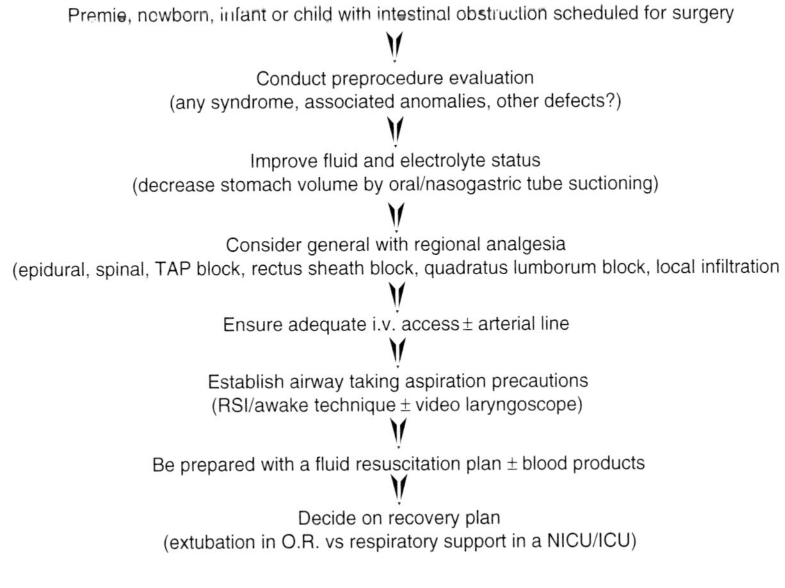

**Fig. 43.1** General principles of care during intestinal obstruction

Premie, newborn, infant or child with intestinal obstruction scheduled for surgery
↓
Conduct preprocedure evaluation
(any syndrome, associated anomalies, other defects?)
↓
Improve fluid and electrolyte status
(decrease stomach volume by oral/nasogastric tube suctioning)
↓
Consider general with regional analgesia
(epidural, spinal, TAP block, rectus sheath block, quadratus lumborum block, local infiltration
↓
Ensure adequate i.v. access ± arterial line
↓
Establish airway taking aspiration precautions
(RSI/awake technique ± video laryngoscope)
↓
Be prepared with a fluid resuscitation plan ± blood products
↓
Decide on recovery plan
(extubation in O.R. vs respiratory support in a NICU/ICU)

# References

1. Glover DM, Barry FM. Intestinal obstruction in the newborn. Ann Surg. 1949;130(3):480–509.
2. Juang D, Snyder CL. Neonatal bowel obstruction. Surg Clin North Am. 2012;92(3):685–711, ix–x.
3. Gangopadhyay AN, Pandey V. Anorectal malformations. J Indian Assoc Pediatr Surg. 2015;20(1):10–5.
4. de Blaauw I, Wijers CH, Schmiedeke E, Holland-Cunz S, Gamba P, Marcelis CL, et al. First results of a European multi-center registry of patients with anorectal malformations. J Pediatr Surg. 2013;48(12):2530–5.
5. Peña A, Hong A. Advances in the management of anorectal malformations. Am J Surg. 2000;180(5):370–6.
6. Kimura K, Loening-Baucke V. Bilious vomiting in the newborn: rapid diagnosis of intestinal obstruction. Am Fam Physician. 2000;61(9):2791–8.
7. Mustafawi AR, Hassan ME. Congenital duodenal obstruction in children: a decade's experience. Eur J Pediatr Surg. 2008;18(2):93–7.
8. Dalla Vecchia LK, Grosfeld JL, West KW, Rescorla FJ, Scherer LR, Engum SA. Intestinal atresia and stenosis: a 25-year experience with 277 cases. Arch Surg. 1998;133(5):490–6; discussion 6–7.
9. Stollman TH, de Blaauw I, Wijnen MH, van der Staak FH, Rieu PN, Draaisma JM, et al. Decreased mortality but increased morbidity in neonates with jejunoileal atresia; a study of 114 cases over a 34-year period. J Pediatr Surg. 2009;44(1):217–21.
10. van der Doef HP, Kokke FT, van der Ent CK, Houwen RH. Intestinal obstruction syndromes in cystic fibrosis: meconium ileus, distal intestinal obstruction syndrome, and constipation. Curr Gastroenterol Rep. 2011;13(3):265–70.
11. Ziegler MM. Meconium ileus. Curr Probl Surg. 1994;31(9):731–77.
12. Westfal ML, Goldstein AM. Pediatric enteric neuropathies: diagnosis and current management. Curr Opin Pediatr. 2017;29:347.
13. Seashore JH, Touloukian RJ. Midgut volvulus. An ever-present threat. Arch Pediatr Adolesc Med. 1994;148(1):43–6.
14. Strouse PJ. Disorders of intestinal rotation and fixation ("malrotation"). Pediatr Radiol. 2004;34(11):837–51.
15. Kapfer SA, Rappold JF. Intestinal malrotation-not just the pediatric surgeon's problem. J Am Coll Surg. 2004;199(4):628–35.
16. Newman B, Koppolu R, Murphy D, Sylvester K. Heterotaxy syndromes and abnormal bowel rotation. Pediatr Radiol. 2014;44(5):542–51.
17. Powell DM, Othersen HB, Smith CD. Malrotation of the intestines in children: the effect of age on presentation and therapy. J Pediatr Surg. 1989;24(8):777–80.
18. Hajivassiliou CA. Intestinal obstruction in neonatal/pediatric surgery. Semin Pediatr Surg. 2003;12(4):241–53.
19. Marsicovetere P, Ivatury SJ, White B, Holubar SD. Intestinal intussusception: etiology, diagnosis, and treatment. Clin Colon Rectal Surg. 2017;30(1):30–9.
20. Mehendale S, Kumar CP, Venkatasubramanian S, Prasanna T. Intussusception in children aged less than five years. Indian J Pediatr. 2016;83(10):1087–92.
21. Jiang J, Jiang B, Parashar U, Nguyen T, Bines J, Patel MM. Childhood intussusception: a literature review. PLoS One. 2013;8(7):e68482.
22. Paul SP, Candy DCA, Pandya N. A case series on intussusceptions in infants presenting with listlessness. Infant. 2010;6(5):174–7.
23. Lochhead A, Jamjoom R, Ratnapalan S. Intussusception in children presenting to the emergency department. Clin Pediatr (Phila). 2013;52(11):1029–33.
24. Murat I, Humblot A, Girault L, Piana F. Neonatal fluid management. Best Pract Res Clin Anaesthesiol. 2010;24(3):365–74.
25. van den Heuvel I, Wurmb TE, Bottiger BW, Bernhard M. Pros and cons of etomidate—more discussion than evidence? Curr Opin Anaesthesiol. 2013;26(4):404–8.
26. Eger EI 2nd, Saidman LJ. Hazards of nitrous oxide anesthesia in bowel obstruction and pneumothorax. Anesthesiology. 1965;26:61–6.
27. Orhan-Sungur M, Apfel C, Akca O. Effects of nitrous oxide on intraoperative bowel distension. Curr Opin Anaesthesiol. 2005;18(6):620–4.
28. Goeller JK, Bhalla T, Tobias JD. Combined use of neuraxial and general anesthesia during major abdominal procedures in neonates and infants. Paediatr Anaesth. 2014;24(6):553–60.
29. Long JB, Joselyn AS, Bhalla T, Tobias JD, De Oliveira GS Jr, Suresh S, et al. The use of neuraxial catheters for postoperative analgesia in neonates: a multicenter safety analysis from the Pediatric Regional Anesthesia Network. Anesth Analg. 2016;122(6):1965–70.
30. Bhalla T, Shepherd E, Tobias JD. Neonatal pain management. Saudi J Anaesth. 2014;8(Suppl 1):S89–97.
31. Gandy RC, Wang F. Should the non-operative management of appendicitis be the new standard of care? ANZ J Surg. 2016;86(4):228–31.
32. Lopez JJ, Deans KJ, Minneci PC. Nonoperative management of appendicitis in children. Curr Opin Pediatr. 2017;29:358.
33. Kabir SA, Kabir SI, Sun R, Jafferbhoy S, Karim A. How to diagnose an acutely inflamed appendix; a systematic review of the latest evidence. Int J Surg. 2017;40:155–62.
34. Dudley GS. Paralytic ileus as a complication of acute appendicitis. Ann Surg. 1926;84(5):729–34.
35. Liu Y, Seipel C, Lopez ME, Nuchtern JG, Brandt ML, Fallon SC, et al. A retrospective study of multimodal analgesic treatment after laparoscopic appendectomy in children. Paediatr Anaesth. 2013;23(12):1187–92.
36. Niraj G, Searle A, Mathews M, Misra V, Baban M, Kiani S, et al. Analgesic efficacy of ultrasound-guided transversus abdominis plane block in patients undergoing open appendicectomy. Br J Anaesth. 2009;103(4):601–5.
37. Abdulhai SA, Glenn IC, Ponsky TA. Incarcerated pediatric hernias. Surg Clin North Am. 2017;97(1):129–45.
38. Wiener ES, Touloukian RJ, Rodgers BM, Grosfeld JL, Smith EI, Ziegler MM, et al. Hernia survey of the section on surgery of the American Academy of Pediatrics. J Pediatr Surg. 1996;31(8):1166–9.
39. Smith J, Fox SM. Pediatric abdominal pain: an emergency medicine perspective. Emerg Med Clin North Am. 2016;34(2):341–61.

# Anesthesia for Epidermolysis Bullosa

Eric Wittkugel and Ali Kandil

## Introduction

According to the National EB Registry (NEBR), which compiled data from 1986 to 2002, the prevalence of EB was approximately 11 per million and the incidence was approximately 20 per million live births. Specifically, during this same time period, the incidence rates for EB by subtype were as follows: eight per million live births for EB simplex; three per million live births for junctional EB; and three per million live births for recessive dystrophic EB [1–3]. Although quite rare, these patients are living longer lives because of more comprehensive, multi-disciplinary care which is centered on nutrition, dental and wound care, pain management, and mental health [4–8]. The onus is on the anesthesia provider to not only ensure the optimal preoperative condition of the patient, but to understand the important role of the anesthesia provider in the perioperative experience of these patients.

In order to properly understand the anesthetic implications and considerations, it is imperative to understand the different types of EB and how their different phenotypes impact their care. EB is both a genetically and phenotypically heterogeneous group of inherited mechanobullous diseases characterized by weakness in the structural integrity of epithelial tissue and marked by blistering that can range from minor to debilitating. There are more than 20 genes responsible for encoding structural proteins which form the intraepidermal adhesion and dermoepidermal anchoring apparatus within the basement membrane of the skin and mucosa. Ultimately, defects in these genes that code for these structural proteins lead to basement membrane fragility, lack of adhesion and proliferation, barrier dysfunction, and ultimately, tissue dehiscence [9–11]. In this chapter, we will focus on the three major subtypes of EB: EB simplex (EBS); junctional EB (JEB); and dystrophic EB (DEB).

1. *Epidermolysis Bullosa Simplex (EBS)*
   EBS is the most common type of EB, accounting for 75–80% of all cases in the Western world [12]. EBS is characterized by intraepidermal blistering both, within the basal keratinocytes or above the level of the basal keratinocytes. By and large, EBS exhibits autosomal dominant inheritance, with extremely rare recessive variants. In most cases of EBS, these autosomal dominant mutations occur in the *KRT5* and *KRT14* genes encoding keratins, resulting in tissue cleavage [13]. Of the three major types of EB, EBS is certainly the most benign. However, EBS itself exhibits a spectrum of manifestations

E. Wittkugel, M.D. (✉) · A. Kandil, D.O., M.P.H.
Anesthesia and Pediatrics, Cincinnati Childrens Hospital Medical Center, Cincinnati, OH, USA
e-mail: eric.wittkugel@cchmc.org; ali.kandil@cchmc.org

and is broken down into three subtypes: EBS-localized, EBS-generalized severe, and EBS-generalized intermediate.

(a) EBS-localized

Localized EBS is the mildest and most common form of EB and it presents between infancy and third decade of life. Initial symptoms are characterized by trauma-induced blistering at the palms and soles. Oral ulcers can occur during infancy secondary to friction from bottle feeding, however this usually resolves with age. Further, these patients have normal dentition and hair and do not exhibit scarring from their blisters [14].

(b) EBS-generalized severe

Generalized severe EBS is the most severe form of EBS. It presents at birth with diffuse friction-induced blistering. Generalized severe EBS can present spontaneously with clustered blisters on the trunk or neck. Involvement of the oral mucosa is most common. Further, these patients can present with nail shedding, hair loss, hyperkeratosis of the palms and soles. Blisters usually heal without scarring, but they can result in change in pigmentation. Generalized severe EBS is worse during infancy and tends to improve with age. These patients may present with extracutaneous features like laryngeal stenosis, which though rare, can increase mortality and become an important consideration in anesthetic management [15].

(c) EBS-generalized intermediate

Generalized intermediate EBS is similar to generalized severe EBS, although more mild. In this subtype, the blistering begins at birth, but is generally mild and specifically involves the hands, feet, and extremities. Hair, teeth and nails are normal and blisters heal without scarring. The changes in pigmentation that result at the blister site are also less severe [15].

2. *Junctional Epidermolysis Bullosa*

Junctional epidermolysis bullosa (JEB) is caused by autosomal recessive mutations in the laminin genes, which compromises the structural integrity of the lamina lucida and superior lamina densa of the basal membrane [16]. This type of EB is associated with high mortality early in life despite aggressive interventions. Blisters and erosions may occur in all stratified squamous epithelial tissues, including oral, gastrointestinal, respiratory and genitourinary mucosa [17, 18]. Strictures and obstructions resulting from healing of mucosal lesions are associated with significant morbidity and mortality. Upper airway injury may occur spontaneously following coughing, crying, or upper respiratory infections. Commonly, JEB patients develop laryngotracheal stenosis and can have complete airway obstruction, a major cause of mortality in these patients. The risk of death in these patients is approximately 45% by age 1 and 60% by age 15 [19, 20].

3. *Dystrophic Epidermolysis Bullosa*

Dystrophic epidermolysis bullosa (DEB) is characterized by blistering of the skin and mucosal membranes that heal with scarring. This type of EB is caused by mutations in a gene responsible for the integrity of the alpha-1 chain of type VII collagen, the main constituent of anchoring fibrils which anchor the epidermal basement membrane to the dermis. Since type VII collagen is also expressed in non-cutaneous stratified epithelia, blistering also occurs in the mucous membranes and upper third of the esophagus [21–23]. DEB is further classified as recessive (RDEB) and dominant (DDEB). The subtype that poses the most significant anesthetic challenges is the RDEB subtype, the most severe form of DEB. Characterized by blistering at birth, these patients' skin is traumatized by even the mildest mechanical insult. Pseudosyndactyly is due to repeated stress and blistering to the hands and feet and is one of the hallmarks of RDEB [24]. Oral, esophageal, and anal mucosa are also affected with scarring. Notably, limited mouth opening, dystrophic teeth, poor mobility of the tongue and esophageal strictures contribute to malnutrition, which perpetuates poor wound healing and disease progression. Malnutrition may result in severe anemia, failure to thrive, and delayed puberty [25]. Anemia is usually caused by decreased absorption and ingestion of iron, blood loss from chronic wound breakdown, and skin turnover. EB produces a chronic inflammatory state, which can stunt erythropoiesis [26]. Anemia, especially in the setting of severe malnutrition has a significant impact on overall well-being, causing malaise, decreased exercise tolerance, loss of appetite and impaired wound healing. Despite iron supplementation, many of these patient remain severely anemic with hemoglobin levels below 8 g/dL, at times necessitating blood transfusion before surgical procedures [24]. The leading cause of death in this population is squamous cell carcinoma [27].

An association between RDEB and dilated cardiomyopathy has been appreciated for at least 25 years, but a common mechanism of disease has not emerged. The absence of type VII collagen is responsible for all cases of RDEB [28], and disruption of extracellular matrix is known to lead to cardiomyopathy in both animal models and patients [29]. Although its absence has not been proven to impact the heart, the normal function of type VII collagen may serve as a modifier of factors that regulate cardiovascular remodeling. The etiology of cardiomyopathy in RDEB is often multifactorial. These patients may take cardiotoxic medications like amitryptiline, a tricyclic antidepressant used for depression, chronic pain and insomnia. In addition to the cardiomyopathy from chronic carnitine and selenium deficiency in these patients [30], these cardiotoxic medications may worsen ventricular dysfunction [28, 31, 32]. In patients with RDEB, especially those with severe malnutrition and those who are taking cardiotoxic medications, consider obtaining a recent preoperative echocardiogram. A number of EB centers perform screening echocardiograms on an annual basis.

## Anesthetic Challenges and Perioperative Management

From these three major variants of epidermolysis bullosa, it is clear that these patients present a myriad of anesthetic challenges. We will now address some of these anesthetic concerns, namely the most effective ways to communicate with the patients and families, place standard monitors, manage the airway, obtain vascular access, and provide perioperative analgesia (Table 44.1). Patients with EB

**Table 44.1** Safe and effective management of patients with epidermolysis bullosa

| | |
|---|---|
| 1. Communication | Patient and parental expectations must be communicated. Preoperative consult is helpful to establish what has worked in the past and to address specific concerns. Planning is crucial |
| 2. Equipment, standard monitoring | Aquaphor, non-adhesive bandages, clip on pulse oximetry, non-adhesive EKG leads, padding for the face, bed, and blood pressure cuff |
| 3. Induction of anesthesia | Premedication with oral midazolam if feasible, gentle induction with sevoflurane or incremental dosing of ketamine, dexmedetomidine or propofol. Maintain spontaneous respiration |
| 4. Vascular access | After mask induction in young children, preoperatively in older children if possible. Consider ultrasound |
| 5. Airway management | Mask ventilation is usually easy. Oropharyngeal airways and laryngeal mask airways may cause trauma. Nasopharyngeal airways may be utilized safely. Direct laryngoscopy becomes more challenging with age. Fiberoptic intubation is good route to minimize trauma (nasal). Lubrication of devices is imperative |
| 6. Analgesia | Multimodal approach is critical. IV acetaminophen, ketamine, dexmedetomidine, local anesthesia (if possible), short and long acting opioid analgesics. Regional anesthesia has been safely employed |

may present for any type of surgery, but certain procedures are more frequent than others, including esophageal balloon dilation for esophageal strictures, dental rehabilitation, plastic surgery for pseudosyndactyly, excision of squamous cell carcinomas, and wound care (both dressing changes and whirlpool treatments for skin debridement) [33–36]. The grace and gentleness with which these issues are handled are especially important in these patients who often have repeated visits to the operating room.

1. *Communication*
   Effective communication is one of the central tenets in successful perioperative anesthetic management. In patients with EB, communication is especially important since they are often appropriately anxious about surgical and anesthetic procedures which may result in painful trauma to the skin and mucous membranes. Listening carefully to patients and their parents about current state of the skin, mucous membranes and eyes, and about what has worked well during previous anesthetics, will allow the anesthesia provider to minimize the risk of further trauma and provide a safe anesthetic. Frequently, these patients have anesthetic regimens that have been effective in the past and their expectation is that the next anesthetic will be similarly effective. However, progression of disease, differences in surgical procedures, and variations in anesthetic technique among providers may challenge these expectations.
2. *Standard Monitoring and Protective Measures*
   The fragile skin and mucous membranes in patients with EB merit significant preparation and consideration, as the anesthetic, analgesic, and psychologic outcomes depend on careful planning. The operating room should be prepared well ahead of time with not only special padding for the bed, but an egg-crate mattress that is present under the patient throughout the entire perioperative period. The operating room should be adequately warmed and special silicone based non-adhesive material should be available to secure endotracheal tubes, intravenous catheters, and EKG leads.

Direct contact to the skin with adhesive materials must be avoided. Unintentional use of adhesives on the skin can cause severe skin trauma and blistering. The patient must be handled very gently and friction on the skin must be avoided.

Starting with the standard ASA monitors (EKG, pulse oximetry, end tidal carbon dioxide monitoring, non-invasive blood pressure monitoring, and temperature monitoring), special precautions are mandatory. There are several options for the EKG monitoring, which include using needle electrode EKG leads or removal of adhesive from standard EKG leads and affixing them to the patient with a non-adhesive dressing (Mepitel® or Mepitac®, Molnlycke Health Care). Oxygen saturation should be monitored with a non-adhesive pulse oximeter, either the clip-type or a Velcro-type. Non-invasive blood pressure monitoring can be performed by placing the blood pressure cuff over a few layers of cotton padding wrapped around the extremity (Fig. 44.1).

After monitors are delicately placed, the next step is to ensure any procedures (mask-ventilation, intubation, vascular access) performed do not result in skin trauma. Prior to mask-ventilation, the application of petrolatum ointment to the provider's gloves and the face mask prior to touching the patient is helpful in protecting the face. An alternative technique is to place a silicone-based foam dressing (such as Mepilex® Transfer, Molnlycke Health Care) under the face mask and on points where the provider's fingers contact the face (Fig. 44.2). Another important consideration is protection of the eyes from corneal abrasion. Tape should not be placed on the delicate skin of eyelids. Methylcellulose ophthalmic drops or gel should be generously applied to the eyes. If the patient's eyelids are not scarred open, moist gauze can gently be placed over the eyes for further protection.

3. *Induction of Anesthesia and Vascular Access*
   Induction of anesthesia in patients with EB is a crucial beginning to safe airway

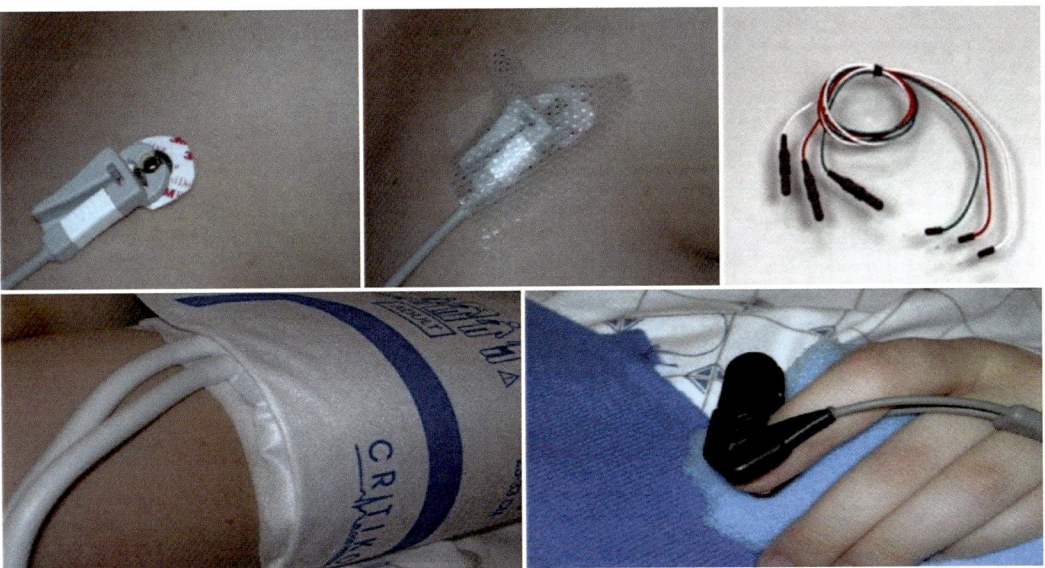

**Fig. 44.1** Standard non-invasive monitors (ECG, BP cuff, pulse oximeter)

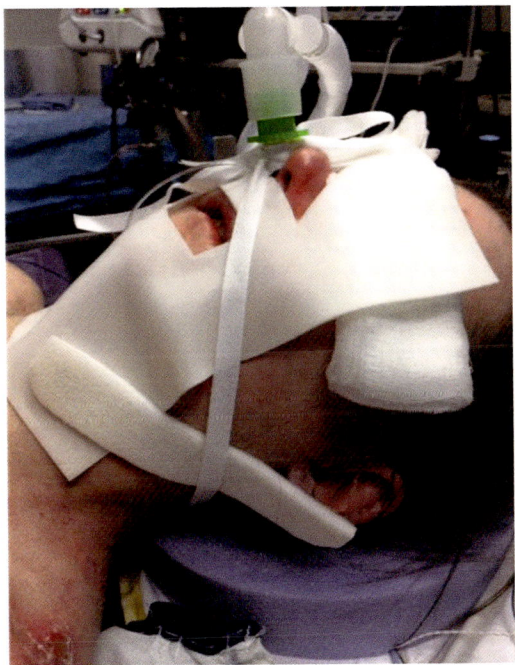

**Fig. 44.2** Nasotracheal intubation with protective padding on face

management. Premedication with oral midazolam helps facilitate a smooth anesthetic induction with minimal anxiety, movement or restlessness. Intramuscular ketamine can also be used, but care must be taken to avoid skin trauma while administering the injection. Depending on the facility, parental presence may be possible to help allay the patient's fears during induction. Gentle inhalational induction with nitrous oxide followed by sevoflurane is a standard approach to induction of anesthesia in children. In patients with EB, care must be taken to keep the patient spontaneously breathing until the intravenous catheter is placed. Since vascular access can be a challenge in the young child with EB, IV placement after mask induction is preferred, using ultrasound if needed. In older cooperative patients who tolerate an awake IV, ultrasound is frequently employed to facilitate access. The tourniquet is generally placed over cotton padded wrap to prevent trauma to the skin, and the IV catheter is secured using a non-adhesive dressing (Mepitac® or Mepiform®, Molnlycke Health Care). In these patients, induction can be accomplished intravenously using incremental doses of propofol, ketamine, dexmedetomidine, and inhaled volatile agents. Muscle relaxants can be administered as needed. Once the airway has been established, anesthesia can be maintained with volatile agents or total intravenous anesthesia.

4. *Airway Management*

Depending on the type of EB, traditional airway management can range from straightforward to very difficult. In patients with EB simplex, airway management is generally routine and direct laryngoscopy is acceptable. However, in patients with junctional EB or recessive dystrophic EB after the first several years of life, airway management becomes increasingly challenging [37]. As these patients approach adolescence, progressive scarring of the mouth often results in limited mouth opening and necessitates fiberoptic intubation. Nasotracheal fiberoptic intubation is an oft-employed route as it avoids traumatizing the lips, tongue, and oropharynx. Careful preparation should be undertaken in order to optimize success and minimize trauma. The endotracheal tube should be warmed, softened and lubricated, the nose should be topicalized with a vasoconstrictive agent like oxymetazoline or phenylephrine, and to the extent possible, the smallest acceptable size endotracheal tube should be employed to avoid friction in the nares and nasopharynx. An added advantage to employing a nasotracheal intubation is that the endotracheal tube can be secured more securely than an oral endotracheal tube (Fig. 44.2). The endotracheal tube can be secured with cloth ties or with nonadhesive silicone based tape (Mepitac®). Given the limitations in mouth opening, laryngeal mask airways (LMAs) are more difficult to delicately place in patients with EB and although they have been used safely, are rarely feasible in patients with advanced cases of EB [38]. One of the most utilized forms of airway management is mask ventilation with volatile anesthetics. If the face is carefully protected, this may serve as the safest and least traumatic form of airway management for appropriate cases. A spontaneously breathing patient with a natural airway and a mask often can tolerate procedures like retrograde esophageal dilatations and wound debridement.

5. *Perioperative Analgesia and Postoperative Management*

Patients with EB, especially older patients are frequently on chronic opioid regimens that mandate higher narcotic doses intraoperatively. A fine balance between sufficient analgesia and a spontaneously breathing patient is often hard to achieve and merits creativity and a multimodal approach. The use of ketamine, dexmedetomidine, intravenous acetaminophen, as well as opioid analgesia can make these patients' experiences more tolerable. In addition to intravenous analgesia, regional anesthesia is not contraindicated in patients with EB and can be an important part of their management. The use of regional anesthesia decreases the need for airway instrumentation and avoidance of trauma to their lips, teeth, tongue and oropharynx. The challenge is to have the appropriate level of cooperation from the patient. Oftentimes in children, this is not possible and a combination of general and regional anesthesia may be employed.

Awake extubation, if indicated, is the safest mechanism for concluding a general anesthetic, to reduce the risk of aspiration of bloody oral secretions from the friable oral mucosa, and to minimize the need for placing the mask on the face after extubation. While perioperative bullae formation may occur in the oropharynx, significant postoperative airway obstruction from these events is rare. Depending on the type of procedure being performed, outpatient surgery is possible, given a straightforward anesthetic course and a period of close observation postoperatively.

## Conclusion

The challenges an anesthesiologist faces when dealing with patients with epidermolysis bullosa are abundant. However, a thoughtful approach enables safe and effective perioperative management. At our institution, several mechanisms have been put in place to standardize care of these patients. It is very important to have an anesthesia consult for these patients to obtain information about the extent of their disease, the previous anesthesia experiences and preferences, their airway management and their perioperative analgesia. Additionally, we have created an EB kit containing all the necessary supplies: non-adhesive bandages dressings for securing the endotracheal tube and intravenous catheters, cushioning materials, lubricants (both for skin and eyes), EKG electrodes and pulse oximetry probes. We always have the airway cart in the room throughout the case, equipped with flexible fiberoptic and video laryngoscopes. Finally, we have a pain service dedicated to the perioperative analgesic management of these patients. The perioperative algorithm for EB patients is readily available on our departmental webpage as a reference for all anesthesia providers. Ultimately, management of patients with EB can be performed safely and a positive perioperative experience can be achieved with careful pre-anesthetic evaluation and attention to detail throughout the anesthetic.

# References

1. Fine JD. Inherited epidermolysis bullosa. Orphanet J Rare Dis. 2010;5:12.
2. Fine JD, Johnson LB, Suchindran C, et al. The National Epidermolysis Bullosa Registry. In: Fine JD, Bauer EA, McGuire J, Moshell A, editors. Epidermolysis bullosa: clinical, epidemiologic, and laboratory findings of the National Epidermolysis Bullosa Registry. Baltimore: The Johns Hopkins University Press; 1999.
3. Fine JD. Epidemiology of inherited epidermolysis bullosa based on incidence and prevalence estimates from the National Epidermolysis Bullosa Registry. JAMA Dermatol. 2016;152:1231.
4. El Hachem M, Zambruno G, Bourdon-Lanoy E, et al. Multicentre consensus recommendations for skin care in inherited epidermolysis bullosa. Orphanet J Rare Dis. 2014;9:76.
5. Fine JD, Johnson LB, Weiner M, Suchindran C. Impact of inherited epidermolysis bullosa on parental interpersonal relationships, marital status and family size. Br J Dermatol. 2005;152:1009.
6. Pope E, Lara-Corrales I, Mellerio J, et al. A consensus approach to wound care in epidermolysis bullosa. J Am Acad Dermatol. 2012;67:904.
7. Goldschneider KR, Lucky AW. Pain management in epidermolysis bullosa. Dermatol Clin. 2010;28:273.
8. Colomb V, Bourdon-Lannoy E, Lambe C, et al. Nutritional outcome in children with severe generalized recessive dystrophic epidermolysis bullosa: a short- and long-term evaluation of gastrostomy and enteral feeding. Br J Dermatol. 2012;166:354.
9. Van Den Heuvel I, Boschin M, Langer M, Frosch M, Gottschalk A, Ellger B, Hahnenkamp K. Anesthetic management in pediatric patients with epidermolysis bullosa: a single center experience. Edizioni Minerva Med. 2013;79(7):727–32.
10. Goldschneider K, Lucky AW, Mellerio JE, Palisson F, del Carmen Viñuela Miranda M, Azizkhan RG. Perioperative care of patients with epidermolysis bullosa: proceedings of the 5th international symposium on epidermolysis bullosa, Santiago Chile, December 4–6, 2008. Pediatr Anaesth. 2010;20:797–804.
11. Samol NB, Wittkugel E. Epidermolysis bullosa. I In: Goldschneider KR, Davidson A, Wittkugel E, Skinner A, editors. Clinical pediatric anesthesia, a case-based handbook. New York: Oxford Press; 2012. p. 650–60.
12. Abu Sa'd J, Indelman M, Pfendner E, et al. Molecular epidemiology of hereditary epidermolysis bullosa in a middle eastern population. J Invest Dermatol. 2006;126:777.
13. Lane EB, McLean WH. Keratins and skin disorders. J Pathol. 2004;204:355.
14. Sprecher E. Epidermolysis bullosa simplex. Dermatol Clin. 2010;28:23.
15. Prodinger C, Diem A, Bauer JW, Laimer M. [Mucosal manifestations of epidermolysis bullosa: clinical presentation and management]. Hautarzt. 2016;67:806.
16. Fine JD, Bruckner-Tuderman L, Eady RA, et al. Inherited epidermolysis bullosa: updated recommendations on diagnosis and classification. J Am Acad Dermatol. 2014;70:1103.
17. Miosge N, Kluge JG, Studzinski A, et al. In situ-RT-PCR and immunohistochemistry for the localisation of the mRNA of the alpha 3 chain of laminin and laminin-5 during human organogenesis. Anat Embryol (Berl). 2002;205:355.
18. Hamill KJ, Paller AS, Jones JC. Adhesion and migration, the diverse functions of the laminin alpha3 subunit. Dermatol Clin. 2010;28:79.
19. Fine JD, Johnson LB, Weiner M, Suchindran C. Cause-specific risks of childhood death in inherited epidermolysis bullosa. J Pediatr. 2008;152:276.
20. Fine JD. Premature death in EB. In: Fine JD, Hintner H, editors. Life with epidermolysis bullosa (EB): etiology, diagnosis, multidisciplinary care and therapy. New York: Springer; 2008. p. 197.
21. Varki R, Sadowski S, Uitto J, Pfendner E. Epidermolysis bullosa. II. Type VII collagen mutations and phenotype-genotype correlations in the dystrophic subtypes. J Med Genet. 2007;44:181.
22. Bruckner-Tuderman L. Dystrophic epidermolysis bullosa: pathogenesis and clinical features. Dermatol Clin. 2010;28:107.
23. Dang N, Murrell DF. Mutation analysis and characterization of COL7A1 mutations in dystrophic epidermolysis bullosa. Exp Dermatol. 2008;17:553.
24. Fine JD, Mellerio JE. Extracutaneous manifestations and complications of inherited epidermolysis

bullosa: part II Other organs. J Am Acad Dermatol. 2009;61:387.
25. Martinez AE, Allgrove J, Brain C. Growth and pubertal delay in patients with epidermolysis bullosa. Dermatol Clin. 2010;28:357.
26. Annicchiarico G, Morgese MG, Esposito S, et al. Proinflammatory cytokines and antiskin autoantibodies in patients with inherited epidermolysis bullosa. Medicine (Baltimore). 2015;94:e1528.
27. Fine JD, Johnson LB, Weiner M, et al. Epidermolysis bullosa and the risk of life-threatening cancers: the National EB Registry experience, 1986-2006. J Am Acad Dermatol. 2009;60:203.
28. Lara-Corrales I, Mellerio JE, Martinez AE, Green A, Lucky AW, Azizkhan RG, Murrell DF, Agero AL, Kantor PF, Pope E. Dilated cardiomyopathy in epidermolysis bullosa: a retrospective, multicenter study. Pediatr Dermatol. 2010;27:238–43.
29. Spinale FG. Myocardial matrix remodeling and the matrix metalloproteinases: influence on cardiac form and function. Physiol Rev. 2007;87:1285–342.
30. Maron BJ, Towbin JA, Thiene J, et al. Contemporary definitions and classification of cardiomyopathies. An American Heart Association scientific statement from the Council on Clinical Cardiology, Heart Failure and Transplantation Committee; Quality of Care an Outcomes Research and Functional Genomics and Translational Biology Interdisciplinary Working Groups; and Council on Epidemiology and Prevention. Circulation. 2006;113:1807–16.
31. Sidwell RU, Yates R, Atherton D. Dilated cardiomyopathy in dystrophic epidermolysis bullosa. Arch Dis Child. 2000;83:59–63.
32. Taibjee SM, Ramani P, Brown R, et al. Lethal cardiomyopathy in epidermolysis bullosa associated with amitriptyline. Arch Dis Child. 2005;90:871–2.
33. Lin AN, Lateef F, Kelly R, Rothaus KO, Carter DM. Anesthetic management in epidermolysis bullosa: review of 129 anesthetic episodes in 32 patients. J Am Acad Dermatol. 1994;30:412–6.
34. Azizkhan RG, Stehra W, Cohen AP, Wittkugel E, Farrell MK, Lucky AW, Hammelman BD, Johnson ND, Racadio JM. Esophageal strictures in children with recessive dystrophic epidermolysis bullosa: an 11-year experience with fluoroscopically guided balloon dilation. J Pediatr Surg. 2006;41(1):55–60.
35. Griffin RP, Mayou BJ. The anaesthetic management of patients with dystrophic epidermolysis bullosa. Anaesthesia. 1993;48:810.
36. Mellerio JE, Weiner M, Denyer JE, et al. Medical management of epidermolysis bullosa: proceedings of the IInd international symposium on epidermolysis bullosa, Santiago, Chile, 2005. Int J Dermatol. 2007;46:795–800.
37. Samol NB, Wittkugel E. Epidermolysis bullosa. In: Davis PJ, Cladis FP, Motoyama EK, editors. Smith's anesthesia for infants and children. 8th ed. Philadelphia: Elsevier Mosby; 2016. p. 1257–60.
38. Fröhlich S, O'Sullivan E. Airway management in adult patients with epidermolysis bullosa dystrophica: a case series. Anaesthesia. 2011;66:842–3.

# Anesthesia for Children with Cerebral Palsy

## Ilana Fromer and Kumar Belani

## Introduction

Cerebral Palsy (CP) is the most common movement disorder in children with world-wide prevalence estimated to be between 1.5 and 4 per 1000 live births. One U.S. surveillance study of children from birth to age 8 found the rate of CP to be 3.1 per 1000 indicating approximately 1/300 children in the U.S. have CP [1, 2]. Although the prevalence of CP appears to have remained constant over the last 20 years, a 2016 Cochrane review suggests that due to newer neonatal interventions and advances in obstetrical care, the incidence and severity of CP may be decreasing [3]. Nevertheless, patients with CP are still commonly encountered in anesthesia practice. With the myriad of treatments and surgical interventions presently available these patients, particularly children, are frequently exposed to anesthesia and carry significant perioperative risks—as high as 63.1% according to a recent study [4]. This chapter will focus on important perioperative considerations during the care of a pediatric patient with CP. Table 45.1 provides a summary of anesthesia considerations in children with Cerebral palsy.

I. Fromer, M.D. (✉)
K. Belani, M.B.B.S., M.S., F.A.C.A., F.A.A.P.
Department of Anesthesiology,
University of Minnesota,
Masonic Children's Hospital,
Minneapolis, MN, USA

Cerebral palsy (CP) is best described by Shepherd and associates [3] as an "umbrella term" with five key elements namely: permanency, movement and or posture problems including motor related issues secondary to interference by an abnormality or lesion that is non-progressive, but occurred in the developing fetal or immature brain, and appearing in early childhood. Most common manifestations include weakness, poor muscle control and diminished muscle tone that primarily effect movement and posture. These are often accompanied by disturbances of sensation, perception, cognition, communication, and behavior [4].

For the practicing anesthesiologist, patients with CP can present a challenge, as no two patients will exhibit the same manifestation of the disease. Furthermore, patients with CP often require multiple surgical interventions. Perioperative concerns for a child with cerebral palsy will vary with the severity of the disease as well as other associated medical problems [5].

## Definition and Diagnosis

Cerebral palsy results from injury to the developing cerebral motor cortex. It can happen in utero, at birth, or within the first 2 years of life (see Fig. 45.1). The result of this injury is both permanent and static meaning the lesion itself will not

**Table 45.1** Summary of anesthesia considerations in children with cerebral palsy

| Plan/preparation/adverse events | Reasoning/management |
|---|---|
| If deep sedation without intubation is planned, have back up device for positive pressure ventilation available for immediate use. In addition, all emergency drugs including muscle relaxant must be readily available | Desaturation from hypoventilations may occur as a result of chronic lung disease and/or scoliosis. Laryngospasm as a result of copious secretions can present and lead to rapid desaturation and hypoxia |
| Preprocedural evaluation<br>– Aspiration<br>– Airway<br>– Cognitive impairment<br>– Medications/seizures<br>– Anxiety<br>– Latex allergy | Patients are usually taking several daily medications which can interact with anesthetic medications |
| Positioning—padding and support | Contractures and poor nutrition leading to minimal subcutaneous fat can lead to skin breakdown and nerve damage |
| Intraoperative management<br>– Inhalational or IV induction<br>– Inhalation or TIVA maintenance<br>– Regional anesthetics | All inhaled and IV anesthetic medications are safe for use. Decreased requirement of volatile anesthetics (minimum alveolar concentration). Neuraxial and regional blocks are also safe and helpful. If poor cognitive status awake blocks may not be possible. Only experienced providers should place blocks in asleep patients |
| Postoperative management and discharge considerations<br>– Pain<br>– Spasms<br>– Seizures<br>– PONV | Due to poor cognitive function patients may not be able to express pain—Family can be very helpful in interpreting child's needs. Preoperative medications such as seizure meds and antispasmodics should be restarted as soon as possible as abrupt discontinuation of some may cause withdrawal symptoms |

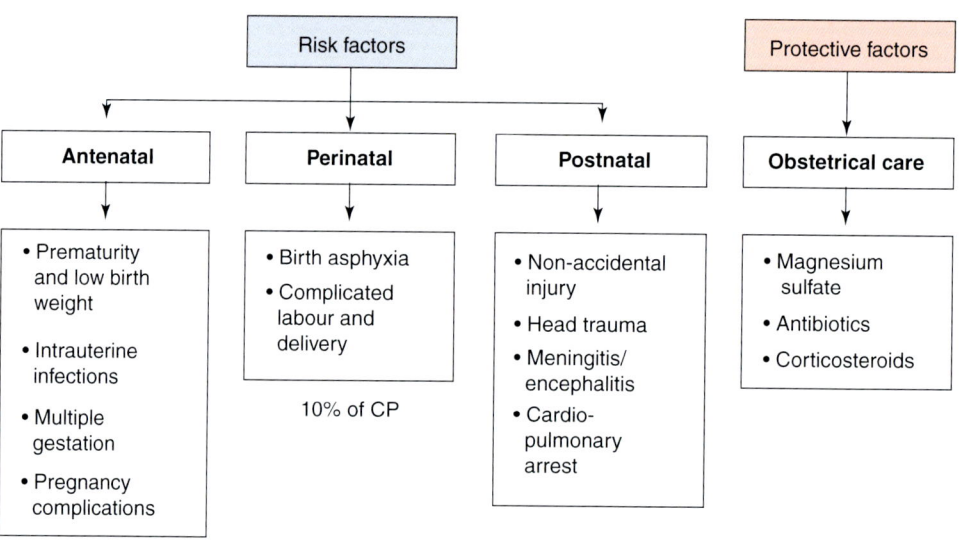

**Fig. 45.1** Antenatal associations are linked in the majority of children with cerebral palsy. Perinatal injury is reported in the others and rarely a postnatal cause. The timely use of magnesium sulfate, antibiotics and corticosteroids in the mother may help to reduce the occurrence of cerebral palsy (from: ophys.org/cerebral-palsy/cp-riskfactors-2/) (Posted December 16, 2012 by Eric Wong)

change over time although the clinical manifestations may change as the child grows [6]. The manifestations and severity vary based on the location and degree of the initial insult to the developing brain and/or spinal cord, ranging from mild motor impairment to whole-body impairment including mental retardation [6]. As cerebral palsy is a term used to describe a spectrum of related CNS syndromes and lesions, it is most easily classified according to the predominant handicap in terms of motor abnormality and extremity/extremities affected. The motor defect may be classified as spastic, ataxic, athetoid/dyskinetic, and mixed. CP can further be organized by degree of body involvement—diplegia (significant leg involvement with little effect on the arms), hemiplegia (involvement of the ipsilateral arm and leg), and quadriplegia (involvement of all four limbs) [6, 7]. Spastic cerebral palsy is the most common subtype comprising 70% of CP patients.

Diagnosis of cerebral palsy necessitates a complete history and physical examination including a detailed account of perinatal events and a general movement assessment (GMA). The GMA measures spontaneous movements in infants less than 4 months old and has been shown to be the most sensitive and specific test for CP currently available [8]. Diagnosis is typically made by 2 years of age although children displaying milder forms may be diagnosed at an older age. Once a child is diagnosed with CP additional neuroimaging tests may be done to assess the degree of the CNS insult [6].

## Treatment

Although the lesion(s) in cerebral palsy are non-progressive, the condition is not curable and the degree of impairment can become more severe over time. Treatment involves an integrated multi-disciplinary approach of medical, surgical, and physical therapy teams that aim at maximizing the child's independence and improving quality of life. Although medical therapy with drugs such as baclofen and diazepam are intended to moderate spasticity and prevent contractures with the aim of decreasing the need for surgical intervention, they can have considerable side effects and must be introduced early for overall effectiveness. Muscular injections of botulinum toxin type A—better known as Botox—is also a widely used treatment for spasticity with the goal of preventing presynaptic release of acetylcholine, thereby causing a functional denervation of the muscle. Orthopedic and neurosurgical interventions such as casting (for improving and maintaining range of motion) and dorsal rhizotomy (to reduce spasticity) are also common and effective [9]. Additionally, more invasive surgeries involving limb lengthening and correction of spinal deformities are also performed. Many are also on anticonvulsants for treatment of seizures.

## Anesthetic Considerations: Preoperative Assessment

Particular problems with respect to patients with CP are variable and as such preoperative considerations should be determined by both the severity of the disease and associated medical conditions. A detailed medical and surgical history should be conducted as many of these patients have had multiple surgeries in the past. All current medications and doses should be clearly reported including but not limited to anti-convulsants, anti-spasmodics, anti-reflux, and pain medications. Of particular note baclofen should not be abruptly stopped as it can lead to withdrawal symptoms. Dantrolene and baclofen use can also cause weakness.

It is also important to ensure that patients continue to receive their anti-epileptic medications as up to 30% of cerebral palsy patients experience seizures [5]. Preoperative labs and studies will vary based on the patient's particular medical ailments and medications as well as the type of procedure and/or anesthesia performed.

During physical exam careful attention should be paid to respiratory function, as both reactive airway disease and chronic pneumonia from aspiration are common. Additionally, many have spinal deformities or severe scoliosis. Careful attention to the extent of deformity should be noted as it may have positioning implications during the surgical procedure. Although the airway will usually appear grossly normal, contractures of the head and neck may require careful positioning during tracheal intubation [5]. It is also important to note that impaired swallowing paired with hyperactive salivary glands may cause copious secretions, limiting visualization of the glottis during laryngoscopy [4].

Because many of these children have difficulty communicating and have previously undergone numerous surgeries and procedures usually under anesthesia, preoperative anxiety may be an unavoidable issue. These cases should warrant premedication with oral or IV midazolam, if applicable [5].

These children have commonly undergone numerous operative procedures and cases of severe reaction to latex have been reported [10]. A history of latex allergy should be discussed with each patient and family during the preoperative evaluation.

## Anesthetic Considerations: Intraoperative Care

Induction of anesthesia may be achieved via the intravenous or inhalational route. Both have advantages and disadvantages and may be challenging due to lack of cooperation and communication difficulties. Often IV access is difficult and may not be the best option for induction if the child does not already have an intravenous catheter or a port in place [7]. If IV induction is planned, all commonly used agents are appropriate although one study from Turkey suggests that non-communicative/nonverbal children with CP required less propofol to obtain the same BIS values compared to otherwise healthy children [11]. Increased drooling has been described to interfere with smooth and safe inhalational induction in children with cerebral palsy [7]. Premedicating these children with an antisialagogue is recommended.

Airway management is usually contingent on the type of procedure to be performed as well as upon patient positioning during the procedure. When clinically appropriate, mask ventilation and laryngeal mask airway are suitable options, although many prefer to routinely use tracheal intubation.

Maintenance of anesthesia depends upon local preference and can be provided with the standard anesthetic drugs and techniques. Inhaled anesthetics, muscle relaxants (both non-depolarizing and depolarizing), opioids, local anesthetics, and hypnotics have all been used safely. It is important to note, however, that children with CP and severe mental retardation require a lower minimum alveolar concentration (MAC) of inhalational anesthetics than healthy children [12].

Although the mechanism is still not clear, it has been shown that children with cerebral palsy demonstrate resistance to vecuronium regardless of whether or not they are taking anticonvulsant medications [13]. Monitoring of the neuromuscular block with a twitch monitor will aid in achieving the desired effect. Alternatively, despite worries that succinylcholine is not appropriate for use in children with CP, studies show that although these children are slightly more sensitive to succinylcholine, it is not enough to be clinically significant [14]. The fear that succinylcholine in children with cerebral palsy will produce a substantive hyperkalemic response is also unfounded as their muscles were never fully developed or functionally innervated and will not have an upregulation of acetylcholine receptors.

Due to contractures and a scoliotic vertebral column, epidural or spinal needle placement can be challenging. However, if performed carefully by an experienced provider while the patient is sedated or anesthetized, neuraxial anesthetics can provide a safe and valuable option for use in children with cerebral palsy whether in juxtaposition with general anesthesia or as the sole anesthetic [7, 15]. Peripheral nerve blocks are also beneficial [16]. A recent study out of Japan found that children with CP who received a popliteal block for lower limb surgery had decreased sevoflurane requirements during surgery and decreased paracetamol use in the PACU [17]. Epidural catheters and peripheral nerve catheters have the added benefit of being continued into the postoperative period for help with pain control and muscle spasm.

Heat loss during general anesthesia is an important concern as thermoregulation can be difficult in children with CP, underscoring the importance of monitoring core temperature throughout the procedure. These children have little subcutaneous fat for insulation and may not be able to shiver due to neurocognitive dysfunction [5]. It is well-known that with the onset of general anesthesia there is a redistribution of heat from the core to the periphery. This is unavoidable and thus it is necessary to diminish its effects to the best of our abilities by pre-warming the operating room prior to induction, humidifying airway gases, using a safe patient warming method during surgery, and limiting exposure of the patient during positioning and/or performance of the anesthetic for the diagnostic or surgical procedures [5, 7]. By the same token, children may experience intraoperative hyperthermia from upper body warming while surgery on both lower extremities is being conducted in these children and orthopedic tourniquets are activated on both the thighs. This happens because the area available for heat redistribution is significantly reduced by the application of the tourniquets.

Positioning can often be challenging in children with cerebral palsy due to contractures and lack of subcutaneous fat requiring padding of pressure points. One needs to be vigilant to avoid pressure sores and unintended nerve compression especially during lengthy surgeries.

## Anesthetic Considerations: Pain Management and Postoperative Care

Intraoperative and postoperative pain management is a key aspect of care for children with cerebral palsy as insufficient analgesia during and immediately after surgery can trigger increased postoperative muscle tone and muscle spasm [17]. Many of these children suffer from chronic pain at baseline which must be adequately gauged prior to exposure to a painful surgical procedure. In addition, many of these patients are unable to conceptualize or communicate their pain because of an intellectual disability, making pain assessment even more difficult. These factors can frequently lead to inadequate analgesia [18, 19]. Often parents and caregivers are the best at assessing and managing their child's pain and are a great resource in the postoperative period. If a child has severe cognitive dysfunction, parent-controlled analgesia may be helpful in a closely monitored setting.

Lower limb and spinal surgeries are some of the more common surgeries undertaken in CP patients. Regional anesthetics as mentioned earlier are both useful for postoperative pain management as well as preventing muscle spasms as the latter are known to aggravate both pain and distress postoperatively [17]. Additionally, regional and local anesthetics also offer the added benefit of reducing opioid-induced constipation that many of these children are prone to due to lack of mobility and decreased fluid intake [18]. Minimizing inhaled anesthetics and opioids will also decrease the risk for post-operative nausea and vomiting (Table 45.1).

It is important to note that post-operative complications are not uncommon in children with severe cerebral palsy and neurologic impairment, often leading to delayed recovery and a prolonged hospital stay. Understanding both the intraoperative and postoperative risk factors is essential when speaking with and advising families and caregivers [4, 20].

## References

1. Christensen D, Van Naarden Braun K, Doernberg NS, Maenner MJ, Arneson CL, Durkin MS, et al. Prevalence of cerebral palsy, co-occurring autism spectrum disorders, and motor functioning—Autism and Developmental Disabilities Monitoring Network, USA, 2008. Dev Med Child Neurol. 2014;56(1):59–65.
2. Rosenbaum P, Paneth N, Leviton A, Goldstein M, Bax M, Damiano D, et al. A report: the definition and classification of cerebral palsy April 2006. Dev Med Child Neurol Suppl. 2007;109:8–14.
3. Shepherd E, Middleton P, Makrides M, McIntyre S, Badawi N, Crowther CA. Neonatal interventions for preventing cerebral palsy: an overview of Cochrane systematic reviews (Protocol). Cochrane Database Syst Rev. 2016;(10):1–12.

4. Wass CT, Warner ME, Worrell GA, Castagno JA, Howe M, Kerber KA, et al. Effect of general anesthesia in patients with cerebral palsy at the turn of the new millennium: a population-based study evaluating perioperative outcome and brief overview of anesthetic implications of this coexisting disease. J Child Neurol. 2012;27(7):859–66.
5. Lerman J. Perioperative management of the paediatric patient with coexisting neuromuscular disease. Br J Anaesth. 2011;107(Suppl 1):i79–89.
6. Koman LA, Smith BP, Shilt JS. Cerebral palsy. Lancet. 2004;363(9421):1619–31.
7. Wongprasartsuk P, Stevens J. Cerebral palsy and anaesthesia. Paediatr Anaesth. 2002;12(4):296–303.
8. Bosanquet M, Copeland L, Ware R, Boyd R. A systematic review of tests to predict cerebral palsy in young children. Dev Med Child Neurol. 2013;55(5):418–26.
9. Novak I, McIntyre S, Morgan C, Campbell L, Dark L, Morton N, et al. A systematic review of interventions for children with cerebral palsy: state of the evidence. Dev Med Child Neurol. 2013;55(10):885–910.
10. Delfico AJ, Dormans JP, Craythorne CB, Templeton JJ. Intraoperative anaphylaxis due to allergy to latex in children who have cerebral palsy: a report of six cases. Dev Med Child Neurol. 1997;39(3):194–7.
11. Saricaoglu F, Celebi N, Celik M, Aypar U. The evaluation of propofol dosage for anesthesia induction in children with cerebral palsy with bispectral index (BIS) monitoring. Paediatr Anaesth. 2005;15(12):1048–52.
12. Frei FJ, Haemmerle MH, Brunner R, Kern C. Minimum alveolar concentration for halothane in children with cerebral palsy and severe mental retardation. Anaesthesia. 1997;52(11):1056–60.
13. Hepaguslar H, Ozzeybek D, Elar Z. The effect of cerebral palsy on the action of vecuronium with or without anticonvulsants. Anaesthesia. 1999;54(6):593–6.
14. Theroux MC, Brandom BW, Zagnoev M, Kettrick RG, Miller F, Ponce C. Dose response of succinylcholine at the adductor pollicis of children with cerebral palsy during propofol and nitrous oxide anesthesia. Anesth Analg. 1994;79(4):761–5.
15. Onal O, Apiliogullari S, Gunduz E, Celik JB, Senaran H. Spinal anaesthesia for orthopaedic surgery in children with cerebral palsy: analysis of 36 patients. Pak J Med Sci. 2015;31(1):189–93.
16. Ozkan D, Gonen E, Akkaya T, Bakir M. Popliteal block for lower limb surgery in children with cerebral palsy: effect on sevoflurane consumption and postoperative pain (a randomized, double-blinded, controlled trial). J Anesth. 2017;31:358.
17. Maranhao MV. Anesthesia and cerebral palsy. Rev Bras Anestesiol. 2005;55(6):680–702.
18. Nolan J, Chalkiadis GA, Low J, Olesch CA, Brown TC. Anaesthesia and pain management in cerebral palsy. Anaesthesia. 2000;55(1):32–41.
19. Ghai B, Makkar JK, Wig J. Postoperative pain assessment in preverbal children and children with cognitive impairment. Paediatr Anaesth. 2008;18(6):462–77.
20. Lipton GE, Miller F, Dabney KW, Altiok H, Bachrach SJ. Factors predicting postoperative complications following spinal fusions in children with cerebral palsy. J Spinal Disord. 1999;12(3):197–205.

# Anesthesia for Nuss Procedures (Pectus Deformity)

## Vanessa A. Olbrecht

## Introduction

Pectus excavatum, one of the most common chest wall deformities, occurs in about 0.8–0.14% of the population, or approximately 1 in every 300–400 births, and has a prevalence of 2.6% in children between the ages of 7 and 14 years [1–3]. It accounts for 90% of all chest wall deformities and is a defect in embryonic development that begins when the ribs fail to fuse properly with the sternum beginning around the 35th day of gestation [3]. Although it is a congenital anomaly, many children do not manifest visible symptoms until after 1 year of age. The deformity is characterized by a depression of the sternum and costal cartilages 3–7 on each side of the chest resulting in a reduction of the anterior-posterior diameter of the chest [4]. Patients with pectus excavatum may also have sloped ribs, a pot belly and rounded shoulders, all of which become more pronounced as the child ages [3]. About 40% of pectus deformities are familial in nature but no specific genetic defect has yet been identified; however, there is strong evidence to suggest that the pectus deformity may result from an autosomal recessive trait [5]. The defect occurs most often in males in a ratio of approximately 4:1 [5]. There is sometimes an association between pectus excavatum and connective tissue disorders, including Marfan syndrome (5–8%) and Ehlers-Danlos syndrome (3%); the majority, however, are idiopathic [4]. While many argue that pectus excavatum is merely a cosmetic defect that has no influence on cardiopulmonary function, the aesthetic defect alone has been associated with mood and anxiety disorders, including suicidal ideation [4, 6]; many others, however, argue that over time, the defect can cause significant cardiopulmonary dysfunction [7–10]. As a child with pectus excavatum develops, the dorsal deviation of the sternum and costal cartilages create a funnel-shaped deformity of the chest that can result in progressive compression of the heart and lungs leading to compressive/restrictive symptoms [11]. Specific symptoms can include: ventricular compression [12], cardiac arrhythmias [13, 14] and restrictive ventilator defects [13].

First described in 1594 by Bauhinus, pectus excavatum has been recognized for hundreds of years [15]. In the 1800s, treatment for the deformity consisted of fresh air, breathing exercises, aerobic activity and lateral pressure [16]. It was not until 1949 that Dr. Ravitch first described a surgical repair of pectus excavatum [17]. His repair involved an open technique to mobilize the sternum via resection of the bilateral costal cartilages and a sternal osteotomy [18]. In 1956, Wallgren and Sulamaa modified the technique by placing a bar through the distal end of the sternum and, in 1961, Adkins and Blades placed the bar behind in lieu of through the sternum [19].

V. A. Olbrecht, M.D., M.B.A.
Department of Anesthesia and Pediatrics,
Cincinnati Children's Hospital Medical Center,
Cincinnati, OH, USA
e-mail: Vanessa.Olbrecht@cchmc.org

Nevertheless, several problems remained with these surgical treatments: the development of acquired asphyxiating chondrodystrophy (secondary to damage to the cartilaginous growth centers due to extensive rib resection and sternal isolation) and recurrence. In the late 1980s, Donald Nuss began developing the Nuss procedure, a minimally invasive technique that places a convex bar under the sternum with little to no resection of the costal cartilages and, by 1998, Nuss and his colleagues reported their 10-year experience with the procedure [1]. Since then, many modifications have been made to the surgery but the basic, minimally invasive surgical repair, remains the standard of care.

## Clinical Presentation and Pathophysiology

Patients with pectus excavatum present with a wide range of symptoms, from physiologically normal to significant cardiopulmonary symptoms. When symptomatic, they often present during adolescence. From 1949 to the late 1990s, surgeons felt that the younger the patient the better as the surgical repair would be easier for both the surgeon and patient and result in improved cosmetic results [5]. However, this opinion has shifted with most surgeons preferring to wait to perform a repair until puberty or later [5]. Because pectus excavatum is a progressive deformity, it can progress rapidly during growth and this progression can be even more pronounced during puberty, resulting in a more complex and more asymmetric deformity and, therefore, a much more complex repair [5].

As a result of worsening depression of the sternum and costal cartilages with associated narrowing of the anterior-posterior diameter of the chest, many patients experience chest pain, fatigue, recurrent respiratory infections, asthma symptoms, dyspnea, heart murmurs and cardiac dysrhythmias [4]. The most common symptoms on presentation include: dyspnea on exertion and a decreased exercise tolerance [4]. In addition to physical manifestations, patients may also exhibit psychological issues, including depression, social aversion, suicidal ideation and poor body image [5]. Psychological trauma, both in and out of school, may occur [20].

## Considerations for Repair

Surgery is the cornerstone for correction of pectus excavatum. The decision as to when to operate remains a careful decision weighing many factors, including the patient's symptoms, signs of respiratory and/or cardiac dysfunction and patient choice [11].The severity of the pectus defect can be determined objectively using the Haller index which is obtained by dividing the lateral diameter of the chest by the antero-posterior diameter; a pectus is defined as severe when the Haller index is greater than 3.35 (normal value: 2.56) [21]. Although there is no consensus for the best age at repair, the mean age has shifted from 6 to 15 years, before the chest wall is fully ossified and is still pliable for repair, resulting in a durable and stable surgical repair [5, 22]. In the past, surgeons felt that the optimal time for repair was in younger children as their chest wall was much more pliable. Both Ravitch and Nuss corrected patients primarily between 4 and 6 years and 3–5 years of age, respectively [1, 18]. Surgical repair can be challenging in very young patients as children are much more active and can inadvertently sustain trauma [1]. Furthermore, rib growth after early repair can be impaired and, with a Ravitch procedure, can result in acquired asphyxiating chondrodystrophy [1]. On the other hand, repairs in older patients can technically be more difficult with longer operating times and higher rates of blood loss [1]. However, by waiting until after the growth spurt is complete, the likelihood of recurrence of the defect is lower. Special considerations exist in patients with concomitant connective tissue disease. These patients often have soft bones and generally require two bars to more equally distribute pressure over a wider area [1]. In those with Marfan and Ehlers-Danlos syndrome, the incidence of recurrence may be higher [23]; however, when properly corrected, outcomes may be equivalent to similarly aged patients [24].

Surgical repair is recommended when patients fulfill certain criteria. Specifically, surgery is generally offered when the patient fulfills two or more of the following criteria:

(a) Severe and progressive deformity with associated symptoms (i.e. dyspnea on exertion, decreased exercise tolerance, chest pain);
(b) A Haller index greater than 3.25 and cardiac compression or displacement on chest CT;
(c) Pulmonary function studies that show restrictive or obstructive ventilator defects;
(d) Cardiac evaluation demonstrating cardiac compression or displacement, mitral valve prolapse, arrhythmias, or murmurs;
(e) Previous failed open or closed repair [5].

In those patients who are asymptomatic or who have only a mild/moderate deformity, conservative management tends to be recommended. Conservative management is composed of a two-prong approach:

(a) Deep breathing with breath holding exercises and a posture program; patients are also encouraged to participate in aerobic activities;
(b) Vacuum bell therapy, requiring a 1–2 year commitment [5].

## Preoperative Anesthetic Assessment

The focus of preoperative assessment must be on the cardiopulmonary system. Work-up begins with a thorough history and physical examination. The severity of the pectus defect can be estimated using caliper measurements of the distance from the deepest depression of the sternum to the top of the rib cage and serial measurements can help keep track of the progress of the deformity over time [3]. Cardiac auscultation may reveal a characteristic murmur or click, signaling mitral valve prolapse, a cardiac abnormality found in about 20% of patients with pectus excavatum [2]. In addition, other symptoms should raise suspicion for associated connective tissue disorders, including the presence of scoliosis, flat feet, joint hypermobility, an arm span 1.05 times greater than height, a high-arched palate and certain craniofacial features (i.e. elongated skull, downward slanting eyes and receding jaw) [3].

Chest CT is the preferred diagnostic study to better define a patient's pectus deformity. The chest CT allows for quantification of the pectus defect through the measurement of the Haller index as well as to identify the presence of cardiac depression and/or displacement [3]. It may also detect any underlying pulmonary infection [25]. Further cardiac investigation may be done using electrocardiogram (EKG) and/or echocardiography (ECHO). EKG can help to identify any underlying cardiac dysrhythmias whereas an ECHO can assess for atrial and ventricular compression, particularly of the right heart [3]. While cardiac function is often normal at rest, it may become restricted during exercise secondary to sternal compression and displacement of the heart; right ventricular emptying is often reduced compared to normal controls [26, 27]. While cardiac MRI may be used to assess cardiac function, this is not yet typically part of the pre-operative assessment. Although not considered necessary, pulmonary function testing (PFTs) may reveal a restrictive ventilator defect on spirometry as well as ventilation-perfusion abnormalities, even in patients with normal exercise capacity [10, 28, 29]. In one review of 557 patients presenting for pectus repair, the authors found that about 26% of patients had a forced vital capacity (FVC) of less than 80% and 32% had a forced expiratory volume in 1 s ($FEV_1$) of less than 80% [30].

Of note, it is also important to assess patients for allergies to metal, including nickel and cobalt, as 10–15% of the population has sensitivity to metals to avoid placing a bar to which the patient has a reaction [11].

## Intraoperative Considerations

The Nuss procedure is the current operation most widely used to repair pectus excavatum. It is a minimally invasive surgery that involves inserting a custom-made metal bar under the sternum, affixing it laterally to the ribs and flipping the bar to elevate the sternum [1]. Many corrections can be done with a single bar but more severe cases require two or even three bars for repair. The Nuss repair, as compared to the open Ravitch approach, is thought to result in less scarring, decreased blood loss, shorter operative time, smaller incisions, less dissection and a lower risk of infection [3, 31]. However, because of the instantaneous surgical correction of the sternum, this operation is associated with significant postoperative pain [32]. A meta-analysis done comparing outcomes between patients undergoing the Ravitch versus the Nuss procedure found no significant differences in total complication rates between the two operations in the pediatric population [31]. Although the majority of patients will undergo a Nuss procedure for this repair, recurrent cases or patients with very complex anatomy may still be candidates for the open approach [3].

Prior to beginning surgery, it is important to obtain adequate intravenous (IV) access and a type and screen. In addition, a decision needs to be made with regard to postoperative pain management (discussed in the next section). If an epidural is to be placed, in older patients, this can be done in a sitting position with mild to moderate sedation; in younger patients that are unable to remain still, the epidural can be placed following induction of general anesthesia. Epidural placement is usually targeted for the T5 to T7 level, allowing the tip to lie close to the dermatomal distribution of the incision but not too high to avoid symptoms of Horner's syndrome (miosis, partial ptosis and/or enophthalmos). Following catheter placement, a test dose of 0.1 mL/kg (up to 3 mL) of 1.5% lidocaine with 1:200,000 epinephrine should be used to verify extra-vascular placement. The epidural can be bolused thereafter with local anesthetic with or without adjuvant (i.e. opioid or clonidine) and can be dosed intraoperatively, either with a continuous infusion or intermittent boluses every 60–90 min. Following loading, it is not uncommon to see a decrease in heart rate and blood pressure of 10–20%.

Standard anesthetic monitoring is used, including a 3-lead EKG and pulse oximetry, along with general endotracheal anesthesia. At our institution, we place one large-bore IV in addition to a smaller IV but an arterial catheter is not routinely used. We opt to place an arterial catheter if the patient is undergoing a redo operation or if there is significant cardiac dysfunction noted on preoperative testing. Nitrous oxide is generally avoided as it may increase the size of a pneumothorax. A foley catheter is typically placed and left in postoperatively. While some surgeons may request single lung ventilation to obtain better visualization, the majority of procedures are done with two lung ventilation with the surgeon using carbon dioxide insufflation to create an artificial pneumothorax [33]. Perioperative transesophageal ECHO (TEE) has been reported to monitor the heart during bar insertion and manipulation [34–36]; however, this is not routine practice.

Patient positioning is an important element during this repair. In order to facilitate bar placement through the left lateral chest wall incision at the point of maximal sternal displacement, the patient's arms must be abducted, which places the patient at risk of brachial plexus injury [37]. In addition, some surgeons place a vertical roll between the scapulae to further push the patient's chest forward, further increasing the risk of injury. Fox and colleagues have suggested a positioning strategy which may help minimize risk of such brachial plexus injury [37].

Although rare, serious complications during a Nuss repair can occur, including: hemothorax, vascular injuries, liver perforation, right ventricular perforation, lung parenchymal laceration, cardiac arrhythmias, hypotension secondary to cardiac compression and bleeding due to intercostal artery injury [1, 38–40]. Residual pneumothorax is quite common, occurring in over half of the cases, but with very few requiring chest tube placement and 95% resolving on their own [39, 41]. While the majority of cardiac and pericardial injury have been reported prior to the adoption of thoracoscopy, anesthesia providers must nevertheless remain vigilant for these major complications by closely monitoring the patient's vital signs and what is happening on the operative field [38]. However, they must also be aware of the more common things that are seen during the surgery. It is not uncommon to see cardiac arrhythmias during mediastinal dissection [41]. In addition, bilateral thoracoscopy with carbon dioxide insufflation, while making conditions safer for dissection and bar placement, can result in issues with hypotension and bradycardia. Following bar placement and securement, temporary suctioning of the pleural spaces accompanied by anesthesia-mediated Valsalva maneuver is used to evacuate the pneumothoraces in the chest. A chest X-ray should be performed at the end of the case while still in the operating room under anesthesia to evaluate for the presence of persistent pneumothorax, hemothorax, mediastinal emphysema, pleural effusion or bar displacement [41]. Some surgeons decrease the incidence of residual pneumothorax by leaving a tube in the chest until the lateral chest wall incisions are closed. At that time, the patient is placed in the Trendelenberg position and positive pressure ventilation with positive end-expiratory pressure is used with the chest tube to water seal. The chest tubes are then removed during an inspiratory hold when no more bubbles are seen in the water seal chamber.

During emergence from anesthesia, it is also important to avoid coughing or straining. Some practitioners advocate the use of deep extubation to avoid a tumultuous wake-up, thereby decreasing the risk of developing subcutaneous emphysema which occurs due to forcible expulsion of a residual pneumothorax [17].

## Postoperative Pain Management

The greatest issue faced by patients undergoing repair of pectus excavatum is pain and successful pain management is a must to optimize patient satisfaction and decrease complication rates [32]. Pain during this surgery results not only from incisional pain but more importantly, from musculoskeletal pain secondary to pectus bar insertion and flipping leading to significant trauma to the costochondral cartilage. In addition to pain, many patients experience anxiety related to the procedure and pain therefore a focus to alleviate and treat anxiety both pre- and postoperatively is important [5]. Preoperative preparation and knowledge is fundamentally important as it may not just help to decrease anxiety but may also improve overall pain outcomes [42]. Aggressive physical therapy and early ambulation should be emphasized [42]. In general, children under the age of 12 recover much faster than older patients; while children often require narcotic pain medication for less than 1 week after surgery and are able to discontinue all pain medications by 2–3 weeks, the same is not true of older patients [5]. Adults may require narcotics for several weeks and often remain on adjuvant pain medications for 1 month or longer [5]. In addition, older teenage and adult patients face the risk of developing chronic pain [43].

Many different strategies have been utilized to optimize analgesia in this population, including systemic opioids via patient-controlled analgesia (PCA), non-steroidal anti-inflammatory agents (NSAIDs), regional anesthesia (epidural, paravertebral blocks and intercostal nerve blocks) and even hypnosis [32]. Ketamine may be considered as an adjuvant to any of these analgesic regimens [17]. Many institutions utilize a combination of different modalities, such as epidural analgesia with opioids (fentanyl, morphine, hydromorphone, oxycodone), NSAIDs (ketorolac, ibuprofen), acetaminophen and muscle relaxants (methocarbamol, diazepam, cyclobenzaprine); some centers even add long-acting opioids such as methadone and neuropathic agents such as gabapentin or pregabalin. There is still great debate in the literature regarding optimal pain management therapy for these patients. A recent retrospective review cited multimodal therapy with a single intra-operative dose of methadone for optimal analgesia [44]. However, this study was fraught with issues and may indeed not represent the best therapeutic modality [45]. The greatest debate that exists in pectus repair surgery is the best analgesic modality for these patients. Despite several large series showing that our current pain control regimens are adequate, there is yet to be a clear determination on optimal strategy, particularly in the debate between PCA and epidural [8, 46, 47]. Because of this debate, there is division as to preference for PCA or epidural among practitioners. While several studies have

**Table 46.1** Dosing considerations of ropivacaine and adjuvants

| Intraoperative dosing | | Postoperative infusion | |
|---|---|---|---|
| *Bolus volume*: 0.05 × weight in kg × dermatomal levels of coverage desired or 0.3 mL/kg<br>*Maximum bolus dose usually ~ 10 mL* | | *Rate*: 0.2–0.4 mL/kg/h<br>*Maximum rate usually 10–12 mL/h* | |
| Local anesthetic | Adjuvant | Local anesthetic | Adjuvant |
| Ropivacaine 0.2% | Fentanyl 1 µg/kg<br>Hydromorphone 7–8 µg/kg<br>Clonidine 1 µg/kg | Ropivacaine 0.125%, 0.15% or 0.2% | Fentanyl 2.5–5 µg/mL<br>Hydromorphone 3–5 µg/mL<br>Morphine 25–50 µg/mL<br>Clonidine 0.5–1 µg/mL |

When making dosing decisions, one must calculate maximum dose of local anesthetic based on patient weight to avoid toxicity (0.4 mg/kg/h). Typical rates of adjuvants include: Fentanyl 1 µg/kg/h, hydromorphone 1 µg/kg/h, morphine 2.5 µg/kg/h and clonidine 0.2 µg/kg/h

shown that patients with thoracic epidurals have improved pain control along with improved postoperative ventilation and pulmonary toilet, the results are mixed [46, 48–50]. Several other studies demonstrate no benefit to epidural over PCA [47, 51–53]. Because of the risks associated with epidurals, particularly spinal cord injury, some centers have shifted to utilizing a PCA over an epidural as there is no clear defined benefit of regional analgesia [39].

If an epidural is chosen, it is placed in the thoracic region of the spine, as detailed earlier. The epidural is usually left in place for several days postoperatively. Epidural opioids may be added to the infusion to help improve the quality of the block [54]; alternatively, clonidine may be added to help optimize analgesia while reducing opioid-related side effects such as nausea and pruritus while maintaining the ability to use systemic opioids as adjuvant therapy [55]. The table below shows typical dosing regimens for perioperative epidural analgesia.

When an epidural is utilized, the transition from regional analgesia to parenteral opioids is often challenging. Some practitioners advocate the addition of a PCA even when patients have epidurals to assist with this transition, especially in older teenage patients [56].

An alternative to epidural analgesia is the paravertebral block. Paravertebral blocks have been commonly used to manage pain following thoracic surgery, particularly in thoracotomy patients [57]. Bilateral paravertebral blocks have been used in pediatric patients and have shown efficacy in postoperative pain management in pediatric patients undergoing the Nuss procedure, resulting in equivalent opioid consumption and pain scores when compared to epidurals [58]. Paravertebral catheters may be an alternative to epidural analgesia if regional analgesia is sought. However, larger volumes of local anesthetic are required to maintain an effective block and this may be an issue in younger patients due to toxicity; in addition, there is also potential risk of local anesthetic toxicity in a highly vascular space [11]. Intercostal nerve blocks may also be considered as an adjuvant to multimodal therapy and has been used in the pediatric population undergoing Nuss repair [59]; however, further study is needed prior to recommending this technique. Dosing considerations of ropivacaine and adjuvants are provided in Table 46.1.

## Outcomes Following Repair

To optimize outcomes after repair it is important for patients to abstain from physical activities, sports, heavy lifting and sleeping on their backs for a minimum of 6 weeks [5]. After 6 weeks, patients may slowly return to normal activities and, by 3 months, they may resume competitive sports with the exception of those that run the risk of significant chest wall trauma (i.e. football, rugby, hockey and boxing) [5]. Patients should continue deep breathing exercises twice daily and aerobic activity until the bar is removed [5]. Patients maintain regular follow-up with the surgeon at 3–6 month intervals for at least 2 years [3]. The bar(s) remain in place for 2–4 years (3 is optimal) to minimize the

**Table 46.2** Summary of anesthesia considerations for the repair of pectus excavatum

| Plan/preparation/adverse events | Reasoning/management |
|---|---|
| Preprocedural evaluation<br>  History and physical exam<br>  Haller index calculation<br>  Chest CT<br>  EKG<br>  ECHO<br>  PFTs | Focus is on understanding the degree of cardiopulmonary compromise relating to the pectus deformity to properly prepare for surgery |
| Position<br>  Typically placed with arms out and above head with possibly a vertical shoulder roll between the scapulae | Caution must be taken to protect the extremities against brachial plexus injury by using padding and avoiding greater than 90° angles in the joints |
| IV access<br>  1 smaller bore IV<br>  1 large-bore IV | A smaller IV is usually placed prior to induction. A large-bore IV is placed in case of hemorrhage. Arterial access is generally not required unless the patient is returning for re-operation or has significant cardiac dysfunction |
| Anesthesia<br>  General endotracheal anesthesia<br>  Regional anesthesia | General endotracheal anesthesia is required, usually with double lung ventilation; single lung ventilation may be required by the surgeon at which point a left-sided double lumen endotracheal tube may be necessary. Nitrous oxide is generally avoided<br>Thoracic epidural placement is commonly performed to help optimize postoperative pain management. Epidural placement most commonly occurs with mild to moderate sedation prior to the induction of general anesthesia. Paravertebral blocks may also be utilized and placed prior to induction |
| Procedural adverse events<br>  Hypotension<br>  Hemorrhage<br>  Cardiac arrythmias | The most severe complication that may occur during the procedure is also luckily the most uncommon: Major cardiovascular injury resulting in severe hemorrhage. Care must be taken to monitor for vital sign changes and signs of bleeding |
| Postoperative adverse events<br>  Pneumothorax<br>  Hemothorax<br>  Inadequate pain control | Providers should have a low threshold to obtain a chest X-ray postoperatively to assess for complications |
| Post-discharge considerations<br>  Pain control<br>  Avoid physical activity for 6 weeks<br>  Avoid competitive sports for ≥3 months<br>  Continue deep breathing exercises 2× daily | As indicated |

risk of recurrence [39]. The most common significant complication in this population is bar displacement requiring surgical repositioning, occurring to date in about 1% of patients in the largest series published [39]. Recurrence rates vary among studies but have been quoted to be about 2–10% in the literature [3]. Several studies report a nearly 95% patient satisfaction rate after surgery [3]. Although the role of surgery in the management of pectus excavatum has remained somewhat controversial, many patients report improvement in pulmonary function, exercise capacity, body image and even quality of life and the minimally invasive approach has essentially become standard of care in the last decade [9, 38, 60–67] (Table 46.2).

# References

1. Nuss D, Kelly RE Jr, Croitoru DP, Katz ME. A 10-year review of a minimally invasive technique for the correction of pectus excavatum. J Pediatr Surg. 1998;33(4):545–52.
2. Croitoru DP, Kelly RE Jr, Goretsky MJ, Lawson ML, Swoveland B, Nuss D. Experience and modification

update for the minimally invasive Nuss technique for pectus excavatum repair in 303 patients. J Pediatr Surg. 2002;37(3):437–45.
3. Abdullah F, Harris J. Pectus excavatum: more than a matter of aesthetics. Pediatr Ann. 2016;45(11):e403–e6.
4. Valenti FBC, Mariani R, et al. Anesthetic management for pediatric correction of pectus excavatum with NUSS technique. Pediatr Anesth Crit Care J. 2014;2(2):3.
5. Nuss D, Obermeyer RJ, Kelly RE Jr. Pectus excavatum from a pediatric surgeon's perspective. Ann Cardiothorac Surg. 2016;5(5):493–500.
6. Ji Y, Liu W, Chen S, Xu B, Tang Y, Wang X, et al. Assessment of psychosocial functioning and its risk factors in children with pectus excavatum. Health Qual Life Outcomes. 2011;9:28.
7. Kelly RE Jr, Lawson ML, Paidas CN, Hruban RH. Pectus excavatum in a 112-year autopsy series: anatomic findings and the effect on survival. J Pediatr Surg. 2005;40(8):1275–8.
8. Kelly RE Jr, Shamberger RC, Mellins RB, Mitchell KK, Lawson ML, Oldham K, et al. Prospective multicenter study of surgical correction of pectus excavatum: design, perioperative complications, pain, and baseline pulmonary function facilitated by internet-based data collection. J Am Coll Surg. 2007;205(2):205–16.
9. Malek MH, Berger DE, Marelich WD, Coburn JW, Beck TW, Housh TJ. Pulmonary function following surgical repair of pectus excavatum: a meta-analysis. Eur J Cardiothorac Surg. 2006;30(4):637–43.
10. Malek MH, Fonkalsrud EW, Cooper CB. Ventilatory and cardiovascular responses to exercise in patients with pectus excavatum. Chest. 2003;124(3):870–82.
11. Patvardhan C, Martinez G. Anaesthetic considerations for pectus repair surgery. J Visualized Surg. 2016;2(12):76.
12. Coln E, Carrasco J, Coln D. Demonstrating relief of cardiac compression with the Nuss minimally invasive repair for pectus excavatum. J Pediatr Surg. 2006;41(4):683–6; discussion 6.
13. Haller JA Jr, Loughlin GM. Cardiorespiratory function is significantly improved following corrective surgery for severe pectus excavatum. Proposed treatment guidelines. J Cardiovasc Surg. 2000;41(1):125–30.
14. Kelly RE Jr. Pectus excavatum: historical background, clinical picture, preoperative evaluation and criteria for operation. Semin Pediatr Surg. 2008;17(3):181–93.
15. Brown A. Pectus excavatum (funnel chest). J Thorac Surg. 1939;9:164.
16. Simon NL, Kolvekar T, Kolvekar SK. History. In: Kolvekar SK, Pilegaard H, editors. Chest wall deformities and corrective procedures. New York: Springer; 2015. p. 13–6.
17. Mavi J, Moore DL. Anesthesia and analgesia for pectus excavatum surgery. Anesthesiol Clin. 2014;32(1):175–84.
18. Ravitch MM. The operative treatment of pectus excavatum. Ann Surg. 1949;129(4):429–44.
19. Haller AJ Jr, Katlic M, Shermeta DW, Shaker IJ, White JJ. Operative correction of pectus excavatum: an evolving perspective. Ann Surg. 1976;184(5):554–7.
20. Van Horne BS, Moffitt KB, Canfield MA, Case AP, Greeley CS, Morgan R, et al. Maltreatment of children under age 2 with specific birth defects: a population-based study. Pediatrics. 2015;136(6):e1504–12.
21. Haller JA Jr, Shermeta DW, Tepas JJ, Bittner HR, Golladay ES. Correction of pectus excavatum without prostheses or splints: objective measurement of severity and management of asymmetrical deformities. Ann Thorac Surg. 1978;26(1):73–9.
22. Pawlak K, Gasiorowski L, Gabryel P, Galecki B, Zielinski P, Dyszkiewicz W. Early and late results of the Nuss procedure in surgical treatment of pectus excavatum in different age groups. Ann Thorac Surg. 2016;102(5):1711–6.
23. Ellis DG, Snyder CL, Mann CM. The 're-do' chest wall deformity correction. J Pediatr Surg. 1997;32(9):1267–71.
24. Olbrecht VA, Nabaweesi R, Arnold MA, Chandler N, Chang DC, McIltrot KH, et al. Pectus bar repair of pectus excavatum in patients with connective tissue disease. J Pediatr Surg. 2009;44(9):1812–6.
25. Iseman MD, Buschman DL, Ackerson LM. Pectus excavatum and scoliosis. Thoracic anomalies associated with pulmonary disease caused by Mycobacterium avium complex. Am Rev Respir Dis. 1991;144(4):914–6.
26. Fonkalsrud EW, Bustorff-Silva J. Repair of pectus excavatum and carinatum in adults. Am J Surg. 1999;177(2):121–4.
27. Mocchegiani R, Badano L, Lestuzzi C, Nicolosi GL, Zanuttini D. Relation of right ventricular morphology and function in pectus excavatum to the severity of the chest wall deformity. Am J Cardiol. 1995;76(12):941–6.
28. Cahill JL, Lees GM, Robertson HT. A summary of preoperative and postoperative cardiorespiratory performance in patients undergoing pectus excavatum and carinatum repair. J Pediatr Surg. 1984;19(4):430–3.
29. Blickman JG, Rosen PR, Welch KJ, Papanicolaou N, Treves ST. Pectus excavatum in children: pulmonary scintigraphy before and after corrective surgery. Radiology. 1985;156(3):781–2.
30. Goretsky MJ, Kelly RE Jr, Croitoru D, Nuss D. Chest wall anomalies: pectus excavatum and pectus carinatum. Adolesc Med Clin. 2004;15(3):455–71.
31. Kanagaratnam A, Phan S, Tchantchaleishvili V, Phan K. Ravitch versus Nuss procedure for pectus excavatum: systematic review and meta-analysis. Ann Cardiothorac Surg. 2016;5(5):409–21.
32. Densmore JC, Peterson DB, Stahovic LL, Czarnecki ML, Hainsworth KR, Davies HW, et al. Initial surgical and pain management outcomes after Nuss procedure. J Pediatr Surg. 2010;45(9):1767–71.
33. Molins L, Fibla JJ, Perez J, Vidal G. Chest wall surgery: Nuss technique for repair of pectus excavatum

in adults. Multimed Man Cardiothorac Surg. 2007; 2007(102):mmcts 2004 000315.
34. Becmeur F, Ferreira CG, Haecker FM, Schneider A, Lacreuse I. Pectus excavatum repair according to Nuss: is it safe to place a retrosternal bar by a transpleural approach, under thoracoscopic vision? J Laparoendosc Adv Surg Tech A. 2011;21(8):757–61.
35. Park SY, Park TH, Kim JH, Baek HK, Seo JM, Kim WJ, et al. A case of right ventricular dysfunction caused by pectus excavatum. J Cardiovasc Ultrasound. 2010; 18(2):62–5.
36. Bouchard S, Hong AR, Gilchrist BF, Kuenzler KA. Catastrophic cardiac injuries encountered during the minimally invasive repair of pectus excavatum. Semin Pediatr Surg. 2009;18(2):66–72.
37. Fox ME, Bensard DD, Roaten JB, Hendrickson RJ. Positioning for the Nuss procedure: avoiding brachial plexus injury. Paediatr Anaesth. 2005;15(12): 1067–71.
38. Hebra A, Swoveland B, Egbert M, Tagge EP, Georgeson K, Othersen HB Jr, et al. Outcome analysis of minimally invasive repair of pectus excavatum: review of 251 cases. J Pediatr Surg. 2000;35(2): 252–7; discussion 7–8.
39. Kelly RE, Goretsky MJ, Obermeyer R, Kuhn MA, Redlinger R, Haney TS, et al. Twenty-one years of experience with minimally invasive repair of pectus excavatum by the Nuss procedure in 1215 patients. Ann Surg. 2010;252(6):1072–81.
40. Umuroglu T, Bostanci K, Thomas DT, Yuksel M, Gogus FY. Perioperative anesthetic and surgical complications of the Nuss procedure. J Cardiothorac Vasc Anesth. 2013;27(3):436–40.
41. Futagawa K, Suwa I, Okuda T, Kamamoto H, Sugiura J, Kajikawa R, et al. Anesthetic management for the minimally invasive Nuss procedure in 21 patients with pectus excavatum. J Anesth. 2006;20(1):48–50.
42. Kehlet H, Wilmore DW. Multimodal strategies to improve surgical outcome. Am J Surg. 2002;183(6): 630–41.
43. Olbrecht VA, Arnold MA, Nabaweesi R, Chang DC, McIltrot KH, Abdullah F, et al. Lorenz bar repair of pectus excavatum in the adult population: should it be done? Ann Thorac Surg. 2008;86(2):402–8; discussion 8–9.
44. Singhal NR, Jones J, Semenova J, Williamson A, McCollum K, Tong D, et al. Multimodal anesthesia with the addition of methadone is superior to epidural analgesia: a retrospective comparison of intraoperative anesthetic techniques and pain management for 124 pediatric patients undergoing the Nuss procedure. J Pediatr Surg. 2016;51(4):612–6.
45. Moore DL, Mavi R, Mecoli M, Sadhasivam S. Response to multimodal anesthesia with the addition of methadone is superior to epidural analgesia. J Pediatr Surg. 2017;52(3):517.
46. Soliman IE, Apuya JS, Fertal KM, Simpson PM, Tobias JD. Intravenous versus epidural analgesia after surgical repair of pectus excavatum. Am J Ther. 2009;16(5):398–403.
47. St Peter SD, Weesner KA, Sharp RJ, Sharp SW, Ostlie DJ, Holcomb GW 3rd. Is epidural anesthesia truly the best pain management strategy after minimally invasive pectus excavatum repair? J Pediatr Surg. 2008; 43(1):79–82; discussion.
48. McBride WJ, Dicker R, Abajian JC, Vane DW. Continuous thoracic epidural infusions for postoperative analgesia after pectus deformity repair. J Pediatr Surg. 1996;31(1):105–7; discussion 7–8.
49. Kavanagh BP, Katz J, Sandler AN. Pain control after thoracic surgery. A review of current techniques. Anesthesiology. 1994;81(3):737–59.
50. Weber T, Matzl J, Rokitansky A, Klimscha W, Neumann K, Deusch E, et al. Superior postoperative pain relief with thoracic epidural analgesia versus intravenous patient-controlled analgesia after minimally invasive pectus excavatum repair. J Thorac Cardiovasc Surg. 2007;134(4):865–70.
51. Gasior AC, Weesner KA, Knott EM, Poola A, St Peter SD. Long-term patient perception of pain control experience after participating in a trial between patient-controlled analgesia and epidural after pectus excavatum repair with bar placement. J Surg Res. 2013;185(1):12–4.
52. Butkovic D, Kralik S, Matolic M, Kralik M, Toljan S, Radesic L. Postoperative analgesia with intravenous fentanyl PCA vs epidural block after thoracoscopic pectus repair in children. Br J Anaesth. 2007;98(5):677–81.
53. St Peter SD, Weesner KA, Weissend EE, Sharp SW, Valusek PA, Sharp RJ, et al. Epidural vs patient-controlled analgesia for postoperative pain after pectus excavatum repair: a prospective, randomized trial. J Pediatr Surg. 2012;47(1):148–53.
54. Yapici D, Atici S, Alic M, Ayan E, Koksel O. Morphine added to local anaesthetic improves epidural analgesia in minimally invasive Nuss operation for pectus excavatum. Br J Anaesth. 2008;100(2):280.
55. Cucchiaro G, Adzick SN, Rose JB, Maxwell L, Watcha M. A comparison of epidural bupivacaine-fentanyl and bupivacaine-clonidine in children undergoing the Nuss procedure. Anesth Analg. 2006; 103(2):322–7, table of contents.
56. Ong CC, Choo K, Morreau P, Auldist A. The learning curve in learning the curve: a review of Nuss procedure in teenagers. ANZ J Surg. 2005;75(6):421–4.
57. Fortier S, Hanna HA, Bernard A, Girard C. Comparison between systemic analgesia, continuous wound catheter analgesia and continuous thoracic paravertebral block: a randomised, controlled trial of postthoracotomy pain management. Eur J Anaesthesiol. 2012; 29(11):524–30.
58. Hall Burton DM, Boretsky KR. A comparison of paravertebral nerve block catheters and thoracic epidural catheters for postoperative analgesia following the Nuss procedure for pectus excavatum repair. Paediatr Anaesth. 2014;24(5):516–20.
59. Lukosiene L, Rugyte DC, Macas A, Kalibatiene L, Malcius D, Barauskas V. Postoperative pain management in pediatric patients undergoing minimally invasive

repair of pectus excavatum: the role of intercostal block. J Pediatr Surg. 2013;48(12):2425–30.
60. Borowitz D, Cerny F, Zallen G, Sharp J, Burke M, Gross K, et al. Pulmonary function and exercise response in patients with pectus excavatum after Nuss repair. J Pediatr Surg. 2003;38(4):544–7.
61. Johnson JN, Hartman TK, Pianosi PT, Driscoll DJ. Cardiorespiratory function after operation for pectus excavatum. J Pediatr. 2008;153(3):359–64.
62. Lam MW, Klassen AF, Montgomery CJ, LeBlanc JG, Skarsgard ED. Quality-of-life outcomes after surgical correction of pectus excavatum: a comparison of the Ravitch and Nuss procedures. J Pediatr Surg. 2008;43(5):819–25.
63. Lawson ML, Mellins RB, Tabangin M, Kelly RE Jr, Croitoru DP, Goretsky MJ, et al. Impact of pectus excavatum on pulmonary function before and after repair with the Nuss procedure. J Pediatr Surg. 2005;40(1):174–80.
64. Sigalet DL, Montgomery M, Harder J, Wong V, Kravarusic D, Alassiri A. Long term cardiopulmonary effects of closed repair of pectus excavatum. Pediatr Surg Int. 2007;23(5):493–7.
65. Sigalet DL, Montgomery M, Harder J. Cardiopulmonary effects of closed repair of pectus excavatum. J Pediatr Surg. 2003;38(3):380–5; discussion −5.
66. Lawson ML, Cash TF, Akers R, Vasser E, Burke B, Tabangin M, et al. A pilot study of the impact of surgical repair on disease-specific quality of life among patients with pectus excavatum. J Pediatr Surg. 2003;38(6):916–8.
67. Krasopoulos G, Dusmet M, Ladas G, Goldstraw P. Nuss procedure improves the quality of life in young male adults with pectus excavatum deformity. Eur J Cardiothorac Surg. 2006;29(1):1–5.

# Pediatric Pain Management

Jennifer Hickman and Jaya L. Varadarajan

## Neurobiology of Pain in Children

Early beliefs of practitioners were that children and neonates either do not feel pain or do not have the same pain experiences as adults [2]. However, this has been proven to be false over the years. It is now known that peripheral and central nervous system structures involved in nociception develop during the second and third trimester of gestation. Furthermore, anatomic and physiologic nociceptive pathways, although still developing, are in place in premature infants as early as 26 weeks of gestation [3]. Thus preterm infants can and do perceive pain comparable to older children [4]. In these preterm or neonatal patients, myelination has not been fully established which means that nociceptive transmission will be slower when compared to an adult, but this slower speed is fully compensated for by the shorter length of nerve layers to pain-modulating centers in the CNS [5]. In addition, synthesis of most neurotransmitters involved in pain modulation occurs early in human development with some as early as the 15th–20th week of gestation [6]. Sherrington Flexion Withdrawal Reflex is the classic nociceptic reflex, and is correlated with the perception of pain. Reflex responses to somatic stimuli are now known to be present at 7–8 weeks. A functional pain system is believed to be in place by 10 weeks. Therefore, based on this knowledge, we now know that neonates and infants do mount a stress response. In addition, the lack of descending modulation in the spinal cord in neonates lowers the threshold to noxious stimuli, creating exaggerated hormonal, metabolic, and immune responses to these insults, thus causing a prolonged hypersensitivity. The long-lasting effects of untreated painful stimuli have been well demonstrated in animal model experimentation. Experimental animals have shown that repetitive neonatal painful experiences may cause long-term or permanent alterations of pain sensation through interference with mechanisms connected to the developmental plasticity of the immature brain [3]. One example of the "memory" of pain is in males circumcised shortly after birth without analgesic procedures, who altered their response to successive pain as evaluated during their vaccinations a few months later [7]. Therefore, children are sensitive and perceive pain regardless of their ability to verbalize it. Practitioners need to be aware of and treat this pain appropriately in the acute setting for not only the immediate elimination of pain, but with the goal of attenuating any long-term consequences later in life.

J. Hickman, M.D. (✉)
Pediatric Anesthesiology, Children's Hospital of Wisconsin, Milwaukee, WI, USA
e-mail: jhickman@mcw.edu

J. L. Varadarajan, M.D.
Anesthesia and Pediatrics, Children's Hospital of Wisconsin, Milwaukee, WI, USA
e-mail: jaya@wi.rr.com

## Pain Assessment

Pain by definition, is a "subjective experience", meaning that the intensity of pain cannot be completely accounted for by the amount of tissue injury as assessed by the provider. Self-report is considered the most reliable and valid estimation of the pain experience so we will explore the assessment tools applicable to children.

It is widely acknowledged that pain in children is often undertreated. The difficulties in assessing pain and lack of knowledge among providers contributes to this. Infants are the most challenging to assess due to their inability to speak; therefore behavioral and physiological measures are used to assess their pain. There is a growing body of literature describing the range of behaviors exhibited in response to painful stimuli [8]. A number of standardized assessment scales have been developed to aid an observer in recognizing and quantifying pain in infants. Despite standardization, the measures are still subject to interpretation which makes them imperfect. Also, the behaviors themselves can be inconsistently expressed by the children. The two most commonly used assessment scales for infants are Neonatal Infant Pain Scale (NIPS) and Faces, Legs, Activity, Cry and Consolability (FLACC).

The Neonatal Infant Pain Scale was developed to discriminate pain response objectively from other distress reactions that infants manifest. This scale uses facial expression, cry, breathing pattern, arm/leg movements and arousal state (Fig. 47.1). Each of these parameters is scored from 0 to 2. Babies with scores greater than 4 require treatment of their pain. This scale is practical and differentiates the severity of pain well on reassessment [9]. The Face, Legs, Activity, Cry and Consolability (FLACC) scale (Fig. 47.2) is similar to the NIPS scale in that it uses behaviors for pain scoring. However, it uses slightly different behaviors. Each behavior on this scale is also scored from 0 to 2. FLACC scores greater than 6 indicate distress and require treatment. A revised version of FLACC is also available that is specifically useful for cognitively impaired children [10].

As children become older and enter school age, they are able to self-report pain. There is a subset of pain assessment scales for this age group. However, younger children (usually less than 8 years), are not yet at a developmental stage to allow for a purely numeric scale for pain reporting so a group of pictorial based pain scales was created, which make minimal cognitive and linguistic demands. These scales include the Faces Pain Scale-Revised by Bieri et al., the Wong-Baker Faces pain scale and the OUCHER

| Pain Assessment | | Score |
|---|---|---|
| **Facial Expression** | | |
| 0 – Relaxed muscles | Restful face, neutral expression | |
| 1 – Grimace | Tight facial muscles; furrowed brow, chin, jaw, (negative facial expression – nose, mouth and brow) | |
| **Cry** | | |
| 0 – No Cry | Quiet, not crying | |
| 1 – Whimper | Mild moaning, intermittent | |
| 2 – Vigorous Cry | Loud scream; rising, shrill, continuous (Note: Silent cry may be scored if baby is intubated as evidenced by obvious mouth and facial movement. | |
| **Breathing Patterns** | | |
| 0 – Relaxed | Usual pattern for this infant | |
| 1 – Change in Breathing | Indrawing, irregular, faster than usual; gagging; breath holding | |
| **Arms** | | |
| 0 – Relaxed/Restrained | No muscular rigidity; occasional random movements of arms | |
| 1 – Flexed/Extended | Tense, straight legs; rigid and/or rapid extension, flexion | |
| **Legs** | | |
| 0 – Relaxed/Restrained | No muscular rigidity; occasional random leg movement | |
| 1 – Flexed/Extended | Tense, straight legs; rigid and/or rapid extension, flexion | |
| **State of Arousal** | | |
| 0 – Sleeping/Awake | Quiet, peaceful sleeping or alert random leg movement | |
| 1 – Fussy | Alert, restless, and thrashing | |

**Fig. 47.1** Neonatal Infant Pain Scale (NIPS) From UCLA David Geffen School of Medicine Department of Anesthesia website

scale. The Faces Pain Scale-Revised is felt to be the most valid and reliable measure of acute pain since an understanding of words or numerical values is not needed [11]. This scale was also revised from the original 7 faces to 6, in order to enhance compatibility with scales that use the 0–10-point metric [12]. The child chooses a face which correlates to a numeric pain score. The Wong-Baker Faces scale is also six faces, however, it is more cartoon like. The child chooses a face which represents their pain, this then correlates to a numeric pain score. This has been validated for use in the ED [13]. However, the Wong-Baker scale has been criticized by some for the pictorial depictions of happiness and sadness at the scale extremes. It is thought that this imposes an affective element to the child's score (i.e. "if my pain were a 5 then I should be crying). This is why Bieri's FPS-R is thought to be superior since it does not depict any type of emotion. The Oucher scale consists of photographs of a child with various facial expressions positioned at regular intervals along a 0–100 vertical numerical scale. It measures pain affect and has been validated in the postoperative setting too. It has also been made with pictures of children from various countries and thus serves children of several nationalities. Children over 8 years of age understand the concept of number and order, and move ahead from the pictorial pain scales to utilize the Visual Analog Scale (VAS) or Verbal Numerical Scale (Fig. 47.3). This is the well-

**Fig. 47.2** Face, legs, activity, cry, consolability scale or FLACC scale

| Face |
|---|
| 0 – No particular expression or smile |
| 1 – Occasional grimace or frown, withdrawn, disinterested |
| 2 – Frequent to constant quivering chin, clenched jaw |
| **Legs** |
| 0 – Normal position or relaxed |
| 1 – Uneasy, restless, tense |
| 2 – Kicking, or legs drawn up |
| **Activity** |
| 0 – Lying quietly, normal position, moves easily |
| 1 – Squirming, shifting back and forth, tense |
| 2 – Arched, rigid or jerking |
| **Cry** |
| 0 – No cry (awake or asleep) |
| 1 – Moans or whimpers; occasional complaint |
| 2 – Crying steadily, screams or sobs, frequent complaints |
| **Consolability** |
| 0 – Content, relaxed |
| 1 – Reassured by occasional touching, hugging or being talked to, distractible |
| 2 – Difficult to console or comfort |

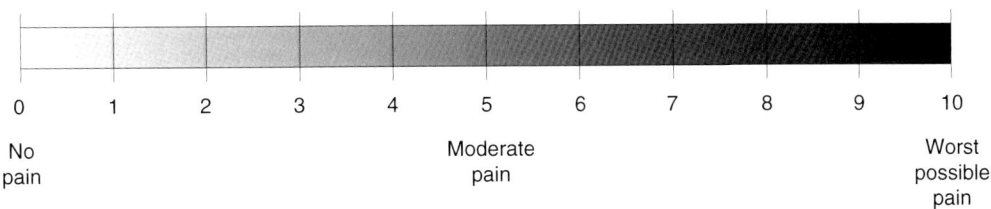

**Fig. 47.3** Verbal numeric scale

known scale of pain from 0 to 10. This scale can either be given to the patient in a verbal fashion asking what number they feel their pain is, or shown to the patient as a pictorial version and have them point to their corresponding pain level.

Despite the widespread use of these pain assessment tools for children and their validation in several settings, there can still be inconsistencies in the reporting of pain by children. There are many factors that can affect the child's reporting. Well-developed coping behaviors may result in the child being perceived to have less pain than they self-report. Disengaging behaviors such as withdrawal, might be viewed as a shy child by the provider instead of one experiencing severe pain. Parents can be helpful in discerning the reasons a child appears calm while reporting severe pain. Children have fewer pain experiences to use as a benchmark. The child's memory of previous pain experiences can affect self-assessment. Children with past pain experiences can respond in one of two ways [14]. They can become accustomed to pain experiences and under report their pain which is common in older patients, or they can become sensitized to pain and have an increased response resulting in higher pain scores. This occurs if the previous pain was severe. Parents can again give insight into past pain experiences to help understand how their child's self-report is affected. Finally, the environment during pain assessment can affect the scoring. It has been shown that a room with less crowding and a lower stress environment is associated with lower pain scores [15]. Also, if the child believes he or she will receive a painful procedure based on their pain rating, the child is less likely to report the full intensity of their pain. Therefore, it is important to take these confounding factors into consideration, when seeking pain scores by self-report from children to obtain an accurate pain assessment.

## Pharmacologic Therapy for Pain

Analgesic pharmacotherapy is the mainstay of pain management. The guiding principle of analgesic therapy is individualization of the therapy for the patient. Through a process of accurate pain assessment, thoughtful drug selection and diligent administration, a balance between pain management and adverse pharmacological effects is achieved.

Growth and developmental differences exist between children and adults which may alter the pharmacokinetics and pharmacodynamics of medications in children. As a result, there are factors that must be considered when treating infants and children. Neonates and infants have a higher percentage of body weight as water and smaller fat and muscle stores compared to adults changing the volume of distribution of some drugs. Children have an anatomically developed liver at birth, but functional maturation is delayed until about 6 months of age. This can affect some drugs metabolized via the liver. The kidneys can have a lower glomerular filtration rate. Plasma concentrations of albumin are lower which may result in greater bioavailability of unbound active drugs increasing the risk of toxicity. Neonates also have an immature blood brain barrier which allows increased passage of certain drugs such as morphine to the brain. Being aware of such differences when treating pain in children and infants will help with drug selection, allowing the practitioner to achieve optimal pain control while minimizing side effects.

## Non-opioid Analgesics

Non-opioid analgesics can be used as the mainstay of treatment for mild to moderate pain or as part of a multimodal plan for more severe pain. Most non-opioid analgesics have a dose-dependent response, they are also limited by a ceiling effect meaning that increasing doses of the drug will not provide an increase in pain relief. Therefore, although often insufficient as the sole treatment for severe pain, these medications are useful in combination with opioids, and can help reduce the opioid requirement which in turn, decreases the adverse effects of the opioid.

Acetaminophen is the most common antipyretic and non-opioid analgesic used in children. It is a unique drug in that, like NSAIDs it weakly inhibits peripheral cyclooxygenase activity but has its primary site of action centrally, where it is a potent antipyretic and mild analgesic, believed to block prostaglandin production [16]. Acetaminophen is available in a wide variety of formulations alone, in combination with decongestants or cold remedies, and in combination with opioids for pain relief. When using formulations and mixtures, it is necessary to pay attention to the total daily dose as the overdose potential is high in children. Acetaminophen comes in oral, rectal and IV formulations. The recommended oral dosing is 15 mg/kg every 4 h and should not exceed 75 mg/kg/day for children. Liver function does not approach adult levels until 6 months of age so the respective daily dosages are 60 mg/kg/day for term infants and 45 mg/kg/day for preterm infants. Acetaminophen can be given orally before surgery. Both gastric fluid volume and pH were unchanged after it was administered orally 90 min before the induction of anesthesia [17]. Rectal absorption is slow and somewhat variable. A single rectal dose of 30–40 mg/kg produces plasma concentrations that are generally in the effective range and not in a range of hepatotoxicity [18]. With these doses, there is a slow decline in plasma concentrations. Based on a 24-h kinetic study, it was recommended that initial does of 35–40 mg/kg rectally be followed by subsequent doses of 20 mg/kg every 6 h [18]. If a large rectal dose is to be followed by oral dosing, it is also recommended that the first oral dose be given no sooner than 6 h after the initial rectal dose. IV acetaminophen is available in the US in a 10 mg/mL solution and should be administered over 15 min with a dosing of 15 mg/kg every 6 h. The maximum daily dose is the same as for oral administration. Analgesic onset after IV acetaminophen occurs in 15 min and antipyresis in 30 min. This fast onset is explained by the drug penetrating the blood brain barrier and yielding detectable concentrations in the CSF within 5 min and peaking within 57 min [19].

NSAIDs (Nonsteroidal anti-inflammatory drugs) are commonly used as part of a multimodal treatment plan and act by reversible inhibition of cyclooxygenases. Cyclooxygenase enzymes convert arachidonic acid to prostanoids. Except for newborns in whom the half-life is longer, the pharmacodynamics and pharmacokinetics of NSAIDs in children are not much different than adults. Children also appear to have a lower incidence of renal and gastrointestinal side effects than adults [20]. Ibuprofen has been well studied and has been used for many years in pediatrics. A large controlled, randomized, double blinded study reported a greater decrease in VAS pain scores with ibuprofen than with acetaminophen or codeine in children presenting to the emergency department with acute pain after musculoskeletal trauma [21]. The usual dosing of ibuprofen is 10 mg/kg every 6–8 h with a maximum daily dose of 40 mg/kg. Ketorolac is an NSAID that is available for IV use. Vetter et al. demonstrated that the administration of a single dose of 0.8 mg/kg of ketorolac reduced the need for self-administered opioid analgesia by approximately 30% in the first 12 h after surgery [22]. There have been multiple studies demonstrating that ketorolac provides postoperative analgesia comparable to opioids in children of all ages. Dosing for ketorolac is 0.3–0.5 mg/kg IV every 6 h. The benefit to using ketorolac is that the reduced opioid use results in fewer opioid-related side effects such as respiratory depression, sedation, and itching. However, as with all NSAIDs it carries risks of platelet dysfunction, GI bleeding, and kidney dysfunction. Ketorolac is known to decrease renal blood flow and many recommend that the course be limited to 48–72 h. If exceeding 72 h is necessary, checking the patient's renal function is recommended. A meta-analysis of the use of NSAIDs for postoperative pain included 27 studies and compared 567 children who received NSAIDs to 418 children who did not [23]. This study found that the use of NSAIDs decreased opioid requirement in the PACU for the first 24 h postoperatively. Therefore, in the absence of contraindications, it has been recommended that NSAIDs be used as part of a multimodal regimen to manage pain and decrease opioid use in children [23] (Fig. 47.4).

| Drug | Dose (mg/kg) and Route | Frequency (h) | Maximum Dose per Day (mg/kg) |
|---|---|---|---|
| Acetaminophen | | | |
|   Infant >32 weeks PCA | 20 PR, 10–15 PO | Every 12 | 60 |
|   Neonate | 20 PR, 10–15 PO | Every 8 | 75 |
|   Infant | 30 PR then 20 PR, 10–15 PO | Every 6 | 75 |
|   Child | 20 PR, 10–15 PO | Every 4–6 | 100 |
| Ibuprofen | 10–15 | Every 6–8 | 40 |
| Indomethacin | | | |
|   Infants >7 days | 0.2 | Every 12 | 0.6 |
|   Children >2 years | 0.5–1 | Every 6–12 | 4 (150–200 mg/day) |
| Naproxen | | | |
|   Children >2 years | 5–7 PO | Every 8–12 | 20 (1000 mg/day) |
| Ketorolac | | | |
|   Infants >44 weeks PCA | 0.5 IV (max 30 mg) | Every 6 | 5-d maximum 2 (120 mg/day) |
| Celecoxib | | | |
|   Children >12 y/between 40 and 50 kg | 100 mg/dose | Every 12 | 200 mg/day |
|   Children >12 y/>50 kg | 200 mg/dose | Every 12 | 400 mg/day |

**Fig. 47.4** NSAIDs—pediatric dosing guidelines

| Drug | Dose (mg/kg) and Route | Frequency (h) | Comments |
|---|---|---|---|
| Morphine | 0.05–0.1 IV | 3–4 | Reduce infant dosing |
| | 0.2–0.4 PO | 3–4 | Immediate release |
| Hydromorphone | 0.01–0.02 IV | 3–4 | |
| | 0.04–0.08 PO | 4–6 | |
| Oxycodone | 0.05–0.15 PO | 4–6 | Elixir often unavailable, metabolism similar to codeine |
| Hydrocodone | 0.1–0.2 PO | 4–6 | Often combined with NSAID, metabolism similar to codeine |
| Codeine | 0.5–1 PO | 4–6 | 7–10% are nonresponders |
| Tramadol | | | |
|   child >20 kg | 1–2 PO | 4–6 | Avoid if seizure potential. Maximum dose 8 mg/kg/day |

**Fig. 47.5** Opioids—pediatric dosing guidelines

## Opioid Analgesics

Opioids are the mainstay of treatment for moderate to severe pain (Fig. 47.5). The decisions guiding opioid selection are based on the formulation and pharmacokinetics of each drug in this class. The three main opioid receptors, mu, kappa and delta, are found throughout the spinal cord and brain with a few located in the periphery. Mu receptor agonism produces the classic opioid effects of analgesia, euphoria, and cough suppression along with side effects that include respiratory depression, constipation, nausea, tolerance and dependence. Two delta receptors produce weak spinal analgesia and mild convulsions. Kappa 1–4 receptors produce sedation, analgesia and dysphoria [24]. Opioids are eliminated through hepatic metabolism by cytochrome P-450, and conjugation to make water soluble metabolites for renal excretion. The elimination of opioids is therefore, dependent on both renal and hepatic function. In neonates, both renal and hepatic function are diminished, reaching adult hepatic function levels by 6 months of age and adult renal clearance by 8–12 months of age [25]. In children between the ages of 2–6 years of age, the hepatic metabolic clearance is increased because the liver is proportionally larger than in children of other ages. This could require an increase in opioid dose or frequency of administration to attain optimal analgesia.

Morphine is considered the gold standard or prototype opioid. Potency comparisons of all other opioids are in relation to morphine. It can be delivered by many routes. The elimination half-life is 2 h in children. However, in the first week of life, the elimination half-life of morphine is more than twice as long as in older children, and even longer in premature infants. Fentanyl and sufentanil also have diminished hepatic metabolism in premature and term neonates.

Hydromorphone is a semisynthetic derivative of morphine that is five times more potent. It has a longer duration of action of 4–6 h and half-life of 3–4 h as compared to morphine. There are anecdotal reports that the side effects of nausea and itching are reduced in comparison to morphine. It also does not have any clinically significant metabolites like morphine, and is therefore safe in patients with liver or renal dysfunction. Despite the fact that there are very few studies of the use of hydromorphone in children, it does remain common practice to use hydromorphone when the side effects from morphine are too great.

Fentanyl is also used in children, primarily in the perioperative or ICU setting. It has a rapid onset of action and is ideal for episodes of rapidly escalating pain. Fentanyl is 80–100 times more potent than morphine. It is also metabolized by the liver. It has a shorter half-life than morphine; however, its context sensitive half-life increases exponentially during a chronic infusion as a result of growing tissue storage. This can be an issue for children on long term infusions as it could result in gradual respiratory depression. Like morphine, fentanyl has a half-life that is twice as long in neonates compared to older children putting them at risk for accumulation [26].

Codeine is a weak opioid agonist with a potency 1/10th that of morphine, but 10% of the drug is metabolized to morphine via the CYP2D6 pathway, the resultant morphine having 200 times greater affinity for the mu receptor. The CYP2D6 enzyme has a large variety of polymorphisms. In the USA, 7–10% of whites are poor metabolizers of codeine by CYP2D6 and received little to no analgesic benefit [27]. Conversely, 3% of whites and up to 40% of individuals of North African descent are ultra-rapid metabolizers and will have plasma levels of morphine up to 50% higher than normal when given codeine. This can have the consequence of respiratory depression when children who are rapid metabolizers are given codeine. Therefore, the FDA has recommended that children under 12 years of age not receive codeine, and that adolescents aged 12–18 years not be given codeine if they have other underlying comorbidities such as sleep apnea, obesity or lung disease. There has also been a case report of mortality in a breast feeding infant of a CYP2D6 ultra-rapid metabolizing mother who was using codeine, making it a safety concern for use of codeine in breast-feeding mothers.

Tramadol is a synthetic codeine analog and an atypical opioid analgesic that works via two complementary mechanisms. One is via weak mu opioid receptor agonism, and the other is via inhibition of serotonin and norepinephrine uptake. It is also believed to be an alpha-2 agonist with some action on cholinergic receptors. It is 1/5th as potent as morphine. Because it only has weak mu agonism, it does not have the same extent of adverse side effects that pure opioids do such as itching, respiration depression and nausea. Tramadol has previously been used for children in ambulatory surgery, both as the primary analgesic and when transitioning from IV opioids to oral analgesics. Tramadol can lower the seizure threshold and should not be used in children with head trauma or a history of seizures, or in combination with other drugs that lower the seizure threshold. The FDA has recently mandated that children under 12 not receive Tramadol. It has also mandated that children under 18 who have undergone tonsillectomy and adenoidectomy not receive Tramadol for pain, due to risk of respiratory complications including death, and recommends against its use in adolescents between 12 and 18 years of age, who are obese and have conditions such as obstructive sleep apnea or severe lung disease.

Patient controlled analgesia (PCA) pumps are utilized in both babies and older children. Most children 5–6 years of age are able to understand and push the demand button themselves. When the child is cognitively unable to understand the concept a nurse/parent controlled PCA is utilized. These PCAs that are controlled by a parent, or nurse have been found to be safe [28].

| | PCA DOSING GUIDELINES | | | | |
|---|---|---|---|---|---|
| DRUG | DEMAND DOSE (µg/kg) | LOCKOUT INTERVAL (min) | BASAL INFUSION (µg/kg/h) | 1-HOUR LIMIT (µg/kg) | PRN IV RESCUE DOSE (µg/kg) |
| Morphine | 20 | 8–10 | 0–20 | 100 | 50 |
| Hydromorphone | 4 | 8–10 | 0–4 | 20 | 10 |
| Fentanyl | 0.5 | 6–8 | 0–0.5 | 2.5 | 0.5–1.0 |
| Nalbuphine | 20 | 8–10 | 0–20 | 100 | 50 |

**Fig. 47.6** Used with permission, From: Kraemer W, Rose J. Acute Pain Management in Children. In: Basics of Pediatric Anesthesia, Ed. Litman, RS. 2016

Morphine is the most common opioid used in PCAs for children. However, hydromorphone and fentanyl are also used. In setting up a PCA for children, it is controversial whether a basal or background infusion should be added. Berde et al. have shown that a basal or background infusion is safe and reduces the incidence of severe episodes of postoperative pain. When deciding if a basal infusion would be beneficial there needs to be consideration of the dose to be used, surgical severity and anticipated recovery, and the child's comorbid conditions; once implemented, vigilant monitoring is essential to ensure safety. Figure 47.6 illustrates appropriate dosing guidelines for a pediatric PCA. Patient monitoring while on a PCA is imperative to prevent adverse outcomes. The Anesthesia Patient Safety Foundation (APSF) recommends the use of continuous respiratory monitoring (minimally pulse oximetry and a continuous measure of respiratory rate) for children receiving PCA, neuraxial, or serial doses of parenteral opioids. APSF also recommends that reliable alerting methods such as audible alarms, central stations or pagers be used to ensure a timely response to a deteriorating respiratory status. It must also be understood that pulse oximetry can only detect hypoventilation if the patient is breathing room air, supplemental oxygen may in fact delay early detection. Oximetry is a measure of oxygenation, not ventilation. Side-stream sampling of end-tidal $CO_2$ via a nasal cannula detects respiratory depression earlier and more frequently than does pulse oximetry or periodic checks of respiratory rate in adults who are receiving opioids via PCA [29]. There is not similar data for children; however, there is data that supports using capnography in children undergoing sedation in the ER and ICU to detect respiratory events that would be unrecognized by pulse oximetry [30]. Despite the utility of capnography cannulas, they can be difficult to keep on children. Therefore, despite the limitations of electronic monitoring and cannulas, it has been reported that the use of computerized physician order entry and involvement of a pediatric pain team improved compliance with routine monitoring and increased the likelihood of early identification of adverse events [31].

## Analgesic Adjuvants

In addition to opioids and NSAIDs, there are medications that provide pain relief via alternative mechanisms. The original use for many of these medications was for treatment of neuropathic or chronic pain, but they have been found to be useful when used in combination with NSAIDs and opioids, for acute pain management that is challenging to treat.

Gabapentin and pregabalin exert their analgesic effect by binding the alpha-2-delta-1 subunit of voltage-dependent calcium channels. Previously used for chronic and neuropathic pain, their use is now advocated as part of a multimodal perioperative pain regimen for children. A dose of 15 mg/kg of gabapentin before spine fusion in children improved pain control and reduced the amount of morphine used [32]. Gabapentin is tolerated well. However, it does have the side effect of sedation which needs to be monitored when given with opioids. The dose does have to be modified in patients with compromised kidney function, but not liver function.

Alpha-2 adrenergic agonists work both centrally and peripherally by inhibiting norepinephrine release in nociception pathways. Clonidine does work best as an adjuvant to opioids and NSAIDs [33]. It is also a good adjuvant for regional techniques. A dose of 1 µg/kg can increase the duration of a single shot caudal. Clonidine can also be added as an adjuvant to an epidural solution to allow for a decreased amount of opioid to be used which then optimizes analgesia but reduces the incidence of adverse effects. While the analgesic effects are positive, the adverse effects of clonidine are sedation, hypotension and bradycardia. Therefore, cardiorespiratory monitoring of patients receiving clonidine is important.

## Epidural Pain Therapy

Epidural pain management techniques are effective techniques for postoperative pain control. However, these procedures are not without risk. Children are less likely to cooperate with positioning, and sitting still during epidural placement, so the majority are placed under general anesthesia. There are certain anatomic considerations to be aware of when doing these procedures. The spinal cord at birth is found to terminate at L3 and the dura at S3-4. At 1 year, this changes to the cord termination being located at L1-2 and the dura at S2. Children have softer spinal ligaments and their vertebrae are cartilaginous, which makes them easily penetrable. The epidural space is less densely packed so injectate spreads easily. When deciding whether one of these procedures is necessary and beneficial to the patient, a careful risk benefit analysis needs to be considered.

Single shot caudal epidural injection is the most widely employed technique for pain management in children. Depending on the volume injected, it can have a dermatomal distribution ranging from T10-S5, making it a useful mode of pain relief for a variety of procedures. The most common approach is to place the block before the surgical incision. This allows for the block to be part of the maintenance of anesthesia, allowing less volatile anesthetic use, and facilitating rapid comfortable emergence from anesthesia. Caudal injections can also be used as the sole anesthetic in premature infants undergoing lower extremity or perineal procedures. The median duration of analgesia produced by a single caudal dose of bupivacaine 0.25% with epinephrine 1:200,000, at 1 mL/kg is about 5–6 h. However, the duration of block can vary among patients. It should be emphasized that a single-shot caudal injection does not guarantee the total absence of pain postoperatively. Caudal injection of opioid alone can also be used for post-operative pain control. Caudal morphine provides longer analgesia than bupivacaine alone, and extends analgesia beyond the lumbosacral dermatomes. It can be used for thoracic and upper abdominal procedures [34]. The use of caudal morphine has the benefit of not causing motor and autonomic blocks. It was also found to be superior to systemic opioid administration in a study of children undergoing orchidopexy [35]. Though caudal morphine can provide prolonged pain relief, the ventilatory response to carbon dioxide can remain depressed for up to 24 h after administration. Therefore, patients who receive caudal morphine should be monitored closely, and it should not be used in the outpatient setting.

Continuous epidural infusion via a catheter in the thoracic or lumbar spine is an excellent method for analgesia for infants and children undergoing major thoracic, abdominal or pelvic procedures. It provides a "balanced" anesthetic and preemptive analgesia when placed prior to incision. It can also facilitate early extubation after major procedures, as well as improved pulmonary function postoperatively. Epidurals in infants and younger children are often placed after induction of general anesthesia with the child in the lateral decubitus position. However, depending on the age and cooperation of the child, epidural catheters can be placed with the child awake or with minimal sedation. Despite the positioning and the short distance to the epidural space in infants and children, there is often good landmark identification and easy placement by standard loss of resistance techniques. In spite of the ease of landmark identification, there can be complications with epidural placement in children. These complications are similar to the complications in adults and can be, but are not limited to, failure of the block, unilateral pain control, intravascular injection of local anesthetic, nerve injury, or dural puncture. Epidural infusions are most effective when the catheter tip is positioned in close proximity to the dermatomes involved in the surgery. Once the catheter is placed, an infusion of bupivacaine or ropivicaine is initiated to achieve pain control. There are early reports of children and infants having convulsions from continuous infusions of bupivacaine [36]. These cases were determined to be due to toxic levels of bupivacaine. Based on further clearance studies, current recommendation is to keep the infusion rates such that cumulative infusion rates of bupivacaine be below 0.4 mg/kg/h in older infants and children, and below 0.2 mg/kg/h for neonates and infants in the first few months of life. Neuraxially administered opioids have a synergistic analgesic effect when combined with local anesthetics. Due to the hydrophilic nature of hydromorphone, there is a slight preference to using hydromorphone for postoperative analgesia for surgical procedures involving multiple dermatomes. Because of the higher cephalad spread of hydromorphone and thereby greater risk of respiratory depression, the use of hydromorphone should be restricted to infants over the age of 6 months. Morphine, Fentanyl, and hydromorphone are the most commonly used opioids in epidural analgesia. Morphine offers no particular advantage over hydromorphone, and is associated with higher incidence of side effects, especially pruritus. All neuraxially administered opioids can cause side effects including nausea, vomiting, respiratory depression, urinary retention, pruritus, sedation, and constipation. Clonidine can also be added to the epidural such that doses of 0.1–0.3 μg/kg/h are delivered.

## Non-pharmacological Pain Treatments

Cognitive behavioral therapy (CBT) is the most commonly researched and supported psychological treatment for the management of pediatric pain. CBT used for pain problems is based on the understanding that pain is a complex biopsychosocial experience shaped by not only the pathophysiology, but also by the individual's thoughts, feelings and behaviors. In CBT, children are taught cognitive strategies to identify and restructure the illogical, or maladaptive thoughts they may have related to their pain. The behavioral strategies are ones that allow the child to relearn adaptive functioning patterns instead of continuing to be nonfunctioning. The goals of CBT for pain include gaining a sense of control over pain, reducing fear of pain, enhancing functioning, increasing mood, and eliminating feelings of hopefulness. CBT is widely used as part of a multidisciplinary approach in the treatment of chronic pain conditions, but also has a place in management of acute pain in the hospital setting, especially when all other pharmacologic methods are failing.

Distraction is also a powerful tool to use in treating pediatric pain. This method shifts the child's attention away from the pain toward a more enjoyable, engaging stimulus. Such techniques can include blowing bubbles, video gaming, reading stories, or movie watching to name a few. A child life specialist is often well versed in distraction techniques for children. These are professionals who promote effective coping through play, preparation, education and self-expression activities. Having a child life specialist as part of the care team can be extremely beneficial in the treatment of the child's pain.

## Summary

Infants and children do experience pain after procedures and need it addressed in a proactive manner. Pain management in children has evolved in a positive way and made significant strides over the last 20 years which allows physicians to better meet the pain needs of children. The assessment and treatment of acute pediatric pain requires knowledge and effort on the part of the physicians and other providers who care for this population of pediatric patients. Being well-informed about the various multimodal options available to treat acute pain, as well as the side effects of each modality is imperative; this aids the physician in tailoring the pain management strategy in an individualized way for each patient, allowing for optimal pain control, with minimal side effects. An optimized pain plan can have positive effects not only on the procedure outcome, but also on patient satisfaction, and the psychological reaction of these children to future procedures.

## References

1. Cunliffe M, Roberts SA. Pain management in children. Curr Anaesth Crit Care. 2004;15(4–5):272–83.
2. Purcell-Jones G, Dormon F, Sumner E. Paediatric anaesthetists' perceptions of neonatal and infant pain. Pain. 1988;33(2):181–7.
3. Loizzo A, Loizzo S, Capasso A. Neurobiology of pain in children: an overview. Open Biochem J. 2009;3:18–25.
4. Anand KJ, Sippell WG, Aynsley-Green A. Randomised trial of fentanyl anaesthesia in preterm babies undergoing surgery: effects on the stress response. Lancet. 1987;1(8524):62–6.
5. Molliver ME, Kostovic I, van der Loos H. The development of synapses in cerebral cortex of the human fetus. Brain Res. 1973;50(2):403–7.
6. Charnay Y, Paulin C, Chayvialle JA, Dubois PM. Distribution of substance P-like immunoreactivity in the spinal cord and dorsal root ganglia of the human foetus and infant. Neuroscience. 1983;10(1):41–55.
7. Taddio A, Katz J, Ilersich AL, Koren G. Effect of neonatal circumcision on pain response during subsequent routine vaccination. Lancet. 1997;349(9052):599–603.
8. Drendel AL, Kelly BT, Ali S. Pain assessment for children: overcoming challenges and optimizing care. Pediatr Emerg Care. 2011;27(8):773–81.
9. Suraseranivongse S, Kaosaard R, Intakong P, Pornsiriprasert S, Karnchana Y, Kaopinpruck J, et al. A comparison of postoperative pain scales in neonates. Br J Anaesth. 2006;97(4):540–4.
10. Malviya S, Voepel-Lewis T, Burke C, Merkel S, Tait AR. The revised FLACC observational pain tool: improved reliability and validity for pain assessment in children with cognitive impairment. Paediatr Anaesth. 2006;16(3):258–65.
11. Bieri D, Reeve RA, Champion GD, Addicoat L, Ziegler JB. The Faces Pain Scale for the self-assessment of the severity of pain experienced by children: development, initial validation, and preliminary investigation for ratio scale properties. Pain. 1990;41(2):139–50.
12. Hicks CL, von Baeyer CL, Spafford PA, van Korlaar I, Goodenough B. The Faces Pain Scale-Revised: toward a common metric in pediatric pain measurement. Pain. 2001;93(2):173–83.
13. Garra G, Singer AJ, Taira BR, Chohan J, Cardoz H, Chisena E, et al. Validation of the Wong-Baker FACES Pain Rating Scale in pediatric emergency department patients. Acad Emerg Med. 2010;17(1):50–4.
14. von Baeyer CL, Marche TA, Rocha EM, Salmon K. Children's memory for pain: overview and implications for practice. J Pain. 2004;5(5):241–9.
15. Shavit I, Kofman M, Leder M, Hod T, Kozer E. Observational pain assessment versus self-report in paediatric triage. Emerg Med J. 2008;25(9):552–5.
16. Anderson BJ. Paracetamol (acetaminophen): mechanisms of action. Pediatr Anesth. 2008;18(10):915–21.
17. Anderson BJ, Rees SG, Liley A, Stewart AW, Wardill MJ. Effect of preoperative paracetamol on gastric volumes and pH in children. Pediatr Anesth. 1999;9(3):203–7.
18. Birmingham PK, Tobin MJ, Fisher DM, Henthorn TK, Hall SC, Cote CJ. Initial and subsequent dosing of rectal acetaminophen in children: a 24-hour pharmacokinetic study of new dose recommendations. Anesthesiology. 2001;94(3):385–9.
19. Kumpulainen E, Kokki H, Halonen T, Heikkinen M, Savolainen J, Laisalmi M. Paracetamol (acetaminophen) penetrates readily into the cerebrospinal fluid of children after intravenous administration. Pediatrics. 2007;119(4):766–71.
20. Lesko SM, Mitchell AA. An assessment of the safety of pediatric ibuprofen. A practitioner-based randomized clinical trial. JAMA. 1995;273(12):929–33.
21. Clark E, Plint AC, Correll R, Gaboury I, Passi B. A randomized, controlled trial of acetaminophen, ibuprofen, and codeine for acute pain relief in children with musculoskeletal trauma. Pediatrics. 2007;119(3):460–7.
22. Vetter TR, Heiner EJ. Intravenous ketorolac as an adjuvant to pediatric patient-controlled analgesia with morphine. J Clin Anesth. 1994;6(2):110–3.
23. Michelet D, Andreu-Gallien J, Bensalah T, Hilly J, Wood C, Nivoche Y, et al. A meta-analysis of the use of nonsteroidal antiinflammatory drugs for pediatric postoperative pain. Anesth Analg. 2012;114(2):393–406.
24. Kraemer FW. Treatment of acute pediatric pain. Semin Pediatr Neurol. 2010;17(4):268–74.
25. Berde CB, Sethna NF. Analgesics for the treatment of pain in children. N Engl J Med. 2002;347(14):1094–103.
26. Collins C, Koren G, Crean P, Klein J, Roy WL, MacLeod SM. Fentanyl pharmacokinetics and hemodynamic effects in preterm infants during ligation of patent ductus arteriosus. Anesth Analg. 1985;64(11):1078–80.
27. Gasche Y, Daali Y, Fathi M, Chiappe A, Cottini S, Dayer P, et al. Codeine intoxication associated with ultrarapid CYP2D6 metabolism. N Engl J Med. 2004;351(27):2827–31.
28. Monitto CL, Greenberg RS, Kost-Byerly S, Wetzel R, Billett C, Lebet RM, et al. The safety and efficacy of

parent-/nurse-controlled analgesia in patients less than six years of age. Anesth Analg. 2000;91(3):573–9.
29. Fu ES, Downs JB, Schweiger JW, Miguel RV, Smith RA. Supplemental oxygen impairs detection of hypoventilation by pulse oximetry. Chest. 2004;126(5):1552–8.
30. Hart LS, Berns SD, Houck CS, Boenning DA. The value of end-tidal CO2 monitoring when comparing three methods of conscious sedation for children undergoing painful procedures in the emergency department. Pediatr Emerg Care. 1997;13(3):189–93.
31. Wrona S, Chisolm DJ, Powers M, Miler V. Improving processes of care in patient-controlled analgesia: the impact of computerized order sets and acute pain service patient management. Paediatr Anaesth. 2007;17(11):1083–9.
32. Rusy LM, Hainsworth KR, Nelson TJ, Czarnecki ML, Tassone JC, Thometz JG, et al. Gabapentin use in pediatric spinal fusion patients: a randomized, double-blind, controlled trial. Anesth Analg. 2010;110(5):1393–8.
33. Tryba M, Gehling M. Clonidine—a potent analgesic adjuvant. Curr Opin Anaesthesiol. 2002; 15(5):511–7.
34. Rosen KR, Rosen DA. Caudal epidural morphine for control of pain following open heart surgery in children. Anesthesiology. 1989;70(3):418–21.
35. Wolf AR, Hughes D, Wade A, Mather SJ, Prys-Roberts C. Postoperative analgesia after paediatric orchidopexy: evaluation of a bupivacaine-morphine mixture. Br J Anaesth. 1990;64(4):430–5.
36. Agarwal R, Gutlove DP, Lockhart CH. Seizures occurring in pediatric patients receiving continuous infusion of bupivacaine. Anesth Analg. 1992; 75(2):284–6.

# Pulmonary Hypertension

Benjamin Kloesel and Kumar Belani

## Introduction

Pulmonary hypertension (PH) is the result of a variety of disease pathomechanisms that ultimately causes an increased resting mean pulmonary artery pressure. The increased pressure, over time, exerts stress on the right ventricle and pulmonary vasculature, that is physiologically designed as a low-pressure system. Pulmonary vascular injury ensues and triggers abnormal cellular growth, inflammation and fibroproliferative changes.

Incidence and prevalence rates are difficult to establish due to significant disease heterogeneity—an epidemiologic study from the Netherlands reported an average incidence of 63.7 cases per million children per year [1]. PH-related hospital admissions have increased over time and the mortality associated with those admissions is higher compared to hospitalizations not associated with PH [2]. For the practicing anesthesia provider, children with PH will require careful assessment and management during the perioperative period because compared to all children undergoing general anesthesia, the rates of cardiac arrest during and after anesthesia and surgery are 20-fold higher in individuals diagnosed with PH [3].

B. Kloesel, M.D., M.S.B.S. (✉)
K. Belani, M.B.B.S., M.S., F.A.C.A., F.A.A.P.
Department of Anesthesiology,
University of Minnesota, Masonic Children's
Hospital, Minneapolis, MN, USA
e-mail: bkloesel@umn.edu

It is important to point out that adult and pediatric PH are quite different in many ways, including genetics, natural history and responsiveness to drug therapies. Also, persistent pulmonary hypertension of the newborn should be considered a separate disease.

## Definition and Diagnosis

In-utero, the pulmonary vasculature is constricted (e.g. pulmonary vascular resistance [PVR] is high) and supports only minimal flow as the majority of blood ejected into the main pulmonary artery is shunted into the systemic circulation via the ductus arteriosus. Shortly after birth, with alveolar gas expansion, the pulmonary vasculature dilates and PVR drops precipitously, reaching adult levels at 2–3 months of age. As such, PH is defined as resting mean pulmonary artery pressure equal to or exceeding 25 mmHg. Pediatric PH is currently classified using the same system that is applied to adult patients (WHO classification with five groups) [4], although experts recommend a transition to the Panama classification system (ten categories) [5], which is more specific to pediatric patients. The latter classification system was released by the pulmonary vascular research institute which also provides a more detailed definition of their preferred term, pulmonary vascular hypertensive disease (PVHD): mean pulmonary artery pressure (mPAP) > 25 mmHg and pulmonary vascular resistance index (PVRI) > 3 Wood Units/m$^2$ for biventricular circulations; and PVRI > 3 WU/m$^2$ or transpulmonary gradient > 6 mmHg even if mPAP < 25 mmHg for univentricular circulations after palliative cavopulmonary anastomosis [5].

Echocardiography is considered the best initial non-invasive screening test and can provide a myriad of information including systolic pulmonary artery pressure (sPAP), right ventricular systolic pressure, mean pulmonary artery pressure (mPAP), end-diastolic pulmonary artery pressure, right ventricular systolic function, right ventricular strain, right ventricular volume, right ventricle-to-left ventricle diameter ratio and right atrium/ventricle dimensions [6]. In regards to adverse events in pediatric patients undergoing surgery under anesthesia, the ratio of either mean pulmonary artery pressure to mean systemic artery pressure or systolic pulmonary artery pressure to systolic systemic blood pressure can be used for risk stratification: values >0.75 are associated with a higher risk. The ratio can also be used to further define PH: <0.7 subsystemic PH; 0.7–1.0 systemic PH; >1.0 suprasystemic PH. Other risk factors for major complications include: calculated RVSP >64 mmHg, presence of syncope or dizziness, and idiopathic PAH [7]; elevated mean right atrial pressure [8]; and suprasystemic PAP, heritable PAH, decreased RV function, decreased pulmonary capacitance index, and treatment naïveness [9]; suprasystemic PH, young age, home oxygen use, encroaching of the hypertensive RV on the left heart leading to left ventricular restriction and functional impairment ("septal bowing" on echo) [10].

Right heart catheterization can confirm the diagnosis and provide additional useful information including severity, response to vasodilator therapy and exclusion of other treatable causes.

## Treatment

Treatment of pulmonary hypertension aims at reducing symptoms, improving quality of life and retarding clinical deterioration. Even though mortality has decreased with the institution of PH-targeted medical therapy, a cure cannot be achieved without definitive surgical care, namely lung transplantation. Other surgical interventions (such as atrial septostomy, Potts shunt, pulmonary artery denervation) are being continuously examined for their potential of palliation. Supportive treatment of pulmonary hypertension includes supplemental oxygen, anticoagulation, diuretics, digitalis and mineralocorticoid receptor antagonists (spironolactone, eplerenone). Calcium channel blockers are prescribed if the patient exhibits a positive response during acute vasoreactivity testing. Pulmonary artery hypertension-targeted therapy includes medications that act on three major pathways: NO/cGMP pathway (sildenafil [oral, intravenous], tadalafil [oral]), endothelin pathway (Bosentan [oral], Ambrisentan [oral]) and prostacyclin pathway (Epoprostenol [intravenous], Trepostinil [intravenous, subcutaneous, inhaled], Iloprost [intravenous, inhaled]). Other medications that are frequently employed in the critical care setting include milrinone, levosimedan and inhaled nitric oxide [11].

## Anesthetic Considerations: Perioperative Care

Prior to induction of anesthesia, a well-formulated plan should be established. During review of preoperative tests, particular attention needs to be paid to the presence of atrial or ventricular communications. If such a communication is present, air bubble precautions should be employed.

If the patient is on long-term medications that address PH, care should be taken to continue those agents in the perioperative period. Intravenous agents require special consideration: continuous infusions of prostacycline or iloprost should never be interrupted. If any problems with the pre-existing access (typically a peripherally inserted central catheter or Broviac catheter) arise through which the medications are delivered, a peripheral intravenous catheter (PIV) should be expeditiously inserted and therapy resumed as soon as possible as the half-life of some of those agents is rather short (epoporostenol = 4 min; treprostinil = 4.5 h).

The sympathetic stimulation from pre-induction PIV access or even mask induction bears the risk of an increase in PVR. Consequently, adequate anxiolysis and sedation can be very valuable. Routinely used agents include benzodiazepines (midazolam, 0.5–1 mg/kg by mouth, up to 20 mg) and ketamine (3–8 mg/kg by mouth). Dexmedetomidine and clonidine are other alternatives.

Hypovolemia from preoperative fasting can compromise right ventricular preload, thus, if intravenous access is available, a pre-induction fluid bolus should be considered (10–15 cc/kg).

Induction of anesthesia can be achieved via the intravenous or inhalational route. Both approaches have advantages and disadvantages. Intravenous induction requires vascular access and allows immediate intervention in case of hemodynamic instabilities or airway problems. Propofol, an otherwise frequently used induction agent, must be used with caution and preferably titrated to effect. Its significant actions on peripheral vascular resistance can jeopardize right ventricular coronary perfusion, especially in patients with right ventricular hypertrophy. Etomidate is an alternative induction agent that maintains cardiac contractility and has no significant effects on SVR and PVR [12]. The main concern with use of etomidate is its suppressive effect on adrenal cortisol production by inhibition of 11-β-hydroxylase. Ketamine is frequently used due to its ability to maintain systemic and pulmonary vascular resistance. Its use appears to be safe in children with pulmonary hypertension [8, 13, 14].

Inhalation induction is a possibility but tricky because it carries significant risks: (a) loss of the airway from obstruction or laryngospasm during induction will quickly lead to hypoxemia and hypercapnia, thus increasing pulmonary vascular resistance and possibly resulting in pulmonary hypertensive crisis or right ventricular ischemia; (b) in the uncooperative and inadequately sedated child, agitation will prolong induction and may also result in increases in pulmonary vascular resistance; (c) volatile agents are potent vasodilators and higher induction doses may result in a decrease in systemic vascular resistance, systemic hypotension and possible right ventricular ischemia.

Volatile anesthetics are associated with clinical pulmonary vasodilation and are therefore a good choice for maintenance of a general anesthetic [15, 16].

Nitrous oxide mildly depresses cardiac output and decreases heart rate and mean blood pressure but has no significant effects on PVR [17]. It can therefore be considered for induction or awake PIV placement, but the potential for hypoxia from delivery of a hypoxic gas-mixture should be kept in mind.

Dexmedetomidine can be used in multiple ways, this includes premedication, as an adjunct during general anesthesia and for peri- and post-procedural sedation. A study by Friesen et al. investigated dexmedetomidine loading in children with pulmonary hypertension. The group confirmed a significant increase in systemic vascular resistance but did not find any increases in pulmonary vascular resistance [18].

Opioids are an integral part of the anesthetic to blunt sympathetic responses to laryngoscopy, incision and other noxious stimuli. Fentanyl has been shown to have no effects on PVR [19]. Depending on the length and invasiveness of the procedure, a variety of different opioids may be employed. Care should be taken to avoid over-narcotization due to the risk of hypoventilation after extubation with subsequent hypercapnia. For this reason, remifentanil is the preferred opioid.

The anesthesiologist needs to weigh benefits and risks of both induction choices and tailor the anesthetic to each individual case. If an inhalational induction is chosen, a sufficient level of sedation will greatly aid in the induction process.

Intraoperative monitoring should include standard American Society of Anesthesiologists (ASA) monitors. Electrocardiography monitoring should be extended to include five leads in order to increase the likelihood of ischemia detection. The threshold of using invasive blood pressure monitoring should be low, although certain shorter, less invasive procedures or diagnostic exams can be performed with non-invasive blood pressure monitoring. Continuous capnography is essential in the care of these patients as it aids in ensuring normocarbia (to avoid PVR increases from hypoventilation) and can help detect sudden decrease in pulmonary blood flow.

For procedures with limited invasiveness and an uneventful anesthesia course, the child can be extubated in the operating room. Recovery often occurs in an intensive care unit setting in order to closely monitor hemodynamics, but patients with milder forms of PH undergoing diagnostic procedures or smaller surgical procedures can be transported to the postanesthesia recovery unit.

Patients with PH remain at higher risk for adverse events in the postoperative period. It is important to note that almost 50% of postoperative cardiac arrests are triggered by respiratory events because the patient with PH is especially vulnerable to hypercarbia secondary to hypoventilation and/or airway obstruction resulting in rapid increases in PVR. Hence, close monitoring of the respiratory status and judicious use of respiratory depressants, such as narcotics and sedatives, is paramount. Table 48.1 summarizes pertinent aspects of anesthetic care for patients with pulmonary hypertension.

## Anesthetic Considerations: Pulmonary Hypertensive Crisis

A feared complication in patients with PH is the development of a pulmonary hypertensive crisis. Various stimuli can lead to a sudden increase in PVR with subsequent right ventricular failure. More precisely, an increase in right ventricular afterload causes an increase in end-diastolic volume and a decrease in right ventricular stroke volume and cardiac output. In the setting of ventricular interdependence, stroke volume from the left ventricle is reduced by decreased preload from reduced right ventricular stroke volume and increases in right ventricular end-diastolic vol-

**Table 48.1** Essential points summarizing care of newborns, children and adolescents with pulmonary hypertension

| Plan/preparation/adverse events | Reasoning/management |
|---|---|
| • If deep sedation without intubation is planned, have back up device for positive pressure ventilation available for immediate use<br>• In addition, all emergency drugs including muscle relaxant must be readily available | • Hypoxia and hypercapnia as a result of inadequate spontaneous ventilation lead to an increase in pulmonary vascular resistance and may cause right ventricular failure |
| • For patients receiving PAH-modifying drugs by intravenous infusion, care must be taken to continue those drugs perioperatively. A dedicated line should be used and interruptions in medication delivery should be avoided | • PAH-modifying drugs administered by the intravenous route have significant effects on the pulmonary vasculature. Interruptions in delivery can have detrimental effects |
| • Pulmonary hypertensive crisis—triggers | • Hypoxia<br>• Hypercapnia<br>• Acidosis<br>• Pain<br>• Tracheal suctioning<br>• Hypothermia<br>• Fever<br>• Interruption of prostanoid infusion<br>• Arrhythmias<br>• Pulmonary infections<br>• Pulmonary embolism<br>• Myocardial ischemia/infarct |
| • Pulmonary hypertensive crisis—treatment | • Hyperventilation<br>• $FiO_2 = 100\%$<br>• Deepen anesthetic<br>• Avoid bradycardia<br>• Sodium bicarbonate to correct acidosis<br>• Treat arrhythmias<br>• Medications:<br>  – Inhaled nitric oxide<br>  – Inhaled postanoid (iloprost)<br>  – Intravenous prostanoid (epoprostenol)<br>  – Intravenous sildenafil<br>  – Inodilators (milrinone); may need to be combined with vasopressor (vasopressin, norepinephrine, epinephrine) if systemic hypotension occurs<br>• VA/VV-ECMO |

ume cause a septal shift towards the left side. Pulmonary hypertensive crises can progress into a vicious cycle (Fig. 48.1): the increased right ventricular end-diastolic volume increases wall tension which, in turn, decreases coronary perfusion. Ischemia and myocardial infarct can occur; this worsens right ventricular function and introduces a potential downward spiral [20].

Triggers for pulmonary hypertensive crises include noxious stimuli (pain from surgical incisions, laryngoscopy), hypoxemia, hypercapnia, acidemia, hypothermia, fever and interruption of prostanoid infusion [21, 22]. Avoidance or rapid recognition and treatment of those factors are the best methods to prevent the occurrence of pulmonary hypertensive crises.

If a patient with PH suffers a perioperative acute pulmonary hypertensive crisis, prompt recognition and treatment are of utmost importance as rapid decompensation towards cardiac arrest can occur. In the intubated patient, hyperventilation with an $FiO_2$ of 100% should be instituted. The anesthetic should be deepened to protect the patient from noxious stimuli that can provoke progression of the pulmonary hypertensive crisis. Inhaled nitric oxide (20–40 ppm) will decrease PVR with minimal systemic effects. If hemodynamic support is required, inodilators such as milrinone and dobutamine can reduce PVR and support cardiac contractility. Acidosis should be corrected with sodium bicarbonate [22].

Children with newly diagnosed PH that are treatment-naïve have the highest risk for developing pulmonary hypertensive crises due to their highly reactive pulmonary vasculature. In contrast, patients with longstanding, chronic PH on therapy develop progressive right ventricular hypertrophy and strain, placing them at higher risk for right ventricular ischemia secondary to coronary hypoperfusion [3].

## Outcomes

While PH is an indisputable factor that leads to an increase in morbidity and mortality during sedation and general anesthesia, it appears that specialized

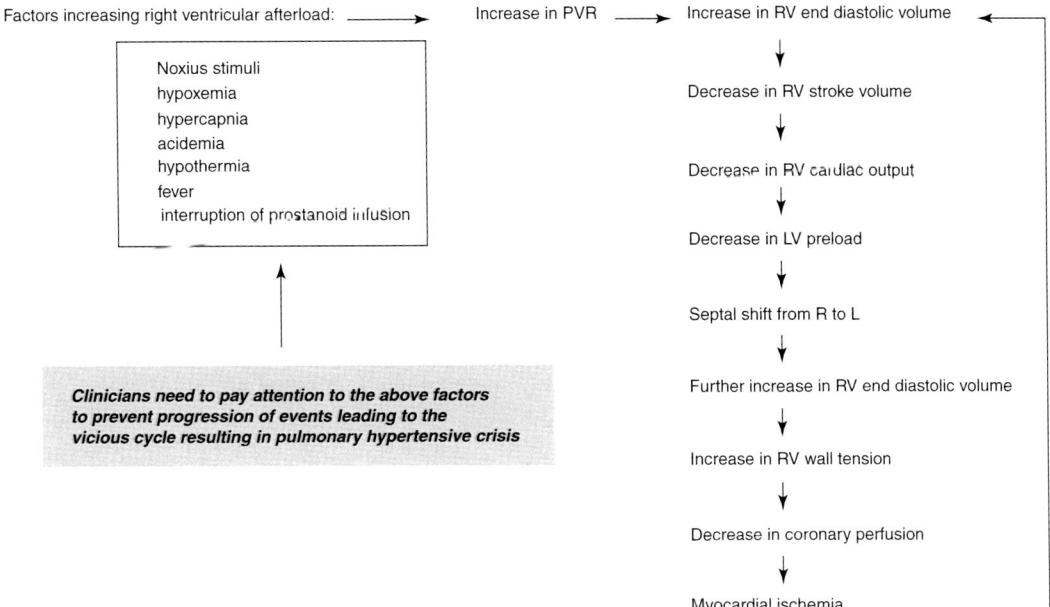

**Fig. 48.1** Modifiable factors in the perioperative period that cause an increase in pulmonary vascular resistance that may precipitate pulmonary hypertensive crisis. Increases in pulmonary vascular resistance can quickly trigger a vicious cycle as myocardial ischemia leads to further increases in right ventricular end-diastolic volume and a decrease in right ventricular cardiac output

centers with dedicated pediatric anesthesiologists familiar with this disease can limit the risks and improve outcomes. Data from the MAGIC registry documented a low adverse event rate with no periprocedural deaths during 177 cardiac catheterizations in children with PH [23].

## References

1. van Loon RL, Roofthooft MT, Hillege HL, ten Harkel AD, van Osch-Gevers M, Delhaas T, et al. Pediatric pulmonary hypertension in the Netherlands: epidemiology and characterization during the period 1991 to 2005. Circulation. 2011;124(16):1755–64.
2. Frank DB, Crystal MA, Morales DL, Gerald K, Hanna BD, Mallory GB Jr, et al. Trends in pediatric pulmonary hypertension-related hospitalizations in the United States from 2000-2009. Pulm Circ. 2015;5(2):339–48.
3. Chau DF, Gangadharan M, Hartke LP, Twite MD. The post-anesthetic care of pediatric patients with pulmonary hypertension. Semin Cardiothorac Vasc Anesth. 2016;20(1):63–73.
4. Ivy DD, Abman SH, Barst RJ, Berger RM, Bonnet D, Fleming TR, et al. Pediatric pulmonary hypertension. J Am Coll Cardiol. 2013;62(25 Suppl):D117–26.
5. Cerro MJ, Abman S, Diaz G, Freudenthal AH, Freudenthal F, Harikrishnan S, et al. A consensus approach to the classification of pediatric pulmonary hypertensive vascular disease: report from the PVRI pediatric taskforce, Panama 2011. Pulm Circ. 2011;1(2):286–98.
6. Koestenberger M, Friedberg MK, Nestaas E, Michel-Behnke I, Hansmann G. Transthoracic echocardiography in the evaluation of pediatric pulmonary hypertension and ventricular dysfunction. Pulm Circ. 2016;6(1):15–29.
7. Taylor CJ, Derrick G, McEwan A, Haworth SG, Sury MR. Risk of cardiac catheterization under anaesthesia in children with pulmonary hypertension. Br J Anaesth. 2007;98(5):657–61.
8. Williams GD, Maan H, Ramamoorthy C, Kamra K, Bratton SL, Bair E, et al. Perioperative complications in children with pulmonary hypertension undergoing general anesthesia with ketamine. Paediatr Anaesth. 2010;20(1):28–37.
9. Bobhate P, Guo L, Jain S, Haugen R, Coe JY, Cave D, et al. Cardiac catheterization in children with pulmonary hypertensive vascular disease. Pediatr Cardiol. 2015;36(4):873–9.
10. Taylor K, Moulton D, Zhao XY, Laussen P. The impact of targeted therapies for pulmonary hypertension on pediatric intraoperative morbidity or mortality. Anesth Analg. 2015;120(2):420–6.
11. Hansmann G, Apitz C. Treatment of children with pulmonary hypertension. Expert consensus statement on the diagnosis and treatment of paediatric pulmonary hypertension. The European Paediatric Pulmonary Vascular Disease Network, endorsed by ISHLT and DGPK. Heart. 2016;102(Suppl 2):ii67–85.
12. Dhawan N, Chauhan S, Kothari SS, Kiran U, Das S, Makhija N. Hemodynamic responses to etomidate in pediatric patients with congenital cardiac shunt lesions. J Cardiothorac Vasc Anesth. 2010;24(5):802–7.
13. Williams GD, Philip BM, Chu LF, Boltz MG, Kamra K, Terwey H, et al. Ketamine does not increase pulmonary vascular resistance in children with pulmonary hypertension undergoing sevoflurane anesthesia and spontaneous ventilation. Anesth Analg. 2007;105(6):1578–84, table of contents.
14. Williams GD, Friesen RH. Administration of ketamine to children with pulmonary hypertension is safe: pro-con debate: pro argument. Paediatr Anaesth. 2012;22(11):1042–52.
15. Friesen RH, Williams GD. Anesthetic management of children with pulmonary arterial hypertension. Paediatr Anaesth. 2008;18(3):208–16.
16. Laird TH, Stayer SA, Rivenes SM, Lewin MB, McKenzie ED, Fraser CD, et al. Pulmonary-to-systemic blood flow ratio effects of sevoflurane, isoflurane, halothane, and fentanyl/midazolam with 100% oxygen in children with congenital heart disease. Anesth Analg. 2002;95(5):1200–6, table of contents.
17. Hickey PR, Hansen DD, Strafford M, Thompson JE, Jonas RE, Mayer JE. Pulmonary and systemic hemodynamic effects of nitrous oxide in infants with normal and elevated pulmonary vascular resistance. Anesthesiology. 1986;65(4):374–8.
18. Friesen RH, Nichols CS, Twite MD, Cardwell KA, Pan Z, Pietra B, et al. The hemodynamic response to dexmedetomidine loading dose in children with and without pulmonary hypertension. Anesth Analg. 2013;117(4):953–9.
19. Hickey PR, Hansen DD, Wessel DL, Lang P, Jonas RA. Pulmonary and systemic hemodynamic responses to fentanyl in infants. Anesth Analg. 1985;64(5):483–6.
20. Kaestner M, Schranz D, Warnecke G, Apitz C, Hansmann G, Miera O. Pulmonary hypertension in the intensive care unit. Expert consensus statement on the diagnosis and treatment of paediatric pulmonary hypertension. The European Paediatric pulmonary vascular disease network, endorsed by ISHLT and DGPK. Heart. 2016;102(Suppl 2):ii57–66.
21. Shukla AC, Almodovar MC. Anesthesia considerations for children with pulmonary hypertension. Pediatr Crit Care Med. 2010;11(2 Suppl):S70–3.
22. Del Pizzo J, Hanna B. Emergency Management of Pediatric Pulmonary Hypertension. Pediatr Emerg Care. 2016;32(1):49–55.
23. Hill KD, Lim DS, Everett AD, Ivy DD, Moore JD. Assessment of pulmonary hypertension in the pediatric catheterization laboratory: current insights from the Magic registry. Catheter Cardiovasc Interv. 2010;76(6):865–73.

# Anesthesia Considerations in a Premie

Arundathi Reddy and Edwin A. Bowe

## Introduction

Preterm neonates are subclassified as mild preterm (32–36 weeks), very preterm (28–31 weeks) and extremely preterm (<28 weeks) [1]. Preterm neonates can also be classified by weight as low birth weight (LBW) < 2500 g, Very Low Birth Weight (VLBW) < 1500 g, and Extremely Low Birth Weight (ELBW) < 1000 g; some describe infants weighing < 750 g as micropremies. In this chapter, we will discuss patient factors and anesthetic considerations in preterm neonates.

## Patient Factors

### Neurologic

**Intracranial Hemorrhage**: The most common type of intracranial hemorrhage in a preterm infant is intraventricular hemorrhage (IVH) also known as germinal matrix hemorrhage (GMH); subdural, subarachnoid and cerebellar hemorrhages may also occur. The incidence of IVH is inversely proportional to gestational age and birth weight and is a significant cause of morbidity and mortality. IVH originates in the germinal matrix, which is located between the caudate nucleus and the thalamus, below the ependymal lining of the ventricles. The pathogenesis of the IVH includes a combination of germinal matrix fragility and disturbances in cerebral blood flow [2]. Risk factors include lack of prenatal care and antenatal steroid therapy, prematurity, respiratory distress syndrome (causing hypoxia, hypercarbia, and requiring mechanical ventilation), pneumothorax, hemodynamic instability and disturbed autoregulation of cerebral blood flow, acidosis, sepsis, anemia, aggressive fluid resuscitation, changes in serum osmolarity, presence of a large patent ductus arteriosus (PDA), thrombocytopenia and possibly vaginal birth. IVH severity has been classified from Grade 1 (which consists of bleeding confined to the periventricular area) to Grade 3 (in which more than 50% of the ventricle is filled with blood). Grade 4 is associated with hemorrhage extending into the brain parenchyma. Neurodevelopment outcomes vary with the grade of IVH. Survivors with IVH requiring ventriculoperitoneal shunts for post hemorrhagic hydrocephalus had severe neurologic impairment [3] while those with IVH grade I and II had less severe neurologic sequelae.

**Pain and the Preterm Infant**: The gestational age at which these preemies begin to experience pain is still unclear. The neuroanatomical pathways necessary for nociception are developed by 23 weeks of gestation and some articles report that pain is observable in fetuses as early as 18 weeks of gestation [4, 5]. With mainly pre-

A. Reddy, M.B., B.S. (✉) · E. A. Bowe, M.D.
Department of Anesthesiology, University of Kentucky Medical Center, Lexington, KY, USA

Kentucky Children's Hospital, Lexington, KY, USA
e-mail: aredd2@uky.edu; edwin.bowe@uky.edu

clinical studies showing neurodegenerative changes in the brain following exposure to anesthetic agents, there have been concerns regarding the use of anesthesia in infants and children below 3 years of age. Conversely, historical studies reported decreased morbidity and mortality and improved postoperative outcome when anesthesia is provided to preterm infants undergoing surgery. In December 2016, the United States Food and Drug Administration (FDA) issued a warning that repeated or lengthy use of general anesthetic and sedation drugs for surgeries or procedures in children younger than 3 years of age or in pregnant women during their third trimester may affect the development of children's brains. However, until there are alternatives to medications currently used for anesthesia and analgesia, compliance with the FDA warning would require that anesthesia be administered only to children less than 3 years of age for surgical procedures required to treat urgent or life-threatening conditions, and then only for the shortest duration possible.

**Respiratory Drive**: Ventilatory control systems are physiologically immature in preemies and any neurological insults like IVH can diminish respiratory drive [6]. The ventilatory response to hypoxia is biphasic, with an initial transient increase in respiratory rate and tidal volume that lasts for 1–2 min followed by a late, sustained decline in spontaneous ventilation and possible apnea [7]. Exposure to anesthetic agents also produces ventilatory depression and, along with immature diaphragmatic musculature, increased chest wall compliance, and decreased pharyngeal muscle tone, results in an increased risk of hypoxia, hypercapnia and apnea in the post-operative period. Therefore, these preemies need to be monitored for post-operative apnea and bradycardia.

**Retinopathy of Prematurity**: ROP is a disease affecting preterm neonates. With increasing survival of these patients, ROP is one of the leading causes of blindness in children. Retinal vascular development begins around 16–18 weeks of gestation and is fully developed by 40–44 weeks of gestational age. The fetal oxygen tension of 25–50 mmHg is conducive for the normal development of these vessels. Preterm birth disrupts this development and results in the formation of abnormal retinal vasculature. While prematurity and the exposure of the infant to supplemental oxygen are the main risk factors for the development of ROP, other risk factors include low levels of insulin-like growth factor-1 (IGF-1), reduced vascular endothelial growth factor, low birth weight, anemia, poor nutrition, hyperglycemia, administration of insulin, and sepsis as well as conditions like necrotizing enterocolitis, IVH, respiratory distress syndrome, bronchopulmonary dysplasia, and congenital cardiac anomalies. Reduction in the incidence of ROP would include better prenatal care to reduce the incidence of prematurity, reduction of risk factors that disrupt normal retinal vascularization, and restriction of supplemental oxygen by targeting $SpO_2$ saturations between 89 and 94%. Conventional treatment involves laser ablation of the abnormal retinal vessels but newer approaches using IGF-1 and vascular endothelial growth factor (VEGF) inhibitors have shown promising results [8].

## Cardiac

**Reversal to Transitional Circulation**: *In utero* oxygenated blood flows from the placenta via the ductus venosus to the inferior vena cava (IVC) and into the right atrium where it is preferentially shunted via the foramen ovale to the left atrium. Blood entering the left atrium flows into the left ventricle where it is preferentially distributed to the brain and coronary arteries. Blood returning via the superior vena cava (SVC) has a lower oxygen content than blood in the IVC and is preferentially distributed to the right ventricle. *In utero* pulmonary vascular resistance is very high and the majority of blood ejected by the right ventricle is shunted from the main pulmonary artery via the ductus arteriosus to the aorta; very little blood flows through the pulmonary circulation. Some of the postductal blood flow in the aorta returns to the placenta, where it is oxygenated; the remainder perfuses the kidneys, abdominal organs, and lower extremities [9]. The two primary changes that occur after birth are a decrease in pulmonary vascular resistance (precipitated both by ventilation of the lungs and an increase in alveolar oxygen tension), and an increase in systemic vascular resistance (caused by clamping of the umbilical cord). The combination of the decrease in pulmonary vascular resistance and the increase in systemic vascular resistance result in functional closure of the foramen ovale (due to a decrease in right atrial pressure secondary to a decrease in pulmonary vascular resistance and an increase in left atrial pressure secondary to increased pulmonary blood flow) and of the ductus arteriosus (due to a relative equalization of pressures in the aorta and pulmonary artery). It's important to understand that although the ductus arteriosus and foramen ovale are functionally closed due to changes in the pulmonary artery/aorta and right atrium/left atrium respectively, increases in pulmonary artery pressure or decreases in aortic pressure may result in a return to fetal circulation. If that occurs, the increase in pulmonary vascular resistance may make it difficult to increase pulmonary blood flow, the factor that is essential to improve oxygenation.

**Patent Ductus Arteriosus (PDA)**: Failure of the ductus arteriosus to close results in persistent shunting of blood between systemic and pulmonary circulations. In term infants, the ductus arteriosus functionally closes by 3 days of life, but in preterm infants, this closure is related to gestational age. At 7 days of life, the ductus remains open in 65% of very preterm and 87% of extremely preterm infants. Shunting of blood through the PDA, also known as "ductal steal," is essentially shunting left to right from the aorta into the pulmonary arteries. Clinically significant shunting can result in pulmonary congestion, pulmonary edema and worsening respiratory distress. Systemic hypoperfusion from moderate to severe ductal steal has been correlated with reduced cerebral blood flow and oxygenation and with reduced celiac artery flow. Some of the comorbidities associated with PDA in premies include pulmonary edema, bronchopulmonary dysplasia (BPD), necrotizing enterocolitis, cardiac failure, IVH, prolonged ventilatory support, and increased length of hospital stay [10, 11]. Conversely, if pulmonary vascular resistance is increased (secondary to hypoxemia, hypercarbia, acidosis, or hypothermia), blood flow through the PDA may become right-to-left. A right-to-left shunt through the ductus may result in decreased pulmonary blood flow with consequent hypoxemia. Echocardiography is the "gold standard" for assessing the magnitude (diameter, shunt volume) of a PDA, but there is no agreement on what constitutes a hemodynamically significant ductus. The current trend in PDA management is conservative management without intervention. Pharmacologic closure with indomethacin or ibuprofen has been successful in producing closure of the ductus in up to 98% of patients, but complications include renal dysfunction, gut ischemia, and platelet dysfunction. Ibuprofen has been used both prophylactically (on day 3 of life) and therapeutically. Ibuprofen is associated with oliguria, increased levels of bilirubin, and gastrointestinal hemorrhage. Studies are also being conducted on the use of acetaminophen. Studies, admittedly small in number, comparing the effects of these three drugs have failed to document any difference in efficacy, complications, or long-term outcomes. Surgical ligation of the ductus arteriosus is now performed only in cases of failure of medical management. Conflicting studies report increased survival but also increased morbidity (generally considered to be pneumothorax, chylothorax, BPD, ROP, and neurodevelopmental problems) but it's not clear how much of a role the increased survival plays in those outcomes.

**Pulse Oximetry Probe Placement**: $SpO_2$ monitoring in the preterm infants is necessary to diagnose and manage both hypoxia and hyperoxia. Preterm infants have a dynamic circulation, which can convert to fetal circulation. Placement of two probes, one to detect oxygen saturation of preductal blood and the other to detect oxygen saturation of postductal blood, may be useful to provide information about changes in blood flow through the ductus arteriosus. Values obtained from a probe placed on the right upper extremity or the head (for example the earlobe) clearly reflects preductal blood. Conversely, probes placed on the lower extremities sample postductal blood. Values obtained from a probe placed on the left hand may not reliably reflect preductal blood; a study comparing results obtained from the right hand, left hand, and a foot showed that there was a trend for values obtained from probes placed on the left hand to be lower than for samples obtained from the right hand [12].

## Respiratory

**Respiratory Distress Syndrome**: Human lung development can be divided into five stages. The embryonic phase (26 days to 6 weeks gestation), the pseudoglandular phase (6–16 weeks gestation), the canalicular phase (16–28 weeks gestation), the saccular phase (28–36 weeks gestation) and the alveolar phase (36 weeks gestation to 4 years of age). Alveoli start to form in the saccular phase, but mature alveoli are not present until 36 weeks of gestation, resulting in preterm infants having a significant alteration in their pulmonary function and physiology. Preemies also have a highly compliant chest wall [13] with immature diaphragmatic muscles. Production of surfactant, necessary to reduce surface tension in the alveoli, begins around the 20th to the 24th week of gestation and reaches adequate levels by 36 weeks of gestation. Decreased levels of surfactant result in diffuse alveolar atelectasis. The structural immaturity of the alveoli along with surfactant deficiency results in Respiratory Distress Syndrome (RDS) of the newborn, previously referred to as hyaline membrane disease. The incidence of RDS is inversely proportional to gestational age. A structurally and functionally immature lung along with well-perfused but atelectatic alveoli, results in intrapulmonary shunt and consequent hypoxmia with the potential for persistent fetal circulation (i.e., right-to-left shunting through the foramen ovale and the ductus arteriosus). There is a marked reduction in both static and dynamic pulmonary compliance resulting in an increased work of breathing. These infants present with respiratory distress, manifested by tachypnea, grunting, nasal flaring, retractions and cyanosis, at or soon after birth. Fortunately, the outcomes in infants with RDS have markedly improved with the use of antenatal glucocorticoid therapy along with modern ventilation techniques and administration of exogenous surfactant [14].

**Bronchopulmonary Dysplasia (BPD)**: BPD, a form of chronic lung disease involving lung parenchyma and small airways, is associated with prematurity. Other contributing factors for the development of BPD include oxygen toxicity, mechanical ventilation, systemic and pulmonary infections, inflammation, late surfactant deficiency, presence of a PDA, pulmonary edema, poor nutritional status and a possible genetic component [15, 16].

**Oxygen Requirement**: Oxygen should be treated as a drug and the lowest possible concentration should be used to achieve an "optimal" oxygen saturation in the preterm neonate. New studies have shown that the use of supplemental oxygen to target a $SpO_2$ concentration between 85% and 89% have resulted in increased mortality compared to use of supplemental $O_2$ to maintain a $SpO_2$ concentration between 91% and 95%. The number and duration of hypoxemic episodes should be reduced and $SpO_2 > 95\%$ should be avoided in infants treated with supplemental $O_2$ to prevent $O_2$ toxicity [17, 18].

## Renal

Nephrogenesis is not completed until 36 weeks of gestation hence preterm neonates continue to develop new nephrons after birth. Consequently, premature infants have fewer nephrons than those infants born at term. Glomerular filtration rate (GFR) increases after birth, doubling by the second week and tripling by the third month of age. The fractional excretion of sodium in the very preterm infants is high and, coupled with alterations in the sodium-potassium ATPase pump, they lose sodium and may develop hyponatremia [19, 20]. Immature renal tubular function coupled with reduced GFR and incomplete nephrogenesis, reduces the ability of these infants to concentrate urine and makes them more susceptible to both dehydration and fluid overload, hence frequent assessments of both sodium and free water requirements are critical in these preterm neonates. Maturation of the kidneys is complete around 18–24 months of age.

**Table 49.1** Daily fluid requirements of preterm infants (mL/kg)

| Age | 750–1000 g | 1000–1250 g | 1250–1500 g | 1500–2000 g |
|---|---|---|---|---|
| 1 day | 85 | 75 | 70 | 60 |
| 2–3 days | 105 | 95 | 80 | 75 |
| 4–7 days | 130 | 120 | 105 | 95 |

## Fluid Distribution and Requirements

Total body water is greater in premature neonates (900 mL/kg) compared to term neonates (850 mL/kg) with most of this difference being attributed to an increase in extracellular fluid volume. A decrease in total body water, especially extracellular fluid volume, contributes to a decrease in weight, averaging about 10% in term neonates and 15% in premature neonates, in the first 24–48 h of life. Daily fluid requirements (mL/kg) of preterm infants vary not only with the age (in terms of day of life), but also with birthweight (Table 49.1) [21]. Other conditions, (e.g., phototherapy, thermal environment) can result in an increase in these requirements.

## Hematologic

The estimated blood volume is greater in premature neonates (100 mL/kg) than in term neonates (90 mL/kg). Management of the umbilical cord after birth can have a significant impact on blood volume and complications in premature neonates. Delayed clamping (defined as 30–180 s after delivery) and/or milking of the umbilical cord (generally defined as "stripping" a 30 cm segment of the umbilical cord 2 to 4 times prior to cord clamping) have been shown to result in the transfusion of up to 22 mL/kg of blood [22] and a decreased incidence of blood transfusion, intraventricular hemorrhage, and necrotizing enterocolitis [23] in premature neonates.

## Hepatic

Hepatic function and albumin synthesis are reduced in a premature compared to a term neonate. This results in decreased metabolism and increased unbound portions of drugs.

## Temperature

The thermoneutral environment is the ambient temperature at which the oxygen demand is minimal and temperature regulation is achieved through non-evaporative physical processes. Preterm infants are highly susceptible to hypothermia since they have a large surface area to body weight ratio, decreased amounts of subcutaneous fat, and immature epidermis with poor keratinization resulting in high evaporative heat loss. Studies have shown hypothermia to be a cause of morbidity and mortality in preterm infants [24, 25]. Hypothermia has been associated with respiratory distress, hypoxia, metabolic acidosis, coagulation defects, increased incidence of intraventricular hemorrhage, and reversion to fetal circulation with worsening of pulmonary hypertension. The use of radiant heaters, increasing ambient temperature and wrapping these infants in polyethylene film reduces heat loss and prevents hypothermia.

## Anesthetic Considerations

**Vascular Access**: Obtaining vascular access is a challenge in preemies; peripheral veins are small and poorly supported by surrounding soft tissue. These infants, especially those born < 28 weeks gestation, usually require parental nutrition. Some form of central venous line is commonly used to minimize the risk of complications from administration of hypertonic solutions through peripheral intravenous catheters (IVs). Usually an umbilical venous catheter is placed through the umbilical vein shortly after birth. Peripherally inserted central catheters (PICC) lines are inserted in the peripheral veins in the extremities. These catheters are long and have a very small lumen and thereby are prone to thrombosis; continuous heparin infusion may be used to prevent thrombosis in these lines [26]. Sometimes, percutaneous central venous catheters (PCVC's) are placed directly into the internal jugular, subclavian or femoral veins.

**Catheter Sizes and Flow Characteristics**: 24G catheter is the most frequently used PIV catheter in preterm infants. Flow rate varies with the catheter diameter (gauge) and length.

**Vein Finders**: Devices are available which use near infrared light or infrared light to help visualize superficial peripheral veins. Transilluminators like VeinViewer™ and Accuvein™, use near infrared light (NIR) spectroscopy and devices like the VeinLite™ and Venoscope™ use infrared light to help visualize the superficial peripheral veins to aide venous access. Ultrasound guidance to access both peripheral and central veins are also used, with some studies showing a higher first attempt success rate [27].

**Tracheal Tubes**: Tracheal intubation in preterm infants is a common procedure. While cuffed tracheal tubes (TT) are being used increasingly in infants and children, their use in infants <3 kg is not recommended by the manufacturer. The use of the appropriate size TT and the correct depth of insertion are vital for ventilation. Recommendations are provided in Tables 49.2 and 49.3 [28].

**Table 49.2** Recommended ETT length to the nearest half-centimeter by corrected gestation (gestation at birth plus postnatal age) and actual weight at the time of intubation

| ETT length at lips (cm) | Corrected gestation (weeks) | Actual weight (kg) |
|---|---|---|
| 5.5 | 23–24 | 0.5–0.6 |
| 6.0 | 25–26 | 0.7–0.8 |
| 6.5 | 27–29 | 0.9–1.0 |
| 7.0 | 30–32 | 1.1–1.4 |
| 7.5 | 33–34 | 1.5–1.8 |
| 8.0 | 35–37 | 1.9–2.4 |
| 8.5 | 38–40 | 2.5–3.1 |
| 9.0 | 41–43 | 3.2–4.2 |

This is the initial length to which the tube should be inserted, followed by a chest radiograph to check its position. The tube length should then be adjusted to align its tip with the thoracic vertebrae T1–T2 (Reprinted with permission from Kempley ST, Moreiras JW, Petrone FL, Endotracheal tube length for neonatal intubation. Resuscitation, 2008-06-01, Vol 77(3); 369–373)

**Table 49.3** Recommended endotracheal tube and laryngoscope blade size for preterm infants

| Weight of the infant | Size of the ETT | Miller | Mac |
|---|---|---|---|
| <1 kg | 2.5 | 0 | 0 |
| 1–3 kg | 3 | 0 | 0 |
| >3 kg | 3.5–4 | 1 | 1 |

## Anesthesia Circuits

**Types**: Historically neonates were anesthetized using open, non-rebreathing circuits (e.g., Mapleson D) because of concerns about increased resistance imposed by valves and the turbulent flow through soda lime. While open systems provide the advantages of decreased dead space and reduced air flow resistance compared to circle systems, this is accomplished at the expense of increased loss of heat and humidity. Furthermore, use of an open circuit results in increased cost (due to increased use of volatile anesthetic agent) and increased atmospheric pollution by volatile anesthetic agents.

**Mechanical Ventilation**: If the decision is made to use mechanical ventilation, there are essentially no advantages for an open circuit over a circle system. The only adaptions to an adult circuit would be the use of a smaller reservoir bag and tubing with a smaller internal diameter. For several reasons mechanical ventilation is indicated in most premature neonates undergoing surgery

1. **Surgical Factors**: Most surgical procedures performed on premature neonates involve pathology in the chest or abdomen.
2. **Patient Factors**: Maintenance of adequate spontaneous ventilation is unlikely in the face of the immature respiratory drive, increased chest wall compliance, and the likelihood of decreased lung compliance.
3. **Pharmacologic Factors**: Anesthetic agents have a disproportionate impact on the respiratory drive of neonates in general (and premature neonates in particular).
4. **Equipment factors**: Even in the presence of an open circuit the presence of a TT will result in an increase in airway resistance.

**Ventilator Adaptations**: Modern anesthesia workstations use ventilators that compensate for the tubing compliance/compression volume and the fresh gas flow rate.

1. **Fresh Gas Flow**: Consider the situation of an older anesthesia machine with a ventilator that does not compensate for fresh gas flow. If the fresh gas flow rate is 6 L/min, 100 mL is added to the circuit each second. If the ventilator rate is set at 30 breaths/min with an inspiratory to expiratory ratio of 1:2, each inspiration will last 2/3rds of a second. Since the fresh gas flows throughout the respiratory cycle, including during inspiration, with a fresh gas flow rate of 6 L/min, approximately 65 mL of gas will be added to the circuit during the inspiratory phase. This volume will be *in addition to* the preset tidal volume. In other words the fresh gas flow rate alone will result in a tidal volume many times the appropriate tidal volume for a 1 kg premature neonate. Obviously the magnitude of this effect can be mitigated by using lower fresh gas flow rates, but even with a fresh gas flow rate of 250 mL/min (the minimum oxygen flow rate permitted on many anesthesia machines) the fresh gas flow rate will add almost 3 mL to the preset tidal volume.
2. **Compression Volume**: In 1983 tests were undertaken to measure the compression volume of commonly used anesthesia circuits [29]. The results revealed that even in the absence of a heated humidifier, in plastic adult circuits the average compression volume of an adult plastic circuit was approximately 7 mL/cm $H_2O$ of pressure and the average compression volume of a pediatric plastic circuit was approximately 5 mL/cm$H_2O$. This means that even using a pediatric circuit if the peak inspiratory pressure was 20 cm$H_2O$, approximately 100 mL was not being delivered to the patient because of compression volume.
3. **Ramifications**: Imagine using an old anesthesia machine which did not allow pressure-limited ventilation and trying to deliver a tidal volume of 7 mL when the fresh gas flow rate adds 3 mL to the preset tidal volume and more than 100 mL of the preset tidal volume will be lost due to tubing compliance. In that situation the only way to determine the adequacy of ventilation is through auscultation of the chest and evaluating a combination of the peak inspiratory pressure and the visible chest excursion. Despite the fact that modern anesthesia workstations not only permit pressure-limited ventilation but also compensate for fresh gas flow rate and compression volume, appropriate anesthesia care dictates auscultation of the chest and evaluation of chest excursion and peak inspiratory pressure each time mechanical ventilation is initiated in a neonate.

## Drug Administration

1. **Volatile Anesthetic Agents**: The minimal alveolar concentration of volatile anesthetic agents is about 20% lower for neonates less than 32 weeks of postconceptual age than for term neonates. The increased airway irritability in response to desflurane makes it a poor choice for a child with BPD. Nitrous oxide is rarely indicated in preemies, in part because the high concentrations necessary to achieve a significant effect are not feasible in neonates who require supplemental oxygen and in part because the fact that the solubility of nitrous oxide results in expansion of air filled spaces (e.g., interstitial emphysema, necrotizing enterocolitis) which are common in preemies.
2. **Distribution**: The increase in total body water and decrease in fat content of the premature neonate have ramifications for drug administration. Decreased albumin synthesis results in larger portions of "free" drugs
3. **Metabolism**: Decreases in hepatic enzymes result in decreased drug metabolism.
4. **Excretion**: Decreased renal function results in decreased elimination, examples include:
    (a) **Opioids**: The volume of distribution of fentanyl is increased in preemies compared to adults. The elimination half-life of fentanyl is increased from 2–3 h in children to 6–32 h in preemies. Similarly

the elimination half-life of morphine is increased from 2–4 h in adults to 6–16 h in premature neonates. These changes have been attributed to decreased levels of plasma proteins, decreased renal excretion due to immature renal function, and decreased levels of CPY450 3A4 enzyme. Increased intraabdominal pressure associated with surgical repair of an abdominal wall defect is associated with an additional increase in elimination half-life which is generally attributed to decreased hepatic blood flow. In contrast the elimination half-life of remifentanil appears to be the same in preemies as in older children and adults.

(b) **Propofol**: Several authors report that administration of 1–3 mg/kg of propofol resulted in prolonged hypotension, decreased cardiac output, and hypoxia. This response is generally attributed to the development of pulmonary hypertension and a reversion to fetal circulation. Compared to older children, premature neonates experience prolonged sedation with propofol. This effect has been attributed to reduced redistribution due to decreased fat and muscle tissue as well as reductions in drug clearance

## References

1. Younge N, Goldstein RF, Bann CM, Hintz SR. Survival and neurodevelopment outcomes among periviable infants. N Engl J Med. 2017;376:617–28.
2. Ballabh P. Intraventricular hemorrhage in premature infants: mechanism of disease. Pediatr Res. 2010;67(1):1–8.
3. Adams-Chapman I, Hansen NI, Stoll BJ, Higgins R. Neurodevelopmental outcome of extremely low birth weight infants with post hemorrhagic hydrocephalus requiring shunt insertion. Pediatrics. 2008;121(5):1167–77.
4. Derbyshire SW. Can Fetuses feel pain? BMJ. 2006;332:909–12.
5. Giannakoulopoulos X, Sepulveda W, Kourtis P, Glover V, Fisk NM. Fetal plasma cortisol and β-endorphin response to intrauterine needling. Lancet. 1994;344:77–81.
6. Carroll JL, Agarwal A. Development of ventilatory control in infants. Paediatr Respir Rev. 2010;11:199–207.
7. Nock ML, Difiore JM, Arko K, Martin RJ. Relationship of the ventilatory response to hypoxia with neonatal apnea in preterm infants. J Pediatr. 2004;144(3):291–5.
8. Wallace DK. Anti-VEGF treatment for ROP: which drug and what dose? J AAPOS. 2016;20(6):476–8.
9. Murphy PJ. The fetal circulation. Contin Edcu Anaesth Crit Care Pain. 2005;5(4):107–12.
10. Laughon MM, Simmons MA, Bose CL. Patency of the ductus arteriosus in premature infant: is it pathologic? Should it be treated? Curr Opin Pediatr. 2004;16(2):146–51.
11. Thébaud B, Lacaze-Mazmonteil T. Patent ductus arteriosus in premature infants: a never closing act. Paediatr Child Health. 2010;15(5):267–70.
12. Ruegger C, Bucher HU, Mieth RA. Pulse oximetry in the newborn: is the left hand pre- or post-ductal? BMC Pediatr. 2010;10:35–41.
13. Collin AA, McEvoy C, Castile RG. Respiratory morbidity and lung function in preterm infants of 32 to 36 weeks' gestational age. Pediatrics. 2010;126(1):115–28.
14. Polin RA, Carlo WA, Committee on Fetus and Newborn, American Academy of Pediatrics. Surfactant replacement therapy for preterm and term neonates with respiratory distress. Pediatrics. 2014;133(1):156–63.
15. Poggi C, Giusti B, Gozzini E, Sereni A. Genetic contributions to the development of complications in preterm neonates. PLoS One. 2015;10(7):e0131741.
16. Merrill JD, Ballard RA, Cnaan A, Hibbs AM. Dysfunction of pulmonary surfactant in chronically ventilated premature infants. Pediatr Res. 2004;56(6):918–26.
17. Stenson B, Brocklehurst P, Tarnow-Mordi W. Increased 36-week survival *with* high oxygen saturation target *in* extremely preterm infants. N Engl J Med. 2011;364(17):1680–2.
18. Darlow BA, Morley CJ. Oxygen saturation targeting and bronchopulmonary dysplasia. Clin Perinatol. 2015;42(4):807–23.
19. Musso CG, Ghezzi L, Ferraris J. Renal physiology in newborns and old people: similar characteristics but different mechanisms. Int Urol Nephrol. 2004;36(2):273–6.
20. Gregory GA, Brett C. Neonatology for anesthesiologists. In: Davis P, Cladis F, editors. Smith's anesthesia for infants and children. 9th ed. Philadelphia: Elsevier; 2016. p. 513–70.
21. Oh W. Fluid and electrolyte therapy in low birth weight infants. Pediatr Rev. 1980;1:313.
22. Yao AC, Lind J, Tiisala R, Michelsson K. Placental transfusion in the premature infant with observation on clinical course and outcome. Acta Paediatr Scand. 1969;58(6):561–6.
23. Rabe H, Diaz-Rossello JL, Duley L, Dowswell T. Effect of timing of umbilical cord clamping and other strategies to influence placental transfusion at preterm birth on maternal and infant outcomes. Cochrane Database Syst Rev. 2012;(8):CD003248.

24. Laptook AR, Salhab W, Bhaskar B, Neonatal Research Network. Admission temperature of low birth weight infants: predictors and associated morbidities. Pediatrics. 2007;119(3):e643–9.
25. Chang HY, Sung YH, Wang SM, Lung HL. Short and long term outcomes in very low birth weight infants with admission hypothermia. PLoS One. 2015;10(7):e0131976.
26. Mehta S, Connors AF, Danish EH, Grisoni E. Incidence of thrombosis during central venous catheterization of newborns, a prospective study. J Pediatr Surg. 1992;27(1):18–22.
27. Giris KK. Ultrasound guidance versus transillumination for peripheral intravenous cannulation in pediatric patients with difficult venous access. Egyptian J Cardiothorac Anesth. 2014;8(1):39–44.
28. Kempley ST, Moreiras JW, Petrone FL. Endotracheal tube length for neonatal intubation. Resuscitation. 2008;77(3):369–73.
29. Coté CJ, Petkau AJ, Ryan JF, Welch JP. Wasted ventilation measured in vitro with eight anesthetic circuits with and without in-line humidification. Anesthesiology. 1983;59(5):442–6.
30. Moutquin JM. Classification and heterogeneity of preterm birth. BJOG. 2003;110 Suppl 20:30–3.
31. Anand KJ, Sippell WG, Aynsley-Green A. Randomised trial of fentanyl anaesthesia in preterm babies undergoing surgery: effects on the stress response. Lancet. 1987;1(8524):62–6.
32. Jevtovic-Todorovic V, Hartman RE, Izumi Y, Benshoff ND. Early exposure to common anesthetic agents causes widespread neurodegeneration in the developing rat brain and persistent learning deficits. J Neurosci. 2003;23:876–82.
33. Hellström A, Smith LE, Dammann O. Retinopathy of prematurity. Lancet. 2013;382(9902):1445–57.

# Anesthesia for Ex-Utero Intra-Partum Procedures

## 50

Magdy Takla, Irwin Gratz, and Bharathi Gourkanti

## Introduction

The Ex Utero Intrapartum Treatment (EXIT) is a novel surgical technique that has become increasingly popular as a life-saving fetal surgical procedure in recent years. Previously known as Operation on Placental Support (OOPS) and Airway Management on Placental Support (AMPS), the EXIT is now the procedure of choice for fetal airway management [1, 2].

The EXIT allows therapeutic interventions on the fetus while preserving fetoplacental circulation and, therefore, maintaining oxygenation [3].

In both OOPS and EXIT procedures, the uteroplacental circulation is maintained by leaving the umbilical cord intact. However, during its early use no attempts were made to prevent normal uterine contractions throughout the procedure [4].

The first report of the OOPS procedure was published by Norris in 1989. He described a case of a preterm fetus with a large neck mass that was prenatally diagnosed as a cervical teratoma. The fetus, however did not survive [2, 4]. Later, in 1997, Mychaliska et al. standardized the procedure and provided guidelines. He also coined the acronym EXIT and described the first series of eight successfully treated cases [4, 5]. It is speculated that approximately a thousand fetal surgeries were performed in the United States in 2012, and the number of these interventions continue to rise steadily [4].The procedure consists of a partial cesarean section with simultaneous maintenance of placental circulation as a way to preserve fetal gas exchanges during the establishment of a definitive airway through direct laryngoscopy, bronchoscopy, or tracheostomy. The anesthetic approach is significantly different from a conventional cesarean section and involves a deep volatile anesthesia with maximum uterine relaxation, preservation of uteroplacental blood flow and fetal anesthesia.

The success of an EXIT depends on a rigorous strategic planning with involvement of a multi-disciplinary team where the anesthesiologist often takes the leadership role.

## Indications

The EXIT procedure was initially used for the reversal of tracheal occlusion in a fetus with prenatally diagnosed severe congenital diaphragmatic hernia (CDH) by performing an in-utero tracheal clip application during pregnancy. However, as anesthesiology and surgical techniques have advanced in the recent years, the indications have also expanded drastically [4].

Today, the most common indications for the EXIT procedure are fetal neck masses and

M. Takla, M.D. · I. Gratz, D.O.
B. Gourkanti, M.D. (✉)
Cooper Medical School Rowan University, Cooper University Hospital, Camden, NJ, USA
e-mail: takla-magdy@CooperHealth.edu;
gourkanti-bharathi@cooperhealth.edu

congenital high airway obstruction syndrome (CHAOS). Other indications can be classified on the basis of the type of lesion, diagnosis, or the goal of the procedure [6] (Table 50.1).

## EXIT-to-Airway Procedure (Fig. 50.1)

If intubation is not possible, fetal tracheostomy can be performed with or without resection of the mass. This approach is commonly used in patients with fetal neck masses, tracheal atresia or congenital high airway obstruction syndrome CHAOS.

## EXIT-to-Resection Procedure

If tracheostomy is not feasible due to anatomic distortion, neck or lung masses may be resected on placental support.

## EXIT-to-ECMO (Extracorporeal Membrane Oxygenation) Procedure

In cases of severe congenital diaphragmatic hernia CDH or severe cardiac abnormality, sudden discontinuation of placental circulation will lead to fetal hypoxia. The risk of hypoxia can be reduced by gradually switching the fetus from placental circulation to the extracorporeal bypass.

## EXIT-to-Separation Procedure

This approach allows rapid control of the airway in cases where surgery is indicated for survival (e.g., in conjoined twins) [6].

The EXIT procedure has also been successfully performed in twin pregnancy, when one of the fetuses had a large neck mass [4].

**Table 50.1** Indications of ex-utero intrapartum procedure (EXIT)

| |
|---|
| Cervical lymphangioma (cystic hygroma) |
| Lingual/pharyngolaryngeal lymphangioma |
| Cervical/thoracic teratoma |
| Epignathus (developed fetal organs arising from basi-sphenoid) |
| Laryngeal and tracheal atresia/stenosis (CHAOS) |
| Congenital thyroid goitre |
| Tongue tumour |
| Severe micrognathia |
| Conjoined twins |
| Embryonic rhabdomyosarcoma |
| Cervical neuroblastoma |
| Plunging ranula |

**Graham**, John M., **Scadding**, Glenis, **Bull**, Peter D. (Eds.), Pediatric ENT (springer) with permission

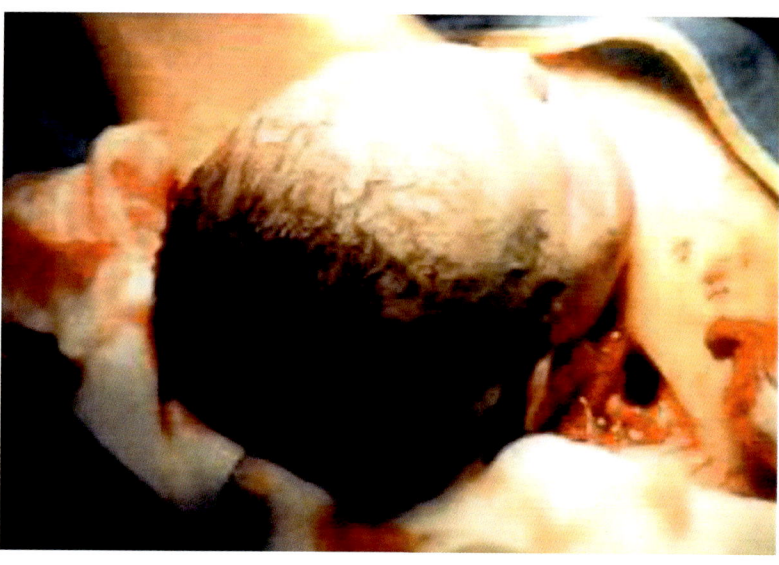

**Fig. 50.1** Baby's upper body delivered during EXIT procedure. Graham, John M., Scadding, Glenis, Bull, Peter D. (Eds.), Pediatric ENT (springer) with permission

## Physiology of EXIT

The EXIT procedure success can be attributed to improved understanding and management of maternofetal physiology and consequently the ability to take advantage and manipulate certain parameters to achieve an ideal state. In the EXIT procedure, complete uterine relaxation is of primary importance throughout the duration of ureteroplacental support preserving maternal-fetal gas exchange at the placental interface. This ensures fetal oxygenation and potentially avoids fetal hypoxia. Inhaled anesthetic agents are preferred for the following reasons:

1. The EXIT procedure often requires delivering the fetal head and shoulder through the incision (Fig. 50.2); this is quite difficult with a low transverse uterine segment incision.
2. The surgical procedure of the fetus may undergo, and will benefit from, adequate anesthesia that it receives via transplacental transfer.
3. The oxygenation is dependent on uterine perfusion and relaxed uterus. Any alteration in mean arterial pressure or increase in uterine tone will affect fetal oxygen delivery.

The understanding of maternal physiological hemodynamic changes during pregnancy and delivery is paramount to ensuring a good outcome. It is important to realize that the uterine vasculature lacks autoregulation, and blood flow is entirely pressure-dependent. Inhalational anesthesia maximally dilates the uterine vessels and fetal blood flow can be compromised. Maternal hemodynamic measurements (Fig. 50.3) may not accurately reflect the uteroplacental circulation [7].

Regional anesthesia is the rule for routine obstetric anesthesia practice. General anesthesia with inhalational agents is the technique of choice for patients undergoing EXIT, but exposes the mother to surgical and postpartum risk without providing any health benefit directly to her. General anesthesia has inherent risks that that are greatly exacerbated by pregnancy. The increased morbidity of general anesthesia is predominately due to failure of tracheal intubation. The incidence of failed intubation during obstetric general anesthesia has been reported to range from 1 in 390 to 1 in 443 cases [8] A high risk of aspiration due to decrease of gastroesophageal sphincter pressure, upward and anterior displacement of

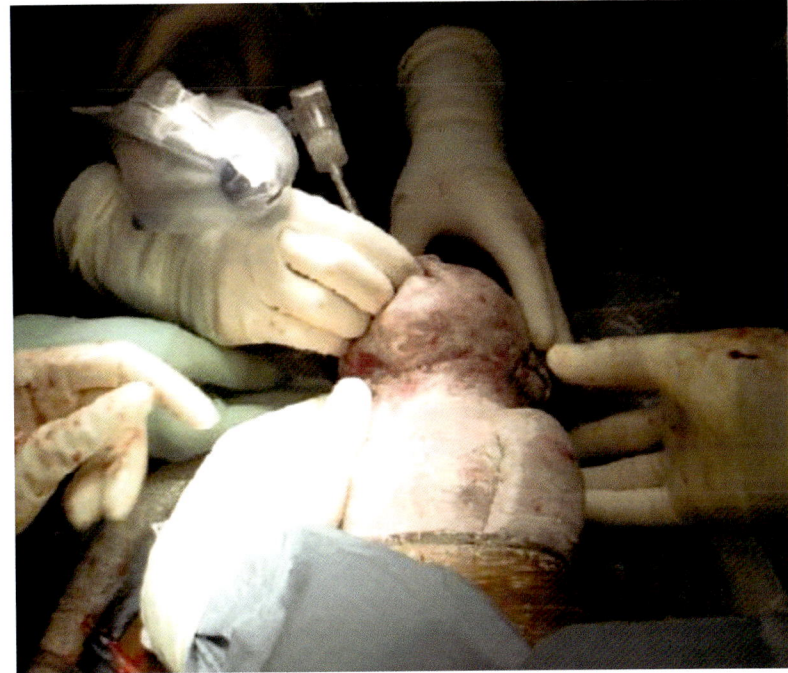

**Fig. 50.2** Confirmation of successful intubation with a neonatal carbon dioxide colorimetric device during an *ex utero* intrapartum treatment procedure

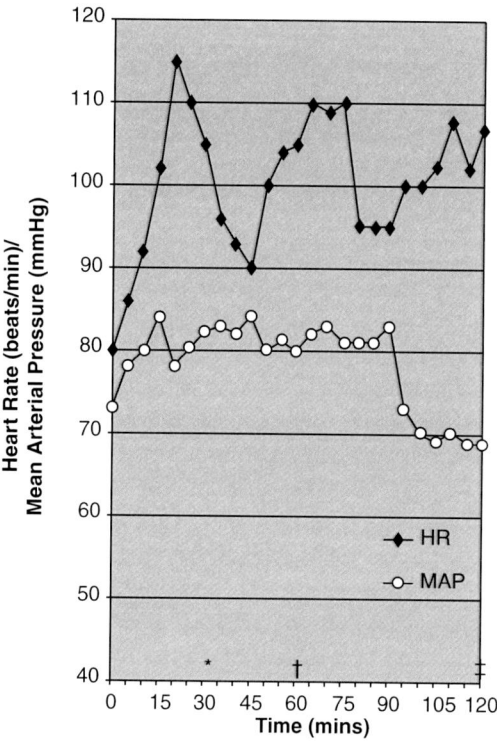

**Fig. 50.3** Maternal hemodynamic data during the intraoperative period (starting from induction of anesthesia to completion of surgery). *HR* heart rate, *MAP* Mean Arterial Pressure, * uterine incision, _ termination of placental support and neonatal delivery, _ neonatal intubation under bronchoscopic guidance. Alexander Butwick, FRCA Æ Pedram Aleshi, MD Æ, Imad Yamout, MD [Obstetric hemorrhage during an exit procedure for severe fetal airway obstruction] Hémorragie obstétricale pendant une procédure de traitement ex utero intrapartum en raison d'une obstruction grave des voies respiratoires du foetus. Can J Anesth/J Can Anesth (2009) 56:437–442. DOI 10.1007/s12630-009-9092-z. Received: 26 November 2008/Revised: 3 March 2009/Accepted: 5 March 2009/Published online: 25 April 2009. _ Canadian Anesthesiologists' Society 2009; 2- Canadian Journal of Anesthesia, March 2007, 54:218. Case series: Combined spinal epidural anesthesia for Cesarean delivery and ex utero intrapartum treatment procedure. Ronald B. George, Abigail H. Melnick, Erin C. Rose, Ashraf S. Habib. ports/Case Series. Accepted: 31 October 2006. DOI: 10.1007/BF03022643. Cite this article as: George, R.B., Melnick, A.H., Rose, E.C. et al. Can J Anesth (2007) 54: 218. doi:10.1007/BF03022643

the stomach. Also exists In addition, decreases Functional Residual Capacity (FRC) making hypoxemia more likely. For these reasons, rapid sequence induction after adequate preoxygenation is preferred.

## Preoperative Considerations

Accurate prenatal diagnosis is the key to good planning. The most common and widely used tool in the prenatal period is the ultrasound. If there is difficulty in visualization an MRI can be used as it has good soft tissue resolution and has an advantage in determining the severity of airway obstruction in CHAOS.

CHAOS and large neck masses are the most common indications for EXIT procedure [6]. Fetal demise in cases of CHAOS was inevitable in the past, but survival rates have significantly improved with the emergence of the EXIT procedure. Currently, all viable fetuses with CHAOS can be attempted for an EXIT delivery [9]. Hence recognition of the defect through prenatal imaging and evaluation of fetal trachea-laryngeal obstruction has become increasingly important [10].

The pathophysiology of CHAOS results from trapping of pulmonary secretions in the bronchopulmonary tree. That leads to hyperinflation of the lungs and increase in the intrathoracic pressure. Subsequently, cardiac output becomes compromised which may result in nonimmune fetal hydrops. These findings can be easily visualized on an MRI (Figs. 50.4 and 50.5).

The EXIT procedure requires maternal laparotomy and hysterotomy. If maternal health is significantly endangered by these interventions, EXIT procedure should not be performed [11].

Maternal risk must be weighed against the potential advantage to the neonate, particularly in cases where other severe anomalies or genetic defects are present. A morphologic and genetic diagnosis is important to ensure that the procedure is not performed on a fetus that has additional lethal anomalies [7].

The success of the EXIT procedure depends on rigorous strategic planning with involvement of a multidisciplinary team [1, 4]. The team should consist of at least the following: two pediatric surgeons, one otolaryngologist, one maternal-fetal medicine physician, one obstetrician, one neonatologist, two anesthesiologists (one for the mother and one for the baby), an ECHO technician, and two scrub technicians Table 50.2 [12].

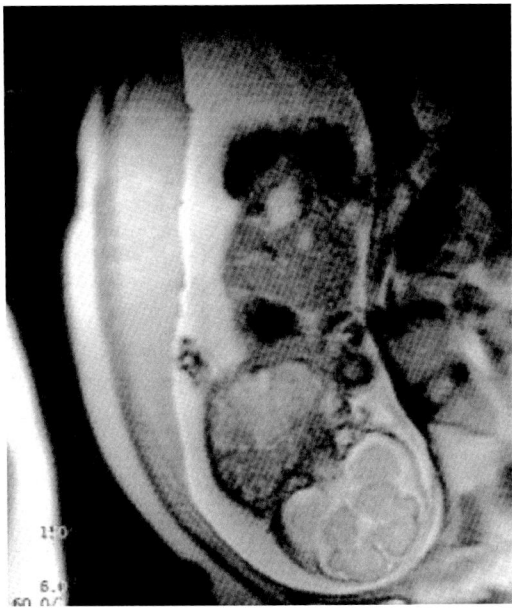

**Fig. 50.4** Fetal thyroid teratoma (MRI). **Graham**, John M., **Scadding**, Glenis, **Bull**, Peter D. (Eds.), Pediatric ENT (springer) with permission

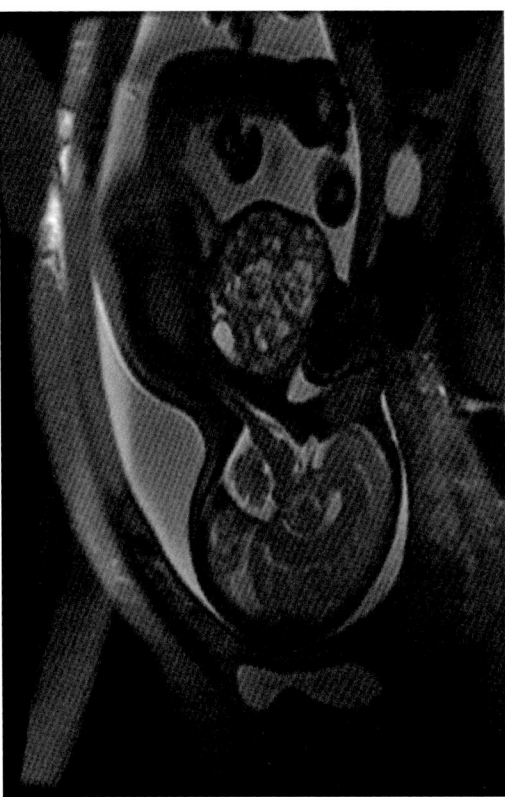

**Fig. 50.5** Fetal magnetic resonance imaging scan taken at 28 weeks gestation revealing an encapsulated cervical mass measuring 9 cm 9.6 cm 9.7 cm arising from the right anterolateral region of the fetal neck

**Table 50.2** Multidisciplinary ex-utero intrapartum treatment (EXIT) team

| |
|---|
| Foetal Medicine Consultant |
| Specialist Radiologist |
| Obstetrician |
| Obstetric Anaesthetist |
| Paediatric Otolaryngologist |
| Paediatric Surgeon |
| Paediatric Anaesthetist |
| Neonatal Intensivists |
| Theatre Nurses and Neonatal Nurses |
| Operating Department Assistants |

**Graham**, John M., **Scadding**, Glenis, **Bull**, Peter D. (Eds.), Pediatric ENT (springer) with permission

An obstetrician will perform the cesarean section. The anesthesiologist is a crucial member of the team as there needs to be an optimum balance between maintaining uterine relaxation and maternal vital parameters. This balance is crucial to ensure that uteroplacental circulation is optimally maintained until fetal airway is established. The procedure may be prolonged in order to establish a fetal airway. A second anesthesiologist should be available to provide both neonatal resuscitation and anesthesia. The pediatric and ENT surgeons help the neonatologist to secure the airway and this may require resection of a neck mass or the aspiration of a cystic lesion. Once the airway is established the surgical team will decide if a primary surgical procedure is required. The geneticist plays a very important role in the preoperative case conference to ensure that chromosomal or other structural abnormalities and syndromes are excluded in order to have an informed discussion with the parents regarding the appropriateness of the EXIT procedure and also the possible long-term outcome for the baby.

The team must ensure that the procedure is not carried out when there are other lethal anomalies. The parents must be aware of the diagnosis, management and the potential future implications. Maternal risks must be weighed against potential advantages to the neonate, particularly in cases where other abnormalities are present. The final outcome will depend on the primary lesion and its severity although the presence of other abnormalities may also play a role. The parents should be made aware of the long-term morbidity that may be associated with some conditions and this is especially important in CHAOS where long term tracheostomy, chronic breathing problems and multiple operations like tracheal reconstruction can have a profound influence on the life of the newborn and other family members. A fetal medicine specialist is important in the antenatal diagnosis and planning. They may also have a role in the operating room to scan and help locate the trachea in case of difficult intubations. The operating room needs to be large enough to accommodate two sets of operating teams—the team that delivers the baby and the team that secures the airway. Each member of the team should be aware of their respective roles and the blood bank must be informed in case blood transfusion is required for postpartum hemorrhage.

Careful planning and set-up, local guidelines, protocols and continuous audit of the results are vital in ensuring a smooth procedure and in obtaining good results.

Polyhydramnios is a consequence of fetal airway anomalies for which most EXIT procedures are performed [13]. The ultrasound is important in ruling out or detecting polyhydramnios and placenta localization, as these have a direct bearing on the success of the EXIT procedure. The recent advances in ultrasound diagnostic technology as D3 and D4 ultrasound has significantly improved the prenatal diagnosis of structural abnormalities.

If there is polyhydramnios, it is better to do an amnioreduction before the EXIT procedure. This is to prevent placental separation and cord prolapse due to the sudden release of large amounts of amniotic fluid on incising the uterus. The polyhydramnios can also flatten out the placenta and this can make the mapping of the lower margin of the placenta difficult.

A detailed obstetric history should be obtained, particularly if amnioreduction was done previously, the volume of fluid withdrawn and details of uterine contractions must be documented.

A detailed history of preterm labor provides insight into the degree of uterine irritability and may indicate the need for additional tocolytic agents during the EXIT procedure. The final diagnosis of an abnormality/abnormalities will decide the way forward depending on the short-term and long-term outcomes to such fetuses. A thorough discussion will then take place with the parents and a treatment plan can be made.

The preoperative visit also provides an avenue to alleviate the patient's anxiety. The importance of a good airway examination and plans for airway management should be established at this time.

## Intraoperative Considerations

### The Procedure

Although the EXIT procedure is done at the time of an elective cesarean section, the basic principles of the EXIT procedure and cesarean section are different (Table 50.3). Anesthesia for cesarean sections is mostly regional, whereas general anesthesia has been the mainstay for EXIT procedures in order to achieve a deep plane of anesthesia to keep the uterus relaxed. Fetal analgesia and anesthesia are not required during a cesarean section but they are required for an EXIT procedure. There is a deliberate attempt to maintain the intrauterine volume during an EXIT procedure until the baby is delivered but there is no such need in a cesarean section. A multidisciplinary team is a prerequisite for the success of

**Table 50.3** Cesarean section vs. EXIT

|  | Cesarean section | EXIT |
|---|---|---|
| Type of anesthesia | Regional | General |
| Anesthetic plane | Avoid fetal depression | Deep for uterine relaxation |
| Uterine tone | Minimal relaxation with rapid return of hypertonic uterus | Maximum relaxation for fetal surgical procedure |
| Intra-uterine warming | Not required | Required |

Modified (Ref. [14])

an EXIT procedure. Therefore, the procedure is generally done at around 37–38 weeks' gestation, unless there are maternal or fetal indications to deliver the baby earlier. An elective procedure ensures that all members of the multidisciplinary team are present and this is crucial for a good outcome.

## Anesthesia

As with any cesarean section, the patient should be positioned with a left lateral tilt to minimize aortocaval compression and to enable maximum blood flow to the uterus and placenta. Preoxygenation followed by rapid sequence intubation with propofol, fentanyl, and succinylcholine is performed in order to secure the mother's airway. The entries of alternate drugs like Rocuronium and remifentanil can be substituted as required. Sugammadex reversal of Rocuronium can be employed when needed in situations of cannot intubate and cannot ventilate events. Following tracheal intubation, an ultrasound of the fetus is repeated to confirm fetal well-being and to verify position. The specific goals of anesthesia are to provide maximum uterine relaxation and fetal oxygenation. Uterine relaxation is an important component of the anesthetic management and this prevents premature separation of the placenta and therefore the interruption of fetal blood flow and interruption of uteroplacental gas exchange. The dose of volatile anesthetics is significantly more for the EXIT procedure compared to a routine cesarean section. General anesthesia with high concentrations of volatile agents provides the necessary uterine relaxation for partial delivery of the fetus and prevents placental delivery while also providing fetal anesthesia by transplacental passage, which might help in fetal surgery [15].

Different centers have their own protocols for the induction and maintenance of anesthesia during the procedure. The doses of these volatile anesthetics are usually kept at around 2–2.5 times the minimal alveolar concentration (MAC), as determined by the end tidal concentration. This is higher and almost double than that required for a cesarean section. Unlike in a classic cesarean section, anesthesia induction is done early to attain good uterine relaxation and the baby is not delivered as quickly as in a cesarean section. Desflurane is a good halogenated agent for this purpose as maternal blood levels can be adjusted rapidly from very high concentrations to low concentrations and this helps in maintaining the uterine tone at a desirable level [16].

This is helpful in rapidly reversing the effects once the fetal airway is established to avoid postpartum hemorrhage that can result from prolonged uterine relaxation.

A recent retrospective study by Boat et al. found that early institution of high concentrations of volatile agents for long periods of time before hysterotomy was performed resulted in the development of intraoperative fetal bradycardia, especially when desflurane was used as the maintenance agent. Based on their findings, the authors of this study suggest the utilization of supplemental intravenous anesthesia with propofol and remifentanil until just before the hysterotomy incision is made, at which point high volatile anesthetic concentrations are used to achieve the desired uterine relaxation [17].

Recently the EXIT procedure has been performed under combined spinal epidural (CSE) anesthesia. The procedure is done by placing an epidural catheter and administering bupivacaine, fentanyl and morphine intrathecally. Uterine relaxation with regional anesthesia has been reported to be adequate for the EXIT procedure. Tocolytic agents (nitroglycerin, magnesium and or terbutaline) can be used for uterine relaxation. Nitroglycerin is the most common tocolytic. A loading dose of **nitroglycerin** of about 100–500 µg i.v. followed by an infusion at a rate of 1–20 µg/kg per min keeps the uterus adequately relaxed [18].

The role for **nitroglycerin** is probably more when regional anesthesia is preferred over general anesthesia, as the uterine relaxing effects of regional techniques are lower than that of a general anesthetic. Maternal hypotension is a serious risk and needs to be countered by the judicious use of I.V. fluids and vasopressors with close monitoring. Vasopressors are preferred to volume expansion in this situation to minimize the risk of pulmonary edema. In view of this, invasive maternal monitoring is widely used. Phenylephrine may be a better choice as a vasopressor than ephedrine in this situation because it may reduce the incidence of fetal acidosis [19].

A phenylephrine infusion may also achieve better control of maternal blood pressure and may be more useful in preventing hypotension. Fetal oxygenation may be further optimized by delivering at least 50% oxygen to the mother [19].

Many centers however, give 100% oxygen at 6 L/min to the mother, although 50% oxygen has been shown to maintain adequate gas exchange at the uteroplacental interface. Some institutions add preoperative indomethacin to maintain uterine relaxation [20].

The anesthesiologist plays a major role in maintaining an optimum balance between uterine relaxation and maternal blood pressure. The goal is to maintain an adequate placental circulation until the airway is established in the neonate before the baby is separated from the mother. The basic anesthetic principles include an understanding of the physiological changes of pregnancy, good maternal and fetal surveillance, and using drugs with a known safety profile.

## Uterine Incision

The site and size of the uterine incision depends on placental location and the degree of exposure required, which depends on the indication for the procedure and the type of fetal abnormality. Large incisions and more exposure will be required in cases of large neck masses. To avoid damage to the placenta a careful mapping of the placental edges by ultrasound should be performed. This prevents the obstetrician from injuring the placenta during the incision. Uterine incisions have even been made on the posterior uterine wall to avoid the placenta and ensure adequate exposure. Skin incisions are almost always transverse but a vertical incision may be required on the uterus in some circumstances. Making the uterine incision and partially delivering the baby while trying to maintain placental circulation poses two problems. The first is that the fetus is exposed to the colder extrauterine environment which can make neonatal resuscitation difficult. Secondly the amniotic fluid escapes upon uterine entry, reducing the intrauterine volume causing the uterus to contract and the placenta to separate. The above issues can be countered by running a warm solution of Ringer Lactate solution continuously into the uterus [21, 22]. The warm Ringers Lactate also prevents the umbilical cord vessels from going into spasm.

## Fetal Anesthesia

The baby's head and arms are delivered. While the fetus remains attached to the placenta, which serves as life support, the surgical team performs the necessary procedures to stabilize the baby. Monitors are placed on the baby and IV access is obtained. A dedicated pulse oximeter should be utilized on the fetus. Fetal saturations of 70% are normal, and fetal oxygen saturation over 40% should be maintained [23]. Continuous fetal echocardiography has also been described to detect fetal bradycardia and decreased myocardial contractility.

Fetal resuscitation equipment is listed in Table 50.4.

The neonatologist, the pediatric surgeon and the ENT surgeon should establish the airway by laryngoscopy, bronchoscopy, and tracheostomy or by resecting the neck mass. Aspiration of pleural effusions or a hydrothorax can also be done if necessary. Fetal anesthesia may be necessary when invasive or time consuming procedures may be required at delivery. Non-depolarizing muscle relaxants can be directly injected into the fetus if immobilization is required. Rocuronium 0.5 mg/kg or Vecuronium 0.2 mg/kg, fentanyl 10–15 μg/kg and atropine 20 μg/kg intramuscularly has been used to prevent movements that may hinder the process of establishing an airway or proceed with complex procedures. If the procedure is prolonged, umbilical artery catheterization is essential for I.V. access. Once the airway is established and secured, surfactant can be

**Table 50.4** Equipment for resuscitation

| Equipment |
| --- |
| Laryngoscope & Miller-MAC blades |
| ETT size 2.5/3 mm |
| Fibro-optic tower |
| Pulse oximeter monitor |
| End-tidal carbon dioxide indicator |
| 24/25 gauge I.V. catheter |
| N/S flush |
| Self-reinflating bag valve mask connected to oxygen source |
| Penrose drain |
| *Fetal medication* |
| Atropine 0.02 mg/kg X2 |
| Fentanyl 0.01 µg/kg X2 |
| Rocuronium 0.5 mg/kg X1 |
| Albumin 10 mL syringe X2 |
| Saline 10 mL syringe X2 |
| *Resuscitation medication* |
| Calcium gluconate/chloride 30 mg/kg |
| Epinephrine 1 µg/kg |

given through the endotracheal tube in case of pre-term babies and this helps to improve outcome. The baby is then completely delivered and handed over to the neonatologist. The umbilical cord blood gas values have been shown to be normal and this provides the evidence that the fetomaternal gas exchange is not adversely affected during the procedure [24].

## Maternal Complications

Uterine atony and postpartum hemorrhage are the main concern due to the induced deep uterine relaxation. As soon as the baby is delivered, uterotonics should be given to keep the uterus contracted. The concentration of the halogenated anesthetics should be reduced to help keep the uterus contracted. An oxytocin infusion at a rate of 10 units per hour should be given for 4 h and it may be necessary to give 250–500 µg of ergometrine I.M or I.V. and/or 250 µg of carboprost (prostaglandin F2 alpha) in addition as an intramuscular or intramyometrial injection. Specially designed uterine staplers with absorbable staples will reduce bleeding from the uterine incision edges during prolonged uterine atony [25]. If this is not available, a continuous stitch can be put around the incised uterine edges. In a series of 31 patients, Bouchard et al. [24] reported an average estimated blood loss of about 850 mL. There was one case of uterine scar dehiscence in a subsequent pregnancy in this series. The risk of scar dehiscence or uterine rupture can be higher in a subsequent pregnancy following EXIT procedure due to the possibility for unusual sites of the uterine incision in an attempt to avoid the placenta. Noah and co-workers [26] compared the complication rate of 34 EXIT procedures with 32 matched controlled caesarean deliveries. The operating time was longer and the estimated blood loss was higher in the EXIT group. As operating times were longer than in a cesarean section, wound infection rates were higher but the postoperative stay and hematocrit levels were not statistically different from that in a caesarean section. Other post-operative maternal complications include coagulopathy or deep venous thrombosis.

## Neonatal Outcome

Neonatal outcome depends on the primary diagnosis, the extent of airway distortion and the severity of associated anomalies. Although many case reports and small case series have been published, there are not many large case series. Low statistical power negatively affects the likelihood that a nominally significant finding actually reflects a true effect. The largest series was reported by Hirose and co-workers [25]. In the 10-year period between 1993 and 2003, 52 EXIT procedures were performed by the above group. The EXIT procedure was initially done and developed to reverse tracheal occlusion carried out *in utero* in fetuses with congenital diaphragmatic hernia (CDH). Initially, tracheal occlusion was done by clipping the trachea and so the EXIT procedure involved removal of the clip followed by establishing an airway. Tracheal clipping and removal can be associated with nerve and tracheal injury. Therefore tracheal occlusion is now done by using an endotracheal balloon. The balloon is placed through a bronchoscope and removed and an airway is then established during the EXIT procedure. EXIT procedure was performed for reversal of tracheal occlusion in 45 cases, of which 30 had a clip removal and 15 had bronchoscopy and balloon removal. Five cases had the procedure for fetal neck masses. One of these cases underwent a 2.5-h neck mass resection followed by intubation while on placental support, one was intubated and three had a tracheostomy. In another two cases, the procedure was performed for congenital high airway obstruction syndrome (CHAOS) and both had a tracheostomy. Of the 52 babies, 51 were born alive and 27 (52%) were alive at 1-year follow-up. All deaths occurred in the group with CDH but this could be because of the serious nature of the primary pathology. Average operating time on placental support was 45 ± 25 min, average gestational age at delivery was 31.95 ± 2.55 weeks and average maternal blood loss was 970 ± 510 mL. There were no maternal deaths. Some 35 of the 45 women who underwent fetal surgery for CDH *in utero* followed by an EXIT procedure attempted a further pregnancy and 31 had subsequent live births. In the series by Bouchard and co-workers [24], 31 women underwent EXIT procedure at an average gestational age of 34 weeks (range 29–40 weeks). The main indications were airway obstruction from a fetal neck mass (13 cases) and for reversal of tracheal occlusion from *in utero* clipping (13 cases). The mean duration of uteroplacental bypass (from uterine incision to umbilical cord clamping) was 30.3 ± 14.7 min (range 8–60 min). No fetus experienced hemodynamic instability during the procedure. Only one death occurred during an EXIT procedure because of inability to secure an airway secondary to extensive involvement by a lymphangioma. Long-term follow-up was not reported in this study.

Fetal complications include loss of placental circulation, inability to intubate, bleeding, tension pneumothorax, and death. Decrease or loss of the placental blood flow is a consequence of maternal hypotension which could be caused by administration of anesthetic agents or/and blood loss.

## Summary

The EXIT procedure is a novel surgical technique that has become increasingly popular secondary to improvements in the antenatal diagnosis of congenital malformations that require therapeutic or life-saving fetal surgical procedures. A partial cesarean section is performed with simultaneous maintenance of placental circulation to preserve fetal gas exchange, while a definitive fetal airway is established through direct laryngoscopy, bronchoscopy, tracheostomy or resection of the neck mass. The most common indications for EXIT procedure are fetal neck masses, lung and mediastinal masses, congenital high airway obstruction syndrome, congenital diaphragmatic hernia and congenital heart diseases. Prenatal imaging techniques like MRI and USG are used to diagnose and evaluate the severity of fetal trachea-laryngeal obstruction. The anesthetic management of these procedures varies greatly and a variety of strategies have been described, both general and regional techniques have been utilized but the major concepts remain the same. The anesthetic goals involve providing anesthesia to ensure maximum uterine relaxation, preservation of uteroplacental blood flow and fetal anesthesia. The most common anesthetic technique is rapid sequence induction and general anesthesia with high concentrations of inhalational agents, which helps to maintain the necessary uterine relaxation for partial delivery of the fetus and prevents placental delivery while simultaneously providing fetal anesthesia by the trans-placental route. Meticulous hemodynamic monitoring is pivotal to ensure adequate fetal oxygen delivery. Non-depolarizing muscle relaxants injected into the fetus provide adequate immobilization for establishing an airway or doing more complex procedures. Intravenous access is established through umbilical artery catheterization for prolonged procedures. Surfactant administered through the endotracheal tube improves postnatal outcome in pre-term babies. Common maternal complications of the EXIT procedure include uterine atony, post-partum hemorrhage, surgical wound infections, coagulopathy and deep venous thrombosis, while fetal complications comprise loss of placental circulation, failure to intubate, bleeding, tension pneumothorax, and death. The success of the EXIT procedure depends on a rigorous strategic planning with involvement of a multidisciplinary team where the anesthesiologist often takes the leadership role. Careful planning and set-up, local guidelines, protocols and continuous audit of the results are vital in ensuring a smooth procedure and in obtaining good results.

## References

1. Marquesa MV, Carneiroa J, Adrianob M, Lanca F. Anesthesia for ex utero intrapartum treatment: renewed insight on a rare procedure. Braz J Anesthesiol. 2015;65(6):525–8.
2. Filipchuk D, Avdimiretz L. The ex utero intrapartum treatment (EXIT) procedure for fetal head and neck masses. AORN. 2009;90(5):661–72.
3. García-Díaz L, de Agustín JC, Ontanilla A, et al. EXIT procedure in twin pregnancy: a series of three cases from a single center. BMC Pregnancy Childbirth. 2014;14:252.
4. Nnamani N. From 'OOPS to EXIT': a review of the origins and progression of ex utero intrapartum treatment. J Anesth Clin Res. 2015;6(7):540.
5. Chiu HH, Hsu WC, Shih JC, Tsao PN, Hsieh WS, Chou HC. The EXIT (ex utero intrapartum treatment) procedure. J Formos Med Assoc. 2008;107(9):745–8.
6. Dighe MK, Peterson SE, Dubinsky TJ, Perkins J, Cheng E. EXIT procedure: technique and indications with prenatal imaging parameters for assessment of airway patency. Radiographics. 2011;31(2):511–26.
7. Chinnappa V, Halpern SH. The ex utero intrapartum treatment (EXIT) procedure: maternal and fetal considerations. Can J Anaesth. 2007;54(3):171–5.
8. Kinsella SM, Winton AL, Mushambi MC, et al. Failed tracheal intubation during obstetric general anaesthesia: a literature review. Int J Obstet Anesth. 2015;24(4):356–74.
9. Derderian SC, Hirose S. Fetal surgery for congenital high airway obstruction. Medscape. 2013 Aug 15.
10. Courtier J, Poder L, Wang Z, Westphalen AC, Yeh BM, Coakley FV. Fetal tracheolaryngeal airway obstruction: prenatal evaluation by sonography and MRI. Pediatr Radiol. 2010;40(11):1800–5.
11. Jelin EB, Jelin AC. Fetal surgery for congenital pulmonary airway malformation. Medscape.2013 Jan 30.
12. Goldsmith JP, Karotkin E. Assisted ventilation of the neonate. 5th ed. New York: Elsevier; 2010. 656 p.
13. Tonni G, Granese R, Martins Santana EF, et al. Prenatally diagnosed fetal tumors of the head and neck: a systematic review with antenatal and postnatal outcomes over the past 20 years. J Perinat Med. 2017;45(2):149–65. https://doi.org/10.1515/jpm-2016-0074.
14. Garcia PJ, Olutoye OO, Ivey RT, Olutoye OA. Case scenario: anesthesia for maternal-fetal surgery: the ex utero Intrapartum therapy (EXIT) procedure. Anesthesiology. 2011;114(6):1446–52.
15. Gaiser RR, Cheek TG, Kurth CD. Anesthetic management of cesarean delivery complicated by ex utero intrapartum treatment of the fetus. Anesth Analg. 1997;84(5):1150–3.
16. Restrepo CE, Gomez ME, Puerta JJ, Upegui A. Anaesthesia for the EXIT procedure: the value of fast track anesthesia. Int J Obstet Anesth. 2006;15:S43.
17. Boat A, Mahmoud M, Michelfelder EC, et al. Supplementing desflurane with intravenous anesthesia reduces fetal cardiac dysfunction during open fetal surgery. Paediatr Anaesth. 2010;20(8):748–56. https://doi.org/10.1111/j.1460-9592.2010.
18. George RB, Melnick AH, Rose EC, Habib AS. Case series: combined spinal epidural anesthesia for cesarean delivery and ex utero intrapartum treatment procedure. Can J Anaesth. 2007;54(3):218–22.
19. Haydon ML, Gorenberg DM, Nageotte MP, et al. The effect of maternal oxygen administration on fetal pulse oximetry during labor in fetuses with nonreassuring fetal heart rate patterns. Am J Obstet Gynecol. 2006;195(3):735–8.
20. Hirose S, Harrison MR. The ex utero intrapartum treatment (EXIT) procedure. Semin Neonatol. 2003;8(3):207–14. Review.
21. Baker PA, Aftimos S, Anderson BJ. Airway management during an EXIT procedure for a fetus dysgnathia complex. Paediatr Anaesth. 2004;14(9):781–6.
22. Schwartz DA, Moriarty KP, Tashjian DB, et al. Anesthetic management of the exit (ex utero intrapartum treatment procedure). J Clin Anesth. 2001;13(5):387–91.
23. Marwan A, Crombleholme TM. The EXIT procedure: principles, pitfalls, and progress. Semin Pediatr Surg. 2006;15:107–15.
24. Bouchard S, Johnson MP, Flake AW, et al. The EXIT procedure: experience and outcome in 31 cases. J Pediatr Surg. 2002;37(3):418–26.
25. Hirose S, Farmer DL, Lee H, Nobuhara KK, Harrison MR. The ex utero intrapartum treatment procedure: looking back at the EXIT. J Pediatr Surg. 2004;39(3):375–80; discussion 375–80.
26. Noah MM, Norton ME, Sandberg P, Esakoff T, Farrell J, Albanese CT. Short term maternal outcomes that are associated with the EXIT procedure as compared with caesarean delivery. Am J Obstet Gynecol. 2002;186(4):773–7.

# Part IV

## Obstetric Anesthesia

# Anesthesia for Cesarean Delivery

Carrie M. Polin, Ashley A. Hambright, and Patrick O. McConville

## Introduction

Cesarean section continues to be the most common surgery worldwide. The rate of abdominal delivery has risen since the mid 1990s and includes women of all ages, ethnicities and geographical areas. Rising rates of primary cesarean sections are fueling an increase in total abdominal deliveries. Primary cesarean sections accounted for 50% of the increasing rate between 2003 and 2009, and the majority of those were subjective indications such as arrest of labor and non-reassuring fetal heart tones. Other contributing factors to rising primary cesarean section rates include suspected macrosomia, preeclampsia, multiple gestation, maternal request, maternal-fetal conditions, and other obstetric conditions [1] (Table 51.1).

Vaginal birth after cesarean section (VBAC), while an option to decrease the incidence of abdominal delivery, is infrequently used. The rate had declined since the mid 1990s but has more recently started to increase [2].

## Operative Techniques

While a variety of incisions can be used for cesarean section, the most commonly utilized are the Pfannenstiel incision for the skin and a lower segment transverse incision for the uterus. The Pfannenstiel skin incision is preferred by obstetricians for better cosmetic appearance, greater strength, and less postoperative pain [3]. This is usually followed by a low transverse uterine incision which is associated with less blood loss, less risk of rupture in future pregnancies, less need for bladder dissection, and easier reapproximation [4].

Vertical skin and uterine incisions can be made when rapid delivery is necessary. These incisions are also preferred when a transverse incision may not provide adequate exposure. Vertical incisions may be low vertical or high vertical (classical). Low vertical incisions may be used for unusual fetal positions and have a slightly increased risk of uterine dehiscence or rupture in subsequent pregnancies compared to low transverse incisions. Classical incisions carry even higher rates of future uterine dehiscence or rupture [5, 6], but may be necessary in some cases.

---

C. M. Polin, M.D. (✉) · A. A. Hambright, M.D.
P. O. McConville, M.D.
Department of Anesthesiology, University of Tennessee Medical Center, Knoxville, TN, USA
e-mail: cpolin@utmck.edu; ahambright@utmck.edu; pmcconvi@utmck.edu

**Table 51.1** Summary of anesthesia considerations in patients undergoing cesarean delivery

| Plan/preparation/adverse events | Reasoning/management |
|---|---|
| Patient preparation | |
|   Lab work | – Platelet count, type and screen, Hct at discretion of anesthesiologist |
|   Aspiration prophylaxis | – H2-receptor antagonists, metoclopramide, nonparticulate antacids |
| Spinal anesthesia | – Most commonly used for routine, scheduled cesarean delivery<br>– Reliable, quick, most dense neurologic block<br>– Performed at L3–4 or L4–5 interspace<br>– T4 level of anesthesia with local anesthetics (see Table 51.2)<br>– Additives<br>  – opioids to increase quality of analgesia and decrease postoperative pain<br>  – clonidine and epinephrine to prolong duration |
| Epidural anesthesia | – Most commonly used in conversion of labor epidural to epidural for cesarean delivery<br>– Local anesthetics added to increase density of block and extend to T4 level (see Table 51.3)<br>– Allows for titration and slower onset of sympathectomy<br>– Allows for prolongation of block by re-dosing if surgical times are extended<br>– Requires larger amount of local anesthetic than spinal |
| General anesthesia | – Most commonly used for emergency cesarean sections<br>– Rapid sequence induction with propofol (2–2.5 mg/kg), succinylcholine (1–1.5 mg/kg)<br>– Opioid administration prior to delivery controversial<br>  – likely beneficial to administer on induction to patients with pre-eclampsia<br>– Volatile anesthetics decreased to 0.5 MAC following delivery with addition of $N_2O$ or propofol infusion to decrease uterine atony |
| Regional anesthesia adverse events | |
|   – Maternal hypotension | – IV fluids, L uterine displacement, vasopressors |
|   – High block/Total spinal anesthesia | – Vasopressors, IV fluids, airway management, amnestic agent |
|   – Local anesthetic systemic toxicity | – ACLS with small doses of epinephrine (10–100 mcg); lipid emulsion 1.5 mL/kg over 1 min |
|   – Post Dural puncture headache | – Gold standard epidural blood patch |
|   – Neurologic complications | – Neurosurgical consultation/MRI for suspected epidural abscess or hematoma |
| General anesthesia adverse events | |
|   – Failed intubation | – Adequate assessment and planning, emergency airway devices present |
|   – Aspiration pneumonitis | – Prevention by using nonparticulate antacids, rapid sequence induction |
|   – Intraoperative awareness | – Prevention by end tidal anesthetic monitoring and depth of anesthesia monitoring |

Abbreviations: *Hct* hematocrit, *MAC* minimum alveolar concentration, *IV* intravenous, *ACLS* advanced cardiovascular life support, *MRI* magnetic resonance imaging

## Patient Preparation

A focused history and physical examination should be conducted prior to anesthetic care. Additional labs and more rarely imaging may be requested depending on the findings from the history and physical. The decision to require platelet counts or other labs are at the discretion of the anesthesiologist and should be individualized. Blood product availability for cesarean section should be considered in high-risk cases. For routine cases, the decision whether or not to require a type and screen should be determined by the anesthesiologist.

While regional anesthesia is the preferred method for cesarean section, discussion should include the initiation of general anesthesia with all patients. Risks and benefits involved with both regional and general anesthesia should be discussed with the patient, and equipment needed to initiate either technique should be readily available. Regardless of technique used, standard ASA monitors should be applied [7].

Obstetrical patients have a greater incidence of gastroesophageal reflux disease late in pregnancy compared to non-parturients. Before cesarean section, NPO guidelines should be followed as per any elective surgery. Medications to mitigate the risks of aspiration including H2-receptor antagonists, antacids, and metoclopramide should be considered. H2-receptor antagonists and antacids have been shown to increase gastric pH, and metoclopramide is associated with reduced nausea and vomiting [8–15]. Improved outcome studies however are not available, and therefore the use of these medications is variable.

## Anesthesia Techniques

*Spinal anesthesia*: Spinal anesthesia is performed by introducing a small gauge needle in a lower lumbar interspace, advancing the needle until there is return of cerebrospinal fluid (CSF), and injecting a local anesthetic into the intrathecal space. For the procedure, the patient is either in the sitting or lateral position. After the medication is injected, the needle is removed, and the patient is positioned supine with left uterine displacement.

The spinal needle is typically inserted in the L3–4 or L4–5 interspace which is below the termination point of the spinal cord at the L1–2 interspace. Insertion of the spinal needle should be at least one level below the end of the spinal cord in order to decrease the risk of neurological trauma. The L3–4 interspace has historically been identified by palpation of the spine at the level of the superior aspect of the iliac crests; however, this landmark has been found to be inaccurate in 40–60% of patients, and providers are often one level higher than anticipated [16]. To minimize the risk of spinal cord damage, the lowest palpated interspace should be used. The use of ultrasound has recently been described to help in identifying interspaces and/or in locating midline in parturients [17].

A T4 level of anesthesia should be obtained to prevent patient discomfort during the cesarean section. Pregnancy is associated with an increased sensitivity to local anesthetics so approximately 30% less medication is needed to produce similar levels compared to non-pregnant patients [18]. Hyperbaric bupivacaine 0.75% in dextrose 8.25% is a common medication used for cesarean delivery. It provides a block with an average time to two-segment regression of 90–120 min [18]. Lidocaine may also be used, however its duration is shorter. Intrathecal lidocaine has also been associated with transient neurological syndrome. See Table 51.2 for common dosages of intrathecal local anesthetics for cesarean section.

Opioids may be combined with the local anesthetic to increase the quality of analgesia intraoperatively and/or postoperatively. Intrathecal fentanyl has a fast onset of 5 min, a duration of action of 2–4 h, and can be given to decrease visceral pain during the cesarean section. Doses of 10–20 mcg are commonly added to the local anesthetic. Sufentanil 10–20 mcg can alternatively be added for intraoperative analgesia. It has an onset of 5 min and duration of action of 3–5 h. Morphine, 100–200 mcg, can be administered in addition to fentanyl or sufentanil. Intrathecal morphine has a longer time to onset of 30–40 min, and thus will not provide much intraoperative analgesia; however, it has a prolonged duration and can provide pain relief for 12–27 h following the cesarean section. All neuraxial opioids can have side effects including urinary retention, reactivation of herpes simplex labialis virus, and pruritis. Neuraxial morphine is poorly lipophilic and is more likely to spread rostrally caus-

**Table 51.2** Intrathecal local anesthetics for cesarean section

|  | Concentration | Dose (mg) | Duration (min) |
| --- | --- | --- | --- |
| Bupivacaine | 0.5–0.75% | 7.5–15 | 90–120 |
| Lidocaine | 2–5% | 75 | 45–75 |

ing side effects of delayed respiratory depression, nausea and vomiting.

A disadvantage of spinal anesthesia is the inability to extend the time of the block once it is placed. For patients who may have a prolonged cesarean section, additives can be combined with the local anesthetic to prolong the blockade or a combined spinal-epidural technique may be utilized. Clonidine 75–100 mcg can be added to intrathecal bupivacaine and fentanyl to prolong the block. The addition of 75 mcg of intrathecal clonidine has been found to prolong a two-segment regression of the block by 16–40 min [19]. Clonidine has side effects of hypotension and sedation. Epinephrine 0.2 mg added to bupivacaine can also enhance the quality of and prolong the blockade. All medications injected into the intrathecal space should be preservative free to avoid arachnoiditis and neurotoxicity.

*Epidural anesthesia*: Epidural anesthesia is routinely used for cesarean sections in patients who were previously laboring with an epidural and deemed necessary for a cesarean section. It is important that the dilute labor analgesia block is converted to a dense surgical anesthesia block for the cesarean section. Several medications can be added to increase the density of the block and raise the level to T4 in order to provide adequate surgical anesthesia. The local anesthetics typically used to dose epidurals for cesarean delivery are lidocaine, bupivacaine, ropivacaine, and chloroprocaine. Doses for these medications can be found in Table 51.3.

Three percent chloroprocaine has the advantage of providing the fastest onset, which can be useful in urgent or emergent cesarean deliveries. It also has limited transfer to the fetus due to rapid metabolism by maternal pseudocholinesterase and can be safely administered in situations with fetal distress. Although the risk of ion trapping is less with chloroprocaine when compared to lidocaine [20], it has been shown that there is minimal fetal uptake of local anesthetics and no difference in fetal outcomes when local anesthetics are administered via epidural for emergency cases [21]. Because of chloroprocaine's fast regression, however, it typically needs to be redosed every 30 min. Epidural morphine has also been found to be less effective following administration of chloroprocaine. This effect can be mitigated by administering epidural morphine 30 min prior to chloroprocaine administration [22].

Two percent lidocaine is another common medication used for cesarean section. The addition of sodium bicarbonate (1 mL per 10 mL lidocaine) can increase the speed of onset to near that of chloroprocaine. Epinephrine (5 mcg/mL) can also be added to lidocaine to increase the density of the block and prolong the duration.

Bupivacaine has the slowest onset, which can be advantageous in situations when it is important to maintain cardiac stability. Sodium bicarbonate cannot be added to bupivacaine to increase the speed of onset because a precipitate will form. Bupivacaine provides the longest block duration and will rarely need to be redosed during a cesarean section.

The addition of epidural opioids to the local anesthetic mixture provides increased intraoperative and postoperative pain relief. Fentanyl 50–100 mcg and sufentanil 20–30 mcg both have an onset of 5–10 min and duration of 2–4 h when given in the epidural space. Epidural morphine 3–5 mg can be given for postoperative pain relief. It has on onset of 30–60 min, and provides 12–27 h of analgesia.

*General anesthesia*: General anesthesia for cesarean sections may be necessary due to contraindications to neuraxial anesthesia, patient

**Table 51.3** Epidural local anesthetics for cesarean section

|  | Concentration | Dose (mg) | Duration (min) | Max dosage (mg/kg) |
|---|---|---|---|---|
| Bupivacaine | 0.5% | 50–100 | 90 | 3 |
| Ropivacaine | 0.5–0.75% | 100–150 | 90 | 3 |
| Chloroprocaine | 2–3% | 600–800 | 25–35 | 12 |
| Lidocaine | 2% | 300–400 | 45–60 | 4.5 (7 with epi) |
| Mepivacaine | 2% | 300–400 | 45–60 | 4.5 (7 with epi) |

preference, or time constraints. Because of concerns of aspiration with decreased lower esophageal tone, parturients should receive a rapid sequence induction (RSI) with cricoid pressure. To minimize the exposure of the fetus to the anesthetics, the patient should be prepped, draped and the surgeons ready for incision after the airway is secured.

The most common agent for induction in the United States is currently propofol. Propofol (2–2.5 mg/kg) has a fast onset, short duration, and decreases the cardiovascular response to intubation. Hypotension can occur with induction of anesthesia with propofol, however uterine blood flow remains unchanged in animal models [23]. In patients with hemodynamic instability, ketamine (1–1.5 mg/kg) or etomidate (0.3 mg/kg) can be alternatively used for induction. Ketamine has sympathomimetic effects, which make it an ideal agent in patients with hypotension from moderate hypovolemia. It is recommended to administer a benzodiazepine with ketamine to prevent postoperative delirium. Ketamine in high doses can lead to neonatal depression and uterine hypertonia [24].

For neuromuscular paralysis, either succinylcholine or a larger dose of rocuronium (1–1.2 mg/kg) should be used. Succinylcholine (1–1.5 mg/kg) is typically used for RSI because of its fast onset and short duration. Rocuronium had historically been avoided due to its prolonged blockade following an RSI dose. With the availability of suggamadex, rapid reversal of rocuronium can now be achieved if intubation is unsuccessful or at the end of surgery.

Opioid administration to parturients on induction of general anesthesia is controversial. Opioids cross the placenta and have the ability to lead to respiratory depression in the neonate. Withholding opioids on induction, however, can lead to an increased maternal hemodynamic response with intubation and increased risk of intraoperative awareness [25]. The maternal hemodynamic response to intubation can be detrimental in parturients with severe preeclampsia leading to an increased risk of stroke [26]. Remifentanil is a short acting opioid that is rapidly metabolized in maternal and fetal circulation. It has been shown to decrease the hemodynamic response to intubation and surgery in parturients [27]. A dose of 0.5 mcg/kg on induction decreased the hypertensive and tachycardic response to intubation in patients with preeclampsia, while causing only transient neonatal respiratory depression. Higher doses of remifentanil were associated with maternal hypotension [28]. If not given on induction, opioids should be administered to the patient after delivery of the infant.

Following intubation, volatile anesthetics can be administered. Although the minimum alveolar concentration (MAC) of volatile anesthetics is reduced in pregnancy, a MAC of at least 0.7–0.8 should be administered to prevent intraoperative awareness [29]. All volatile anesthetics cause a dose dependent decrease in uterine tone [30, 31]. To prevent uterine atony, following delivery, the concentration of volatile anesthetics should be reduced to 0.5 MAC and supplemented with either nitrous oxide or a propofol infusion.

*Anesthetic methods advantages and disadvantages*: Single shot spinal anesthesia has become the most common method for providing anesthesia for scheduled cesarean sections [32]. Compared to other techniques for regional anesthesia, it is reliable, has a quick onset, and is easy to perform in most cases [33, 34]. Difficult cesarean sections or the addition of a tubal ligation however may outlast the duration of the spinal in some cases. Likewise, morbidly obese patients can have exaggerated responses to single injections, and the lack of a catheter to titrate or continue dosing is a limitation [35]. Epidural catheters used either alone or in conjunction with a combined spinal-epidural, as well as continuous spinal catheters to allow for titration and may be more useful in such cases where prolonged anesthesia is required.

Epidural catheters are most commonly used for unplanned cesarean sections when patients present from the labor and delivery floor requiring an abdominal delivery. Epidural anesthesia does not require dural puncture, allows for continuous titratable intraoperative anesthesia, and is a method for providing postoperative analgesia. Patients with potential hemodynamic instability from congestive heart failure or stenotic valvular heart disease may better tolerate the slower onset anesthesia. Disadvantages of epidurals include a greater total amount of drug required and the potential for less reliability than spinal anesthesia [36].

Combined spinal-epidural anesthesia is a preferred method by some for the rapid onset of a spinal anesthetic combined with the ability to augment anesthesia with an epidural catheter. A significant disadvantage however is the delayed verification of a functional epidural catheter.

Continuous spinal anesthetics have regained interest in recent years with the U.S. Food and Drug Administration (FDA) approval of medium-sized 24 gauge catheters. They are smaller than traditional epidural catheters, yet larger than the micro catheters previously banned by the FDA in 1992. Continuous spinals ideally offer the reliability of a spinal combined with the ability to titrate with a catheter. Differences in ease of placement and reliability when compared to epidurals and single shot spinals are still unknown. Complications of rare events such as infection and neurological injury are difficult to compare and require large-scale studies.

General anesthesia for cesarean section, while the most common method used years ago has fallen out of favor due to higher rates of morbidity and mortality [37–39]. Blood loss, aspiration of gastric contents, failed intubation in the mother, and neonatal complications are concerns with general endotracheal anesthesia in parturients. General anesthesia may be advantageous, however, in some cases including emergency cesarean section. A simulation study compared the speed of spinal versus general anesthesia in onset and found that general anesthesia was the fastest on average. The limiting factor of the spinal is the unpredictable time needed for a spinal block to develop after injection [40]. Other indications for general anesthesia for cesarean section include patients with contraindications to neuraxial anesthesia, planned ex utero intrapartum treatment (EXIT) procedures where profound uterine relaxation may be needed following delivery, or failed neuraxial anesthesia.

## Complications of Neuraxial Anesthesia Techniques

*Maternal hypotension*: Maternal hypotension is the most frequent complication from neuraxial techniques used for cesarean delivery. Hypotension occurs secondary to the sympathetic blockade and decreased systemic vascular resistance after initiation of neuraxial blockade. Several factors influence the severity of hypotension: the type of neuraxial blockade (spinal/epidural), maternal positioning, and the presence of maternal labor. The clinical impact of this hypotension varies. Spinal anesthesia is associated with a more rapid and pronounced sympathetic blockade, whereas an epidural has the potential for a more gradual onset of blockade and the avoidance of sudden hypotension.

Maternal hypotension has both maternal and neonatal affects. Hypotension leading to insufficiency of uteroplacental perfusion can cause fetal acidosis, fetal hypoxia, and neonatal injury. Hypotension can also lead to maternal complications, such as nausea and vomiting, altered mental status, and cardiac arrest. Recognition and prompt treatment of maternal hypotension can avoid these outcomes.

Prevention and treatment of hypotension include intravenous fluids, left uterine displacement, and vasopressor therapy. Co-loading with crystalloid (15 mL/kg) at the time of spinal placement has been shown to be more effective than preloading for the prevention of maternal hypotension, however neither has been shown to completely prevent hypotension without the need for vasopressors [41]. Colloid has been shown to be superior to crystalloid solutions in preventing hypotension, but has an increased risk of anaphylaxis and higher cost [42–44]. Left uterine displacement helps reduce aortocaval compression and improve venous return. Vasopressor boluses or titrated infusions can be used to treat hypotension. Both ephedrine and phenylephrine bolus medications are safe and effective when administered in the appropriate setting. Routine administration of a phenylephrine infusion (100 mcg/min) in combination with a crystalloid co-load at the time of spinal placement has been shown to be an effect method of preventing hypotension [45].

*High block/total spinal anesthesia*: High block or total spinal anesthesia can occur secondary to excessive spread of local anesthetic in the intrathecal space or epidural space, or an unintentional administration of an epidural dose into the intrathecal or subdural space. A study published in 2014, evaluating serious complications in obstetrics, reported an incidence of high neuraxial blockade of 1:4336 [46]. Caution should be used when administering local anesthetics in an epidural catheter after an unintentional dural puncture using a large bore needle. The practitioner should also be aware of the possibility of a high spinal if a spinal block is performed after a failed epidural as imaging studies have shown compression of the dural sac and reduction of CSF volume after injection of saline into the epidural space [47]. Though it is not uncommon for a parturient to report mild dyspnea after neuraxial blockade, indicators of a high neuraxial blockade include a weak hand grip, respiratory depression, impaired phonation, difficulty swallowing, unconsciousness, bradycardia, severe hypotension, and cardiovascular collapse. Treatment includes vasopressor therapy, intravenous fluid administration, and left uterine displacement. Airway management is important and endotracheal intubation may be necessary to maintain adequate oxygenation, ventilation, and prevent aspiration. During this event, the patient might remain aware; therefore, it is important to administer an amnestic agent while the patient is intubated.

*Failed regional block*: Failure of regional technique can be due to an inadequate dose of local anesthetic, maldistribution of local anesthetic, or failure of injection into the intrathecal or epidural space. Failed spinals are less common than failed epidural techniques, at 0.5–2% vs. 2–12% [48–50].

There are several risk factors associated with the failure to convert a lumbar epidural used for labor analgesia to a surgical anesthetic block for cesarean delivery. These include: number of top-up doses, enhanced urgency for cesarean section, and care provided by a non-obstetric anesthesiologist [51].

*Local anesthetic systemic toxicity*: Local anesthetic systemic toxicity (LAST) can be caused by inadvertent intravenous injection of local anesthetic. Precautions should be taken whenever there is administration of local anesthetics. Resuscitation equipment and lipid emulsion should be readily available. Several steps can be taken to reduce the incidence of LAST: aspiration of epidural catheter prior to any injection, test dosing the epidural catheter, and fractionated dosing. Intravascular injection may be indicated by a patient reporting tinnitus, dizziness, metallic taste or perioral paresthesia, palpitations or increased heart rate if epinephrine used in the test dose. Accidental intravenous dosing of local anesthetic leading to toxicity can present as seizures, myocardial depression, and cardiovascular collapse. If LAST occurs, it is important to get help, maintain a clear airway, and ensure adequate oxygenation and ventilation. If seizure activity is present, treatment with an anticonvulsant, such as a benzodiazepine, is indicated. Early administration of lipid emulsion should be considered, dosed 1.5 mL/kg over 1 min, followed by 0.25 mL/kg/min for at least 10 min [52]. Advanced Cardiac Life Support should be initiated in the event of cardiovascular collapse; vasopressin use is not recommended in this clinical situation. Using smaller doses of epinephrine (10–100 mcg) is preferred. Cardiopulmonary bypass should also be considered. Recommended maximum doses of local anesthetics can be found in Table 51.3.

*Post dural puncture headache*: Incidence of post dural puncture headache (PDPH) is determined by the size and type of the needle, with incidence falling with the use of smaller gauge needles and needles with a non-cutting bevel. Risk factors that place the parturient at increased risk are female gender, age, and reduced epidural pressure after delivery. The incidence of PDPH after unintentional dural puncture using a 16–17 gauge needle can range from 40–80%; however, using a 25 gauge pencil point needle can drastically reduce the incidence to <1–2%. Several treatment options are available. If symptoms are mild, hydration and analgesics can be used to treat the discomfort. Caffeine has been used in treating PDPH symptoms; however, the effects are typically transient. Caffeine also has risks, such as precipitating seizures and tachyarrhythmias. For more severe headaches, the gold standard is an epidural blood patch. Autologous blood is injected using aseptic technique into the patient's epidural space, near the site of the dural puncture. Other techniques have also been described in treatment of PDPH such as adrenocorticotropin hormone, theophylline, gabapentin, hydrocortisone, and sphenopalatine blocks, though studies remain small and data is limited.

*Neurologic complications*: The risk of permanent neurologic injury following neuraxial blockade, though rare, does exist. Transient neurologic injury is more common and typically resolves within a few months to a year. Neurologic injury can occur secondary to lithotomy position, instrumentation, or by compression of the fetal head. Pressure or any trauma to neural elements by the needle or catheter will illicit pain and should prompt the provider to stop actions immediately and redirect placement. Anesthetics should never be injected where there is persistent paresthesia.

Epidural abscess and meningitis are rare but serious complications of neuraxial anesthesia. The Serious Complication Repository Project developed by the Society of Obstetric Anesthesia and Perinatology to determine anesthetic risk in the obstetric population found the risk of epidural abscess or meningitis to be 1:62,866 [46]. Strict adherence to aseptic technique is important to limit risk of infection. Symptoms of epidural abscess include progressive neurologic deficit, severe back pain, and/or fever. Meningitis can have similar presenting symptoms as PDPH (headache, neck stiffness, and photophobia). It is important to distinguish the two by history and physical that focuses on any signs or symptoms of infection as a delay in diagnosis can be life-threatening. Epidural hematoma also presents with progressive neurologic deficit. The presence of coagulopathy places patients at an increased risk of epidural hematoma formation. The incidence of epidural hematoma in obstetric population is 1:251,463 [46]. It is important to have high clinical suspicion for abscess/hematoma as rapid diagnosis and treatment is paramount for avoidance of permanent neurologic injury. Neurosurgical consultation should be obtained and diagnosis confirmed with MRI. Surgical decompression is at the discretion of the neurosurgeon, with potential for medical management for cases without spinal compression.

## Complications of General Anesthesia

Anesthesia related maternal mortality is highest during cesarean delivery under general anesthesia secondary to failed intubation, inadequate oxygenation, inadequate ventilation, or pulmonary aspiration. Incidence of failed intubation increases during pregnancy because of certain anatomical changes that occur: fat deposition, mucosal edema, and difficulty in optimizing patient position. Management of a difficult airway starts with adequate assessment and planning. Emergency airway devices should be present and attention paid to the optimal positioning of the parturient, especially those that are obese.

The risk of aspiration is increased during pregnancy secondary to decreased lower esophageal sphincter tone and increased incidence of gastroesophageal reflux. The incidence of aspiration has declined secondary to increased use of neuraxial techniques for cesarean delivery. The risk of aspiration can be reduced by following NPO guidelines [53], using nonparticulate antacids, and applying effective cricoid pressure at time of induction to prevent regurgitation into the hypopharynx.

Cesarean delivery under general anesthesia has a high risk for intraoperative awareness. Factors contributing to this include the lack of premedication and the use of low dose of volatile agents. Though pregnancy lowers anesthetic requirements, administration of 0.5 MAC volatile anesthetic may not provide adequate depth of anesthesia to prevent awareness/recall. End tidal anesthetic monitoring as well as depth of anesthesia monitoring should be used.

## References

1. Barber EL, Lundsberg L, Belanger K, Pettker CM, Funai EF, Illuzzi JL. Contributing indications to the rising cesarean delivery rate. Obstet Gynecol. 2011;118(1):29–38.
2. Data from National Vital Statistics. Data from Martin JA, Hamilton BE, Ventura SJ, Osterman MJ, Mathews TJ. Births: final data for 2011 Natl Vital Stat Rep. 2013;62(2):1–90.
3. Cunningham FG, Leveno K, Bloom S, et al. Williams obstetrics. 24th ed. New York: McGraw-Hill Education; 2014.
4. Dahlke JD, Menndez-Figueroa H, Rouse DJ, et al. Evidence-based surgery for cesarean delivery; an updated systematic review. Am J Obstet Gynecol. 2013;209:294.
5. Patterson LS, O'Connell CM, Baskett TF. Maternal and perinatal morbidity associated with classic and inverted T cesarean incisions. Obstet Gynecol. 2002;100:633.
6. Magann EF, Chauhan SP, Bufkin L, et al. Intra-operative haemorrhage by blunt versus sharp expansion of the uterine incision at caesarean delivery; a randomized clinical trial. BJOG. 2002;109:448.
7. Standards for Basic Anesthetic Monitoring (Approved by ASA House of Delegates 10/21/86 and last amended 10/20/2010.
8. Dewan DM, Floyd HM, Thistlewood JM, Bodard TD, Spielman FJ. Sodium citrate pretreatment in elective cesarean section patients. Anesth Analg. 1985;64:34–7.
9. Jasson J, Lefevre G, Tallet F, Talafre ML, Legagneux F, Conseiller C. Oral administration of sodium citrate before general anesthesia in elective cesarean section. Effect on pH and gastric volume. Ann Fr Anesth Reanim. 1989;8:12–8.
10. Ormezzano X, Francois TP, Viaud JY, Bukowski JG, Bourgonneau MC, Cottron D, Ganansia MF, Gregoire FM, Grinand MR, Wessel PE. Aspiration pneumonitis prophylaxis in obstetric anaesthesia: comparison of effervescent cimetidine-sodium citrate mixture and sodium citrate. Br J Anaesth. 1990;64:503–6.
11. Wig J, Biswas GC, Malhotra SK, Gupta AN. Comparison of sodium citrate with magnesium trisilicate as pre-anaesthetic antacid in emergency caesarean sections. Indian J Med Res. 1987;85:306–10.
12. Lin CJ, Huang CL, Hsu HW, Chen TL. Prophylaxis against acid aspiration in regional anesthesia for elective cesarean section: a comparison between oral single-dose ranitidine, famotidine and omeprazole assessed with fiberoptic gastric aspiration. Acta Anaesthesiol Sin. 1996;34:179–84.
13. O'Sullivan G, Sear JW, Bullingham RE, Carrie LE. The effect of magnesium trisilicate mixture, metoclopramide and ranitidine on gastric pH, volume and serum gastrin. Anaesthesia. 1985;40:246–53.
14. Qvist N, Storm K. Cimethidine pre-anesthetic. A prophylactic method against Mendelson's syndrome in cesarean section. Acta Obstet Gynecol Scand. 1983;62:157–9.
15. Mishriky BM. Metoclopramide for nausea and vomiting prophylaxis during and after caesarean delivery: a systematic review and meta-analysis. Br J Anaesth. 2012;108:374–83.
16. Broadbent CR, Maxwell WB, Ferrie R, et al. Ability of anaesthetists to identify a marked lumbar interspace. Anaesthesia. 2000;55(11):1122–6.
17. Talati C, Arzola C, Carvalho JC. The use of ultrasonography in obstetric anesthesia. Anesthesiol Clin. 2017;35(1):35–58.
18. Lussos SA, Datta S. Anesthesia for cesarean delivery part I: general considerations and spinal anesthesia. Int J Obstet Anesth. 1992;1:79–91.
19. Benhamou D, Thorin D, Brichant JF, Dailland P, Milon D, Schneider M. Intrathecal clonidine and fentanyl with hyperbaric bupivacaine improves analgesia during cesarean section. Anesth Analg. 1998;87:609–13.
20. Philipson EH, Kuhnert BR, Syracuse CD. Fetal acidosis, 2-chloroprocaine, and epidural anesthesia for cesarean section. Am J Obstet Gynecol. 1985;151:322–4.
21. Gaiser RR, et al. Epidural lidocaine for cesarean delivery of the distressed fetus. Int J Obstet Anesth. 1998;7:27–31.
22. Toledo P, McCarthy RJ, Ebarvia MJ, Huser CJ, Wong CA. The interaction between epidural 2-chloroprocaine and morphine: a randomized controlled trial of the effect of drug administration timing on the efficacy of morphine analgesia. Anesth Analg. 2009;109(1):168–73.
23. Rucklidge M. Up-to-date or out-of-date: does thiopental have a future in obstetric general anaesthesia? Int J Obstet Anesth. 2013;22:175–8.
24. Nayar R, Sahajanand H. Does anesthetic induction for cesarean section with a combination of ketamine and thipentone confer any benefits over thiopentone or ketamine alone? A prospective randomized study. Minerva Anestesiol. 2009;75:185–90.
25. Panditt JJ, Andrade J, Bogod DG, et al. The 5th National Audit Project (NAP5) on accidental awareness during general anesthesia: summary of main findings and risk factors. Anaesthesia. 2014;69:1089–101.
26. Huang CJ, Fan YC, Tsai PS. Differential impacts of modes of anaesthesia on the risk of stroke among preeclamptic women who undergo caesarean delivery: a population-based study. Br J Anaesth. 2010;105:818–26.
27. Heesen M, Klohr S, Hofmann T, et al. Maternal and foetal effects of remifentanil for general anaesthesia in parturients undergoing caesarean section: a systematic review and meta-analysis. Acta Anaesthesiol Scand. 2013;57:29–36.
28. Park BY, Jeong CW, Jang EA, et al. Dose-related attenuation of cardiovascular responses to tracheal intubation by intravenous remifentanil bolus in severe preeclamptic patients undergoing caesarean delivery. Br J Anaesth. 2011;106:82–7.

29. Robins K, Lyons G. Intraoperative awareness during general anesthesia for cesarean delivery. Anesth Analg. 2009;109:886–90.
30. Munson ES, Embro WJ. Enflurane, isoflurane, and halothane and isolated human uterine muscle. Anesthesiology. 1977;46(1):11–4.
31. Yildiz K, Dogru K, Dalgic H, et al. Inhibitory effects of desflurane and sevoflurane on oxytocin-induced contractions of isolated pregnancy human myometrium. Acta Anaesthesiol Scand. 2005;49(9):1355–9.
32. Bucklin BA, Hawkins JL, Anderson JA, et al. Obstetric anesthesia workforce survey: twenty-year update. Anesthesiology. 2005;103:645–53.
33. Riley ET, Cohen SE, Marcario A, et al. Spinal versus epidural anesthesia for cesarean section: a comparison of time efficiency, costs, charges, and complications. Anesth Analg. 1995;80:709–12.
34. Fettes PD, Jansson JR, Wildsmith JA. Failed spinal anaesthesia: mechanisms, management, and prevention. Br J Anaesth. 2009;102:739–48.
35. Brodsky JB, Lemmens HJ. Regional anesthesia and obesity. Obes Surg. 2007;17(9):1146–9.
36. Kinsella SM. A prospective audit of regional anesthesia failure in 5080 cesarean sections. Anaesth. 2008;63(8):822–32.
37. Clark SL, Belfort MA, Dildy GA, et al. Maternal death in the 21st century: causes, prevention, and relationship to cesarean delivery. Am J Obstetric Gynecol. 2008;199:36.
38. Hawkins JL, Koonin LM, Palmer SK, et al. Anesthesia-related deaths during obstetric delivery in the United States, 1979,1990. Anesthesiology. 1997;86:277–84.
39. Hawkins JL, Chang J, Palmer SK, et al. Anesthesia-related maternal mortality in the United States: 1979-2002. Obstet Gynecol. 2011;117:69–74.
40. Kathirgamanathan A, Douglas MJ, Tyler J, Saran S, Gunka V, Preston R, Kliffer P. Speed of spinal vs general anaesthesia for category-1 caesarean section: a simulation and clinical observation-based study. Anaesthesia. 2013;68(7):753–9.
41. Oh AY, Hwang JW, Song IA, et al. Influence of the timing of administration of crystalloid on maternal hypotension during spinal anesthesia for cesarean delivery: preload versus coload. BMC Anesthesiol. 2014;14:36.
42. Banerjee A, Stocche RM, Angle P, et al. Preload or coload for spinal anesthesia for elective cesarean delivery: a meta-analysis. Can J Anaesth. 2010;57:24.
43. Dyer RA, Farina Z, Jouber IA, et al. Crystalloid preload versus rapid crystalloid administration after induction of spinal anesthesia (coload) for elective cesarean section. Anaesth Intensive Care. 2004;32:351–7.
44. Morgan PJ, Halpern SH, Tarshis J. The effect of an increase of central blood volume before spinal anesthesia for cesarean delivery: a qualitative systematic review. Anesth Analg. 2001;92:997.
45. Ngan Kee WD, et al. Prevention of hypotension during spinal anesthesia for cesarean delivery. Anesthesiology. 2005;103:744–50.
46. D'Angelo R, Smiley RM, Riley ET, et al. Serious complications related to obstetric anesthesia: the serious complication repository project of the Society for Obstetric Anesthesia and Perinatology. Anesthesiology. 2014;120:1505–12.
47. Higuchi H, et al. Effects of epidural saline injection on cerebrospinal fluid volume and velocity waveform. Anesthesiology. 2005;102:285–92.
48. Pan PH, Bogard TD, Owen MD. Incidence and characteristics of failures in obstetric neuroaxial analgesia and anesthesia: a retrospective analysis of 19,259 deliveries. Int J Obstet Anesth. 2004;13:227–33.
49. Tortosa JC, Parry NS, Mercier FJ, Mazoit JX, Benhamou D. Efficacy of augmentation of epidural analgesia for caesarean section. Br J Anaesth. 2003;91:532–5.
50. Kinsella SM. A prospective audit of regional anaesthesia failure in 5080 caesarean sections. Anaesthesia. 2008;63:822–33.
51. Bauer ME, et al. Risk factors for failed conversion of labor epidural analgesia to cesarean delivery anesthesia: a systemic review and meta-analysis of observational trials. Int J Obstet Anesth. 2012;21:294–309.
52. Neal JM, Bernards CM, Butterworth JF 4th, et al. ASRA practice advisory on local anesthetic systemic toxicity. Reg Anesth Pain Med. 2010;35:152.
53. American Society of Anesthesiologists Task Force on Obstetric Anesthesia. Practice guidelines for obstetric anesthesia: an updated report by the American Society of Anesthesiologist Task Force on Obstetric Anesthesia. Anesthesiology. 2007;106:843–63.

# Anesthesia for Non-delivery Obstetric Procedures

52

John C. Coffman, Blair H. Herndon, Mitesh Thakkar, and Kasey Fiorini

## Introduction

Obstetric anesthesia providers most commonly provide either labor analgesia or cesarean delivery anesthesia, though there are a number of other obstetric procedures that also require anesthesia care. This chapter highlights the surgical and anesthetic considerations of the most common non-delivery obstetric procedures.

## Postpartum Tubal Sterilization

### Introduction

Tubal sterilization is a frequently used method of providing permanent contraception. These procedures are commonly performed following vaginal delivery or in conjunction with cesarean delivery, being estimated to follow 8–9% of live births in the United States [1]. The postpartum period is advantageous because the patient is already admitted to the hospital and there is easier surgical access to the fallopian tubes for the first few days postpartum given the uterine fundus remains enlarged to approximately the level of the umbilicus [2, 3]. Though sterilization failure can occur [4], this should be considered an irreversible procedure and thus obstetricians typically begin the discussion and consent process prior to labor and delivery to help ensure the patient is making a well-informed decision. Providers should also remain aware of other insurance, state or federal regulations regarding sterilization consent and adopt processes to ensure prenatal consents are obtained at the appropriate time and are available at the time of delivery [5]. Previous reports have noted a range of approximately 30–50% of patients desiring postpartum tubal sterilization do not undergo the procedure [6–9], and one report observed that almost half of women with unfulfilled requests became pregnant within the following year [6]. It is important to make efforts to complete these postpartum tubal sterilization procedures in patients with valid consents in order to reduce future unintended pregnancies and the significant costs associated with them [5, 10].

### Surgical Considerations

Provider and patient preferences, institutional practices, availability of personnel, patient *nil per os* (NPO) status, and other individual patient factors may all play a role in the timing of postpartum tubal sterilization procedures after delivery. These procedures should not be performed at a

J. C. Coffman, M.D. (✉) · B. H. Herndon, M.D.
M. Thakkar, M.D. · K. Fiorini, M.D.
Department of Anesthesiology, The Ohio State University Wexner Medical Center, Columbus, OH, USA
e-mail: john.coffman@osumc.edu; blair.herndon@osumc.edu; mitesh.thakkar@osumc.edu; kasey.fiorini@osumc.edu

time when staffing may be limited or care to other patients may be compromised [2, 11]. Postpartum tubal sterilization in the immediate postpartum period (within 8 h after delivery) may be considered in healthy patients that had an uncomplicated vaginal delivery. Delaying the procedure beyond the immediate postpartum period may be indicated in cases of postpartum hemorrhage, maternal fever, concerning neonatal status, or other circumstances [2]. Some obstetricians prefer to perform sterilization procedures 8–24 h after delivery given that the risk of uterine atony and postpartum bleeding is lessened and longer assessment of the newborn is possible.

In the postpartum period, the fallopian tubes can be readily accessed via a small infraumbilical minilaparotomy incision that is extended down through the parietal peritoneum [3]. Postpartum sterilization most commonly involves a partial salpingectomy, for which several different methods have been described including the Pomeroy, Parkland, Uchida and Irving [3]. Lower incidence of sterilization failure and subsequent pregnancy have been observed if partial salpingectomy is performed compared to clip sterilization [4]. Overall, tubal sterilization procedures are a safe and effective means of providing permanent contraception, as there is typically minimal blood loss and major morbidity has rarely been reported for any type of tubal sterilization procedure [12].

## Anesthetic Considerations and Management

*Preoperative evaluation:* Anesthesia providers may already be familiar with patients undergoing postpartum sterilization if they received care during the labor and delivery period, though the medical and anesthetic history should be reevaluated prior to the surgical procedure. Anesthesia providers should review estimated blood loss at the time of delivery, postpartum vital signs, lab values, maternal NPO status and determine the condition of the newborn. The presence of ongoing hemorrhage, orthostatic symptoms, fever or other signs of infection, or concerns regarding the neonate may all impact the timing of a tubal sterilization procedure and may even necessitate postponement until after hospital discharge. The *Practice Guidelines for Obstetric Anesthesia* recommends that patients not have intake of solid food for at least 6–8 h (depending on the type of food) prior to a postpartum tubal sterilization procedure [11]. Gastric emptying can be delayed during labor and in postpartum patients that received parenteral opioids during labor [11, 13], and it is also recommended that providers consider administering some form of aspiration prophylaxis (oral non-particulate antacid, IV famotidine or IV metoclopramide) [11].

*Epidural anesthesia:* The anesthetic technique selected should be individualized, though *Practice Guidelines for Obstetric Anesthesia* recommends that neuraxial techniques be considered over general anesthesia for most cases [11]. Epidural anesthesia is commonly chosen for patients that have indwelling epidural catheters that were effective in providing labor analgesia. Previous investigators have reported a range of 74–92% rates of successful labor epidural reactivation for postpartum tubal sterilization anesthesia [14–17]. The potential for epidural anesthesia failure and possible need for a repeat neuraxial procedure or general anesthesia should be discussed with patients preoperatively. Anesthesia providers should be aware that epidural anesthesia failure may be more likely when the tubal sterilization procedure is performed at longer post-delivery intervals [11, 14–16]. For example, Vincent and Reid observed that 95% of patients had successful reactivation of the epidural catheter for postpartum tubal sterilization anesthesia if the procedure occurred less than 4 h after delivery, compared to 67% successful reactivation if surgery was >4 h after delivery [14]. Goodman and Dumas observed 90–95% successful labor epidural reactivation if tubal sterilization occurred within 24 h of delivery, compared to 80% successful reactivation if surgery was >24 h after delivery [15]. Prior to performing epidural anesthesia, it is important to ensure that the epidural catheter and dressing remains intact and the catheter remains secured close to the skin marking at which it was initially placed (usually within 1–2 cm). It is also important to aspirate the epidural catheter and administer a test dose (1.5–2% lidocaine with 1:200,000 epinephrine 3 mL) to rule out intravascular or intrathecal migration of the epidural catheter. Local anesthetic choices may vary according to provider preferences and length of operative times in different practices. 2% lidocaine with 1:200,000 epinephrine or 3% 2-chloroprocaine 15–20 mL are commonly selected and administered in 5 mL increments every 3–5 min [14–16], while monitoring the patient's vital signs and the onset of motor and sensory blockade during epidural dosing. Some authors recommend a sensory blockade up to the T4 dermatomal level for effective anesthesia [18], though sensory blockade up to T6 provides effective anesthesia in many cases [16]. Epidural fentanyl 50–100 mcg may also be administered to supplement the local anesthetic and improve the quality of anesthesia. Addition of sodium bicarbonate to the local anesthetic (ex. add 8.4% sodium bicarbonate 1 mL to 3% 2-chloroprocaine 10 mL) may also be considered, as pH-adjustment has been shown to shorten the onset of neuroblockade and may also improve the quality of epidural anesthesia [19–21]. Epidural morphine 2 mg has been shown to improve analgesia after postpartum tubal sterilization and reduce need for supplemental oral analgesics compared to a control group [22]. It is recommended that providers consider patient discharge timing when making decisions to administer long-acting neuraxial opioids.

*Spinal anesthesia:* Spinal anesthesia is commonly chosen for patients that did not have labor epidural analgesia or had ineffective labor epidural analgesia. Anesthesia providers should be aware that higher doses of spinal medication may be required to achieve satisfactory surgical blockade compared to term parturients undergoing cesarean delivery [23, 24]. Local anesthetic selection may differ according to provider preference or expected operative duration. Hyperbaric bupivacaine 10–12 mg has been reported to be an effective dosing range in multiple different investigations [23–25]. Spinal lidocaine 75 mg may also be effectively utilized [26], though some providers avoid spinal lidocaine due to concerns of transient neurologic symptoms despite the low risk of this complication in obstetric patients. Spinal fentanyl 10–15 mcg is commonly administered along with local anesthetic to improve the quality of intraoperative anesthesia and provide early post-operative analgesia. Spinal morphine 50–100 mcg has also been administered for postpartum tubal sterilization procedures [24, 25, 27]. Habib et al. observed that spinal morphine 50 mcg improved postoperative pain relief and reduced consumption of oral analgesics compared to a saline control group [27]. Anesthesia providers should be aware of the potential for spinal-induced hypotension, though the incidence spinal-induced hypotension and vasopressor requirements during postpartum tubal sterilization are reduced compared to term women undergoing cesarean delivery [23–25].

*General anesthesia:* General anesthesia is often reserved for patients that have contraindications to neuraxial anesthesia or those who have inadequate neuraxial anesthesia. Similar to general anesthesia for cesarean delivery, rapid sequence induction and endotracheal intubation are recommended for postpartum tubal sterilization procedures performed under general anesthesia. Anesthesia providers should be aware that the incidence of failed intubation in pregnancy is greater than the general population [28]. The Mallampati class may increase over the course of pregnancy due to capillary engorgement of the oropharyngeal and upper airway mucosa [29], and during the course of labor further increases in Mallampati class as well as decreased oropharyngeal and upper airway volumes have been observed [30]. Many of these airway changes may begin to resolve in the postpartum period, though providers should still be aware of the potential for difficult airway management and have appropriate backup equipment available (smaller endotracheal tube sizes, laryngeal mask airways, video laryngoscopy, etc.). Propofol (1.5–2 mg/kg) and succinylcholine (1 mg/kg) are commonly used as induction medications for these procedures, though other medications may be considered depending on the individual patient characteristics. Succinylcholine has been observed to prolong neuromuscular blockade in the postpartum period by approximately 3 min compared to term pregnant and non-pregnant patients [31], and the effect of succinylcholine may be further prolonged if the patient has received metoclopramide given it inhibits plasma cholinesterase activity [32]. If nondepolarizing muscle relaxants are used for induction or muscle relaxation during the surgical procedure, it is recommended that short acting medications (rocuronium) be selected given the short operative duration. The duration of rocuronium has also been observed to be prolonged in the postpartum period compared to non-pregnant women [33], and thus it should be dosed incrementally while monitoring neuromuscular blockade with a peripheral nerve stimulator. Postpartum tubal sterilization procedures are typically delayed if there are preoperative concerns for uterine atony or postpartum hemorrhage, though anesthesia providers should remain aware that volatile anesthetic agents can contribute to uterine relaxation and bleeding complications, particularly in the immediate postpartum period. Prior to extubation, it is recommended that patients demonstrate protective airway reflexes, are able to follow simple commands, and neuromuscular blockade is fully reversed.

---

Postpartum Tubal Sterilization—Key Points

- Permanent sterilization in the post-partum period is logistically more favorable than scheduling another procedure as an outpatient.
- The fallopian tubes are easily accessible via minilaparotomy due to the enlarged uterus.
- Preoperative fasting for 6–8 h is necessary, as well as medical optimization, in the setting of post-delivery procedures.
  - Fluid and blood product resuscitation should be completed as necessary.
  - The procedure may need to be delayed in the setting of postpartum hemorrhage, maternal fever, concerning neonatal status, or other circumstances.
- In-situ labor epidurals are commonly dosed for anesthesia. Greater success with labor epidural reactivation has been observed if the tubal sterilization is performed closer to the time of delivery.
  - Commonly utilized: 2% lidocaine with 1:200,000 epinephrine (15–20 mL) or 3% 2-chloroprocaine (15–20 mL) given incrementally. Some providers add sodium bicarbonate, epidural fentanyl (50–100 mcg) and/or epidural morphine (1–2 mg).
- Spinal anesthesia doses for adequate blockade may be higher than doses required for cesarean section.
  - Commonly utilized: Spinal bupivacaine 10–12 mg or lidocaine 75 mg. Some providers include spinal fentanyl (10–15 mcg) and/or spinal morphine (50–100 mcg).
- Providers should consider the planned timing for hospital discharge when administering long-acting neuraxial opioids.
- General anesthesia may be required for those unable to receive neuraxial anesthesia.
  - Rapid sequence induction and endotracheal intubation are recommended, and providers should recognize there is increased potential for failed intubation compared to the general population.
  - There is potential for increased risk of aspiration in the postpartum period, and administering some form of aspiration prophylaxis is recommended.
  - There is potential for prolonged duration of action of certain drugs (e.g., succinylcholine, rocuronium) and volatile anesthetics may contribute to uterine relaxation and bleeding complications.

---

# External Cephalic Version

## Introduction

Breech presentation, in which the fetal buttocks or feet lie closest to the cervix, is estimated to occur in 3–4% of term pregnancies [34]. Management options in cases of breech presentation may depend on patient preferences and the expertise of the obstetrician, and include planned cesarean delivery, vaginal breech delivery or an attempt at external cephalic version (ECV). Previous studies have observed an increased risk of perinatal morbidity and mortality with planned vaginal breech delivery compared to cesarean delivery [35, 36], which led to high rates of cesarean delivery in some practices [37–39]. It should be noted that that based on subsequent trials, the American

College of Obstetricians and Gynecologists (ACOG) committee opinion is that planned breech delivery may be reasonable at institutions with appropriate management protocols and clinician expertise [40]. However, cesarean delivery is preferable to many obstetrician providers due to diminishing experience with vaginal breech deliveries [40]. Cesarean delivery is an option in cases of breech presentation, though it has been associated with increased maternal morbidity compared to vaginal birth [41, 42], and may also place the woman at higher risk for complications in subsequent pregnancies.

Given the potential risks of vaginal breech and cesarean modes of delivery, it is also important for providers to discuss the possibility of ECV procedures with patients. ECV involves the manual application of pressure over the patient's abdomen to attempt to convert a breech or shoulder presentation to a cephalic presentation, and if successful, ECV will improve the chances of vaginal delivery [34].

## Surgical Considerations

It is recommended that obstetricians assess and document the fetal presentation beginning at 36 weeks gestation, and if breech presentation is found then ECV attempt should be offered assuming there are no contraindications [34]. The timing of the ECV procedure may differ according to patient and provider preferences. Preterm ECV (prior to 37 weeks) has been associated with higher success rates [43–45], but ECV in this interval has been associated with increased incidence of spontaneous reversion [43] and may also increase the rate of preterm birth compared to ECV after 37 weeks [44, 45]. ACOG management guidelines state that ECV after at least 37 weeks gestation is preferable given that spontaneous version will have likely occurred by this time, risk of spontaneous reversion after ECV will be lessened and the risks of potential preterm birth are avoided [34]. In addition to discussing the timing of ECV, patients should also be counseled regarding other potential complications of ECV. More common risks include patient discomfort during the procedure and transient fetal heart rate changes (4.7%), while more rare complications include: emergency cesarean delivery (0.35%), rupture of membranes (0.22%), umbilical cord prolapse (0.18%), vaginal bleeding (0.34%), placental abruption (0.18%), fetomaternal transfusion (0.9%) or even fetal demise (0.19%) [46].

Fetal ultrasound should be performed on the day of the ECV procedure to confirm the fetus remains breech. A fetal non-stress test should also be performed before and after ECV to ensure the heart tracing is reactive and there are no signs of fetal distress [34]. During ECV attempts, it is common to encounter fetal heart rate changes, which are usually transient and resolve when manual application of pressure is discontinued [34, 46]. Fetal heart tones should be intermittently checked between ECV attempts to ensure no fetal distress is present, and if fetal distress is noted then further ECV attempts should be delayed or stopped depending on the clinical circumstances. ECV should be performed in centers which cesarean delivery can be readily accomplished given that persistent fetal distress or other complications during ECV can lead to emergent cesarean delivery [34, 46].

Several factors can influence the success rate of ECV and should be considered when counseling individual patients. Factors that have been observed to reduce the rate of successful ECV include nulliparity, maternal obesity, anterior placental location, low amniotic fluid volume, engagement of the breech presenting part, uterine anomalies, and a non-relaxed uterus [47, 48]. Obstetricians commonly administer a tocolytic (e.g., terbutaline) to provide uterine relaxation. Tocolytic parenteral beta stimulants have been shown to increase the number of cephalic presentations for labor and reduce the number of cesarean deliveries [49]. Also, successful ECV is more likely with regional anesthesia in combination with a tocolytic compared to a tocolytic alone [49].

## Anesthetic Considerations and Management

A complete anesthetic assessment including review of medical history, anesthetic history, significant events or changes during pregnancy, current lab values, medications, vital signs and NPO status should be completed prior to the ECV procedure. Providers should ensure that the patients have not had intake of solid foods for at least 6–8 h (depending on the type of food), and also have not had clear liquids for at least 2 h prior to the procedure. Peripheral IV access should be established and patient consent for anesthesia care should be obtained. Some obstetricians and patients may prefer to attempt ECV without anesthesia involvement, though a preoperative anesthetic assessment should still be completed and consent obtained in the event that an emergent cesarean delivery becomes necessary. It is also important to confirm the obstetric plan prior to ECV, as the type of neuraxial procedure (epidural, spinal or combined spinal-epidural (CSE)) may differ if the obstetric plan is for hospital discharge after ECV versus immediate cesarean delivery if ECV is unsuccessful or immediate induction of labor (IOL) if ECV is successful.

One goal of anesthesia for ECV procedures is to provide pain relief, as maternal discomfort can be significant with application of abdominal pressure by the obstetrician during ECV. Inhaled nitrous oxide (50:50 N2O/O2 mixture) and IV opioids (e.g., remifentanil infusion 0.1 mcg/kg/min ± 0.1 mcg/kg rescue boluses) have been shown to improve pain relief compared to no analgesic intervention, though have not been shown to increase the ECV success rates [50–52]. A study directly comparing inhaled nitrous oxide with remifentanil infusion 0.1 mcg/kg/min (with remifentanil 0.1 mcg/kg rescue boluses as needed) noted improved pain relief in patients receiving remifentanil, though no difference in ECV success rate was observed and mild adverse events were greater in those receiving remifentanil [53]. IV opioid analgesia has been shown to be inferior to neuraxial blockade with both anesthetic and analgesic doses of local anesthetic [52, 54].

In addition to providing maternal comfort, there is strong evidence that neuraxial blockade facilitates successful ECV [55–57]. For example, a meta-analysis reported that ECV success with regional anesthesia was 59.7% compared to 37.6% in patients receiving IV or no analgesia [55]. Improved relaxation of abdominal wall muscles has been observed even with analgesic doses of local anesthetic [54], and neuraxial anesthesia has been shown to reduce the applied force necessary for successful ECV [58]. It is important to distinguish between anesthetic and analgesic doses of local anesthetic for ECV procedures, as anesthetic doses are more likely to improve the success of ECV [56, 57]. A previous meta-analysis compared anesthetic doses (defined as local anesthetic dosing capable of producing motor blockade) to analgesic doses of local anesthetic [56]. These authors reported that anesthetic doses almost doubled the likelihood of successful ECV compared to no anesthesia (RR = 1.95; 95% CI = 1.46–2.60; $P < 0.001$), while analgesic doses did not result in significant improvement in ECV success compared to IV or no analgesia (RR = 1.18; 95% CI = 0.94–1.49; $P = 0.15$) [56].

Neuraxial anesthesia to an approximate sensory blockade level of T6 has been targeted by several past investigators, as this level of blockade will help ensure patient comfort, abdominal muscle relaxation, and will also likely provide adequate anesthesia if emergent cesarean delivery becomes necessary due to fetal compromise [52, 59–63]. The type of neuraxial anesthesia and dosing regimens selected vary according to provider preferences and can depend on the obstetric plan of care. Epidural blockade has been effectively utilized for ECV anesthesia using 2% lidocaine ± 1:200,000 epinephrine 15–20 mL [59–61, 64], which providers should administer incrementally (e.g., 5 mL every 3–5 min) while checking motor and sensory blockade between doses. Epidural fentanyl 50–100 mcg may also be administered to supplement the local anesthetic and help improve the quality of anesthesia [64]. Spinal blockade with spinal bupivacaine 7.5–10 mg or lidocaine 45–60 mg has also been described for ECV anesthesia [52, 61–63], and spinal fentanyl 10–15 mcg may also be combined with the local anesthetic to improve the quality of anesthesia [52, 61]. CSE anesthesia may be also considered for ECV procedures. CSE can offer the advantages of avoiding the need for a repeat neuraxial procedure if the plan is for IOL or cesarean section immediately following the ECV attempt (depending on the outcome), and an indwelling epidural catheter also allows for additional dosing if the patient is uncomfortable during ECV or possible cesarean delivery. Lastly, it is important to note that neuraxial anesthesia has also been shown in several investigations to be effective in facilitating successful ECV after failed primary ECV attempts without anesthesia, which should be considered when counseling and caring for patients [52, 58, 61, 65].

---

**External Cephalic Version (ECV)—Key Points**

- Management options in cases of breech presentation include planned cesarean delivery, vaginal breech delivery or an attempt at ECV.
- Vaginal breach deliveries may be associated with increased perinatal morbidity and mortality, and cesarean delivery is associated with increased maternal morbidity compared to a vaginal birth.
  - If breech presentation is documented after 36 weeks gestation, ECV attempt should be offered assuming there are no contraindications.
  - Successful ECV and conversion of a breech or shoulder presentation to a cephalic presentation improves the chance of vaginal delivery.
- Per ACOG, optimal timing for ECV attempt is 37 weeks gestation.
  - Non-stress test should be performed before and after, with intermittent fetal heart monitoring throughout.
- The most common risks are patient discomfort during the procedure and transient fetal heart rate changes, but rare complications including emergent delivery are possible.
- Reduced chance of ECV success with nulliparity, maternal obesity, anterior placental location, low amniotic fluid volume, engagement of the breech presenting part, uterine anomalies, and a non-relaxed uterus.
- Pre-operative assessment should be completed even if anesthesia is not involved in the ECV as there is always a risk of fetal distress and emergent delivery.
  - IV access should be established and patients should adhere to standard NPO guidelines.
  - ECV should be performed in centers which cesarean delivery can be readily accomplished.
- IV opioids and inhaled nitrous oxide have been used to provide patient analgesia during ECV, but have not been shown to improve ECV success rates.
- Neuraxial anesthesia with anesthetic dosing sufficient to produce motor blockade and a T6 sensory blockade level significantly improves patient comfort and the ECV success rate compared to no anesthesia or IV analgesia.
  - Neuraxial blockade with only analgesic dosing of local anesthetic improves maternal comfort, but has not been shown to increase the rate of ECV success.
  - Spinal, Epidural and CSE have all been used successfully. The plan of patient care after successful or unsuccessful ECV should be discussed with obstetrician, as this may alter the anesthetic.
  - Commonly utilized: Epidural 2% lidocaine ± 1:200,000 epinephrine 15–20 mL, administered incrementally. May also consider epidural fentanyl 50–100 mcg.
  - Commonly utilized: Spinal bupivacaine 7.5–10 mg or lidocaine 45–60 mg. May also consider spinal fentanyl 10–15 mcg.

---

## Cerclage

### Introduction

Cervical insufficiency is defined by ACOG as "the inability of the uterine cervix to retain a pregnancy in the second trimester" [66]. An obstetric history of unexplained second trimester pregnancy losses may suggest cervical insufficiency, though a more definitive clinical diagnosis is made when painless cervical dilation and bulging fetal membranes are observed in the second trimester without the presence of uterine contractions or other factors such as bleeding or infection [66, 67]. The etiology of cervical insufficiency is poorly understood, though potential contributing factors include cervical trauma from prior surgical procedures or a previous vaginal birth, genetic pre-disposition, congenital abnormities of the reproductive tract, maternal *in utero* exposure to diethylstilbestrol, or intraamniotic inflammation [66–69]. Non-invasive treatments such as activity restriction, bed rest or pelvic rest have not been shown to be effective [66]. Surgical treatment with transvaginal or transabdominal cerclage to prevent pregnancy loss or preterm birth may be indicated for some patients depending on their obstetric history, physical exam and ultrasound findings [66, 67, 70].

## Surgical Considerations

Current ACOG recommendations are that cerclage procedures be performed in the second trimester before fetal viability has been achieved [66]. Prophylactic cerclage placement may be considered based on a patient history of one or more second trimester losses or previous cerclage placement related to painless cervical dilation, and are generally inserted at 13–14 weeks gestation [66, 71]. Cerclage placement is also recommended if there is a patient history of preterm birth (<34 weeks gestation) accompanied by short cervical length (<25 mm) on ultrasound exam prior to 24 weeks gestation, as cerclage placement in this setting has been observed to reduce the incidence of preterm birth [66, 71]. It should be noted that cerclage placement has not been shown to be beneficial in patients with short cervical length (<25 mm) without a prior preterm birth, and cerclage placement in twin pregnancies with short cervical length (<25 mm) may increase the risk of preterm birth [66, 72]. Emergent or rescue cerclage placement may be recommended based on physical exam findings of painless cervical dilation in the midtrimester [66, 71]. Emergency cerclage in well-selected patients has been shown to prolong pregnancy and improve neonatal outcomes compared to expectant management [73].

Obstetricians should ensure there are not uterine contractions, signs of bleeding or infection prior to performing cerclage procedures. Ultrasound is also performed prior to cerclage placement to confirm fetal viability and detect any major congenital anomalies [71]. Cerclage is most commonly performed with transvaginal techniques (McDonald or Shirodkar), though transabdominal cerclage placements are sometimes recommended. The most common transvaginal technique is the McDonald cerclage, which involves insertion of a simple purse-string suture at the cervicovaginal junction [66]. The Shirodkar procedure is technically more difficult and involves dissection of the bladder and rectum away from the cervix in order to place a submucosal suture closer to the internal cervical os [66]. The superiority of one transvaginal cerclage technique has not been clearly established, and many providers favor McDonald technique given the relative ease of insertion and removal [66, 74, 75]. Transabdominal cervicoisthmic cerclage may be a considered in patients with cervical insufficiency that have anatomic limitations preventing transvaginal cerclage placement or if there is history of failed second trimester transvaginal cerclage. Laparatomy and laparoscopic approaches have been described for abdominal cerclage placement, and are usually performed prior to pregnancy or at 10–14 weeks gestation [66].

Cervical cerclage complication rates may differ depending on the timing and patient circumstances at the time of the procedure, though in general there is low incidence of complications. For example, one report cited an overall complication rate of 0.6% for patients undergoing history-indicated or ultrasound-indicated cerclage placement [76]. Obstetricians should counsel patients regarding the potential for rupture of membranes, vaginal or cervical lacerations, chorioamnionitis, and suture displacement [66, 71]. There is typically minimal blood loss associated with cerclage procedures, though providers should recognize the potential for greater blood loss with Shirodkar or transabdominal cerclage procedures.

Transvaginal cerclage removal is recommended at 36–37 weeks gestation for patients in which vaginal delivery is anticipated, though earlier removal of the cerclage may be indicated in cases of preterm labor, preterm premature rupture of membranes or other circumstances [66, 71]. McDonald cerclage removal can often be accomplished in the outpatient office setting, though patient discomfort may necessitate anesthesia care for cerclage removal in the operating room. A Shirodkar cerclage is more likely to require anesthesia care for removal in the operative setting. If cesarean delivery is planned, providers may consider delaying transvaginal cerclage removal until the time of delivery [66, 71]. Transabdominal cerclage removal can also be done at the time of cesarean delivery, though many providers will leave it in place if the patient wishes to have future pregnancies.

## Anesthesia Considerations and Management

Preoperatively, anesthesia providers should assess the patient's medical and obstetric history, establish IV access, ensure NPO status, review available lab values and consider administering aspiration prophylaxis. The type of cerclage procedure planned (McDonald, Shirodkar, transabdominal), anticipated surgical duration, and the potential need for uterine relaxation should be discussed preoperatively with the obstetricians since these factors can impact the anesthetic management. There are relatively few published reports on anesthesia for cerclage procedures, though spinal, epidural and general anesthesia have all been described.

Many providers and patients prefer neuraxial anesthesia for cerclage and other procedures during pregnancy when possible, as this approach avoids need for instrumentation of the maternal airway and minimizes fetal exposure to anesthesia medications. Though it should be noted that no anesthesia medications have been clearly demonstrated to be toxic in humans [77, 78]. Among studies that have compared general and neuraxial anesthesia for cerclage procedures, no differences have been observed in obstetric outcomes [79, 80]. Yoon et al. compared general to spinal anesthesia in patients undergoing Shirodkar cerclage placement during the midtrimester (15–16 weeks gestation), and observed no differences in oxytocin levels, post-operative uterine activity, fetal loss before 20 weeks gestation, or preterm delivery between study groups [79]. Crawford et al. performed a retrospective comparison of patients receiving general anesthesia to neuraxial anesthesia (spinal or epidural) for cerclage procedures and reported no difference in fetal outcomes of inevitable abortion or low birth weight [80]. A recent retrospective study observed that spinal anesthesia slightly prolonged the patient time in the operating room and in the post-anesthesia care unit (PACU), though patients receiving general anesthesia were more likely to require opioid or non-opioid analgesics in PACU [81].

The type of neuraxial procedure performed, level of sensory blockade required, and local anesthetic dosing may depend on the type of cerclage procedure. For transvaginal cerclage placements and removals, it is important to ensure sensory blockade from T10-S4 to ensure patient comfort with vaginal speculum placement and cervical manipulations. Transabdominal cerclage placement will likely require sensory blockade up to T4-T6 to provide effective anesthesia. Spinal anesthesia for cerclage placement or removal is most commonly selected, though epidural anesthesia has been reported [80, 82]. Epidural or CSE techniques may be useful if a longer surgical duration is anticipated (e.g., Shirodkar or transabdominal cerclage) or if a cerclage removal is to be followed by labor, since an indwelling epidural catheter can later be dosed in these circumstances. Epidural blockade can be accomplished with 3% 2-chloroprocaine or 2% lidocaine with 1:200,000 epinephrine 10–15 mL, injected incrementally while monitoring the onset of motor and sensory blockade. Epidural fentanyl 50–100 mcg can also be administered to augment the surgical blockade.

Spinal anesthesia provides rapid, reliable onset of a dense surgical block and there are typically short operative times that do not require repeated dosing of an epidural catheter [77]. The dose of local anesthetic may depend on the type of cerclage procedure and anticipated surgical duration, though hyperbaric bupivacaine 6–10 mg is commonly used to provide surgical anesthesia for transvaginal cerclage placements and removals. Spinal lidocaine 40–50 mg may also be considered, though spinal lidocaine has been noted to increase incidence of transient neurologic symptoms (TNS), especially for procedures in the lithotomy position [77, 83, 84]. Fentanyl 10–15 mcg is commonly co-administered with spinal local anesthetic to enhance the surgical block. When deciding on a dose of local anesthetic, anesthesia providers should also consider the gestational age at the time of surgery. Lee et al. performed spinal anesthesia with bupivacaine 7 mg in pregnant women undergoing second trimester cerclage placement and in non-pregnant women undergoing perianal surgery. They observed a greater extent of sensory blockade in the second trimester of pregnancy compared to non-pregnant women (11 vs. 8 dermatomes blocked, respectively) [85]. A separate investigation noted that bupivacaine 7 mg resulted in a higher level of sensory blockade and increased incidence of hypotension in women undergoing late second trimester (22 weeks gestation) compared to early second trimester cerclage (13 weeks gestation) [86]. For cerclage removal procedures at term, greater block height and incidence of hypotension should be anticipated from a given dose of spinal local anesthetic compared to preterm women [87]. Left uterine displacement positioning is recommended for procedures after 18 weeks gestation in order to minimize incidence of hypotension and help maintain uteroplacental perfusion.

General anesthesia is generally not favored, though may be considered if there are contraindications to neuraxial anesthesia or if providers wish to use volatile anesthetic agents to aid in uterine relaxation. Past reports have described general anesthesia for cerclage procedures with tracheal intubation, laryngeal mask airways, face mask assisted ventilation and IV sedation with a natural airway [79, 81]. Endotracheal intubation is currently performed for cerclage procedures in many practices given concerns for increased aspiration risk associated with pregnancy, particularly for procedures in the late second trimester. Uterine relaxation with halogenated volatile agents may decrease intrauterine pressure and be helpful in reducing the bulging fetal membranes during an emergency cerclage procedure, though this potential benefit should be weighed against the potential for increases in intrauterine pressure due to coughing on the endotracheal tube [77]. Neuraxial anesthesia with incremental doses of IV nitroglycerin may also be effective in providing uterine relaxation [77, 88]. Providers may also consider other strategies for helping reduce bulging fetal membranes during rescue cerclage procedures: administration of a tocolytic, trendelenberg or high dorsal lithotomy positioning, backfilling the bladder, amnioreduction, and other surgical maneuvers [73]. For patients receiving general anesthesia, prophylactic IV anti-emetics should be considered to reduce chances of post-operative nausea and vomiting, as this can also result in acute increases in intrauterine pressure.

Pudendal nerve blocks by the obstetrician have also been described for McDonald cerclage placements, and were reported to provide effective pain relief during the procedure [89]. This technique may be considered as an option in some patient cases, though there may often be a lack of provider experience and it may not provide adequate anesthesia for every patient.

| Cerclage—Key Points |
|---|
| • Cervical insufficiency is successfully treated with transvaginal or transabdominal cerclage to prevent pregnancy loss or preterm birth. Placement recommended in the following situations:<br>  – History of second trimester losses, or previous cerclage related to painless cervical dilation.<br>  – History of preterm birth (<34 weeks) and short cervical length (<25 mm).<br>  – Painless cervical dilation in midtrimester.<br>• Cerclage removal is recommended at 36–37 weeks gestation, or possibly earlier in the setting of preterm premature rupture of membranes or preterm labor.<br>• Preoperative assessment, establishing of IV access and ensuring appropriate NPO status are all necessary.<br>• Neuraxial anesthesia is generally preferred over general anesthesia to avoid need for airway instrumentation and minimize fetal exposure to anesthetics.<br>  – Studies have not shown any difference in obstetric outcomes when comparing neuraxial and general anesthesia for cerclage procedures.<br>• Spinal anesthesia is most commonly utilized, but epidural and CSE techniques may be useful in approaches that require longer surgical duration.<br>  – Endotracheal intubation and general anesthesia is favored over heavy sedation due to aspiration risk associated with pregnancy, especially in the late second trimester.<br>  – General anesthesia may be selected given uterine relaxation with halogenated volatile agents may decrease intrauterine pressure and be helpful in reducing the bulging fetal membranes, though coughing on the endotracheal tube or post-operative vomiting will increase intrauterine pressure.<br>• The type of cerclage and surgical approach will dictate anesthetic requirements. Epidural or CSE techniques may be considered if longer surgical duration is anticipated.<br>  – Transvaginal placements and removals require a T10-S4 sensory blockade<br>     Commonly utilized: spinal bupivacaine 6–10 mg. May also include fentanyl 10–15 mg to enhance surgical block.<br>  – Transabdominal placements require T4-T6 sensory blockade.<br>• Anesthesia providers should consider gestational age when dosing spinal medications. Pregnant women (even in the second trimester) have a decreased local anesthetic requirement compared to non-pregnant women.<br>  – For cerclage removals done close to term, one should expect greater spinal block height and incidence of hypotension compared to spinal anesthesia for procedures in the second trimester.<br>     Utilize left uterine displacement after 18 weeks gestation. |

## D&C and D&E

### Introduction

Dilation and curettage (D&C) refers to the process of removing the endometrial lining of the uterus by suction and sampling associated lesions. In obstetric patients, D&C procedures may be indicated in cases of incomplete or missed abortions or for the treatment of retained products of conception in the postpartum period [90, 91]. Dilation and evacuation (D&E), while similar in procedure, involves greater cervical dilation and the use of surgical instruments for uterine evacuation and typically is employed beyond the gestational age of 13–15 weeks when fetal ossification has already occurred or in patients with molar pregnancy that want to preserve fertility [90]. Unfortunately patients can present with intrauterine fetal demise even late into the second trimester, and studies have shown D&E to be safer and more efficacious when compared to induced abortion in cases of second trimester fetal death or significant fetal anomalies [92, 93]. Specifically, retrospective studies have observed that D&E in the second trimester has been associated with decreased risk of infection requiring IV antibiotics [92], and also reduced risk of retained tissue requiring D&C or manual removal of the placenta compared to management with induced abortion [93].

## Surgical Considerations

The timing of D&C or D&E procedures during pregnancy often range from the second trimester to the postpartum period, and the urgency of the procedure may depend on the presence of ongoing hemorrhage and other patient factors. A case by case assessment of preoperative blood loss and the intraoperative bleeding risk should be made. Preoperative complete blood count (CBC), coagulation studies, and blood typing with antibody screening and possible crossmatching should be ordered as indicated [77, 90, 91]. In addition to the gestational age and the presence of bleeding, the surgical and anesthetic approaches may also depend on the degree of cervical dilation, NPO status, and patient preferences.

Obstetricians should counsel patients on the potential for associated procedural complications, including hemorrhage, infection, cervical laceration, uterine perforation, and retained products of conception [77, 90, 91, 94]. In cases of D&E being performed for molar pregnancies, providers should also be aware of the potential for excessive uterine size for gestational age, preeclampsia, hyperemesis gravidarum, anemia, hyperthyroidism, trophoblastic embolization and cardiorespiratory distress [95]. Some of these associated medical conditions may require patient optimization prior to surgery [95].

## Anesthetic Considerations and Management

Every anesthetic begins with a comprehensive history and physical examination, review of lab values, and a goal-directed discussion amongst physician providers and the patient regarding the procedure and anesthetic planning. D&C and D&E may be carried out either in the operating room or in a procedure specific site, though patient specific factors should be incorporated into this decision. IV access needs should be tailored to each individual patient but consists of at least one adequately running peripheral IV [77, 94]. The need for central venous access, arterial line blood pressure monitoring or other emergency resuscitation equipment are typically not necessary, though should be considered in cases of significant hemorrhage or hemodynamic instability. Positioning for the procedure is in dorsal lithotomy, so care must be taken to ensure adequate padding of extremities against stirrups to prevent postoperative neuropathy.

The choice of anesthetic technique often depends on a number of factors, including the indication for the procedure, gestational age, fetal ossification, cervical dilation, NPO status, patient anxiety and the presence of ongoing hemorrhage or hemodynamic stability. In hemodynamically stable patients with adequate cervical dilation, the procedure may be deemed possible with simple curettage and suction. In these circumstances, the option of paracervical blockade with dilute local anesthetic (e.g., 1% lidocaine or 1% 2-chloroprocaine) combined with intravenous sedation (e.g., IV midazolam 1–2 mg, IV fentanyl 50–100 mcg or low doses of IV induction agents) may be employed [77, 90, 94]. Typically administered by the obstetrician, paracervical blockade does carry the risk of local anesthetic toxicity upon accidental intravascular injection or systemic absorption of local anesthetic. Should this technique be used in cases where dilation is necessary, providers should be aware of the risks of concomitant vasovagal reactions and greater patient discomfort during cervical dilation [90, 94]. Neuraxial or general anesthesia will likely be necessary to ensure patient comfort with advancing gestational age in which greater degrees of cervical dilation are required.

General anesthesia may be favored in circumstances of patient emotional distress, significant bleeding, sepsis or hemodynamic instability. In the anxious patient consideration should be given to administration of preoperative anxiolytic, and a general anesthetic may even be requested [77, 90]. Rapid sequence induction and endotracheal intubation should be performed if the patient has a full stomach. Propofol (1.5–2 mg/kg) and succinylcholine (1 mg/kg) are commonly selected for IV induction, though etomidate or ketamine may be favored in the presence of significant bleeding or hemodynamic instability [90]. Transient uterine relaxation with a volatile agent may be beneficial for removal of retained placenta in postpartum patients [91], though generally in D&E cases it is recommended to maintain volatile anesthetic below 0.5 MAC along with nitrous oxide in order to diminish the effect on uterine relaxation and potential for increased bleeding [77, 90]. Uterotonics should be immediately available for administration. Anesthesia providers may also consider propofol infusion to maintain anesthesia rather than inhalational agents, as this approach has been observed to reduce the blood loss during general anesthesia for D&E procedures [96, 97].

Neuraxial anesthesia may also be considered for D&E cases with the potential for greater patient discomfort assuming there are no contraindications such as coagulopathy, sepsis or hemodynamic compromise. Operative times are typically short, and spinal anesthesia with hyperbaric bupivacaine 6–10 mg with fentanyl 10–15 mcg is usually sufficient to produce sensory blockade from T10-S4. Anesthesia providers should remain aware that a given dose of spinal bupivacaine will produce a greater extent of sensory blockade with advancing gestation [85–87]. Spinal lidocaine 40–50 mg may also be considered, though many providers avoid spinal lidocaine for procedures in the lithotomy position given the increased incidence of TNS [83, 84]. In cases of postpartum hemorrhage due to placental retention, an already properly functioning labor epidural can often be utilized as the primary anesthetic by incrementally dosing 2% lidocaine with 1:200,000 epinephrine or 3% 2-chloroprocaine 10–15 mL to achieve a T10-S4 sensory blockade. Women in the postpartum period without a functioning epidural catheter can also be considered for a short-acting spinal anesthetic, assuming there are no contraindications [94]. IV nitroglycerine 100–200 mcg may assist in providing transient uterine relaxation to aid with removal of a retained placenta in postpartum patients not under general anesthesia [91, 98, 99].

| Dilation and Curettage (D&C), Dilation and Evacuation (D&E)—Key Points |
|---|
| • The timing of D&C and D&E procedures can vary, as does the urgency and associated procedural complications.
• Preoperative evaluation should consider the degree of bleeding and cervical dilation, uterine and cervical integrity, presence of retained products of conception or infection.
• D&E procedures may be performed in cases of molar pregnancies that want to preserve fertility. In these patients, providers should be aware of the potential for excessive uterine size for gestational age, preeclampsia, hyperemesis gravidarum, anemia, hyperthyroidism, trophoblastic embolization and cardiorespiratory distress. Some of these conditions may necessitate preoperative optimization or additional postoperative monitoring.
• A single peripheral large bore IV is sufficient access for most cases. Central venous catheter or invasive hemodynamic monitoring may be indicated for cases with significant hemorrhage.
• Anesthetic techniques commonly employed:
  – Paracervical blockade (typically by surgeon) with IV sedation: 1–2 mg of midazolam ± fentanyl 50–100 mcg or low doses of IV induction agents.
  – Neuraxial anesthesia requires a T10-S4 sensory blockade: spinal hyperbaric bupivacaine 6–10 mg ± fentanyl 10–15 mcg or incremental dosing of epidural 2% lidocaine with 1:200,000 epinephrine 10–15 mL is usually sufficient.
  – General anesthesia may be favored in circumstances of emotional distress, significant ongoing hemorrhage, sepsis or hemodynamic instability. Consider rapid sequence induction and endotracheal intubation.
• Uterine relaxation with incremental doses of nitroglycerine 100–200 mcg or volatile anesthetic may assist with removal of retained placenta.
• Uterotonics should be immediately available for D&C and D&E cases. |

## Fetal Procedures

### Introduction

Antenatal diagnosis is being made for an increasing number of fetal conditions, some of which may require treatment before birth. Fetal interventions performed during pregnancy vary widely in complexity and include fetal surgeries, ex utero intrapartum therapy (EXIT) procedures and minimally invasive procedures [77, 100–102].

### Surgical Considerations

Open (hysterotomy-based) and endoscopic fetal surgeries are mostly performed in the second or early third trimester, while EXIT procedures are performed near term and involve securing the fetal airway or completing a surgical intervention prior to umbilical cord clamping at the time of delivery [77, 100–102]. Generally, fetal surgeries and EXIT procedures are complex and involve coordination among obstetricians, anesthesiologists, pediatric surgeons and other specialists. The scope of this discussion is limited to the more common minimally invasive fetal procedures performed by obstetricians that may require anesthesia care.

For minimally invasive fetal interventions, obstetricians typically gain access to the fetus or other intrauterine structures through the abdominal and uterine walls. Common examples include fetal blood sampling, intrauterine transfusion and fetoscopic laser photocoagulation procedures [77, 101, 102]. Fetal blood sampling and possible transfusion are indicated if the fetus is determined to be at risk for severe fetal anemia due to maternal alloimmunization and transplacental passage of antibodies resulting in hemolytic disease in the fetus [103]. Fetoscopic laser photocoagulation of placental anastomoses may be indicated in advanced cases of twin-twin transfusion syndrome (TTTS) that can occur in monochorionic diamniotic twin pregnancies [104]. There are other fetal conditions and types of minimally invasive interventions that may be indicated before birth, though the considerations for anesthetic management are similar for many of these procedures.

### Anesthesia Considerations and Management

The details and anticipated duration of the procedure should be determined preoperatively, as well as the potential for maternal or fetal pain and the need for fetal immobility. The anesthetic technique will depend on these factors as well as patient and provider preferences.

General anesthesia has been utilized for fetoscopic laser photocoagulation procedures, and this approach provides maternal and fetal anesthesia, assists with fetal immobility, and provides uterine relaxation in cases requiring more extensive surgical manipulation of the uterus [101, 105]. However, many practitioners prefer to avoid general anesthesia during pregnancy when possible, and either neuraxial or local anesthetic techniques are favored for minimally invasive fetal procedures in many practices [77, 101, 102, 106–109]. Neuraxial anesthesia (spinal, epidural or CSE) provides dense sensory block and may be preferable for procedures with the potential for greater difficulty or maternal discomfort [77, 101, 106]. Epidural or CSE techniques offer the potential advantage of being able to dose the indwelling catheter in more prolonged procedures. Sensory blockade up to T4 has been suggested for surgeries associated with uterine manipulation [101], though the level of sensory blockade required may vary depending on the procedure. Local anesthesia, commonly combined with IV sedation, has also been successfully employed for procedures such as intrauterine transfusion or laser photocoagulation of aberrant fetal vessels [108, 109].

It is important to recognize that neuraxial and local anesthetic techniques will not reduce fetal movements or provide fetal anesthesia, which is important in reducing the fetal stress response to noxious stimuli [101, 110]. Minimally invasive procedures involving non-innervated tissues such as the placenta or umbilical cord may not require fetal anesthesia or analgesia, though fetal immobility may still be necessary to complete the procedure [101, 102]. Procedures involving the fetus itself will require treatment to block fetal responses to nociceptive stimulation and provide fetal immobility [101, 102]. IV medications may be given to aid with maternal sedation and analgesia, and transplacental passage of these medications helps minimize fetal movements and provide fetal anesthesia. To accomplish these goals, maternal administration of benzodiazepines (e.g., IV midazolam 1–2 mg), opioids (e.g., IV fentanyl 50–100 mcg or remifentanil 0.1–0.2 mcg/kg/min), and sometimes low-dose induction agents may be selected [101, 102, 105–108, 111]. IV remifentanil infusion may be preferable in minimally invasive fetal procedures as it has been observed to provide effective maternal sedation, reliable fetal immobilization, and these effects are quickly reversible at the end of the procedure given that remifentanil is quickly metabolized in both the mother and the fetus [106, 107, 112]. Close maternal monitoring and supplemental oxygen is recommended if any form of maternal sedation is administered, and providers should remain aware the many IV sedation and analgesic medications will reduce the fetal heart rate variability. Providers may also consider fetal intramuscular or cord administration of opioids (e.g., fentanyl 10 mcg/kg) and muscle relaxants (e.g., vecuronium 0.2 mg/kg) to provide fetal anesthesia and immobility [101, 102].

Fetal assessment in minimally invasive procedures is often limited to fetal heart rate monitoring and visual assessment of fetal movements on ultrasound imaging [101]. Fetal procedures can result in fetal distress or complications prompting emergent cesarean delivery if the fetus is viable, and appropriate preparations should be made [101].

---

Fetal Procedures—Key Points
- Minimally invasive fetal interventions can be performed under general, neuraxial or local anesthesia with IV sedation—neuraxial and local anesthesia are generally preferred in most cases.
- Preoperative planning should consider the type of procedure and anticipated duration, the potential for maternal and neonatal pain, and determine the need for fetal immobility.
- General anesthesia will provide maternal and fetal anesthesia, fetal immobility, and uterine relaxation for cases potentially requiring more extensive uterine surgical manipulation.
- Neuraxial anesthesia (spinal, epidural or CSE) may be preferable for procedures anticipated to have greater surgical difficulty or likelihood to produce maternal discomfort.
  - Epidural and CSE techniques are advantageous for cases with potentially longer surgical times.
  - A T4 sensory blockade level is suggested for procedures involving uterine manipulation.
- Local anesthesia combined with maternal sedation is adequate for many minimally invasive fetal procedures.
- Neuraxial and local anesthetic techniques provide maternal comfort, though will not reduce fetal movements or provide fetal anesthesia, and are thus commonly combined with IV sedation and analgesic medications. Commonly utilized medications for maternal sedation, fetal anesthesia, and fetal immobility include: low dose benzodiazepines (IV midazolam 1–2 mg), opioids (IV fentanyl 50–100 mcg or remifentanil 0.1–0.2 mcg/kg/min), or low doses of IV induction agents.
  - Remifentanil infusion may be preferable given it has been observed to provide effective maternal sedation, reliable fetal immobilization, and the effects are quickly reversible at the end of the procedure.
  - Close maternal monitoring and supplemental oxygen are recommended if IV sedation or analgesia is administered.
  - Fetal intramuscular or cord administration of opioids and muscle relaxants may also be considered to provide fetal anesthesia and immobility.
- Fetal procedures should be performed in settings which cesarean delivery can be readily accomplished if the fetus is viable, as procedure complications or fetal distress may necessitate emergent delivery.

## References

1. Chan LM, Westhoff CL. Tubal sterilization trends in the United States. Fertil Steril. 2010;94:1–6.
2. Bucklin BA, Smith CV. Postpartum tubal ligation: safety, timing, and other implications for anesthesia. Anesth Analg. 1999;89:1269–74.
3. Moss C, Isley MM. Sterilization: a review and update. Obstet Gynecol Clin N Am. 2015;42:713–24.
4. Peterson HB, Xia Z, Hughes JM, Wilcox LS, Tylor LR, Trussell J. The risk of pregnancy after tubal sterilization: findings from the U.S. Collaborative Review of Sterilization. Am J Obstet Gynecol. 1996;174:1161–8.
5. Committee on Health Care for Underserved Women. Committee opinion no. 530: access to postpartum sterilization. Obstet Gynecol. 2012;120:212–5.
6. Thurman AR, Janecek T. One-year follow-up of women with unfulfilled postpartum sterilization requests. Obstet Gynecol. 2010;116:1071–7.
7. Albanese A, French M, Gossett DR. Request and fulfillment of postpartum tubal ligation in patients after high-risk pregnancy. Contraception. 2016. [Epub ahead of print].
8. Seibel-Seamon J, Visintine JF, Leiby BE, Weinstein L. Factors predictive for failure to perform postpartum tubal ligations following vaginal delivery. J Reprod Med. 2009;54:160–4.
9. Zite N, Wuellner S, Gilliam M. Failure to obtain desired postpartum sterilization: risk and predictors. Obstet Gynecol. 2005;105:794–9.
10. Trussell J. The cost of unintended pregnancy in the United States. Contraception. 2007;75:168–70.
11. Practice Guidelines for Obstetric Anesthesia: An Updated Report by the American Society of Anesthesiologists Task Force on Obstetric Anesthesia and the Society for Obstetric Anesthesia and Perinatology. Anesthesiology 2016;124:270–300.
12. Lawrie TA, Kulier R, Nardin JM. Techniques for the interruption of tubal patency for female sterilisation. Cochrane Database Syst Rev. 2016;8:CD003034.
13. O'Sullivan GM, Sutton AJ, Thompson SA, Carrie LE, Bullingham RE. Noninvasive measurement of gastric emptying in obstetric patients. Anesth Analg. 1987;66:505–11.
14. Vincent RD Jr, Reid RW. Epidural anesthesia for postpartum tubal ligation using epidural catheters placed during labor. J Clin Anesth. 1993;5:289–91.
15. Goodman EJ, Dumas SD. The rate of successful reactivation of labor epidural catheters for postpartum tubal ligation surgery. Reg Anesth Pain Med. 1998;23:258–61.
16. Powell MF, Wellons DD, Tran SF, Zimmerman JM, Frölich MA. Risk factors for failed reactivation of a labor epidural for postpartum tubal ligation: a prospective, observational study. J Clin Anesth. 2016;35:221–4.
17. Viscomi CM, Rathmell JP. Labor epidural catheter reactivation or spinal anesthesia for delayed postpartum tubal ligation: a cost comparison. J Clin Anesth. 1995;7:380–3.
18. Hawkins JL. Postpartum tubal sterilization. In: Chestnut DH, editor. Obstetric anesthesia principles and practice. 5th ed. Philadelphia: Elsevier Saunders; 2014. p. 540.
19. Stevens RA, Chester WL, Schubert A, Brandon D, Grueter JA, Zumrick J. pH-adjustment of 2-chloroprocaine quickens the onset of epidural anaesthesia. Can J Anaesth. 1989;36:515–8.
20. Lam DT, Ngan Kee WD, Khaw KS. Extension of epidural blockade in labour for emergency Caesarean section using 2% lidocaine with epinephrine and fentanyl, with or without alkalinisation. Anaesthesia. 2001;56:790–4.
21. Capogna G, Celleno D, Costantino P, Muratori F, Sebastiani M, Baldassini M. Alkalinization improves the quality of lidocaine-fentanyl epidural anaesthesia for caesarean section. Can J Anaesth. 1993;40:425–30.
22. Marcus RJ, Wong CA, Lehor A, McCarthy RJ, Yaghmour E, Yilmaz M. Postoperative epidural morphine for postpartum tubal ligation analgesia. Anesth Analg. 2005;101:876–81.
23. Abouleish EI. Postpartum tubal ligation requires more bupivacaine for spinal anesthesia than does cesarean section. Anesth Analg. 1986;65:897–900.
24. Teoh WH, Ithnin F, Sia AT. Comparison of an equal-dose spinal anaesthetic for caesarean section and for post partum tubal ligation. Int J Obstet Anesth. 2008;17:228–32.
25. Kwok SC, Teoh WH, Ithnin F. Effect of sitting position on equal-dose spinal anaesthetic for caesarean section and post-partum tubal ligation. Acta Anaesthesiol Scand. 2014;58:743–50.
26. Huffnagle SL, Norris MC, Leighton BL, Arkoosh VA, Elgart RL, Huffnagle HJ. Do patient variables influence the subarachnoid spread of hyperbaric lidocaine in the postpartum patient? Reg Anesth. 1994;19:330–4.
27. Habib AS, Muir HA, White WD, Spahn TE, Olufolabi AJ, Breen TW. Intrathecal morphine for analgesia after postpartum bilateral tubal ligation. Anesth Analg. 2005;100:239–43.
28. Samsoon GL, Young JR. Difficult tracheal intubation: a retrospective study. Anaesthesia. 1987;42:487–90.
29. Pilkington S, Carli F, Dakin MJ, Romney M, De Witt KA, Doré CJ, Cormack RS. Increase in Mallampati score during pregnancy. Br J Anaesth. 1995;74:638–42.
30. Kodali BS, Chandrasekhar S, Bulich LN, Topulos GP, Datta S. Airway changes during labor and delivery. Anesthesiology. 2008;108:357–62.
31. Leighton BL, Cheek TG, Gross JB, Apfelbaum JL, Shantz BB, Gutsche BB, Rosenberg H. Succinylcholine pharmacodynamics in peripartum patients. Anesthesiology. 1986;64:202–5.
32. Kao YJ, Tellez J, Turner DR. Dose-dependent effect of metoclopramide on cholinesterases and suxamethonium metabolism. Br J Anaesth. 1990;65:220–4.

33. Pühringer FK, Sparr HJ, Mitterschiffthaler G, Agoston S, Benzer A. Extended duration of action of rocuronium in postpartum patients. Anesth Analg. 1997;84:352–4.
34. American College of Obstetricians and Gynecologists' Committee on Practice Bulletins—Obstetrics. Practice Bulletin No. 161: External Cephalic Version. Obstet Gynecol. 2016;127:e54–61.
35. Hannah ME, Hannah WJ, Hewson SA, Hodnett ED, Saigal S, Willan AR. Planned caesarean section versus planned vaginal birth for breech presentation at term: a randomised multicentre trial. Term Breech Trial Collaborative Group. Lancet. 2000;356:1375–83.
36. Rietberg CC, Elferink-Stinkens PM, Brand R, van Loon AJ, Van Hemel OJ, Visser GH. Term breech presentation in The Netherlands from 1995 to 1999: mortality and morbidity in relation to the mode of delivery of 33824 infants. BJOG. 2003;110:604–9.
37. Hartnack Tharin JE, Rasmussen S, Krebs L. Consequences of the Term Breech Trial in Denmark. Acta Obstet Gynecol Scand. 2011;90:767–71.
38. Rietberg CC, Elferink-Stinkens PM, Visser GH. The effect of the Term Breech Trial on medical intervention behaviour and neonatal outcome in The Netherlands: an analysis of 35,453 term breech infants. BJOG. 2005;112:205–9.
39. Martin JA, Hamilton BE, Sutton PD, Ventura SJ, Menacker F, Munson ML. Births: final data for 2002. Natl Vital Stat Rep. 2003;52:1–113.
40. ACOG Committee on Obstetric Practice. ACOG Committee Opinion No. 340. Mode of term singleton breech delivery. Obstet Gynecol. 2006;108:235–7.
41. Pallasmaa N, Ekblad U, Gissler M. Severe maternal morbidity and the mode of delivery. Acta Obstet Gynecol Scand. 2008;87:662–8.
42. Liu S, Liston RM, Joseph KS, Heaman M, Sauve R, Kramer MS, Maternal Health Study Group of the Canadian Perinatal Surveillance System. Maternal mortality and severe morbidity associated with low-risk planned cesarean delivery versus planned vaginal delivery at term. CMAJ. 2007;176:455–60.
43. Kornman MT, Kimball KT, Reeves KO. Preterm external cephalic version in an outpatient environment. Am J Obstet Gynecol. 1995;172:1734–8.
44. Hutton EK, Hannah ME, Ross SJ, Delisle MF, Carson GD, Windrim R, Ohlsson A, Willan AR, Gafni A, Sylvestre G, Natale R, Barrett Y, Pollard JK, Dunn MS, Turtle P, Early ECV2 Trial Collaborative Group. The Early External Cephalic Version (ECV) 2 Trial: an international multicentre randomised controlled trial of timing of ECV for breech pregnancies. BJOG. 2011;118:564–77.
45. Hutton EK, Hofmeyr GJ, Dowswell T. External cephalic version for breech presentation before term. Cochrane Database Syst Rev. 2015;7:CD000084.
46. Grootscholten K, Kok M, Oei SG, Mol BW, van der Post JA. External cephalic version-related risks: a meta-analysis. Obstet Gynecol. 2008;112:1143–51.
47. Kok M, Cnossen J, Gravendeel L, van der Post J, Opmeer B, Mol BW. Clinical factors to predict the outcome of external cephalic version: a metaanalysis. Am J Obstet Gynecol. 2008;199:630.e1–7.
48. Kok M, van der Steeg JW, van der Post JA, Mol BW. Prediction of success of external cephalic version after 36 weeks. Am J Perinatol. 2011;28:103–10.
49. Cluver C, Gyte GM, Sinclair M, Dowswell T, Hofmeyr GJ. Interventions for helping to turn term breech babies to head first presentation when using external cephalic version. Cochrane Database Syst Rev. 2015;2:CD000184.
50. Burgos J, Cobos P, Osuna C, de Mar CM, Fernández-Llebrez L, Astorquiza TM, Melchor JC. Nitrous oxide for analgesia in external cephalic version at term: prospective comparative study. J Perinat Med. 2013;41:719–23.
51. Muñoz H, Guerra S, Perez-Vaquero P, Valero Martinez C, Aizpuru F, Lopez-Picado A. Remifentanil versus placebo for analgesia during external cephalic version: a randomised clinical trial. Int J Obstet Anesth. 2014;23:52–7.
52. Khaw KS, Lee SW, Ngan Kee WD, Law LW, Lau TK, Ng FF, Leung TY. Randomized trial of anaesthetic interventions in external cephalic version for breech presentation. Br J Anaesth. 2015;114:944–50.
53. Burgos J, Pijoan JI, Osuna C, Cobos P, Rodriguez L, Centeno Mdel M, Serna R, Jimenez A, Garcia E, Fernandez-Llebrez L, Melchor JC. Increased pain relief with remifentanil does not improve the success rate of external cephalic version: a randomized controlled trial. Acta Obstet Gynecol Scand. 2016;95:547–54.
54. Sullivan JT, Grobman WA, Bauchat JR, Scavone BM, Grouper S, McCarthy RJ, Wong CA. A randomized controlled trial of the effect of combined spinal-epidural analgesia on the success of external cephalic version for breech presentation. Int J Obstet Anesth. 2009;18:328–34.
55. Goetzinger KR, Harper LM, Tuuli MG, Macones GA, Colditz GA. Effect of regional anesthesia on the success rate of external cephalic version: a systematic review and meta-analysis. Obstet Gynecol. 2011;118:1137–44.
56. Lavoie A, Guay J. Anesthetic dose neuraxial blockade increases the success rate of external fetal version: a meta-analysis. Can J Anaesth. 2010;57:408–14.
57. Sultan P, Carvalho B. Neuraxial blockade for external cephalic version: a systematic review. Int J Obstet Anesth. 2011;20:299–306.
58. Suen SS, Khaw KS, Law LW, Sahota DS, Lee SW, Lau TK, Leung TY. The force applied to successfully turn a foetus during reattempts of external cephalic version is substantially reduced when performed under spinal analgesia. J Matern Fetal Neonatal Med. 2012;25:719–22.
59. Schorr SJ, Speights SE, Ross EL, Bofill JA, Rust OA, Norman PF, Morrison JC. A randomized trial of epidural anesthesia to improve external cephalic version success. Am J Obstet Gynecol. 1997;177:1133–7.
60. Carlan SJ, Dent JM, Huckaby T, Whittington EC, Shaefer D. The effect of epidural anesthesia on safety

60. and success of external cephalic version at term. Anesth Analg. 1994;79:525–8.
61. Cherayil G, Feinberg B, Robinson J, Tsen LC. Central neuraxial blockade promotes external cephalic version success after a failed attempt. Anesth Analg. 2002;94:1589–92.
62. Weiniger CF, Ginosar Y, Elchalal U, Sharon E, Nokrian M, Ezra Y. External cephalic version for breech presentation with or without spinal analgesia in nulliparous women at term: a randomized controlled trial. Obstet Gynecol. 2007;110:1343–50.
63. Weiniger CF, Ginosar Y, Elchalal U, Sela HY, Weissman C, Ezra Y. Randomized controlled trial of external cephalic version in term multiparae with or without spinal analgesia. Br J Anaesth. 2010;104:613–8.
64. Mancuso KM, Yancey MK, Murphy JA, Markenson GR. Epidural analgesia for cephalic version: a randomized trial. Obstet Gynecol. 2000;95:648–51.
65. Neiger R, Hennessy MD, Patel M. Reattempting failed external cephalic version under epidural anesthesia. Am J Obstet Gynecol. 1998;179:1136–9.
66. American College of Obstetricians and Gynecologists. ACOG Practice Bulletin No.142: Cerclage for the management of cervical insufficiency. Obstet Gynecol. 2014;123:372–9.
67. Owen J, Mancuso M. Cervical cerclage for the prevention of preterm birth. Obstet Gynecol Clin N Am. 2012;39:25–33.
68. Warren JE, Silver RM, Dalton J, Nelson LT, Branch DW, Porter TF. Collagen 1Alpha1 and transforming growth factor-beta polymorphisms in women with cervical insufficiency. Obstet Gynecol. 2007;110:619–24.
69. Lee SE, Romero R, Park CW, Jun JK, Yoon BH. The frequency and significance of intraamniotic inflammation in patients with cervical insufficiency. Am J Obstet Gynecol. 2008;198:633.e1–8.
70. Debbs RH, Chen J. Contemporary use of cerclage in pregnancy. Clin Obstet Gynecol. 2009;52:597–610.
71. Wood SL, Owen J. Vaginal cerclage: preoperative, intraoperative, and postoperative management. Clin Obstet Gynecol. 2016;59:270–85.
72. Berghella V, Odibo AO, To MS, Rust OA, Althuisius SM. Cerclage for short cervix on ultrasonography: meta-analysis of trials using individual patient-level data. Obstet Gynecol. 2005;106:181–9.
73. Naqvi M, Barth WH Jr. Emergency cerclage: outcomes, patient selection, and operative considerations. Clin Obstet Gynecol. 2016;59:286–94.
74. Odibo AO, Berghella V, To MS, et al. Shirodkar versus McDonald cerclage for the prevention of preterm birth in women with short cervical length. Am J Perinatol. 2007;24:55–60.
75. Wood SL, Owen J. Cerclage: Shirodkar, McDonald, and Modifications. Clin Obstet Gynecol. 2016;59:302–10.
76. Drassinower D, Poggi SH, Landy HJ, Gilo N, Benson JE, Ghidini A. Perioperative complications of history-indicated and ultrasound-indicated cervical cerclage. Am J Obstet Gynecol. 2011;205:53.e1–5.
77. Aaronson J, Goodman S. Obstetric anesthesia: not just for cesareans and labor. Semin Perinatol. 2014;38:378–85.
78. Reitman E, Flood P. Anaesthetic considerations for non-obstetric surgery during pregnancy. Br J Anaesth. 2011;107(Suppl 1):i72–8.
79. Yoon HJ, Hong JY, Kim SM. The effect of anesthetic method for prophylactic cervical cerclage on plasma oxytocin: a randomized trial. Int J Obstet Anesth. 2008;17:26–30.
80. Crawford JS, Lewis M. Nitrous oxide in early human pregnancy. Anaesthesia. 1986;41:900–5.
81. Ioscovich A, Popov A, Gimelfarb Y, Gozal Y, Orbach-Zinger S, Shapiro J, Ginosar Y. Anesthetic management of prophylactic cervical cerclage: a retrospective multicenter cohort study. Arch Gynecol Obstet. 2015;291:509–12.
82. Schumann R, Rafique MB. Low-dose epidural anesthesia for cervical cerclage. Can J Anaesth. 2003;50:424–5.
83. Beilin Y, Zahn J, Abramovitz S, Bernstein HH, Hossain S, Bodian C. Subarachnoid small-dose bupivacaine versus lidocaine for cervical cerclage. Anesth Analg. 2003;97:56–61.
84. Gaiser RR. Should intrathecal lidocaine be used in the 21st century? J Clin Anesth. 2000;12:476–81.
85. Lee GY, Kim CH, Chung RK, Han JI, Kim DY. Spread of subarachnoid sensory block with hyperbaric bupivacaine in second trimester of pregnancy. J Clin Anesth. 2009;21:482–5.
86. Lee MH, Son HJ, Lee SH, et al. Comparison of spread of subarachnoid sensory block and incidence of hypotension in early and late second trimester of pregnancy. Korean J Anesthesiol. 2013;65:322–6.
87. James KS, McGrady E, Patrick A. Combined spinal-extradural anaesthesia for preterm and term caesarean section: is there a difference in local anaesthetic requirements? Br J Anaesth. 1997;78:498–501.
88. Cousins LM, Pue A. Nitroglycerin facilitates therapeutic cerclage placement. J Perinatol. 1996;16:127–8.
89. McCulloch B, Bergen S, Pielet B, Keller J, Elrad H. McDonald cerclage under pudendal nerve block. Am J Obstet Gynecol. 1993;168:499–502.
90. Arendt KW. Problems of early pregnancy. In: Chestnut DH, editor. Obstetric anesthesia principles and practice. 5th ed. Philadelphia: Elsevier Saunders; 2014. p. 345–55.
91. Taslimi MM, El-Sayed Y, Carvalho B, Coleman L. In: Jaffe RA, editor. Anesthesiologist's manual of surgical procedures. 4th ed. Philadelphia: Lippincott Williams and Wilkins; 2009. p. 837–43.
92. Edlow AG, Hou MY, Maurer R, Benson C, Delli-Bovi L, Goldberg AB. Uterine evacuation for second-trimester fetal death and maternal morbidity. Obstet Gynecol. 2011;117:307–16.
93. Bryant AG, Grimes DA, Garrett JM, Stuart GS. Second-trimester abortion for fetal anomalies or fetal death: labor induction compared with dilation and evacuation. Obstet Gynecol. 2011;117:788–92.

94. Kodali BS, Segal S. Non-delivery obstetric procedures. In: Datta S, editor. Obstetric anesthesia handbook. 5th ed. New York: Springer; 2010. p. 360–2.
95. Berkowitz RS, Goldstein DP. Current management of gestational trophoblastic diseases. Gynecol Oncol. 2009;112:654–62.
96. Kumarasinghe N, Harpin R, Stewart AW. Blood loss during suction termination of pregnancy with two different anaesthetic techniques. Anaesth Intensive Care. 1997;25:48–50.
97. Hall JE, Ng WS, Smith S. Blood loss during first trimester termination of pregnancy: comparison of two anaesthetic techniques. Br J Anaesth. 1997;78:172–4.
98. Chedraui PA, Insuasti DF. Intravenous nitroglycerin in the management of retained placenta. Gynecol Obstet Investig. 2003;56:61–4.
99. Riley ET, Flanagan B, Cohen SE, Chitkarat U. Intravenous nitroglycerin: a potent uterine relaxant for emergency obstetric procedures. Review of literature and report of three cases. Int J Obstet Anesth. 1996;5:264–8.
100. Sviggum HP, Kodali BS. Maternal anesthesia for fetal surgery. Clin Perinatol. 2013;40:413–27.
101. Brusseau R, Mizrahi-Arnaud A. Fetal anesthesia and pain management for intrauterine therapy. Clin Perinatol. 2013;40:429–42.
102. Van de Velde M, De Buck F. Fetal and maternal analgesia/anesthesia for fetal procedures. Fetal Diagn Ther. 2012;31:201–9.
103. Society for Maternal-Fetal Medicine (SMFM). Electronic address: pubs@smfm.org, Mari G, Norton ME, Stone J, Berghella V, Sciscione AC, Tate D, Schenone MH. Society for Maternal-Fetal Medicine (SMFM) Clinical Guideline #8: the fetus at risk for anemia—diagnosis and management. Am J Obstet Gynecol 2015;212:697–710.
104. Society for Maternal-Fetal Medicine, Simpson LL. Twin-twin transfusion syndrome. Am J Obstet Gynecol. 2013;208(1):3–18.
105. Myers LB, Watcha MF. Epidural versus general anesthesia for twin-twin transfusion syndrome requiring fetal surgery. Fetal Diagn Ther. 2004;19:286–91.
106. Van de Velde M, Van Schoubroeck D, Lewi LE, Marcus MA, Jani JC, Missant C, Teunkens A, Deprest JA. Remifentanil for fetal immobilization and maternal sedation during fetoscopic surgery: a randomized, double-blind comparison with diazepam. Anesth Analg. 2005;101:251–8.
107. Missant C, Van Schoubroeck D, Deprest J, Devlieger R, Teunkens A, Van de Velde M. Remifentanil for foetal immobilisation and maternal sedation during endoscopic treatment of twin-to-twin transfusion syndrome: a preliminary dose-finding study. Acta Anaesthesiol Belg. 2004;55:239–44.
108. Morimoto Y, Yoshimura M, Orita H, Matayoshi H, Nagamizo D, Sakabe T, Nakata M. Anesthesia management for fetoscopic treatment of twin-to-twin transfusion syndrome. Masui. 2008;57:719–24.
109. Cooley S, Walsh J, Mahony R, Carroll S, Higgins S, McParland P, McAuliffe F. Successful fetoscopic laser coagulation for twin-to-twin transfusion syndrome under local anaesthesia. Ir Med J. 2011;104:187–90.
110. Fisk NM, Gitau R, Teixeira JM, Giannakoulopoulos X, Cameron AD, Glover VA. Effect of direct fetal opioid analgesia on fetal hormonal and hemodynamic stress response to intrauterine needling. Anesthesiology. 2001;95:828–35.
111. Han G, Li L, Tian Y, Xue H, Zhao P. Influences of different doses of midazolam on mother and fetus in fetoscopic surgery for twin-to-twin transfusion syndrome. Pharmacology. 2015;96:151–4.
112. Kan RE, Hughes SC, Rosen MA, Kessin C, Preston PG, Lobo EP. Intravenous remifentanil: placental transfer, maternal and neonatal effects. Anesthesiology. 1998;88:1467–74.

# Anesthesia and Major Obstetric Hemorrhage

## 53

Tekuila Carter, Yasser Sakawi, and Michelle Tubinis

## Introduction

Globally, the maternal mortality rate (MMR; number of maternal deaths per 100,000 live births) has declined from 282 in 1990 to 196 in 2015. However in the United States, the MMR has increased from 16 in 1990 to 26 in 2015. Maternal hemorrhage is the leading cause of maternal mortality for almost all age groups worldwide (see Fig. 53.1) [1].

Maternal hemorrhage is on the rise in the United States due to the increasing incidence of postpartum hemorrhage. Evidence indicates that uterine atony is largely the cause for this increase. A study by Callaghan et al. found an increase in PPH from 2.3% in 1994 to 29% in 2006 and an increase in PPH caused by uterine atony from 1.6% in 1994 to 2.4% in 2006 [2].

## Types of Hemorrhages and Etiologies

### Antepartum Hemorrhage

Antepartum hemorrhage (APH) is defined as bleeding from the genital tract after 24 weeks of gestation and occurs with an estimated incidence of 5.9–6.5% for singleton pregnancies [3]. There are several etiologies for antepartum hemorrhage. The most significant morbidity and mortality is caused by placenta previa and placental abruption. Although a source of concern is the health of the mother, antepartum hemorrhage has a higher risk for fetal mortality than maternal mortality [3].

### Placenta Previa

When the placental attachment overlies the endocervical os, placenta previa is the diagnosis. This occurs at an incidence of 4 in 1000 pregnancies [4]. Although previously classified as complete, partial, or marginal, placenta previa is now defined as any placentation that overlies the cervical os to any degree. The term low-lying placenta is used to define placentation that is near, but not overlying the cervical os [5]. Although MRI can be useful in diagnosis, transvaginal ultrasound is more practical.

The risk factors for placenta previa include uterine scar (i.e. cesarean section, myomectomy), multiparity, advanced maternal age, and large placenta. It is expected that as the rate of cesarean

T. Carter (✉) · Y. Sakawi · M. Tubinis
Department of Anesthesiology and Perioperative Medicine, University of Alabama at Birmingham, Birmingham, AL, USA
e-mail: tcarter@uabmc.edu; ysakawi@uabmc.edu; mtubinis@uabmc.edu

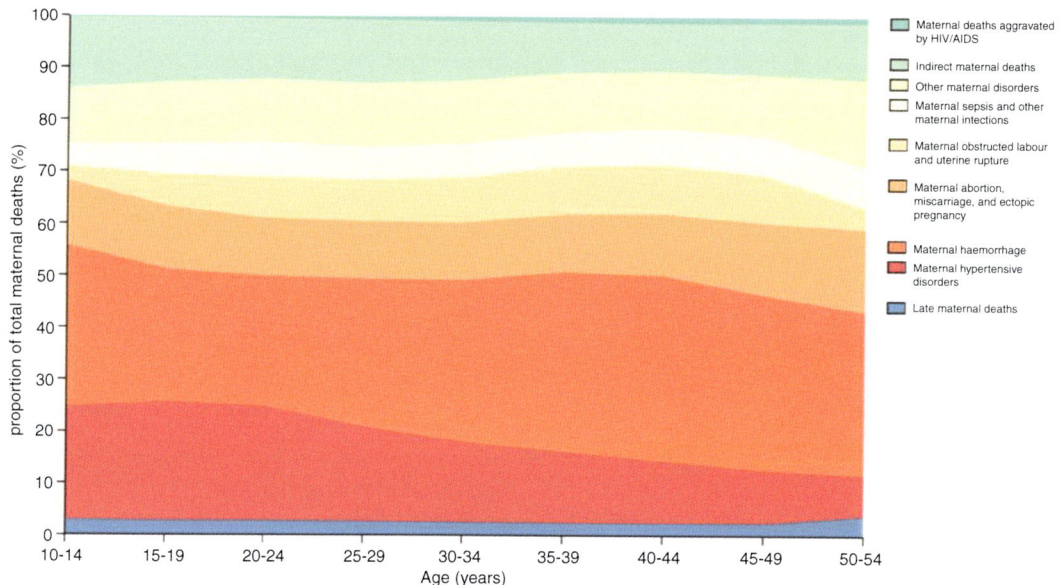

**Fig. 53.1** Global proportion of total maternal deaths by underlying cause and age, 2015. From: Kassebaum NJ, Steiner C, Murray CJL, et al. Global, regional, and national levels of maternal mortality, 1990–2015: a systematic analysis for the Global Burden of Disease Study. Lancet. 2016;388(10053):1775–1812 [1]

deliveries and use of assisted reproductive technology continues to increase, the rate of placenta previa will continue to increase as well [6].

Approximately half of women with placenta previa will experience antepartum hemorrhage, and there is approximately a tenfold increase in risk of antepartum bleeding as compared to patients without placenta previa [7, 8]. These patients are also at an increased risk of need for hysterectomy, need for blood transfusion, ICU admission, disseminated intravascular coagulation (DIC), and infection [8]. Patients with APH and placenta previa may be expectantly managed and observed if the mother and fetus are considered to be stable. However, if the patient or fetal status is not reassuring, obstetric management is to proceed with delivery. Cesarean section is most often required for delivery in patients with placenta previa.

## Placental Abruption

Placental abruption occurs when there is placental separation prior to delivery resulting in hemorrhage under the placental bed. There are significant complications associated with placental abruption as bleeding behind the placental bed can result in consumption of coagulation factors and cause DIC. It is estimated to occur in 1–2% of all pregnancies [9]. Risk factors include cocaine and alcohol use, direct or indirect trauma, hypertensive disorders of pregnancy, premature rupture of membranes, abnormal uterus, multiparity, and advanced maternal age [3]. The diagnosis is often a clinical diagnosis confirmed by abdominal ultrasound.

Obstetric management is dependent upon the degree of abruption, maternal status and gestational age of the fetus. If maternal and fetal status is reassuring and the fetus is premature, expectant management might be appropriate. If maternal and fetal status are reassuring and the fetus is term, vaginal delivery might be appropriate. If the mother is hemodynamically unstable, coagulopathic, or the fetal status is non-reassuring, urgent/emergent cesarean section is usually indicated. Patients typically recover quickly and completely after delivery.

## Uterine Rupture

Uterine rupture is a relatively rare cause for antepartum hemorrhage. The most significant risk factor for uterine rupture is the presence of a uterine scar. This highlights the increased risk of trial of labor after cesarean section, but it can occur in a nulliparous uterus. Other risk factors include uterine manipulation/instrumentation, prolonged labor/induction, fetopelvic disproportion, grand multiparity (>5 pregnancies), congenital anomalies, trauma, and connective tissue disorders [10]. The presentation of uterine rupture is frank hemorrhage with fetal distress and loss of uterine tone. Patients may have epidural breakthrough pain out of proportion to contractions or become hemodynamically unstable secondary to blood loss into the abdominal cavity. The most reliable indicator of uterine rupture is loss of fetal heart tones. Uterine rupture represents a true obstetric emergency, necessitating emergent exploratory laparotomy for delivery and uterine repair with possible arterial ligation and hysterectomy.

## Postpartum Hemorrhage

Despite advances in modern medicine, postpartum hemorrhage (PPH) remains a significant source of maternal morbidity and mortality. Several definitions have been proposed for PPH but none are comprehensive. Traditionally, PPH has been defined as blood loss within the first 24 hours greater than 500cc following a vaginal delivery and greater than 1000cc following a cesarean section. It is difficult to objectively and accurately quantify blood loss with evidence showing that it is usually underestimated [21]. For this reason, a post-delivery decrease in hematocrit of 10% is accepted as a more accurate means to diagnose PPH [11]. There are several etiologies for postpartum hemorrhage, including but not limited to, uterine atony, retained placenta, placenta accreta, uterine inversion, genital trauma, and coagulopathy. PPH complicates approximately 3% of pregnancies, which has increased since the 1990s due to an increase in uterine atony [12].

### Uterine Atony

Uterine atony occurs when the uterus fails to contract normally following delivery resulting in significant blood loss. An atonic uterus is often referred to as "boggy" or soft. Uterine atony is the number one cause of PPH in the first 24 hours, accounting for 80% of PPH [12]. Common risk factors include conditions that over distend the uterus, hypertensive disorders of pregnancy, and prolonged or augmented labor. As discussed previously, the rates of uterine atony are increasing, likely secondary to the increase in number of cesarean sections, multiple gestation births, and advanced maternal age women giving birth [12]. Treatment for uterine atony starts with the use of uterotonic agents (see Table 53.1).

### Retained Placenta

The World Health Organization (WHO) defines retained placenta as incomplete expulsion of the placenta within 30 minutes of delivery [13]. Risk

**Table 53.1** Uterotonic drugs

| Drug | Drug class | Dose and route | Side effects | Increased risk for complications |
|---|---|---|---|---|
| Oxytocin (Pitocin) | Synthetic oxytocin | 10–40 units/500–1000 mL infusion Or 10 units IM | Tachycardia, hypotension, N/V, Water intoxication | None |
| Methylergonovine (Methergine) | Ergot alkaloid | 0.2 mg IM | HTN, Arteriolar constriction, N/V, Headache | HTN, Preeclampsia, CAD |
| 15-Methylprostaglandin (Carboprost/Hemabate) | Prostaglandin | 0.25 mg IM | Bronchospasm, Flushing, Diarrhea, N/V | Pulmonary HTN, Reactive airway disease |
| Misoprostol (Cytotec) | Prostaglandin | 600–1000 mcg rectally | Diarrhea, abdominal pain | None |

Abbreviations: *IM* intramuscular, *HTN* hypertension, *N/V* nausea and vomiting, *CAD* coronary artery disease factors include history of retained placenta, preterm delivery, previous uterine surgery, grand multiparity, preeclampsia, repeat miscarriages, and prolonged use of oxytocin [14]. The WHO recommends a conservative approach to delivery of the placenta by waiting another 30 min in patients with no acute hemorrhage. If the placenta is not delivered after an hour, it is up to the clinician to decide further treatment [13]. Further treatment includes manual removal of the placenta. If manual removal is not successful, dilation and curettage may be necessary.

## Placenta Accreta

The diagnosis of placenta accreta is made when any part of the placenta invades the uterine wall and cannot be separated from it [15]. Placenta accreta can be divided into three types. Placenta accreta vera, which occurs the most, has no decidual layer between the placenta and the uterine myometrium. Placenta increta exists when the placenta invades the uterine myometrium. Placenta percreta exists when the placenta invades the uterine myometrium, uterine serosa, and can continue to invade adjacent structures like the bladder. Placenta percreta is the most severe and occurs the least [15].

Risk factors include any procedure or condition that damages the myometrium, including cesarean section and placenta previa. When those two risk factors are combined, the percentage of patients with placenta accreta dramatically increases from 3% with previa and one prior cesarean section, 11% with two prior, 40% with three prior, and 61% with four prior [5]. Estimated blood loss can range from 2 to 7.8 L, often with associated morbidity [5].

The American Congress of Obstetricians and Gynecologists (ACOG) recommends planned delivery at a tertiary hospital with an experienced multidisciplinary team and resources to manage massive hemorrhage [15]. Although ACOG recommends that most patients with accreta are treated with a preterm cesarean hysterectomy without the attempt to remove the placenta from the uterus, there is no consensus on the timing, obstetric care, or surgical management of placenta accreta. A treatment plan should be individualized for optimum outcomes for the patient and fetus [15].

## Uterine Inversion

Uterine inversion can cause severe postpartum hemorrhage. It can progress from an inverted fundus to a completely everted uterus. Risk factors include uterine atony, uterine abnormalities, placenta accreta, aggressive fundal pressure or umbilical cord traction, and fundal placental implantation. Treatment is to replace the uterus to its normal position. While there are several methods described to do this, it can be difficult to accomplish. While the obstetrician is attempting to replace the uterus, oxytocin or any other uterotonics should be discontinued, adequate IV access should be obtained to prepare for massive blood loss, and tocolytics should be considered if the uterus is contracted [16]. General anesthesia with volatile agents may be required to relax the uterus if initial attempts are unsuccessful.

## Genital Trauma

Genital trauma includes lacerations and hematomas. Both types are described based on the location of the trauma. Trauma can occur anywhere along the birth canal including, external genitalia, vagina, cervix, and perineum. Treatment depends on the severity of the trauma, the area damaged, and stability of the patient. Most do not require treatment or receive minor treatment. Minor treatments include repair of the lacerations or incision and evacuation of hematomas. Perineal hematomas can be the most dangerous and may require exploratory laparotomy. Estimated blood loss is often inaccurate and treatment is sought after significant undetected blood loss. Vigilance is the key to successful early treatment.

## Coagulopathy

Inherited bleeding disorders, such as von Willebrand disease, are rare. However, complications of pregnancy can cause coagulopathy, including hemolysis, elevated liver enzymes, and low platelet count (HELLP) syndrome, placental abruption, intrauterine fetal demise, and amniotic fluid embolism [17]. Coagulopathy can also be a complication of excessive bleeding and treatment of hemorrhage. If coagulopathy is suspected, laboratory tests, including CBC, PT, PTT, and fibrinogen, should be obtained and treatment should be based on the lab results and/or clinical judgment. Fibrinogen levels of less than 2 g/L are independently associated with an increased risk of severe PPH and should be treated with cryoprecipitate or fibrinogen concentrates [18].

## Prevention of Morbidity and Mortality

Most of the morbidity and mortality related to maternal hemorrhage has been determined to be preventable [19, 20]. Early recognition, prevention of bleeding, preparation, and early appropriate treatment have been identified as areas of improvement for prevention of these adverse outcomes.

## Early Recognition

Patients should be risk stratified for bleeding on admission to labor and delivery. Based on their risk, appropriate laboratory testing should be ordered. Table 53.2 is an example of a quick admissions risk assessment to determine the need for blood products. Scheduled repeat risk assessments should be done throughout admission due to the potential for change in maternal condition.

Visual estimation of blood loss has been shown to be an inaccurate indicator of actual blood loss [21, 22]. Providers tend to underestimate the amount of blood loss and this underestimation gets larger as the amount of blood loss increases. Quantitative measurements can improve the accuracy of blood loss estimation. These include weighing blood saturated materials, using separate canisters for amniotic fluid, and using drapes with graded markers. Everyone on the obstetric team should receive regular training in formal quantitative measurements of blood loss to maintain their skills [23]. A new tablet application that measures hemoglobin concentration in blood soaked objects, like sponges, and canisters filled with bloody fluids might make estimating blood loss more objective [24].

## Prevention of Bleeding

Obstetric patients should be optimized during the antepartum period. For example, if they are anemic, consider starting iron replacement, erythropoietin, or transfusing blood products in severe cases. All patients, especially high risk patients, should be counseled on their risk of bleeding for both vaginal and cesarean delivery. Interdisciplinary planning for scheduled cesarean delivery should be considered for high risk patients that are unlikely to successfully deliver vaginally. A discussion on the patient's desire to receive blood products, and desire for future pregnancies should be done prior to the day of delivery.

**Table 53.2** Sample admission risk assessment and recommended laboratory test (from the University of Alabama at Birmingham massive transfusion protocol)

|  | Low (type and screen) | Medium (type and screen) | High (type and cross) |
|---|---|---|---|
| Admission | No previous uterine incision<br>Singleton pregnancy<br>≤4 previous vaginal births<br>No known bleeding disorder<br>No history of PPH | Prior cesarean birth(s) or uterine surgery<br>Placenta previa W/no evidence of accreta<br>Multiple gestation<br>>4 previous vaginal births<br>Low lying placenta<br>History of previous PPH<br>Large uterine fibroids<br>Estimated fetal weight >4 kg<br>Morbid obesity | Placenta previa W/prior C/S<br>Diagnosed or suspected placenta accreta or percreta<br>Hematocrit <21 and 1 or more med/high risk factors<br>Platelets <50,000<br>Active bleeding on admission<br>Known coagulopathy |

During the peripartum period, high risk patients should have increased surveillance with constant monitoring of vital signs, urine output, and mental status. They should also have at least two large bore intravenous catheters. Intra-arterial internal iliac balloon placement should be considered in high risk patients, such as known placenta accreta with a desire for fertility preservation. ACOG recommends administration of oxytocin after the delivery of the anterior shoulder of the fetus or after the placenta is delivered [17]. This active management of the third stage of labor often includes controlled traction on the cord and bimanual uterine massage.

## Preparation

Development of a multidisciplinary care team protocol, including OB/GYN, anesthesiology, blood bank, operating and labor room nurses, neonatology, and interventional radiology, is important to reduce maternal morbidity [25]. The logistics from triggering the multidisciplinary response team to each member's responsibilities should be established. An obstetric hemorrhage cart, kit, and/or tray should be assembled (see Table 53.3). The development of a maternal massive transfusion protocol (MTP) can reduce delays in treatment. Trauma studies show that MTPs can also reduce multiple organ failure and other complications of massive transfusion [26]. An example of a local MTP from the University of Alabama-Birmingham is depicted in Fig. 53.2. Multidisciplinary team practice drills are also important not only for everyone to practice working together but also to expose latent errors or forgotten details.

## Appropriate Management

### Obstetric Management

First line treatments are oxytocin and bimanual compression of the uterus. Second line treatments usually consist of other uterotonics (see Table 53.1). Other treatments include tamponade techniques of packing with gauze, fluid filled foley catheters or specialized balloons, ligation of uterine vessels, compression sutures, or peripartum hysterectomy. Arterial embolization is another option in a stable patient with continued bleeding.

**Table 53.3** Example items for OB Hemorrhage Cart, Kit, and Tray. Modified from OB Hemorrhage Toolkit V 2.0 | California Maternal Quality Care Collaborative [Internet]. Cmqcc.org. 2017 [cited 26 February 2017]. Available from: https://www.cmqcc.org/resources-tool-kits/toolkits/ob-hemorrhage-toolkit

| Example items for OB Hemorrhage Cart, Kit, and Tray |
|---|
| **OB Hemorrhage Medication Kit: Available in L&D and Postpartum Floor refrigerator** |
| Pitocin 10–40 units per 500–1000 mL NS 1 bag |
| Hemabate 250 mcg/mL 1 ampule |
| Cytotec 200 mcg tablets 5 tabs |
| Methergine 0.2 mg/mL 1 ampule |
| **OB Hemorrhage Tray: Available on Postpartum Floor** |
| IV start kit |
| 16 gauge Angiocath |
| 1 liter bag lactated ringers |
| IV tubing |
| Sterile speculum |
| Urinary catheter kit |
| Flash light |
| Lubricating jelly |
| Assorted sizes sterile gloves |
| Lab tubes: red, blue, tiger top |
| **OB Hemorrhage Cart** |
| Set of vaginal retractors (long right angle) |
| Sponge forceps (minimum: 2) |
| Sutures (for cervical laceration repair and B-Lynch) |
| Vaginal packs |
| Uterine balloon |
| Multiple size banjo curettes |
| Several sizes |
| Long needle holder |
| Uterine forceps |
| Bright task light on wheels behind ultrasound machine |
| Diagrams depicting various procedures (e.g. B-Lynch, uterine artery ligation, balloon placement) |

### Anesthetic Management

The type of anesthesia for any cause of maternal hemorrhage depends on the stability of the patient, the level of anesthesia needed, the urgency of treatment, and the presence of preexisting neuraxial anesthesia. However, there are

## OB BLOOD PRODUCT PROTOCOL

**PRE OP**

Screen all patients for hemorrhage risk:
Low, Medium and High risk
Discuss risk of transfucion
**Verify Type and Screen-if patient has POSITIVE ANTIBODIES they should be Type & Crossed for 1-2 Units PRBCs

For patients who decline blood products:
Notify OB provider for POC
Early consult with anesthesia
Review consent for refusal of blood products

**ADMISSION**

| LOW (TYPE AND SCREEN) | MEDIUM (TYPE AND SCREEN) | HIGH (TYPE AND CROSS) |
|---|---|---|
| NO PREVIOUS UTERINE INCISION | PRIOR CESAREAN BIRTH(S) OR UTERINE SURGERY | PLACENTA PREVIA W/ PRIOR C/S |
| SINGLETON PREGNANCY | PLACENTA PREVIA W/ NO EVIDENCE OF ACCRETA | DIAGNOSED OR SUSPECTED PLACENTA ACCRETA OR PERCRETA |
| ≤ 4 PREVIOUS VAGINAL BIRTHS | MULTIPLE GESTATION | HEMATOCRIT <21 AND 1 OR MORE |
| NO KNOWN BLEEDING DISORDER | > 4 PREVIOUS VAGINAL BIRTHS | MED/HIGH RISK FACTORS |
| NO HISTORE OF PP HEMORRHAGE | LOW LYING PLACENTA | PLATELETS < 50,000 |
|  | HISTORY OF PREVIOUS PP HEMORRHAGE | ACTIVE BLEEDING ON ADMISSION |
|  | LARGE UTERNE FIBROIDS | KNOWN COAGULOPATHY |
|  | ESTIMATED FETAL WEIGHT > 4 KG |  |
|  | MORBID OBESITY |  |

**OP PREP**

| Make sure T&S is current | Have current T&S<br>Notify OB/Anesthesia of risk factors for hemorrhage and mceive POC | BLOOD BANK NOTIFIED: Signed forms to BB<br>IF > 1500 mL BLOOD LOSS ANTICIPATED<br>MDs to order Type & Screen w/# of units needed<br>Call Blood Bank with pt name, MR# and # of units ordered<br>Request the BB place the blood in a cooler for transport<br>Designate one person to go to the BB to retrieve cooler<br>*Make sure to take a stamped green card to BB for pick up |
|---|---|---|

**GIVING BLOOD IN OR**

| When Giving blood with NO TYPE AND CROSS | When Giving blood NON-EMERGENTLY: | When Giving blood from cooler: |
|---|---|---|
| Call blood bank and state the need for Emergency Release Blood with pt's name, MR# and # of units Ordered<br>Obtain the 'EMERGENCY RELEASE OF BLOOD /BLOOD COMPONENTS' form (in WPACU)<br>Stamp and fill out appropriately<br>Tube to Blood Bank #770<br>BB will call when blood is sent<br>Verify the correct products have been sent<br>Give blood to anesthesia<br>Verify blood with anesthesia<br>Sign and return the sheet that came with the blood to the BB | MUST HAVE TYPE & CROSS ORDER!<br>Have MD order blood<br>Call the blood bank to notify them of the patient and MR# and how many units are needed, to be tubed to WPACU #881<br>Stamp a green sheet and tube to the blood bank (tube#770)<br>Indicate number of units on green card<br>BB will call when blood is sent<br>Verify the correct products have been sent<br>Give blood to anesthesia<br>Verify blood with anesthesia<br>Sign and return the sheet that is sent with blood to BB | Verity blood with anesthesia<br>Document in Surginet what was given<br>**IF BLOOD REMAINS IN THE COOLER AFTER THE CASE, IT MUST BE RETURNED TO BB WITHIN 6 HOURS! |

**EMERGENCY**

WHAT TO DO WHEN IN AN EMERGENCY WHEN PATIENT HAS NO T&S OR T&C
The CB Attending/Anesthesia Attending activates the "MASSIVE TRANSFUSION PROTOCOL"
Call the blood bank (6-8911) and states which MD has activated the protocol,
what area needs the cooler and how many coolers/number of units are needed (max of 2).
Cooler contairs 6U PRBCs, 4FFP, 1Platelet/Cryo (separate order for ayo)
Designated person goes to blood bank with STAMPED GREEN SHEET
Make sure labs have been sent for T&S/T&C
MDs should order 4 Units PRBCs to BS as needed to stay ahead
Verify Blood with anesthesia and return any unused blood to BB in the cooler within 6 hours
*Make sure to call Blood Bank when MD's DEACTIVATE MASSIVE TRANSFUSION PROTOCOL!

**PREPLANNED OR BLOOD ADMIN**

| FOR PLACENTA ACCRETA<br>Early consult with Anesthesia<br>Orders for pt to be Type & Crossed for 4 U PRBS, 2 FFP and 1 Platelets (Or specific orders)<br>Alert Main PACU/ICU about possible transfer of pt<br>*TREAT MULTIPLE RISK FACTORS AND HIGH RISK<br><br>ALL PERCRETAS AND OTHER HIGHLY COMPLICATED CASES WILL BE PERFORMED IN MAIN OR | Notify OB/Anesthesia of patient arrival; obtain orders for Type and Cross<br>Notify Main PACU/ICU of patient arrival if a bed is to be reserved<br>Call the Blood Bank with patient's name, MR, and if of units ordered<br>*TELL THE BLOOD BANK THE BLOOD WILL NEED TO BE IN A COOLER FOR TRANSPORT TO THE OR TO BE ON STANDBY<br>Designate one person to walk to the blood bank to obtain cooler<br>**Take a stamped green sheet to the Blood Bank for pick up!<br>Alert anesthesia when cooler of blood is in the OR<br>Verify Blood with anesthesia<br>***THe OR RN IS RESPONSIBLE FOR MAKING SURE THE COOLER ALONG WITH ANY UNUSED BLOOD IS RETURNED TO THE BB WITHIN 6 HOURS!!!! |
|---|---|

**Fig. 53.2** University of Alabama at Birmingham massive transfusion protocol

advantages and disadvantages of neuraxial and general anesthesia. The decision for either should be individualized (see Table 53.4). Preoperative assessment prior to the day of delivery is helpful to develop an anesthetic plan for the planned vaginal and cesarean section delivery. A contingency plan in the event that an emergency cesarean section is needed should also be developed. In a patient that is at risk for hemorrhage or is currently experiencing peripartum hemorrhage, the need for adequate intravenous access cannot be understated. In these cases, a minimum of two large bore peripheral intravenous catheters should be placed. If it is anticipated that there will be significant blood loss and need for large volume resuscitation, such as in placenta percreta, central venous access may be appropriate and should be considered.

## Anesthetic Management for Vaginal Delivery

In patients who the obstetric team have deemed eligible for vaginal delivery, neuraxial anesthesia is appropriate if there are no contraindications for placement. For high risk patients, as is the case with low-lying placenta or patients with coagulation disorders, advanced monitoring should be considered. Intra-arterial blood pressure monitoring or the use of non-invasive cardiac monitors can be helpful, especially in the event that an emergent cesarean hysterectomy should occur.

## Anesthetic Management for Cesarean Delivery

In patients with high risk of hemorrhage, a cesarean section may be planned to ensure a well-prepared multidisciplinary team approach to the care of the patient and delivery of the newborn.

For planned cesarean sections, there are many aspects to consider when deciding whether general or neuraxial anesthesia is more appropriate (see Table 53.4). If large volumes of blood loss are anticipated, such as in placenta percreta, general anesthetics may be a more appropriate choice. If urgent or emergent cesarean section is needed, the stability of the patient and fetus will often determine the anesthetic choice. General anesthesia is the anesthetic of choice with unstable hemorrhaging patients.

The decision for post-operative destination is dependent on patient stability and status of labs. A patient that is coagulopathic or unstable will likely necessitate an ICU admission.

**Table 53.4** Risk and benefits of neuraxial versus general anesthesia

| Neuraxial | General |
|---|---|
| • Reduced mortality rate | • Avoid patient discomfort |
| • Avoid airway related GA risk | • Avoid patient and/or family member distraction from patient care |
| • Less fetal drug exposure | • Increased risk of difficult airway and aspiration |
| • Opportunity to see fetus and have family member present | • Risk of code on induction |
| • Reduced blood loss | • May increase risk of uterine atony with use of volatile agents |
| • Faster recovery | • Secured airway |
| • Better postop analgesia | • Better management of hemodynamic instability |
| • Always a risk of needing to go to GA in the middle of surgery | • Placement of invasive monitors easier |

*GA* general anesthesia

## References

1. Kassebaum NJ, Steiner C, Murray CJL, et al. Global, regional, and national levels of maternal mortality, 1990-2015: a systematic analysis for the Global Burden of Disease Study 2015. Lancet. 2016;388(10053):1775–812.
2. Callaghan W, Kuklina E, Berg C. Trends in postpartum hemorrhage: United States, 1994–2006. Am J Obstet Gynecol. 2010;202(4):353.e1–6.
3. Giordano R. Antepartum haemorrhage. J Perinat Med. 2010;4(1):12–6.
4. Faiz Ananth C. Etiology and risk factors for placenta previa: an overview and meta-analysis of observational studies. J Matern Fetal Neonatal Med. 2003;13(3):175–90.
5. Silver R. Abnormal Placentation: Placenta previa, Vasa Previa, and Placenta Accreta. Obstet Gynecol. 2015;126(3):654–68.

6. Romundstad L, Romundstad P, Sunde A, et al. Increased risk of placenta previa in pregnancies following IVF/ICSI; a comparison of ART and non-ART pregnancies in the same mother. Hum Reprod. 2006;21(9):2353–8.
7. Fan D, Wu S, Liu L, Xia Q, Wang W, Guo X, et al. Prevalence of antepartum hemorrhage in women with placenta previa: a systematic review and meta-analysis. Sci Rep. 2017;7:40320.
8. Crane J, Van der Hof M, Dodds L, Armson BA, Liston R. Maternal complications with placenta previa. Am J Perinatol. 2000;17(2):101–5.
9. Ananth C, Wilcox AJ. Placental abruption and perinatal mortality in the United States. Am J Epidemiol. 2001;153(4):332–7.
10. Vilchez G, Dai J, Kumar K, Lagos M, Sokol R. Contemporary analysis of maternal and neonatal morbidity after uterine rupture: a nationwide population-based study. J Obstet Gynaecol Res. 2017.
11. Kominiarek MA, Kilpatrick SJ. Postpartum hemorrhage: a recurring pregnancy complication. Semin Perinatol. 2007;31:159–66.
12. Bateman BT, Berman MF, Riley LE, Leffert LR. The epidemiology of postpartum hemorrhage in a large, nationwide sample of deliveries. Anesth Analg. 2010;110(5):1368–73.
13. WHO recommendations for the prevention and treatment of postpartum haemorrhage. Geneva: World Health Organization; 2012.
14. Endler M, Grünewald C, Saltvedt S. Epidemiology of retained placenta. Obstet Gynecol. 2012;119(4):801–9.
15. American College of Obstetricians and Gynecologists. Committee Opinion No. 529: placenta accreta. Obstet Gynecol. 2012;120(1):207–11.
16. Mirza F, Gaddipati S. Obstetric Emergencies. Semin Perinatol. 2009;33(2):97–103.
17. ACOG Practice Bulletin No. 76: postpartum hemorrhage. Obstet Gynecol 2006;108(4):1039–48.
18. Cortet M, Deneux-Tharaux C, Dupont C, Colin C, Rudigoz R, Bouvier-Colle M, et al. Association between fibrinogen level and severity of postpartum haemorrhage: secondary analysis of a prospective trial. Br J Anaesth. 2012;108(6):984–9.
19. Berg C, Harper M, Atkinson S, Bell E, Brown H, Hage M, et al. Preventability of pregnancy-related deaths. Obstet Gynecol. 2005;106(6):1228–34.
20. McClure J, Cooper G, Clutton-Brock T. Saving Mothers' lives: reviewing maternal deaths to make motherhood safer: 2006-8: a review. Br J Anaesth. 2011;107(2):127–32.
21. Bose P, Regan F, Paterson-Brown S. Improving the accuracy of estimated blood loss at obstetric haemorrhage using clinical reconstructions. BJOG. 2006;113(8):919–24.
22. Lertbunnaphong T, Lapthanapat N, Leetheeragul J, Hakularb P, Ownon A. Postpartum blood loss: visual estimation versus objective quantification with a novel birthing drape. Singap Med J. 2016;57(06):325–8.
23. Toledo P, Eosakul S, Goetz K, Wong C, Grobman W. Decay in blood loss estimation skills after web-based didactic training. Simul Healthc. 2012;7(1):18–21.
24. Sharareh B, Woolwine S, Satish S, Abraham P, Schwarzkopf R. Real time intraoperative monitoring of blood loss with a novel tablet application. Open Orthop J. 2015;9(1):422–6.
25. Eller A, Bennett M, Sharshiner M, Masheter C, Soisson A, Dodson M, et al. Maternal morbidity in cases of placenta accreta managed by a multidisciplinary care team compared with standard obstetric care. Obstet Gynecol. 2011;117(2, Part 1):331–7.
26. Cotton B, Au B, Nunez T, Gunter O, Robertson A, Young P. Predefined massive transfusion protocols are associated with a reduction in organ failure and postinjury complications. J Trauma. 2009;66(1):41–9.

# Anesthesia for Medical Termination of Pregnancy

Patricia Dalby and Erica Coffin

## Introduction

Termination of pregnancy is one of the most emotionally charged procedures. It is also one of the most commonly performed procedures worldwide. The World Health Organization (WHO) via the Guttmacher Institute estimates that the number of global abortions from 2010 to 2016 averaged 56 million per year. They also report that about 25% of all pregnancies end with induced abortion, yet only about half of these were performed safely. The WHO states that the elimination of unsafe abortions is a major goal. Between 1990 and 2014, the overall number of abortions per 1000 women of childbearing age in developed countries declined from 46 to 27, while in developing countries there was a non-significant change, from 39 to 37 [1].

In 2013, the Centers for Disease Control (CDC) reported that 664,435 termination procedures were performed in the United States (US). Not included in the report were the states of California, Maryland, Louisiana and West Virginia, indicating that the actual numbers are significantly higher.

The CDC also reports 12.5 induced abortions per 1000 women of childbearing age (between the ages of 15–44) and an abortion ratio of 200 per 1000 live births [2]. According to Guttmacher, the US abortion rate in 2014 was only 14.6 abortions per 1000 women of childbearing age, down 14% from 2011, and the lowest abortion rate ever seen in the US. The year abortion became legal, in 1973, the rate was 16.3 per 1000 live births [3].

The findings from a new study by the Guttmacher Institute and the WHO found that between 1990 and 2014, the overall number of abortions per 1000 women of childbearing age (15–44 years old) in developed countries dropped from 46 to 27, while in developing countries, it changed little, from 39 to 37, a non-significant difference. The study's findings appear in an article, "Abortion incidence between 1990 and 2014: global, regional, and sub-regional levels and trends," by Gilda Sedgh et al., published in The Lancet [4, 5]. This unfortunate trend for developing countries and those with philosophical barriers to abortion, have become the major thrust of the WHO to develop educational materials, a web site, personnel for logistical aide, and a Clinical Practical Handbook for Safe Abortion since 2003 [6].

In the US, the trend has been for termination of pregnancy procedures to be performed earlier in pregnancy, as well as for the increased use of non-surgical (i.e. medical techniques). Currently, an estimated 15% of first term (less than 9 weeks gestational age) abortion procedures in the US are medically induced. The medications most

P. Dalby, M.D. (✉) · E. Coffin, M.D.
Department of Anesthesia, Magee-Womens Hospital of UPMC, Pittsburgh, PA, USA
e-mail: dalbypl@anes.upmc.edu; dalbypl@upmc.edu

commonly used are mifepristone and misoprostol with or without methotrexate. These early medical abortions may still be followed by surgical procedures if the uterine evacuation is incomplete.

Gestational age, the reason for termination (medical necessity or elective), and the facility in which the procedure is performed influence both the choice of anesthetic and procedural technique. We will discuss the preoperative considerations for pregnancy termination, the procedures, the potential early and late complications, and the post-abortion considerations and care. Finally, we will discuss the associated anesthesia controversies. See Table 54.1.

**Table 54.1** Anesthesia for termination of pregnancy

| Pregnancy termination: method and GA | Anesthetic plan/preparation | Reasoning and management | Possible adverse events |
|---|---|---|---|
| Medical termination (49 to 63 days gestation) | 1. Preoperative evaluation<br>2. Ultrasound evaluation<br>3. Pharmacotherapy | 1. Oral analgesics: NSAIDs<br>2. Oral opioid analgesics<br>Sequential hCG to prove termination | 1. Continued pregnancy<br>2. Retained POC<br>3. Growth of pregnancy requiring surgery |
| Surgical terminations | | | |
| First trimester (up to 13 weeks GA) Suction dilation and curettage (D&C) | 1. Preoperative evaluation<br>2. Ultrasound evaluation<br>3. ± Intravenous access<br>4. Type and screen<br>5. Antibiotic prophylaxis | Anesthesia type:<br>1. Local anesthetic paracervical block only<br>2. Conscious IV sedation with paracervical block<br>Sequential hCG to prove termination<br>Rhogam if indicated | 1. Continued pregnancy<br>2. Retained POC<br>3. Uterine perforation<br>4. Cervical laceration<br>5. Bleeding<br>6. Endometritis |
| Second trimester (14–22 weeks GA) dilation and evacuation (D&E) | 1. Preoperative evaluation and lab<br>2. Ultrasound evaluation<br>3. Intravenous access (large bore)<br>4. Perform in institution with surgical resources<br>5. Type and screen<br>6. Antibiotic prophylaxis | Anesthesia type:<br>1. Moderate to deep IV sedation with paracervical block<br>Rhogam if indicated | 1. Retained POC<br>2. Uterine perforation<br>3. Cervical laceration<br>4. Bleeding (hemorrhage)<br>5. Endometritis<br>6. Embolism (thrombotic or amniotic fluid) |
| Late gestational (greater than 19 weeks GA) dilation, evacuation (D&E) Or induction of labor | 1. Preoperative evaluation (lab)<br>2. Ultrasound evaluation<br>3. Large bore IV access<br>4. Type and screen (cross match if anemic)<br>5. After 22 weeks often indication is severe fetal anomalies or maternal life saving<br>6. Perform in institution with surgical resources or hospital<br>7. ± Fetacide prior to procedure (not in USA)<br>8. Cervical preparation techniques imperative<br>9. Antibiotic prophylaxis | Anesthesia type:<br>1. For D&E deep IV sedation or general anesthesia with paracervical block<br>2. Labor analgesia techniques: IV narcotics, nitrous oxide, epidural analgesia, or CSE<br>Rhogam if indicated | 1. Retained POC<br>2. Uterine perforation<br>3. Cervical laceration<br>4. Bleeding (hemorrhage)<br>5. Endometritis<br>6. Embolism (thrombotic or amniotic fluid) |

*GA* gestational age, *hCG* human chorionic gonadotrophin, *NSAIDs* non-steroidal Anti-inflammatory agents, *POC* products of conception

Most early term abortion procedures take place in freestanding clinics or in doctor's offices. Regulations of these facilities vary by state as to what type of equipment that the facility must have. Same day hospitalization is often required for abortion procedures beyond the first trimester, or for women who have comorbid diseases.

## Preoperative Considerations

A preoperative history and physical is mandatory, and most facilities still require the use of standard American Society of Anesthesia (ASA) preoperative fasting guidelines. The patient should receive counseling about the appropriate choice of procedure, the risks involved, as well as alternatives such as adoption. Some states in the US legally require that specific topics be discussed as part of preoperative counselling or require a waiting period between counselling and the procedure. Likewise, states differ in who can actually give permission for the abortion. Some require parental consent for minors or a court order for medically necessary termination.

Determination of gestational age is paramount prior to termination. It is based on the woman's last menstrual date, the use of bimanual exam or by ultrasound. Ultrasound is not always available in austere environments; however, the use of ultrasound is helpful in determining the location of the placenta in more advanced pregnancies, the existence of uterine anomalies, and coexisting pregnancies [7].

Common laboratory tests include hematocrit or hemoglobin and Rh(D) immunization status. Blood type should be determined if the patient is anemic and has an advanced gestation. If there has been an intrauterine fetal demise then fibrinogen concentration and coagulation tests should be done. Other testing depends on maternal comorbidities.

Antibiotic prophylaxis as a means to avoid post-abortal endometritis is a common practice but the actual antibiotics prescribed are variable. Doxycycline, metronidazole, and azithromycin are the most common antibiotics used. Sexually-transmitted diseases may be screened in the preoperative period or at the time of the procedure [7, 8].

In most cases, cervical ripening is performed when pregnancies have advanced beyond 12 weeks. Prior to 13 weeks of gestation, the most common procedure used for abortion is the suction dilation and curettage (D&C) with or without cervical preparation. Lesser amounts of suction are required for D&C at earlier gestational ages [8].

After 13 weeks, cervical ripening is usually required to assist with cervical dilation. Cervical dilation is accomplished by the use of progressively larger rigid metal dilators until the os is wide enough for evacuation of uterine contents. Adequate cervical preparation decreases the likelihood of cervical tears and uterine perforation during fetal extraction. Cervical preparation should be initiated 6–48 hours prior to the procedure. Osmotic dilators called laminaria absorb cervical moisture and release endogenous prostaglandins to prepare the cervix. The laminaria need to be placed at least 6 hours before the fetal extraction procedure and should not be retained for more than 2 days because of the increased risk for infection. Misoprostol, which is a prostaglandin E1 analogue, will also soften the cervix if placed hours before the procedure. Mifepristone and isosorbide dinitrate have also been used [8]. Fever and nausea are known side effects of all of the above techniques.

## Medication Induced Pregnancy Termination and Analgesia

Medication-induced abortion may be performed until 63 days of gestation. The use of ibuprofen after the onset of uterine cramping improves pain scores and decreases subsequent analgesic use [7]. Other studies have found that non-steroidal anti-inflammatory agents (NSAIDs) were more efficacious for pain from uterine cramping than acetaminophen-containing analgesics [8]. Several studies have demonstrated that there is no significant improvement in pain when a paracervical block is used [9]. Medically induced second trimester pregnancy terminations are more frequent in countries other than the US. Literature concerning analgesia for these terminations has indicated equivalent analgesia utilizing intravenous patient controlled analgesia modalities compared to that of patient controlled epidural analgesia [9, 10].

## Surgery and Anesthesia

### First Trimester Surgically Assisted Pregnancy Termination

Most surgically assisted abortions at this gestational age are achieved by suction dilation and curettage (D & C) under local anesthesia by paracervical block with or without sedation. Sedation medications are generally limited to narcotics with or without mild anxiolytics. Propofol sedation should be performed only by licensed anesthesia personnel. Cervical preparation is not required before 13–14 weeks of gestation, and the amount of suction required is minimal. A 12-gauge cannula is normally used. Most of these procedures are performed in freestanding outpatient centers, so sedation should be minimal to allow the patient to return home the same day and with a responsible companion. The WHO has looked at alternative providers other than physicians to perform these early pregnancy terminations as a way to increase women's access to safe procedures with overall favorable findings, and no measurable increase in complications [11].

### Second Trimester Termination of Pregnancy

There is a definite need for cervical preparation and surgical intervention when the gestational age of the fetus has progressed to the second trimester. These abortions should be performed in a hospital or in a facility associated with a hospital because of the increased risk of complications. Complications include uterine perforation, cervical lacerations, and hemorrhage. There are several surgical techniques used for this procedure: the most common being the standard dilation and evacuation technique (D&E), which can be performed after cervical preparation and cervical dilation to at least 2–3 cm. The procedure is performed in the lithotomy position with removal of dilators and antiseptic preparation of the cervix. A paracervical block is usually placed, the amniotic fluid drained, and ultrasound used to guide the removal of the products of conception (POC). POC removal is accomplished by forceps and followed by a combination of sharp and suction curettage. Suction D&C may also be used for earlier second trimester terminations up to 14–16 weeks, usually without cervical preparation. There are rare reports of prolonged (2–3 days) intact dilation and extraction (D&X) or even the performance of a hysterotomy for late second term terminations. The latter procedure involves surgical laparotomy and general anesthesia. Anesthesia for the first three surgical techniques is usually provided by sedation or general anesthesia combined with a paracervical block. There is some controversy concerning the efficacy of the paracervical block in the second trimester as well as concern for deep sedation in a woman with pregnancy-induced gastrointestinal changes and an unprotected airway [12, 13].

Neuraxial anesthesia (spinal or epidural) has been used for these procedures but without intravenous sedation does not provide any form of fetal anesthesia [14]. Local anesthetics dosages for subarachnoid dosages include: Hyperbaric mepivacaine 45–60 mg (not available in US), lidocaine 45–50 mg, procaine 100 mg, or bupivacaine 7.5–10 mg will provide adequate coverage and duration for the procedure. Transient Neurologic Symptoms (TNS) following ambulatory spinal anesthesia in the lithotomy position, but pregnant patients may be at lower risk of this complication. A dermatomal level at least to T10 is required to ensure coverage of the pain associated with dilation of the cervix. Fentanyl 10–20 μg may be added to deepen the block and reduce the total dose of local anesthetic required (e.g., 30 mg lidocaine or 5.25 mg bupivacaine). Low-dose epidural analgesia has also been reported but has a longer onset time and the risk of a more profound post-dural puncture headache [15]. Ultrasound guidance is becoming the normal procedure for second trimester and late pregnancy terminations to ensure that all of the amniotic fluid and fetal parts have been removed.

In addition, studies have shown that ultrasound reduces the time needed to perform the terminations, complications from the termination, and is a valuable teaching tool [8].

## Late Gestational Age Termination of Pregnancy

Late gestational age termination is defined as pregnancy termination after 22 weeks. This is the most controversial time period concerning abortion. These late terminations are usually performed for severe fetal anomalies or for the sake of preservation of maternal health. In a few countries, outside of the US, feticide is performed so as not produce a live birth [16, 17]. In 2007 the United States Supreme Court upheld the Partial Birth Abortion Ban Act of 2003, and partial birth abortions are no longer performed. Partial birth abortions consist of delivery of a live fetus until half of the fetus is outside of the mother's body. A lethal maneuver is then performed on the fetus prior to complete delivery of the dead infant. The most common obstetrical technique to induce these late terminations is by induction of labor with prostaglandin administration. Anesthesia is provided with common labor analgesia techniques such as intravenous opioids, the use of nitrous oxide inhalation analgesia, continuous epidurals with low dose local anesthetics, or combined spinal epidural techniques.

## Post-abortion Care

The procedure is considered complete after all of the products of conception have been removed and there is no ongoing bleeding. There are some additional issues that should be addressed in this period concerning maternal iso-immunization against fetal blood cells, the provision of medication to prevent bleeding, infection prevention, recovery from anesthesia, and the institution of birth control methods. Concerning the latter, women may receive Depo-Provera, Implanon, or an intrauterine device (IUD) on the day of the procedure. Women are asked to refrain from placing anything in their vagina for a variable period of time, but at least a week after the procedure.

Most practices prescribe antibiotics to all women who have undergone surgical abortion. Analgesics in the form of mild narcotics or non-steroidal anti-inflammatory agents are prescribed for pain. Prophylactic antiemetic medications are offered. Most centers will observe women who have undergone D&E for at least 60 min for signs of bleeding and recovery from anesthesia. The woman is sent home with discharge instructions in the company of a responsible adult. Uterotonic agents are not usually used prophylactically, as there is no data supporting this use, but are prescribed if there is ongoing hemorrhage or uterine atony [7, 18]. Women who are Rh(D)-negative must be given anti-D immune globulin (Rhogam) to prevent problems with future pregnancies.

## Complications of Abortion

Complications associated with surgical termination of pregnancy include amniotic fluid embolism, infection in the form of endometritis or even sepsis, uterine atony, uterine hemorrhage, uterine perforation, cervical or vaginal lacerations, and anesthetic complications. Permanent infertility may result. Complications are unfortunately common if the woman has undergone an unsafe abortion. Deaths associated with legal safe abortions are less than 1 per 100,000; most of these are a result of terminations at more than 13 weeks gestation [19, 20].

Unsafe abortion occurs when a pregnancy is terminated in a suboptimal environment with minimal or no standards, and/or by persons who are inadequately trained to perform the procedure. Approximately 22 million unsafe abortions are performed globally each year, primarily in developing countries. Many of these could have been prevented by sexual education and contraceptive use. It has been estimated that the annual cost of treating major complications from unsafe abortions is $680 million per year; by the WHO [21].

The risk of complications from terminations increases with the gestational age of the fetus.

Early major complications include hemorrhage, cervical laceration, incomplete abortion, and uterine perforation. These complications may require hospitalization, with additional surgery or intensive care, and occur at a rate of 0.06% [7]. Hemorrhage may be mitigated by the use of uterotonic agents, uterine massage and compression, and blood product transfusion. The worst hemorrhage cases may go on to require pelvic embolization procedures, surgical repair, uterine vessel ligation, and even hysterectomy. General anesthesia is required for the correction of most of these complications and should be performed in an inpatient setting. Severe immediate postoperative pain may signal the development of hematomata and will require surgical evacuation.

Delayed complications (occurring more than 72 hours after the termination procedure) include retained products of conception that may cause ongoing vaginal bleeding or infection. Additional surgical procedures may be required with the provision of sedation or general anesthesia for maternal comfort. The possibility of ongoing or concurrent missed pregnancy requires repeat pregnancy tests within 3–5 days to ensure a decrease in serum human chorionic gonadotrophin (hCG) levels. If serum hCG levels remain elevated, additional procedures will be required.

Anesthesia complications can occur in the form of protracted nausea and vomiting after the procedure, airway and dental damage due to airway instrumentation, post-dural puncture headache from neuraxial anesthesia, and, rarely, pulmonary aspiration [22]. The CDC has reported that anesthesia related complications have accounted for 35% of first trimester abortion-related deaths, while hemorrhage, infection and thromboembolism accounted only for 15% [19].

## Controversial Topics Having to Do with Anesthesia Practices for the Medical Termination of Pregnancy

Appropriate anesthesia for a freestanding outpatient setting is controversial. Generally, if the patient requires deep sedation or general anesthesia, then the increased risk for complications necessitates the use of a surgical center with a recovery room and associated hospital. Categories of women that may need more profound anesthesia are the developmentally delayed, very young or immature women, women with a history of sexual abuse, or women with conditions that might make them at risk for uterine injury, such as cervical stenosis or prior uterine scarring [8]. Women who have profound cardiac or pulmonary comorbidities are recommended to receive their procedure in a hospital setting. This is also true for women who are at increased risk for bleeding, such as those with placenta previa, placenta accreta, or women with known uterine abnormalities that may make the procedure difficult such as fibroids or uterine arterial venous fistula [20].

Another controversy surrounds the efficacy and safety of the paracervical local anesthetic block (usually performed by the proceduralist). The paracervical block is widely used as the sole anesthetic for first trimester terminations or in conjunction with many levels of sedation or general anesthesia for more advanced terminations. Several studies have found the impact of the paracervical block to be minimally helpful, if it all, in reducing intraoperative pain or postoperative analgesic use [9, 23]. Vasopressin may be added to the local anesthetic used for the paracervical block to cause vasoconstriction and thereby decrease bleeding. Systemic absorption of vasopressin may cause maternal hypertension. The paracervical block is not a totally benign procedure; intravascular injections from placement of the block have caused subsequent local anesthetic toxicity. Vasovagal syncope with block placement has resulted in profound bradycardia and atropine should be immediately available.

There is concern about the provision of heavy sedation to the parturient population with an unguarded airway and the proper fasting interval before the termination procedure. Several studies have looked at the practice of intravenous sedation without intubation in women up to 18 weeks gestation and found the incidence of perioperative anesthesia complications to be very low [13, 24]. The provision of deep intravenous sedation in obese women has also been studied. These patients may be prone to airway obstruction, however these studies did not find their risk for anesthesia complications to be greater than for non-obese women [25, 26]. Two studies have looked at the liberalization of fasting policies for these procedures up to 18 weeks' gestation and fortunately found very few complications [27, 28].

One other very controversial issue is that of fetal pain. Many anesthesiologists would choose a neuraxial technique in pregnant women who have fetuses of gestational age greater than the first trimester. However, without the provision of systemic medication to the mother, the fetus probably would not receive any analgesia benefit [14].

## Conclusions About Anesthesia Care for Surgical Termination of Pregnancy

A thorough review of a woman's medical and anesthetic history should be used to formulate an individualized anesthetic plan. Informed consent of anesthesia risks must be presented and include a discussion of the potential for blood transfusion. A skilled provider should perform the procedure in the appropriate setting and taking into account the gestational age of the fetus and the comorbidities of the woman. Procedural complications should be anticipated and appropriate preparations made. Planning for outpatient settings should include logistical considerations for urgent or emergent transfer to a facility with extensive medical capabilities.

## References

1. World Health Organization: Media Center, Preventing unsafe abortion Fact sheet, Updated May 2016. http://www.who.int/mediacentre/factsheets/fs388/en/. Accessed 31 Mar 2017.
2. Center for Disease Control 24/7; Reproductive Health Data and Statistics, MMWR: Abortion Surveillance—United States, 2013. https://www.cdc.gov/reproductivehealth/data_stats/. Accessed 31 Mar 2017.
3. May 2016 Fact Sheet: Induced Abortion World Wide Global Incidence and Trends. https://www.gutmacher.org/fact-sheet/induced-abortion-worldwide/. Accessed 31 Mar 2017.
4. Sedgh G, Singh S, Shah IH, et al. Induced abortion: incidence and trends worldwide from 1995 to 2008. Lancet. 2012;379:625–8.
5. Pazol K, Zane SB, Parker WY, et al. Abortion surveillance-United States, 2008. MMWR Surveill Summ. 2011;60:1–5.
6. Rasch V. Unsafe abortion and postabortion care—an overview. Acta Obstet Gynecol Scand. 2011;90:692–700.
7. Steinauer J. Overview of Pregnancy Termination. https://www.uptodate.com/contents/overview-of-pregnancy-termination. Accessed 31 Mar 2017.
8. Prager SW, Oyer DJ. Second-trimester surgical abortion. Clin Obstet Gynecol. 2009;52(2):179–87.
9. Andersson IM, Benson L, Christensson K, Gemzell-Danielsson K. Paracervical block as pain treatment during second-trimester medical termination of pregnancy: an RCT with bupivacaine versus sodium chloride. Hum Reprod. 2016;31(1):67–74.
10. Jackson E, Kapp N. Pain control in first-trimester and second-trimester medical termination of pregnancy: a systemic review. Contraception. 2011;83:116–26.
11. Barnard S, Kim C, Park MH, Ngo C. Doctors or mid-level providers for abortion. Cochrane Database Syst Rev. 2015;7:CD011242.
12. Lazenby GB, Fogelson NS, Aeby T. Impact of paracervical block on postabortion pain in patients undergoing abortion by general anesthesia. Contraception. 2009;80:578–82.
13. Dean G, Jacobs AR, Goldstein RC, Gevirtz CM, Paul ME. The safety of deep sedation without intubation for abortion in the outpatient setting. J Clin Anesth. 2011;23:437–42.
14. Lee SJ, Ralston HJ, Drey EA, et al. Fetal pain: a systematic multidisciplinary review of the evidence. JAMA. 2005;294:947–500.
15. Datta S, Kodali BS, Segal S. Non-delivery obstetric procedures. In: Obstetric anesthesia handbook. New York: Springer; 2010. p. 351–60.
16. Habiba M, Fre MD, Viafora C, et al. The EUROBS Study Group. Late termination of pregnancy: a comparison of obstetricians' experience in eight European countries. BJOG. 2009;116:1240–349.
17. Dibar G, Bemjamou D. Anesthesiologists' practices for late termination of pregnancy: a French national study. IJOA. 2010;19:395–400.
18. Carroll E, Grossman D. Complications from first-trimester aspiration abortion: a systemic review of the literature. Contraception. 2015;92:422–38.
19. Bartlett LA, Berg CJ, Atrash H, et al. Risk factors for legal induced abortion-related mortality in the United States. Obstet Gynecol. 2004;103(4):729–37.
20. Zane S, Creanga AA, Callaghan WM, et al. Abortion-related mortality in the United States 1998–2010. Obstet Gynecol. 2015;126(2):258–65.
21. http://www.who.int/reproductivehealth/topics/unsafe_abortion/magnitude/en/. Accessed 31 Mar 2017.
22. D'Angelo R, Smiley R, Riley ET, Segal S. Serious complications related to obstetric anesthesia—the serious complication repository project of the

society for obstetric anesthesia and perinatology. Anesthesiology. 2014;120:1505–12.
23. Winkler M, Wolters S, Funk A, Rath W. Second trimester abortion with vaginal gemeprost—improvement by paracervical anesthesia? Zentble Gynakol. 1997;119:621–4.
24. Gokale P, Lappen JR, Waters J, Perriera LK. Intravenous sedation without Intubation and the risk of anesthesia complications for obese and non-obese women undergoing surgical abortion: a retrospective cohort study. Anesth Analg. 2016;122:1957–62.
25. Lederle L, Steinauer JE, Kerns JL, et al. Obesity as a risk factor for complication after second trimester abortion by dilation and evacuation. Obstet Gynecol. 2015;126(3):585–92.
26. Murphy LA, Thornburg LL, Betstadt SJ, et al. Complications of surgical termination of second-trimester pregnancy in obese versus non-obese women. Contraception. 2012;86:402–6.
27. Wiebe ER, Byczko B, Kaczorowski J, McLane AL. Can we safely avoid fasting before abortions with low-dose procedural sedation? A retrospective cohort chart review of anesthesia-related complications in 47,748 abortions. Contraception. 2013;87:51–4.
28. Wilson LC, Chen BA, Creinin MD. Low-dose fentanyl and midazolam in outpatient abortion up to 18 weeks of gestation. Contraception. 2009;79:122–8.

# Anesthesia and Hypertensive Emergencies

Oksana Klimkina

## Introduction

Hypertension is defined as a systolic BP (SBP) equal to or above 130 mmHg and diastolic BP (DBP) equal to or above 80 mmHg. It is essential to keep both the SBP and DBP within normal range to support the functions of vital organs. There is strong evidence to support treating hypertensive persons aged 60 years or older to a BP goal of less than 150/90 mmHg and hypertensive persons 30 through 59 years of age to a diastolic goal of less than 90 mmHg [6]. Clinical trials have demonstrated that control of isolated systolic hypertension reduces total mortality, cardiovascular mortality, stroke, and heart failure events [7, 8].

Hypertensive emergencies are characterized by severe elevations in BP >180/120 mmHg complicated by evidence of impending or progressive target organ dysfunction. Patients require immediate BP reduction to prevent or limit target organ damage [9]. Examples of end-organ dysfunction includes acute renal failure, hypertensive encephalopathy, intracranial or subarachnoid hemorrhage, myocardial ischemia or infarction, acute left ventricular dysfunction, acute pulmonary edema, or aortic dissection [10].

Organ dysfunction is not common for DBP <130 mmHg [11].

These emergencies are rarely encountered in the preoperative anesthesia period. In preoperative period, it is important to identify potential risk factors which can cause major intraoperative blood pressure fluctuations. Stimulation of the sympathetic system with initiation of general anesthesia, particularly intubation, can cause significant hypertension. Pain from surgical incision and surgical manipulation as well as discontinuation of antihypertensive drugs before surgery can contribute to intraoperative severe hypertension. Postoperative hypertension is common in patients with essential hypertension. Assessment of adequate analgesia in the postoperative period is necessary together with symptomatic treatment of blood pressure.

## Preoperative Evaluation

Common predictors of perioperative hypertension include a history of hypertension, especially a diastolic blood pressure greater than 110 mmHg, and the type of surgery [12] (Table 55.1). Independent risk factors for mortality following noncardiac surgery include a history of hypertension, a severely limited activity level, and a creatinine clearance of less than 0.83 mL/s [13]. The presence of isolated SBP has been associated with an increase in renal failure or insufficiency, cerebrovascular accident, left ventricular dysfunction,

O. Klimkina
Department of Anesthesiology, College of Medicine, University of Kentucky, Lexington, KY, USA
e-mail: oklim2@uky.edu

and combined adverse outcomes in patients scheduled for elective CABG surgery [14].

Although 90% of patients have idiopathic (essential or primary) hypertension, secondary causes of hypertension such as endocrine tumors, renal, cardiovascular, neurological disease should be considered. The major pathophysiologic causes of hypertension and the perioperative considerations are listed in Table 55.2.

Patients with isolated "white coat" hypertension have not been shown to be at high risk for anesthesia and therefore surgery should not be delayed [9]. Elderly patients with SBP below 160 mmHg should also be considered for surgery, particularly if there is little evidence of end organ damage, as well as patients with episodic hypertension. For patients with chronic hypertension a diastolic BP >80 but <110 mmHg is not considered to be a reason to postpone surgery. One randomized trial demonstrated no benefit for delaying surgery in chronically treated hyperten-

**Table 55.1** Surgical procedures associated with hypertensive emergency

| |
|---|
| Cardiovascular surgery |
| Vascular surgery on aorta and major peripheral vessels (carotid, femoral, renal) |
| Intrathoracic and major abdominal surgeries |
| Craniotomy and intracranial procedures |
| Kidney transplantation and kidney tumor removal |
| Major trauma and severe burns |
| Emergency operation, predominantly in elderly |

**Table 55.2** Etiology of preoperative hypertension

| Etiology of preoperative hypertension | Pathology | Preoperative consideration |
|---|---|---|
| Cardiovascular | Chronic essential hypertension<br>Coarctation of aorta | Continue treatment with chronic antihypertensive drugs Cardiology evaluation |
| Endocrine | Pheochromocytoma<br>Cushing's syndrome/other glucocorticoid excess states<br>Hyperthyroidism<br>Primary hyperaldosteronism and other mineralocorticoid excess states | Medical treatment before surgery with Phenoxybenzamine<br>If surgery non-emergent consider delay and further evaluation<br>Postpone surgery until the patient is euthyroid<br>If surgery non-emergent consider cancellation and further evaluation |
| Renal | Renovascular hypertension (most common cause of secondary hypertension)<br>Chronic kidney disease<br>End Stage Renal Disease<br>Kidney stone | Possible surgical correction or stenting, continue chronic medications<br>Continue chronic medications<br>Consider hemodialysis before surgery if appropriate<br>Control pain/consider urinary tract obstruction |
| Neurological | Increased intracranial pressure<br>Spinal cord injury with autonomic hyperreflexia<br>Familial dysautonomia | Neurosurgical evaluation, consider TIVA<br>Consider neuraxial anesthesia<br>Identify and attempt to remove stressful triggers |
| Obstructive Sleep Apnea | Sodium retention and resistance to antihypertensive therapy | Consider corrective therapy and devices |
| Pregnancy | Preeclampsia | Consult obstetrician, consider regional anesthesia and fetal monitoring if appropriate |
| Pharmacological cause | Withdrawal of antihypertensive medications<br>Clonidine<br>β-blockers<br>Oral contraceptives<br>Chemotherapy drugs | Restart medication/give IV dose<br>Clonidine patch/IM Clonidine<br>β-blocker IV dose (if appropriate)<br>Symptomatic treatment |

sive patients with well-controlled hypertension who presented for noncardiac surgery with DBP between 110 and 130 mmHg and who have had no previous myocardial infarction (MI), unstable or severe angina pectoris, renal failure, pregnancy-induced hypertension, LV hypertrophy, previous coronary revascularization, aortic stenosis, preoperative dysrhythmias, conduction defects or stroke [15]. With fast acting intravenous agents, blood pressure can be quickly controlled.

Patients on chronic antihypertensive therapy should continue their medications before surgery, including the morning of surgery, as it may contribute to fewer intraoperative blood pressure fluctuations [9, 16]. Sudden discontinuation of certain medications (β-blockers, clonidine) was associated with considerable rebound hypertension and risk for perioperative uncontrolled hypertension. Clonidine withdrawal syndrome can simulate the hypertensive crisis of pheochromocytoma, and can result in hypertension, headache, agitation, and tremor. If this cause identified, symptoms can be treated with intramuscular clonidine or with labetalol and methyldopa.

Discontinuation of angiotensin-converting enzyme (ACE) inhibitors and angiotensin receptor blockers (ARBs) on the day of surgery to prevent intraoperative hypotension is usualy recommended. In some studies they have been shown to potentiate the hypotensive effects of anesthetic agents, even data remained inconsistent [17]. The latest 2014 Guideline from the American College of Cardiology and American Heart Association on Perioperative Cardiovascular Evaluation and Management of Patients Undergoing Noncardiac Surgery recommended perioperative continuation of ACE inhibitors and ARBs [18]. Recently published international prospective cohort study found that "withholding ACE inhibitors and ARBs before major noncardiac surgery was associated with a lower risk of death and postoperative vascular events", and the authors of the study recommended to withhold this medications 24 h before surgery [19].

The utility of perioperative β-blocker therapy remains controversial. Beta blockers should be continued in patients undergoing surgery who have been on beta blockers chronically and in the absence of bradycardia or hypotension. β-blockers may be prescribed to the patients with known ischemic heart disease and are at a high risk for perioperative MI, however, therapy should not be started on the day of surgery. This recommendation endorsed by 2014 Guideline on Perioperative Cardiovascular Evaluation and Management of Patients Undergoing Noncardiac Surgery [18]. The optimal timing of initiation and dose of perioperative β-blockade is uncertain, and prospective trials are necessary. However, it is reasonable to begin therapy more than a week before surgery to determine safety and tolerability [20].

In the preoperative setting, patients who present with SBP >180 mmHg or DBP >120 mmHg without end-organ damage and without history of essential or secondary hypertension, should be evaluated. Incidental hypertensive findings may indicate long standing untreated hypertensive disease. In order to establish this several blood pressure measurements should be taken with an appropriately sized cuff. Elective surgery should be postponed and management of patient transferred to primary care team.

When emergent surgery is necessary, uncontrolled blood pressure should be treated to prevent damage of vital organs and limit bleeding. These patients may benefit from regional anesthetic techniques to avoid the risks of general anesthesia.

## Intraoperative Hypertensive Emergencies

Intraoperative severe elevation of blood pressure frequently requires emergent management. Sympathetic activation during the induction of anesthesia and intubation can cause the blood pressure to rise by 20–30 mmHg and the heart rate to increase by 15–20 beats per minute even in normotensive individuals [21]. This response may be more pronounced in patients with untreated hypertension in whom the SBP can increase by 90 mmHg and heart rate by 40 beats per minute. The mean arterial pressure under anesthesia usually decreases secondary to direct effects of the anesthetic, inhibition of the sympathetic nervous system, and loss of the baroreceptor reflex control of arterial pressure. Even small blood pressure elevations during surgery can result in increased risk of post-operative mortality and renal failure, especially during cardiovascular procedures [22]. Significant hypertensive episodes are encountered more frequently during carotid surgery, followed by surgeries involving the abdominal aorta, peripheral vascular procedures, and major abdominal and thoracic surgery (Table 55.1). Patients with chronic hypertension more prone to intraoperative blood pressure fluctuations. DBP greater than110 mmHg immediately before surgery is associated with a number of complications including dysrhythmias, myocardial ischemia and infarction, neurologic complications, and renal failure [21]. Acute intraoperative BP changes and associated physiologic stress with surgical procedures may contribute to adverse perioperative cardiovascular events, including cardiac death, nonfatal myocardial infarction, and nonfatal cardiac arrest [23].

Hypertensive episodes that occur after tracheal intubation, surgical incision and surgical stimulation usually be treated with increasing the depth of anesthesia or administering an opioidor antihypertensive drugs. Causes of hypertension as endobronchial intubation, hypercarbia (hypoventilation, soda lime exhaustion, inadequate fresh gas flow), light anesthesia due to failure to deliver anesthetic agent should be promptly excluded [24]. An inappropriate size of blood pressure cuff, erroneous position and calibration of the arterial line transducer should be also considered as causes of intraoperative hypertension.

The most effective management of crisis is prevention. A thorough history, including the evaluation of the patient's data, type and duration of surgical intervention, presence of preoperative primary or secondary hypertension, can help establish the intraoperative target for blood pressure control. Potential intraoperative sources of hypertensive emergency and possible complications are presented in Table 55.3.

**Table 55.3** Intraoperative causes and complications of hypertensive crisis

| Cause/complication | Symptoms | Emergent treatment | Comments |
|---|---|---|---|
| Acute ischemia, myocardial infarction, congestive heart failure | Hypertension followed by hypotension, tachycardia, arrhythmia, ECG changes with ST depression/elevation, acute pulmonary edema, cardiac arrest | NTG, β-blockers for pressure and heart rate control, if appropriate Inotropic support if indicated | Avoid β-blockers in acute CHF, particularly with low ejection fraction Consider invasive monitoring, TEE |
| Acute aortic dissection | Hypertension, tachycardia, ST segment changes on ECG if dissection propagates retrograde to coronary arteries | NTG, SNP, and Esmolol for BP and HR control to prevent propagation of dissection Goal is to decrease force of LV contraction | Vasodilators may cause reflex tachycardia Consider invasive monitoring, TEE |
| Autonomic hyperreflexia | Hypertension, bradycardia, arrhythmias, pulmonary edema, myocardial ischemia, possible cerebral hemorrhage | Increase depth of anesthesia, α-adrenergic blockers, direct vasodilators, SNP | Consider neuraxial block before surgery |
| Thyroid storm | Hypertension, tachycardia, hyperpyrexia | Esmolol infusion, cooling, hydration, IV Propranolol | Consider Propylthiouracil by NG tube |
| Pheochromocytoma | Severe hypertension which may be resistant to SNP and NTG Severe bradycardia or severe tachycardia, arrhythmia, myocardial ischemia | SNP, NTG, Phentolamine, Fenoldopam, Nicardipine, Labetatol with caution | Unopposed α-adrenergic stimulation following injection of β-blockers can induce vasospasm and potentiate HTN Consider neuroaxial block before surgery and invasive BP monitoring |

| Cause/complication | Symptoms | Emergent treatment | Comments |
|---|---|---|---|
| Carcinoid crisis | Profound flushing, bronchospasm, tachycardia, and broad fluctuation in blood pressure | α-adrenergic blockers, Labetalol | Hypertension can be resistant to conventional therapy, consider IV boluses of Octreotid |
| Cocaine abuse | Hypertension, tachycardia, arrhythmia, coronary spasm following by cardiac ischemia, rare pulmonary hemorrhage | NTG, Phentolamine Labetalol is controversial | Unopposed α-adrenergic stimulation following injection of selective β-blockers can induce vasospasm and potentiate HTN Consider regional anesthesia for surgery |
| Intracranial hemorrhage | Hypertension greater than 160/90 mmHg Symptoms depend on degree of brain damage, mass effect and increased ICP May be diagnosed in early postoperative period | If suspected, treatment of hypertension should be aggressive to prevent extent of bleeding SNP, Esmolol, Labetalol Hydralazine Nicardipine | Evaluate coagulation status Consider to monitor ICP if appropriate Vascular neurosurgery may be needed for temporary occlusion of bleeding vessel |
| Significant surgical stimulation | Extreme surgical traction, excessive gas insufflations, pressure on tissues and organs causing severe hypertension and tachycardia Prolonged tourniquet time | Stop stimulation until blood pressure is controlled Consider tourniquet deflation, watch time of tourniquet inflation | |

Abbreviations: *NTG* nitroglycerin, *SNP* sodium nitroprusside, *CHF* congestive heart failure, *TEE* transesophageal echocardiography, *ICP* intracranial pressure, *NG* nasogastric tube

## Pharmacological Management of Intraoperative Hypertension

Antihypertensive pharmacological treatment for hypertensive emergency should be started after other reversible causes of rapidly increased BP have been excluded. These include pain, hypoxia, hypercarbia, agitation, bladder distension, excessive surgical stimulation, and hypervolemia. Appropriate analgesia and sedation should be considered before initiation of antihypertensive therapy. Volume status should be assessed as intravascular volume depletion can increase sympathetic activity [22]. The choice of drug will depend on the clinical presentation, underlying cause, presence of side effects or contraindications and pharmacological properties. The ideal agent for treatment of hypertensive emergencies should be fast acting, easily titratable, predictable, safe and accessible. Pharmacotherapy for hypertensive crisis involves a wide variety of agents with different mechanisms of action and pharmacologic properties.

Intravenous drugs for acute management of hypertensive emergency, mechanism of action and adverse effects are presented in Table 55.4.

## Special Considerations

In the acute setting, the treatment goal is to decrease blood pressure by no more than 25% [9]. Advancing these guidelines, Varon and Marik [25] suggested the immediate goal of therapy in hypertensive emergencies to reduce DBP by 10–15%, or to approximately 110 mmHg, over a period of 30–60 min. Sodium and volume depletion can be significant, and gentle volume expansion with IV saline solution will serve to restore organ perfusion and prevent an rapid decline in blood pressure during antihypertensive treatment. This goal decreases the likelihood of over aggressive control, which may result in target organ

**Table 55.4** Intravenous drugs for acute management of hypertensive emergency

| Drug | Mechanism of action | Dose/time of action | Adverse effects |
|---|---|---|---|
| Sodium Nitroprusside | **Nitrovasodilator** Donator of NO | 0.3–0.5 mcg/kg/min infusion with max dose of 8–10 mcg/kg/min Onset of action is 1–2 min, plasma half-life is 3–4 min | Decrease coronary, renal, cerebral perfusion May increase ICP Cyanide toxicity with large doses and prolong usage Avoid in pregnancy, and in patients with hepatic or renal insufficiency |
| Nitroglycerine | **Nitrovasodilator** Donator of NO Produces more venous than arterial dilation | 0.5–1 mcg/kg/min infusion with max dose 100 mcg/min Onset of action is 3–5 min, plasma half-life is 2–7 min | Can cause reflex tachycardia, may increase ICP Methemoglobinemia reported if used >24 h |
| Esmolol | **Adrenergic inhibitor** Selective β1-blocker | Loading dose 0.5–1 mg/kg, then 50–300 mcg/kg/min infusion Onset of action is 1–2 min, plasma half-life is 9 min | May cause hypotension, bradycardia Avoid for patients with greater than first degree heart block, CHF, bronchospasm |
| Labetalol | **Adrenergic inhibitor** Selective α1 and nonselective β-blocker | Loading dose 20 mg, with boluses 20–80 mg q 10 min with max dose 300 mg. Infusion rate 0.5–2 mg/min Onset of action is 2–5 min, plasma half-life is 5–8 h | May cause hypotension Avoid for patients with greater than first degree heart block, CHF, COPD, asthma |
| Phentolamine | **Adrenergic inhibitor** Nonselective α-blocker | Bolus 5–20 mg IV, repeat every 5–15 min if needed Onset of action is 1–2 min, plasma half-life when given IV is 19 min | Drug used to treat hypertensive emergency related to catecholamine excess May cause prolonged hypotension, tachycardia, cardiac arrhythmias |
| Nicardipine | **Calcium Channel Blocker** Dihydropyridine | 5–15 mg/h IV infusion Onset of action is 5–20 min, plasma half-life is 45 min to 14 h with long term infusion | Contraindicated for patients with severe aortic stenosis May cause significant reduction in diastolic BP |
| Clevidipine | **Calcium Channel Blocker** Dihydropyridine | 2–16 mg/h IV infusion Onset of action is 2–4 min, plasma half-life is 1–15 min | Contraindicated for patients with egg or soy allergy, defective lipid metabolism and severe aortic stenosis |
| Fenoldopam | **Dopamine D1-receptor selective agonist** | 0.1 mcg/kg/min infusion with max dose 1.6 mcg/kg/min Onset of action is 4–5 min, plasma half-life is 5 min | Caution in patient with glaucoma or increased intraocular pressure May cause hypokalemia |
| Hydralazine | **Direct vasodilator** | 10 mg IV bolus with max dose 40 mg Onset of action is 5–20 min, plasma half-life is 2–4 h | Can cause reflex tachycardia, ischemia in patient with CAD, increase ICP Avoid in patients with dissecting aneurysms |

hypoperfusion. Patients with chronic hypertension have cerebral and renal perfusion autoregulation shifted to a higher range. The brain and kidneys are particularly prone to hypoperfusion if blood pressure is lowered too rapidly [25].

There are some emergent situation when blood pressure should be treated more assertively.

## Aortic Dissection

Aortic dissection with hypertension is associated with a 1-year mortality rate of 70–90% and a 5-year mortality rate of nearly 100%. In aortic dissection target organ damage occurs in the form of retrograde dissection into the heart, involvement of aortic branches, and endothelial injury [23]. If suspected, acute aortic dissection should be treated promptly to reduce SBP to 100–120 mmHg within about 20 min of diagnosis, or to the lowest level without compromise perfusion of target organs (heart, brain, kidney). β-blocker (esmolol) treatment should be initiated first to reduce the force of cardiac contraction, to achieve heart rate of 60–70 beats/min, and control the rate of rise of the aortic pressure (dP/dt), immediately followed by vasodilators (Clevidipine or Sodium Nitroprusside) for emergent control of systemic blood pressure.

## Intracranial Hemorrhage (ICH)

The perioperative course of patients undergoing intracranial procedures is frequently complicated by the incidence of systemic hypertension. Intraoperatively, acute hypertensive episodes may occur during brain manipulation, but more often are produced by events such as administration of epinephrine-containing local anesthetic, head-pin application, periosteal dissection, and emergence. When cerebral autoregulation is disturbed, blood flow passively increases with blood pressure. This in turn can increase intracranial pressure or cause breakdown of the blood–brain barrier with resultant transudation of intravascular fluid. Bleeding and signs of encephalopathy develop. After intracranial surgery, acute hypertension may also increase morbidity and mortality by exacerbating cerebral edema, raising intracranial pressure (ICP) [26]. More than 90% of patients who have ICH have acute hypertension, typically greater than 160/90 mmHg. Elevated blood pressure is associated with expansion of hematoma and poor outcomes. Blood pressure should be reduced aggressively in a controlled fashion to achieve a reduction of blood pressure without compromise of cerebral perfusion.

The guidelines for antihypertensive therapy in patients with acute stroke may be used in the first few hours of treatment of ICH [27]. SNP used for SBP >230 and DBP >140 mmHg, intravenous β-blockers and Diltiazem can be used for SBP >180 but <230 mmHg and DBP >105 but <149 mmHg. Antihypertensive therapy can be postponed if SBP <180 mmHg and DBP <105 mmHg. If ICP monitoring is present, cerebral perfusion pressure should be kept at >70 mmHg (CPP = MAP-ICP).

## Pheochromocytoma

Pheochromocytoma is a tumor arising from chromaffin cells in the adrenal medulla or in other paraganglia of the sympathetic nervous system. Clinical presentation depends on excessive secretion of norepinephrine, epinephrine or dopamine into the circulation. Patients with predominantly norepinephrine-secreting tumors present with hypertension, often severe and refractory to conventional therapy, and patients with predominantly epinephrine- (and dopamine-) secreting tumors present with tachycardia, palpitations, and panic attacks [28]. Preparation for the elective surgery with a diagnosed tumor is well described in literature. It is takes at least 2 weeks of treatment with α-blockers (Phenoxybenzamine or Doxazosin) initiated first followed by β-blockers (Propranolol) started several days before the planned surgical intervention for patients with tachycardia and arrhythmias to prevent hypertension during surgery. It is strongly recommended that β-blockers should never be started before the α-blockers since blockade of vasodilatory peripheral β-adrenergic receptors with unopposed α-adrenergic stimulation can potentiate hypertension.

The intraoperative incidental presentation of the pheochromocytoma represents a significant challenge for anesthesiologists due to severe hypertensive crisis. Blood pressure can dramatically rise at any time during the anesthetic or surgical management (intubation, line placement, incision etc.). Aggressive and immediate BP control needed to prevent life-threatened complications including significant reductions in cardiac output, left ventricular systolic dysfunction, and tachyarrhythmia. Immediate treatment should include increasing the depth of anesthesia, and rapid administration direct arterial vasodilators

(SNP and NTG) to reduce preload. Both drugs have a fast onset of action and are easily titratable. In resistant cases, nicardipine and fenoldopam have been successfully used [29]. To control heart rate, a short-acting β-blocker (esmolol) can be used. Magnesium sulfate has been increasingly used for hemodynamic control during the pheochromocytoma resection. This potent vasodilator inhibits catecholamine release by direct inhibition of their receptors and is a strong calcium antagonist [29].

## Acute Postoperative Hypertension

Acute postoperative hypertension has been defined as an SBP above 190 mmHg and/or DBP above 100 mmHg on two consecutive readings after surgical intervention [22].

Hypertensive episodes may started as soon as 20–30 min in postoperative period and may last up to 2 h [30]. Postoperative hypertension is precipitated by peripheral vasoconstriction, catecholamine release and reduced baroreceptor sensitivity. Hypoventilation, hypoxia, hypercarbia, anxiety and inadequate pain control after anesthesia may grossly contribute to development of hypertensive episodes in this period. Any patient with absence of this risk factors and significant increase of SBP >180 mmHg and DBP >110 mmHg after surgery should be treated with antihypertensive medications to achieve blood pressure level <130/80 mmHg. Patients with untreated hypertension have an increased risk of myocardial ischemia, myocardial infarction, arrhythmias, pulmonary edema, cerebrovascular accidents, and risk of bleeding [22]. Myocardial ischemia most commonly occurs in the postoperative period and may present hours to days after the surgical procedure. There are no strong recommendations for choice of antihypertensive drugs in the postoperative period; however, common drug classes include β-blockers (esmolol, labetalol) and calcium channel blockers (nicardipine). Patients on chronic antihypertensive therapy should resume their usual medication when it is appropriate. For those who are not able to take oral medication, a corresponding intravenous dose should be chosen.

## References

1. World Health Organization. Global status report on Non-communicable diseases 2010. Geneva: World Health Organization; 2011; http://www.who.int/nmh/publications/ncd_report_full_en.pdf.
2. Sung Sug (Sarah) Yoon; Cheryl D. Fryar; Margaret D. Carroll. Hypertension Prevalence and Control Among Adults: United States, 2011–2014 NCHS Data Brief No. 220, November 2015.
3. Causes of Death 2008 [online database]. Geneva: World Health Organization. http://www.who.int/healthinfo/global_burden_disease/cod_2008_sources_methods.pdf.
4. Lim SS, Vos T, Flaxman A, Danaei G, et al. A comparative risk assessment of burden of disease and injury attributable to 67 risk factors and risk factor clusters in 21 regions, 1990-2010: a systematic analysis for the Global Burden of Disease Study 2010. Lancet. 2012;380(9859):2224–60.
5. Laslett L. Hypertension. Preoperative assessment and perioperative management. West J Med. 1995;162(3):215–9.
6. James PA, Oparil S, Carter BL, Pharm D, et al. Evidence-based guideline for the management of high blood pressure in adults. Report from the Panel Members Appointed to the Eighth Joint National Committee (JNC 8). JAMA. 2014;311(5):507–20. https://doi.org/10.1001/jama.2013.284427.
7. Kostis JB, Davis BR, Cutler J, Grimm RH Jr, Berge KG, Cohen JD, et al. Prevention of heart failure by antihypertensive drug treatment in older persons with isolated systolic hypertension. SHEP Cooperative Research Group. JAMA. 1997;278:212–6.
8. SHEP Cooperative Research Group. Prevention of stroke by antihypertensive drug treatment in older persons with isolated systolic hypertension. Final results of the Systolic Hypertension in the Elderly Program (SHEP). JAMA. 1991;265:3255–64.
9. Chobanian AV, Bakris GL, Black HR, et al. The seventh report of the Joint National Committee on prevention, detection, evaluation and treatment of high blood pressure. JAMA. 2003;289(19)
10. Aggarwal M, Khan IA. Hypertensive crisis: hypertensive emergencies and urgencies. Cardiol Clin. 2006;24(1):135–46.
11. Varon J. Treatment of acute severe hypertension: current and newer agents. Drugs. 2008;68:283–97.
12. Khuri SF, Daley J, Henderson W, Barbour G, Lowry P, Irvin G, Gibbs J, Grover F, Hammermeister K, Stremple JF, et al. The National Veterans Administration Surgical Risk Study: risk adjustment for the comparative assessment of the quality of surgical care. J Am Coll Surg. 1995;180(5):519–31.

13. Browner WS, Li J, Mangano DT. In-hospital and long-term mortality in male veterans following noncardiac surgery. The Study of Perioperative Ischemia Research Group. JAMA. 1992;268(2):228–32.
14. Aronson S, Boisvert D, Lapp W. Isolated systolic hypertension is associated with adverse outcomes from coronary artery bypass grafting surgery. Anesth Analg. 2002;94(5):1079–84.
15. Weksler N, Klein M, Szendro G, et al. The dilemma of immediate preoperative hypertension: to treat and operate, or to postpone surgery? J Clin Anesth. 2003;15:179–83.
16. Goldberg ME, Larijani GE. Perioperative hypertension. Pharmacotherapy. 1998;18(5):911–4.
17. Wolf A, McGoldrick KE. Cardiovascular Pharmacotherapeutic Considerations in Patients Undergoing Anesthesia. Cardiol Rev. 2011;19(1):12–6.
18. Fleisher LA, et al. 2014 ACC/AHA guideline on perioperative cardiovascular evaluation and management of patients undergoing noncardiac surgery: executive summary. J Am Coll Cardiol. 2014;64(22):e77–137.
19. Roshanov PS, Rochwerg B, Patel A, et al. Withholding versus continuing angiotensin-converting enzyme inhibitors or angiotensin II receptor blockers before noncardiac surgery. Anesthesiology. 2017;126:16–27.
20. Smilowitz NR, Berger JS. Perioperative management to reduce cardiovascular events. Circulation. 2016;133:1125–30.
21. Wolfsthal SD. Is blood pressure control necessary before surgery? Med Clin North Am. 1993;77:349.
22. KM Soto-Ruiz, WF Peacock, J Varon. Perioperative hypertension: diagnosis and treatment. Neth J Crit Care 2011;15(3).
23. Aronson S. Perioperative hypertensive emergencies. Curr Hypertens Rep. 2014;16:448.
24. Paix AD, Runciman WB, Horan BF, Chapman MJ, Currie M. Crisis management during anaesthesia: hypertension. Qual Saf Health Care. 2005;14(3):e12.
25. Varon J, Marik PE. Perioperative hypertension management. Vasc Health Risk Manag. 2008;4(3):615–27.
26. Basali A, Mascha EJ, Kalfas I, Schubert A. Relation between perioperative hypertension and intracranial hemorrhage after craniotomy. Anesthesiology. 2000;93:48–54.
27. Hsieh PC, et al. Current updates in perioperative management of intracerebral hemorrhage. Neurosurg Clin N Am. 2008;19(3):401–14.
28. Prys-Roberts C. Phaeochromocytoma-recent progress in its management. Br J Anaesth. 2000;85:44–57. https://doi.org/10.1093/bja/85.1.44.
29. Ramakrishna H. Pheochromocytoma resection: Current concepts in anesthetic management. J Anaesthesiol Clin Pharmacol. 2015;31(3):317–23.
30. Gal TJ, Cooperman LH. Hypertension in the immediate postoperative period. Br J Anaesth. 1975;47:70.

# Part V

# Neuroanesthesia

# Supratentorial Masses: Anesthetic Considerations

## 56

Marc D. Fisicaro, Amy Shah, and Paul Audu

## Introduction

Brain tumors constitute the majority of neurosurgical pathology that presents for surgery. Tumors vary from benign meningiomas to the aggressive malignant gliomas. Eighty percent of brain tumors are located in the supratentorial fossa, the remaining 20% are located in the posterior fossa.

Neurosurgical anesthesia is a delicate balance between providing adequate cerebral perfusion and optimizing surgical conditions while compensating for underlying neuropathology. Thorough understanding of neurological physiology and how it is affected by anesthetic techniques are imperative for the safe and effective care of the neurosurgical patient.

## Pathophysiology

The brain uses approximately 20% of available oxygen for normal function, making regulation of blood flow and oxygen delivery critical for survival. Cerebral blood flow (CBF) is directly related to cerebral perfusion pressure and carbon dioxide. Cerebral perfusion pressure (CPP) is the difference between the Mean Arterial Pressure (MAP) and Intracranial Pressure (ICP). This pressure gradient drives cerebral blood flow (CBF) and therefore oxygen and metabolite delivery. Autoregulation maintains a constant cerebral blood flow despite changes in cerebral perfusion pressures. Autoregulation is effective between pressures from 50 to 150 mmHg, however, autoregulation can be altered by anesthesia, tumors, bleeding and hypertension. Above and below this limit, autoregulation is lost and cerebral blood flow becomes dependent on mean arterial pressure. When CPP falls below the lower limit of autoregulation, cerebral ischemia occurs. Carbon dioxide content (PaCO2) also directly affects cerebral blood flow, such that hypercapnia causes marked dilation of cerebral arteries and arterioles and increased blood flow, whereas hypocapnia causes constriction and decreased blood flow. Over a range of PaCO2 values of 20–80 mmHg, for each 1 mmHg increase or decrease in PaCO2 there a 3–5% increase or decrease in CBF [1]. Additionally, CPP rises very quickly in response to an increase in the cerebral metabolic rate (CMRO2) as well. Once the CMRO2 diminishes to minimal levels, the CPP is dependent on MAP. CBF <20 mL/100 g/min will cause ischemia unless CPP is restored or CMRO2 is decreased. Patients who undergo neurosurgery have varying intracranial pathologies as well as different systemic diseases. Edema, acidosis, and hypoxia are some of the most common consequences of brain disorders. All of which can impair autoregulation,

M. D. Fisicaro, M.D. (✉) · A. Shah, M.D.
Sydney Kimmel Medical School, Thomas Jefferson University Hospital, Philadelphia, PA, USA

P. Audu, M.D.
Cooper University Medical Center,
Camden, NJ, USA
e-mail: audu-paul@cooperhealth.edu

CO2 reactivity, and CMRO2, highlighting the importance of strict blood pressure control and respiratory management.

Intracranial Pressure is the pressure inside the skull and therefore in the brain and cerebrospinal fluid (CSF). It is kept stable between a range of 7–15 mmHg. The cranium is incompressible and has a fixed volume. The Monro-Kellie hypothesis (Fig. 56.1) states that because the cranium has a fixed volume, the volume of CSF (10%), blood (5%) and brain (85%) must remain constant [2, 3]. The increase in one compartment can only be compensated by decreasing the content of one or both of the remaining two. An increase in ICP is likely to cause severe harm if it rises too high and can become fatal if left untreated. Any increase or decrease in blood flow will directly affect intracranial pressure. Causes of increased ICP include mass effect, generalized brain swelling, increases in venous pressure, obstruction of CSF outflow/absorption, and increased CSF production. In the case of supratentorial tumors, increased intracranial pressure is caused by mass lesion itself and edema of the surrounding brain tissues.

An increase in ICP can cause ischemia by decreasing CPP. As the ICP approaches the level of the mean systemic pressure, cerebral perfusion falls. The physiological response to a fall in CPP is to increase the systemic blood pressure and dilate cerebral blood vessels to increase CBF. This increase in CBF results in increased cerebral blood volume, which in turn increases ICP, lowering CPP further, resulting in a vicious cycle. This results in the widespread reduction in cerebral flow and perfusion, eventually leading to ischemia and brain infarction and ultimately, herniation.

As ICP increases most patients typically present with a headache, nausea, seizures altered mental state, or blurry vision. Retinal hemorrhages indicate a very high ICP. Also, patients with increased ICP may present with altered breathing patterns; an ominous sign. As ICP continues to increase, CBF decreases which cause a systemic sympathetic response that increases MAP and can cause bradycardia and an increased cardiac output known as a Cushing's reflex. This reflex is an attempt to restore cerebral perfusion. However, this response can cause cerebral vasodilation which causes an increase in intracranial volume and pressure which can lead to ischemia or herniation. Tumors and their surrounding vasogenic edema increase the volume of the brain. A decrease in either CSF or blood volume is necessary to compensate, as the brain has itself, limited ability to compensate. Modulation of CBF through hyperventilation and use of intravenous anesthetics is an effective way to manage ICP. Other techniques include 15-degree head elevation to ensure adequate cerebral venous and CSF drainage, as well as the administration of osmotic diuretics such as Mannitol or hypertonic saline. In the setting of intracranial hypertension, diuretics and hypertonic saline increase blood plasma osmolarity which enhances water flow from the brain and spinal cord to interstitial fluid and plasma. Hyperventilation to decrease PaCO2 of the intubated patient is effective for a limited time. A ventricular drain can be placed to drain CSF. Hypotension should be avoided to prevent secondary insults.

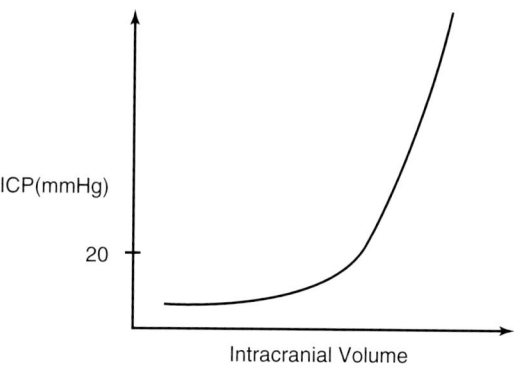

**Fig. 56.1** Relationship between intracranial pressure and intracranial volume

## Preoperative Assessment

Preoperative assessment of patients undergoing craniotomies for tumors is vital. In addition to a complete history and physical examination, a thorough neurological evaluation is necessary for the formulation of an anesthetic plan and safe perioperative patient management. The neurological exam determines the extent and location of the neurologic lesion and its documentation allow for postoperative comparison. The examination should include the patient's level of consciousness and a physical examination to assess the function of the sensory and motor systems and evaluation of cranial nerves. The neurological exam should focus on the presence of increased intracranial pressure. Nausea, somnolence, headaches, and seizures may be signs of increased ICP.

Patients with supratentorial tumors can present with variable symptoms depending on the type of tumor, tumor size, and tumor location. Types of tumors include meningiomas, gliomas, cysts, and epidermoids. During the evaluation of the patient with a supratentorial tumor, it may be helpful to review imaging to ascertain characteristics of the tumor such as vascularity, size, location, and radiologic evidence of increased ICP, such as collapsed ventricles or midline shift.

Any antiplatelet or anticoagulation medications should be noted. In addition, current medications should be obtained, paying special attention to antiepileptics, steroids, antihypertensives, and hypoglycemia agents. The use of prophylactic anticonvulsants for craniotomies in seizure naïve primary brain tumors remains controversial [4]. Currently, there is no recommendation for their use. As with all anesthesia preoperative assessments, an airway examination including head and neck range of motion, history of fusion or trauma, spinal stenosis, and rheumatoid arthritis is required to determine the difficulty of intubation and positioning. Routinely patients should have an electrocardiogram, a complete blood count, basic metabolic panel, coagulation parameters and type and screen done preoperatively. Additional studies may be performed depending on the patient's past medical history.

## Anesthesia for Brain Tumor Surgery

The goal of the anesthesiologist during intracranial surgery is to maintain adequate perfusion and oxygenation to the brain, assist in optimization of surgical conditions for resection, accommodate intraoperative neuromonitoring, and provide rapid emergence to facilitate immediate neurological exam.

In addition to maintaining hemodynamic stability, it is imperative to select an anesthetic technique that will maintain CPP without further increasing ICP. Preoperative anxiolytics for patients are essential. It has been reported in the literature that more than 50% of patients experience anxiety prior to their surgery [5]. But, premedication should carefully be chosen on an individual case basis, as patients with underlying neuropathology may be extremely sensitive to benzodiazepines and opioids. Proper selection of induction and maintenance drugs can achieve this goal. With the exception of ketamine, all intravenous induction agents decrease the cerebral metabolic rate and cerebral blood flow, making them ideal choices for the neurosurgical patient. Opioids are commonly given in conjunction with the Intra Venous (IV) agents to suppress airway reflexes, and to attenuate the hemodynamic response to airway manipulation. As long a mean arterial pressure is maintained, opioids have little effect on cerebral physiologic parameters. Fentanyl, alfentanil, and remifentanil are all used for rapid effect. Remifentanil, an ultrashort-acting opioid, can be used for induction but should be administered by infusion, with or without an initial bolus, to avoid abrupt offset and resultant hypertension and tachycardia. In addition to opioids, intravenous lidocaine is often given to also blunt the response to airway manipulation. Neuromuscular blocking agents (NMBA) are routinely given to facilitate tracheal intubation. NMBA have no effect on neurophysiology. Succinylcholine may be chosen to assist in Rapid Sequence Intubation (RSI). Succinylcholine may transiently increase ICP but this effect can be ameliorated by administering a defasciculating dose of NMBA prior to succinylcholine.

The positioning of patients during craniotomies is often difficult, time consuming and if done improperly can lead to physiologic and pathological consequences. Direct compression of neural soft tissue may result in ischemia and tissue damage. Even low grade stretching of nerves has been shown to cause neuropathy [6, 7]. Supine positioning requires padding of all bony joints, such as elbows, heels, and hands. Extreme head and neck positioning can lead to nerve injury as well as obstruction of jugular venous draining which can lead to increased ICP. Lateral decubitus positioning can cause plexopathy secondary to excessive stretching from arm abduction greater than 90° to external rotation and posterior shoulder displacement. The weight of the chest in the lateral position can compress the lower shoulder and axilla putting pressure on the axillary neurovascular bundle. Placing a chest roll caudal to the dependent axilla can relieve this pressure. Prone positioning can lead to hemodynamic changes such as an increase in systemic vascular resistance and pulmonary vascular resistance and a decrease in stroke volume and cardiac index. Prone positioning increases the risk of blindness due to increased intraocular pressure while lying prone [8]. The position that is fraught with the most complications is the sitting position craniotomy. Some of the serious consequences of this position are pneumocephalus, quadriplegia, peripheral nerve injury and venous air embolism (VAE) [1].

VAE occurs when there is a negative pressure gradient between the right atrium and the veins at the operative site. This negative pressure entrains air into the vasculature. The amount of air entrapped, the rate of its accumulation, and patient's position (when the head is above the level of the heart) determine the severity of the VAE. Even small amounts of venous air can cause serious complications. Consequences of VAE include hypotension, arrhythmias, desaturation, pulmonary hypertension, Cerebro Vascular Accident (CVA), and cardiac arrest. Trans Esopahgeal Echocardiography (TEE) is the most sensitive test for diagnosing a VAE, however, its use can be awkward and cumbersome during sitting craniotomies. Precordial Doppler is the most sensitive non-invasive test. The Doppler is placed on the third intercostal space on the right parasternal. When a VAE occurs it sounds like a continuous machine-like sound. If a VAE is suspected treatment includes hemodynamic support, flooding the surgical field with saline, placing the patient in left lateral decubitus with Trendelenburg positioning to place the surgical site below the level of the heart, 100% oxygen, and an attempt to remove the air with aspiration from a Central Venous Pressure (CVP) line.

The anesthetic technique chosen for maintenance of anesthesia depends on several factors including patients' preexisting medical history, presence and severity of increased intracranial pressure, need for intraoperative surgical monitoring, and the need to optimize the brain relaxation to improve surgical conditions. A balanced anesthetic is often necessary to maintain normal cerebral physiology as volatile inhalational anesthetics can affect cerebral physiology (Table 56.1). Although they

**Table 56.1** Summary of effects of inhalational and intravenous anesthetics

| Anesthetic agent | Cerebral blood flow | Cerebral metabolic rate | Intracranial pressure |
|---|---|---|---|
| Isoflurane | +[a] | − − | +[a] |
| Sevoflurane | +[a] | − − | +[a] |
| Desflurane | +[a] | − − | +[a] |
| Propofol | − − | − − | − − |
| Etomidate | − − | − − | − − |
| Barbituates | − − | − − | − − |
| Ketamine | ++ | + | + |
| Opioids | = | = or − | = |
| Dexmedetomidine | − | = or − | = |
| Benzodiazepines | − | − | = or − |

[a]CBF and ICP do not increase until MAC 1.0

decrease cerebral metabolic rate, they increase cerebral blood flow and can hamper cerebral autoregulation. Also, inhalational agents can interfere with intraoperative neuromonitoring. It is common to use a combination of inhalational agents with or without nitrous oxide supplemented with opioids. For patients with significantly elevated ICP, a total intravenous anesthetic is indicated.

Minimizing hemodynamic fluctuations intraoperatively is essential in maintaining adequate CPP. In extremes of MAP, the brain is unable to compensate for changes in perfusion pressure. Consequently, CBF changes proportionally with changes in mean arterial pressure. This can put the brain tissue at risk for either ischemia- at low perfusion pressures- or edema and/or hemorrhage at high pressures [9]. An appropriate MAP range should be determined for each individual patient based on patient factors- patients' pre-morbid baseline blood pressure, existing co-morbidities and intracranial pathology. Patients suffering from an ischemic stroke, traumatic brain injury or systemic hypertension may have altered cerebral autoregulation [10]. In such patients, the lower limit of cerebral autoregulation was increased [11, 12]. In patients with elevated ICP, it is imperative to increase the MAP to ensure adequate cerebral perfusion.

Normovolemia aids in maintaining adequate cerebral perfusion pressure. Too much fluid can cause cerebral edema and too little can decrease cerebral perfusion pressure and cause systemic hypotension. The goal is therefore to maintain an even fluid balance. If mannitol is given to improve operative conditions, fluids should be administered to match urine output with proper adjustments made to compensate for bleeding. Crystalloid solutions are preferred over colloid; albumin has been shown to worsen long-term outcomes in traumatic brain injuries [13].

It is not uncommon to administer diuretics such as mannitol or furosemide or steroids such as dexamethasone to improve surgical conditions. Hyperventilation to a $PaCO_2$ of 30–35 mmHg can also help for a limited time. The brain can become "tight" or swell during the procedure. It may be necessary to relax or "shrink" the brain to avoid ischemia due to swelling and mechanical retraction. By reducing cerebral edema surgeons are able to operate without using excessive retraction and lessen local areas of ischemia. Sometimes it may be imperative to aggressively diurese patients intraoperatively for better surgical conditions but it can lead to hyponatremia, hypokalemia, and serum osmolarity imbalance.

Intraoperative electroencephalography (EEG) and evoked potential monitoring during craniotomy may be used depending on the location of the tumor. At higher concentrations, inhalational agents may interfere with neuromonitoring. In this case, a mixed IV and inhalational technique or Total Intra Venous Anesthesia (TIVA) may be chosen. If motor evoked potentials are to be monitored, NMBA should be avoided.

Following intracranial neurosurgery, rapid emergence from general anesthesia is the goal. It is imperative that the patient cooperates with a neurologic exam soon after the surgery is completed to evaluate the patient for possible postoperative complications such as hematoma, herniation, cerebral edema, or ischemia [14]. The effects of residual anesthesia may complicate the clinical picture and delay the diagnosis and treatment of a developing intracranial pathology. Delayed emergence may result in unnecessary medical testing such as emergency Computerised Tomogram (CT) scan or cerebral angiogram. Also, the lingering effects of general anesthesia can place these patients at increased risk for aspiration, airway obstruction, hypoxia, and hypercapnia. Such secondary injuries in a patient with neurological pathology can be devastating [14].

Emergence times from anesthesia vary. Individual patient differences can account for a wide range of emergence times. Reported mean times to awakening and orientation range from 8 to 61 min [15]. Although the clinical definition of delayed emergence may vary, difficulty awakening after 15 min from the cessation of general anesthesia has been accepted as prolonged awakening [14]. The causes of delayed awakening can be divided into several categories; drug factors, neurologic factors, and metabolic factors. The most common reason for delayed awakening after craniotomy is considered to be effects of drugs or anesthetics. These include anesthetic adjuncts, premedication, and opioids. After the lingering effects of general anesthesia have been ruled out, other factors that independently cause delayed emergence must be investigated. These factors are age, metabolic abnormalities, and epilepsy.

Although rapid emergence from anesthesia is beneficial, it is not without risks. Recovery from anesthesia is a time of tremendous physiological stress for the patient. Postoperative physiologic stress can be caused by pain, hypothermia, discomfort secondary to the endotracheal tube, or external stimulation during awakening [16]. All of these contribute to increased oxygen consumption, heart rate, and blood pressure. Hypertension can be the most dangerous of these side effects. The occurrence of emergence hypertension has been reported to be as high as 90% in neurosurgical patients [17]. The most serious consequence of postoperative hypertension is the formation of an intracranial hematoma, cerebral edema, and emergence delirium [18]. To avoid and treat postoperative hypertension, intravenous antihypertensive agents should be readily available. These include esmolol, labetalol, and nicardipine. In a study comparing labetalol and nicardipine for the control of emergence hypertension after craniotomy, the nicardipine-treated group experienced a higher incidence of hypotension and tachycardia than the labetalol group. The combination of diltiazem and nicardipine is effective, with the advantage of inducing less tachycardia than nicardipine alone [19].

In addition to postoperative hypertension, emergence can be associated with other side effects. The best way to manage early emergence is to properly prepare. First, hypothermia needs to be avoided as it causes shivering which will then cause an increase in oxygen consumption cardiac output and blood pressure [16]. To avoid postoperative shivering, efforts should be taken throughout the case to maintain normothermia, such as forced air heat and maintaining room temperature. Next, patient's pain needs to be well controlled. Pain is also associated with increased heart rate, blood pressure, and oxygen consumption. Short-acting opioids such as remifentanil have been used to promote rapid emergence from anesthesia, but they have caused an increase in postoperative hypertension, most likely due to the lack of postoperative analgesia [16]. A low dose fentanyl infusion has been shown to be an effective technique for achieving the early awakening after craniotomy and prevention of emergence hypertension [20]. Nausea and vomiting are also common after intracranial surgery. A prophylaxis against postoperative nausea and vomiting is often indicated. Ondansetron is safe and has few side effects but is only partially effective. Droperidol may also be used and it is both safe and effective, but repeated doses may cause sedation.

Despite the use of short-acting anesthetics such as propofol and remifentanil, emergence in the neurosurgical patient may not be rapid. The differential diagnosis of a protracted emergence can be long, but it is imperative that a diagnosis is made quickly to ensure proper treatment.

The most common cause of delayed emergence from general anesthesia remains medications and anesthetic agents. Pharmacological effects depend on dose, absorption, distribution, metabolism, excretion and context sensitive half-life of a drug. Emergence from volatile agent anesthesia depends upon pulmonary elimination of the drug and Minimum Alveolar Concentration (MAC). Pulmonary elimination is determined by alveolar ventilation. Alveolar hypoventilation delays recovery from anesthetic agents by lengthening the time taken to exhale the volatile agent [21]. Extremes of age have an effect on the duration of drugs that affect the central nervous system such as anesthetics, opioids, and benzodiazepines. It has been suggested that total dose and recovery time from intravenous anesthesia (propofol and remifentanil) are more determined by patient age than by body weight [22]. In addition to an increased sensitivity, older patients tend to have a slower circulation time and decreased creatinine clearance which can also increase the duration of action of drugs. Close monitoring of depth of anesthesia and neuromuscular blockade, avoidance of benzodiazepines, and the substitution of non-steroidal analgesic agents should all be considered as preventive of prolonged sedation in geriatric patients [23]. Residual neuromuscular blockade results in paralysis which may be perceived as unresponsiveness though the patient is conscious and aware. A large number of pharmacological interactions with neuromuscular blocking agents prolong neuromuscular block, by interfering with calcium, a second messenger involved in acetylcholine release. Benzodiazepines are used for anxiolysis and premedication, co-induction facilitates the hypnotic and sedative properties of other agents. Benzodiazepines potentiate the central nervous system depressant effects of anesthetic and analgesic drugs and may delay emergence from anesthesia. Benzodiazepines combined with high dose opioids can have a pronounced effect on respiratory depression, producing hypercapnia and coma [21].

Certain underlying metabolic disorders such as hypoglycaemia, severe hyperglycaemia, electrolyte imbalance especially hyponatremia, hypoxia, hypercapnia, central cholinergic syndrome, chronic hypertension, liver disease, hypoalbuminemia, uremia and severe hypothyroidism may also be responsible for delayed recovery after anesthesia.

Severe hypothermia may lead to reduced conscious level. A core temperature of less than 33 °C has a marked anesthetic effect itself and will potentiate the Central Nervous System (CNS) effects of anesthetic drugs. In addition, hypothermia reduces the MAC value of inhalational agents, antagonises muscle relaxant reversal and limits drug metabolism. The direct hypothermic effects on brain tissue are compounded by the cardiovascular and respiratory disturbance at less profound degrees of hypothermia. Cardiac output decreases with a decrease in temperature and cardiac arrhythmias may occur. Low cardiac output affects circulation and drug pharmacokinetics as well as tissue perfusion [21].

Once the above causes are ruled out, it is then necessary to evaluate the patient for neurological factors that may be contributing to delayed emergence. Cerebral hypoxia will result in a reduced level of consciousness and may first present itself as delayed emergence.

# References

1. Gracia I, Fabregas N. Craniotomy in sitting position: anesthesiology management. Curr Opin Anesthesiol. 2014;27(5):474–83.
2. Kumaresan A, Kasper E, Bose R. Anesthetic management of supratentorial tumors. Int Anesthesiol Clin. 2015;53(1):74–86.
3. Mokri B. The Monro–Kellie hypothesis applications in CSF volume depletion. Neurology. 2001;56(12):1746–8.
4. Sayegh ET, Fakurnejad S, Oh T, Bloch O, Parsa AT. Anticonvulsant prophylaxis for brain tumor surgery: determining the current best available evidence: a review. J Neurosurg. 2014;121(5):1139–47.
5. Perks A, Chakravarti S, Manninen P. Preoperative anxiety in neurosurgical patients. J Neurosurg Anesthesiol. 2009;21(2):127–30.
6. Nilsson UG. Intraoperative positioning of patients under general anesthesia and the risk of postoperative pain and pressure ulcers. J Perianesth Nurs. 2013;28(3):137–43.
7. Dawson DM, Krarup C. Perioperative nerve lesions. Arch Neurol. 1989;46(12):1355–60.
8. Kamel I, Barnette R. Positioning patients for spine surgery: avoiding uncommon position-related complications. World J Orthop. 2014;5(4):425.
9. Lassen NA. Cerebral blood flow and oxygen consumption in man. Physiol Rev. 1959;39(2):183–238.
10. Czosnyka M, Smielewski P, Piechnik S, Steiner LA, Pickar JD. Cerebral autoregulation following head injury. J Neurosurg. 2001;95(5):756–63.
11. Schwarz S, Georgiadis D, Aschoff A, Schwab S. Effects of induced hypertension on intracranial pressure and flow velocities of the middle cerebral arteries in patients with large hemispheric stroke. Stroke. 2002;33(4):998–1004.
12. Strandgaard S. Autoregulation of cerebral blood flow in hypertensive patients. The modifying influence of prolonged antihypertensive treatment on the tolerance to acute, drug-induced hypotension. Circulation. 1976;53(4):720–7.
13. SAFE Study Investigators, Australian and New Zealand Intensive Care Society Clinical Trials Group, Australian Red Cross Blood Service, George Institute for International Health, Myburgh J, Cooper DJ, Finfer S, Bellomo R, Norton R, Bishop N, Kai Lo S, Vallance S. Saline or albumin for fluid resuscitation in patients with traumatic brain injury. N Engl J Med. 2007;357(9):874.
14. Schubert A, Mascha E, et al. Effect of cranial surgery and brain tumor size on emergence from anesthesia. Anesthesiology. 1996;85:513–21.

15. From RP, Warner DS, Todd MM, Sokol MD. Anesthesia for craniotomy: a double blind comparison of alfentinal, fentanyl, and sufentanil. Anesthesiology. 1990;73:896–904.
16. Bruder NJ. Awakening management after neurosurgery for intracranial tumours. Curr Opin Anaesthesiol. 2002;15(5):477–82.
17. Muzzi DA, Black S, Losasso TJ, Cucchiara RF. Labetalol and esmolol in the control of hypertension after intracranial surgery. Anesth Analg. 1990;70:68–71.
18. Basali A, Mascha EJ, Kalfas I, Schubert A. Relation between perioperative hypertension and intracranial hemorrhage after craniotomy. Anesthesiology. 2000;93:48–54.
19. Kross R, Ferri E, Leung D, et al. A comparative study between a calcium channel blocker (nicardipine) and a combined alpha-beta-blocker (labetalol) for the control of emergence hypertension during craniotomy for tumor surgery. Anesth Analg. 2000;91:904–9.
20. Bhagat H, Dash HH, Bithal PK, Chouhan RS, Pandia MP. Planning for early emergence in neurosurgical patients: a randomized prospective trial of low-dose anesthetics. Anesth Analg. 2008;107(4):1348–55.
21. Sarangi S. Delayed awakening from anesthesia. Internet J Anaesthesiol. 2009;19(1).
22. Herminghaus A, Löser S, Wilhelm W. Anesthesia for geriatric patients: Part 2: anesthetics, patient age and anesthesia management. Anaesthesist. 2012;61(4):363–74.https://doi.org/10.1007/s00101-012-1985-5.
23. Frost E. Differential diagnosis of delayed awakening from general anesthesia: a review. Middle East J Anaesthesiol. 2014;22(6):537–48.

# Anesthetic Management for Posterior Fossa Surgery

## 57

Naginder Singh

## Introduction

The most common indications for surgery in the posterior fossa are [1]:

- Debulking or excision of brain tumors of the cerebellum, cerebello-pontine angle or brainstem
- The correction of anomalies affecting the craniovertebral junction (most commonly the Arnold-Chiari malformations)
- The emergency relief of pressure on the brainstem which may be caused by hydrocephalus or hemorrhage
- The treatment of aneurysms and arteriovenous malformations arising from the vertebrobasilar circulation
- Decompression of cranial nerves from vascular anomalies (in particular, cranial nerves V, VII and IX)

The surgical approach to access structures within the posterior fossa is typically by way of a sub-occipital craniectomy and this can be either midline or paramedian.

An understanding of the anatomy of the structures contained in the posterior fossa, their physiological function, the commonly encountered pathology and how these can be affected by surgery affords the basis for optimal perioperative care. Equally important are the practical aspects of monitoring, positioning and postoperative care which are also considered in this chapter.

## Anatomy

The tentorium cerebelli is a reflection of meningeal dura that separates the occipital lobes superiorly from the contents of the posterior fossa that lie inferiorly. Anteriorly, the posterior fossa is bound by the dorsum sellae (part of the sphenoid bone) and the clivus (the anterior most part of the occipital bone), laterally by the petrous part of the temporal bone and by the occipital bone posteriorly and inferiorly. The foramen magnum is situated at the base of the occipital bone and is the largest opening in the posterior fossa. The posterior fossa contains the cerebellum, brainstem (comprising the midbrain, pons and medulla) and lower cranial nerve nuclei. The transverse and sigmoid venous sinuses traverse the posterior fossa and merge at the confluence of

N. Singh, M.A. (Cantab) M.B.B.S., F.R.C.A
Queen Elizabeth Hospital, University Hospitals Birmingham NHS Foundation Trust,
Birmingham, UK
e-mail: naginder.singh@doctors.org.uk

sinuses. The cerebral aqueduct and fourth ventricle lie within the brainstem and so the normal flow of cerebrospinal fluid (CSF) can be obstructed within the posterior fossa resulting in acute hydrocephalus. Even a small mass effect within the posterior fossa can rapidly be fatal due to the very limited space and consequent pressure applied to the brainstem.

## Physiology of the Brainstem

The brainstem is composed of the midbrain, pons and medulla. The brainstem contains:

- The respiratory center, responsible for the regulation of breathing
- The cardiovascular center that regulates heart rate and blood pressure
- The reticular activating system that mediates consciousness

Also contained within the brainstem are the cranial nerve nuclei (except for cranial nerves I and II) as well as the ascending and descending tracts between the brain and spinal cord which decussate in the medulla. Lesions or surgical injury to posterior fossa structures can therefore result in impaired consciousness and respiration, altered control of heart rate and blood pressure, focal neurology (contralateral limb signs, ipsilateral cranial nerve signs) and a compromised ability to protect the airway (due to impaired gag and cough reflexes).

## Pathology

Posterior fossa pathology is highly varied (detailed in Table 57.1) but the most common indications for surgery are for tumor excision or to evacuate hemorrhage causing brainstem compression. In brief, pathology encountered in the posterior fossa can be categorised as; tumors, cysts, lesions involving the cranial nerves or the vasculature and congenital or acquired anomalies affecting the craniocervical junction [2]. These pathologies are detailed further in the table below (adapted with permission [2]).

**Table 57.1** Posterior fossa pathologies

| 1. **Tumors** |
|---|
| (a) Axial tumors |
|     Medulloblastoma |
|     Metastatic tumors |
|     Cerebellar astrocytoma |
|     Brainstem glioma |
|     Ependymoma |
|     Choroid plexus papilloma |
|     Dermoid tumors |
|     Hemangioblastoma |
| (b) Cerebellopontine angle tumors |
|     Schwannoma |
|     Meningioma |
|     Glomus jugulare tumor |
|     Acoustic neuroma |
| 2. **Cysts** |
| Epidermoid cyst |
| Arachnoid cyst |
| 3. **Vascular malformations** |
| Posterior cerebellar artery aneurysm |
| Vertebral/vertebrobasilar aneurysm |
| Basilar tip aneurysm |
| AV malformations |
| Cerebellar hematoma |
| Cerebellar infarction |
| 4. **Craniocervical abnormalities** |
| (a) Atlanto-occipital instability |
|     Congenital |
|     Acquired |
| (b) Atlanto-axial instability |
|     Congenital |
|     Acquired |
| (c) Arnold-Chiari malformations |
| 5. **Cranial nerve lesions** |
| Trigeminal neuralgia (CN V) |
| Hemifacial spasm (CN VII) |
| Glossopharyngeal neuralgia (CN IX) |

## Anesthesia Considerations

### Preoperative Evaluation

In addition to routine preoperative evaluation, it is also important to assess and to document the patient's neurological condition and to review up to date neuroimaging. A comprehensive neurological examination is particularly relevant when neurology has recently changed or is evolving. A plan that includes the practicalities of intraoperative care can then be made in consultation with the neurosurgical team. Preoperative evaluation should be supplemented with the following specific aspects that are of particular relevance to posterior fossa surgery.

Pathology affecting posterior fossa structures can result in a reduced level of consciousness or impaired airway reflexes and therefore, carries an associated risk of aspiration of gastric contents. In the acute setting, patients may already be intubated and ventilated on arrival or they may require a period of sedation and ventilation post-operatively. Performing an early tracheostomy may be considered if airway compromise is thought likely to persist in the postoperative period [3].

Dehydration and malnutrition can develop acutely, particularly in patients with posterior fossa tumors as oral intake may have been inadequate pre-operatively. As such, an assessment of fluid balance, hydration status and the correction of abnormalities of serum electrolytes should be done pre-operatively. Monitoring trends of central venous pressure (CVP) using a central line or the use of cardiac output monitoring intra-operatively may be utilized to aid optimal fluid management.

A thorough airway assessment is advisable, particularly in patients undergoing surgery at the craniovertebral junction who may present challenges for airway management due to cervical spine instability or restricted neck movements. Careful consideration should also be given to patients' existing injuries as well as disability or deformities which may influence decisions regarding intra-operative positioning.

## Positioning

Posterior fossa surgery can be done in the supine, prone, lateral, park-bench or sitting positions [4]. Meticulous attention is required when positioning patients so as to ensure an appropriate degree of neck flexion (to avoid hyper-flexion), optimal cerebral venous drainage and the prevention of compression to vulnerable peripheral nerves and pressure points. This is particularly important because posterior fossa surgery can often be several hours in duration.

## Sitting

Although often advantageous from a surgical perspective, use of the sitting position now seems to be declining and this is likely to be due to its associated complications (see below) which can be life-threatening and include a significant risk of venous air embolism [5]. Its advantages include good surgical access for midline pathology as well as a reduction in intracranial pressure and cerebral venous pressure. Potential complications include a reduction in cerebral perfusion pressure, reduced venous return and a limited ability for anaesthetised patients to physiologically compensate for the consequent hypotension [6]. These changes can be compounded by extremes of age, concurrent comorbidity and acute illness. Careful patient selection, appropriate fluid loading, the use of vasopressors and the maintenance of an adequate cerebral perfusion pressure are therefore important in avoiding cerebral ischemia. The need for intraoperative cardiopulmonary resuscitation or to address dislodgement of the airway require a prompt return to the supine position. Venous air embolism can result from the combination of open venous sinuses through which air entrainment can occur and the significant pressure gradient produced in the sitting position. The propagation of air emboli to the systemic circulation via any right to left shunt such as a patent foramen ovale (PFO) may result in stroke. In many centers cardiac defects including PFO are therefore, routinely screened for using echocardiography and interventionally corrected prior to undertaking posterior fossa surgery [7].

## Supine

The supine position, with the head turned to face the contralateral side is useful for accessing cerebello-pontine angle tumors including acoustic neuromas. Lateral rotation of the table, the use of a shoulder roll under the ipsilateral shoulder and head-up tilt can facilitate surgical access but note that elevation of the head is likely to reduce cerebral perfusion pressure.

## Prone

The prone position is the most commonly used position for posterior fossa surgery but presents several challenges to the anesthesiologist and for the neurosurgical team as a whole. An opening that leaves the chest and abdomen relatively free is a consistent feature of commonly used frames for prone positioning to allow unimpeded excursion of the diaphragm to aid mechanical ventilation and to produce a reduction in intracerebral venous pressure. In obese patients, the logistics of turning prone, ensuring adequate ventilation and the avoidance of pressure related nerve injuries can be especially challenging. Ophthalmic injuries are a recognized complication after non-ocular surgery and include the very rare risk of postoperative visual loss (POVL) [8]. Ischemic optic neuropathy and central retinal artery thrombosis are postulated as likely causes. While prone positioning and posterior fossa surgery are not independent risk factors for ophthalmic complications, external pressure on the eyes and hypotension can occur, are often implicated in POVL and should be diligently avoided. Achieving the prone position and maintaining safe anesthesia also requires care and attention to avoid dislodging the endotracheal tube, invasive lines and monitoring some of which may be briefly removed and then reapplied once prone.

### Lateral/Park-Bench

As with supine and prone positioning, lateral positioning may, for some operations offer a suitable alternative to the sitting position and therefore, the advantage of avoiding its associated complications. The ipsilateral forearm can lie supported and is easily accessible. The lateral position is useful from a surgical perspective, where lesions are unilateral and/or laterally located e.g. in one cerebellar hemisphere.

The park-bench position is a variation of lateral positioning offering better access to midline structures as compared with standard lateral positioning. In the park-bench position, the patient lies semi-prone with the head flexed and turned to face towards the floor. Both lateral and park bench positions allow gravity assisted drainage of blood and CSF and both may also be suitable alternatives to the prone position in selected patients.

## Monitoring

### Routine Monitoring

Standard monitoring includes pulse oximetry, ECG, capnography, non-invasive blood pressure at induction and the measurement of core temperature. Invasive measurement of arterial blood pressure is routinely used intra-operatively on account of the potential for hemodynamic fluctuation. Placing the arterial pressure transducer at the level of the external auditory meatus during sitting position is recommended to allow an accurate calculation of cerebral perfusion pressure. A central venous catheter placed in the right internal jugular vein is often sited to allow assessment of volume status and for the use of vasoactive medications if required. If the tip of the central venous catheter is sufficiently close to or advanced into the right atrium it may be possible to aspirate air in the event of venous air embolism (discussed further below). A urinary catheter and hourly measurement of urine output is essential given that surgery is often prolonged.

### Advanced Monitoring

The integrity of the motor and sensory tracts can be monitored using motor evoked potentials (MEPs) and somatosensory evoked potentials (SSEPs) by a trained neurophysiologist or assistant where spinal cord perfusion could be compromised or mechanical injury is a possibility. The use of volatile agents interferes with the measurement of SSEPs while muscle relaxation will inhibit motor activity (and therefore, hamper MEPs) and so a total intra-venous anesthesia (TIVA) technique is best suited in these circumstances [9]. TIVA comprises target controlled infusions of propofol and remifentanil delivered with pre-programmed pumps that utilize mathematrical algorithms based on age, gender, height and weight to deliver user defined concentrations. Where TIVA is used, the use of electro-encephalogram (EEG) based depth of anesthesia monitors such as BIS (bispectral index) or EEG entropy is recommended [10] to allow tailored dosing as well as providing an assessment of anaesthetic depth. Where there is an appreciable risk, monitoring for venous air embolism should be considered and the various methods are detailed in the following section.

## Complications

### Venous Air Embolism (VAE)

Air entrainment into the venous circulation can occur whenever an operative site is higher than the level of the right atrium and is made more likely by a significant pressure gradient. The incidence of VAE in the sitting position for posterior fossa surgery is made more frequent by the combination of the steep head up position and relatively non collapsible veins/venous sinuses through which air entrainment can occur [6]. It is important to note however, that VAE can potentially occur during any procedure involving vascular access and anesthesiologists should therefore maintain a high index of suspicion under these circumstances.

The clinical manifestations of VAE differ greatly according to the volume and speed at which air is entrained. VAE may be asymptomatic and therefore, it may be undetected if a small volume of air is entrained or by contrast, it may cause cardiac arrest if a large volume of air is rapidly entrained. More commonly, tachycardia, dysrhythmias and hypoxemia are apparent with VAE. A large volume of air causes an air-lock in the right atrium and therefore impedes both venous return and right ventricular outflow resulting in acute pulmonary hypertension and cardiovascular collapse which rapidly leads to cardiac arrest.

It is likely that multiple small VAE occur regularly and invariably in patients undergoing posterior fossa surgery with steep head-up or in the sitting position. The volume of air that is detectable varies considerably according to the monitoring modality that is used. The most practical monitor is end tidal capnography, since this is routinely used and falls responsively with any reduction in cardiac output. The most sensitive monitor is transesophageal echocardiography which can detect volumes of air as small as 0.02 mL/kg, this is followed by precordial doppler and transcranial doppler (both 0.05 mL/kg), end-tidal capnography (0.5 mL/kg) and the precordial stethoscope (1.5 mL/kg) [5].

Fluid loading, leg elevation and the use of positive end expiratory pressure (PEEP) can increase cerebral venous pressure and are therefore employed as strategies in preventing VAE. In some centers, military antishock trousers or a 'G suit' are used elevate venous pressure in patients undergoing sitting craniotomies [11]. Trendelenburg positioning while the head remains elevated reduces the gradient for air entrainment and fluid balance can be optimally tailored using trends in central venous pressure or cardiac output monitoring. Equally, meticulous surgical technique and the liberal use of saline soaked swabs and bone wax to bony openings to prevent air entrainment are recommended.

The management of VAE is largely supportive and should involve simultaneous resuscitative measures as well as attempts to remove air already entrained and the prevention of further air entrainment. Resuscitation should follow an airway, breathing, circulation approach and in the event of cardiac arrest, cardiopulmonary resuscitation should be commenced promptly. When VAE is suspected, the surgical field should immediately be flooded with saline, again making use of saline soaked swabs and bone wax as needed. Cardiovascular support using fluids and vasopressors and transient jugular vein compression can also aid resuscitation and prevent further air entrainment. Air aspiration via a right internal jugular vein central line or a dedicated air aspiration catheter in the left lateral reverse Trendelenburg position can be attempted where a large volume of air may be causing an air lock in the right atrium. Clearly, the practicalities of achieving this position in a patient with an open operative field and ongoing resuscitation are very challenging.

### Macroglossia

Airway oedema and macroglossia are associated with prolonged prone or lateral positioning due to obstruction of venous and lymphatic drainage of the tongue with neck flexion. The potential for airway obstruction is compounded in young children where the tongue is relatively large. A period of post-operative ventilation should be considered to allow macroglossia time to subside.

### Hemorrhage

Hypertension at emergence, at the point of extubation and in the post-operative period should be avoided as with all neuroanesthesia but this is especially important following posterior fossa surgery as bleeding and the formation a hematoma can rapidly lead to a deterioration and fatality. As such, the proactive management of hypertension is warranted to maintain a systolic blood pressure of <160 mmHg with the use of a beta-blocker or nitrate infusion as necessary.

### Pneumocephalus

Entrainment of air into the cranial cavity following a dural incision is inevitable and steps should be taken to minimize this, primarily through surgical technique but also by avoiding the use of nitrous oxide. Pneumocephalus can however be compounded after closure of the cranial wound by cerebral oedema and re-expansion of the brain when osmotherapy has been used e.g. mannitol, creating an acute elevation in ICP and this is termed tension pneumocephalus. If untreated, tension pneumocephalus can rapidly lead to brainstem compression, tonsillar herniation and cardiac arrest. Patients with pneumoceaphlus may present with delayed recovery, confusion, agitation, convulsions or neurological deficit and these clinical features should prompt urgent investigation with a CT scan. Conservative management with a high inspired concentration of oxygen increases the absorption rate of post-craniotomy pneumocephalus [12] but when it is severe, burr-hole evacuation may be necessary.

### Postoperative Care

Following uneventful posterior fossa surgery in patients without any compromising pre-operative neurological defect, the aim should be to wake and to extubate at the end of surgery in order to facilitate recovery and an early assessment of neurology. Once extubated, postoperative care should be in a high dependency area where routine neurological observations can be conducted. The judicious use of opiate analgesia [13] and routine use of anti-emetic agents is recommended toward the end of surgery.

The most critical post-operative complications are detailed above but other possible complications include hydrocephalus, respiratory compromise, injury to the cranial nerves, peripheral nerves or spinal cord all of which also warrant early clinical review and investigation. At worst, spinal cord injury can result in quadriplegia and this is thought to be due to over flexion of the neck causing compression and ischemia of the spinal cord, which is particularly compounded by hypotension. Meticulous care and attention to neck positioning and the avoidance of hypotension are therefore, the mainstay of its prevention perioperatively.

If there has been extensive hemorrhage or surgery involving manipulation of the brainstem or lower cranial nerves, a deferred extubation should be considered. There is the potential for airway compromise following posterior fossa surgery owing to any combination of airway edema, a depressed level of consciousness and bulbar palsy.

In the post-operative period, it is prudent to maintain a low threshold for investigation of any significant clinical deterioration with serial neuroimaging and physician review.

### Pediatric Considerations

Brain tumors are the most common solid tumors of childhood and two thirds arise in the posterior fossa compared with only one third of adult brain tumors [14]. Management of anesthesia for pediatric posterior fossa surgery should combine the principles of both pediatric anesthesia and neuroanesthesia. Of note, the dural venous pressure is higher in children and this is likely to account for a lower incidence of VAE [15]. The pediatric airway owing to its anatomy is more readily obstructed and as such where macroglossia or airway edema are apparent, a lower threshold for a deferred extubation may be considered. Intra-operative blood loss should be accurately measured and replaced. Given the increased potential for hypothermia in children on account of the relatively large surface area of the head, care should be taken in maintaining normothermia.

## References

1. Greenberg MS. Handbook of neurosurgery. 7th ed. New York: Thieme Publishers; 2010.
2. Jagannathan S, Krovvidi H. Anaesthetic considerations for posterior fossa surgery. Contin Educ Anaesth Crit Care Pain. 2014;14(5):202–6.
3. Jessop ZM, Kane AD, Menon DK. The role of early tracheostomy in patients with posterior fossa haemorrhage in neurocritical care. J Intensive Care Soc. 2012;13(4):293–6.
4. Veenith T, Absalom AR. Anaesthetic management of posterior fossa surgery. In: Matta BF, Menon DK, Smith M, editors. Core topics in neuroanaesthesia and neurointensive care. Cambridge: Cambridge University Press; 2011. p. 237–45.
5. Mirski MA, Lele AV, Fitzsimmons L, Toung TJK. Diagnosis and treatment of vascular air embolism. Anesthesiology. 2007;106:164–77.
6. Porter JM, Pidgeon C, Cunningham AJ. The sitting position in neurosurgery: a critical appraisal. Br J Anaesth. 1999;82:117–28.
7. Fathi A-R, Eshtehardi P, Meier B. Patent foramen ovale and neurosurgery in sitting position: a systematic review. Br J Anaesth. 2009;102(5):588–96.
8. Edgcombe H, Carter K, Yarrow S. Anaesthesia in the prone position. Br J Anaesth. 2008;100(2):165–83.
9. Pajewski TN, Arlet V, Phillips LH. Current approach on spinal cord monitoring: the point of view of the neurologist, the anesthesiologist and the spine surgeon. Eur Spine J. 2007;16(Suppl 2):115–29.
10. Depth of anaesthesia monitors—Bispectral Index (BIS), E-Entropy and Narcotrend-Compact M. National Institute of Clinical Excellence. 2012. https://www.nice.org.uk/guidance/DG6. Accessed 3 March 2018.
11. Webber S, Andrzejowski J, Francis G. Gas embolism in anaesthesia. Br J Anaesth. 2002;2(2):53–7.
12. Gore PA, Maan H, Chang S, Pitt AM, Spetzler RF, Nakaji P. Normobaric oxygen therapy strategies in the treatment of postcraniotomy pneumocephalus. J Neurosurg. 2008;108(5):926–9.
13. Morad A, Winters B, Stevens R, White E, et al. The efficacy of intravenous patient-controlled analgesia after intracranial surgery of the posterior fossa: a prospective, randomized controlled trial. Anesth Analg. 2012;114(2):416–23.
14. Furay C, Howell T. Paediatric neuroanaesthesia. Contin Educ Anaesth Crit Care Pain. 2010;10:172–6.
15. Harrison EA, Mackersie A, McEwan A, Facer E. The sitting position for neurosurgery in children: a review of 16 years' experience. Br J Anaesth. 2002;88(1):12–17.

# Anesthetic Management of Cerebral Aneurysm Surgery (Intracranial Vascular Surgeries)

## Mohammed Asif Arshad and Paul Southall

## Cerebral Aneurysms

### Epidemiology

Cerebral aneurysms are acquired outpouchings of cerebral arteries secondary to haemodynamic stresses and turbulent flow. Overall Prevalence is 3.2% with a higher incidence in women, those with a family history of cerebral aneurysms or subarachnoid haemorrhage and in patients with polycystic kidneys [1]. Most occur at bifurcations with 80–85% occurring in the anterior circulation.

### Presentation

The cerebral aneurysms are often incidental findings [2] but also present in several ways including a headache, bitemporal hemianopia, bilateral lower limb weakness, opthalmoplegia (intercavernous internal carotid artery aneurysm) and symptoms of brainstem dysfunction (posterior circulation aneurysms) [3, 4]. The most common and devastating presentation is in the form of a sub arachnoid haemorrhage (SAH).

In addition to SAH, aneurysms can also present as intra-parenchymal, subdural (2–5%) and intraventricular bleeds (13–28%).

### Investigation and Management

Symptomatic aneurysms (with a high risk of rupture based on site, size and progression) are referred for treatment. Treatment options are radiological coiling or surgical clipping and the optimum management is decided on a patient by patient basis by a multidisciplinary team taking into account aneurysm characteristics and patients' comorbidities. The optimal management of un-ruptured asymptomatic aneurysms is controversial and the risk of rupture needs to be balanced against the risks of major neurosurgical intervention [5].

### Prognosis

The prognosis of treated un-ruptured aneurysms is good. If patients undergo endovascular coiling, they are typically in hospital for shorter period compared to neurosurgical clipping, for which, recovery to full activity takes between 4 and 6 weeks. The prognosis of ruptured aneurysms is much poorer as described below.

M. A. Arshad, F.R.C.A., F.F.I.C.M., M.R.C.P. (✉)
P. Southall, F.R.C.A.
Queen Elizabeth Hospital, Birmingham, UK
e-mail: asif.arshad@cantab.net;
paul.southall@doctors.org.uk

## Subarachnoid Haemorrhage (SAH)

### Epidemiology

The incidence of SAH is 8–10 per 100,000 per year with a peak age of 60.

Seventy-five percent of non-traumatic SAH are caused by cerebral aneurysms with the remainder being caused by AV malformations, arterial dissections, vasculitis or tumours. In some cases the cause remains unknown [6].

### Presentation

Risk factors for aneurysm rupture causing SAH are female sex, Japanese or Finnish descent, size and location of aneurysms, hypertension, smoking and cocaine abuse [7]. Patients typically present with a sudden onset of severe occipital headache often described as a 'thunderclap' headache, 'the worst headache of my life' or 'like being hit in the back of the head with a baseball bat'. A SAH headache is often associated with nausea, vomiting, neck rigidity and photophobia [8]. Depending on the severity of the SAH, there can be associated focal neurological deficit, transient or prolonged loss of consciousness, photophobia, meningism and seizures. SAH is preceded by a sentinel headache, a warning headache occurring a few weeks before, in as many as 40% of patients [9].

### Investigation and Diagnosis

As well as the routine investigations listed in Table 58.1, the mainstay of diagnosis is a rapid unenhanced CT head. Modern CT scanners pick up 98% of SAH within 12 h and 93% within 24 h as blood is rapidly absorbed from the subarachnoid space. If there is a high degree of clinical suspicion, a lumbar puncture should be performed looking for red cells in the cerebrospinal fluid (CSF) and xanthochromia which is a yellow discoloration of the CSF representing metabolised haemoglobin in the CSF [10].

**Table 58.1** Routine investigations in suspected SAH

| Investigation | Reason |
|---|---|
| Full blood count Coagulation screen | Assess Hb and look for any coagulopathy |
| Serum urea and electrolytes | Electrolyte abnormalities for example hyponatraemia can be associated with SAH |
| Serum glucose | Hyperglycaemia, associated with poor outcome |
| Serum magnesium | Hypomagnesaemia, common and associated with poor outcome after SAH |
| Chest X-ray | Non cardiogenic pulmonary oedema and aspiration |
| 12-lead ECG | Cardiac arrhythmias and ischaemia common after SAH due to sympathetic surge |

**Table 58.2** World federation of neurosurgeons grading of subarachnoid haemorrhage [11]

| Grade | GCS | Motor deficit |
|---|---|---|
| I | 15 | Absent |
| II | 13–14 | Absent |
| III | 13–14 | Present |
| IV | 7–12 | Present or absent |
| V | <7 | Present or absent |

Once the diagnosis of SAH is made, further investigations are required to identify a ruptured aneurysm or identify another cause. CT angiography is the most commonly used investigation but others include MRI angiography and direct catheter angiography (digital subtraction angiography) [6].

### Grading

There are many different grading systems for SAH and commonly used ones include the World Federation of Neurosurgeons (WFNS) grading (Table 58.2) and the Fisher grading (Table 58.3). The WFNS grading is easy to use and relies on clinical parameters so is reliable and reproducible. The fisher grading grades SAH based on the volume, character and distribution of blood. It is thought to be the best predictor of vasospasm and risk of overall outcome.

**Table 58.3** Fisher grading of SAH [12]

| Grade | CT findings | Risk of symptomatic vasospasm |
|---|---|---|
| 1 | No subarachnoid or intraventricular haemorrhage (IVH) detected | 21% |
| 2 | Diffuse thin <1 mm SAH with no clots | 25% |
| 3 | Localised clots and/or layers of blood >1 mm in thickness with no IVH | 37% |
| 4 | Diffuse or no subarachnoid blood, but with intracerebral or intraventricular clots | 31% |

**Table 58.4** Complications of SAH

| Complication | Prevention | Treatment |
|---|---|---|
| Re-bleeding<br>• 8%<br>• Highest risk in first 72 h | Secure aneurysm as soon as possible [13]<br>Aim systolic BP = 140 until aneurysm secured [21–23] | Supportive neuroprotective measures |
| Vasospasm | Nimodipine<br>Euvolaemia<br>Avoid hypotension | Hypertension once aneurysm secured<br>Euvolaemia |
| Hydrocephalus | | External ventricular drainage |
| Arrhythmias | | Treat underlying cause<br>Correct electrolyte abnormalities<br>Consider antiarrhythmics |
| Cardiomyopathy<br>• Reduced LV function<br>• Takusobo Cardiomyopathy<br>• Neurogenic stunned myocardium | Minimise sympathetic stimulation<br>Effective analgaesia | Supportive therapy with inotropes and vasopressors |
| Neurogenic pulmonary oedema | | O2<br>CPAP<br>Judicious use of nitrates and diuretics due to risks of vasospasm |
| Electrolyte disturbances<br>• SIADH or cerebral salt wasting possible<br>• Hyponatraemia common | | Supportive<br>Correct electrolyte disturbance<br>Keep euvolemic |

## Management

The management of SAH is to find the underlying cause and then

- treat the cause as soon as possible (if aneurysmal secure the aneurysm within 72 h) [13]
- reduce the risk of re-bleeding
- prevent vasospasm and
- monitor for complications (Table 58.4).

The rest of the management is supportive.

## Coiling vs. Clipping

Interventional coiling or surgical clipping are the treatment options for aneurysmal SAH and choice of technique depends upon many factors including patients' comorbidities, anatomy, location of the aneurysm and local expertise.

The International Subarachnoid Aneurysm Trial (ISAT) was a prospective international multicentre RCT comparing surgical clipping vs. radiological coiling with a primary endpoint of death or dependency at 1 year [14]. The results were published in 2002 and showed coiling to have a lower death/dependency rate (23.5%) than surgical clipping (30.9%). However, the rate of rebleeding at 1 year was higher in the coiling group (2.6%) than the clipping group (1%) [14]. Five year follow up also showed a better mortality rate with coiling (11%) vs. clipping (14%) [15]. However the ISAT trial had some limitations particularly in relation to recruitment. Out of 9559 screened only 2143 were recruited. In addition 97% of patients had anterior circulation aneurysms, 92% had aneurysms <1 cm in size and 88% of patients had WFNS grade I–II SAH. Patients >70 years of age were also excluded. These limitations raise concerns about whether these results can be generalised to all patients with aneurysmal SAH. Due to these concerns ISAT II, another multicentre RCT comparing coiling vs. clipping, started recruiting in 2012 and is due to finish in 2024. The study design has been modified from ISAT to represent patients over the age of 70, patients with WFNS grade III/IV SAH, posterior circulation and middle circulation aneurysms and aneurysms >1 cm in size.

In summary there is evidence that coiling has a lower rate of death and dependency at year 1 than clipping but this difference decreases over time at least partly due to a higher rebleed risk with coiling [15]. Younger patients may benefit from the reduced rebleeding rate that clipping provides. Currently practice varies and the choice of technique depends upon local expertise and MDT discussion between neurosurgeons and interventional radiologists.

## Complications

Potential complications from SAH are listed in the table below. Vasospasm and rebleeding are common complications with significant associated morbidity and are discussed in more detail below.

## Vasospasm

Cerebral vasospasm may occur when cerebral vessels are exposed to blood in the subarachnoid space. It occurs in 60–70% of bleeds typically 4–14 days post SAH. As most aneurysms are located around the circle of Willis and this is the most common location for aneurysmal rupture, the large proximal blood vessels supplying the brain are most at risk of vasospasm.

Vasospasm causes a reduction in blood vessel diameter thereby decreasing cerebral blood flow (CBF) resulting in secondary ischaemic injury. Vasospasm is one of the most common causes of morbidity and mortality following SAH. Approximately 70% of aneurysmal SAH patients will demonstrate angiographic evidence of vasospasm. However only 40% will have clinical symptoms, approximately 30% will have delayed ischaemic injury and up to 20% of patients will die or have severe neurological deficits as a result of vasospasm [16]. Once vasospasm occurs, it lasts between 2 and 3 weeks. Diagnosis of vasospasm can be made clinically in patients who have an unexplained drop in GCS or new neurological deficit several days post aneurysmal SAH that cannot be explained by re-bleeding or hydrocephalus both of which can be ruled out with an uncontrasted CT head. Other investigations which can help with the diagnosis of vasospasm include transcranial Doppler velocities, CT angiography, CT brain perfusion scan and direct catheter angiography.

Management of vasospasm includes preventative measures with regular oral nimodipine (calcium channel blocker) from day 1 of SAH, euvolaemia and avoiding hypotension. Doses of nimodipine must not be missed even if this means a nasogastric tube needs to be placed or an IV infusion of nimodipine needs to be commenced. Nimodipine is the only treatment modality that has been shown systematically to improve outcome in aneurysmal SAH and is generally well tolerated [17].

In confirmed vasospasm 'triple H' therapy (THT) is often used to prevent ischaemia becoming infarction. THT is a combination of hypertension, hypervolemia and haemodilution. The logic behind the therapy is that a higher driving pressure of more dilute less viscous blood will enhance cerebral blood flow through the vasospastic arteries. This is generally achieved by using a vasopressor aiming for a systolic of 180 or a mean of 110–130, ensuring a 3 L fluid intake and aiming for a haematocrit of 30–35%. However although THT is widely practiced and has a theoretical foundation it has never been shown to significantly improve outcome in vasospasm associated with SAH. In addition there have been significant reports of adverse effects [16].

Various combinations of THT have been used. Raabe et al. [18] performed a retrospective review of 45 patients with aneurysmal SAH associated vasospasm looking at cerebral oxygenation during periods of hypervolemia alone, moderate induced hypertension in euvolemic states or aggressive hypervolemic hypertension. They found that moderate induced hypertension (perfusion pressure of approximately 90) in euvolemic patients increased cerebral oxygenation in 90% of cases. This was much better than hypervolemia alone (12%) and aggressive hypervolemic hypertension (60%). This study also showed significant rate of adverse effects with aggressive hypervolemic hypertension (50%) vs. euvolemic moderate hypertension (8%).

Muench et al. [19] showed in a prospective observational study that hypervolemic haemodilution neither increased cerebral blood flow nor cerebral oxygenation. THT increased CBF but not cerebral oxygenation. Only euvolemic hypertension increased both CBF and cerebral oxygenation.

A retrospective study looking at over 350 patients showed that hypervolemia and hypertension resulted in higher rates of pulmonary oedema, sepsis and mortality than euvolaemia, optimisation of cardiac output and moderate hypertension [20].

Although nimodipine is instituted as a prophylactic measure for all non-traumatic SAH, the benefits of **prophylactic** THT are controversial. Some studies have shown that THT actually induces vasospasm [20].

In summary although several studies have shown increased cerebral blood flow and oxygenation with hypertension, no study has convincingly demonstrated the benefits of hypervolemia or haemodilution on cerebral blood flow. Despite increased cerebral blood flow and cerebral oxygenation no aspect of THT has yet been shown to improve clinical outcome. There have however been multiple studies showing clinical adverse effects of THT. As such current practice is shifting away from THT towards euvolemic hypertension [4]. Other novel therapies including intra-arterial vasodilators and mechanical devices augmenting cerebral blood flow are currently showing physiological promise.

## Rebleeding

Rebleeding significantly increases mortality in SAH. The two main strategies to reduce the risk of rebleeding are aimed at early control of the aneurysm and blood pressure (BP) control prior to securing the aneurysm. A systematic review has confirmed early control of ruptured aneurysms improves clinical outcome [13].

Optimal blood pressure (BP) management prior to securing the aneurysm always leads to debate amongst clinicians. The cerebral perfusion pressure needs to be high enough to perfuse vulnerable areas of brain to prevent secondary brain injury, particularly in the setting of raised ICP following SAH. However hypertension also increases the risk of rebleeding from an unsecured aneurysm. There have now been several studies including two RCTs (INTERACT-2 and ATACH II) that have looked at lowering blood pressure to 140 systolic vs. 180 systolic in the setting of intracerebral haemorrhage. Both RCTs found no difference in mortality or disability rates between the two groups [21, 22]. Another physiological study looked at perfusion in the vulnerable penumbra in patients with intracerebral haemorrhage in whom the BP was lowered to 150 mmHg compared with 180 mmHg and did not find any reduction in perfusion in the vulnerable penumbra [23]. Although these studies did not specifically look at aneurysmal SAH as a result of these studies, it has been concluded that BP can be safely lowered to around 140 mmHg without adverse neurological and mortality consequences in the setting of aneurysmal SAH. Current practice is to aim for a systolic BP of 140 mmHg until the aneurysm is secured.

## Prognosis

Advancing age, impaired consciousness on admission (WFNS grading) and larger volume of blood on CT scan (Fisher Grading) are associated with worse prognosis.

Despite modern advances in care, 50% of patients die within 4 weeks with the majority (70%) dying from the initial bleed often within the first 24 h and 30% dying from re-bleeding and other complications detailed above. Re-bleeding in particular carries a very poor prognosis with 64% of patients dying from the first re-bleed and 96% from a second re-bleed. Only about 30% of all patients will survive without neurological deficits highlighting the need for optimal management to improve prognosis [6].

## Anesthesia for the Treatment of Cerebral Aneurysms

### Pre operative Assessment

Careful preop assessment is required in addition to a standard preop visit with particular attention to potential complications of SAH as mentioned above

#### Cardiovascular
- Baseline BP to assess safe levels of hypotension
- Arrhythmias or any evidence of cardiomyopathy
- Any evidence of fluid overload
- Starting Haemoglobin
- Coagulopathy or anticoagulants

#### Respiratory
- Any evidence of aspiration, atelectasis or pulmonary oedema

#### Renal
- Renal function—likely to have had significant doses of contrast
- Electrolyte disturbances particularly hyponatraemia should be corrected gradually prior to theatre

#### Neurological
- Assessment of how aneurysm or SAH if present has affected neurology
- Seizures and how well controlled these are
- Detailed neurological exam as a baseline
- Presence of EVD and if this is draining

### Investigations
- Full blood count
- Clotting
- Chest x-ray
- ECG
- ECHO if suspicion of cardiomyopathy in SAH (This should not delay urgent aneurysm controlling surgery)

### Optimisation
- Correct anaemia
- Correct coagulopathy
- Correct electrolyte abnormalities
- Thorough explanation of process to relieve anxiety
- Consider premedication with benzodiazepine to relieve anxiety
- Cross match 2 units of blood.

## Anesthesia for Clipping of Intracranial Aneurysms

### Goal Throughout Surgery

**Avoid increase in aneurysm transmural pressure to prevent rupture/bleeding**. The risk of rupture primarily depends upon the transmural pressure across the aneurysm i.e. the mean arterial pressure—CSF pressure. Therefore minimise sudden increases in blood pressure (BP) and sudden decreases in CSF pressure. Times when BP is prone to suddenly increasing is at laryngoscopy, at the time of pinning the skull, at the time of skin incision and at the time of bone flap resection. Times of sudden drop in CSF pressure include craniotomy, drainage of CSF and mannitol prior to dura opening. Once the dura is opened, the CSF space is essentially open to the atmosphere and the pressure fluctuates much less.

### Monitoring and Lines
- **Invasive arterial monitoring** ideally prior to induction but definitely prior to intubation to minimise sudden changes in BP and risk of aneurysm rupture

- **Neurophysiological monitoring**
  - Electroencephalogram (EEG)/Somatosensory evoked potential (SSEP)/Motor evoked potentials (MEP)/brainstem auditory evoked potentials (BEAP) to guide when clipping is leading to detrimental effect on neurology
  - Not validated or have an evidence base as yet [4]
- Central venous line
- Be prepared for massive haemorrhage. Wide bore venous access is mandatory.

## Induction

The goals of induction are to have a cardio-stable induction minimising any elevation or significant drop in BP. Avoiding hypotension reduces risk of vasospasm and secondary cerebral ischaemia and avoiding hypertension reduces the risk of aneurysm rupture and re-bleeding. As long as this goal is achieved, the drugs used are less important. Remifentanil/Propofol Total Intra Venous Anesthesia (TIVA) is a good choice as it is very easily titratable to haemodynamics.

## Maintenance

**Positioning:** most commonly patients are positioned supine for anterior circulation and lateral for posterior circulation aneurysms.

**Generic neuroprotective measures:** Avoid hyperthermia and hyperglycaemia. Ensure good oxygenation, ventilation and avoid any obstruction of venous return. Discuss seizure prophylaxis with neurosurgical team.

**Brain relaxation.** Brain relaxation, i.e. keeping the brain slack improves surgical exposure minimising the need for surgeons to use retraction which can compromise cerebral perfusion to the areas where the retractors are placing pressure. Brain relaxation is best achieved by good oxygenation, normocapnia, ensuring there is no impairment to venous drainage, slight head up, using TIVA with propofol. As an adjunct to these basic measures osmotic diuretics (mannitol and furosemide) can be used. In SAH, these have to be used with caution as they may exacerbate vasospasm induced cerebral ischaemia by causing hypovolaemia. Finally CSF drainage can be undertaken via a lumbar drain or a ventricular drain to improve surgical access. However if this is done prior to the opening of the dura, the CSF pressure will drop increasing the transmural pressure across the aneurysm potentially causing a rupture or re-bleed.

**Cerebral protection during clipping:** The feeding vessels are often temporarily occluded to aid dissection and limit effects of any rupture during surgical clipping of the aneurysm. During this time the perfusion to the brain supplied by that feeding vessel will abruptly be reduced. In order to protect this vulnerable part of the brain, blood pressure must be elevated to levels comparable with pre operative levels in order to allow collateral flow to the at risk brain. This is done with vasopressors and ensuring euvolaemia. In addition, occlusion of the feeding vessel should be kept to less than 20 min as longer periods are associated with worse outcomes [24]. Cerebral monitoring may help detect any periods of brain hypo perfusion.

### Intraoperative Rupture of Aneurysm

As discussed above the unprotected aneurysm could rupture at several stages during surgery. Managing intraoperative rupture requires teamwork and good communication between surgeon and anaesthetist. Prior to dura opening, recognition of aneurysmal rupture may be difficult in an anaesthetised patient. Haemodynamic changes could be seen with arrhythmias and hypertension and there may be some swelling at the site of surgery. Rupture prior to dura opening is normally caused by changes in aneurysm transmural pressure. After dura opening, the majority of ruptures are caused during dissection of the aneurysm.

Management of a ruptured aneurysm includes managing massive haemorrhage, discussing with the surgeon re BP targets and providing the surgeon with optimum operating conditions in order to control the bleeding. In some cases this involves temporary significant hypotension. Adenosine induced temporary cardiac standstill has also been safely and successfully used [25]. Other measures include general neuroprotective measures namely good oxygenation, hyperventilation, avoiding hyperthermia, normoglycaemia and ensuring no impediment to venous return of the head and neck.

## Emergence

Early emergency is recommended to allow continual neurological evaluation as the best way of diagnosing any complications. A smooth emergence is the aim avoiding coughing, bucking, vomiting and hypertension.

## Radiological Coiling

Often done through the groin and can take several hours through which the patient has to remain completely still. All cases are done under general anaesthesia for this reason. The principles for anaesthesia for coiling are the same as for surgical clipping with particular attention to haemodynamics and transmural pressure. The patients are normally very stable and as the incision is small, there is minimal post op pain and patients have a short stay in hospital.

However, aneurysmal rupture during coiling can be catastrophic as with a closed cranium and arterial bleeding, significant cerebral ischaemia and brain damage can occur. Unless angiographic control of the bleeding can be quickly obtained, patients would need to go to theatre for a decompressive craniectomy and ventricular drainage. In this situation, lowering the blood pressure with vasodilators should be avoided and other methods used such as anaesthetic boluses.

## Post operative Period

Patients are admitted to intensive care post clipping or coiling of aneurysms due to the high risk of complications (Table 58.4) and the need to identify complications early and manage them rapidly.

## Conclusion

Intracranial aneurysms and aneurysmal subarachnoid haemorrhage is a significant health burden with high mortality and morbidity. Advancing age, reduced conscious level and volume of blood on CT are poor prognostic indicators. CT head followed by a lumbar puncture is required in order to avoid misdiagnosis. Treatment is aimed at early control of the aneurysm and treatment of any complications to minimise delayed cerebral ischaemia. Treatment choice is shifting towards coiling following the results of the ISAT trial but there are currently still situations where clipping is appropriate. Anaesthetic considerations for coiling or clipping include reducing risk of aneurysm rupture/rebleed, reducing the risk of secondary brain damage, management of aneurysm rupture if it does occur and optimising surgical operating conditions with brain relaxation.

## References

1. Vlaq MHM, Algra A, Brandenburg R, Rinkel GJ. The Prevalence of unruptured intracranial aneurysms, with emphasis on sex, age, comorbidity, country and time period: a systemic review and meta-analysis. Lancet Neurol. 2011;10:626–36.
2. Vernooij MW, Arfan Ikram M, Tanghe HL, et al. Incidental findings on brain MRI in the general population. N Engl J Med. 2007;357:1821–8.
3. Keedy A. An overview of intracranial aneurysms. Mcgill J Med. 2006;9(2):141–6.
4. D'Souza S. Aneurysmal subarachnoid hemorrhage. J Neurosurg Anesthesiol. 2015;27(3):222–40.
5. Lecours M, Gelb AW. Anesthesia for the surgical treatment of cerebral aneurysms. Rev Colomb Anestesiol. 2015;43(Supl1):45–51.
6. Al-Shahi R, White PM, Davenport RJ, Lindsay KW. Subarachnoid haemorrhage. Br Med J. 2006;333:235–40.
7. Wermer MJ, van der Schaaf IC, Algra A, Rinkel GJ. Risk of rupture of unruptured intracranial aneurysms in relation to patient and aneurysm characteristics: an updated meta-analysis. Stroke. 2007;38(4):1404–10. Epub 2007 Mar 1.
8. Suarez JI, Tarr RW, Selman WR. Aneurysmal subarachnoid hemorrhage. N Engl J Med. 2006;354: 387–96.

9. Ostergaard JR. Headache as a warning symptom of impending aneurysmal subarachnoid haemorrhage. Cephalalgia. 1991;11(1):53–5.
10. Manno EM. Subarachnoid hemorrhage. Neurol Clin. 2004;22(2):347–66.
11. Teasdale GM, Drake CG, Hunt W, et al. A universal subarachnoid hemorrhage scale: report of a committee of the World Federation of Neurosurgical Societies. J Neurol Neurosurg Psychiatry. 1988;51(11):1457.
12. Fisher CM, Kistler JP, Davis JM. Relation of cerebral vasospasm to subarachnoid hemorrhage visualized by computerized tomographic scanning. Neurosurgery. 1980;6(1):1–9.
13. de Gans K, Nieuwkamp DJ, Rinkel GJ, et al. Timing of aneurysm surgery in subarachnoid hemorrhage: a systematic review of the literature. Neurosurgery. 2002;50(2):336–40; discussion 340–2.
14. Molyneux A, Kerr R, Stratton I, Sandercock P, et al. International Subarachnoid Aneurysm Trial (ISAT) Collaborative Group. International Subarachnoid Aneurysm Trial (ISAT) of neurosurgical clipping versus endovascular coiling in 2143 patients with ruptured intracranial aneurysms: a randomised trial. Lancet. 2002;360(9342):1267–74.
15. Molyneux AJ, Kerr RS, Birks J. Risk of recurrent subarachnoid haemorrhage, death, or dependence and standardised mortality ratios after clipping or coiling of an intracranial aneurysm in the International Subarachnoid Aneurysm Trial (ISAT): long-term follow-up. Lancet Neurol. 2009;8(5):427–33.
16. Dabus G, Nogueira RG. Current options for the management of aneurysmal subarachnoid hemorrhage-induced cerebral vasospasm: a comprehensive review of the literature. Interv Neurol. 2013;2(1):30–51.
17. Pickard JD, Murray GD, Illingworth R, et al. Effect of oral nimodipine on cerebral infarction and outcome after subarachnoid haemorrhage: British Aneurysm Nimodipine Trial. BMJ. 1989;298:636–42.
18. Raabe A, Beck J, Keller M, et al. Relative importance of hypertension compared with hypervolemia for increasing cerebral oxygenation in patients with cerebral vasospasm after subarachnoid hemorrhage. J Neurosurg. 2005;103:974–81.
19. Muench E, Horn P, Bauhuf C, et al. Effects of hypervolemia and hypertension on regional cerebral blood flow, intracranial pressure, and brain tissue oxygenation after subarachnoid hemorrhage. Crit Care Med. 2007;35:1844–51.
20. Kim DH, Haney CL, van Ginhoven G. Reduction of pulmonary edema after SAH with a pulmonary artery catheter-guided hemodynamic management protocol. Neurocrit Care. 2005;3:11–5.
21. Anderson CS, Heeley E, Huang Y, et al. Rapid blood-pressure lowering in patients with acute intracerebral hemorrhage. N Engl J Med. 2013;368:2355–65.
22. Qureshi AI, Palesch YY, Barsan WG, et al. Intensive blood-pressure lowering in patients with acute cerebral hemorrhage. N Engl J Med. 2016;375:1033–43.
23. Butcher KS, Jeerakathil T, Hill M, et al. The intracerebral hemorrhage acutely decreasing arterial pressure trial. Stroke. 2013;44(3):620–6.
24. Woertgen C, Rothoerl RD, Albert R, et al. Effects of temporary clipping during aneurysm surgery. Neurol Res. 2008;30(5):542–6.
25. Guinn NR, McDonagh DL, Borel CO, et al. Adenosine-induced transient asystole for intracranial aneurysm surgery: a retrospective review. J Neurosurg Anesthesiol. 2011;23(1):35–40.

# Anesthetic Considerations for Surgical Resection of Brain Arteriovenous Malformations

## Catalin Ezaru

## Pathophysiology of Arteriovenous Malformations

AVM are defects in cerebral vasculature development leading to the formation of shunts between the high-pressure arterial and the low-pressure venous systems without an intervening normal capillary bed. Congenital factors but also active angiogenic and inflammatory processes can contribute to the formation of AVMs.

The primary characteristic of cerebral circulation in patients with untreated AVMs is the diversion of flow thorough the path of least resistance (the AVM itself), bypassing the normal arteriolar and capillary system in the adjacent normal tissue. This can lead to chronic cerebral hypotension and potential for ischemia (cerebral steal). However, few patients with unruptured AVMs present with ischemia and neurologic deficits despite the presence of cerebral hypotension in the adjacent brain areas. This indicates that autoregulatory capacity is maintained in these territories. In fact, it has been observed that the lower limit of autoregulation has shifted to the left, similar (but in the opposite direction) to the effect observed in patients with chronic systemic hypertension. This phenomenon called "adaptive autoregulatory displacement" [1] may explain why brain areas adjacent to AVMs maintain autoregulatory capacity even below normal brain blood pressure (50–70 mmHg).

Similarly, the phenomenon of normal perfusion pressure breakthrough (NPPB) or cerebral dys-autoregulation has been described when brain swelling (often sudden and severe) occurs after the resection of AVM. Cerebral hyperemia is believed to occur due to increased blood flow through the previously hypotensive areas adjacent to (now removed) AVM, assuming those vessels have lost autoregulatory capacity and are chronically vasodilated. The evidence supporting the existence of NPPB is limited and several observations contradict this theory such as the left shift on the autoregulation curve encountered in the hypotensive areas (indicating intact autoregulation) and maintenance of the vascular reactivity to carbon dioxide [2]. The main clinical implication is that if brain swelling occurs after the resection of AVM it should not be automatically attributed to NPPB before other correctable causes (such as bleeding) are ruled out.

## Clinical Presentation and Risk Assessment in Patients with Arteriovenous Malformations

AVMs typically present between ages 10 and 45. The most common clinical presentation and cause of morbidity is spontaneous intracranial hemorrhage (ICH) with signs and symptoms related to

C. Ezaru, M.D.
University of Pittsburgh School of Medicine,
Veterans' Affairs Hospital Pittsburgh,
Pittsburgh, PA, USA
e-mail: EzaruC@anes.upmc.edu

increased intracranial pressure (headache, focal neurologic deficits, altered consciousness). They can also present with mass effect (large AVM, hematoma) or seizure activity. Many AVMs are discovered incidentally after brain imaging.

ICH associated with AVMs typically occurs intra-parenchymal or intraventricular in contrast to subarachnoid hemorrhage due to cerebral aneurysms which may explain the infrequent occurrence of vasospasm in patients with AVMs.

Prognosis depends on multiple factors: AVM size, location, deep venous drainage, clinical presentation. The risk factors associated with natural evolution of AVMs (spontaneous bleeding) may overlap with factors that increase the risk of intervention but they are not the same. For example, larger size will increase the risk for surgical resection but smaller AVMs have greater risk of spontaneous bleeding due to higher intravascular pressure.

The system most commonly used to assess the risk of surgical resection is the Spetzler-Martin grading scale [3] based on the AVM size, vascular anatomy, and location (see Table 59.1). The total grade is obtained by the addition of points in each category and the maximum grade is 5. Typically, grade 3 and higher lesions portend an increased surgical risk but other factors may also need to be considered. For example, the Spetzler-Martin scale defines eloquence anatomically—neurologic deficits related to brain areas affected by AVM. However, the presence of AVM can lead to relocation of certain brain functions to a different region (functional eloquence) and preoperative imaging with functional MRI may be helpful to better define the neurologic impact and potential risk.

**Table 59.1** Spetzler-Martin grading scale for AVM

| Graded feature | Points |
|---|---|
| **AVM size** | |
| – Small (<3 cm) | 1 |
| – Medium (3–6 cm) | 2 |
| – Large (>6 cm) | 3 |
| **Pattern of venous drainage** | |
| – Superficial only | 0 |
| – Deep | 1 |
| **Eloquence of adjacent brain** | |
| – Non-eloquent | 0 |
| – Eloquent | 1 |

## Treatment Options in Patients with Arteriovenous Malformations

There are three treatment options for patients with AVM: endovascular embolization, radiosurgery and microsurgical excision. Conservative/expectant management can also be considered for asymptomatic lesions and those deemed high-risk for intervention. The main goals for treatment of AVMs are protection against ICH and maximizing the neurological function. Due to the nature of disease, a cooperative multidisciplinary approach with staged interventions is frequently employed.

Endovascular embolization is typically the first step in the treatment of large AVMs in preparation for radiosurgery or surgical excision. The main goal of preoperative embolization is to occlude vessels that may be difficult to control surgically thereby facilitating AVM excision and reducing blood loss. One potential advantage might be allowing surrounding brain regions to adapt to the circulatory changes. Embolization alone is rarely curative.

Radiosurgery involves the precise delivery of radiation to the target using a stereotactic frame leading to endothelial cell proliferation and progressive closure of the vessels. It is useful for smaller AVMs and those located in deep brain areas. The main drawback is the long time needed for complete obliteration of the AVM to occur (1–3 years) during which time the patient is still exposed to the risk of bleeding.

Surgical excision is indicated for accessible lesions preferably located in noneloquent areas (low grade as defined by Spetzler-Martin scale) and is commonly preceded by endovascular embolization. AVM surgery is rarely an emergency procedure unless there is an immediate need to evacuate an intracranial hematoma.

## Anesthetic Management for Resection of AVMs

Anesthetic management follows the general goals of neurovascular anesthesia: close hemodynamic monitoring, maintenance of cerebral perfusion pressure (CPP), minimize the chance of bleeding, and readiness to treat sudden massive hemorrhage. The management concerns are then similar to patients with aneurysms although the risk of intraoperative rupture is much lower for AVMs.

## Preoperative Evaluation

Preoperative evaluation is largely dependent on the clinical presentation. Patients undergoing elective resection of AVM may have already undergone other procedures (endovascular embolization) that required anesthesia and allowed more time for optimization of chronic medical conditions. Patients presenting with ICH, neurologic deficits, or seizures may require a more urgent surgical intervention. Factors to be considered include: size of AVM (potential for blood loss), location of AVM (eloquent brain areas), the potential impact of neurologic dysfunction, neurophysiologic monitoring and vascular access.

## Intraoperative Management

### Monitoring and Vascular Access

In addition to standard monitors (electrocardiogram, pulse oximeter, end-tidal carbon dioxide), intra-arterial catheters are routinely used to allow for close hemodynamic monitoring. Additional benefits include frequent blood sampling to monitor blood gases (if hyperventilation and hypocarbia are employed) and electrolytes. AVMs have a much lower risk of rupture compared to aneurysms so placement of the arterial catheter prior to induction of general anesthesia may not be as important. However, avoidance of acute hypertension still remains a fundamental goal for any neurovascular procedure in order to minimize the risk of bleeding and brain edema.

The use of a central venous catheter can be considered for fluid replacement (in case of inadequate peripheral access), infusion of vasoactive drugs or if the potential for venous air embolism is significant (to allow for therapeutic aspiration of air). Monitoring of the central venous pressure (CVP) to guide fluid management should not be the primary reason for placement of a central catheter as multiple studies have demonstrated a poor relationship between CVP and circulating blood volume and between static CVP and volume responsiveness [4]. Systolic pressure and pulse pressure variations derived from arterial pressure waveform analysis may be better predictors of intravascular volume responsiveness [5, 6].

Overall, adequate preparation for significant intraoperative operative blood loss is extremely important. This should include adequate communication with the surgeon, large-bore intravenous access (peripheral or central), availability of blood products and cell salvage capabilities.

Various neurophysiologic monitoring techniques may be used similar to surgery for aneurysms including electroencephalogram (EEG), somatosensory and motor evoked potentials. EEG can be helpful during periods of flow interruption or to guide administration of agents that reduce cerebral metabolic requirements (barbiturate induced burst suppression). Techniques monitoring direct cerebral blood flow and jugular venous saturation have been described but are not used routinely. Direct transduction of intravascular pressures in the operating field may help the surgeon differentiate between arterial and venous vessels of the AVM and allow for venous clipping during the resection.

### Anesthetic Technique

There is no evidence that one anesthetic technique is superior to others as long as the general goals of neurovascular anesthesia are observed: maintain adequate CPP and prevent increases in the ICP. Increased ICP is typically not an issue for the patient presenting for elective surgery but that can change during the operation so it may be prudent to use anesthetic agents that do not increase cerebral blood flow (CBF) and/or decrease cerebral metabolic requirements (CMR). Communication with the neurosurgeon throughout the perioperative period is critical as conditions can change abruptly. If the goal is to extubate the patient at the end of the operation to perform a neurologic exam, the anesthetic technique and plan for rapid, smooth emergence should be tailored accordingly.

Premedication with benzodiazepines such as midazolam is acceptable as long as the patient is neurologically intact and if it does not interfere with emergence. Induction of anesthesia can be achieved with any of the intravenous agents commonly in use (propofol, etomidate, thiopental). The potential for anesthetic-induced hypotension which may lead to decreased CPP is ever present during any anesthetic but especially so during induction. Some practitioners prefer etomidate due to its limited inhibition of sympathetic system and decreased likelihood of hypotension; however, tachycardia and hypertension may ensue. Some data suggest that etomidate may worsen focal cerebral ischemia during aneurysm clipping [7]. Regardless of which drug or combination of drugs is used for induction, adequate monitoring (including placement of intra-arterial catheter prior to induction in select patients) and availability of short-acting vasoactive medications are paramount for precise manipulation of hemodynamic parameters.

Maintenance of anesthesia can be accomplished with intravenous agents, opioids, inhalational drugs, or a combined technique. There is no strong evidence that any particular anesthetic agent has cerebral protective effect (except barbiturates as discussed below). Traditionally, intravenous agents have been favored because of their ability to decrease both CMR and CBF (with the notable exception of ketamine which has the opposite effects). Inhalational agents are also acceptable since they reduce CMR but they have the potential for increasing CBF when used in higher doses. While this is likely not significant in the majority of cases, it may need to be considered in certain situations when additional brain relaxation is required.

Barbiturates are the only anesthetic drugs proven to have additional cerebral protective effect [8]; however, the overall outcome does not appear to be affected in patients undergoing AVM resections. They are not used routinely because of the adverse hemodynamic effects (hypotension) and delayed emergence. Barbiturates use varies institutionally but they are probably best reserved for situations when prolonged arterial occlusion is likely or signs of ischemia develop on EEG.

## Brain Protection

Maintenance of CPP to ensure adequate perfusion and collateral flow, and good brain relaxation to facilitate surgical access and minimize retractor pressures are the main goals of intervention. Factors contributing to cerebral damage can be broadly divided into two main categories: anatomic and physiologic. Anatomical factors are typically related to the neurosurgeon: direct vascular injury (bleeding, ischemia), brain retraction, direct disruption of brain tissue. Physiological factors are the ones more likely to be under the control of anesthesiologists: adequate brain relaxation and reduction in brain volume, maintenance of CPP and O2 delivery, avoidance of hyperglycemia and hypo-osmolarity. These factors can act in synergistic fashion towards a deleterious neurologic outcome—for example, small amount of brain retraction coupled with modest decrease in perfusion pressure.

All the usual techniques for brain relaxation can be used for surgical resection of AVMs as dictated by clinical picture and practitioners' preference (see Table 59.2). Adequate head

**Table 59.2** Brain protection strategies

| | |
|---|---|
| Relaxed brain | • Adequate head position<br>• Osmotic diuretics<br>• Mild hypocapnia<br>• Avoidance of sudden increases in airway pressure (coughing, bronchospasm, airway obstruction)<br>• Avoidance of cerebral vasodilators (volatile anesthetics, nitroprusside, calcium channel blockers)<br>• Cerebrospinal fluid drainage |
| Controlled hemodynamics | • Normovolemia<br>• Optimal cerebral perfusion pressure |
| Fluids and electrolytes | • Normovolemia<br>• Avoid hypo-osmolarity<br>• Avoid reduction in colloid oncotic pressure<br>• Normo- to mild hyperglycemia |
| Temperature | • Mild hypothermia |
| Controlled emergence | • Avoidance of acute hypertension<br>• Avoidance of sudden increases in airway pressure (coughing, straining, airway obstruction) |

Adapted with permission from Young WL, Talke P, Lawton MT: Anesthetic considerations for surgical resection of brain arteriovenous malformations. In Cottrell and Young's Neuroanesthesia, Philadelphia: Mosby Elsevier, 2010. 264–277 position (slightly elevated, avoid extreme flexion and rotation) will promote venous drainage. Osmotic diuretic therapy with mannitol is widely used to facilitate exposure and reduce retractor pressures; mannitol may have additional protective effects in areas with impaired CBF. Hypocapnia, traditionally a staple of neuroanesthesia due to reduction in CBF, is now used much less frequently due to concerns for vasoconstriction and potential ischemia. Cerebral vasodilators (such as inhalational anesthetics in higher doses) should be discontinued when additional brain relaxation is needed. Sudden increases in intrathoracic pressure (coughing, airway obstruction etc.) can lead to increased ICP and should be prevented or promptly addressed.

## Fluid Management

The fundamental principles for patients undergoing resection of AVM are the same as for other intracranial procedures: (1) maintain normovolemia and (2) avoid reductions in serum osmolarity. In addition, (3) avoidance of hyperglycemia and (4) prevention in reduction of colloid oncotic pressure may also be advantageous but available supporting evidence is less conclusive.

Maintaining normovolemia is the mainstay of modern neurosurgical practice and the foundation of maintaining normal MAP and CPP. Reduction in serum osmolarity can result in brain edema [9]. There is little evidence that the choice of fluid can influence the patient outcome as long as the above mentioned goals are observed. Crystalloid solutions such as normal saline, lactated Ringer, and Plasma-lyte are the fluids most commonly used intraoperatively (Table 59.3). Normal saline (0.9% NaCl) is misleadingly named as its composition is quite different from the normal (physiologic) plasma. It can cause hyperchloremic acidosis when administered in large volumes. Lactated Ringer is hypoosmolar (273 mOsm/L) and slightly acidic (pH 6.5) but remains popular among clinicians despite those apparent flaws. Plasma-Lyte has the composition that most closely resembles "physiologic" plasma (ph, osmolarity and main electrolytes) so it is the author's crystalloid fluid of choice, even more so in the setting of large fluid volume administration.

In addition to maintaining normovolemia and normal serum osmolarity, it may be important to avoid reductions in colloid oncotic pressure (COP). The role of COP in the formation of brain edema is much less important when compared to serum osmolarity changes (and not well documented), but it can be a contributor in certain situations when the blood-brain barrier is disrupted [10]. The majority of elective uncomplicated cases do not require administration of colloid solutions since the fluid requirements are generally modest and the likelihood of reducing COP is low.

The evidence regarding glucose management is controversial [11]. It is believed that increased plasma glucose can aggravate cerebral ischemia, but other data suggest that the injured brain may require "extra sweetness" (meaning that the brain may become "hypoglycemic" during an acute ischemic episode). A common sense approach would be to avoid glucose-containing fluids unless there is a specific indication. Maintaining plasma glucose between 140 and 180 mg/dL [12] appears to be a reasonable if somewhat arbitrary target as the potential for hypoglycemia in an anesthetized patient should not be overlooked.

**Table 59.3** Comparison between composition of plasma and crystalloid solutions

| Fluid | Osmolality (mOsm/L) | pH | Electrolytes (mEq/L) | | | | | Buffers |
|---|---|---|---|---|---|---|---|---|
| | | | Na | Cl | K | Ca | Mg | |
| *Plasma* | 290 | 7.4 | 140 | 104 | 4 | 5 | 2 | *Bicarbonate (25)* |
| Plasma-Lyte | 294 | 7.4 | 140 | 98 | 5 | – | 3 | Acetate (27) Gluconate (23) |
| 0.9% sodium chloride (normal saline) | 308 | 5.0 | 154 | 154 | – | – | – | – |
| Lactated Ringer's | 273 | 6.5 | 130 | 109 | 4 | 3 | – | Lactate (28) |

## Hemodynamic Control

The most obvious goal for patients undergoing AVM surgery (and all of intracranial procedures) is maintaining optimal CPP. The difficulty arises in defining "optimal" as this can vary based on the clinical situation, patients' characteristics, and practitioner's preferences. Communication with the surgeon is extremely important in establishing goals and thresholds for intervention. Even in patients presenting with asymptomatic AVM, adjacent brain areas may be marginally perfused and highly dependent on maintaining collateral perfusion pressure. Preoperative and intraoperative events (such as mass effect, hemorrhage, retractor pressure) can lead to ischemia and make maintaining perfusion pressure even more critical. As a general rule, CPP should be maintained at normal or even high-normal levels unless induced hypotension is necessary to control hemorrhage. There is no best anesthetic technique suited to achieve this goal but factors to be considered include: adequate monitoring (intra-arterial catheter with the transducer located at the brain level for accurate measurement of MAP and CPP), resuscitation capabilities (intravenous access and blood products), minimizing or countering the hypotensive effects of anesthetic agents while maintaining adequate anesthesia and patient immobility.

Induced hypotension may be needed during AVM resection if significant hemorrhage ensues. This is more likely to occur for AVMs with deep arterial supply and the acute reduction in blood pressure can facilitate surgical hemostasis. Direct vasodilators such as sodium nitroprusside are very effective to induce hypotension but may have potential deleterious effects on perfusion of adjacent brain areas (which may be maximally vasodilated). Barbiturate therapy (thiopental) may be used as an adjuvant for induced hypotension but also for their CMR-reductive and cerebral protective capabilities. As always, communication between surgeon and anesthesiologist is paramount in order to best respond to a rapidly evolving clinical situation.

## Hypothermia

Numerous laboratory studies have showed that mild hypothermia (32–34 °C) can reduce neurologic injury associated with ischemia which led to widespread use in neurovascular procedures. However, recent multicenter trials failed to show benefits in humans [13, 14]. Significant side effects can be associated with the use of (even mild) hypothermia: cardiac dysrhythmias, coagulation impairment, delayed emergence due to diminished drug metabolism, shivering and hypertension accompanying emergence if the patient has not been fully rewarmed. Based on the available evidence and potential for side effects, routine use of hypothermia is not recommended. The decision to use mild hypothermia is selective and local, typically when the risk of intraoperative ischemia is judged to be high and the surgeons are comfortable with the possibility of delayed emergence precluding immediate postoperative examination.

## Emergence from Anesthesia

When planning for emergence, the first question to be answered by anesthesiologist and surgeon is whether the patient is a good candidate for rapid emergence to facilitate early neurologic examination. A complicated intraoperative course, massive fluid resuscitation, preexisting neurologic deficits may be indications for postoperative sedation and ventilation. Regardless of the timing and location of emergence (operating room or intensive care unit), the same general principles of intracranial procedures apply: avoidance of acute hypertension, coughing and straining. Arterial hypertension can contribute to intracranial bleeding and edema formation. Coughing and straining lead to sudden increases of intrathoracic pressure that is transmitted to cerebral circulation with the same potential damaging consequences: increased ICP, bleeding, and edema formation.

There are many approaches used to achieve those goals although no single "best" technique is suitable for all patients. Opioids are helpful in suppressing cough (blunting effect of the airway reflexes) as long as their use is compatible with return of spontaneous ventilation at the end of procedure. Early discontinuation of volatile agents may be helpful to avoid the "neither here nor there" phase (patient starting to emerge and cough due to presence of endotracheal tube but not meeting criteria for extubation yet). If volatile agents are discontinued, low-dose nitrous oxide and propofol can be used to maintain anesthesia until the conclusion of surgery. Lidocaine can be used to suppress cough during emergence; instillation through a modified endotracheal tube appears more effective than intravenous administration [15]. Short acting vasoactive medications should be available to treat hypertension and tachycardia; beta blockers such as labetalol or esmolol may be preferred over direct vasodilators like nitroprusside due to lack of effect on CBF. Dexmedetomidine may be a useful adjuvant due to its sympatholytic and sedative effects allowing for patient's arousal to perform neurologic exam while minimizing the potential hypertensive response.

## Postoperative Period

Avoidance of bleeding and brain swelling remain the principal goals in the immediate postoperative period. An intraoperative or postoperative angiogram may be performed to confirm complete resection or if bleeding is suspected. Postoperative care varies but maintenance of optimal CPP and prevention of postoperative hypertension are of utmost importance due to the concern that the dysautoregulating brain adjacent to the resected AVM will develop edema or hemorrhage.

### Conclusion

Despite their rare occurrence, AVM can be a significant cause of morbidity and mortality in neurosurgery. Good communication between anesthesiologist and neurosurgeon, proper understanding of the pathophysiology and patient's characteristics, adequate preparation and continuous vigilance are paramount in ensuring a favorable outcome.

## References

1. Kader A, Young WL. The effects of intracranial arteriovenous malformations on cerebral hemodynamics. Neurosurg Clin N Am. 1996;7:767–81.
2. Young WL, Talke P, Lawton MT. Anesthetic considerations for surgical resection of brain arteriovenous malformations. In: Cottrell and Young's Neuroanesthesia. Philadelphia: Mosby Elsevier; 2010. p. 264–77.
3. Spetzler RF, Martin NA. A proposed grading system for arteriovenous malformations. J Neurosurg. 1986;65:476–83.
4. Marik PE, Baram M, Vahid B. Does central venous pressure predict fluid responsiveness? A systematic review of the literature and the tale of seven mares. Chest. 2008;134:172–8.
5. Perel A. Automated assessment of fluid responsiveness in mechanically ventilated patients. Anesth Analg. 2008;106:1031–3.
6. Berkenstadt H, Margalit N, Hadani M, et al. Stroke volume variation as a predictor of fluid responsiveness in patients undergoing brain surgery. Anesth Analg. 2001;92:984–9.
7. Hoffman WE, Charbel FT, Edelman G, et al. Comparison of the effect of etomidate and desflurane on brain tissue games and pH during prolonged middle cerebral artery occlusion. Anesthesiology. 1998;88:1188–94.
8. Patel PM, Drummond JC, Lemkuil BP. Cerebral physiology and the effects of anesthetic drugs. In: Miller's Anesthesia. Philadelphia: Saunders Elsevier; 2015. p. 387–422.
9. Tommasino C, Moore S, Todd MM. Cerebral effects of isovolemic hemodilution with crystalloid or colloid solutions. Crit Care Med. 1988;16:862–8.
10. Drummond JC, Patel PM, Cole DJ, et al. The effect of reduction of colloid oncotic pressure, with and without reduction of osmolality, on post-traumatic cerebral edema. Anesthesiology. 1998;88:993–1002.
11. Drummond JC, Patel PM, Lemkuil BP. Anesthesia for neurologic surgery. In: Miller's Anesthesia. Philadelphia: Saunders Elsevier; 2015. p. 2158–99.
12. Finfer S, Chittock DR, Su SY, et al. Intensive versus conventional glucose control in critically ill patients. N Engl J Med. 2009;360:1283–97.
13. Todd MM, Hindman BJ, Clarke WR, et al. Mild intraoperative hypothermia during surgery for intracranial aneurysm. N Engl J Med. 2005;352:135–45.
14. Clifton GL, Valadka A, Zygun D, et al. Very early hypothermia induction in patients with severe brain injury (the National Acute Brain Injury Study: Hypothermia II): a randomised trial. Lancet Neurol. 2010;10:131–9.
15. Gonzalez RM, Bjerke RJ, Drobycki T, et al. Prevention of endotracheal tube-induced coughing during emergence from general anesthesia. Anesth Analg. 1994;79:792-795.

# Awake Craniotomy

Ronan Mukherjee and Mohammed Al-Tamimi

## Introduction

Awake Craniotomy (AC) is a technique which has gained popularity since it's conception in the 1800s. With its initial indication being for the treatment of epilepsy, we are now seeing its use in,

- Tumour resection surgery,
- Arteriovenous malformations,
- Mycotic aneurysms,
- Deep Brain Stimulation in Parkinson's Disease and
- Obsessive Compulsive Disorder

AC predated the history of currently known anesthesia. Since ancient times people have used trepanation to treat seizures and remove "evil air" [1], with the discovery of local anesthetics by Koller in 1884 possibly facilitating its' evolution into the technique we know today [2].

Anesthesia for AC was initially delivered by neurosurgeons with local anesthetics only. Davidoff and Penfield added sedation to local anesthesia in the middle of 1930s, the latter using sedation after brain testing, with the introduction of GA In 1953 by Pasquet [3].

The more recognisable change, came after the development of propofol in the 1990s [4]. Due to its rapid onset and redistribution, its use is ideal in AC. Further to this, the advantageous properties of the ultra-short opioid Remifentanil has also secured its place in modern techniques.

AC can be divided into three phases; the *initial phase* is the craniotomy, exposing the brain. This can be performed either awake, with sedation or asleep, as you can imagine this is one of the most stimulating parts of the procedure. Fortunately, there is no benefit to keeping the patient awake for this part, therefore General Anesthesia is more frequently used. The *second phase* is that of tumor resection. It is here that cortical mapping needs to be performed to identify and avoid eloquent areas of the brain, this requires an awake and cooperative patient. The *final phase* is hemostasis and closure of Dura, bone flap and skin. Similarly, as in the initial phase, there is no real merit to keeping the patient awake with many anesthetists again inducing General Anesthesia to assure patient comfort and satisfaction.

Being awake allows the use of cortical mapping to maximise excision/resection of disease, whilst minimising post-operative neurological deficit. Cortical mapping utilises direct electrical stimulation of the cortex to identify functional areas thus preventing iatrogenic injury during surgery [5]. Stimulation of the Broca's and Wernicke's areas of speech and language inhibits or slows speech, while stimulation of the sensory and motor areas increases sensation or alters the motor function to the corresponding areas. For

R. Mukherjee, F.R.C.A. (✉) · M. Al-Tamimi, M.D.
University Hospital Birmingham, Birmingham, UK
e-mail: ronan.mukherjee@doctors.org.uk

successful neurophysiological monitoring, the patient is required to be fully awake to engage in conversation for assessment of speech, as well as to cooperate and perform tasks for motor assessment.

There are different techniques for awake craniotomies depending on the surgeon, anesthetist and institutional preference.

There is no evidence suggesting the superiority of a technique over others. Familiarity with a specific technique is an important factor for success and good outcome.

## Pre-operative Evaluation

### Patient Selection

To maximise the success of AC and minimise conversion to GA, patient selection is paramount. Good candidates are generally cooperative adults who are able to communicate however, there are several case reports of successful awake craniotomies in children.

The selected patients must be prepared both psychologically and physically in the pre-operative period (Table 60.1).

The benefit of AC in aphasic patients and those with profound weakness is questionable, therefore these patients are generally excluded. Communication is a prerequisite for AC however, those with language barrier may have a translator to facilitate the process.

Lack of cooperation is an absolute contraindication for AC, also patients with anxiety disorders like claustrophobia may experience panic attacks during the procedure that can cause failure of the procedure and/or severe complications.

Physically, those patients who are unable to lie still for long periods of time may cause early abandonment of the procedure. This may include the morbidly obese, pregnant and those with chronic back or body pain.

Meetings with the Neurosurgeons and Anesthetists are arranged to assess suitability and discuss what to expect on the day. Many centers also offer a preoperative visit to the theatre to allow familiarisation with the environment helping to establish a rapport with the patient and hence cooperation during the procedure.

**Table 60.1** Indications and contraindications for AC

| |
|---|
| **Indications** |
| • Tumour resection |
| • Excision of vascular malformations |
| • Excision of epileptic foci |
| • Deep brain stimulation |
|   – Parkinson's disease |
|   – Obsessive compulsive disorder |
| **Contraindications** |
|  **Absolute** |
| • Patient refusal |
| • Unable to communicate |
|   – Language barrier |
|   – Learning difficulty |
|   – Age <11 (10) |
| • Unable to cooperate |
|   – Confusion |
|   – Anxiety |
|   – Inability to lie still/flat |
|  **Relative** |
| • Co-morbidity |
|   – Obesity |
|   – Pregnancy |
|   – Difficult airway |
|   – Chronic cough |
|   – Severe lung disease |
|     Chronic Obstructive Airways Disease |
|     Obstructive Sleep Apnoea |

## Anaesthetic Considerations

A standard anesthetic assessment should be performed, including documentation of existing neurological deficits or seizure activity. The presence of significant comorbidity requires careful assessment to determine suitability for AC as well as pre-operative optimisation.

There are no investigations specific to AC, basic investigations should be performed as per those for craniotomy under general anesthesia. Serum antiepileptic levels may worth checking prior to the day of operation.

## On the Day

### Theatre Layout

Attention is required to balance the need for unhindered assessment of speech and motor functions against both anesthetic and surgical access to the patient. The layout also largely depends on tumor position, with the majority of cases performed in the supine or lateral position and occasionally semi-sitting for occipital tumors.

When considering the positioning of theatre equipment, it is crucial to maintain line of sight so that the neurophysiologists may assess function. Drapes should be applied in a way that keeps the patients face clearly visible for both communication and airway management on emergence.

A thorough Multidisciplinary team brief will enable an agreeable solution.

### Monitoring

Standard levels of monitoring usually are recommended. The use of Depth of Anesthesia monitoring is questioned, with some studies recommending its use, and others circumspect given its potential limitations in neurological pathology [6].

All peripheral lines should be inserted into the opposite site of the test limbs. The patient must be kept warm intraoperatively to avoid hypothermia and shivering. The use of catheters must be carefully thought out as they may cause intraoperative discomfort. The use of convenes in male patients can avoid this issue, if unavoidable, liberal use of local anesthetic lubricants can help.

### Emergency Drugs and Equipment

Different airway equipment of different sizes must be prepared and checked for immediate use. Drugs including antiepileptics, antiemetics, analgesics, antihypertensives and inotropes should also be available in the operating room.

### Anaesthetic Technique

As alluded to previously, there are three phases of an AC and the anaesthetic for each phase may vary. Patients can be kept awake throughout with a Local Anaesthetic Scalp Block, patients can be sedated (Monitored Anesthesia Care) or general anesthetic can be induced for the first and/or third stages (Asleep-Awake-Asleep or Asleep-Awake-Awake).

### Scalp Block [7]

An effective scalp block is vital to anesthesia for awake craniotomy, it provides analgesia in the awake phase and consequently hemodynamic stability by attenuating response to pain.

Seven nerves from both sides of the scalp are identified and blocked individually. A ring block can also be done but it requires a larger volume of drug with higher risk of local anesthetic toxicity.

Bupivicaine, levobupivicaine and ropivicaine are the most commonly used drugs. A mix of both short and faster acting local anesthetics can be used to speed onset of the block. The addition of epinephrine to the mixture minimises bleeding from the surgical wound, prolongs the local anesthetic effect and hence decreases systemic absorption and risk of toxicity.

### Anatomy of Scalp Block (Fig. 60.1)

1. **Supraorbital Nerve**
   - Origin: Trigeminal nerve, V1 distribution
   - Supply: Forehead and anterior part of the scalp
   - How to block: Palpate supraorbital notch, inject 4 mL of LA above the eyebrow line
   - Possible complications: None

**Fig. 60.1** Scalp neuroanatomy

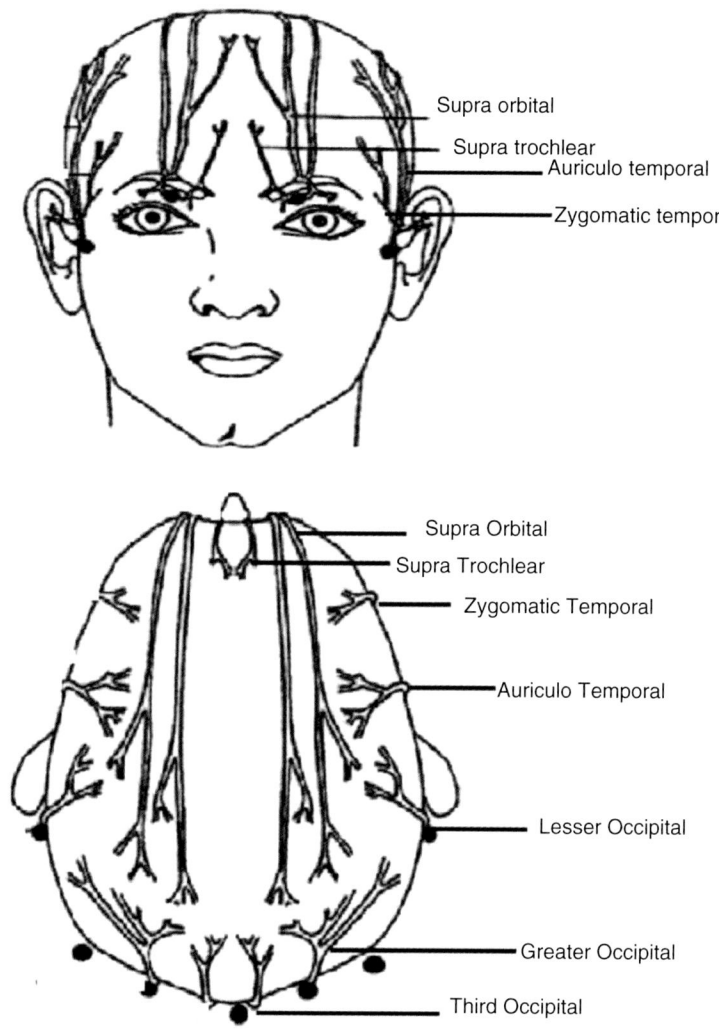

2. **Supratrochlear Nerve**
   - Origin: Trigeminal nerve, V1 distribution
   - Supply: Forehead and anterior part of the scalp
   - How to block: Medial to the supraorbital injection site
   - Possible complications: None
3. **Zygomaticotemporal Nerve**
   - Origin: Trigeminal nerve, V2 distribution
   - Supply: Small area of forehead and temporal area
   - How to block: Deep and superficial infiltration to the temporalis muscle, from the edge of the supraorbital margin to the distal aspect of the zygomatic arch
   - Possible complications: None
4. **Auriculotemporal Nerve**
   - Origin: Trigeminal nerve, V3 distribution
   - Supply: Temporal area, auricle and scalp above auricle
   - How to block: one centimeter anterior to the auricle
   - Possible complications: intra-arterial injection into the superficial temporal artery.
5. **Lesser Occipital Nerve**
   - Origin: a branch of C2 or C3 nerve roots
   - Supply: scalp in the lateral area of the head posterior to the auricle
   - How to block: L.A infiltration behind the auricle starting from the top-down to the auricular lobule then continue to infiltrate

from the superior nuchal line to the greater occipital nerve
 – Possible complications: None
6. **Greater Occipital Nerve**
 – Origin: C2 nerve root
 – Supply: Posterior part of the scalp, can also supply the scalp at the top of the head and over the auricle
 – How to block: medial to the occipital artery
 – Possible complications: Intra-arterial injection of L.A
7. **Greater Auricular Nerve**
 – Origin: C2 or C3 nerve roots
 – Supply: skin over the parotid gland and mastoid process, and the auricle
 – How to block: inject L.A at about 2 cm posterior to the auricle at the level of the tragus
 – Possible complications: None

## Monitored Anesthesia Care (MAC)

Monitored Anesthesia Care is defined by the American Society of Anesthesiologists (ASA) as a planned procedure utilising local anesthetic with sedation and analgesia. The level of sedation is adjusted according to the level of procedural stimulation. At the beginning, the patient is deeply sedated to facilitate a scalp block, insertion of vascular access, head pinning and craniotomy. It is then lightened or stopped for neurophysiological testing and deepened again for closure.

**Advantages**
- Doesn't require invasive airway
- Smooth and quick emergence from sedation

**Disadvantages**
- Uncontrolled airway
- Risk of hypoxia and/or hypercapnia
- Requires experience in sedation technique

## Asleep-Awake-Asleep (SAS)

General anesthesia is induced with Total Intravenous Anesthesia technique, with Propofol and Remifentanil being the most commonly used agents although volatile anesthetics can be used.

Laryngeal Mask Airways (LMA) are most commonly used for airway management as they are well tolerated and allow spontaneous breathing. Endotracheal Tubes (ETT) can also be used but potentially require muscle relaxation and may cause coughing whilst in Mayfield pins. The LMA/ETT is then replaced with a Hudson face mask during the "awake" stage, capnography should be continued at this stage if sedation/analgesia is continued.

On completion of the test, patient can either be put back into general anesthesia with definitive airway or only sedation.

**Advantages**
- Better control of airway and ventilation.
- Less stressful for the patient, anaesthetised during the painful procedures.

**Disadvantages**
- Airway manipulation may be stimulating.
- Relative slower wakening for intraoperative brain testing.
- The risk of intraoperative nausea and vomiting associated with volatile anesthetic.

## Anaesthetic Agents

### Propofol
Commonly used and familiar to most anesthetists, this familiarity allows for safe and effective titration of sedation with a Target Controlled Infusion (TCI).

### Remifentanil
An ultra-short acting opioid, Remifentanil is also commonly used and at low doses will provide analgesia with minimal sedation. Its profound analgesic effect.

### Dexmedetomidine
An $\alpha 2$ agonist which causes sedation, analgesia and anxiolysis, its rapid pharmacokinetics and titratability providing ideal conditions for AC. Suggested doses; load with 1 mcg/kg

followed by an infusion of between 0.2–0.7 mcg/kg/h [8].

## Complications

### Airway Complications

Airway management is determined by anesthetic technique. In Asleep-Awake-Asleep (SAS) for instance, an LMA or ETT is placed during the initial asleep stage with option of LMA re-insertion after awake stage. Oxygen delivery is maintained by Hudson face mask throughout monitored anesthesia technique and during awake stage of SAS. Airway management can be very challenging with the head fixed with pins, therefore difficult airway is a contraindication to awake craniotomy.

Airway complications include failure of airway devices like LMA leading to hypoxia and hypercarbia. Other complications documented are upper airway obstruction, aspiration of gastric contents, hyperventilation and apnea.

### Seizures

Electrical stimulation of the cortex during testing is the main trigger of seizures with Local Anesthetic toxicity and low serum levels of antiepileptics other potential causes. Focal seizures are the most common, but generalised seizures can occur. This usually responds to cold saline irrigation. Sometimes antiepileptic drugs are required in recurrent and resistant cases. Some drugs like benzodiazepines may prolong sedation and delay brain testing. Patients are advised to take their regular antiepileptic drugs in the morning on the day of surgery.

### Nausea and Vomiting

This is a common complication due to both intracranial pathology and potential surgical manipulation around the Chemoreceptor Trigger Zone. Not only is this an issue due to patient discomfort but vomiting whilst pinned will cause movement and can risk neck injury. Different classes of antiemetics are sometimes required to control nausea.

### Pain

Pain is mainly caused by head pin fixation, scalp incision, craniotomy and opening of dura. Analgesia of the surgical field relies on effective scalp block. In addition to remifentanil infusion, other classes of analgesics may be considered if needed. Prolonged immobility can cause discomfort or pain distant from surgical site, for this reason, attention is needed when positioning the patient ensuring pressure points are well padded and joints well supported. Urinary catheters, as mentioned above, can cause pain or discomfort. This can be mitigated by the use of convenes or extra Local Anesthetic gel on insertion.

### Cerebral Oedema

Cerebral oedema often accompanies intracranial lesions, manipulation and traction of brain tissue causes or aggravates this swelling. This can manifest as tight brain or temporary postoperative focal neurology.

### Conclusion

AC is a procedure that is growing in popularity and clinical indication, given its superior patient safety and post-operative recovery profile. Anesthesia for AC requires skill and experience for effective delivery, yet there is currently no consensus on the exact anesthetic recipe. A thorough multi-disciplinary approach is paramount to ensure appropriate patient selection, preparation and ultimately satisfaction.

## References

1. July J, Manninen P, Lai J, Yao Z, Bernstein M. The history of awake craniotomy for brain tumor and its spread into Asia. Surg Neurol. 2009;71:621–53.
2. Bulsara KR, Johnson J, Villavicencio A. Improvements in brain tumor surgery: the modern history of awake craniotomies. Neurosurg Focus. 2005;18:e5.
3. De Castro J, Mundeleer P. Anesthésie sans barbituriques. La neuroleptanalgésie. Anesth Analg. 1959;16:1022.
4. Silbergeld DL, Mueller WM, Colley PS, Ojemann GA, Lettici E. Use of propofol (Diprivan) for awake craniotomies: technical note. Surg Neurol. 1992;38:271–2.

5. Krieg SM, Shiban E, Droese D, Gempt J, Buchmann N, Pape H, Ryang YM, Meyer B, Ringel F. Predictive value and safety of intraoperative neurophysiological monitoring with motor evoked potentials in glioma surgery. Neurosurgery. 2012;70:1060–70; discussion 1070–1.
6. Stevanovic A, Rossaint R, Veldeman M, Bilotta F, Coburn M. Anaesthesia management for awake craniotomy: systematic review and meta-analysis. PLoS One. 2016;11(5):e0156448. https://doi.org/10.1371/journal.pone.0156448.
7. Costello TG, Cormack JR. Anaesthesia for awake craniotomy: a modern approach. J Clin Neurosci. 2004;11:16–9.
8. Ard JL Jr, Bekker AY, Doyle WK. Dexmedetomidine in awake craniotomy: a technical note. Surg Neurol. 2005;63:114–7.

# Functional Brain Surgery (Stereotactic Surgery, Deep Brain Stimulation)

**61**

Ilyas Qazi and Hannah Church

## Introduction

Functional stereotactic surgery as originally pioneered by Swedish neurosurgeon Lars Leksell, involves image-guided sophisticated targeting of smaller and deeper brain structures. Since the early 1980s there have been significant technological advances in the field of functional neurosurgery [1].

Deep Brain stimulation (DBS), as a minimally invasive surgical treatment modality has revolutionized the treatment of patients with refractory movement disorders including Parkinson's disease, essential tremors, dystonia and Tourette's syndrome. DBS has also been utilized as a modulatory treatment strategy for intractable chronic pain conditions, management of refractory epilepsy and alleviation of psychiatric ailments, namely, refractory depression and obsessive-compulsive disorders [2, 3].

The origins of DBS can be traced back to the evolving surgical treatment options for movement disorders, particularly Parkinson's disease [4]. DBS was approved as an adjunctive treatment in 2002 by the US Food and drug administration (FDA) for reducing symptoms that were not adequately controlled by medications in levodopa-responsive advanced Parkinsonian patients [5].

I. Qazi, F.R.C.A. (✉) · H. Church, F.R.C.A.
Queen Elizabeth Hospital, Birmingham, UK
e-mail: hannahchurch@doctors.net.uk

## Parkinson's Disease (PD)

Parkinson's disease is the second most common age-related progressive neurodegenerative disorder after Alzheimer's disease. An estimated seven to ten million people worldwide suffer from PD. The prevalence of the disease ranges from 41 people per 100,000 in the fourth decade of life to more than 1900 people per 100,000 among those 80 years and older.

The diagnosis of Parkinson's disease is based mainly on the patient's presenting clinical features. The cardinal diagnostic features include motor signs such as resting tremors, muscle rigidity and bradykinesia. The most common initial presenting symptom is an asymmetric resting tremor in one of the upper extremities. Patients may then notice a progressive worsening of their axial posture, slowness of movement and gait instabilities with typically shorter strides during ambulation [6].

Besides the motor symptoms, other clinical features include sensory abnormalities, sleep disturbances, cognitive impairment, anxiety, depression and autonomic instability. Some of the non-motor symptoms such as decreased olfaction, rapid eye movement (REM) behaviour disorder (RBD), memory impairment, constipation, urinary urgency and excessive daytime sleepiness may precede the motor features of PD.

## Pathophysiology

Parkinson's disease results from a dysfunction in the motor and non-motor neural circuits within the basal ganglia. There is a loss of striatal dopaminergic neurons in the pars compacta region of the substantia nigra which results in an imbalance between acetylcholine-induced excitation and dopaminergic inhibition of the striatum [7].

While excessive inhibition of the thalamus and brainstem nuclei result from increased excitation; motor symptoms such as akinesia, rigidity and tremor occur as a consequence of cortical motor system suppression. Inhibition of the brain stem motor areas lead to gait abnormalities and postural instability.

The non-motor features of PD likely result from non-dopaminergic changes in the central nervous system (CNS), as also from changes in the dopaminergic neurons outside these pathways.

## Pharmacologic Treatment

Pharmacological treatment in PD is aimed at reinstating the balance between the CNS neurotransmitters dopamine and acetylcholine [8]. In the later stages of the disease, as pharmacological therapy becomes less effective, there is progressive neurological deterioration which can have a negative impact on patient's quality of life.

Dopaminergic drugs are highly effective in controlling the motor manifestations of PD. The mainstay of pharmacological treatment is with dopamine agonists such as Levodopa, considered to be a dopamine precursor within the CNS.

Carbidopa, a commonly co-administered drug is a carboxylase inhibitor, that impedes peripheral metabolism of Levodopa thereby enhancing its CNS availability.

Rotigotine, a non-ergoline, is another dopamine agonist that is available in the form of once daily transdermal patches.

Apomorphine, is the only dopamine agonist that is available as a parenteral preparation and is generally used as a rescue therapy in PD.

Nausea and vomiting are commonly encountered side effects of treatment with dopaminergic drugs and frequently require anti-emetic therapy.

Monoamine oxidase (MAO) B inhibitors e.g. Selegiline prevent degradation of dopamine within the CNS.

Amantadine, an antiviral medication, has a role in treatment of mild PD, although its mechanism of action is uncertain.

Anticholinergics e.g. benzotropine may improve tremor and rigidity and can be offered as a second line treatment in PD.

## Special Considerations in PD

Besides routine anesthetic considerations in patients with PD undergoing DBS, there are certain disease-specific issues which can have an impact on peri-operative anaesthetic management and outcomes (Table 61.1).

## Deep Brain Stimulation System

Deep brain stimulation as compared to permanent surgical lesioning techniques such as Pallidotomy and thalamotomy, is advantageous in being reversible, programmable, non-destructive and with a better patient safety profile [9, 10].

DBS involves targeted placement of stimulator electrodes within the deeper brain parenchymal structures. The most common targets for movement disorders are the ventralis intermedius nucleus (Vim), the subthalamic nucleus (STN) and the internal globus pallidus (GPi) [11].

The subthalamic nucleus (STN) is now considered to be the preferred target for DBS in Parkinson's disease [12]. STN stimulation provides good symptom control of primary motor features, including rigidity, tremor, akinesia, bradykinesia, gait disturbances, motor fluctuations, and levodopa-induced dyskinesia in advanced Parkinson's disease.

**Table 61.1** Peri-operative implications in patients with Parkinson's disease

| Peri-operative issues in PD | Anaesthetic implications |
|---|---|
| Pharyngeal and laryngeal dysfunction | Airway complications such as laryngospasm, aspiration and inability to manage secretions |
| Poor cough, recurrent chest infection, and rigidity-induced restrictive lung disease | Respiratory complications are more common |
| Dysphagia, poor nutrition, immuno-compromised states | Malnutrition, anaemia, metabolic imbalances, increased risk of infections |
| Autonomic instability | Peri-operative risk of hypotension, hypovolemia, arrhythmias and temperature dysregulation |
| Existing dementia and depression | May impede intraoperative communication and cooperation, risk of postoperative delirium is increased |
| Severe tremor and abnormal posturing | Difficult vascular access, monitoring and positioning |
| Treatment with dopaminergic medications | Drug interactions in the perioperative period |
| With-holding of anti-Parkinsonian medications during DBS | Effects on motor symptom control |
| Use of anticholinergic medications such as—antiemetics (e.g., metoclopramide, prochlorperazine) and antipsychotic medications (e.g., haloperidol) | May worsen the symptoms of PD and should be avoided |

## Mechanism of Action

Deep-brain stimulation changes the firing rate and pattern of individual neurons in the basal ganglia and in most cases, is able to inhibit neuronal cells and excite neural fibres that are closest to the implanted electrode [13]. The electrical current delivered acts at synapses and activates neighbouring astrocytes to alter calcium homeostasis and promote local release of neurotransmitters (e.g. glutamate and adenosine). The therapy is also known to increase blood flow and stimulate neurogenesis. All these effects occur collectively across a large neural network, extending beyond local neuronal cell bodies and axons located around the electrical field.

Deep-brain stimulation thus, by the virtue of its effects on multiple thalamo-cortical circuits, downstream pathways, and other brain parenchymal structures is able to exert a significant influence on the electrical, chemical, and neural networks within the brain tissue [14]. However, it remains uncertain as to how these influences lead to modification of the symptoms of Parkinson's disease; hence, the benefits of this modality of treatment have been established more or less empirically.

## Components of the DBS System

To achieve effective functional stimulation a combined approach of imaged based localisation of the target, and neurophysiology assessment of the precise placement is required [15].

There are four main components to the DBS system;

1. Multicontact quadripolar intracranial electrodes, which are inserted surgically via a burr hole into the targeted brain parenchymal sites,
2. A plastic ring and cap seated onto a burr hole to fix the electrodes to the skull,
3. An extension cable that is tunnelled subcutaneously under the skin of the scalp and the neck to the anterior chest wall or abdomen, and is connected to
4. A single or a dual channel internal pulse generator (IPG), implanted in a surgically fashioned subcutaneous pocket.

## Surgical Technique

As the initial localisation of the intended target is imaged based, the patient is first imaged after placement of a stereotactic frame—this is usually an MRI performed under GA [16]. Frameless systems are available with the predictable decrease in accuracy weighed up against the improvement in patient experience [17]. The patient is then transferred to theatre, whilst localisation of intended target is performed by the neurosurgeon [18]. A burr hole is created and the electrodes are inserted under constant neurophysiological monitoring. The ideal placement is confirmed by an agreement of intended anatomical location and confirmatory neurophysiology.

The procedure is either performed unilaterally, or bilaterally depending on the condition being treated. If bilateral placement of electrodes is required, the electrodes are joined via an extension cable under the scalp. The wires are then tunnelled subcutaneously through the neck and attached to a pulse generator, that is typically implanted into the chest in the infra-clavicular area. DBS procedures can either be performed on the same day as a one-stage technique or may be performed as a two-staged procedure. With the two-staged DBS technique, the first stage would involve target localisation and insertion of DBS electrodes and the second stage would entail internalisation of the electrodes and connection to the internal pulse generator and the battery unit in a separate sitting. The pulse generator's battery usually lasts 2–5 years and needs to be changed along with the generator. The battery change is most commonly done under local anaesthesia.

## Anesthetic Management

### Pre-operative Evaluation and Management

A successful peri-operative outcome is dependent on appropriate patient selection and careful assessment carried out at a multi-disciplinary level [19]. This multidisciplinary team should typically comprise a neurosurgeon, neuroanesthetist, neurologist, neuropsychologist, neurophysiologist and a nurse specialist. A pragmatic and an individualized risk vs. benefits analysis should be conducted before offering patients the surgical option of DBS. It is important that a holistic approach is undertaken in identifying and addressing not just the medical issues surrounding the patient's care but also tackling any psychosocial issues.

DBS surgery can be considered to be clinically indicated for Parkinson's disease when the patient develops severe tremors, dyskinesia and rigidity, intolerance to medication or 'off periods' with moderate to severe motor fluctuation. Although, currently there is no clear consensus on the best timing for surgery, there is evidence to suggest that, PD patients with disabling motor symptoms who exhibit responsiveness to levodopa treatment are more likely to benefit from DBS surgery [20].

Exclusions to DBS surgery include severe cognitive impairment, major behavioural disorders, significant cardiorespiratory and medical comorbidities. Increasing patient age is predictive of increased clinical risk and poorer peri-operative outcome.

The aim of pre-operative assessment is to identify the extent of clinical severity of patient's symptoms, coexisting medical conditions, history of alcohol and substance abuse, claustrophobia and previous inability to tolerate sedation. A thorough pre-operative assessment helps to recognise potential problems e.g. poorly controlled hypertension, clotting disorders, etc., that can contribute to increased surgical risks and would need optimisation prior to surgery.

It is absolutely vital to assess the patient's motivational state and ability to co-operate with the procedure before planning an awake technique, as the procedure entails several hours of immobilisation and intra-operative functional testing. A detailed discussion with the patient regarding the steps of the procedure is crucial for overall success of the procedure. Need for invasive monitoring is determined based on the severity of existing co-morbidities and intra-operative patient position, for e.g. monitoring for venous air embolism in sitting position.

A thorough airway assessment and planning is important to avoid airway related complications, especially when the stereotactic frame is in situ.

Anti-Parkinsonian medications are generally withheld pre-operatively to facilitate intra-operative functional testing in an 'off-drug state' during DBS. It is imperative for the clinical team to be wary of the side-effects secondary to abrupt, but planned withdrawal of these medications. Premedication drugs such as benzodiazepines and other sedatives are largely avoided as they may interfere with intra-operative electrophysiological recordings and interpretation of the tremor disorder during DBS.

## Anesthetic Technique and Intra-operative Management

The anesthetic technique is usually tailored to meet the following objectives-intra-operative patient comfort, optimisation of the surgical field, facilitation of electrophysiological and functional testing during target localisation, and timely diagnosis and management of complications. The anesthetic techniques commonly employed include Awake (local anesthetic) technique with or without sedation, Asleep-awake-asleep technique and complete general anesthetic techniques, with no clear consensus on the superiority of any one technique over another [21].

### Awake Technique
An awake technique allows real time assessment of motor symptom changes in response to deep brain stimulation which in essence, is used as a guide for placement of stimulator electrodes. Intra-operative monitoring of vital parameters (HR, ECG, BP, SpO2, EtCO2) may be challenging in the presence of a severe movement disorder. Beat-to-beat monitoring of invasive blood pressure may be beneficial in patients with labile blood pressure requiring vasoactive drugs for BP control. Ensuring adequate patient comfort during positioning, maintaining good communication, providing constant motivation and reassurance, temperature control, use of a sheath catheter as an alternative to urinary catheterisation are some of the important measures in improving patient compliance during this otherwise stressful procedure. Administration of a local anesthetic Scalp block prior to the placement of a head frame alleviates intra-operative pain and augments patient wellbeing. Surgical draping should allow access to patient's face, arms and legs.

To improve patient relaxation, a titrated IV sedation technique with Propofol [22] e.g. a targeted controlled infusion (TCI), can be utilised during the stages of surgical incision and burr hole creation until the commencement of brain mapping and electrophysiological recording. Propofol permits easy titratability due to a rapid onset and offset effect, secondary to a more conducive pharmacokinetic profile. Use of benzodiazepines as sedatives is actively discouraged, as they can inhibit Micro-electrode recording (MER) signals and interfere with motor responses during DBS. Dexmedetomidine, an α2-adrenoreceptor agonist, is a highly useful agent for IV sedation with minimal respiratory depressant effects. Due its analgesic and antihypertensive properties, dexmedetomidine has shown to attenuate the hemodynamic stress response to pinning, surgical incision and craniotomy. In a low-dose infusion (0.3–0.6 μg/kg/h) it does not seem to attenuate motor responses during DBS and has no effect on MERs [23, 24]. With an awake technique, backache can be a substantial problem for patients undergoing lengthy DBS procedures. Spinal opioids e.g. intrathecal hydromorphone, have been reported to provide pain relief without abolishing electrophysiologic recordings [25].

### General Anesthetic Technique
General anesthesia (GA) may be used as a comprehensive technique on its own or as part of an Asleep-awake-asleep technique. A comprehensive GA technique is used in children and adults who are severely dystonic or are unable to tolerate the procedure awake due to concurrent anxiety and or psychiatric disorders [26]. DBS procedures planned under general anesthesia, would need securing of the airway before insertion of the head frame, due to restricted airway access after the frame application. Concerns regarding lack of intra-operative assessment and abolition of MERs leading to suboptimal placement of DBS electrodes under general anesthesia have been raised [27]. A small number of studies

have failed to demonstrate a co-relation between the type of anesthesia utilised and surgical outcomes following DBS [28].

Regardless of the anesthetic technique chosen, it is absolutely imperative that the neuroanesthetist pays attention to detail, maintains a state of thorough vigilance and careful patient monitoring and appropriately manages any problems encountered during the procedure with a team based approach.

## Intra-operative Complications

Based on the data available, the incidence of intra-operative complications has been variously quoted between 5 and 16% [29].

Hypertension is a frequent intraoperative complication and is usually related to patient distress, pain, anxiety and/or poor pre-operative BP control. Titrated doses of analgesics e.g. Remifentanil and IV antihypertensives e.g. Labetalol can be used to treat the acute surges in BP.

Potential loss of airway during the awake technique can occur as a consequence of oversedation and can easily lead to significant airway compromise and risk of aspiration. This is further compounded by the presence of stereotactic head frame making airway access difficult. Rapid control of the airway with a supraglottic airway device, such as LMA, I-gel® or even a swift disengagement of the head frame to allow airway access can be potentially lifesaving during an airway crisis.

Other notable neurological complications include intracranial haemorrhage, seizures, venous air embolism, pneumocephalus, changes in neurological status such as confusion, speech deficits and or limb weakness.

## Post-operative Concerns

Post-operative monitoring of neurological complications is mandatory even in patients receiving limited intra-operative anesthesia for stereotactic procedures, as it can significantly impact patient outcomes.

Akinetic rigid states may develop in the immediate post-operative period and may need activation of the DBS stimulator. Anti-Parkinsonian medications should be re-instituted as early as possible to avoid aggravation and fluctuation of motor symptoms as this can further confound neurological signs and impede patient's ability to clear secretions secondary to respiratory muscle weakness.

## Patients with DBS System Presenting for a Non-DBS Related Procedure

Patients with deep brain stimulators may present for non-DBS related surgery [30]. DBS systems like other Implantable devices such as pacemakers, Automated Implantable Cardioverter-defibrillators (AICD) may interact with monitoring equipment e.g. ECG, resulting in artefacts and recording errors. Medical equipment such as electrocautery, short-wave diathermy devices and peripheral nerve stimulators may interfere with the functioning of DBS systems. Unlike cardiac pacemakers, some deep brain stimulators may be turned off depending on the severity of the patient's symptoms. In these cases, symptom control would then be reliant on timely commencement and appropriate titration of oral medications.

Electrocautery devices may adversely impact the performance of the DBS system through inadvertent reprogramming, as a result of electrical interference. They may also induce electrical burns to the neural tissues at the DBS site [31], hence switching off the DBS device should be preferably undertaken before the use of electrocautery. Bipolar diathermy is safer in comparison to a monopolar cautery when used at lower energy levels and in short pulses [32]. If a monopolar assembly is used the grounding pad should be placed as far away as possible from the DBS system.

The safety of use of external and internal cardiac defibrillators with a DBS system in situ has yet to be established. If an external defibrillator is used, it is advisable to apply the electrode gel pads at a site distant to the DBS pulse generator.

The safety of DBS devices in patients undergoing Magnetic Resonance Imaging (MRI) [33] and electroconvulsive therapy (ECT) will need careful evaluation, adoption of relevant safety measures, and adherence to the manufacturer's guidelines. The deep brain stimulation system should be working, and the leads and extensions should be intact and undamaged to avoid the risk of neural injury. If the DBS device was switched off during the MRI it would need to be turned back on post imaging. If the device was programmed in bipolar mode and remained on during the MRI, the original DBS settings may need to be restored.

# References

1. Miocinovic S, Somayajula S, Chitnis S, Vitek JL. History, applications, and mechanisms of deep brain stimulation. JAMA Neurol. 2013;70:163–71.
2. Sharma M, Naik V, Deogaonkar M. Emerging applications of deep brain stimulation. J Neurosurg Sci. 2016;60(2):242–55.
3. Williams NR, Okun MS. Deep brain stimulation (DBS) at the interface of neurology and psychiatry. J Clin Invest. 2013;123(11):4546–56.
4. Benabid AL, Pollak P, Louveau A, et al. Combined (thalamotomy and stimulation) stereotactic surgery of the VIM thalamic nucleus for bilateral Parkinson disease. Appl Neurophysiol. 1987;50:344–6.
5. Okun MS. Deep-brain stimulation for Parkinson's disease. N Engl J Med. 2012;367:1529–38.
6. Davie CA. A review of Parkinson's disease. Br Med Bull. 2008;86(1):109–27.
7. DeMaagd G, Philip A. Parkinson's disease and its management: part 1: disease entity, risk factors, pathophysiology, clinical presentation, and diagnosis. P T. 2015;40(8):504–32.
8. Massano J, Bhatia KP. Clinical approach to Parkinson's disease: features, diagnosis, and principles of management. Cold Spring Harb Perspect Med. 2012;2(6):a008870.
9. Venkatraghavan L, Luciano M, Manninen P. Anesthetic management of patients undergoing deep brain stimulator insertion. Anesth Analg. 2010;110:1138–45.
10. Larson PS. Deep brain stimulation for movement disorders. Neurotherapeutics. 2014;11(3):465–74.
11. Kocabicak E, Temel Y, Hollig A, et al. Current perspectives on deep brain stimulation for severe neurological and psychiatric disorders. Neuropsychiatr Dis Treat. 2015;11:1051–66.
12. Benabid AL, Torres N. New targets for DBS. Parkinsonism Relat Disord. 2012;18:S21–3.
13. Johnson MD, Miocinovic S, McIntyre CC, Vitek JL. Mechanisms and targets of deep brain stimulation in movement disorders. Neurotherapeutics. 2008;5:294–308.
14. Grant R, Gruenbaum SE, Gerrard J. Anaesthesia for deep brain stimulation: a review. Curr Opin Anaesthesiol. 2015;28:505–10.
15. Scharpf DT, Sharma M, Deogaonkar M, et al. Practical considerations and nuances in anesthesia for patients undergoing deep brain stimulation implantation surgery. Korean J Anesthesiol. 2015;68:332–9.
16. Venkatraghavan L, Manninen P. Anesthesia for deep brain stimulation. Curr Anesthesiol Rep. 2016;6(3):233–43.
17. Sharma M, Rhiew R, Deogaonkar M, et al. Accuracy and precision of targeting using frameless stereotactic system in deep brain stimulator implantation surgery. Neurol India. 2014;62:503–9.
18. Sharma M, Deogaonkar M. Accuracy and safety using intraoperative O-arm during placement of deep brain stimulation electrodes without electrophysiological recordings. J Clin Neurosci. 2016;27:80–6.
19. Erickson KM, Cole DJ. Anesthetic considerations for awake craniotomy for epilepsy and functional neurosurgery. Anesthesiol Clin. 2012;30:241–68.
20. Yeoh TY, Manninen P, Kalia SK, Venkatraghavan L. Anesthesia considerations for patients with an implanted deep brain stimulator undergoing surgery: a review and update. Can J Anesth. 2017;64:308–19.
21. Chen SY, Tsai ST, Lin SH, et al. Subthalamic deep brain stimulation in Parkinson's disease under different anesthetic modalities: a comparative cohort study. Stereotact Funct Neurosurg. 2011;89:372–80.
22. Kim W, Song IH, Lim YH, et al. Influence of propofol and fentanyl on deep brain stimulation of the subthalamic nucleus. J Korean Med Sci. 2014;29(9):1278–86.
23. Kwon WK, Kim JH, Lee JH, et al. Microelectrode recording (MER) findings during sleep-awake anesthesia using dexmedetomidine in deep brain stimulation surgery for Parkinson's disease. Clin Neurol Neurosurg. 2016;143:27–33.
24. Martinez-Simon A, Alegre M, Honorato-Cia C, et al. Effect of dexmedetomidine and propofol on basal ganglia activity in Parkinson disease: a controlled clinical trial. Anesthesiology. 2017;126(6):1033–42.
25. Bindu B, Bithal PK. Anaesthesia and deep brain stimulation. J Neuroanaesthesiol Crit Care. 2016;3:197–204.
26. Chen T, Mirzadeh Z, Chapple K, et al. "Asleep" deep brain stimulation for essential tremor. J Neurosurg. 2015;27:1–8.
27. Mann JM, Foote KD, Garvan CW, et al. Brain penetration effects of microelectrodes and DBS leads in STN or GPi. J Neurol Neurosurg Psychiatry. 2009;80:794–7.

28. Moro E, Lozano AM, Pollak P, et al. Long-term results of a multicenter study on subthalamic and pallidal stimulation in Parkinson's disease. Mov Disord. 2010;25:578–86.
29. Fenoy FJ, Simpson RK Jr. Risks of common complications in deep brain stimulation surgery: management and avoidance. J Neurosurg. 2014;120:132–9.
30. Venkatraghavan L, Chinnapa V, Peng P, Brull R. Non-cardiac implantable electrical devices: brief review and implications for anesthesiologists. Can J Anaesth. 2009;56:320–6.
31. Nutt JG, Anderson VC, Peacock JH, et al. DBS and diathermy interaction induces severe CNS damage. Neurology. 2001;56:1384–6.
32. Poon CC, Irwin MG. Anaesthesia for deep brain stimulation and in patients with implanted neurostimulator devices. Br J Anaesth. 2009;103:152–65.
33. Larson PS, Richardson RM, Starr PA, Martin AJ. Magnetic resonance imaging of implanted deep brain stimulators: experience in a large series. Stereotact Funct Neurosurg. 2008;86:92–100.

# Perioperative Management of Adult Patients with Severe Head Injury

## 62

Adam Low

## Introduction

Traumatic brain injury is a significant public health concern as is a leading cause of both death and disability worldwide [1]. The disability associated with traumatic brain injury, reduced contribution to society and associated care costs rightly make the peri-operative management of adult patients with severe head injury an important area of practice. Public health campaigns in the last 20 years have focussed on improving road safety as well as car safety profile as the young male injured in a road traffic collision dominated the public health statistics for major trauma and traumatic brain injury. Traumatic brain injury nevertheless remains the most common cause of death in those <40 years [2]. However, it is also worth noting that a change in demographic and mechanism of injury for patients suffering major trauma has been noted, with increasingly elderly patients presenting with higher injury severity scores associated with falls <2 m, compared to the young male patient with major trauma secondary to road traffic collisions who were the main demographic and mechanism for major trauma 20 years ago [3]. That said, road traffic collision remains an important cause of head injury in the developing world, with the World Health Organisation predicting that traumatic brain injury and road traffic collisions will be the leading cause of disease and injury worldwide by 2020 [4]. This presents specific challenges to clinicians responsible for perioperative management of adult patients with severe head injury beyond the traditional aim of preventing secondary injury occurring.

## Epidemiology and Pathophysiology of Traumatic Brain Injury

The initial mechanism of injury and primary traumatic injury to the brain will be the predominant cause of morbidity and disability. However, meticulous attention to clinical parameters is mandated to prevent and minimise secondary injury to vulnerable surrounding structures by ensuring adequate supply of oxygenated blood, preventing seizures/maintaining normothermia and preventing hyper or hypoglycaemia.

Table 62.1 details the common causes of traumatic brain injury (and severe traumatic brain injury) and reported incidence according to published literature.

As mentioned in the introduction, there is an increasing proportion of cases in the elderly demographic associated with falls (typically <2 m).

Whatever the mechanism of injury, a force applied to the cranium results in either fracture to the skull vault, or acceleration deceleration of the brain tissue against the vault with associated

A. Low, MbCHB, F.R.C.A. Dip IMC
University Hospital Birmingham, Birmingham, UK
e-mail: adam.low@uhb.nhs.uk

**Table 62.1** Reported causes of traumatic brain injury (moderate-severe) from a large European review [5] and audit data for England and Wales [6]

| Mechanism of injury | Male: female ratios | Proportion of all reported head injuries |
|---|---|---|
| Road traffic collision | 1.46–2.7:1.0 | 55.3% (48–58.9%) |
| Falls | 3.2:1.0 | 51.8% (47–62%) |
| Assaults | 2.1:1.0 | 8% (4–12%) |
| Other | | 6% (3–8%) |

Note that different studies use different diagnostic criteria for severity grading. The estimated incidence for traumatic brain injury was 326 per 100,000 with a mortality rate between 3 per $10^5$ and 18.3 per $10^5$ [5]

diffuse axonal injury, with or without associated haemorrhage. The injured brain tissue is prone to oedema, excitotoxicity and cell death, with associated risk of raised intra-cranial pressure. The tissue around the injured brain is vulnerable to injury and cell death (secondary brain injury), and subsequent medical and surgical management is aimed at reducing the likelihood of this. It is probably a little over-simplistic to consider things in term of primary then secondary brain injury. We should thus consider traumatic brain injury as a progressive disease where the pathophysiological result of initial injury interplay and are aggravated by secondary insults as and when they arrive.

Anaesthetists may be involved in the resuscitation, stabilisation, operative management and ongoing care of traumatic brain injured patients, and so a sound knowledge is mandated with meticulous attention to detail. The overall management of these patients requires a multidisciplinary approach incorporating: emergency medicine, intensive care, neurosurgery, microbiology, physiotherapy, dietitians and rehabilitation medicine.

One of the difficulties is actually defining what a severe head injury is. Simplistically it can be considered as a Glasgow Coma Score (GCS) <8 after initial resuscitation, but this is still subject to individual clinician interpretation of the best score, and takes no account of mechanism of injury or radiological findings. Table 62.2 summarises some possible methods of defining severity of head injury. Injury profiles that subject the patient to high energy transfers to the cranium, associated with a dropping GCS or GCS <8, seizures, radiological changes and indications for intra-cranial pressure monitoring (see below) suggest severe head injury. Again caution is mandated when dealing with elderly patients, who are prone to lower force injuries (e.g. falls) and who have comparatively higher presenting GCS for comparably severe anatomical injury severity compared to younger patients [7]. Any drop in motor score of the GCS indicates high likelihood of a severe traumatic brain injury in those over 65. Elderly patients however do have comparatively good outcomes from management in a Neurosurgical centre, and account should be taken of this when triaging patients in the pre-hospital phase.

The Mayo System is a newer classification of traumatic brain injury that takes account all of the factors in Table 62.2 as well as the neuroimaging findings [8]:

- Possible traumatic brain injury: blurred vision, confusion, dizziness, focal neurological symptoms and headache or nausea.
- Probable traumatic brain injury: any of: loss of consciousness up to 30 min, post traumatic

**Table 62.2** Demonstrates some of the different classification systems for severity of traumatic brain injury

| Grading system | Mild | Moderate | Severe |
|---|---|---|---|
| Glasgow Coma Score (GCS) | 13–15 | 9–12 | <8 |
| Duration of loss of consciousness/fluctuation in mental state | <30 min | 30 min to 6 h | >6 h |
| Post traumatic amnesia (interval from injury until the patient is orientated and can form new memory) | <24 h | 1–7 days | >7 days |

These are subjective, depending upon the assessors interpretation and have their limitations. Some may consider a patient with a GCS of 13 for example to have a greater incidence of morbidity and therefore unsuitable to be classified as "mild". Injury may also be classified by aetiology: blunt, penetrating or blast, or by radiological findings: diffuse or focal

amnesia up to 24 h, depressed or linear skull fracture with the dura intact.
- Definite moderate—severe traumatic brain injury: loss of consciousness over 30 min, post traumatic amnesia beyond 24 h, worst GCS in the first 24 h of <13, evidence of haematoma/contusion/brain stem involvement on neuroimaging and a penetrating injury.

## Secondary Brain Injury Prevention

These appear very simple on paper, but the reality is that this is not always the case, especially in the context of polytrauma. Despite this, each merits attention and ongoing monitoring/optimisation:

- Avoidance of hypoxia
- Avoidance of hypotension
- Avoidance of hypo and hypercarbia
- Maintenance of adequate cerebral perfusion pressure (CPP)
- Minimising cerebral metabolic rate
- Avoidance of hyper and hypoglycaemia
- Control of intracranial pressure (ICP)

Conducting randomised controlled trials into optimal prevention of secondary injury is ethically difficult, so recommendations are based on observational studies, some historic and expert consensus opinion. The IMPACT study, a meta-analysis of 8721 patients suggested that hypoxia and hypotension had significant impact on outcome at 6 months post injury [9].

## Hypoxia

A single episode of hypoxia following primary injury is poorly tolerated and associated with worse outcome. Maintenance of satisfactory oxygen saturation warrants careful attention, and in cases of moderate-severe injury consideration given to securing the airway and ventilating, ensuring adequate oxygenation. There has been increased focus in recent years on targeting brain tissue oxygen (pb-O2), monitored by PET scanning or microdialysis, as well as monitoring ICP or CPP. Observational studies suggest a survival benefit [10] in severe traumatic brain injury. Concerns have been raised about the risk of free radical formation with hyperoxia, with poorer short term outcomes, though the evidence base for this is not yet robust. A pragmatic solution is to rationalise oxygen delivery titrated to arterial blood gas analysis of PaO2 10–13 kPa in line with international guidelines relevant to your country of practice, or to achieve satisfactory pb-O2. The Brain Trauma Foundation recommend maintaining saturations >90%.

## Hypotension and Maintaining Adequate CPP

A single episodes of hypotension following injury are associated with increased mortality (three times compared to normotensive patients) and duration of hypotension was inversely related to functional outcome [11]. Hypotension can be related to ongoing blood loss, drug administration to facilitate airway management, or administration of mannitol. However, hypotension does not just occur in the initial resuscitation and stabilisation: there is a 32–65% incidence during emergency decompressive craniectomy [12], associated with worse outcome. The following specific risk factors for hypotension [12, 13] are worth bearing in mind:

- Low admission GCS
- Pre-operative tachycardia and hypertension
- CT findings of sub-dural haematoma of multiple foci of injury
- Longer duration of anesthesia
- Bilateral dilated pupils

The earliest possible ascertainment of invasive blood pressure monitoring is advisable as will allow prompt recognition and active management of hypotension of a trend in blood pressure suggestive of risk of hypotension. The arterial line transducer should be zeroed at the level of the tragus to allow accurate measurement of CPP once ICP monitoring is established. This change means that a target CPP of 60 mmHg rather than 50 mmHg as previously aimed for is more appropriate. Resuscitation should initially be with warmed crystalloid to maintain normovolaemia depending on injury pattern and bleeding status. Some centres advocate the use of hypertonic saline in the resuscitation phase for intravascular expansion and cerebral oedema management. This should be given ideally via a central line with close observation of plasma sodium (should not exceed 150 mmol/L). Early supplementation of blood products may be required. Transfusion trigger will depend upon individual patient factors, but remember an adequate haemoglobin is required to deliver oxygen to vulnerable brain tissue. Haemoglobin values of <70 g/L definitely warrant transfusion. Traumatic brain injury is a risk factor for coagulopathy and this, as well as the effects of anticoagulants/anti-platelet drugs should be considered and addressed according to local protocols/specialist advice.

The use of vasopressors or inotropes will facilitate improving haemodynamic values with ongoing volume resuscitation. Choice of drug will depend on patient factors (co-morbidities and injury pattern) and clinician preference. The Brain Trauma Foundation recommend maintaining a Mean Arterial Pressure (MAP) of >80 having initially resuscitated to a systolic pressure over 90 mmHg, European guidelines suggest targeting a MAP of 85. In the absence of ICP monitoring, this ensures a CPP >50 mmHg.

## Hypo and Hypercarbia

The arterial concentration of carbon dioxide is related to cerebral vessel diameter and therefore cerebral blood flow as illustrated in Fig. 62.1.

In the past, this has been used to treat raised ICP by hyperventilating patients. This has now been shown on PET scan imaging to have a global impact on cerebral blood flow predisposing to hypoxia. It is now accepted practice to aim for normocapnia (PaCO2 4.5–5 kPa) and this should be calibrated to the end tidal CO2 reading at the earliest opportunity to ascertain the arterial-alveolar carbon dioxide gradient. Hyperventilating patients should be reserved as a last resort at times of critical ICP.

## Minimising Cerebral Metabolic Rate

This is achieved by adequate sedation, analgesia and prevention of seizures or hyperthermia. Choice of sedation agent (and opiate where appropriate) will depend upon drug availability, user familiarity and unit protocols. In the acute phase the aim of sedation is to allow for adequate

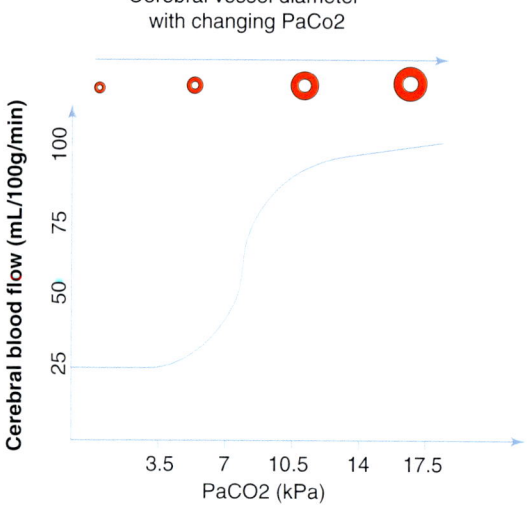

**Fig. 62.1** A graphical illustration of how the cerebral wall diameter and cerebral blood flow change with increasing levels of arterial carbon dioxide

nursing care, synchronisation with mechanical ventilation without coughing, reduce cerebral metabolic rate and medically manage ICP. Depth of anesthesia monitoring may be helpful, especially if neuromuscular blocking drugs are required as well. This makes sense since the risk associated with over sedation is primarily hypotension (a possible reason why barbiturate induced coma is rarely used in clinical practice now). However, the role of depth of anesthesia monitoring in severe traumatic brain injury has yet to be clearly established, or indeed incorporated in national guidance.

Any patient with a depressed skull fracture or temporal injury warrant prophylactic anticonvulsant with either Levetiracetam (1 g loading dose then 500 mg BD) or phenytoin (15–18 mg/kg loading then 200 mg TDS/dosage according to serum levels to maintain therapeutic range).

## Endocrine Considerations

Both hyper and hypoglycaemia have been shown to have an adverse outcome in severe traumatic brain injury. Brain is the most metabolically active organ in the body reflected by the fact that while it is only 3% of total body weight, it receives 15% of the cardiac output. Healthy brain does not tolerate hypoxia or hypoglycaemia well as cannot compensate with anaerobic respiration. This is also true of brain tissue at risk of secondary injury. It is therefore essential to maintain an adequate supply of glucose, ideally utilising the enteral route with NG feeding, or if this is not possible via total parenteral nutrition (TPN). However, hyperglycaemia predisposes to metabolic acidaemia and potential free radical formation with resultant neuronal death. The stress response to injury or polytrauma will result in relative insulin resistance, and therefore hyperglycaemia, warranting active management with a variable rate insulin infusion, but extra care must be taken to ensure hypoglycaemia does not occur.

The CRASH study [14] showed an increased mortality in traumatic brain injured patients treated with glucocorticoids. However, it is important to remember that 76% of patients with head injury suffer pituitary insufficiency [15], the risk increasing with severity of injury. Unexplained persistent hypotension may be due to pituitary insufficiency and should prompt a short synacthen test and where appropriate steroid supplementation.

## Control of ICP

The Brain Trauma Foundation recommendations for ICP monitoring are summarised in Table 62.3. It is worth remembering that there is no clear evidence of reduced mortality or morbidity associated with ICP monitoring [16], and therefore warrants a multi-disciplinary approach on an individual case basis. The fourth edition of the guidelines [17] acknowledges that there is no firm evidence base for the recommendations of who to institute ICP monitoring in, but recognises patients at risk of raised intra-cranial pressure.

ICP monitoring can be achieved via a surgically sited bolt, or via an external ventricular drain (EVD) if this has been sited. EVDs have the additional advantage of allowing CSF drainage that may facilitate management of ICP in the acute phase. The following simple interventions should not be overlooked in the management of raised ICP:

- 30° head up positioning (additional ventilator benefits but watch out for hypotension on initial positioning)
- Early removal of cervical spine immobilisation collars if used based on low suspicion on

**Table 62.3** Brain Trauma Foundation recommendations for ICP monitoring

| Indication for ICP monitoring | Salvageable patients with severe TBI<br>GCS 3–8 post resuscitation with abnormal CT<br>Severe TBI with a normal CT scan and >2 of:<br>– Age > 40<br>– Unilateral motor posturing<br>– Bilateral motor posturing<br>– SBP < 90 mmHg |
|---|---|

injury on initial radiology (trauma series CT or MRI spine)
- Loose endotracheal tube ties or holder
- Avoidance on internal jugular vein central lines (subclavian preferable)
- Adequate sedation while maintaining CPP
- Laxatives to avoid straining

Ongoing research is being done looking at brain tissue oxygenation via parenchymal catheters (inserted via a ICP bolt) and microdialysis catheters to monitor parenchymal tissue metabolites. These monitoring modalities are yet to be validated. Near infra-red spectroscopy has also been investigated as a non-invasive technique of monitoring regional brain tissue oxygen saturation. However, their use against established ICP monitors is yet to be validated, though NIRS is more sensitive than jugular venous saturations that has predominantly been used in the research setting.

In the context of ongoing raised ICP the following can be considered:

- Barbiturate coma. This is now rarely used but sedation should be optimised without causing hypotension. Barbiturates should be considered on a case by case basis.
- Surgical management: decompressive craniectomy or CSF drainage via EVD. The Rescue-ICP trial randomised patients after initial simple measures to control ICP including EVD, but in whom ICP remained over 25 mmHg for 1–2 h to either decompressive craniectomy with ongoing medical therapy or continued medical therapy with the option of adding in a barbiturate. The results showed reduced mortality in the decompressive craniectomy group but worse incidence of persistent vegetative state and disability [18].
- Hyperosmolar medication: hypertonic saline or mannitol. These should only be considered as bridging therapies to surgical intervention of CSF drainage or decompressive craniectomy to prevent herniation of tissue due to raised ICP. Mannitol and hypertonic saline draw fluid into the intravascular space which reduces overall tissue volume, reduces haematocrit and improves micocirculatory blood flow to vulnerable brain tissue. Mannitol may also have the additional benefit of free radical scavenging. However the benefits are only transient.

## Other Treatments

There have been recent international trials looking at different treatment interventions in the management of severe traumatic brain injury, including administration of progesterone, therapeutic hypothermia and erythropoietin. Unfortunately the SYNAPSE trail (a phase 3 randomised controlled trial) investigating progesterone administration within 8 h of injury versus placebo showed no difference in mortality or Glasgow outcome scale [19]. Frustratingly the concept of therapeutic hypothermia in traumatic brain injury makes sense in terms of reducing cerebral metabolic rate, matching cerebral blood flow with metabolic demand, reducing cerebral oedema and stabilising the blood brain barrier. These benefits were evident in animal models, but unfortunately have not translated into a robust clinical evidence base. Indeed the Euro-Therm trial was stopped early because of safety concerns in the intervention group [20]. Some clinicians will still consider mild systemic hypothermia as a last ditch rescue therapy for refractory raised ICP. The EPO-TBI was a multicentred randomised controlled trial with patients randomised within 24 h of injury to sub-cut erythropoietin or placebo looking at Glasgow outcome score at 6 months as primary end point [21]. Again, unfortunately there was no statistical difference between the two cohorts and there was no evident difference in mortality either.

## Conduct of Anesthesia in Severe Traumatic Brain Injury

### History

Consideration should be given to the mechanism of injury and potential for other injuries. This may include reviewing trauma CT images. Do spinal injury precautions need to be taken when moving the patient or at intubation? What are the patients co-morbidities? Are they regularly on anti-coagulants and do actions need to be taken to reverse the effects of these with Prothrombin complex concentrate and/or vitamin K? Collateral history may be required from relatives, primary care physician or reviewing hospital records.

## Investigations

Baseline haemoglobin and clotting profile are useful to know, as patients with severe traumatic brain injury are at risk of coagulopathy. You should have a low threshold for doing a 12 lead ECG as arrhythmias during the perioperative period are possible depending on anatomical site of brain injury and resultant oedema.

## Induction

Authors personal preference is to attain invasive blood pressure monitoring before induction of anesthesia wherever feasible. This minimises the risk of hypotension following induction of anesthesia and active management of the hypertensive response to laryngoscopy. In isolated head injury cases one can use a propofol/remifentanil target controlled infusion for induction with 1.2 mg/kg rocuronium with neuromuscular blockade monitoring using acceleromyography for quantification of train of four. Thirty degrees head up is maintained for ICP as well as reduce the risk of aspiration. Any reduction in blood pressure is treated with a peripheral vasoconstrictor to a target MAP >85, until central venous access is secured. A reinforced endotracheal tube has the advantage of minimising risk of tube kinking with head turning or lateral positioning but will need changing for ongoing ventilator support on intensive care or if MRI imaging is required. Central venous access should be attained.

Maintenance can either be with target controlled infusions of propofol and remifentanil or volatile with an opiate infusion depending upon personal experience. Depth of anesthesia monitoring is recommended with total intravenous anesthesia. Urethral catheterisation is essential to assist in monitoring and if Mannitol/hypertonic saline have been or may be used. Consider prophylactic anti-convulsant if not already given. This may be discussed as part of the WHO surgical checklist time out.

Careful attention should be paid to pressure areas and positioning to avoid neuropraxia. Mechanical compression devices will help to reduce the risk of venous thromboembolism since low molecular weight heparin risks haematoma expansion. Active warming is necessary to maintain normothermia.

If intra-operative bleeding is encountered the an anti-fibrinolytic such as Tranexamic acid can be given as a bolus followed by infusion. The role of prophylactic tranexamic acid has yet to be ascertained. Point of care testing with Thromboelastography may be helpful where available in the context of coagulopathy to guide blood product administration.

## Post-op

The patient should be transferred intubated and ventilated to neurocritical care with ongoing sedation and analgesia and full monitoring, for continuation of prevention of secondary injury.

## Future Developments

There is current interest in the role of biomarkers for brain injury and whether assays correlate to severity of injury. Trials are currently underway. The role of prophylactic tranexamic acid to minimise haematoma expansion and risk of death or disability is being investigated in a randomised controlled trial of tranexamic acid versus placebo. The aim is to recruit 10,000 patients by the end of 2017.

## References

1. Faul M, Xu L, Wald MM, Coronado VG. Traumatic brain injury in the United States: emergency department visits, hospitalizations, and deaths. Atlanta: Centers for Disease Control and Prevention, National Center for Injury Prevention and Control; 2010.
2. National Institute for Health and Clinical Excellence: Guidance. Head injury: triage, assessment, investigation and early management of head injury in children, young people and adults. London: National Institute for Health and Care Excellence (UK); 2014.
3. Kehoe A, Smith JE, Edwards A, Yates E, Lecky F. The changing face of major trauma in the UK. Emerg Med J. 2015;32:911–5. https://doi.org/10.1136/emermed-2015-205265.
4. Dinsmore J. Traumatic brain injury: an evidence based review of management. Contin Educ Anaesth Crit Care Pain. 2013;13(6):189–95.
5. Peeters W, Van Den Bande R, Polinder S, Brazinova A, Steyerberg EW, Lingsma HF, et al. Epidemiology of traumatic brain injury in Europe. Acta Neurochir (Wien). 2015;157(10):1683–96.
6. Lawrence T, Helmy A, Boumra O, et al. Traumatic brain injury in England and Wales: prospective audit of epidemiology, complications and standardised mortality. BMJ Open. 2016;6(11):e012197. https://doi.org/10.1136/bmjopen-2016-012197.
7. Kehoe A, Smith JE, Boumara O, Woodford M, Lecky F, Hutchinson PJ. Older patients with traumatic brain injury present with higher GCS score than younger patients for a given severity of injury. Emerg Med J. 2016;33:381–5.
8. Malec JF, Brown AW, Leibson CL, Flaada JT, Mandrekar JN, Diehl NN, et al. The mayo classification system for traumatic brain injury severity. J Neurotrauma. 2007;24(9):1417–24.
9. McHugh GS, Engel DC, Butcher I, Steyerberg EW, Lu J, Mushkudiani N, et al. Prognostic value of secondary insults in traumatic brain injury: results from the IMPACT study. J Neurotrauma. 2007;24:287–93.
10. Nangunoori R, Maloney-Wilensky E, Stiefel M, Park S, Kofke A, Levine JM, et al. Brain tissue oxygen-based therapy and outcome after severe traumatic brain injury: a systematic literature review. Neurocrit Care. 2012;17(1):131–8.
11. Pietropaoli JA, Rogers FB, Shackford SR, Wald SL, Schmoker JD, Zhuang J. The deleterious effects of intraoperative hypotension on outcome in patients with severe head injuries. J Trauma. 1992;33:403–7.
12. Sharma D, Brown MJ, Curry P, Noda S, Chesnut RM, Vavilala MS. Prevalence and risk factors for intraoperative hypotension during craniotomy for traumatic brain injury. J Neurosurg Anesthesiol. 2012;24:178–84.
13. Algara NN, Sharma D. Perioperative management of traumatic brain injury. Curr Anesthesiol Rep. 2016;6:193–201.
14. Edwards P, Arango M, Balica L, Cottingham R, El-Sayed H, Farrell B, et al. Final results of MRC CRASH, a randomised placebo-controlled trial of intravenous corticosteroid in adults with head injury outcomes at 6 months. Lancet. 2005;365:1957–9.
15. Klose M, Juul A, Struck J, Morgenthaler NG, Kosteljanetz M, Feldt-Rasmussen U. Acute and long term pituitary insufficiency in traumatic brain injury: a prospective single centre study. Clin Endocrinol. 2007;4:598–606.
16. Yuan Q, Wu X, Sun Y, Yu J, Li Z, Du Z, et al. Impact of intracranial pressure monitoring on mortality in patients with traumatic brain injury: a systematic review and meta-analysis. J Neurosurg. 2015;122(3):574–87.
17. Carney N, Totten AM, O'Reilly C. Guidelines for the management of severe traumatic brain injury. 4th ed. Brain Trauma Foundation 2016 at: https://braintrauma.org/uploads/03/12/Guidelines_for_Management_of_Severe_TBI_4th_Edition.pdf.
18. Hutchinson PJ, Kolias AG, Timofeev IS, Corteen EA, Czosnyka A, Timothy J, et al. Trial of decompressive craniectomy for traumatic intracranial hypertension. N Engl J Med. 2016;375:1119–30.
19. Skolnick SE, Maas AI, Narayan RK, van der Hoop RG, MacAllister T, Ward JD, et al. A clinical trial of progesterone for severe traumatic brain injury. N Engl J Med. 2014;371:2467–76.
20. Andrews PJD, Sinclair HL, Rodriguez A, Harris BA, Battison CG, Rhodes JK, et al. Hypothermia for intracranial hypertension after traumatic brain injury. N Engl J Med. 2015;373:2403–12.
21. Nichol A, French C, Little L, Haddad S, Presneill J, Arabi Y, et al. Erythropoietin in traumatic brain injury (EPO-TBI): a double blind randomised controlled trial. Lancet. 2015;386:2499–506.

# Part VI

# Vascular Anesthesia

# Anaesthesia for Endovascular Aortic Aneurysm Repair (EVAR)

## Milad Sharifpour and Salman Hemani

## Abdominal Endovascular Aneurysm Repair (EVAR)

Approximately 65% of aortic aneurysms occur in the abdomen, with 80% arising below the renal arteries [1, 2]. Smoking is the greatest risk factor for abdominal aortic aneurysms (AAA), with hypertension, hyperlipidemia, and a family history also being contributing factors. Abdominal aortic aneurysms (AAA) are more common in men than women, and most are discovered incidentally during workup for other pathologies [3]. Surgical intervention is not warranted until the diameter of the aorta is greater than 5 centimeters (cm). However, given the high mortality associated with ruptured AAAs (approximately 80% mortality), early surgical intervention is recommended for painful aneurysms, those complicated by embolic phenomena, and/or in cases where the aneurysm is rapidly expanding.

First introduced in 1991, EVAR was developed as an alternative approach to conventional open surgical AAA repair in an attempt to decrease the high morbidity and mortality associated with open repair. Additionally, advantages of EVAR were touted as decreased length of stay, and lower hospital and patient cost. After several years of clinical practice, endovascular repair has demonstrated several benefits over the more invasive open repair. These include shorter operative times, decreased blood loss and need for transfusion, and faster patient recovery. Endovascular approach also avoids the large hemodynamic swings associated with aortic cross clamping and unclamping which minimizes intraoperative hemodynamic perturbations, distal tissue ischemia, and end-organ damage. Overall, this leads to lower rates of perioperative morbidity and mortality. The reported mortality for EVAR is 1.7% in patients considered fit to undergo open surgical repair versus 9% in those identified as high-risk for open surgical approach [4]. Compared to open AAA repair, EVAR is associated with lower short-term morbidity and mortality. Long-term mortality however, is similar between both groups as demonstrated in the EVAR 1 and 2 Trials [4, 5]. Additionally, as compared to open repair, patients undergoing EVAR are at increased risk for requiring re-intervention.

Classification of thoracoabdominal aortic aneurysms is based on the location of the aneurysmal sac within the aorta and is defined by the Crawford Classification System (Table 63.1) [6].

Important surgical considerations for EVAR include favorable aneurysmal anatomy, with particular attention to the length of the aortic neck. The aortic neck should be at least 1.5 centimeters (cm) long in order to provide a stable proximal landing zone for the graft. The graft has to be sufficiently long to extend into the iliac arteries

M. Sharifpour, M.D., M.S. · S. Hemani, M.D. (✉)
Department of Anesthesiology, Emory University, Atlanta, GA, USA
e-mail: milad.sharifpour@emoryhealthcare.org; shemani@emory.edu

**Table 63.1** Crawford classification [6]

| Extent | Description |
|---|---|
| I | Aneurysmal sac occurs between the left subclavian and the renal arteries |
| II | Aneurysmal sac occurs after the left subclavian arterial take-off and extends distally to the aortic bifurcation |
| III | Aneurysmal sac extends from the mid-descending aorta to the aortic bifurcation |
| IV | Aneurysmal sac involves most (or all) of the abdominal aorta including the celiac artery, and may or may not involve the infrarenal segment |

should the aneurysmal sac extend past the aortic bifurcation.

The aorta is accessed via bilateral femoral artery cut-downs. Subsequently, the synthetic graft is introduced through the common femoral artery and positioned over the aneurysmal sac under fluoroscopic guidance. An alternative approach involves catheterizing the brachial or the subclavian artery to gain access. Surgical time varies due to the complexity of the patient's anatomy, ease of access to the vascular bed, location of the aneurysm and the need for a fenestrated graft. Typically, a 2–6 h case is expected.

## Preoperative Evaluation and Considerations

### Cardiac

The primary purpose of the preoperative clinic visit is to medically optimize patients, particularly those at highest risk for perioperative complications. The prevalence of coronary artery disease (CAD) approaches nearly 50% in patients undergoing vascular surgery. As such, preoperative optimization is of utmost importance to minimize the risk of myocardial ischemia, arrhythmia, and decompensated heart failure. Beta-blockers are routinely continued perioperatively in patients who are on chronic beta-blocker therapy, with exception to those who have severe bradycardia (HR < 50 beats per minute) or hypotension [7]. Patients naïve to beta-blocker therapy can be considered for initiation when undergoing high risk vascular surgery, especially if they have ≥3 revised cardiac risk index (RCRI) risk factors. RCRI risk factors include: history of ischemic heart disease, congestive heart failure, diabetes mellitus requiring insulin therapy, chronic kidney disease, or cerebrovascular disease. However, de novo beta blockade should be titrated minimally 7 days (ideally 30 days) prior to elective surgery to adjust for bradycardia and hypotension. The goal heart rate for patients on beta-blockers is between 60 and 80 bpm. The clinician should avoid starting beta-blocker therapy day of surgery, as it can increase the risk of death and stroke [8, 9]. Chronic statin therapy should be continued. Initiation of statin therapy is reasonable in patients undergoing vascular surgery because it has been demonstrated that this family of medications reduce major adverse cardiac events particularly in vascular surgery patients [7, 10, 11].

Given their high risk of CAD and or PAD, many vascular patients present on dual antiplatelet therapy (DAPT) with aspirin (ASA) and a thienopyridine. Particularly following recent (<1 year) coronary stenting, DAPT is necessary to reduce future cardiac risk and in-stent thrombosis. DAPT, when prescribed for indications outside of acute coronary syndrome (ACS), requires shorter waiting periods prior to proceeding with elective surgery. Guidelines recommend that elective surgery should be postponed at least 1-month after bare metal stent (BMS) deployment or 6–12 month following drug-eluting stent (DES) placement. When placed in the setting of ACS, the suggested wait period prior to elective surgical intervention, for both BMS and DES, is 12 months [12]. If surgery is necessary before the recommended waiting period, continuation of aspirin should be highly considered, and antiplatelet therapy should be restarted as soon as possible postoperatively [12].

In the absence of an active cardiac condition (unstable angina, myocardial infarction in the past month, decompensated CHF, severe valvular disease, or significant arrhythmia), further non-invasive testing is dictated by the patient's functional capacity and presence of clinical risk factors. Asymptomatic patients able to achieve activity level equivalent to four or more metabolic equivalents (METs), do not benefit from further cardiac testing. It is reasonable to perform exercise stress testing in patients with elevated risk (≥3 of the following: History of ischemic heart disease, compensated or prior CHF, diabetes mellitus requiring insulin therapy, chronic kidney disease, cerebrovascular disease) and unknown functional capacity if the result will change preoperative disease management [13]. All patients undergoing major vascular surgery, including AAA repair, should have a 12-lead electrocardiogram (ECG).

## Pulmonary

Chronic obstructive lung disease (COPD) is common in this patient population due to the high association between cigarette smoking and AAA. Cessation of smoking decreases cardiovascular, respiratory, cerebrovascular, and wound-related complications [14, 15]. Tobacco use remains the most significant risk factor for aneurysm development, expansion, and rupture. Chronic obstructive pulmonary disease is an independent risk factor for operative mortality after AAA repair. As such, room air arterial blood gas (ABG) and pulmonary function tests (PFTs) may be considered in those with history of symptomatic COPD. If COPD is severe and poorly controlled, formal pulmonary consult is recommended to optimize medical therapy that may provide benefit for both short- and long-term prognosis. The quality of evidence supporting preoperative pulmonary testing is moderate at best. Although the presence of COPD is associated with higher morbidity [16], abnormal preoperative PFTs and ABG values are not predictive of a poor outcome after aneurysm repair [17].

## Renal

The prevalence of chronic kidney disease varies between 3 and 20% in patients undergoing AAA repair, therefore assessment of baseline renal function is imperative. Strategies to minimize the risk of kidney injury include cessation of nephrotoxic agents (NSAIDs, aminoglycosides), minimizing intravenous contrast load, and pre-hydration with intravenous crystalloid solutions prior to the procedure in patients at risk [18]. There is no compelling evidence that the use of N-acetylcysteine or sodium bicarbonate solutions reduce the risk of contrast-induced nephropathy (CIN) in patients undergoing EVAR [19].

## Intraoperative Management

Endovascular AAA repair is most often performed under general or neuraxial anesthesia. Consideration for the use of neuraxial anesthesia needs to include a detailed review of the patient's anti-platelet and anti-coagulant medications, as often these will preclude safe epidural use. Guidelines published by the American Society of Regional Anesthesiology (ASRA) should be followed [20]. Monitored anesthetic care (MAC) may be considered in those patients whose risk under general anesthesia (GA) is high, and who are not suitable candidates for epidural placement. When MAC is used, the surgical team must infiltrate the femoral cut down sites with local anesthetic to ensure patient comfort. Additionally, the anesthesiologist should be prepared to induce general anesthesia (GA) if conversion to an open procedure is required. There is no evidence to suggest improved outcomes when comparing neuraxial anesthesia versus GA versus MAC supplemented with local infiltration [21].

The advantages of GA include a secure patient airway, increased patient comfort for those who are not able to lie supine for prolonged periods on a rigid radiology suite or hybrid operating room table, and the easy ability to provide prolonged breath holds to improve fluoroscopic image quality. Neuraxial anesthesia is advantageous in a select population of patients with poor respiratory function. Avoiding endotracheal intubation and the subsequent atelectasis associated with GA reduces the risk of postoperative pulmonary complications [22].

Intraoperative management of patients undergoing EVAR must focus on hemodynamic stability with particular attention to coronary perfusion in order to minimize the risk of myocardial ischemia. Additionally, the anesthesiologist must ensure adequate end-organ perfusion (with particular attention to the spine and the kidneys), manage intravascular volume, maintain normothermia, and correct electrolyte abnormalities and coagulopathy.

## Monitors

In addition to the standard ASA monitors, an invasive arterial catheter is recommended for close blood pressure monitoring. The decision to place the arterial catheter prior to induction depends on the patient's general condition and should be considered on an individual basis. Monitoring central venous pressure and pulmonary artery pressure is not necessary unless indicated by the patient's comorbidities. Bladder catheterization is necessary to monitor urine output. Transesophageal echocardiography (TEE) can be utilized to monitor volume status, bi-ventricular function, and wall motion abnormalities.

## Preparation

Considering the risk of intraoperative aneurysm rupture and massive blood loss, two large bore (16 gauge or larger) peripheral intravenous lines are placed for these procedures. A central line may be indicated if infusion of vasoactive medications is anticipated or, if patient anatomy is significantly complex that stent deployment is complicated with risk of hemorrhage or rupture. The patient should have 2–4 type and cross-matched units of blood available prior to incision.

## Induction and Maintenance

General anesthesia may be induced with a variety of agents. Commonly, a balanced anesthetic consisting of propofol, a short acting opioid (ex: fentanyl), and a neuromuscular blocking agent are used for induction. A low dose vasopressor infusion or controlled bolus dosing during induction can attenuate the hypotension associated with the decrease in systemic vascular resistance (SVR) that can occur with propofol. It is important however, to avoid uncontrolled hypertension during direct laryngoscopy to minimize the risk of aneurysm rupture. Short acting agents such as esmolol, nitroglycerin, and nitroprusside should be readily available to blunt the hemodynamic response to direct laryngoscopy. Anesthesia is maintained with a mixture of volatile anesthetic, nitrous oxide, and oxygen. Total intravenous anesthesia (TIVA) is also an appropriate anesthetic option. The surgical stimulation is minimal compared to more invasive open surgery; small doses of opioids are titrated throughout the case to allow for post-operative pain relief. A low dose vasopressor infusion is commonly used to maintain the MAP near baseline value.

Following the exposure of the femoral arteries, baseline activated clotting time (ACT) is measured and intravenous (IV) heparin is administered. Target ACT value for EVAR is approximately 2.0–2.5 times the baseline measurement (approximately 250–300 s). Activated clotting time is measured 3–5 min following the initial dose, and every 30 min thereafter [23]. During stent deployment, the aorta is temporarily occluded, resulting in a sudden increase in left ventricular afterload and the patient's blood pressure.

Due to the high incidence of chronic renal impairment in patients undergoing EVAR, it is important to maintain adequate intravascular volume and renal perfusion, and to minimize IV contrast dye during the case.

## Postoperative Care

Depending on the location of the aneurysmal sac and difficulty of the repair, patients may be admitted directly to an intensive care or a step-down unit, or they may be appropriate for the post-anesthesia care unit with subsequent discharge to surgical ward. If continuous hemodynamic monitoring, vasoactive infusions, and/or regular lower extremity neurovascular checks are indicated, an increased level of post-operative care should be pursued.

While most patients resume a clear liquid or normal diet on the night of surgery, patients should continue to receive IV hydration in order to attenuate the risk of CIN. According to a recent prospective cohort study, the incidence of patients developing acute kidney injury following elective EVAR is 18.8% [24]. Management includes optimizing intravascular volume and cardiac output, avoiding nephrotoxic drugs, and treating any underlying causes that could reduce renal perfusion [25]. There is minimal postoperative pain associated with EVAR and pain is most often managed with oral analgesics.

Given the numerous abdominal aortic vessels providing arterial blood flow to the mesentery, stents deployed above or near the celiac, superior mesenteric and/or inferior mesenteric artery require close monitoring to ensure that blood flow to the bowel is not decreased or disrupted. Unexpected hypotension, increasing lactate levels or elevated liver enzymes, and loose or bloody bowel movements should be immediately investigated. Any delay in detection can lead to bowel ischemia.

An extensive list of possible complications that occur during or following EVAR is listed in Table 63.2.

## Thoracic Endovascular Aortic Repair (TEVAR)

Thoracic aneurysms are categorized according to their location relative to the aortic arch. Ascending aneurysms arise distal to the aortic valve and terminate near the aortic arch. Those that arise in the arch itself are considered aortic arch aneurysms, and those located distal to the arch progressing into the descending aorta are labeled descending aortic aneurysms.

Similar to an EVAR, the endovascular approach to a thoracic aortic aneurysm attempts to occlude the aneurysmal sac through an arterial cut down and the deployment of a stent. Adequate proximal and distal neck lengths (minimally 1.5 cm) are required to allow for successful graft anchoring [26].

**Table 63.2** Complications associated with EVAR/TEVAR

| Complications | Management |
|---|---|
| *Intraoperative* | |
| Spinal cord ischemia | Increase BP, insertion of a lumbar drain/increase drainage, notify surgeons |
| Bowel ischemic | Emergent return to OR for revascularization or bowel resection |
| Femoral cut down site hemorrhage | Correction of coagulopathies, surgical repair |
| Retroperitoneal hemorrhage | Correction of coagulopathies, IR embolization vs. open surgical repair |
| Vessel damage | Open surgical repair |
| Ruptured aneurysm | Emergent surgical repair |
| Conversion to open repair | Induction of general anesthesia, supportive care |
| Failure of the stent to deploy | |
| Stent deployment in an incorrect position | Endovascular versus open surgical retrieval |
| *Postoperative* | |
| Endoleak | See Table 63.3 |
| Neurologic impairment | Neurology consult, induced hypertension |
| Myocardial ischemia | ASA, IV heparin infusion, increase coronary perfusion pressure, cardiology consult |
| Renal failure | Optimization of intravascular volume, supportive care |
| Hypothermia | Rewarming |

**Table 63.3** Types of endoleak

| Endoleak type | Description |
|---|---|
| Type I | Inadequate seal of the endograft either at the proximal or distal end |
| Type II | Filling of the aneurysmal sac or sealed space between the graft and the aorta with blood |
| Type III | Structural defect in the graft or a space between two consecutive grafts; may include a hole in the graft |
| Type IV | Graft fabric or porosity leak |
| Type V | Aneurysmal expansion without an identifiable leak |

After induction of anesthesia, the patient is placed either in a supine or right lateral decubitus position. Management is similar to that of patients undergoing EVAR. However, anesthetic considerations must additionally account for the anatomy of the thoracic aorta, most notably the take-off of several important branches to the head, arms and spine.

## Preoperative Considerations

### Medical Optimization

Please refer to the section on EVAR; medical optimization for TEVAR patients includes the same considerations.

### Imaging

Preoperative imaging using computed tomography angiography (CTA) for TEVAR outlines the curvature of the thoracic aorta and determines the involvement of aortic branches. Identification of the location of the artery of Adamkiewicz is necessary to plan for spinal cord perfusion and minimize the risk of ischemia.

### Pre-operative Considerations for Left Subclavian Artery Stent (LSA) Placement

As discussed previously, a sufficient length of proximal aorta is needed to secure the graft. In the aortic arch, the ability to create this distance is limited and may require coverage of the LSA. Revascularization of the LSA may be required before TEVAR and pre-operative identification of these patients is mandated. Patients with prior CABG with left internal mammary artery (LIMA) graft and those with a left arm arteriovenous fistula often undergo carotid-subclavian bypass prior to TEVAR.

## Intraoperative Management

### Monitors

In addition to standard ASA monitors, an arterial line, and central venous access are recommended. Additional monitoring with TEE or pulmonary artery catheter is dictated by the patient's comorbidities. Intraoperative TEE can provide valuable information about cardiac function and volume status.

It is imperative to pay close attention to spinal perfusion. In most individuals, the artery of Adamkiewicz arises from the T8-T12 vertebral segments. Graft deployment to this region in the aorta may compromise blood flow to the spinal cord. Currently, somatosensory evoked potentials (SSEP) and motor evoke potentials (MEP) are used to monitor spinal cord function intraoperatively. Neuromonitoring requires special equipment and trained personnel, while evidence regarding its effectiveness is inconclusive [27, 28]. If intraoperative neuromonitoring is utilized, TIVA is the preferred anesthetic as volatile agents depress the amplitude of evoked potentials. Opiates and/or dexmedetomidine are suitable anesthetic adjuncts as they minimize the changes in SSEPs and MEPs. Additionally, to reduce the risk of spinal cord ischemia, a lumbar drain may be placed pre- or post-operatively to drain cerebrospinal fluid and improve spinal cord perfusion [28]. Cerebral perfusion and oxygenation can be continuously monitored using transcutaneous near-infrared spectroscopy or transcranial cerebral oximetry. Transcranial Doppler measures the velocity of blood flow in large cerebral vessels and can detect cerebral microemboli. These monitoring modalities are particularly relevant during TEVAR because of the close proximity of the graft landing zone to the cerebral blood vessels, and the risk of microemboli dislodgement during graft deployment. However, the advantage of additional monitoring for cerebral microemboli without a clear rescue intervention remains unclear [29].

### Induction and Maintenance

General anesthesia can be induced using a similar technique as that used for EVAR. Anesthesia is maintained with a mixture of volatile anesthetic, nitrous oxide, and oxygen. Alternatively, a TIVA using a combination of propofol and an opioid can be used.

Once arterial access is obtained, the stent is advanced over a guide wire, with the aid of a sheath and dilator, under fluoroscopic guidance. Maintaining adequate blood pressure throughout the case promotes blood flow to collateral vessels of the spine. Graft coverage of the LSA can decrease blood flow to the spine; the posterior spinal artery arises from the left vertebral artery, which is a branch of the LSA. Vigilance by the anesthesia team optimizes forward flow to the spinal cord when graft placement reduces spinal perfusion. Following stent deployment, a MAP of 90–110 mmHg improves cord perfusion pressure. Lumbar drain (cerebral spinal fluid) pressure should be transduced and fluid (CSF) drained to maintain a spinal cord perfusion pressure > 70 mmHg. Recommendations vary but a CSF pressure of 8–12 mmHg is a reasonable intraoperative target.

Blood pressure is often lowered to a MAP of 50–60 mmHg in anticipation of stent deployment in order to prevent inadvertent downstream deployment of the graft caused by a high blood pressure. After successful deployment, the blood pressure can be increased to the baseline value or higher to maintain end organ perfusion. While the femoral artery is accessed, heparin may be administered as a continuous infusion targeting an ACT 2.0–2.5 times the baseline value. Following the removal of the delivery sheath heparin is stopped and is slowly reversed with protamine. The artery used for access is repaired prior to the end of the procedure.

## Postoperative Care

Patients undergoing TEVAR should recover in an ICU or step-down monitored unit. Hourly lower extremity neurovascular checks should be performed. If a lumbar drain is in place, it should be monitored and drained on hourly basis. In addition to the increased risk of spinal cord ischemia, patients undergoing TEVAR are also at increased risk for intestinal ischemia. Lactic acid levels, blood gases, and electrolytes and liver enzymes should be monitored on regular basis.

Please refer to Table 63.2 for a list of potential complications after TEVAR.

## References

1. Aggarwal S, Qamar A, Sharma V, Sharma A. Abdominal aortic aneurysm: a comprehensive review. Exp Clin Cardiol. 2011;16:11–5.
2. Harikrishnan K, Chieh GLH, Khan SA, Karthekeyan RB, Sharad SS. Anesthetic considerations for endovascular abdominal aortic aneurysm repair. Ann Card Anaesth. 2016;19:132–41.
3. Dua A, Kuy S, Lee CJ, Upchurch GR, Desai SS. Epidemiology of aortic aneurysm repair in the United States from 2000 to 2010. J Vasc Surg. 2014;59:1512–7.
4. Greenhalgh RM, et al. Endovascular aneurysm repair and outcome in patients unfit for open repair of abdominal aortic aneurysm (EVAR trial 2): randomized controlled trial. Lancet. 2005;365:2187–92.
5. Greenhalgh RM, et al. Endovascular aneurysm repair and outcome in patients unfit for open repair of abdominal aortic aneurysm (EVAR trial 1): randomized controlled trial. Lancet. 2005;365:2179–86.
6. Crawford ES, Coselli JS. Thoracoabdominal aneurysm surgery. Semin Thorac Cardiovasc Surg. 1991;3:300–22.
7. Fleisher LA, Fleischmann KE, Auerbach AD, Barnason SA, Beckman JA, et al. 2014 ACC/AHA guidelines on perioperative cardiovascular evaluation and management of patients undergoing noncardiac surgery: executive summary. J Am Coll Cardiol. 2014;64:2373–405.
8. Devereaux PJ, Yang H, Yusuf S, Guyatt G, Leslie K, et al. Effects of extended-release metoprolol succinate in patients undergoing non-cardiac surgery (POISE trial): a randomized controlled trial. Lancet. 2008;371:1839–47.
9. Flu WJ, van Kuijk JP, Chonchol M, Winkel TA, Verhagen HJ, Bax JJ, Poldermans D. Timing of preoperative Beta-blocker treatment in vascular surgery patients: influence on post-operative outcome. J Am Coll Cardiol. 2010;56:1922–9.
10. Kertai MD, Bountioukos M, Boersma E, Bax JJ, Thomson IR, et al. Aortic stenosis: an underestimated risk factor for perioperative complications in patients undergoing noncardiac surgery. Am J Med. 2004;116:8–13.
11. Molnar AO, Coca SG, Devereaux PJ, Jain AK, Kitchlu A, et al. Statin use associated with a lower incidence of acute kidney injury after major elective surgery. J Am Soc Nephrol. 2011;22:939–46.
12. Levine GN, Bates ER, Bittl JA, Brindis RG, Fihn SD, et al. 2016 ACC/AHA guideline focused update on duration of dual antiplatelet therapy in patients with coronary artery disease. J Am Coll Cardiol. 2016;68(10):1082–115.
13. Lee TH, Marcantonio ER, Mangione CM, Thomas EJ, Polanczyk CA, et al. Derivation and prospective validation of a simple index for prediction of cardiac risk of major noncardiac surgery. Circulation. 1999;100:1043–9.

14. Mills E, Eyawo O, Lockhart I, Kelly S, Wu P, Ebbert JO. Smoking cessation reduces perioperative complications: a systematic review and meta-analysis. Am J Med. 2011;124:144–54.
15. Grønkjær M, Eliasen M, Skov-Ettrup LS, Tolstrup JS, Christiansen AH, et al. Preoperative smoking status and postoperative complications: a systematic review and meta-analysis. Ann Surg. 2014;259:52–71.
16. Axelrod DA, Henke PK, Wakefield TW, Stanley JC, Jacobs LA, et al. Impact of chronic obstructive pulmonary disease on elective and emergency abdominal aortic aneurysm repair. J Vasc Surg. 2001;33:72–6.
17. Upchurch GR, Proctor MC, Henke PK, Zajkowski P, Riles EM, et al. Predictors of severe morbidity and death after elective abdominal aortic aneurysmectomy in patients with chronic obstructive pulmonary disease. J Vasc Surg. 2003;37:594–9.
18. Roger R, Bell RM, Hausenloy DJ. Contrast induced nephropathy following angiography and cardiac interventions. Heart. 2016;0:1–11. https://doi.org/10.1136/heartjnl-2014-306962.
19. Fishbane S. N-Acetylcysteine in the prevention of contrast-induced nephropathy. Clin J Am Soc Nephrol. 2008;3:281–7.
20. Horlocker TT, Wedel DJ, Rowlingson JC, Enneking FK, Kopp SL, et al. Regional anesthesia in the patient receiving antithrombotic or thrombolytic therapy: American Society of Regional Anesthesia and Pain Medicine Evidence-Based Guidelines (Third Edition). Reg Anesth Pain Med. 2010;35:64–101.
21. Kothandan H, Chieh GLH, Khan SA, Karthekeyan RB, Sharad SS. Anesthetic considerations for endovascular abdominal aortic aneurysm repair. Ann Card Anaesth. 2016;19:132–41.
22. van Lier F, van der Geest PJ, Hoeks SE, van Gestel YR, Hol JW, et al. Epidural analgesia is associated with improved health outcomes of surgical patients with chronic obstructive pulmonary disease. Anesthesiology. 2011;115:315–21.
23. Bowers J, Ferguson JJ. The use of activated clotting times to monitor heparin therapy during and after interventional procedures. Clin Cardiol. 1994;17:357–61.
24. Saratzis A, Melas N, Mahmood A, Sarafidis P. Incidence of acute kidney injury (AKI) after endovascular abdominal aortic aneurysm repair (EVAR) and impact on outcome. Eur J Vasc Endovasc Surg. 2015;49:534–40.
25. Borthwick E, Ferguson A. Perioperative acute kidney injury: risk factors, recognition, management, and outcomes. BMJ. 2010;341:c3365.
26. Fann JI, Mitchel RS, Kaiser C, Kee ST, Dake MD, van der Starre PJA. Vascular surgery. In: Jaffe RA, Schmiesing CA, Golianu B, editors. Anesthesiologist's manual of surgical procedures. Philadelphia: Lippincott; 2014. p. 406–61.
27. Fok M, Mason A. The use of neuromonitoring in descending and thoraco-abdominal aortic aneurysm surgery: literature review. International Conference on Sensing Technology; 2014. p. 174–78.
28. Fok M, Jafarzadeh F, Sancho E, Abello D, Rimmer L, et al. Is there any benefit of neuromonitoring during descending and thoracoabdominal aortic aneurysm repair? Innovations (Phila). 2015;10:342–8.
29. Shah A, Khoynezhad A. Thoracic endovascular repair for acute type A aortic dissection: operative technique. Ann Cardiothorac Surg. 2016;5:389–96.

# Anesthesia for Open AAA

Jimmy C. Yao and Milad Sharifpour

## Introduction

The incidence of abdominal aortic aneurysms (AAA) is nearly 8%, with more than 30,000 deaths each year resulting from ruptured AAAs in the United States [1]. Risk factors for AAA include old age, smoking, male sex, atherosclerotic disease, and family history of AAA. Of these, smoking remains the only modifiable risk factor. Given the high morbidity without intervention, the United States Preventive Services Task Force (USPSTF) recommends AAA screening for all men ages 65–75 years old, even those who have never smoked [2].

Aneurysmal dilation of the aorta is the result of both aging and atherosclerotic plaque buildup. Chronic inflammation and destruction of the connective tissue within the aortic wall leads to the loss of protective layers. While the development of AAA is a multi-factorial process, elastin degradation is the prevailing mechanism by which the aorta dilates [3, 4].

Most AAAs are detected on radiographic imaging as part of routine screening or incidentally during emergency room scans. Given the extremely high mortality of ruptured AAA, it is important for practitioners to be familiar with factors associated with rupture. The best predictors of risk of AAA rupture include the diameter and the rate of expansion of the aneurysm. A vascular surgeon should evaluate those at the highest risk for aneurysm rupture, however medical management is appropriate for many aneurysms. Aneurysms between 4.0 and 5.5 centimeters (cm) in diameter account for more than 90% of all aortic aneurysms in the United States [5] (Table 64.1). Early repair in this cohort, regardless of open or endovascular approach, does not provide a long-term survival benefit [6, 7]. Thus, medical management is recommended in this size range. Annual surveillance is recommended to determine when/if surgical intervention is needed. Broad consensus supports that the risks of elective repair are acceptable for perceived mortality benefit when an aneurysms is 6.0 cm or greater in size. Controversy still exists regarding elective repair of aneurysms 5.5–5.9 cm in diameter. Surgical repair is considered in symptomatic patients, or in those whose aneurysm expands by more than 0.5 cm in 6 months. Aneurysms at 5.5 cm mark the inflection point, at which the risk of rupture equals or surpasses the risk of perioperative mortality.

J. C. Yao, M.D.
Department of Anesthesiology, Emory University School of Medicine, Atlanta, GA, USA
e-mail: jimmy.yao@emory.edu

M. Sharifpour, M.D., M.S. (✉)
Department of Anesthesiology, Emory University Hospital, Emory University School of Medicine, Atlanta, GA, USA
e-mail: milad.sharifpour@emoryhealthcare.org

**Table 64.1** Recommendations for care of abdominal aortic aneurysms based on diameter

| <4 cm | Benign finding |
|---|---|
| 4–5.5 cm | Ultrasound surveillance |
| 5.6–5.9 cm | Consider surgical repair |
| ≥6 cm | Elective surgical repair |
| Increase of >0.5 cm in 6 months | Elective surgical repair |

## Emergent Versus Elective Repair

Perioperative mortality for elective AAA repair is 4–8%. However, that of emergent repair of ruptured AAAs approaches 50%. Accounting for patients whose aneurysms rupture and result in death prior to hospital arrival, the mortality rate for ruptured AAA exceeds 90% [8]. Symptoms of a ruptured aneurysm are non-specific and include back and/or abdominal pain, and vomiting. Abdominal pain in a patient with known AAA or a pulsatile mass must be treated as a dissection or rupture until proven otherwise.

## Open Versus Endovascular Repair

While endovascular aortic repair (EVAR) is becoming a more accepted treatment approach to elective AAA repair, the data supporting EVAR are controversial [9–11]. Patients who undergo EVAR have a higher rate of re-intervention after eliminating those who underwent repair of incisional hernia in the open aortic repair (OAR) group [12]. The greatest benefit of EVAR stems from the superior short-term survival rate compared to OAR. However, this survival benefit is lost as early as 2 years after intervention [13]. Aortic aneurysms can continue to dilate despite successful endovascular intervention. Over time, even properly placed devices can leak, migrate, and fail, requiring re-intervention. The increased mortality in EVAR group is attributed to secondary aneurysm sac rupture and increased cancer-related complications. Elective endovascular repair of AAA may be the most appropriate choice for patients with limited life expectancy and those with high perioperative risk. Studies that compare OAR to EVAR for ruptured, emergent AAAs are not controlled for confounders that likely impact outcomes. The OAR cohort over-represents patients who are unstable on arrival, require immediate operative intervention, and have challenging anatomy. This places the OAR group at a significant disadvantage for achieving better outcomes. The largest multicenter, randomized control trial to date (IMPROVE, 2015) has shown that EVAR does not offer a survival benefit 1 year out when compared to OAR for ruptured AAA [14].

## Preoperative Evaluation

Open AAA repair is responsible for the highest risk of cardiovascular morbidity and mortality among major vascular surgeries. The management and evaluation of patients undergoing elective repair requires the consideration of numerous systems including cardiac, pulmonary, cerebrovascular, and renal.

## Cardiovascular

The prevalence of coronary artery disease (CAD) approaches nearly 50% in this patient population. As such, preoperative optimization is of utmost importance to minimize the risk of myocardial ischemia, arrhythmia, and decompensated heart failure. Chronic beta-blockade is routinely continued perioperatively [15], with exceptions being made under extenuating circumstances such as severe bradycardia (HR < 50 beats per minute) or hypotension. Patients who are naïve to beta-blocker therapy can be considered for initiation when undergoing high risk vascular surgery, especially if the patient has major comorbidities including recent (MI), congestive heart failure, diabetes, renal insufficiency, or cerebrovascular disease. However, de novo beta blockade should be titrated minimally 7 days (ideally 30 days) prior to elective surgery to adjust for bradycardia and hypotension. The goal heart rate for patients on beta-blockers is between 60 and 80 beats per minute. The clinician should avoid starting beta-blocker therapy on the day of surgery, as it can increase the risk of death and stroke [16, 17]. Statins and acetylsalicylic acid (ASA) should be continued in accordance with the ACC/AHA guidelines [15, 18, 19]. Angiotensin converting enzyme inhibitors (ACEI) and angiotensin receptor blockers (ARB) should be held on the day of surgery; 30-day mortality is increased in patients undergoing AAA repair on concomitant ACEI and ARB therapy. Continuation of diuretics on the day of surgery should be considered on an individual basis.

Patients undergoing vascular surgery are more likely to have CAD or previous MI requiring percutaneous intervention. Dual antiplatelet therapy with ASA and an anti-platelet agent following coronary stenting is necessary to reduce future cardiac risk and in-stent thrombosis. Coronary stent placement, for indications outside of acute coronary syndrome (ACS), requires shorter waiting periods prior to proceeding with elective surgery. Guidelines recommend elective surgery is postponed minimally 1-month after bare metal stent (BMS) deployment or 6–12 month following DES placement. Regardless of the type of stent (bare metal or drug eluting stent), when placed for an ACS indication, the suggested wait time prior to elective surgical intervention is 12 months [20]. If surgery is necessary before the recommended waiting period, continuation of aspirin should be highly considered, and anti-platelet agent should be restarted as soon as possible postoperatively.

In the absence of active cardiac condition (unstable angina, MI within the past month, decompensated CHF, severe valvular disease, significant arrhythmias), further non-invasive testing is dictated by the patient's functional capacity and presence of clinical risk factors. Patients able to achieve moderate or high activity level, equivalent to four or more metabolic equivalent units (METs), do not benefit from further preoperative cardiac testing. If functional activity is poor or unknown, the clinician must determine whether any of the five independent clinical risk factors are present (prior MI, compensated or prior CHF, diabetes mellitus, renal insufficiency, cerebrovascular disease). Those with three or more risk factors are considered at increased risk for perioperative cardiac complications, and may benefit from stress testing [21]. All patients undergoing AAA repair, including any other major vascular surgery, should have a 12-lead electrocardiogram (ECG).

## Pulmonary

Obstructive lung disease is common in this patient population due to the high association between cigarette smoking and AAA. Cessation of smoking decreases cardiovascular, respiratory, cerebrovascular, and wound-related complications [22, 23]. Tobacco use remains the most significant risk factor for aneurysm development, expansion, and rupture. Chronic obstructive pulmonary disease (COPD) is an independent risk factor for postoperative mortality following AAA repair. If COPD is severe or symptoms are poorly controlled, formal pulmonary consult is recommended for optimization of medical therapy and assessment of short- and long-term prognosis. Room air arterial blood gas (ABG) and pulmonary function tests (PFTs) can be considered in those with history of symptomatic COPD or long-standing tobacco use to assess severity of lung disease; however the quality of evidence in support of preoperative pulmonary testing is moderate at best. Although the presence of COPD is associated with higher morbidity [24], abnormal preoperative PFTs and ABG values were not predictive of a poor outcome after aneurysm repair [25].

Patients with COPD are particularly vulnerable to postoperative pulmonary complications, especially after major abdominal surgery. Respiratory muscle weakness and abdominal pain together cause reduced lung volumes and atelectasis. Use of epidural analgesia decreases systemic opioid requirements and subsequent risk of respiratory depression. Epidural analgesia carries the additional benefit of significantly reducing the risk of postoperative pneumonia in COPD patients undergoing major abdominal surgery [26]. However, the risk of epidural abscess and the potential for delayed surgery after a bloody epidural attempt must be carefully weighed against the benefits. The American Society of Regional Anesthesia and Pain Medicine (ASRA) guidelines should be followed prior to any neuraxial intervention. Specifically, clopidogrel should be stopped 7 days prior to planned neuraxial anesthesia, and ticagrelor 5–7 days. Aspirin alone can be continued, and does not confer additional risk.

## Renal

Vascular patients are more likely to have co-existing renal disease from long-standing hypertension and diabetes. Therefore assessment of baseline renal function is imperative. Higher baseline serum creatinine, age > 75 years, and hypertension are associated with acute kidney injury following elective open AAA [27]. The incidence of post-operative acute kidney injury (AKI) also varies based on the location of the aneurysm; patients with suprarenal and juxtarenal aneurysms are two times more likely to require post-operative renal replacement therapy than those patients with an infrarenal aneurysm. Emergent repair of a ruptured aortic aneurysm is highly associated with post-operative AKI with up to 75% of these patients suffering acute kidney injury following surgery [28]. Those on dialysis should be dialyzed the day before surgery to decrease risk of volume overload, hyperkalemia, and uremia.

## Neurologic

Patients undergoing vascular surgery are at increased risk for perioperative stroke, delirium, and spinal cord ischemia. Aortic aneurysm repair is an independent risk factor for delirium, a diagnosis that is associated with increased risk of short and long-term mortality, and hospital length of stay. Risk factors for postoperative delirium include advanced age, pre-existing pulmonary and renal disease, cerebrovascular disease, longer operative time, and high perioperative transfusion requirement. Alcohol abuse and smoking remain the few modifiable risk factors for postoperative delirium.

Stroke is two times more common in patients undergoing AAA repair compared to the general surgical population [29]. Morbidity due to permanent neurologic damage remains high and unfortunately, there are few modifiable risk factors to decrease the risk of perioperative stroke. Those with symptomatic carotid stenosis should undergo carotid endarterectomy prior to major vascular surgery. Atrial fibrillation and discontinuation of antiplatelet therapy are two other identifiable risk factors that increase the incidence of perioperative stroke [30].

Spinal cord ischemia is a known risk of aortic repair and merits significant preoperative consideration and planning. Spinal cord malperfusion results in severe morbidity due to irreversible paralysis of the lower limbs when blood flow is limited through the Artery of Adamkiewicz. This predominant radicular artery most commonly arises from segments T9-T12, and is responsible for perfusion to the anterior two thirds of the spinal cord via the anterior spinal artery. Decreased perfusion from prolonged hypotension, or lengthy cross clamp time, places the patient at increased risk for spinal cord ischemia and anterior spinal cord syndrome. A high (proximal) aortic cross clamp further compounds the ischemic insult by hampering the heart's ability to maintain adequate cardiac output, and also creates an unfavorable cerebral spinal fluid pressure gradient due to increased central venous pressure and decreased distal arterial pressure. When aortic aneurysms extend into the thoracic region, cerebrospinal fluid (CSF) drainage is used to improve perfusion pressure to the spinal cord. Placement of a lumbar drain has been shown to decrease spinal cord ischemia, however data supporting its use is limited primarily to thoracic and thoracoabdominal aneurysms [31].

## Endocrine

Diabetic patients scheduled to undergo elective vascular surgery should be well optimized prior to the procedure. A diagnosis of diabetes mellitus increases the risk of death and cardiovascular complications in patients undergoing major vascular procedures. Currently, the literature regarding optimal target glucose range for the perioperative patient is unclear. Although hyperglycemia is associated with adverse outcomes, treatment of hyperglycemia with insulin infusions has not consistently improved outcomes [32]. In addition, elevated preoperative hemoglobin A1c (HbA1c), while predictive of morbidity in non-diabetic patients, was not found to be associated with increased mortality [33]. In both diabetics and non-diabetics, it is beneficial to keep glucose levels below 180 mg/dL. Metformin should be held the day of surgery, and newer sodium-glucose co-transport 2 (SGLT-2) inhibitors at least 24 h prior to surgery. A diagnosis of diabetes alone also warrants further cardiac evaluation preoperatively. Minimally, an electrocardiogram should be obtained, and further stress test or coronary angiography may be completed if it will change pre-operative or surgical management of the patient [15].

## Perioperative Management

Obtaining adequate intravenous (IV) access is essential for intraoperative management given the high propensity for bleeding and need for resuscitation. Minimally, two large bore peripheral IVs (16 gauge or larger) should be placed. An arterial line should be established prior to induction of anesthesia to monitor and prevent large hemodynamic changes with induction. Additionally, the arterial line allows frequent blood sampling. Laboratory blood samples should be obtained prior to surgery including chemistry, hemoglobin, platelet count, activated clotting time (ACT) and/or prothrombin time. Additionally, at least three further blood samples examining these values as well as arterial pH and plasma lactate should be drawn during the case to facilitate resuscitation efforts. The authors recommend vigilant lab monitoring during cross-clamp, following cross-clamp release, and prior to extubation.

A central venous catheter is often established to allow administration of vasoactive drug infusions. While CVP is traditionally used as a measure of intravascular volume status, it is a poor predictor of both volume status and fluid responsiveness [34, 35]. For those with significant right ventricular dysfunction or pulmonary hypertension, a pulmonary artery catheter (PAC) should be considered.

Transesophageal echocardiography (TEE) may be utilized in place of PAC for those with pre-existing poor left (LV) or right ventricular (RV) function, CHF, CAD, or an anticipated high cross clamp. TEE is useful in guiding fluid therapy and can detect cardiac wall motion abnormalities in real-time. Increased afterload following aortic cross-clamp can exacerbate cardiac ischemia, worsen pre-existing regional wall motion abnormalities, and lead to LV failure. It is important to note, however, that there is no gold standard for hemodynamic monitoring during open AAA repair and no data exist that outcomes are improved with use of PAC or TEE.

Resuscitation equipment including rapid infusers should be ready in anticipation of large blood losses. Patients should routinely have four to six units of packed red blood cells cross-matched and readily available. Cell salvage technology can decrease allogenic blood transfusion [36]. Thrombelastography (TEG) or thromboelastometry (ROTEM) seem to reduce perioperative blood loss when used to guide transfusion therapy, however there is insufficient evidence to suggest their use improves morbidity or mortality in severely bleeding patients [37].

The need for CSF drainage, somatosensory- and/or motor-evoked potential monitoring (SSEP and MEP, respectively) should be discussed with the surgeon beforehand, especially if extensive repair is anticipated (i.e. complicated anatomy, aneurysm extending into the thoracic aorta).

## Intraoperative Management

### Induction

Open AAA repair can be performed under general anesthesia, epidural anesthesia, or a combination of both. There are no proven long-term benefits of either form over the other [38, 39]. The addition of neuraxial anesthesia to general anesthesia reduces intraoperative transfusion requirements and the risk of postoperative respiratory failure, and offers superior postoperative pain control. The anesthesiologist must balance adequate depth of anesthesia and analgesia while maintaining stable hemodynamics throughout induction and the duration of the surgery. There are several key stages during open AAA repair that need special consideration from the anesthesiologist, as outlined below in Table 64.2.

A combination of IV anesthetics including propofol, opioids (fentanyl, remifentanil, sufentanil) and muscle relaxants are used to provide stable hemodynamics for laryngoscopy. Blood pressure should be kept within 20% of the baseline value and heart rate < 90 beats per minute. A combination of short acting vasoactive agents such as esmolol, sodium nitroprusside, nitroglycerin, phenylephrine, and norepinephrine need to be available.

**Table 64.2** Unique anesthetic considerations for open abdominal aortic aneurysm repair

| Preoperative evaluation | Common risk factors: MI, CAD, DM, renal dysfunction, tobacco use, COPD, CVA |
|---|---|
| IV access | 2 large bore IV ≥18 g, possible CVC |
| Monitoring | Arterial line, CVC, ±PAC, ±TEE, ±SSEP/MEP, ±lumbar drain |
| Anesthetic plan | GA, epidural, GA + epidural |
| Aortic cross clamp | Ensure adequate heparinization (75–100 units/kg, ACT ≥250 s) immediately prior to cross clamp Renal protection (mannitol, diuretic, etc) Vasodilators available to ↓afterload Maintain preload and CO |
| Aortic unclamping | Correct metabolic derangements, coagulopathy Reverse heparin Rewarm Vasopressors readily available, anticipate ischemic-reperfusion injury Optimize postop pain control, dose epidural when relatively stable hemodynamics |
| Adverse perioperative events | MI due to high incidence of CAD and increased myocardial oxygen demand Renal dysfunction from ATN Hypothermia Spinal cord ischemia Ischemic bowel |

## Maintenance

Fentanyl or sufentanil, in combination with inhaled volatile anesthetics and nitrous oxide maintain adequate anesthesia for the case. A greater proportion of opioids to volatile agent should be considered in patients with poor LV function. The use of an epidural catheter during aortic repair in conjunction with general anesthesia can cause significant hypotension, which is particularly problematic when the cross clamp is released. Infusion of local anesthetic through the epidural is generally avoided until the aorta is unclamped and the patient's hemodynamics and fluid requirements have stabilized. Post-operatively the epidural provides superior pain relief but it has been shown to result in the increased use of IV fluid and vasopressor [40].

## Temperature Management

Preventing hypothermia can be challenging during open AAA repair. Since the lower extremities are hypoperfused during aortic clamping, metabolic demands in the lower body should be kept to a minimum during this time. Forced air warming should only be applied to the upper body until the cross clamp is removed. Hypothermia contributes to development of coagulopathy, delays wound healing, and increases the hospital length of stay [41]. Hypothermia and shivering create an unfavorable oxygen supply to demand ratio, increasing the risk of myocardial ischemia. All IV fluids and blood products should be provided on warmed lines. Warmed fluids placed in the open abdomen will increase a patient's body temperature if other warming techniques are insufficient to keep the body normothermic.

## Renal Protection

Acute kidney injury after AAA is associated with significant morbidity and mortality. Nearly all kidney injury and failure after aortic repair is due to acute tubular necrosis (ATN), secondary to intra-operative hypotension and hypoperfusion. The strongest predictor of postoperative renal dysfunction is preoperative renal insufficiency. Additionally, prolonged operative and cross-clamp time, large volume blood loss, use of vasopressors, and positive fluid balances are the other independent risk factors for postoperative kidney injury [42, 43]. Adequate urine output alone does not predict postoperative renal function, and therefore cannot serve as the sole surrogate for renal perfusion in the perioperative period. While aortic cross-clamp causes significant reduction in renal blood flow, it is important to note that many additional factors contribute to kidney injury. Injury to kidneys can be caused by ischemia-reperfusion injury, intravascular volume depletion, embolization of atherosclerotic plaques, and direct surgical trauma to renal arteries.

While many pharmacologic agents such as mannitol, loop diuretics, and low-dose dopamine are commonly utilized prior to cross clamp in an attempt to protect the kidneys, there is little evidence of improved clinical outcomes [44]. Mannitol is thought to scavenge free radicals, decrease renin secretion, and increase renal prostaglandin synthesis. Loop diuretics and low-dose dopamine are thought to increase renal blood flow and urine output. Use of these agents should prompt careful attention to intravascular volume status since hypovolemia and renal hypoperfusion can increase the risk of kidney injury.

## Surgical Dissection

During the dissection phase, the abdominal aorta is exposed via a transperitoneal or retroperitoneal approach. The goal for this period is to maintain normotension. It is prudent for the practitioner to determine the individual patient's responsiveness to vasopressors and vasodilators during this time because it will guide management when large hemodynamic swings occur during aortic cross clamp- and unclamping. Approximately 5 min prior to aortic cross-clamp, unfractionated heparin is given at a dose of 75–100 units/kg, with goal ACT > 250 s.

## Aortic Clamping

Application of the aortic cross clamp produces sudden and drastic increases in systemic vascular resistance (SVR) and LV afterload. The extent of these hemodynamic changes depends on the proximity of the clamp to the aortic valve, baseline LV function, and the degree of collateral blood flow. Most abdominal aortic repairs involve infra-renal clamping, which induces minimal changes in LV afterload and wall tension. The more proximal the level of the aortic cross clamp, the more significant its impact on the cardiovascular system, with supraceliac clamp inducing the most significant increases in LV filling pressures and afterload. A heart with preserved LV function can withstand large increases in afterload without significant ventricular distention; a heart with decreased ejection fraction and coronary artery disease may not tolerate such hemodynamic disturbances and is at risk to develop ischemia from impaired subendocardial perfusion. In such instances, aortic clamp should be applied deliberately in a slow and controlled fashion. Minimizing the acute increase in LV afterload and wall tension controls the rapid increase in myocardial oxygen demand and may mitigate coronary ischemia. Short acting vasodilator infusions should be readily available to reduce afterload. Nitroglycerin would be preferred in patients with ECG changes or wall motion abnormalities seen on TEE. Selective arterial vasodilators (sodium nitroprusside or nicardipine) also play a role in treating severe hypertension. Increasing the depth of anesthesia can be used to reduce blood pressure. However, volatile agents are not easily titratable and their effect is often unpredictable. Relative hypovolemia, as assessed by TEE or PAC filling pressures, may be beneficial in the period immediately prior to aortic cross-clamping to attenuate hemodynamic shifts associated with cross-clamp. Care must be taken to avoid excessive hypotension since spinal cord perfusion is dependent on collateral flow below the aortic cross clamp.

## Aortic Unclamping

Removal of the aortic cross clamp releases potassium, lactic acid, and other metabolic waste products into the systemic circulation, resulting in a significant decrease in SVR and severe arterial hypotension. Correcting existing metabolic derangements, hypovolemia, and coagulopathy before aortic clamp is removed is imperative. Vasodilators should be discontinued, while vasopressors, inotropes, and calcium chloride should be readily available and administered as needed. In addition to pharmacologic agents, the surgeon can mitigate the severity of hemodynamic changes by releasing the aortic clamp in a gradual and controlled fashion (restoring 25%, 50%, then 75% of flow), such that vasoactive medications have sufficient circulation time to take effect. This also allows quick reapplication of the clamp if metabolic derangement or hypovolemia results in profound instability that mandates immediate treatment before attempting complete cross clamp release. The electrocardiogram should be closely monitored for any changes, particularly signs of hyperkalemia. Rewarming the patient should be initiated as the lower extremities are being reperfused.

The use of protamine to reverse heparin at the completion of repair is not universal and is often based on the surgeon's preference or subjective perception of bleeding at the operative site. Protamine should be infused in a slow and controlled manner, as rapid administration is associated with significant hemodynamic disturbances. While hypotension from histamine release is the most commonly observed phenomenon, anaphylactic shock and catastrophic pulmonary hypertension are rare but serious complications [45]. When comparing patients receiving protamine after major vascular surgery to those who did not, no significant differences in total blood loss, blood product use, and coagulation status were noted [46].

Pain control should be optimized by starting the epidural infusion once hemodynamics are stable. If the patient remains hypotensive, an opioid-only epidural infusion can be substituted for local anesthetic-opioid combination.

## Emergence

Coagulopathy, metabolic derangements, and hypothermia should be corrected prior to emergence. Cross clamp times longer than 30 min, large volumes of blood or crystalloid administration, and poor baseline pulmonary function increase the likeliness that the patient will not meet extubation criteria in the operating room. The same pharmacologic support used during induction to maintain stable hemodynamics should also be available for emergence.

The addition of epidural analgesia to general anesthesia is generally advocated for postoperative pain control as it has been shown to improve pain relief the first three postoperative days [40]. Patients who received epidural analgesia are extubated more quickly than those receiving systemic analgesics. However, epidural anesthesia has not been shown to reduce postoperative mortality.

## Postoperative Considerations

Most patients will be transported to the intensive care unit upon completion of the case for continued cardiac and pulmonary support, as well as hemodynamic and neurologic monitoring. The extent of required pharmacological hemodynamic support, the need for further intravenous fluid and blood product resuscitation, correction of coagulopathy and hypothermia, adequacy of pain control, and other patient-specific cardiac and respiratory concerns should be considered when deciding to extubate.

Patients in this population are at high risk for organ ischemia due to prolonged hypotension or malperfusion due to physical obstruction. Renal function and urine output should be carefully monitored because the development of AKI increases morbidity and mortality [43]. Initiation of dialysis should not be delayed if signs of volume overload, metabolic acidosis, hyperkalemia, or uremia develop. The risk of limb ischemia from reduced lower extremity perfusion necessitates frequent neurovascular checks. Neurologic deficit from spinal cord ischemia (SCI) can be unpredictable and mostly unpreventable due to its multifactorial etiology. There is currently no optimal treatment for SCI, however augmenting spinal cord perfusion pressure can be helpful. Acute bowel ischemia is another rare, but devastating complication after AAA repair. Common symptoms include non-specific cramping abdominal pain and an urge to defecate. Passage of bloody stools, an unexplained decline in postoperative progress, and lactic acidosis are worrisome signs of colonic ischemia [47].

## References

1. Bobadilla JL, Kent KC. Screening for abdominal aortic aneurysms. Adv Surg. 2012;46:101–9.
2. Guirguis JM, Beil TL, Sun X, Senger CA, Whitlock EP. Primary care screening for abdominal aortic aneurysm: an evidence update for the U.S. Preventive Services Task Force. Rockville; 2014.
3. Lindholt J, Ashton H, Heickendorff L, Scott R. Serum elastin peptides in the preoperative evaluation of abdominal aortic aneurysms. Eur J Vasc Endovasc Surg. 2001;22(6):546–50.
4. Dale M, Xiong W, Carson J, Suh M, Karpisek A, Meisdinger T, et al. Elastin-derived peptides promote abdominal aortic aneurysm formation by modulating M1/M2 macrophage polarization. J Immunol. 2016;196(11):4536–43.
5. Lederle F, Wilson S, Johnson G, Reinke D, Littooy FN, Acher C, et al. Immediate repair compared with surveillance of small abdominal aortic aneurysms. N Engl J Med. 2002;346(19):1437–44.
6. Brewster D, Cronenwett J, Hallett J, Johnston K, Krupski W, Matsumura J. Guidelines for the treatment of abdominal aortic aneurysms. J Vasc Surg. 2003;37(5):1106–17.
7. Hollier L, Taylor L, Ochsner J. Recommended indications for operative treatment of abdominal aortic aneurysms. J Vasc Surg. 1992;15(6):1046–56.
8. Upchurch G, Schaub T. Abdominal aortic aneurysm. Am Fam Physician. 2006;73(7):1198–204.
9. The United Kingdom EVAR Trial Investigators. Endovascular versus open repair of abdominal aortic aneurysms. N Engl J Med. 2010;362(20):1863–71.
10. Lederle F, Freischlag J, Kyriakides T, Padberg FJ, Matsumura J, Kohler T, et al. Outcomes following endovascular vs open repair of abdominal aortic aneurysm: a randomized trial. JAMA. 2009;302(14):1535–42.
11. De Bruin J, Baas A, Buth J, et al. Long-term outcome of open or endovascular repair of abdominal aortic aneurysm. N Engl J Med. 2010;362(20):1881–9.
12. Becquemin JP, Pillet JC, Lescalie F, et al. A randomized controlled trial of endovascular aneurysm repair versus open surgery for abdominal aortic aneurysms in low- to moderate-risk patients. J Vasc Surg. 2011;53(5):1167–73.
13. Patel R, Sweeting MJ, Powell JT, Greenhalgh RM, et al. Endovascular versus open repair of abdominal aortic aneurysm in 15 years' follow-up of the UK endovascular aneurysm repair trial 1 (EVAR trial 1): a randomised controlled trial. Lancet. 2016;388:2366–74.
14. IMPROVE Trial Investigators, Braithwaite B, Cheshire N, Greenhalgh R, Grieve R, Hassan T, et al. Endovascular strategy or open repair for ruptured abdominal aortic aneurysm: one-year outcomes from the IMPROVE randomized trial. Eur Heart J. 2015;36(31):2061–9.
15. Fleisher L, Fleischmann K, Auerbach A, Barnason S, Beckman J, Bozkurt B, et al. 2014 ACC/AHA guideline on perioperative cardiovascular evaluation and management of patients undergoing noncardiac surgery. J Am Coll Cardiol. 2014;64(22):e77–e137.
16. POISE Study Group, Devereaux P, Yang H, Yusuf S, Guyatt G, Leslie K, et al. Effects of extended-release metoprolol succinate in patients undergoing non-cardiac surgery (POISE trial): a randomised controlled trial. Lancet. 2008;371(9627):1839–47.
17. Flu W, van Kuijk J, Chonchol M, Winkel T, Verhagen H, Bax J, et al. Timing of pre-operative beta-blocker treatment in vascular surgery patients: influence on post-operative outcome. J Am Coll Cardiol. 2010;56(23):1922–9.
18. Kertai M, Boersma E, Westerhout C, van Domburg R, Klein J, Bax J, et al. Association between long-term statin use and mortality after successful abdominal aortic aneurysm surgery. Am J Med. 2004;116(2):96–103.
19. Molnar A, Coca S, Devereaux P. Statin use associates with a lower incidence of acute kidney injury after major elective surgery. J Am Soc Nephrol. 2011;22(5):939–46.
20. Levin G, Bates E, Bittl J, Brindis R, Fihn S, Fleisher L, et al. 2016 ACC/AHA guideline focused update on duration of dual antiplatelet therapy in patients with coronary artery disease. J Am Coll Cardiol. 2016;68(10):1243–75.
21. Lee TH, Marcantonio ER, Mangione CM, et al. Derivation and prospective validation of a simple index for prediction of cardiac risk of major noncardiac surgery. Circulation. 1999;100(10):1043–9.
22. Mills E, Eyawo O, Lockhart I, Kelly S, Wu P, Ebbert J. Smoking cessation reduces postoperative complications: a systematic review and meta-analysis. Am J Med. 2011;124(2):144–54.
23. Grønkjær M, Eliasen M, Skov-Ettrup L, Tolstrup J, Christiansen A, Mikkelsen S, et al. Preoperative smoking status and postoperative complications: a systematic review and meta-analysis. Ann Surg. 2014;259(1):52–71.
24. Axelrod DA, Henke PK, Wakefield TW, et al. Impact of chronic obstructive pulmonary disease on elective

and emergency abdominal aortic aneurysm repair. J Vasc Surg. 2001;33:72–6.
25. Upchurch GR, Proctor MC, Henke PK, et al. Predictors of severe morbidity and death after elective abdominal aortic aneurysmectomy in patients with chronic obstructive pulmonary disease. J Vasc Surg. 2003;37:594–9.
26. van Lier F, van der Geest PJ, Hoeks SE, et al. Epidural analgesia is associated with improved health outcomes of surgical patients with chronic obstructive pulmonary disease. Anesthesiology. 2011;115:315–21.
27. Grant SW, Grayson AD, Purkayastha D, McCollum CN. What are the risk factors for renal failure following open elective abdominal aortic aneurysm repair? Eur J Vasc Endovasc Surg. 2012;43(2):182–7.
28. Kopolovic I, Simmonds K, Duggan S, et al. Risk factors and outcomes associated with acute kidney injury following ruptured abdominal aortic aneurysm. BMC Nephrol. 2013;14:99.
29. Eldrup N, Budtz-Lilly J, Laustsen J, Bibby B, Paaske WP. Long-term incidence of myocardial infarct, stroke, and mortality in patients operated on for abdominal aortic aneurysms. J Vasc Surg. 2012;55(2):311–7.
30. Selim M. Perioperative stroke. N Engl J Med. 2007;356:706–13.
31. Khan SN, Stansby G. Cerebrospinal fluid drainage for thoracic and thoracoabdominal aortic aneurysm surgery. Cochrane Database Syst Rev. 2012;10:CD003635.
32. NICE-SUGAR Study Investigators, Finfer S, Chittock DR, et al. Intensive versus conventional glucose control in critically ill patients. N Engl J Med. 2009;360(13):1283–97.
33. O'Sullivan CJ, Hynes N, Mahendran B, et al. Haemoglobin A1c (HbA1C) in non-diabetic and diabetic vascular patients. Is HbA1c an independent risk factor and predictor of adverse outcome? Eur J Vasc Endovasc Surg. 2006;32(2):188–97.
34. Marik P, Baram M, Vahid B. Does central venous pressure predict fluid responsiveness? A systematic review of the literature and the tale of seven mares. Chest. 2008;134(1):172–8.
35. Madger S. Understanding central venous pressure: not a preload index? Curr Opin Crit Care. 2015;21(5):369–75.
36. Shantikumar S, Patel S, Handa A. The role of cell salvage autotransfusion in abdominal aortic aneurysm surgery. Eur J Vasc Endovasc Surg. 2011;42(5):577–84.
37. Afshari A, Wikkelsø A, Brok J, et al. Thrombelastography (TEG) or thromboelastometry (ROTEM) to monitor haemotherapy versus usual care in patients with massive transfusion. Cochrane Database Syst Rev. 2011;16(3):CD007871.
38. Licker M, Christoph E, Cartier V, Mugnai D, Murith N, Kalangos A, et al. Impact of anesthesia technique on the incidence of major complications after open aortic abdominal surgery: a cohort study. J Clin Anesth. 2013;25(4):296–308.
39. Ruppert V, Leurs L, Steckmeier B, et al. Influence of anesthesia type on outcome after endovascular aortic aneurysm repair: an analysis based on EUROSTAR data. J Vasc Surg. 2006;44(1):16–21.
40. Guay J, Kopp S. Epidural pain relief versus systemic opioid-based pain relief for abdominal aortic surgery. Cochrane Database Syst Rev. 2016;1:CD005059.
41. Kurz A, Sessler D, Lenhardt R. Perioperative normothermia to reduce the incidence of surgical-wound infection and shorten hospitalization. Study of Wound Infection and Temperature Group. N Engl J Med. 1996;334(19):1209–15.
42. Georgakis P, Paraskevas K, Bessias N, et al. Duration of aortic cross-clamping during elective open abdominal aortic aneurysm repair operations and postoperative cardiac/renal function. Int Angiol. 2010;29(3):244–8.
43. Ellenberger C, Schweizer A, Diaper J, et al. Incidence, risk factors and prognosis of changes in serum creatinine early after aortic abdominal surgery. Intensive Care Med. 2006;32(11):1808–16.
44. Zacharias M, Mugawar M, Herbison GP, Walker RJ, Hovhannisyan K, Sivalingam P, Conlon NP. Interventions for protecting renal function in the perioperative period. Cochrane Database Syst Rev. 2013;(9). Art. No.: CD003590. https://doi.org/10.1002/14651858.CD003590.pub4.
45. Park K. Protamine and protamine reactions. Int Anesthesiol Clin. 2004;42(3):135–45.
46. Dorman B, Elliott B, Spinale F, Bailey M, Walton J, Robison J, et al. Protamine use during peripheral vascular surgery: a prospective randomized trial. J Vasc Surg. 1995;22(3):248–55.
47. Van Damme H, Creemers E, Limet R. Ischaemic colitis following aortoiliac surgery. Acta Chir Belg. 2000;100(1):21.

# Anesthesia for Lower Extremity Bypass

## Jay Sanford and Brendan Atkinson

**Key Concepts** Vascular surgery patients tend toward multiple comorbidities and therefore, are medically challenging patients in the operating room

- The presence of coronary artery disease should be assumed in these patients, and has been proven to be a risk factor that predicts long-term negative outcomes in vascular surgery patients.
- If time affords, a focused but thorough history and physical exam is performed, appropriate lab and diagnostic exams ordered prior to surgery.
- Beta-blockers should be continued in these patients, with the decision to stop ACE/ARB therapy individualized to each patient's clinical scenario.
- Relevant patient anatomy requires review to evaluate the patient's appropriateness for either regional/neuraxial or general anesthesia. Local expertise in either technique is the most important factor determining outcomes [1].
- Standard American Society of Anesthesiologists (ASA) monitors with the addition of an arterial line should be considered in all vascular patients. The addition of further monitors should be made after careful consideration of the patient's comorbid conditions to decide if they confer benefit.
- Minimally, these patients require at least two large bore (18 Gauge) intravenous (IV) lines should the need for intra-operative resuscitation arise. Central venous access may be considered in cases of poor peripheral intravenous access, anticipated significant blood loss, or need for vasoactive medication administration.
- Careful post-operative care must be provided to adequately monitor these patients for untoward outcomes related to underlying medical comorbidities and/or graft disruption and failure.

## Pre-operative Evaluation

Infra-inguinal bypass surgery is performed for a variety of reasons; patients with critical limb ischemia (CLI) are amongst those most commonly presenting for this type surgery. CLI is end stage arterial insufficiency causing chronic tissue hypo-perfusion that is characterized by pain at rest and often leg or foot ulceration or gangrene, Hemodynamic evidence of arterial insufficiency typically in the form of diminished ankle-brachial

J. Sanford, D.O. (✉) · B. Atkinson, M.D.
Department of Anesthesiology, Emory University School of Medicine, Emory University Hospital, Atlanta, GA, USA
e-mail: jay.sanford@emoryhealthcare.org;
breandan.thomas.atkinson@emory.edu

indices and computed tomography angiography (CTA) confirms the diagnosis. The average patient waits over 2 months from onset of symptoms to seek consultation from a vascular surgeon [2]. Depending on the severity of disease, this frequently affords the anesthesiologist, surgeon, and primary care physician minimal time to medically optimize comorbid conditions that impact overall survival and functional outcomes.

Due to the vascular disease burden, a complete review and examination of the cardiovascular, pulmonary, endocrine, and renal systems should be performed.

## Comorbid Disease Management

***Peripheral Arterial Disease:*** Perhaps the most important disease process underlying patients presenting for lower extremity revascularization, is the presence of atherosclerosis. Atherosclerosis is the process of intraluminal plaque formation and deposition within the endothelium which leads to luminal narrowing, a local inflammatory response, and potential for plaque rupture. A focused examination looking for signs of claudication and arterial insufficiency (ulcerations, gangrene, tissue atrophy, cool temperatures) should occur, with careful questioning of the patient regarding their symptoms. Understanding the evolution of a patient's peripheral arterial disease allows the anesthesiologist to appropriately address the potential pitfalls and complications that may arise in the operating room, as well determine patient appropriateness for a regional anesthetic.

***Coronary Artery Disease***: The cardiovascular assessment is merited when evaluating all patients prior to an anesthetic, but perhaps none more so than in vascular surgery. Complications arising from coronary artery disease (CAD) are the leading cause of postoperative morbidity and mortality in patients who undergo surgical treatment of PAD [3]. Numerous investigations have conservatively estimated that 50% of patients with PAD suffer concomitant flow-limiting CAD [3]. Ninety-two percent of patients having undergone lower extremity amputation were found to have significant CAD at the time of autopsy [4]. An original study examining the correlation between CAD and PAD, found an astonishing 30% of patients had sufficiently severe coronary disease to warrant revascularization [5]. While the exact prevalence of clinically significant CAD is unknown, treating all vascular patients as though they have CAD provides safe anesthetic planning.

Prior to elective surgery, a preoperative electrocardiogram (ECG) needs to be completed. The cornerstone of the evaluation of a patient's coronary artery disease burden, is an assessment of functional capacity using metabolic equivalents (METS). Further testing should be done in accordance with the evidence-based guidelines put forth by the American Heart Association and The American College of Cardiology (ACC/AHA) [6, 7].

***Hypertension***: Every effort should be undertaken to determine the patient's disease history, paying careful attention to disease progression, medication regimen, and most importantly signs of end organ damage. Vascular patients often present with elevated baseline blood pressures on the day of surgery, likely related to a number of factors, including requiring them to hold medications central to their regimen, their failure to take antihypertensive medications on the day of surgery, and generalized anxiety with regards to their upcoming procedure. In an urgent/emergent scenario, it is the anesthesiologist's job to determine the best course of treatment for intra-operative blood pressure control. The decision to treat high blood pressure is determined by the patient's history and their past blood pressure range. An acute decrease in blood pressure to normal (140/80 or less) is not appropriate in many patients and may be associated with increased post-operative risk [8]. In elective scenarios, the risk versus benefit of postponing a procedure to attempt better blood pressure control prior to surgery needs to be determined; special consideration should be given to patients with uncontrolled hypertension and and worsening end-organ damage. The ACC/AHA recommends postponing surgeries with blood pressures in excess of 180/110 with signs of end organ damage, until a patient is under better control. Hanada et al. analyzed several studies evaluating pre-operative hypertension and concluded that patients with severe hypertension and signs of end organ damage should have their case delayed to improve perioperative outcomes. However, mild to moderate pre-operative hypertension did not appear to lead to significant morbidity or mortality. Their analysis did uncover that patients with uncontrolled blood pressure have an increased risk for intraoperative hemodynamic instability in those patients, and this may be the most significant impact of hypertension on the vascular surgery patient [9–11].

*Diabetes Mellitus*: Diabetes is of particular concern to the vascular anesthesiologist. Not only is diabetes common in those presenting for vascular surgery, but because the underlying pathophysiology of hyperglycemia increases the risk of post-operative morbidity and mortality. Adverse clinical outcomes associated with poor glucose management include delayed wound healing, increased surgical site infections, and an overall increase in length of stay [12]. While the debate continues over the method of glucose management and thresholds for treatment, it is clear that the detrimental effects of uncontrolled diabetes and stress hyperglycemia impact surgical outcomes. Several professional organizations recommend target blood glucose in all patients of less than 180 mg/dL [13–15]. Monitoring can be done with simple point-of-care finger stick glucometers when feasible, and or arterial sampling in other more invasive cases.

*Tobacco Abuse*: While tobacco abuse has long been shown to have a detrimental effect on the lung parenchyma leading to the development of COPD, the effects of smoking on the vascular system may be overlooked. With prolonged smoking history, patients develop long-standing intravascular inflammatory changes and plaque formation. It is now widely accepted that tobacco abuse has a distinct impact on the endothelial lining of the vascular system, and smoking is intimately linked to the development of PAD [16]. Several studies suggest that tobacco abuse has a greater association with PAD than CAD, and a meta-analysis in 2013 by Lu et al. reinforced this claim [17]. Unsurprisingly, numerous studies corroborate the direct link between amount smoked and prevalence of PAD, with heavy smokers being at the greatest risk [18].

Of all the risk factors for development of arterial disease, smoking tobacco is one of the few modifiable contributors to the disease. Ideally, patients abstain from tobacco use months before surgery, however this is often times not practical or possible. Evidence exists to suggest that even as much as 8 h of abstinence from tobacco use can decrease a patients carboxyhemoglobin levels to near non-smoker levels, and subsequently increase oxygen carrying capacity of hemoglobin. Patients with intermittent claudication can reduce disease progression and reduce the likelihood of undergoing vascular surgery with smoking cessation [19]. Patients who continue to smoke after infra-inguinal bypass graft have three times the rate of graft failure over nonsmokers. Fortunately, graft failure rates in patients who successfully quit smoking trend toward those of nonsmokers, demonstrating the importance of smoking cessation both before and after vascular intervention [20].

## Day of Surgery Medication Management

Decisions regarding medication use on the day of surgery are often left to the anesthesiologist. As such, following formal guidelines is recommended however, reviewing patients on individual basis is imperative particularly in the setting of those using ACEI/ARB anti-hypertensives and/or dual anti-platelet therapy.

*Angiotensin Converting Enzyme Inhibitors and Angiotensin Receptor Blockers:* Among the anti-hypertensive agents, the use of angiotensin converting enzyme inhibitors (ACEI) and angiotensin receptor blockers (ARBS) is controversial in the perioperative period. These medications continue to incite dialogue in regards to their perioperative use, particularly in regard to their perceived propensity to lead to refractory intraoperative hypotension. Case reports and recent studies agree that intraoperative hypotension refractory to the commonly used vasopressors, namely ephedrine and phenylephrine, is more frequently observed in patients continuing their ACEI/ARB therapy on the day of surgery [21–23]. There is limited evidence to suggest that discontinuing these medications prior to surgery reduces post-operative events. Roshanov et al. demonstrated a decrease in 30 days all-cause mortality, stroke, and myocardial injury in patients whose ACEI/ARB therapies were held [24]. The study also demonstrated in this same patient group, episodes of intraoperative hypotension were not as frequent as recorded in the patients taking their ACEI/ARB medications on the day of surgery. This however was not independently associated with mortality or vascular events. With the controversy that exists in regards to these medications, the known/potential risk of intraoperative hypotension must be weighed against the potential benefits provided to the patients by maintaining their anti-hypertensive therapies through the perioperative period. Based on the above discussion, common practice in most institutions is to hold these medications during the perioperative period.

**Beta-Blockade**: Current evidence suggests a mortality benefit related to the continuation of previously prescribed beta-blockers (BB) throughout the perioperative period. Past evidence demonstrated decreased rates of post-operative myocardial infarction and decreased length of stay in patients undergoing infra-renal vascular surgery when these medications were continued [25]. Likewise, research also suggests that starting a beta-blocker naïve patient on therapy during the immediate peri-operative period, is associated with increased post-operative mortality and morbidity. While these recommendations remain the gold standard for management of these medications in the peri-operative period, there may be an evolution of treatment in the near future. Following publication of the 2014 ACC/AHA guidelines, further studies have not shown beta-blockers to reduce all-cause mortality; they do however, appear to reduce rates of non-fatal myocardial infarction/ischemia while increasing the number of non-fatal strokes [25]. To further complicate the picture, a large retrospective cohort study published in the New England Journal of Medicine showed a decrease in death in patients with a high revised cardiac risk index (RCRI) score, while patients with a low RCRI saw possible harm [26]. While further well-designed studies are necessary to elucidate information needed to determine if a change in practice is necessary, continuing beta blocker therapy throughout the perioperative period is currently advised. It is not advisable to initiate treatment with BB prior to non-cardiac surgery without adequate time for titration as this may confer an increased risk of 30-day all-cause mortality [27].

**Statin Therapy**: The importance of statin therapy in vascular surgery patients was demonstrated in the Heart Protection Study [28], demonstrating improved mortality benefit and improved cardiovascular outcomes in patients with PAD. Statins decrease endothelial dysfunction and help stabilize atherosclerotic lesions. As to which statin and what the appropriate dosing regimen should be, this should be determined by a patient's clinical condition, risk factors, and tolerance to statin therapy. Currently patients are divided into either high dose or low dose statin therapy, with high dose therapy withheld for those with the most advanced vascular disease as well as comorbid conditions such as HTN and DM [29].

**Dual Anti-Platelet Therapy (DAPT)**: Vascular patients often present on dual antiplatelet therapy either for primary prevention (i.e., prior to a thromboembolic event) or as secondary prevention (following drug eluting or bare metal stent placement, peripheral vascular bypass, and or post cerebral vascular event). It is important to determine need for these medications in context of the patient's disease burden, and to discuss their continuation with the surgical team and prescribing physician. Risk of bleeding versus risk of in-stent thrombosis/myocardial infarction must be weighed. Often in vascular surgery, DAPT is continued through the perioperative period, because the risk of cardiac event is far higher than the potential for excessive bleeding. Guidelines for management of DAPT specifically for cardiac stents, are available and provide direction for clinicians [30]. In emergent procedures, the anesthesiologist must be prepared for excessive bleeding. Laboratory exams such as platelet functional assays and thromboelastography (TEG) can help determine appropriate therapy. Platelets assist with achieving hemostasis in the face of DAPT, and should be considered in patients undergoing high risk emergent surgeries in which hemostasis is of significant concern.

## Relevant Lower Extremity Anatomy

Knowing the location and duration of patient symptomatology, and relevant patient anatomy, aids the anesthesiologist's decision regarding appropriate anesthetic technique. Distal revascularization or amputation can be accomplished with peripheral blocks or neuraxial technique, whereas more proximal procedures and those that are infra-renal but extensive, may best lend themselves to a general anesthetic. Table 65.1 outlines suggested anesthetic techniques for the most common lower extremity vascular procedures. Further discussion regarding regional anesthesia techniques for this type of surgery can be found in the regional section of this text.

*Vasculature*: As with any procedure, it is important that the anesthesiologist possess a functional understanding of the relevant surgical anatomy in order to anticipate intraoperative patient positioning, estimate potential fluid losses, and to determine the type of anesthesia appropriate for the proposed surgery.

The general approach to lower extremity revascularization is to redirect blood flow from a proximal source (the inflow), past an obstruction, to a distal source (the outflow). Typically, two or more separate incisions are made on the extremity, one for proximal anastomosis and one for the distal "target" artery. In the groin, the surgeon may expose the common femoral, superficial femoral, or deep femoral artery. The axillary artery is also used as the inflow vessel in certain cases. The target artery will depend on the individual patient's disease burden and preoperative imaging obtained to identify candidate arteries for distal anastomosis. For revascularization near the level of the knee, an incision is typically made along the medial aspect of the limb.

The external iliac artery becomes the common femoral artery as it crosses under the inguinal ligament. Due to size and location, it can be an excellent conduit for providing unobstructed inflow for lower extremity revascularization. In the majority of patients, including those with extensive atherosclerotic burden, it is easily palpable just below the inguinal crease. Approximately 2.5–5.0 cm past the inguinal ligament, the common femoral artery divides into the deep femoral (profunda femoris) and superficial femoral artery. The superficial femoral artery continues distally only a few centimeters in its "superficial" location before diving deep beneath the sartorious muscle to enter the adductor canal. Here, it travels alongside the femoral vein and branches of the femoral nerve (particularly the

**Table 65.1** Anesthesthetic techniques for common lower extremity vascular procedures

|  | Epidural/spinal | Femoral/sciatic block | Femoral/popliteal block | General anesthesia | Monitored anesthesia care |
|---|---|---|---|---|---|
| Fem/pop bypass | X | X |  | X | X (with regional) |
| LE AVF | X | X | X | X | X (with regional) |
| Amputations | X (AKA/BKA) | X (AKA/BKA) | X (BKA) | X | X (with regional) |
| Ax/fem bypass |  |  |  | X |  |
| Endoscopic stenting/angioplasty | X |  |  | X | X |

saphenous nerve), before exiting the canal and becoming the popliteal artery just proximal to the knee. Posterior to the knee joint, the popliteal artery may be palpable as it courses alongside the popliteal vein and tibial nerve before bifurcating into the anterior tibial artery and tibioperoneal trunk typically just caudal to the tibial plateau [31]. The anterior tibial artery runs along the tibia and becomes the dorsalis pedis artery, a superficial artery of the ankle that may not be palpable or detectable with Doppler signal, particularly in this patient population. The tibioperoneal trunk is a short segment of artery, typically <3 cm, which further divides into the peroneal and posterior tibial arteries of the lower leg. The peroneal artery is a deep and non-palpable structure that runs along the medial aspect of the fibula. The posterior tibial artery is located along the medial aspect of the lower leg and crosses the ankle posterior to the medial malleolus, where again, it may or may not be palpable or provide Doppler signal.

The saphenous vein is a long and superficial structure that begins its course anterior to the medial malleolus and along the medial aspect of the dorsal foot. It continues proximally, remaining relatively superficial, posteromedial to the tibia and within the medial thigh, allowing it to frequently be easily accessed as a conduit for autologous vein grafting in infra-inguinal bypass procedures. It ends its extensive course by emptying into the femoral vein distal to the inguinal ligament.

*Nervous System*: As infra-inguinal bypass procedures are frequently performed under regional anesthesia, the anesthesiologist must be proficient in such techniques and knowledgeable of nerve anatomy of the lower limbs and their relative distributions. While an understanding of basic lower extremity neuro-anatomy is vital for the anesthesiologist, it is complex will not be discussed in detail within this chapter.

## Intraoperative Management

*Anesthetic Technique*: In a patient population with substantial comorbidities, it is appropriate, to opt for a regional anesthetic, either spinal/epidural or peripheral nerve blockade, when possible. It has been suggested that neuraxial anesthesia offers several benefits over general anesthesia, including decreased catecholamine surge, improved lower extremity blood flow to improve graft patency, lower heart rate variability, diminished hemodynamic swings, and a reduced incidence of post-operative pneumonia [1]. Yet, the evidence does not support the selection of regional anesthesia in this regard. In a large observational analysis of the NSQIP database, patients undergoing 5462 infra-inguinal bypass procedures using general (87%) versus regional (13%) anesthesia were investigated. After comparison, no statistical difference was seen in mortality, morbidity, or length of stay in comparing general anesthesia patients to the regional anesthesia cohort [32].

Studies have demonstrated a decrease in circulating catecholamines for cases done under regional versus general anesthesia, however the reduction in deep venous and arterial graft thrombosis rates remains inconsistent and does not favor one anesthetic method [33, 34]. The Perioperative Ischemia Randomized Anesthesia Trial (PIRAT), did demonstrate an increased risk of graft failure in patients whom underwent infra-inguinal bypass under general anesthesia as opposed to spinal anesthesia [35], but subsequent studies have had difficulty replicating this outcome. With this in mind, the previous claims remain theoretical, and multiple explanations have been offered for this difference. Researchers posit the increased incidence of graft failure rates in the general anesthesia population may be due in part to an elevated serum level of plasminogen activator inhibitor-1, but this remains unproven [36]. Paradoxically, a large multicenter study again using NSQIP data has shown significantly lower rates of 30-day graft patency in patients who underwent spinal rather than general anesthesia. Patency rates in patients receiving epidural versus general anesthesia were not statistically different [1]. Most studies conclude that there is a lack of a statistical difference in study end points between regional and general anesthesia, making recommendation of one technique over the other difficult. Positive patient outcomes seem to be directly correlated to local preference for regional or general anesthesia, not the data proven efficacy of either approach.

Even with the above debate, there appears to have been a shift amongst vascular anesthesiologists and those who care for these patients, towards selection of the anesthetic technique that affords the patient improved functional outcomes. Multiple studies that agree that functional outcomes such as ambulatory status and independent living status, are not necessarily determined by the patency of the graft itself and trips back to the OR. Rather, these functional outcomes seem to be linked to preexisting patient factors. While graft patency and limb salvage is understandably an important endpoint to the surgeon, and may be affected by regional versus general anesthetic technique, preventing a decline in ambulatory status, independence, and of course, avoidance of death, is what is important to the patient and should therefore be the goal of surgeon and the anesthesiologist. Ultimately whichever technique selected, it must afford the patient the best chance of recovering reasonable functional status following intervention.

***Intravenous Access and Monitoring***: While standard ASA monitors are mandated, vascular surgery patients present the potential need to escalate monitoring. With the presence of multiple diseases, intra-operative monitoring of hemodynamics as well as laboratory results may be necessary. Patients undergoing lower extremity vascular cases, regardless of level of complexity, need two large bore (18 gauge or greater) intravenous lines. The addition of an arterial line should be based on the patient's other comorbid diseases that would warrant close hemodynamic monitoring, and also factor the complexity of the surgical repair, risk for bleeding, and need for resuscitation. A pre-induction arterial line should be placed in patients whose medical conditions allow for little hemodynamic perturbation, as induction can produce significant swings in blood pressure and heart rate even under the most controlled situations. While endovascular procedures may appear less invasive, careful attention should be paid to the location of the bypass and the extent of the procedure. Arterial access should be considered if patient disease merits its presence, even in minimally invasive surgeries.

Central venous catheters (CVC) are necessary if the nature of the lower extremity surgery is extensive. While CVC may not be necessary in an endovascular lower extremity stent placement, open procedures on larger vessels may require volume resuscitation that a CVC quickly facilitates. Central venous access, with the option to trend venous pressures, may aid in determining volume status when used in conjunction with hemodynamics, urine output and pulse/systolic pressure variation. Risks and benefits of CVC line placement must be balanced with the potential risks of intraoperative events requiring rapid resuscitation.

Further intra-operative monitoring can be considered based on the patient's medical comorbidities. Adjunct monitors if available, such as, pulse pressure variation, transesophageal echocardiography, cerebral oximetry, bio-impedance monitors, and esophageal Doppler, can and should be considered. In patients whose hemodynamic monitoring may be challenging but necessary, the addition of any of the above monitors gives the anesthesiologist another tool to guide intra-operative decision-making. Goal directed therapy (GDT) to determine intravascular volume and need for resuscitation/fluid administration is becoming a vital component to delivering a safe anesthetic. There is a growing body of evidence that suggests GDT during the operative period in patients at high risk for post-operative complications, has a positive impact on their outcomes. Thus, addition of at least one of the above monitors to assist in guiding fluid therapy is recommended by the authors [37].

The complex medical histories of these patients often requires intra-operative laboratory exams including arterial blood gas monitoring, point-of-care glucose testing, and activated clotting time measurements after the administration of heparin and subsequent protamine. Baseline lab values should be obtained prior to surgery if time affords. Knowledge of a patient's electrolyte status, kidney function, hemoglobin level, and acid base status, will guide the anesthesiologist in the OR during differentphases of the surgery.

***Intra-operative Events***: Of particular importance during lower extremity revascularization is the importance of the reperfusion process and the possibility for hemodynamic instability and derangements in laboratory exams. Distal to the proposed anastomosis anaerobic metabolism prevails, leading to the build-up of toxic metabolites. Additionally, placement of the surgical cross clamp will increase the tissue area in which blood flow and oxygen are limited. Upon removal of the clamp, reperfusion of ischemic tissue occurs, and metabolites (lactate, potassium and inflammatory mediators) are washed into systemic circulation. Careful attention must be paid to a patient's pH, electrolyte status, lactate, and bicarbonate levels throughout the case, particularly prior to and immediately following limb reperfusion. It is necessary for the anesthesiologist to treat abnormalities during this time period as means to mitigate subsequent hemodynamic issues.

## Post-operative

Vascular surgery patients regardless of the method of anesthesia employed should be monitored in the post-anesthesia care unit, or depending on their clinical status, admitted directly to the ICU. Careful attention should be paid to signs of hemorrhage or threatened graft patency. Experienced personnel need to perform frequent neurovascular checks. If at any time it is felt that the patency and integrity of a recently re-vascularized extremity or stent is threatened, the vascular surgery service must be notified at once to determine if re-intervention is needed. Likewise, comorbid disease states must be managed and play heavily into the success of the surgery performed. Blood pressure control is often paramount, as graft patency and surgical success hinges on normol tension. Given the high risk of cardiac events in vascular surgery patients, signs or symptoms of cardiac compromise urge immediate work-up. Management of post-operative glucose remains important because a euglycemia state facilitate wound healing, decreases inflammation, and is associated with a reduction in post-operative complications including stroke and acute kidney injury.

## References

1. Singh N, et al. The effects of the type of anesthesia on outcomes of lower extremity infra-inguinal bypass. J Vasc Surg. 2006;44(5):964–8.
2. Chung J, Bartelson B, et al. Wound healing and functional outcomes after infra-inguinal bypass with reversed saphenous vein for critical limb ischemia. J Vasc Surg. 2006;43:1183–90.
3. Hur D, Kizilgul M, et al. Frequency of coronary artery disease in patients undergoing peripheral artery disease surgery. Am J Cardiol. 2012;110:736–40.
4. Mautner G, Mautner S, et al. Amounts of coronary arterial narrowing by atherosclerotic plaque at necropsy in patients with lower extremity amputation. Am J Cardiol. 1992;70:1143–6.
5. Hertzer N, Beven E, et al. Coronary artery disease in peripheral vascular patients. Ann Surg. 1984;199(2):223–33.
6. Ghadimi K, Thompson A. Update on perioperative care of the cardiac patient for non-cardiac surgery. Curr Opin Anesthesiol. 2015;28:342–8.
7. Fleisher LA, et al. 2014 ACC/AHA guidelines on perioperative cardiovascular evaluation and management of patients undergoing non-cardiac. J Am Coll Cardiol. 2014;64(22):e77–e137.
8. Stepelfeldt WH, Yuan H, Dryden JK, Strehl KE, Cywinski JB, Ehrenfeld JM, Bromley P. The SLUScore: a novel method for detecting hazardous hypertension in adult patients undergoing noncardiac surgical procedures. Anesth Analg. 2017;124(4):1135–52.
9. Fontes ML, Aronson S, et al. Pulse pressure and risk of adverse outcome in coronary bypass surgery. Anesth Analg. 2008;107(4):1122–9.
10. Asopa A, Jidge S, et al. Preoperative pulse pressure and major perioperative adverse cardiovascular outcomes after lower extremity vascular bypass surgery. Anesth Analg. 2012;114:1177–81.
11. Hanada S, Kawakami H, Goto T, Morita S. Hypertension and anesthesia. Curr Opin Anesthesiol. 2006;19:315–9.
12. Duggan E, et al. Perioperative hyperglycemia and management: an update. Anesthesiology. 2017;126(3):547–06.
13. Moghissi ES, Korytkowski MT, DiNardo M, et al. American Association of Clinical Endocrinologists and American Diabetes Association consensus statement on inpatient glycemic control. Diabetes Care. 2009;32(6):1119–31.
14. Joshi GP, Chung F, Vann MA, et al. Scoiety for ambulatory Anesthesia consensus statement on perioperative blood glucose management in diabetic

patients undergoing ambulatory surgery. Anesth Analg. 2010;111:1378–87.
15. Dhartariya K, Levy N, Kivert A, Watson B, Cousins D, Flanagan D, Hilton L, Jairam C, Leyden K, Lipp A, Lobo D, Sinclair-Hammersley M, Rayman G, For the Joint British Diabetes Societies. NHS diabetes guideline for the perioperative management of the adult patient with diabetes. Diabetes UK position statements and care recommendations. Diabetes. 2012;29:420–33.
16. Price JF, Mowbray PI, et al. Relationship between smoking and cardiovascular risk factors in the development of peripheral arterial disease and coronary artery disease: Edinburgh artery study. Eur Heart J. 1999;20(5):344–53.
17. Lu L, Mackay DF, Pell JP. Meta-analysis of the association between cigarette smoking and peripheral arterial disease. Heart. 2014;100:414–23.
18. Willigendael EM, Teijink JA, et al. Influence of smoking on incidence and prevalence of peripheral arterial disease. J Vasc Surg. 2004;40(6):1158–65.
19. Jonason T, Bergstrom R. Cessation of smoking in patients with intermittent claudication. Acta Med Scand. 1987;221:253–60.
20. Willigendael EM, et al. Smoking and the patency of lower extremity bypass grafts: a meta-analysis. J Vasc Surg. 2005;42(1):67–74.
21. Brabant SM, et al. The hemodynamic effects of anesthetic induction in vascular surgical patients chronically treated with angiotensin II receptor antagonists. Anesth Analg. 1999;88:138–1392.
22. Comfere T, Sprung J, Kumar M, et al. Angiotensin system inhibitors in a general surgical population. Anesth Analg. 2005;100:636–44.
23. Bertrand M, Godet G, Meersschaert K, et al. Should the angiotensin II antagonists be discontinued before surgery? Anesth Analg. 2001;92:26–30.
24. Roshanov P, Rochwerg B, et al. Withholding versus continuing angiotensin-converting enzyme inhibitors or angiotensin II receptor blockers before non-cardiac surgery. Anesthesiology. 2017;126:16–27.
25. Bangalore S, Wetterslev J, et al. Perioperative B blockers in patients having non-cardiac surgery: a meta-analysis. Lancet. 2008;372:1962–76.
26. Lindenauer P, Pekow P, et al. Perioperative beta-blocker therapy and mortality after major non-cardiac surgery. N Engl J Med. 2005;353:349–61.
27. Bouri S, et al. Meta-analysis of secure randomized controlled trials of B-blockade to prevent perioperative death in non-cardiac surgery. Heart. 2014;100:456–64.
28. Heart Protection Study Collaborative Group. MRC/BHF heart protection study of cholesterol lowering with simvastatin in 20,536 high risk individuals: a randomized placebo-controlled trial. Lancet. 2002;360:7–22.
29. Conte MS, et al. Society for Vascular Surgery practice guidelines for atherosclerotic occlusive disease of the lower extremities: management of asymptomatic disease and claudication. J Vasc Surg. 2015;61(3):2S–41S.
30. Webster TD, et al. Perioperative management of dual anti-platelet therapy. Hosp Pract. 2016;44(5):237–41.
31. Kil SW, Jung GS. Anatomical variations of the popliteal artery and its tibial branches: analysis of 1242 extremities. Cardiovasc Intervent Radiol. 2009;32(2):233–40.
32. Ghanami RJ, et al. Anesthesia-based evaluation of outcomes of lower-extremity vascular bypass procedures. Ann Vasc Surg. 2013;27:199–207.
33. Parker SD, Breslow MJ, et al. Catecholamine and cortisol responses to lower extremity revascularization: correlation with outcome variables. Crit Care Med. 1995;23:1954–61.
34. Breslow MJ, Parker SD, et al. Determinants of catecholamine and cortisol responses to lower extremity revascularization. The PIRAT study group. Anesthesiology. 1993;79:1202–9.
35. Christopherson R, et al. Perioperative morbidity in patients randomized to epidural or general Anesthesia for lower extremity vascular surgery. Anesthesiology. 1993;79:422–34.
36. Perler BA, et al. The influence of anesthetic method on infra-inguinal bypass graft patency: a closer look. Am Surg. 1995;61(9):784–9.
37. Lobo SM, et al. Clinical review: what are the best hemodynamic targets for non-cardiac surgical patients? Crit Care. 2013;17:210.
38. Fowkes G, et al. Comparison of global estimates of prevalence and risk factors for peripheral artery disease in 2000 and 2010: a systematic review and analysis. Lancet. 2013;382(9901):1329–40.
39. Vascular Events In Noncardiac Surgery Patients Cohort Evaluation (VISION) Study Investigators. Association between postoperative troponin levels and 30-day mortality among patients undergoing non-cardiac surgery. JAMA. 2012;307:2295–304.
40. Siracuse JJ, Meltzer EC, Gill HL, et al. Outcomes and risk factors of cardiac arrest after vascular surgery procedures. J Vasc Surg. 2015;61:197–202.

# Anesthesia for Nephrectomy with Vena Cava Thrombectomy

## 66

Michael A. Evans and Francis A. Wolf

## Introduction

Renal cell carcinoma (RCC) is the most common form of kidney cancer, comprising more than 90% of renal malignancies [1]. Worldwide, RCC is the ninth most common cancer [2, 3] and accounts for 2% of all neoplasms and cancer-related deaths in adults. Major established risk factors include smoking, obesity, and high blood pressure, however genetic factors also contribute [3]. The incidence of RCC varies geographically. In most developed countries, the incidence of RCC is increasing; yet mortality across the population is stable or decreasing [2, 3]. This may be due to the early incidental discovery of small tumors that have not yet metastasized [2, 3]. RCC demonstrates a biological propensity for intravascular extension with formation of venous tumor thrombus (VTT) [4]. An estimated 4–10% of patients with RCC have extension of the tumor into the renal vein or IVC [5] and 1–2% of patients have tumor extension into the right atrium [6]. In rare cases, tumor thrombus can extend through the tricuspid valve into the right ventricle.

The treatment of choice for RCC with VTT is surgical resection. Even in the presence of distant metastases [5], resection has been demonstrated to improve symptoms, quality of life, and prognosis [1, 7, 8]. Surgical resection represents optimal long-term survival benefit for patients who have RCC extending into the vena cava [9], because currently, targeted agents have not been proven effective as neoadjuvant chemotherapy [4]. Expectant management is associated with a median survival of 5 months and 1-year disease-specific survival rate is 29% [10]. Surgical resection results in a 5-year survival rate of 40–64% in the absence of metastatic disease [4, 11] and 50% with metastatic disease [12]. Radical nephrectomy involves the complete resection of Gerota's fascia and its contents (kidney, adrenal gland, perinephric fat) as well as removal of lymphatics and the proximal ureter. Removal of tumor thrombus may require extensive mobilization of the liver, vascular exclusion of the liver, or vascular bypass depending on the degree of thrombus extension. Reconstruction or resection of the IVC may also be necessary.

## Preoperative Considerations

The majority of patients with RCC and VTT are symptomatic and may present with a plethora of symptoms including fatigue, weight loss, hematuria, flank pain, paraneoplastic syndromes, lower extremity edema, ascites, varicocele, caput medusa, Budd Chiari syndrome, deep venous thrombosis (DVT) and pulmonary

M. A. Evans, M.D. · F. A. Wolf, M.D. (✉)
Department of Anesthesiology, Emory University School of Medicine, Emory University Hospital, Atlanta, GA, USA
e-mail: mevans@northwestern.edu;
francis.wolf@emory.edu

embolus (PE). Symptoms are not however associated with negative surgical outcomes. For example, preoperative PE, present in up to 5% of patients upon diagnosis of RCC [6, 13, 14], is not associated with increased 90-day postoperative mortality, tumor recurrence, or cancer-specific mortality [13].

## Pre-operative Imaging

Metastases are present at diagnosis in about one third of patients with RCC and VTT [4], often involving the lung, bones, liver, or brain. Complete imaging evaluation is essential. Computed tomography (CT) of the chest, abdomen, and pelvis should be performed preoperatively; brain imaging is often also performed. Preoperative renal function will influence the use of intravenous contrast and timing should allow appropriate washout prior to surgery. Collateralization of vessels in the presence of venous tumor thrombus can be seen on abdominal imaging, and may herald surgical difficulties and increased blood loss. Bland thrombus may be present below the level of the tumor thrombus, and can at times be extensive.

High-quality imaging defining the extent of VTT is essential for preoperative planning. The cephalad extension of the tumor affects surgical technique as well as the likelihood of needing vascular bypass. Because of the aggressive nature of RCC and potential for tumor thrombus to enlarge rapidly, imaging should be performed within 14 days [15–18], or at most, 30 days of surgery [19]. Magnetic resonance imaging (MRI) has traditionally been recommended, but modern CT imaging has excellent accuracy in describing tumor size and thrombus extent and is an acceptable alternative [20]. In some cases, tumor thrombus invades into the wall of the IVC, necessitating excision of the vessel wall or segmental IVC resection. The risk for vascular invasion is increased if one or more of the following findings are identified on imaging: (1) the IVC diameter is greater than 40 mm [21]; (2) the AP diameter is >18 mm at the level of the renal vein [22]; (3) contrast fails to pass around the tumor thrombus; and (4) MRI shows tumor signal both inside and outside the vessel wall [4]. Color-flow ultrasound is also used to assess attachment of tumor to the caval wall [23].

## Preoperative Evaluation

Preoperative laboratory testing should include a complete blood count, comprehensive metabolic panel including serum calcium, and liver function tests. Coagulation tests are required if liver involvement or hepatic venous congestion is suspected. A blood type and crossmatch should be performed in all patients because of the high risk of bleeding. Doppler ultrasound of the lower extremities should be obtained in patients with symptoms suggestive of DVT. A transthoracic echocardiogram (TTE) can be helpful to evaluate cardiac function and predict tolerance of volume loading prior to IVC clamping. Preoperative stress testing may be indicated in patients with <4 METs or uncertain exercise tolerance, especially if they have risk factors for ischemic heart disease, as per AHA/ACC guidelines [24].

Anticoagulation should be considered in patients with extensive thrombus (complete or near complete IVC occlusion), recent DVT or thromboembolic event, or in those with combined bland and tumor thrombus. Low molecular weight heparin (LMWH) is preferred to warfarin for anticoagulation in patients with malignancy as it is associated with increased overall survival and decreased thromboembolic events [25, 26]. LMWH should be held for at least 24 h prior to surgery.

Preoperative renal artery angioembolization of the affected kidney is performed at some centers. Advocates cite the potential for reduced surgical blood loss from collateral vessels, ability to ligate the renal vein prior to ligation of the artery, and the development of post-embolization perinephric edema that can facilitate dissection [16]. Contrary opinion counters that it is an unnecessary additional procedure with its own risks and complications, including potential delay in definitive surgery due to the high incidence of post-infarction syndrome (fever, pain, hypertension and hyponatremia) [4, 11].

The surgeon and healthcare system are important to patient outcomes, as higher surgical volume is a predictor of decreased short-term mortality [27]. Patients with tumors extending beyond the infrahepatic IVC should have their surgical intervention performed in an experienced center with advanced capabilities including surgical specialists (cardiac, vascular, oncologic or liver transplant), anesthesiologists skilled in intraoperative transesophageal echocardiography (TEE), availability of venovenous bypass if desired, and resources for initiating cardiopulmonary bypass (CPB) including a perfusionist and cardiac surgeon. Cases that are not planned with CPB may require emergent conversion in the event of catastrophic embolism or unanticipated intra-cardiac extension of the thrombus.

## Anatomy, Surgical Technique, and Anesthetic Considerations

RCC tumors with VTT are typically classified according to the level of cephalad extent of the thrombus. Currently, there is no uniform approach to classification, and at least seven different systems have been proposed [28]. In this chapter, the classification system used is one proposed by Blute et al. [6] (Table 66.1 and Fig. 66.1a). Similar to other classifications defining RCC tumors with caval invasion, the hepatic veins represent an important landmark; thrombus extending above the ostia of the hepatic veins typically requires extensive liver mobilization and clamping of the hepatoduodenal ligament (Pringle maneuver) to avoid liver congestion when the IVC is clamped above the tumor thrombus (Fig. 66.1b).

## Surgical Anatomy

Basic knowledge of renal and IVC anatomy is helpful in understanding the surgical steps during vascular clamping. The kidneys are positioned obliquely in the retroperitoneal space. Due to inferior displacement by the liver during development, the right kidney is approximately 1–2 cm lower than the left. The left kidney sits close to the pancreas, spleen and the splenic flexure of the colon. The superior pole of the right kidney lies in close proximity to the liver; caudally, the right kidney is adjacent to the hepatic flexure of the colon. Each kidney is contained within a capsule, surrounded by perinephric fat, and further enclosed by Gerota's fascia, which includes the ipsilateral adrenal gland.

A single artery arising from the abdominal aorta provides renal blood flow. The right renal artery is longer than the left and typically passes behind the vena cava. The right renal vein is 2–4 cm in length and provides venous return from the solitary organ. Comparatively, the left renal vein is 2–3 times longer and additionally collects venous drainage from the left adrenal and gonadal vein, and in some individuals, also from the phrenic and lumbar veins. Variations in renal vascular anatomy are common however and may not follow this typical pattern. Approximately 20% of patients have an additional renal artery and almost 40% have variation in renal vein anatomy [16]. The renal veins drain into the IVC at the L1–L2 level behind the duodenum and the pancreas. The infrahepatic IVC extends a short distance before reaching the lower edge of the liver, where the retrohepatic IVC passes behind the liver either lying in a shallow groove, or within a partial or complete tunnel. As the IVC approaches the diaphragm, it receives the three major hepatic veins (right, left, and middle). In most patients there is a short segment of IVC above the liver and below the caval hiatus of the

**Table 66.1** Classification of tumor thrombus

| Tumor thrombus level | Description |
|---|---|
| 0 | Thrombus is limited to renal vein, detected clinically, or during assessment by pathology after resection |
| I | Thrombus extends into the inferior vena cava, <2 cm above the renal vein |
| II | Tumor thrombus extends into the IVC, >2 cm above the renal vein, but below the hepatic veins |
| III | Thrombus extends to or above the hepatic veins, but below the diaphragm |
| IV | Thrombus extends above the diaphragm (includes intracardiac) |

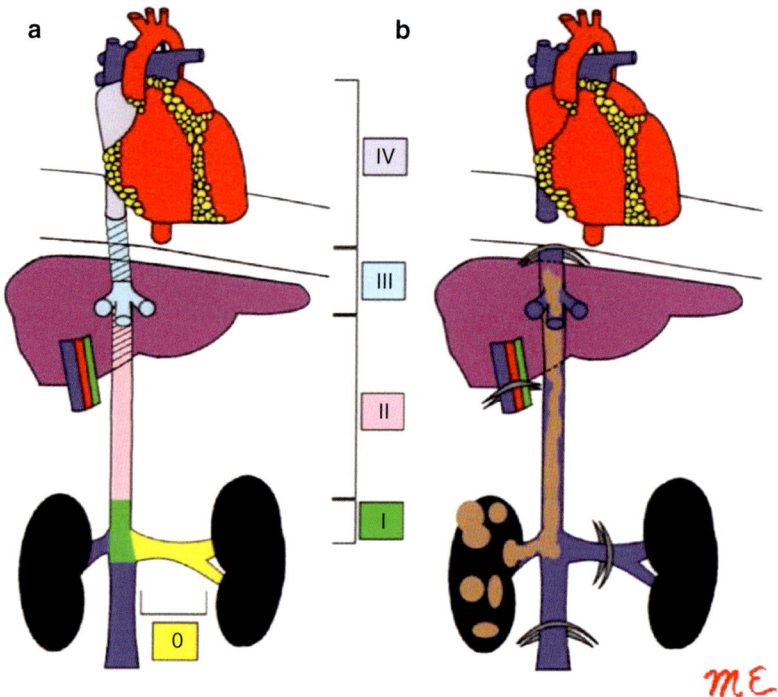

**Fig. 66.1** Classification of tumor thrombus (**a**) and surgical clamp positions (**b**)

diaphragm at the T8 level. The intrathoracic portion of the IVC is about 1 cm long and is mainly contained within the pericardium.

The portal anatomy is relevant to IVC thrombectomy cases because total hepatic vascular exclusion (IVC clamp plus Pringle maneuver) may be required. The porta hepatis contains the hepatic artery, common bile duct, and portal vein. The portal vein is formed from the confluence of the splenic vein, inferior mesenteric and superior mesenteric veins. It includes venous return from the gastrointestinal tract, pancreas, and spleen, while the IVC below the hepatic veins carries venous return from the lower extremities and pelvis via the iliac veins.

## Surgical Technique

Surgical technique varies and is contingent upon the extent of tumor thrombus (Table 66.2). Utilizing tumor thrombus classifications, Blute et al. [6] published an extensive review of 30 years of experience managing nephrectomy and IVC thrombectomy at the Mayo Clinic to delineate the surgical approach at each thrombus level.

Surgical principles include early clamping of the renal artery in the affected kidney, gaining proximal and distal control of the IVC, opening the cava to remove tumor thrombus, performing the nephrectomy, and closing the cavotomy. For higher levels of thrombus, gaining distal control of the IVC may require extensive mobilization of the liver and in some cases a partial clamping of the right atrium. When the cephalad IVC clamp is above the hepatic veins, a Pringle maneuver is typically used to avoid hepatic congestion and allow for cavotomy. Patients with metastatic disease may have resection of metastases during the same procedure. This may require a separate consulting surgical team (e.g. hepatic, thoracic, colorectal).

Some surgeons prefer a thoracoabdominal incision but many use a transabdominal approach via midline laparotomy, subcostal or chevron incision.

**Table 66.2** Summary of surgical approach and considerations by tumor level

| Tumor level | Thrombus extent | Surgical technique and considerations |
|---|---|---|
| 0 | Thrombus limited to renal vein | Radical nephrectomy with resection of renal vein. No IVC intervention |
| I | Thrombus extends into IVC ≤2 cm above the renal veins | Milk tumor out of IVC and into renal vein, clamp renal vein distal to thrombus, oversew caval defect |
| II | Extension into IVC >2 cm above renal veins but below hepatic veins | Dissection of infrahepatic vena cava, limited liver mobilization off IVC, lumbar vein ligation as needed. Superior IVC clamp is inferior to major hepatic veins, other clamps applied to contralateral renal vein and infrarenal IVC |
| III | Extension to or above hepatic veins, but below diaphragm | Intraoperative TEE or sterile ultrasound useful. Can be performed with or without vascular bypass. Liver must be more fully mobilized, exposing the retrohepatic IVC. Pringle maneuver used to meter hepatic inflow. May be possible to milk tumor lower allowing for clamping below hepatic veins. Trial cross-clamp is performed to assess hemodynamic changes |
| IV | Extension above diaphragm | May require cardiopulmonary bypass with or without hypothermic circulatory arrest, or veno-venous bypass if thrombus appears reducible below diaphragm on TEE. Some techniques avoid vascular bypass for mobile tumor thrombus, by gently pulling the right atrium down below the diaphragm before clamping [11] or using a thoracoabdominal approach to control the right atrium [39] |

For procedures requiring CPB the incision is extended to a median sternotomy [4]. Regardless of the type of incision or disease extension in the IVC, ligation of the renal artery in the affected kidney is performed early in the procedure (after mobilizing the kidney medially). Arterial ligation reduces blood loss and decompresses collateral circulation. It can also reduce tumor thrombus size because the renal artery provides significant blood supply to the tumor thrombus.

Patients with Level 0 disease do not require IVC intervention, only radical nephrectomy. Level I tumors generally cause partial IVC occlusion and are most often resected without IVC dissection. After thrombus is sequestered in the renal vein, a vascular clamp is applied. This technique avoids the need for IVC clamping and prevents cephalad embolization of thrombus. Level II tumors may require mobilization of the liver off the IVC in its inferior aspect and ligation of lumbar veins. Once the caudal and cephalad IVC clamps are applied and the contralateral renal vein is clamped, a cavotomy can be performed and the tumor extracted. Before the cavotomy is completely repaired, the IVC is de-aired and flushed clear of debris.

If tumor invades into the wall of the IVC, the vessel wall is resected. A caval patch is typically used when resection results in ≤50% decrease in IVC diameter, and a synthetic tube graft is used when segmental resection of the IVC is necessary. If the cava has been chronically occluded, segmental resection without reconstruction can be performed [4].

### Higher Level Tumor Thrombus and Collaboration with Other Specialties

Level III tumors frequently require extensive liver mobilization to allow full exposure of the infrahepatic, retrohepatic, and suprahepatic IVC. Consultation with vascular, hepatic, or oncologic surgeon with experience in these techniques may be needed. Level IV venous tumor thrombus (extension above the diaphragm) merits consultation with perfusion and cardiothoracic surgery in the event vascular bypass is required. Intracardiac tumor thrombus is often managed with hypothermic circulatory arrest, allowing for full inspection and removal of thrombus from the heart and IVC [29].

## Surgical and Post-operative Complications

Perioperative mortality rates of 2–4.5% [6, 11] are commonly reported, however as high as 10% mortality is quoted in some studies [13, 15, 30]. Early postoperative complications occur in 15–78% of patients [4] with more frequent occurrence in patients with higher thrombus level. Short-term complications include perioperative hemorrhage, PE and DVT. Acute kidney injury (AKI) occurs in greater than 50% of patients, and may require temporary renal replacement therapy or progress to chronic kidney disease and failure [31]. Male gender and caval cross clamp time greater than 20 min are risk factors for postoperative AKI. Blute et al.'s data show that tumor characteristics (stage, grade, fat invasion, involvement of lymph nodes, and distant metastases)—as opposed to extent of tumor thrombus—impact long-term outcomes [6, 32, 33]. Despite a normal creatinine, patients with renal cancer may have reduced renal function. This may account in part, for the increased incidence of renal insufficiency following nephrectomy for cancer compared to nephrectomy for kidney donation [34–36]. IVC and renal vein clamping are without doubt, a major contributing factor for renal injury following nephrectomy with vena cava thrombectomy.

## Anesthetic Considerations

Anesthetic management for radical nephrectomy with vena cava thrombectomy can be challenging due to decreased venous return during IVC clamping, potential for hemodynamic instability and massive hemorrhage. Additionally, in up to 2% of cases, patients experience intraoperative tumor embolization. Coordination and communication between the anesthesiologist and surgeon is paramount to ensure successful patient management. The anesthesiologist should understand the cephalad extent of the tumor thrombus and the likely surgical plan, including plans to clamp the IVC and porta hepatis. The surgeon should inform the anesthesiologist of anticipated clamping and unclamping to ensure that the team is prepared for possible hemodynamic compromise. Table 66.3 provides essentials of providing anesthesia for Nephrectomy with Inferior vena cava thrombectomy.

*Assessment of thrombus with TEE.* Intraoperative TEE can be used as both a monitor and diagnostic medium, particularly in those

**Table 66.3** Key points for nephrectomy with inferior vena cava thrombectomy

| |
|---|
| Surgical resection is the treatment of choice for RCC with venous tumor thrombus, improving outcomes even in the presence of metastatic disease |
| RCC tumors with intravascular extension of tumor thrombus are classified according to the level of cephalad extent of the thrombus. Higher levels of tumor thrombus present greater surgical challenges and risks |
| Surgery for higher level tumor thrombus should be performed at an experienced center with immediate TEE, venovenous bypass, and cardiopulmonary bypass readily available |
| A multidisciplinary team approach is warranted in these cases |
| Complete imaging evaluation is essential for surgical and anesthetic planning, and should be performed close to the time of surgery |
| The anesthetic approach for these cases includes GETA with arterial and large bore central venous lines, cross-matched packed red blood cells, and anticipation of IVC cross-clamping |
| Extension of thrombus above the ostia of the hepatic veins usually necessitates liver mobilization and Pringle maneuver, which can decrease preload and cardiac output by 40–60% when combined with inferior IVC clamping |
| Volume loading prior to IVC clamping helps patients tolerate the decrease in venous return and preload |
| Intraoperative tumor embolization occurs in 2% of cases and carries a 75% mortality risk |
| Tumors extending above the diaphragm may require venovenous or cardiopulmonary bypass |
| A cardiac surgeon, perfusion team, CPB circuit, and cardiothoracic anesthesiologist must be available for level IV tumor resections |
| Perioperative mortality for the surgical procedure ranges from 2 to 10% |

with thrombus extending above the level of the hepatic veins. An alternative or complementary monitoring technique is surgeon-performed sterile intra-abdominal ultrasound, which can be used to assess tumor extent from the field. TEE is useful in case of suspected intraoperative tumor embolization and unexplained hypotension.

*Hemorrhage.* Large collateral blood vessels, vascular abnormalities, and vascular injury may result in massive hemorrhage and the anesthesiologist must be adequately prepared. Invasive blood pressure monitoring and large bore venous access is mandatory. Blood products should be immediately available, checked, and ready to transfuse. Availability of a massive transfusion protocol and use of rapid transfusion devices can be helpful to resuscitate during hemorrhage.

*Vascular clamping.* While patients with occluded or nearly occluded IVC may have developed extensive collateral venous return and tolerate IVC clamping fairly well, other patients manifest a significant decrease in venous return and resultant drop in cardiac output. These effects can be offset by preemptive fluid loading and use of vasoactive medication to support systemic blood pressure. In cases where the cephalad clamp is placed above the hepatic veins, the combination the Pringle maneuver and clamping of the infrarenal IVC results in a decrease of 40–60% in the venous return and cardiac output [37].

*Venovenous bypass.* Select centers use venovenous bypass for higher-level tumor thrombus to enable venous return in patients who are unable to tolerate decreased preload during clamping. To initiate venovenous bypass, the inferior IVC is cannulated below the level of the renal veins with a 16 to 20-Fr intravascular cannula. Blood is routed through the bypass circuit and a centrifugal pump returns flow to a central circulation vein via a large (8–16 Fr) venous cannula, most often placed in the right axillary or internal jugular vein. VVB has also been used in patients with mobile supra-diaphragmatic and intra-atrial tumors as an alternative to cardiopulmonary bypass. Particular to these cases, VVB is associated with fewer complications than CPB and does not require systemic heparinization [6].

*Cardiopulmonary bypass.* Intracardiac tumors often require CPB with or without circulatory arrest. These cases are handled by a cardiothoracic anesthesiology team and cardiac surgeon in collaboration with the urologist and require systemic anticoagulation. Circulatory arrest is required for pulmonary thromboendarterectomy or when a bloodless field is required by the surgeon to ensure full tumor thrombus removal. These cases may also be performed without circulatory arrest and instead, are done on CPB with moderate to deep hypothermia. Intracardiac tumors that are mobile and reducible below the diaphragm may be successfully managed using venovenous bypass or a high clamp without vascular bypass.

*Intraoperative embolization.* Intraoperative embolization of tumor thrombus occurs in up to 2% of cases and is associated with a 75% mortality rate [4]. Risk increases with tumor thrombus level. New hypoxemia may be the presenting sign in the case of smaller thrombi versus acute cardiovascular collapse in the case of a large embolism. Rapid employment of TEE aids in diagnosis. Massive embolism may require emergent sternotomy, systemic heparinization and cardiopulmonary bypass for extraction of the tumor thrombus from the heart and/or pulmonary artery.

## Intraoperative Management

Nephrectomy with IVC thrombectomy is a relatively uncommon complex surgical procedure. The surgical and anesthetic approaches vary according to local practice, expertise and experience. The technique described here represents one approach to these cases.

*Intraoperative monitors and access.* Operations are performed under general endotracheal anesthesia (GETA) with standard induction agents. Neuromuscular blockade is maintained throughout the operation. In addition to standard ASA monitors, an intra-arterial line and central venous access are recommended in all patients. Pulse pressure variability (PPV) and systolic pressure variability (SPV) should be used to assist with fluid management, particularly if TEE is not utilized. In cases where TEE is employed, it provides information about volume and cardiac status, can evaluate tumor thrombus that extends above the level of the hepatic veins, and allows immediate evaluation in cases of suspected intraoperative tumor embolization. Routine use of a pulmonary artery catheter is not required, but should be considered in patients with pulmonary hypertension. In addition to the CVC, peripheral venous access consists of one to two large bore peripheral IVs (16 gauge or larger). The CVC should be 8 French or larger, and provides a rapid infusion port for fluid administration as well as a route for en vasoactive infusions. A rapid transfusion device (Belmont, Level I or other device) should be placed in the operating room for Level III-IV cases. Four to six units of packed red blood cells (PRBCs) are cross-matched and present in the operating room prior to incision in higher-level tumor classification.

*Analgesia*. Approaches to postoperative pain using regional or neuraxial techniques depend on the incision used. Thoraco-abdominal incisions require T7 to T12 dermatomal coverage, whereas flank incisions may only require T9–T11 coverage. An ultrasound-guided four-quadrant transversus abdominis plane (TAP)/rectus sheath block or thoracic epidural can be placed preoperatively. Intravenous ketamine can also be used as an adjunct to decrease postoperative pain and opioid requirements. Opioids are also administered to mitigate post-operative pain.

*Dissection phase*. During mobilization of the liver and IVC dissection, a fluid restriction approach is used unless significant bleeding occurs. This strategy facilitates IVC dissection and liver mobilization and limits bleeding and hepatic congestion. To maintain perfusion to the non-affected kidney, baseline MAP is maintained ±20% or >70 mmHg (whichever is higher) using an infusion of phenylephrine or norepinephrine as needed.

*IVC clamping*. Prior to IVC clamping (and possible Pringle maneuver), balanced crystalloid solution (Plasmalyte/Normosol or Lactated Ringers), colloid (5% albumin), and blood (if indicated) are used to increase preload and mitigate physiologic effects of decreased venous return. Fluid status and administration is assessed by PPV (goal <8%), urine output (goal >0.5 mL/kg), surgeon assessment of IVC tension (subjective direct evaluation) or TEE (gold standard).

*Fluid resuscitation*. Ongoing blood loss is replaced with 5% albumin and packed red blood cells (PRBCs) when the hemoglobin approaches our transfusion threshold (8–9 g/dL in most patients). Fresh frozen plasma (FFP) is transfused after resuscitation reaches ≥4 units of PRBCs. A 1:1 PRBC:FFP ratio is followed for the remainder of the resuscitation. A transfusion of platelets is given after 6 units of PRBCs (goal ratio 1:6) and cryoprecipitate if fibrinogen levels are <100 mg/dL. The hospital's massive transfusion protocol (MTP) is activated in cases of ongoing severe hemorrhage. Frequent assessment of acid-base status and hemoglobin levels is achieved with arterial blood gas testing and periodic coagulation studies (PT/PTT and fibrinogen) plus CBC. If available, thromboelastography (TEG or ROTEM) can play a valuable role in determining component therapy during resuscitation. Blood salvage is not utilized for these procedures, except in rare cases of patients who refuse blood transfusion, due to theoretical concern for cancer spread. This possibility, however, remains controversial [38].

*Post-operative Care*. Many patients are extubated in the operating room and recover in the post-anesthesia recovery unit (PACU) and then the surgical ward. Patients requiring significant resuscitation, or those with continued need for pressor or inotrope therapy, may remain intubated and be cared for in the intensive care unit. Significant fluid shifts into the interstitial space can continue during the first day after surgery and patients require close attention to maintain adequate intravascular volume and perfusion of the remaining solitary kidney. As mentioned, early postoperative complications include intra- or perioperative death (0–7.1%), hemorrhage (0.9–25%), DVT (0–3%), PE (0–4.6%), myocardial infarction (0–7.1%), wound infection (0–2.6%), acute renal failure (0–3.6%), and need for dialysis (0–3.6%), although the incidence of each of these early complications is very low with low-grade tumor thrombus level [6]. It is important to note that longitudinal follow-up of these patients is critical given their high incidence of postoperative renal insufficiency that peaks months to years after resection, as mentioned previously in the *Surgical and Post-Operative Complications* section. Regardless of tumor thrombus level, median length of hospitalization ranges from 7 to 9 days (range 1–31 days); there can be wide inter-patient variability in recovery from this surgical population.

## References

1. Gupta K, Miller JD, Li JZ, Russell MW, Charbonneau C. Epidemiologic and socioeconomic burden of metastatic renal cell carcinoma (mRCC): a literature review. Cancer Treat Rev. 2008;34:193–205.
2. Jonasch E, Gao J, Rathmell WK. Renal cell carcinoma. BMJ. 2014;349:g4797.
3. Hsieh JJ, Purdue MP, Signoretti S, Swanton C, Albiges L, Schmidinger M, et al. Renal cell carcinoma. Nat Rev Dis Primers. 2017;3:17009.
4. Psutka SP, Leibovich BC. Management of inferior vena cava tumor thrombus in locally advanced renal cell carcinoma. Ther Adv Urol. 2015;7:216–29.
5. Lardas M, Stewart F, Scrimgeour D, Hofmann F, Marconi L, Dabestani S, et al. Systematic review of surgical management of nonmetastatic renal cell carcinoma with vena caval thrombus. Eur Urol. 2016;70:265–80.
6. Blute ML, Leibovich BC, Lohse CM, Cheville JC, Zincke H. The Mayo Clinic experience with surgical management, complications and outcome for patients with renal cell carcinoma and venous tumour thrombus. BJU Int. 2004;94:33–41.
7. Chapman E, Pichel AC, et al. BJA Educ. 2015;16:98–101.
8. Kirkali Z, Van Poppel H. A critical analysis of surgery for kidney cancer with vena cava invasion. Eur Urol. 2007;52:658–62.
9. Haferkamp A, Bastian PJ, Jakobi H, Pritsch M, Pfitzenmaier J, Albers P, et al. Renal cell carcinoma with tumor thrombus extension into the vena cava: prospective long-term followup. J Urol. 2007;177:1703–8.
10. Reese AC, Whitson JM, Meng MV. Natural history of untreated renal cell carcinoma with venous tumor thrombus. Urol Oncol. 2013;31:1305–9.
11. Ciancio G, Livingstone AS, Soloway M. Surgical management of renal cell carcinoma with tumor thrombus in the renal and inferior vena cava: the University of Miami experience in using liver transplantation techniques. Eur Urol. 2007;51:988–94; discussion 994–5.
12. Tilki D, Hu B, Nguyen HG, Dall'Era MA, Bertini R, Carballido JA, et al. Impact of synchronous metastasis distribution on cancer specific survival in renal cell carcinoma after radical nephrectomy with tumor thrombectomy. J Urol. 2015;193:436–42.
13. Abel EJ, Thompson RH, Margulis V, Heckman JE, Merril MM, Darwish OM, et al. Perioperative outcomes following surgical resection of renal cell carcinoma with inferior vena cava thrombus extending above the hepatic veins: a contemporary multicenter experience. Eur Urol. 2014;66:584–92.
14. Parekh DJ, Cookson MS, Chapman W, Harrell F Jr, Wells N, Chang SS, et al. Renal cell carcinoma with renal vein and inferior vena caval involvement: clinicopathological features, surgical techniques and outcomes. J Urol. 2005;173:1897–902.
15. Boorjian SA, Sengupta S, Blute ML. Renal cell carcinoma: vena caval involvement. BJU Int. 2007;99:1239–44.
16. Wotkowicz C, Wszolek MF, Libertino JA. Resection of renal tumors invading the vena cava. Urol Clin North Am. 2008;35:657–71; viii.
17. Boorjian SA, Blute ML. Surgery for vena caval tumor extension in renal cancer. Curr Opin Urol. 2009;19:473–7.
18. Woodruff DY, Van Veldhuizen P, Muehlebach G, Johnson P, Williamson T, Holzbeierlein JM. The perioperative management of an inferior vena caval tumor thrombus in patients with renal cell carcinoma. Urol Oncol. 2013;31:517–21.
19. Dominik J, Moravek P, Zacek P, Vojacek J, Brtko M, Podhola M, et al. Long-term survival after radical surgery for renal cell carcinoma with tumour thrombus extension into the right atrium. BJU Int. 2013;111:E59–64.
20. Guzzo TJ, Pierorazio PM, Schaeffer EM, Fishman EK, Allaf ME. The accuracy of multidetector computerized tomography for evaluating tumor thrombus in patients with renal cell carcinoma. J Urol. 2009;181:486–90; discussion 491.
21. Gohji K, Yamashita C, Ueno K, Shimogaki H, Kamidono S. Preoperative computerized tomography detection of extensive invasion of the inferior vena cava by renal cell carcinoma: possible indication for resection with partial cardiopulmonary bypass and patch grafting. J Urol. 1994;152:1993–6; discussion 1997.
22. Zini L, Destrieux-Garnier L, Leroy X, Villers A, Haulon S, Lemaitre L, et al. Renal vein ostium wall invasion of renal cell carcinoma with an inferior vena cava tumor thrombus: prediction by renal and vena caval vein diameters and prognostic significance. J Urol. 2008;179:450–4; discussion 454.
23. Gupta NP, Ansari MS, Khaitan A, Sivaramakrishna MS, Hemal AK, Dogra PN, et al. Impact of imaging and thrombus level in management of renal cell carcinoma extending to veins. Urol Int. 2004;72:129–34.
24. Fleisher LA, Fleischmann KE, Auerbach AD, Barnason SA, Beckman JA, et al. 2014 ACC/AHA guidelines on perioperative cardiovascular evaluation

and management of patients undergoing noncardiac surgery: executive summary. J Am Coll Cardiol. 2014;64:2373–405.
25. Lee AYY. Anticoagulation in the treatment of established venous thromboembolism in patients with cancer. J Clin Oncol. 2009;27:4895–901.
26. Lyman GH, Khorana AA, Falanga A, Clarke-Pearson D, Flowers C, Jahanzeb M, et al. American Society of Clinical Oncology guideline: recommendations for venous thromboembolism prophylaxis and treatment in patients with cancer. J Clin Oncol. 2007;25:5490–505.
27. Yap SA, Horovitz D, Alibhai SMH, Abouassaly R, Timilshina N, Finelli A. Predictors of early mortality after radical nephrectomy with renal vein or inferior vena cava thrombectomy—a population-based study. BJU Int. 2012;110:1283–8.
28. Mandhani A, Patidar N, Aga P, Pande S, Tewari P. A new classification of inferior vena cava thrombus in renal cell carcinoma could define the need for cardiopulmonary or venovenous bypass. Indian J Urol. 2015;31:327–32.
29. Gaudino M, Lau C, Cammertoni F, Vargiu V, Gambardella I, Massetti M, et al. Surgical treatment of renal cell carcinoma with cavoatrial involvement: a systematic review of the literature. Ann Thorac Surg. 2016;101:1213–21.
30. Toren P, Abouassaly R, Timilshina N, Kulkarni G, Alibhai S, Finelli A. Results of a national population-based study of outcomes of surgery for renal tumors associated with inferior vena cava thrombus. Urology. 2013;82:572–7.
31. Shin S, Han Y, Park H, Chung YS, Ahn H, Kim C-S, et al. Risk factors for acute kidney injury after radical nephrectomy and inferior vena cava thrombectomy for renal cell carcinoma. J Vasc Surg. 2013;58:1021–7.
32. Gettman MT, Boelter CW, Cheville JC, Zincke H, Bryant SC, Blute ML. Charlson co-morbidity index as a predictor of outcome after surgery for renal cell carcinoma with renal vein, vena cava or right atrium extension. J Urol. 2003;169:1282–6.
33. Frank I, Blute ML, Cheville JC, Lohse CM, Weaver AL, Zincke H. An outcome prediction model for patients with clear cell renal cell carcinoma treated with radical nephrectomy based on tumor stage, size, grade, and necrosis: the SSIGN score. J Urol. 2002;168:2395–400.
34. Huang WC, Levey AS, Serio AM, Snyder M, Vickers AJ, Raj GV, et al. Chronic kidney disease after nephrectomy in patients with renal cortical tumours: a retrospective cohort study. Lancet Oncol. 2006;7(9):735–40.
35. Najarian JS, Chavers BM, McHugh LE, Matas AJ. 20 years or more of follow-up of living kidney donors. Lancet. 1992;340:807–10.
36. Fehrman-Ekholm I, Duner F, Brink B, et al. No evidence of accelerated loss of kidney function in living kidney donors: results from a cross-sectional follow-up. Transplantation. 2001;72:444–9.
37. Eyraud D, Richard O, Borie DC, Schaup B, Carayon A, Vézinet C, et al. Hemodynamic and hormonal responses to the sudden interruption of caval flow: insights from a prospective study of hepatic vascular exclusion during major liver resections. Anesth Analg. 2002;95:1173–8, table of contents.
38. Davis M, Sofer M, Gomez-Marin O, Bruck D, Soloway MS. The use of cell salvage during radical retropubic prostatectomy: does it influence cancer recurrence? BJU Int. 2003;91:474–6.
39. Patil MB, Montez J, Loh-Doyle J, Cai J, Skinner EC, Schuckman A, et al. Level III-IV inferior vena caval thrombectomy without cardiopulmonary bypass: long-term experience with intrapericardial control. J Urol. 2014;192:682–8.

# Anesthesia for Carotid Endarterectomy

## Abigail Monnig and Gaurav Budhrani

## Introduction

Stroke is now the fifth leading cause of death in the United States, which is a significant decline in the past decade [1]. These trends have been attributed to the increased use of statin and antihypertensive medications. However, carotid artery disease secondary to atherosclerosis still remains a major preventable cause of stroke in the United States. Medical versus surgical management of patients with carotid artery stenosis is based on the following: history of an ischemic event, degree of stenosis, and estimated perioperative risk. A Cochrane database analysis of the North American Symptomatic Endarterectomy Trial, the European Carotid Surgery Trial, and Veterans Administration Cooperative Trial showed benefit to surgical management in patients with severe stenosis (70–99%) without near-occlusion. There was marginal benefit in patients with 50–69% stenosis and no benefit in patients with near occlusion [2]. Rates of carotid endarterectomy (CEA) have actually decreased in recent years as the use of carotid stenting (CAS) has dramatically increased. The Carotid Revascularization Endarterectomy versus Stenting Trial (CREST) showed no overall difference in stroke, myocardial infarction (MI), or death in CEA compared to stenting [3]. However, further statistical analysis of the CREST trial has revealed that patients undergoing CAS or CEA with regional anesthesia had lower risk of periprocedural MI than those undergoing CEA with general anesthesia. The authors advocate that since periprocedural MI is one of the few variables favoring CAS over CEA, regional anesthesia should seriously be considered for patients undergoing CEA [4].

This chapter describes perioperative and intraoperative anesthetic management of patients undergoing CEA. Regional techniques, general anesthetic techniques, and neuromonitoring are described. Refer to Table 67.1 for a summary of anesthetic management for patients undergoing CEA.

A. Monnig, M.D.
Department of Anesthesiology, Emory University School of Medicine, Atlanta, GA, USA
e-mail: abigail.marie.monnig@emory.edu

G. Budhrani, M.D. (✉)
Division of Critical Care Medicine, Department of Anesthesiology, Emory University School of Medicine, Atlanta, GA, USA
e-mail: gaurav.budhrani@emory.edu

## Anatomy, Physiology and Imaging Modalities of Carotid Stenosis

### Anatomy and Physiology of the Carotid Arteries

The common carotid arteries are located bilaterally in the neck and supply blood to the brain, neck and face. The right common carotid originates from the brachiocephalic trunk and the left common carotid is a direct branch from the aortic

**Table 67.1** Summary of anesthetic plan for carotid endarterectomy

| Plan/preparation/adverse events | Reasoning/management |
|---|---|
| Preoperative evaluation<br>  Timing of procedure<br>  Hypertension management<br>  Coronary atherosclerosis/revascularization | Intraoperative HTN management is required; pre-operative management and optimization improves BP control on the day of surgery<br>Consider urgency of CEA before work up for coronary atherosclerosis |
| Position: Supine, arms tucked, shoulder roll | Access to airway may be challenging due to positioning and draping |
| Monitors: Standard ASA with continuous arterial blood pressure monitoring | Hemodynamic instability is common and requires frequent titration of vasoactive substances |
| Regional Anesthesia<br>  Superficial cervical plexus block<br>  Deep cervical plexus block<br>  Intraoperative local infiltration<br>  Dexmedetomidine infusion | Most commonly superficial plexus block with additional local infiltration as needed. Minimize sedation to provide appropriate anxiolysis but avoid heavy sedation to allow for optimal neurologic assessments |
| General Anesthesia<br>  Blunt airway response on induction<br>  TIVA versus volatile versus combination<br>  Vasoactive drugs<br>  Rapid emergence and early evaluation | Prepare for hemodynamic lability and prevent when able. Various types of vasoactive drugs should be immediately available. Consider the neuromonitoring method to be used when choosing maintenance anesthetic. Rapid emergence is critical for accurate neurologic assessment |
| Neurologic monitoring<br>  Awake patient if using regional<br>  EEG is gold standard for general<br>  Consider stump pressure<br>  Consider TCD in post op period | Frequent neurologic checks in the awake patient during carotid cross clamping. Use of EEG has significant limitations but is considered gold standard. Addition of stump pressure to TCD or EEG increases the sensitivity for neurologic deficits. Early studies suggest use of TCD in post op period for embolic events |
| Postoperative considerations<br>  Continued hemodynamic monitoring<br>  Strict treatment of hypertension<br>  Continued neurologic checks | Avoidance of hypertension and prevention of cerebral hyperperfusion syndrome. Neurologic checks to determine hyperperfusion and early stroke detection |

arch. Each common carotid artery is located medially within the carotid sheath along with the internal jugular vein (most lateral) and vagus nerve. The common carotid arteries branch into two divisions at the level of the fourth cervical vertebra. The internal carotid artery (ICA) supplies blood to the brain and the external carotid supplies blood to the face and neck. Eighty to 90% of the cerebral blood supply comes from the ICAs, while the vertebral arteries account for the remainder. The terminal branches of the ICA include the anterior and middle cerebral arteries, which contribute to the circle of Willis. Collateral circulation exists between the two common carotid arteries via the circle of Willis, and in the neck via the thyroid arteries [5, 6].

The carotid sinus, or bulb, is a dilated area at the base of the ICA. Here, baroreceptors participate in pressure regulation via the carotid reflex. The baroreceptors are innervated by a branch of the glossopharyngeal nerve, which synapses centrally with the vagus nerve and leads to modulation in heart rate and myocardial contractility.

The carotid body is a small mass of chemoreceptors located in the bifurcation of the common carotid artery. The chemoreceptors respond primarily to decreases in the partial pressure of oxygen, resulting in an increase in ventilation via the glossopharyngeal and vagus nerves [7].

## Atherosclerosis of the Carotid Arteries

The most common location for carotid artery atherosclerosis is at the bifurcation of the common carotid artery in the region of the carotid sinus. Plaque formation is enhanced secondary to low shear stress along the carotid sinus, as well as from stasis and non-laminar flow at the bifurcation point. Symptoms of stroke and transient ischemic attacks (TIA) are the result of unstable plaques that embolize distally. Alternatively, ischemic stroke can result if adequate collateral pathways do not develop, or if multiple cerebral arteries develop significant stenoses [8–10].

## Imaging of Atherosclerotic Carotid Artery Stenosis

Doppler-ultrasound is the initial imaging modality of choice in symptomatic patients. In addition to determining degree of stenosis, duplex imaging can aid in the characterization of the plaque. Three criteria exist to determine the degree of stenosis: maximum doppler flow velocities, carotid ratio, and area ratio [11]. Peak systolic velocity is the most common criterion for ultrasound determination of disease severity [12]. Limitation of ultrasound exists with near-occlusive plaques, and since full occlusion of the ICA is a contraindication to CEA, further imaging with cerebral angiography may be indicated. Cerebral angiography has the additional benefit of evaluating collateral blood flow and concurrent atherosclerosis. Other imaging modalities include high-resolution MRI and transcranial doppler ultrasound.

## Preoperative Evaluation

Two important distinctions from other vascular surgical candidates need to be considered: (1) the urgency of CEA in symptomatic patients and (2) factors that increase the risk of carotid artery stenosis and stroke.

The benefit of CEA in symptomatic patients with 50–99% carotid stenosis is greatest when performed within 2 weeks of presenting with a TIA or stroke. Ninety-day stroke risk in these patients may be as high as 30%. Additionally, data suggest that the benefit of surgery may actually be lost if surgery is delayed greater than 3 months [13–15].

Factors that increase the risk of carotid artery atherosclerosis include hypertension, tobacco smoking, hyperlipidemia, diabetes mellitus, obesity, metabolic syndrome, and physical inactivity.

Preoperative evaluation in patients presenting for carotid endarterectomy should be tailored to these commonly associated conditions. Although aggressive treatment of hypertension and hyperlipidemia can reduce stroke risk, blood pressure goals should be adjusted in patients with severe carotid artery stenosis or those who are symptomatic. Ideally, patients with hypertension should be stabilized on their antihypertensive agents prior to presenting for CEA. Due to the distinct risk of hemodynamic lability postoperatively, these patients should continue their antihypertensives on the day of surgery, particularly beta-blockers [10, 16–18].

Patients presenting for carotid endarterectomy often have systemic atherosclerosis, including coronary artery disease (CAD). The urgency of CEA should be considered before further testing is ordered. According to the ACC/AHA 2014 guidelines, a validated risk-prediction tool can be useful in predicting the risk of perioperative major adverse cardiac events (MACE). CEA is considered an intermediate risk procedure. The ACC/AHA guidelines propose a stepwise approach to perioperative cardiac assessment for CAD, which includes the estimated perioperative risk of MACE. Patients with greater than 1% risk of MACE and poor or unknown functional capacity should be considered for further testing if coronary revascularization would be an option for the patient. Patients with elevated risk of MACE, who would not be candidates for coronary revascularization, should be recommended for medical therapy rather than surgical management of carotid artery stenosis. Minimally, a 12-lead electrocardiogram can be considered in all patients undergoing CEA [16–18].

## Anesthetic Considerations: Neuromonitoring

### Monitoring for Cerebral Ischemia

Although clinical evidence of stroke after carotid revascularization is uncommon, it is associated with significant morbidity and a nearly threefold increase in future mortality. Stroke following

CEA has been attributed to thromboembolic events from disruption of the plaque and to cerebral hypoperfusion secondary to cross clamping of the carotid artery [19]. During carotid endarterectomy, the carotid artery is temporarily clamped. Collateral flow from the contralateral carotid artery and vertebral arteries via the Circle of Willis maintains cerebral perfusion. Alternatively, the ipsilateral carotid artery can provide blood flow to the brain via a shunt placed by the surgeon. The use of a shunt is controversial, and risks include atheromatous or air emboli, arterial dissection and acute arterial occlusion. Several studies indicate that a shunt increases the surgical difficulty, while other studies suggest that this is true only for surgeons who use shunting selectively rather than routinely. Additionally, it has been shown that approximately 85% of patients tolerate cross-clamping without shunting. Reliable monitoring for cerebral ischemia allows for more conservative, rather than routine use. However, no specific method of monitoring in selective shunting has been proven to produce better outcomes [20–23].

## Awake Patient

Neurologic assessment of the awake patient is considered the gold standard for identification of patients who would benefit from shunt placement. This is done by mental status examination and monitoring for weakness of the contralateral upper and lower extremities. Therefore, the patient's head and contralateral upper extremity should be accessible to the anesthesiologist. Neurologic assessment should occur just prior to a clamp trial and 2 min after cross-clamping the internal carotid artery, with periodic assessments, while the clamp remains in place. Neurologic changes during CEA in the awake patient predict a high risk of postoperative stroke and may indicate the need for a shunt [22, 24–28].

## Electroencephalography

In patients undergoing general anesthesia, several cerebral monitoring methods have been proposed, with electroencephalography (EEG) considered the gold standard approach. Studies indicate that EEG monitoring alone can result in an increased number of false positive and negative detections of acute neurologic changes when compared to the examination of the awake patient [29]. However, EEG use has also been shown to decrease unnecessary shunt use without increasing perioperative stroke rate [30]. EEG, when combined with stump pressure measurements, increases the sensitivity of detecting acute neurologic deficits and the need for shunt placement increases [31]. Stump pressure is measured in the internal carotid artery distal to the clamp and is theorized to represent the pressure within the Circle of Willis [32]. A pressure less than 50 mmHg and abnormal EEG changes have been suggested to represent cerebral ischemia and need for carotid shunt [33].

The electroencephalogram records spontaneous electrical activity of cortical surface cells but fails to capture activity within deeper brain structures [31]. Normal cerebral blood flow is 50 mL/min/100 g brain tissue. Ischemia is apparent on EEG (decreased amplitude or slowed frequency) at cerebral blood flows of less than 20 mL/min. However, the changes in EEG pattern may be delayed [22, 34, 35] and ischemia may not be immediately detected. Studies advocate for shunt insertion when EEG changes are classified as moderate or severe (increase of theta waves >25%, increase in delta waves, or severe flattening of amplitude or isoelectric curve) [36].

Several limitations for the successful implementation of EEG exist: (1) Only superficial cortical structures are monitored by EEG. (2) Detection of regional ischemic events decreases when fewer EEG channels are monitored. (3) A 16-lead EEG requires a skilled technician and continuous observation. (4) Hypocarbia, hypothermia, and deep anesthesia can all mimic changes seen in EEG during ischemia.

## Somatosensory Evoked Potentials (SSEP)

A recent meta-analysis of the diagnostic value of SSEPs during CEA revealed that changes had a strong specificity (91%) but weaker sensitivity (58%) for prediction of perioperative stroke in patients undergoing CEA for symptomatic carotid stenosis [37]. Additionally, neurologic outcome is not improved based on selective shunting guided by changes in SSEPs [38]. Further studies are needed to promote use of SSEPs as the sole neuromonitoring modality for patients undergoing CEA. Similarly to EEG, SSEP requires an expert technician and is affected by anesthetic agents.

## Transcranial Doppler

Transcranial doppler (TCD) is used primarily to detect embolic events. Doppler pulses are used to measure mean blood flow velocity in the middle cerebral artery (MCA) by insonating the MCA through the temporal bone. A doppler microembolic signal has specific characteristics well described by a consensus committee [39]. Several studies have shown that the principal cause of strokes from CEA are thromboembolic in nature, rather than secondary to hyper or hypoperfusion [40–42]. It is suggested that surgeons can use TCD information to alter their surgical technique. One study in particular showed a decrease in rate of stroke with permanent deficit over time with use of TCD monitoring [43]. Incidence of permanent deficit was 7% in the first 100 operations and only 2% in the last 400 operations.

Evidence indicates that most strokes that occur in the perioperative setting following CEA occur after a symptom-free interval. Therefore, some providers advocate for continued use of TCD in the immediate postoperative period to detect further embolic events [41].

## Near-Infrared Spectroscopy

Near-infrared spectroscopy (NIRS) is a noninvasive technique that continuously monitors cerebral oxygen saturation. This technique is simple to use and interpret. However, there is no statistically proven correlation of regional cerebral oxygenation saturation to neurologic dysfunction. Additionally, due to the low sensitivity and specificity, there is no predictable threshold value at which shunt is indicated [44, 45].

## Summary of Monitoring Devices

No specific monitoring method has been shown to improve outcomes of carotid endarterectomy. This may be in part due to the fact that postoperative emboli are the most common cause of perioperative stroke. A recent meta-analysis published in the Canadian Journal of Anesthesia compared various cerebral monitors to regional anesthesia. In this study, the diagnostic odds ratio for cerebral ischemia was highest when a *combination* of stump pressure and either TCD or EEG was used [31]. Again, there is growing body of evidence that TCD monitoring may be useful in the postoperative period as well [41].

## Anesthetic Considerations: General Versus Regional Anesthesia

Anesthetic type is guided by multiple factors including patient characteristics and preference as well and surgeon and anesthesiologist inclination. Ideally, the anesthesiologist should be well versed in both regional and general anesthetic techniques for carotid endarterectomy. Current evidence in the literature to support general versus regional is equivocal.

A Cochrane study published in 2013, pooled data from 14 randomized controlled trials comparing local versus general anesthesia for carotid endarterectomy. The pooled analyses found no statistical difference in the rate of stroke or death at 30 days [46]. The National Surgical Quality Improvement Program (NSQIP) published data in 2012 on outcomes of CEA under general and regional anesthesia. The study found that general anesthesia was an independent risk factor for postoperative myocardial infarction (MI) with an adjusted odds ratio of 2.18 (95% CI, 1.17–4.04). Additionally, the rate of MI was higher in patients with preoperative neurologic symptoms [47]. Data from CREST published in 2016 confirmed a two times higher risk of MI in patients undergoing general anesthesia versus regional, though this was not statistically significant [4].

The major advantage of regional anesthesia is the ability to perform neurologic assessments on the awake patient rather than using monitoring devices such as EEG. The real-time feedback provided by an awake exam, as well as its increased sensitivity and specificity for cerebral ischemia, facilitates selective and accurate need for shunt placement. Additionally, regional anesthesia may be indicated in patients with particular systemic diseases in which general anesthesia is best avoided, such as severe chronic obstructive lung disease.

The disadvantages of regional anesthesia include patient discomfort and risk of urgent conversion to general anesthesia. General anesthesia may be required for patients who are unable to cooperate with neurologic assessments either due to neurocognitive dysfunction or elevated anxiety. In patients unable to tolerate being supine, general anesthesia may be required. Ultimately, the anesthetic approach is specifically tailored to each individual on a case-by-case basis.

## General Anesthesia Techniques

There is no one anesthetic technique favored in the literature. Some considerations include use of intravenous anesthetics with particular neurologic monitoring methods, neuroprotective techniques, and maintenance of hemodynamic stability.

Induction of anesthesia can be performed with a combination of agents such as etomidate or propofol, and fentanyl/lidocaine to blunt airway responsiveness. The anesthesiologist is guided by patient characteristics. A secured airway with endotracheal intubation is encouraged since the patient's airway may be difficult to reach during the operation due to positioning and draping [22, 32].

Maintenance of anesthesia can be accomplished with volatile anesthetics, total intravenous anesthetic or a combination. This decision is largely based on anesthesiologist preference and choice of neuromonitoring method. Nitrous oxide may increase cerebral metabolic rate but has been safely used in combination with volatiles. Sevoflurane is an agent that provides for rapid emergence and early neurologic evaluation of the patient, while also producing a concomitant reduction in cerebral metabolic blood flow and metabolic rate at concentrations of up to 1.0 MAC. At concentrations above 1.0 MAC, there is an uncoupling of this relationship, permitting a regional reduction in blood flow and no further decrease in metabolic rate. Desflurane likely produces a similar profile in the CEA patient but has not been well studied. Sevoflurane generates a dose-dependent increase in latency of SSEPs and a dose-dependent deceleration pattern on EEG. For this reason, some anesthesiologists choose total intravenous anesthetics or a combination of intravenous and volatile agents [22, 32, 48].

Emergence from anesthesia should be rapid for early neurocognitive assessment. Avoidance of long-acting medications is necessary.

## Hemodynamic Monitoring and Management

Carotid endarterectomy may be associated with extreme hemodynamic lability. Patients presenting for CEA often have chronic hypertension making them more prone to hemodynamic fluctuations. The intraoperative manipulation of carotid baroreceptors adds a surgical component contributing to blood pressure changes. Patients undergoing CEA require invasive intra-arterial blood pressure monitoring for rapid detection of hyper- or hypotension, and for attentive titration of vasoactive drugs. Typically, the arterial line should be placed prior to induction of anesthesia [32].

There are several well-known periods of hemodynamic instability during CEA. The first period is during induction of anesthesia (hypotension) and endotracheal intubation (hypertension). Drugs should be slowly titrated during induction, lidocaine and fentanyl should be utilized to blunt airway reflexes. Throughout the procedure, surgical manipulation of the carotid sinus leads to increased sympathetic stimulation and resultant tachycardia/hypertension, Conversely, it may also trigger a parasympathetic outflow surge with resultant bradycardia and hypotension. A prospective study of 20 patients undergoing CEA evaluated the effect of 1% lidocaine injection into the adventitial layer of the artery in the region of the carotid sinus. The study found that the baroreceptor response to intraluminal stretch stimulation was abolished by infiltration of local anesthetic [49].

Placement of the carotid cross-clamp may lead to ipsilateral cerebral ischemia. While the cross clamp is in place, blood pressure should be maintained approximately 20% above the patient's baseline mean arterial pressure to optimize collateral flow. It is common to see hypotension during carotid unclamping. Vasoactive substances should be immediately available for this surgery in order to treat acute hemodynamic derangements [9, 22, 32].

## Regional Anesthesia Techniques

Local or regional anesthesia is described below. This technique is often supplemented by intravenous sedation. However, sedation must be minimized to accurately perform serial neurologic assessments of the patient. A commonly used sedative medication is dexmedetomidine. Two randomized controlled studies determined the sedative effects of dexmedetomidine to be equal to conventional methods of sedation, but demonstrated a decreased in hemodynamic lability in the dexmedetomidine groups [50, 51].

## Local Infiltration

The surgeon can infiltrate local anesthesia throughout the procedure including a superficial field block followed by deeper tissue infiltration as the surgery progresses. This is slow and can be uncomfortable for the patient. Regional techniques are better suited for CEA, but local infiltration remains an option to supplement regional blocks as needed.

## Superficial Cervical Plexus Block

The goal of the superficial cervical plexus block is to deposit local anesthetic near the C2–4 nerve roots. The block is typically performed in the supine or semi-recumbent position with the patient's head turned to the side opposite of the surgical site. Using sterile technique, the needle tip is guided into the plane immediately deep to the sternocleidomastoid muscle, adjacent to the plexus. The block can be performed with or without ultrasound guidance. The plexus is visualized with ultrasound in the plane immediately deep or lateral to the posterior border of the sternocleidomastoid muscle. But if the plexus is not well visualized, infiltration along the posterior border of the sternocleidomastoid is appropriate. Approximately 10–15 mL of local anesthetic is deposited (bupivacaine 0.25% or 0.5% is often used), aspirating intermittently to prevent intravascular injection [28, 32, 52, 53].

Risks of superficial cervical plexus block include intravenous injection of local anesthetic, hematoma, and direct injury to the nerve or surrounding structures. Additional local infiltration by the surgeon may be required during the procedure; the anesthesiologist needs to calculate the total local anesthetic dose allowed and limit further infiltration when maximal doses have been achieved.

## Deep Cervical Plexus Block

Positioning for the deep cervical plexus block is similar to superficial block. Using landmark technique, the transverse processes of the cervical vertebra are marked on the neck. The C1 transverse process is palpated at the level of the mastoid process and the C6 transverse process is palpated at the level of the cricoid cartilage. Ultrasound can assist in determining the location of the transverse processes in patients with more subcutaneous fat. A line is drawn to connect the C1 to C6 transverse processes, and C2–4 transverse processes are marked at equidistance. Next, a needle is inserted until the transverse process is contacted, and then withdrawn 1–2 mm. Three to

5 mL of local anesthetic is injected at each level (C2–4) [52, 54].

The deep cervical plexus block can also be performed under ultrasound guidance. The neck is scanned from the mastoid process to Chassaignac's tubercle (anterior tubercle of the transverse process of C6), visualizing each of the cervical transverse processes. Ultrasound guidance reduces the risk of intra-arterial injection [55].

Complications of the deep cervical plexus block are more frequent than superficial. Phrenic nerve blockade is expected and may be a contraindication to deep plexus block in patients with respiratory disease. Other expected side effects include Horner's syndrome, stellate ganglion block and transient recurrent laryngeal nerve palsy. More serious complications include subarachnoid or epidural injection, intravascular injection and local hematoma.

A prospective study of 1000 blocks for carotid artery surgery found low complication rates for both superficial and deep cervical plexus blocks. Less than 1% of patients had clinical evidence of intravascular injection of local anesthesia. Surgical supplementation of the block was required in half of the cases and conversion to general anesthesia was required in 2.5% of operations [56]. A more recent systematic review of complications related to superficial or deep cervical plexus block by Pandit et al. found that rates or complications were lower in the superficial group, and that there was higher incidence of conversion to general anesthesia in the deep cervical plexus block group [57].

## Cervical Epidural Anesthesia

An epidural catheter is placed at the C6–7 interspace and a dilute solution of local anesthetic is injected. Bilateral cervical and upper thoracic nerve roots are affected. Significant side effects are expected and include hypotension, bradycardia and respiratory insufficiency. Complications include dural tap, epidural hematoma and direct spinal cord damage. Due to the significant risks and side effects, cervical epidural anesthesia is rarely used. A case series by Bonnet et al. reviewed 394 patients with cervical epidurals and found serious complications to include dural puncture (2 patients), epidural venipuncture (6 patients) and respiratory muscle paralysis (3 patients) [32, 55, 58].

## Postoperative Considerations

Postoperatively, continued hemodynamic lability is common, secondary to the disrupted baroreceptor function. Continuous invasive monitoring of blood pressure should be continued in the acute postoperative period until hemodynamic stability is established. Both hypertension and hypotension can be expected [22, 32].

Cerebral hyperperfusion syndrome can result if hypertension is not strictly controlled. The syndrome occurs after blood flow is restored within a previously hypoperfused region. The relative increase in perfusion pressure leads to cerebral edema and hemorrhage, and causes neurologic deficits. The best treatment for cerebral hyperperfusion syndrome is prevention via exact blood pressure management [32].

Stroke is the second most common cause of death following CEA. Major stroke is usually delayed and apparent in the postoperative period. Thus, continued frequent neurologic assessments are required. Analysis of the CREST data suggests that the incidence of minor strokes is highest the day of surgery but few were observed intraoperatively. Major strokes most commonly occur several days after revascularization [19].

Other complications of CEA include cervical hematoma, nerve injury, infection, and carotid restenosis. Cervical hematoma is a serious complication that can lead to nerve palsy or airway compromise. Prevention of cervical hematoma includes reversal of anticoagulation, control of postoperative hypertension, and smooth emergence from general anesthesia. Urgent surgical re-evaluation is required if hematoma is suspected or the patient shows signs of airway compromise [59].

## Authors Preferred Method

In all qualified patients, we prefer to perform carotid endarterectomy under regional anesthesia with superficial cervical plexus block ± deep cervical plexus block. The block is performed preoperatively by a dedicated pain service. Preoperative arterial line is placed and a bolus of dexmedetomidine is begun (usually 0.5 μg/kg over 10 min) as the patient is transferred to the operating room. The patient is positioned supine on the bed with arms tucked at the patient's side. A squeezable noise-making toy is placed in the patient's contralateral hand. Anxiolysis is typically maintained with continuous infusion of dexmedetomidine (0.1–1 μg/kg/h). Strict avoidance of over sedation is required for accurate neurologic assessments throughout the procedure. Additional infiltration of local anesthetic may be required during dissection to the carotid artery. The following vasoactive substances are made immediately available for hemodynamic control: nicardipine infusion, esmolol, labetalol, phenylephrine, and norepinephrine. Neurologic assessments occur just prior to cross-clamp, 2 min after clamp and periodically thereafter—including in the postoperative period. Patients are monitored closely in the post anesthesia care unit with continued management of blood pressure, repeated evaluation of the neck incision for hematoma, and frequent neurologic assessments.

## References

1. Mozaffarian D, Benjamin EJ, Go AS, et al. Heart disease and stroke statistics—2016 update: a report from the American Heart Association. Circulation. 2016;133(4):e38–60.
2. Rerkasem K, Rothwell PM. Carotid endarterectomy for symptomatic carotid stenosis. Cochrane Database Syst Rev. 2011;(4):CD001081.
3. Brott TG, Hobson RW, Howard G, et al. Stenting versus endarterectomy for treatment of carotid-artery stenosis. N Engl J Med. 2010;363(1):11–23.
4. Hye RJ, Voeks JH, Malas MB, et al. Anesthetic type and risk of myocardial infarction after carotid endarterectomy in the Carotid Revascularization Endarterectomy versus Stenting Trial (CREST). J Vasc Surg. 2016;64(1):3–8.e1.
5. Cho L, Mukherjee D. Basical cerebral anatomy for the carotid interventionalist: the intracranial and extracranial vessels. Catheter Cardiovasc Interv. 2006;68:104–11.
6. Layton KF, Kallmes DF, Cloft HJ, et al. Bovine aortic arch variant in humans: clarification of a common misnomer. AJNR Am J Neuroradiol. 2006;27:154102.
7. Gonzalez C, Almaraz L, Obeso A, et al. Carotid body chemoreceptors: from natural stimuli to sensory discharges. Physiol Rev. 1994;74(4):829–98.
8. Glagov S, Zarins C, et al. Hemodynamics and atherosclerosis. Insights and perspectives gained from studies of human arteries. Arch Pathol Lab Med. 1988;112(10):1018–31.
9. Allain R, Marone LK, et al. Carotid endarterectomy. Int Anesthesiol Clin. 2005;43(1):15–38.
10. Grotta JC. Carotid stenosise. N Engl J Med. 2013;369(12):2359–61.
11. de Bray JM, Glatt B. Quantification of atheromatous stenosis in the extracranial internal carotid artery. Cerebrovasc Dis. 1995;5:414–26.
12. Alexandrov AV, Needleman L. Carotid artery stenosis: making complex assessments of a simple problem or simplifying approach to a complex disease? Stroke. 2012;43:627–8.
13. Fairhead JF, Mehta Z, Rothwell PM. Population-based study of delays in carotid imaging and surgery and the risk of recurrent stroke. Neurology. 2005;65(3):371–5.
14. Rothwell PM, Eliasziw M, Gutnikov SA, et al. Endarterectomy for symptomatic carotid stenosis in relation to clinical subgroups and timing of surgery. Lancet. 2004;363:915–24.
15. Gladstone DJ, Oh J, Fang J, et al. Urgency of carotid endarterectomy for secondary stroke prevention: results from the registry of the Canadian stroke network. Stroke. 2009;40:2776–82.
16. Kernan WN, Ovbiagele B, Black HR, et al. AHA/ASA guidelines for the prevention of stroke in patients with stroke or transient ischemic attack: a guideline for healthcare professionals from the American Heart Association/American Stroke Association. Stroke. 2014;45:2160–236.
17. Brott TG, Halperin JL, Abbara S, et al. ASA/ACCF/AHA/AANN/AANS/ACR/ASNR/CNS/SAIP/SCAI/SIR/SNIS/SVM/SVS guideline on the management of patients with extra-cranial carotid and vertebral artery disease: executive summary: a report of the American College of Cardiology Foundation/American Heart Association Task Force on Practice Guidelines, and the American Stroke Association, American Association of Neuroscience Nurses, American Association of Neurological Surgeons, American College of Radiology, American Society of Neuroradiology, Congress of Neurological Surgeons, Society of Atherosclerosis Imaging and Prevention, Society for Cardiovascular Angiography and Interventions, Society of Interventional Radiology, Society of Neuro Interventional Surgery, Society for

Vascular Medicine, and Society for Vascular Surgery. Stroke. 2011;42:e420–63.
18. Fleisher LA, Fleischmann KE, Auerbach AD, et al. 2014 ACC/AHA guideline on perioperative cardiovascular evaluation and management of patients undergoing noncardiac surgery: a report of the American College of Cardiology/American Heart Association task force on practice guidelines. Circulation. 2014;130:e278–333.
19. Hill MD, Brooks W, Mackey A, et al. Stroke after carotid stenting and endarterectomy in the Carotid Revascularization Endarterectomy versus Stenting Trial (CREST). Circulation. 2016;126(25):3054–61.
20. Chongruksut W, Vaniyapong T, Rerkasem K. Routine or selective carotid artery shunting for carotid endarterectomy (and different methods of monitoring in selective shunting). Cochrane Database Syst Rev. 2014;23(6):CD000190.pub3.
21. Gumerlock MK, Neuwelt EA. Carotid endarterectomy: to shunt or not to shunt. Stroke. 1988;19:1485–90.
22. Nicoara A, Swaminathan M. Anesthesia for major vascular surgery. In: Longnecker DE, Brown DL, et al., editors. Anesthesiology. 2nd ed. New York: McGraw Hill Medical; 2012. p. 1009–31.
23. AbuRahma AF, Stone PA, Hass SM, et al. Prospective randomized trial of routine versus selective shunting in carotid endarterectomy based on stump pressure. J Vasc Surg. 2010;51(5):1133–8.
24. Mendonca CT, Fortunato JA, Carvalho CA, et al. Carotid endarterectomy in awake patients: safety tolerability and results. Rev Bras Cardiovasc. 2014;29(4):574–80.
25. Benjamin ME, Silva MB, Watt C, et al. Awake patient monitoring to determine the need for shunting during carotid endarterectomy. Surgery. 1993;114(4):673–81.
26. Davies MJ, Mooney PH, Scott DA, et al. Neurologic changes during carotid endarterectomy under cervical block predict a high risk of postoperative stroke. Anesthesiology. 1993;78(5):829–33.
27. Browse NL, Ross-Russel R. Carotid endarterectomy and the Javid shunt: the early results of 215 consecutive operations for transient ischemic attacks. Br J Surg. 1984;71(1):53–7.
28. Stoneham MD, Knighton JD. Regional anesthesia for carotid endarterectomy. Br J Anaesth. 1999;82:910–9.
29. Stoughton J, Nath RL, Abbott WM. Comparison of simultaneous electroencephalographic and mental status monitoring during carotid endarterectomy with regional anesthesia. J Vasc Surg. 1998;28(6):1014–21.
30. Schneider JR, Droste JS, Schindler N, et al. Carotid endarterectomy with routine electroencephalography and selective shunting: influence of contralateral internal carotid artery occlusion and utility in preventing perioperative strokes. J Vasc Surg. 2002;35:1114–22.
31. Guay J, Kopp S. Cerebral monitors versus regional anesthesia to detect cerebral ischemia in patients undergoing carotid endarterectomy: a meta-analysis. Can J Anaesth. 2013;60(3):266–79.
32. Howell SJ. Carotid endarterectomy. Br J Anaesth. 2007;99:119–31.
33. Calligaro KD, Dougherty MJ. Correlation of carotid artery stump pressure and neurologic changes during 474 carotid endarterectomies performed in awake patients. J Vasc Surg. 2005;42(4):684–9.
34. Boysen G, Engell HC, Pistolese GR, et al. Editorial: on the critical level of cerebral blood flow in man with particular reference to carotid surgery. Circulation. 1974;49(6):1023–5.
35. Pinkerton JA. EEG as a criterion for shunt need in carotid endarterectomy. Ann Vasc Surg. 2002;16(6):756–61.
36. Arnold M, Stursenegger M, Schaffler L, et al. Continuous intraoperative monitoring of middle cerebral artery blood flow velocities and electroencephalography during carotid endarterectomy. Stroke. 1997;28:1345–50.
37. Nwachuku EL, Balzer JR, Yabes JG, et al. Diagnostic value of somatosensory evoked potential changes during carotid endarterectomy: a systematic review and meta-analysis. JAMA Neurol. 2015;72(1):73–80.
38. Wober C, Zeitlhofer J, Aenbaum S, et al. Monitoring of median nerve somatosensory evoked potentials in carotid surgery. J Clin Neurophysiol. 1998;15(5):429–38.
39. Spencer MP, Ackerstaff RGA, Babikian VL, et al. Basic identification criteria of doppler microembolic signals. Stroke. 1995;26:1123.
40. JMJ K, Gijn J, Ackerstaff RGA, et al. Site and pathogenesis of infarcts associated with carotid endarterectomy. Stroke. 1989;20(3):324–8.
41. de Borst GJ, Moll FL, van de Pavoordt HDWM, et al. Stroke from carotid endarterectomy: when and how to reduce perioperative stroke rate? Eur J Vasc Endovasc Surg. 2001;21(6):484–9.
42. Jansen C, Vriens EM, Eikelboom BC, et al. Carotid endarterectomy with transcranial doppler and electroencephalographic monitoring: a prospective study in 130 operations. Stroke. 1993;24(5):665–9.
43. Spencer MP. Transcranial doppler monitoring and cause of stroke from carotid endarterectomy. Stroke. 1997;28(4):685–91.
44. Rigamonti A, Scandroglio M, Minicucci F, et al. A clinical evaluation of near-infrared cerebral oximetry in the awake patient to monitor cerebral perfusion carotid endarterectomy. J Clin Anesth. 2005;17(6):426–30.
45. Samra SK, Dorje P, Zelenock GB, et al. Cerebral oximetry in patients undergoing carotid endarterectomy under regional anesthesia. Stroke. 1996;27:49–55.
46. Vaniyapong T, Chongruksut W, Rerkasem K. Local versus general anesthesia for carotid endarterectomy. Cochrane Database Syst Rev. 2013;(12):CD000126.
47. Leichtle SW, Mouawad NJ, Welch K, et al. Outcomes of carotid endarterectomy under general and regional anesthesia from the American College of Surgeons' National Surgical Quality Improvement Program. J Vasc Surg. 2012;56(1):81.

48. Duffy CM, Basil FM. Sevoflurane and anesthesia for neurosurgery. J Neurosurgical Anesth. 2000;12(2):128–40.
49. Al-Rawi PG, Siguado-Roussel D, Gaunt ME. Effect of lignocaine injection in carotid sinus on baroreceptor sensitivity during carotid endarterectomy. J Vasc Surg. 2004;39(6):1288–94.
50. Bekker AY, Basile J, Gold M, et al. Dexmedetomidine for awake carotid endarterectomy: efficacy, hemodynamic profile, and side effects. J Neurosurg Anesthesiol. 2004;16(2):126–35.
51. MCutcheon CA, Orme RM, Scott DA, et al. A comparison of dexmedetomidine versus conventional therapy for sedation and hemodynamic control during carotid endarterectomy performed under regional anesthesia. Anesth Analg. 2006;102(3):668–75.
52. Spargo JR, Thomas D. Local anesthesia for carotid endarterectomy. Contin Educ Anesth Crit Care Pain. 2004;4(2):62–5.
53. Ultrasound-guided superficial plexus block. The New York School of Regional Anesthesia. 2013. www.nysora.com
54. Cervical plexus block. The New York School of Regional Anesthesia. 2013. www.nysora.com
55. Stoneham MD, Stamou D, Mason J. Regional anesthesia for carotid endarterectomy. Br J Anaesth. 2015;114(3):372–83.
56. Davies MJ, Silbert BS, Scott DA, et al. Superficial and deep cervical plexus block for carotid artery surgery: a prospective study of 1000 blocks. Reg Anesth. 1997;22(5):442–6.
57. Pandit JJ, Satya-Krishna R, Gration P. Superficial or deep cervical plexus block for carotid endarterectomy: a systematic review of complications. Br J Anaesth. 2007;99(2):159–69.
58. Bonnet F, Derosier JP, Pluskwa F, et al. Cervical epidural anaesthesia for carotid artery surgery. Can J Anaesth. 1990;37(3):353–8.
59. Kunkel JM, Gomez ER, Spebar MJ, et al. Wound hematomas after carotid endarterectomy. Am J Surg. 1984;148(6):844–7.

# Anesthesia for AV Fistulas (Upper Extremity)

Kavitha A. Mathew and Joseph V. Schneider

## Introduction

End-stage renal disease (ESRD) is the final stage of chronic kidney disease (CKD) when renal function is irreversibly impaired and dialysis or transplant is required for survival. The decreased glomerular filtration rate and urine production lead to uremia, derangements in plasma volume, decreased elimination of drugs and nitrogenous wastes, reduced synthesis of erythropoietin and inability to maintain plasma pH. Renal replacement therapy via hemo- or peritoneal dialysis is required to maintain these functions. ESRD has an effect on nearly every organ system, and it has a major impact on patient mortality despite dialysis therapy.

The incidence of ESRD is increasing in the United States. Approximately 660,000 patients carried a diagnosis of ESRD in 2015, with newly diagnosed disease affecting greater than 115,000 people in 2013 [1]. The incidence of ESRD has increased tenfold over the last 30 years. Of these patients, 65% are treated with hemodialysis, 30% with renal transplantation and 5% with periotoneal dialysis (PD). While the definitive treatment is renal transplantation, the number of organs available in the transplant pool cannot meet increasing demand. Currently, the average wait time on the renal transplant list is 1.7 years [1].

ESRD is associated with significant morbidity and mortality. The average life expectancy of patients with ESRD is 5.8 years with 22% annual mortality [2, 3]. Approximately 89,000 people in the United States die from ESRD each year [1]. Patients presenting for fistula surgery almost universally suffer from multiple medical comorbidities that require attention in the perioperative period. These patients require input and evaluation from the surgeon, anesthesiologist, nephrologist, and potentially from a cardiologist and endocrinologist as well. Coordinated care among medical specialties optimizes patients presenting for fistula surgery but also illustrates the significant socioeconomic burden of this patient population. The Dialysis Outcomes and Practice Patterns Study (DOPPS), a prospective cohort study coordinated by the National Institute of Health, demonstrates that patients with ESRD account for 1.3% of the Medicare population but account for 7.5% of Medicare spending, totaled at $25.7 billion in 2010 [3].

K. A. Mathew, M.D., M.P.H. (✉)
Emory University School of Medicine,
Atlanta, GA, USA
e-mail: kmathew@emory.edu

J. V. Schneider, M.D., M.S.
Department of Anesthesiology, Emory University School of Medicine, Atlanta, GA, USA
e-mail: jospeh.vincent.schneider@emory.edu

## Arteriovenous (AV) Fistula Surgery

The goal of AV fistula surgery is to provide reliable access to the patient's circulation with minimal complications. The National Kidney

Foundation guidelines for optimal access include the following criteria: vein diameter >6 mm, ability for dialysis flow >600 cc/min and access depth <6 mm [4]. Options for hemodialysis access include central venous access, placement of a graft material between arterial and venous sites (AV graft) and a direct communication between a systemic artery and vein (AV fistula). Of these, AV fistula is preferred due to having the lowest risk of morbidity, mortality, and complications, as well as best long-term patency [5]. The optimal location for placement of the AV fistula or graft is the radial artery and basilic vein. Another commonly used site is the brachial artery and cephalic vein. In patients with prior failed access or poor anatomy, other sites in the arms, lower extremities or central venous access may be considered.

The procedure involves dissection of the pertinent arterial and venous structures; these typically are superficial in location to facilitate easy future access during dialysis sessions. Once exposed, a small dose of intravenous heparin is given (2000–5000 units) prior to clamping the artery and vein. Arteriotomy and venotomy are performed, and the vein is anastamosed to the artery in an end-to-side fashion. Surgical hemostasis is then ensured. If there is a concern regarding residual effect of heparin, a small dose of protamine may be given. The protamine dose is usually less than 50 mg.

## Preoperative Assessment and Optimization

Patients presenting with CKD or ESRD for AV fistula surgery should have a thorough history and physical examination to determine involvement of multiple organ systems. The anesthesiologist must ascertain if further medical optimization is required prior to surgery.

## Cardiovascular

Cardiovascular disease is the most frequent cause of death in this population [6]. Cardiac mortality is 10- to 20-fold greater in those with CKD/ESRD than in age-matched controls without CKD or ESRD [7]. Hypertension is prevalent in 90% of CKD patients. At the time of presentation to a nephrologist, at least 35% of patients have evidence of ischemic disease or prior cardiac event (angina or myocardial infarction) [8]. Exercise tolerance for each patient is determined using metabolic equivalents (METS); in conjunction with the patient's revised cardiac risk index (RCRI) score, high-risk patients are identified [9]. Evaluation should follow the 2014 American College of Cardiology/American Hospital Association (ACC/AHA) guidelines for patients undergoing non-cardiac surgery [10]. For patients with poor or unknown functional capacity and elevated risk, it may be reasonable to perform exercise testing with cardiac imaging if the results will change management. The decision to perform stress testing should not be based solely on a planned general anesthesia (GA) or monitored anesthesia care (MAC) approach. The American Society of Anesthesiology Position Statement on MAC instructs that patients with planned MAC must be evaluated for all aspects of anesthesia, with a clear emphasis on the ability to convert to GA [11]. ESRD patients are often on statins and beta-blockers; the AHA/ACC recommends continuation throughout the perioperative period [10]. It is also reasonable to take angiotensin converting enzyme inhibitors (ACEIs) and angiotensin receptor blockers (ARBs) on the day of surgery. However, studies do demonstrate an increased risk of hypotension with general anesthesia hence these agents may be held at the discretion of the anesthesiologist based on patient risk. If an ACEI/ARB are held on the day of surgery, they should be resumed post-operatively as soon as deemed safe.

Hypertension is the cause of ESRD in nearly 30% of patients. Even in those that suffer ESRD of other etiology, hypertension is almost universally present due to the vascular and endocrine changes associated with disease. Transthoracic echocardiography commonly demonstrates left ventricular hypertrophy and diastolic dysfunction in these patients [12]. These patients are at risk for heart failure perioperatively. The preoperative physical exam should focus on signs of volume overload such as peripheral edema and crackles on pulmonary examination. Although not mandatory, pre-operative electrocardiography (EKG) and echocardiography can help clarify these issues.

A significant portion of ESRD patients has pulmonary hypertension [13]. It is important to assess severity, current therapy and optimization of disease prior to proceeding to the operating room. A select portion of these patients with severe disease will require intraoperative monitoring of pulmonary artery pressures with a pulmonary artery catheter. Alternatively, transesophageal echocardiography provides intraoperative monitoring of right ventricular function and estimated pulmonary artery pressures.

## Pulmonary

Pulmonary evaluation identifies the presence of co-morbid conditions such as smoking, and acute or chronic lung diseases. History and physical exam should evaluate for dyspnea, accessory muscle use and need for supplemental oxygen. Signs and symptoms of impaired oxygenation carry implications for both GA and regional anesthesia (RA) techniques. For those undergoing general anesthesia with endotracheal tube, there is a risk of airway and pulmonary complications including hypoxia during direct laryngoscopy, and prolonged intubation. Should regional anesthesia be chosen, caution needs to be exercised because brachial plexus block can significantly impair respiratory function by causing hemidiaphragm paralysis. Sedatives also need to be used sparingly in those with poor baseline oxygenation because pulmonary reserve is reduced; hypoventilation and hypercarbia can lead to respiratory arrest.

## Hematologic

The anemia associated with CKD is due to iron deficiency and decreased erythropoietin production. The resulting decrease in oxygen carrying capacity can affect overall quality of life, and worsen or exacerbate myocardial ischemia and dysfunction. The Kidney Disease Outcomes Quality Initiative recommends patients should be on erythropoietin-stimulating agents as well as iron supplements to target a goal hemoglobin concentration of 11–12 g/dL [14]. In the perioperative period, there is limited evidence to recommend target hemoglobin. One small, non-randomized prospective observational study found that hemoglobin concentration of less than 8 g/dL was an independent risk factor for primary AVF failure [15]. Additionally, there is risk of bleeding during the procedure because of uremic platelet dysfunction. Perioperative use of desmopressin and platelet products may be clinically indicated [6].

## Renal

For those patients currently requiring dialysis, perioperative planning should include assessment of the timing and adequacy of the dialysis regimen. Table 68.1 outlines pre-operative dialysis related questions to assess in the preoperative period.

Most patients are scheduled for hemodialysis every other day. One can assume that patients presenting for surgery immediately after dialysis are likely volume deplete, whereby patients presenting due for dialysis are at increased risk for intravascular volume overload. Comparing weight before surgery to a patient's known "dry weight" aids in volume assessment. Additionally, a physical exam is paramount to determine volume status. Following volume evaluation, the anesthesiologist must determine risk in relation

**Table 68.1** Preoperative ESRD related questions

| |
|---|
| Type and location of current dialysis access? |
| Frequency of current dialysis? |
| Date of most recent dialysis? |
| Usual daily fluid intake? |
| Usual daily urine output? |
| "Dry" or target weight? |
| Serum urea and creatinine concentrations? |
| Serum potassium concentration on day of surgery? |

to the patient's other comorbidities to assess the safety of an anesthetic. Patient's with severe systolic heart failure or pulmonary arterial hypertension are often less tolerant of volume overload states than those without these co-morbid conditions. Likewise, those with diastolic heart failure poorly manage rapid changes in volume status and/or notable hypo- or hypervolemia.

ESRD patients frequently have abnormalities in electrolyte values such as sodium, potassium and calcium. When evaluating electrolyte disarray, the chronicity of the aberration should be determined. Patients tolerate chronic derangements in electrolyte composition better than acute changes. Hyperkalemia is not uncommon in these patients and can place them at risk for significant dysrhythmias and cardiac arrest if exacerbated perioperatively. Often, providers check serum potassium levels prior to surgery however, clear evidence suggesting this prevents poor outcomes is lacking. Prior doctrine has suggested that a level above 5.5 mEq/L may be reason to cancel elective surgery [16]. However, recent study demonstrates that serum potassium levels >6 mEq/L, as obtained <120 min prior to surgery, did not negatively impact surgical or anesthetic outcomes. Additionally, in patients who underwent surgery with last serum potassium value >6.5 mEq/L (without preoperative recheck), outcomes did not differ from those with lower preoperative potassium levels [17]. It is unclear if ESRD patients need mandatory potassium testing prior to fistula surgery. Current evidence does demonstrate that use of potassium free solutions such as normal saline may actually worsen hyperkalemia and adverse events due to the low pH and metabolic acidosis produced if administered in of large amounts [18, 19].

## Endocrine

Many ESRD additionally suffer from diabetes mellitus (DM). The pathophysiology of diabetes mellitus expands beyond hyperglycemia. It is a multifactorial process which involves oxidative stress, inflammatory cytokines, endothelial dysfunction and altered immune function [20, 21].

The primary organs affected include the brain, liver, kidneys, pancreas, skeletal muscle and adipose tissue. Hyperglycemia has been associated with adverse outcomes such as delayed wound healing, increased infection, end-organ dysfunction (neurologic, cardiovascular, and renal) and death [20]. Surgical patients with hyperglycemia should have target blood glucose levels of 140–180 mg/dL to reduce the occurrence of poor outcomes while minimizing the risks associated with hypoglycemia [20, 22]. There are multiple strategies for day of surgery insulin treatment based on type of diabetes, home medication regimen, and calculated insulin sensitivity. Preoperatively, once daily basal insulin should be reduced to by 20–25% the evening prior to surgery [22]. On the morning of surgery, for those taking twice daily basal insulin, the dose is reduced to 80% of the usual dose [19]. Mixed insulins can be dosed on the morning of surgery at 50% of regular dose if the patient's BG is >120 mg/dL [21, 22]. All home prandial and short-acting insulin should be held while the patient is NPO. Intravenous insulin is preferred delivery route in critically ill patients and is typically administered as a bolus followed by an infusion. For non-critically ill patients, intravenous (IV) insulin is also used, but there is a growing trend in favor of using rapid onset subcutaneous (SC) insulin in this patient population on the day of surgery. Caution needs to be exercised when dosing SC insulin in patients with ESRD because the metabolism of insulin relies on the kidney; those with reduced GFR are sensitive to insulin's effects [21]. There is currently no established threshold of hyperglycemia at which elective surgery should be postponed. Physical exam or laboratory findings consistent with severely altered glucose metabolism (diabetic ketoacidosis, severe dehydration, hyperosmolar hyperglycemic state) should prompt surgical delay [23].

## Gastrointestinal

Patients with ESRD have delayed gastric emptying. This can be further exacerbated by DM and

**Table 68.2** Comorbid conditions in ESRD patients on HD 2003–2008

| Comorbidity | Number | Percentage (%) | Median age (year) |
|---|---|---|---|
| Angina | 1845 | 16.9 | 71.3 |
| Smoking | 1629 | 15.3 | 61.2 |
| Malignancy | 1457 | 13.3 | 72 |
| MI >3 months ago | 1304 | 11.9 | 70.8 |
| Cerebrovascular disease | 1177 | 10.8 | 71.1 |
| Diabetes | 977 | 9.1 | 70.9 |
| Claudication | 957 | 8.7 | 70.6 |
| COPD | 855 | 7.9 | 70.8 |
| CABG/angioplasty | 837 | 7.7 | 69 |
| Angioplasty/vascular graft | 411 | 3.8 | 71.4 |
| Ischemic/neuropathic ulcers | 410 | 3.7 | 62.6 |
| MI <3 months ago | 339 | 3.1 | 70.7 |
| Liver disease | 329 | 3 | 60 |
| Amputation | 248 | 2.3 | 61.3 |

Modified with permission from [5]

obesity. These patients should be considered a "full stomach" regardless of NPO status and appropriate precautions taken (Table 68.2).

## Choice of Anesthetic Technique and Intraoperative Management

There are currently three accepted anesthetic techniques for AV fistula creation: MAC with local anesthesia (LA), GA, and RA. Currently, surgical and anesthetic texts support any of these methods [24]. There are potential and theoretical risks associated with each anesthetic technique. Retrospective studies evaluating outcomes in patients receiving GA vs. MAC or RA demonstrated no difference in complications [25, 26]. The patient's comorbidities are the primary determining factors when formulating an anesthetic plan however, operative location and patient preference also need to be considered.

With regards to anesthetic technique and surgical outcomes, there is a paucity of large, high-quality trials. There is some prospective data that graft patency and flow are greater with regional anesthesia techniques compared to local anesthetic infiltration [27, 28]. There are advantages and disadvantages of each type of anesthetic.

## General Anesthesia

According to the National Surgical Quality Improvement Project data (2007–2010) for patients undergoing new upper extremity AVF creation, 85.2% of 1540 cases were done using GA [29]. Benefits of GA include control of the patient's airway, oxygenation and ventilation. The anesthesiologist can also ensure patient immobility. GA can be a useful technique in patients that are unable to lie flat on an operating table for long periods due to anxiety, chronic pain or musculoskeletal abnormalities. Disadvantages include vasodilatation from anesthetics in a patient that may already be volume deplete and the cardiac depressant effects of volatile agents in those who are at high risk for cardiac event. These patients may require volume administration or inotope/vasopressor use intraoperatively. Additionally, compared to MAC and RA, GA patients often receive medications that rely on renal elimination; these drugs may have prolonged or unpredictable effects in ESRD.

In ESRD patients undergoing GA for AV fistula creation, there are several important considerations. Choice of endotracheal tube versus supraglottic airway should be dictated by the risk of aspiration. Either can be safely used. In the case of supraglottic airway use, the patient often requires airway support if allowed to spontaneously ventilate. Poor tidal volumes and hypoventilation cause respiratory acidosis and promote extracellular potassium shifts as the body's acid-base buffering system compensates via a hydrogen ion/potassium ion exchange. Choice of paralytic for direct laryngoscopy should be dictated by patient risk for aspiration, potassium levels and anticipated length of drug metabolism. Succinylcholine can transiently increase serum potassium levels by up to 0.5 mEq/L. The choice of non-depolarizing neuromuscular blocker for laryngoscopy should be based on consideration for prolonged effects due to renal excretion and elimination. While vecuronium and rocuronium are primarily eliminated through hepatic biotranformation and hepatobiliary excretion, there is a portion (<25%) that is eliminated by the kidney. Cisatricurium, which relies on the chemical process of Hoffman elimination, does not have prolonged effect in ESRD patients. The hemodynamic goals of induction must include avoidance of hypotension, which can be managed with volume administration or vasopressor use. Poorly controlled blood pressure and left ventricular hypertrophy (LVH) are common in these patients. The thickened myocardium may tolerate hypotension poorly. Additionally, diabetic patients often suffer from autonomic dysfunction, placing them at increased risk for refractory hypotension following the induction of anesthesia.

Standard ASA monitors are often sufficient for most patients undergoing fistula or graft creation. In select patients with significant co-morbid conditions, intra-arterial blood pressure monitoring may be indicated. This should be balanced against the potential future need for the artery as an AV fistula site. Often one 18 gauge or larger peripheral intravenous (IV) line is usually sufficient however, in patients with poor peripheral access or significant comorbidities, central access may be warranted.

The patient's blood pressure should be maintained to ensure adequate perfusion to the heart and brain. ESRD patients with LVH require higher blood pressures to ensure coronary perfusion pressure. Fluids need to be balanced to avoid volume overload while also providing sufficient preload to maintain cardiac output and blood pressure. Although normal saline may be used in small volumes, administration of large quantities is avoided due to risk of hyperchloremic acidosis and potential resultant hyperkalemia [18, 19]. As these patients often have diastolic dysfunction and are unable to tolerate volume loading; judicious use of IV fluids is merited.

The AV fistula is most frequently placed superficially and does not typically cause significant pain. Small to moderate doses of narcotics and non-narcotics adjunvants are sufficient for analgesia in non-opioid tolerant patients. Surgeons can also perform a field block with local anesthetic to augment analgesia and minimize narcotics.

Extubation is appropriate in most patients in the operating room however, emergence planning needs to decrease aspiration risk, and ensure return of muscle strength if neuromuscular blockade was used. A train-of-four ratio >0.9 informs the anesthesiologist of adequate reversal and can be measured with an accelerometer. Reversal In ESRD and severed CKD is accomplished most frequently with neostigmine and glycopyrrolate. Sugammadex is not currently recommended for use in patients with severe renal disease [30].

## Regional Anesthesia or Local Infiltration

In addition to increased graft patency, benefits to a regional technique in this patient population include a decline in surgical stress, a reduction in hemodynamic perturbations associated with induction of GA, and faster recovery and post-anesthesia care unit discharge [28, 29]. RA appears to be superior to LA with regards to graft patency [26, 27]. Both RA and LA also have the benefit of avoiding many of the common post-operative adverse effects of GA with volatile anesthetics such as post-operative delirum (may depend on adjunct sedation), nausea and vomiting, and prolonged sedation. Potential concerns when using RA or LA include cardiac and neurologic toxicity secondary to inadvertent intravascular injection of local anesthetic, infection and hematoma.

RA approaches to the brachial plexus most frequently used for upper extremity AV fistula/graft are the supraclavicular, infraclavicular and axillary blocks. The interscalene approach may be employed however, the inferior trunk may not be adequately blocked using this technique. Supplemental block of the ulnar nerve may be needed to assure adequate coverage of the forearm. Ultrasound guidance is recommended; visualization of the inferior trunk may improve the adequacy of the block for forearm surgery. Additionally, for blocks with targets close to the pleura, the use of ultrasound has been shown to reduce the incidence of pneumothorax [31]. If there is concern for the patient's respiratory status, a supraclavicular or interscalene block should be avoided, as the ipsilateral phrenic nerve will be blocked in 50–100% of cases respectively. If the provider elects to use an axillary approach, a separate block must be done to provide optimal surgical anesthesia to the forearm. The musculocutaneous and intercostobrachial nerves are not in the axillary sheath and need to be supplemented for adequate coverage of their sensory distribution. Longer acting local anesthetics such as bupivicaine and ropivicaine can be selected to provide satisfactory surgical anesthesia, particularly in patients with complicated anatomy or anticipated difficult graft/fistula creation. These longer lasting anesthetics also provide post-operative analgesia and increase vessel diameter and blood flow. While there is often excellent dermatomal coverage with regional anesthesia, the surgical team should be prepared to supplement the block in case of imperfect blockade.

## Medication Management

The anesthesiologist must be aware of the pharmacologic considerations for patients in renal failure. Patients with ESRD often have low serum protein levels. This affects medications that are highly protein bound in circulation; low serum albumin levels lead to an increased fraction of free (unbound) drug. Oppositely, the increased volume of distribution often increased the drug dose needed to achieve effect. Careful titration of anesthetics is merited in renal failure because the pharmaco-kinetics and dynamics of anesthetic agents is less predictable.

Sedation is often used to increase patient comfort in the operating room when the surgery is performed under regional block. Many benzodiazepines undergo hepatic metabolism into active metabolites. Following liver conjugation, byproducts are eliminated by the kidney. Benzodiazepines are often highly protein bound; slow titration is recommended in patients with ESRD because low serum protein levels decrease binding and more free drug is available to traverse cell membranes and exert pharmacologic effect.

In patients undergoing surgery under regional anesthesia, the anesthesiologist must always be prepared to convert to general anesthesia in cases of block failure. Often the RA and LA are supplemented with sedation. Judicious sedation is recommended. It is imperative to minimize or avoid medications with prolonged effect in renal failure.

Morphine should be used with caution due to the accumulation of the active metabolite morphine-6-glucuronide and can lead to respiratory depression. Similarly, meperidine should be avoided due to accumulation of the toxic metabolite normeperidine, which has been associated with seizures. Fentanyl, remifentanil, sufentanil, alfentanil do not depend on renal clearance [32].

Although dexmedetomidine pharmacokinetics do not demonstrate significant change in patients with renal impairment, the majority of drug metabolites are renally excreted [33]. At this time, dose reductions in the loading bolus and infusion are appropriate in those with ESRD. Optimal sedation provides anxiolysis yet avoids hypoventilation that may result in hypercarbia, respiratory acidosis, airway obstruction and hypoxia.

## Post-operative Management

Due to the superficial nature of this procedure, post-operative care is usually routine and uneventful. Patients should however, be monitored for return of motor function and sensation (if a block was used), adequate distal pulse and warm extremity. Post-operative surgical complications include graft thrombosis; routine neurovascular monitoring is recommended in the post-anesthesia care unit as means to reliably, and quickly, recognize unexpected changes in the operative extremity. AV fistula maturation typically takes 4–12 weeks following surgery. Long-term complications of AV fistula surgery are rare but, do occur and may require a second surgery to remedy. Median complication rate per 1000 patient days include the following: 0.04 aneurysm development, 0.11 infection, 0.05 steal event, and 0.24 thrombotic event [34]. Primary AV fistula failure occurs in upwards of 30% of patients and is most frequently the result of stenosis, thrombosis or a combination of the two [34].

## Summary

Patients with ESRD presenting for AV fistula surgery are often medically challenging with multiple comorbidities. A thorough preoperative evaluation and optimizations are very important in planning the anesthetic care of these patients. There remains a high potential for perioperative complications, including AV fistula failure. Although historically viewed as equivalent, the type of anesthesia can affect post-operative complications. Ultimately, the optimal anesthetic approach is patient specific and requires a thorough understanding of the available therapeutic options.

## References

1. U.S Renal Data System Annual Report 2015: Atlas of end-stage renal disease in the United States. Centers for Medicare and Medicaid Services. Bethesda, MD: National Institutes of Health, National Institute of Diabetes and Digestive and Kidney Diseases, 2015.
2. U.S Renal Data system USRDS 2008 annual data report: Atlas of end-stage renal disease in the United States. Bethesda, MD: National Institutes of Health, National Institute of Diabetes and Digestive and Kidney Diseases, 2008.
3. Goodkin DA, et al. Association of comorbid conditions and mortality in hemodialysis patients in Europe, Japan, and the United States: the Dialysis Outcomes and Practice Patterns Study (DOPPS). J Am Soc Nephrol. 2003;14:3270–7.
4. National Kidney Foundation. K/DOQI Clinical Practice Guidelines for Vascular Access, 2006 updates. Am J Kidney Dis. 2001;37:S137–81.
5. Hemodialysis Adequacy 2006 Work Group. Clinical practice guidelines for hemodialysis adequacy, update 2006. Am J Kidney Dis. 2006;48(Suppl 1): S2–90.
6. Trainor D, Borthwick E, Ferguson A. Perioperative management of the hemodialysis patient. Semin Dial. 2011;24:314–26.
7. Weiner D, Tighiouart H, Amin M, Stark P, MacLeod B, Griffith J, Sarnak M. Chronic kidney disease is a risk factor for cardiovascular disease and all-cause mortality: a pooled analysis of community-based studies. J Am Soc Nephrol. 2004;15:1307–15.
8. Levin A. Clinical epidemiology of cardiovascular disease in chronic kidney disease prior to dialysis. Semin Dial. 2003;16(2):101–5.
9. Goldman L, Caldera DL, Nussbaum SR, Southwick FS, Krogstad D, Murray B, Burke DS, O'Malley TA, Goroll AH, Caplan CH, Nolan J, Carabello B, Slater EE. Multifactorial index of cardiac risk in noncardiac surgical procedures. N Engl J Med. 1977;297(16):845–50.
10. Fleisher LA, Fleischmann KE, Auerbach AD, Barnason SA, Beckman JA, Bozkurt B, Davila-Roman VG, Gerhard-Herman MD, Holly TA, Kane GC, Marine JE, Nelson MT, Spencer CC, Thompson A, Ting HH, Uretsky BF, Wijeysundera DN. 2014 ACC/AHA guideline on perioperative cardiovascular evaluation and management of patients undergoing noncardiac surgery: executive summary: a report of the American College of Cardiology/American Heart Association Task Force on Practice Guidelines. Circulation. 2014;130(24):2215–45.
11. American Society of Anesthesiologists, Position on Monitored Anesthesia Care (Oct 16, 2013). Accessed from: www.asahq.org/~/media/Sites/ASAHQ/.../position-on-monitored-anesthesia-care.pdf
12. Pecoits-Filho R, Bucharles S, Barberato SH. Diastolic heart failure in dialysis patients: mechanisms, diagnostic approach, and treatment. Semin Dial. 2012;25:35–41.
13. Kawar B, Ellam T, Jackson C, Kiely DG. Pulmonary hypertension in renal disease: epidemiology, potential mechanisms and implications. Am J Nephrol. 2013;37(3):281–90.
14. KDOQI. KDOQI Clinical Practice Guideline and Clinical Practice Recommendations for anemia in chronic kidney disease: 2007 update of hemoglobin target. Am J Kidney Dis. 2007;50:471–530.
15. Khavanin Zadeh M, Gholipour F, Hadipour R. The effect of hemoglobin level on arteriovenous fistula survival in Iranian hemodialysis patients. J Vasc Access. 2008;9(2):133–6.
16. Schonberger RB. Fluid, electrolyte and acid-base disorders. In: Hines RL, Marschall KE, editors.

Stoelting's Anesthesia and co-existing disease. Philadelphia: Saunders (Elsevier); 2012. p. 366.
17. Ehrenfeld JM, Sedykh A, Furman W. Management of potassium abnormalities on the day of surgery: a retrospective review. Abstract presentation. Chicago, IL: American Society of Anesthesiologists; 2011.
18. O'Malley C, et al. A randomized, double-blind comparison of lactated Ringer's solution and 0.9% NaCl during renal transplantation. Anesth Analg. 2005;100:1518–24.
19. Potura E, et al. An acetate-buffered balanced crystalloid versus 0.9% saline in patients with end-stage renal disease undergoing cadaveric renal transplantation: a prospective randomized controlled trial. Anesth Analg. 2015;120:123–9.
20. Evans CH, Lee J, Ruhlman MK. Optimal glucose management in the perioperative period. Surg Clin North Am. 2015;95(2):337–54.
21. Duggan EW, Klopman MA, Berry AJ, Umpierrez G. The Emory University Perioperative Algorithm for the management of hyperglycemia and diabetes in non-cardiac surgery patients. Curr Diab Rep. 2016;16(3):34.
22. Duggan EW, Carlson KT, Umpierrez GE. Perioperative hyperglycemia management, an update. Anesthesiology. 2017;126(3):547–60.
23. Joshi GP, Chung F, Vann MA, Ahmad S, Gan TJ, Goulson DT, et al. Society for ambulatory anesthesia consensus statement on perioperative blood glucose management in diabetic patients undergoing ambulatory surgery. Anesth Analg. 2010;111(6):1378–87.
24. Cronenwett JA. Rutherford's vascular surgery. 8th ed. Philadelphia, PA: Elsevier Inc.; 2014.
25. Solomonson M, Johnson M, Ilstrup D. Risk factors in patients having surgery to create an arteriovenous fistula. Anesth Analg. 1994;79:694–700.
26. Son A, Mannoia K, Herrera A, Chizari M, Hagdoost M, Molkara A. Dialysis access surgery: does anesthesia type affect maturation and complication rates? Ann Vasc Surg. 2016;33:116–9.
27. Aitken E, Jackson A, Kearns R, Steven M, Kinsella J, Clancy M, Macfarlane A. Effect of regional versus local anaesthesia on outcome after arteriovenous fistula creation: a randomised controlled trial. Lancet. 2016;388:1067–74.
28. Sahin L, Gul R, Mizrak A, Deniz H, Sahin M, Koruk S, et al. Ultrasound-guided infraclavicular brachial plexus block enhances postoperative blood flow in arteriovenous fistulas. J Vasc Surg. 2011;54(3):749–53.
29. Siracuse JJ, Gill HL, Parrack I, Huang ZS, Schneider DB, Connolly PH, Meltzer AJ. Variability in anesthetic considerations for arteriovenous fistula creation. J Vasc Access. 2014;15(5):364–9.
30. Bridion (package insert). Whitehouse Station, MJ. Merck & Co., Inc.; 2015.
31. De Tran QH, Clemente A, Doan J, Finlayson RJ. Brachial plexus blocks: a review of approaches and techniques. Can J Anesth. 2007;54(8):662–74.
32. Melzer J. Renal physiology. In: Hemmings HC, Egan TD, editors. Pharmacology and Physiology for Anesthesia. Philadelphia: Saunders (Elsevier); 2013.
33. Precedex (package insert). Lake Forest, IL: Hospira Inc.; 2008.
34. Al-Jaishi AA, Liu AR, Lok CE, Zhang JC, Moist LM. Complications of the arteriovenous fistula: a systematic review. J Am Soc Nephrol. 2017;28:1839–50.

# Trauma Anesthesia

**69**

Michael A. Evans and Richard B. Johnson

## Initial Assessment

The anesthesiologist plays a variety of roles in the spectrum of trauma resuscitation. Initial assessment may occur in the trauma bay, or in some centers, in an emergency department (ED) space that dually functions as a trauma bay and operating room (OR). If the emergency room is separate from the OR, the ED/trauma surgery teams start assessment and initiate all immediate treatment and resuscitation needs. The Advanced Trauma Life Support (ATLS) protocol, developed by the American College of Surgeons, has been adopted in over 50 countries to systematically and rapidly identify life-threatening injuries [3]. The *primary survey* can be remembered with the mnemonic "ABCDE," which lists its components in order of priority:

1. **Airway** and maintenance of cervical spine protection
2. **Breathing** and ventilation
3. **Circulation** with hemorrhage control
4. **Disability**/Neurologic assessment
5. **Exposure** of the patient's body, looking for occult injury and environmental control to limit hypothermia

M. A. Evans, M.D. · R. B. Johnson, M.D. (✉)
Department of Anesthesiology, Emory University Hospital, Emory University School of Medicine, Atlanta, GA, USA
e-mail: michaelevans@emory.edu; richard.benjamin.johnson@emoryhealthcare.org

## Airway

Airway assessment and control is a first priority for all trauma patients. Supplemental oxygen should be applied immediately to augment tissue oxygen delivery and in anticipation of possible airway management. If the patient has not been intubated in the field, the anesthesiology team must assess the airway, oxygenation, and ventilation status quickly to determine need for a secured airway. Multiple considerations determine airway approach, equipment and difficulty. Trauma patients are at an increased risk of aspiration of gastric contents, so if intubation is indicated, rapid sequence intubation should be performed. Two studies evaluating survival in blunt trauma examined aspiration rates. The incidence of aspiration in non-survivors was 20% [4] and 54% [5] respectively. Aspiration has also been correlated with non-survivable injury [4, 6].

An additional predominant airway concern in an acute trauma victim is the possible presence of an unstable cervical spine; caution during airway management is always prudent because more obvious injuries may distract both patient and involved providers, preventing detection of cervical spine damage particularly in conscious patients who are protecting their airway. In the case of an uncertain spine injury, intubation should be performed with the cervical immobilization collar in place, or with an assistant providing in-line stabilization to maintain the cervical spine in a neutral position. The proportion of all trauma patients who suffer a cervical spine injury is 3.7%, and the prevalence in awake and alert trauma patients is 2.8%. Patients in whom a neurological exam cannot be performed, due to obtundation or presence of distracting injury, have an increased risk for cervical spine injury. Upwards of 8% of these patients will suffer cervical spine trauma resulting in instability [7].

Trauma patients may present with conditions that complicate the task of securing an airway. Maxillofacial trauma distorts airway anatomy and can make landmarks difficult to identify and mask ventilation impossible. The face has a complex network of arterial and venous vasculature, and uncontrolled bleeding can result in difficulty obtaining a view with laryngoscopy. In patients with suspected craniofacial injuries, nasotracheal tubes are avoided in the event of potential basilar skull fracture. Direct airway trauma may necessitate a surgical airway due to the impossibility of intubation.

Smoke and fire cause thermal burns to the airway lumen, resulting in blistering, stridor and/or edema. Bronchial or alveolar damage from smoke inhalation affects gas exchange and patient finding range of from cough and dark sputum to frank dyspnea and impending respiratory failure. Studies have demonstrated that benign initial airway exam is not a reliable predictor of impending airway obstruction in those who have been exposed to smoke inhalation [8]. Thermal exposure leads to rapid edema formation and will quickly obstruct normal landmarks. Systemic poisoning with carbon monoxide (CO) and hydrogen cyanide may be initially undetected by providers on primary survey. CO causes tissue hypoxia because its binding affinity to hemoglobin is 200 times that of oxygen and due to the leftward shift of the hemoglobin dissociation curve impairing oxygen release to the tissues.

## Breathing, Oxygenation and Ventilation

Generally, "A," "B," and "C" are performed simultaneously whenever possible. Assessment of a patient's breathing and ventilation includes a survey of the chest to rule out life-threatening conditions. These may include tension pneumothorax, open pneumothorax, cardiac tamponade, flail chest with pulmonary contusion, hemothorax, and outright airway obstruction. The chest wall should be auscultated for breath sounds, and palpated to assess for tracheal deviation and subcutaneous emphysema respectively. If there is high concern for intrathoracic trauma including hemothorax or pneumothorax, evacuation of the pleural space is crucial to protect the lungs from further injury. In the emergent or prehospital setting, needle thoracostomy is performed as a temporizing and lifesaving measure by placing a large-bore angiocath into the second intercostal space in the midclavicular line of the affected hemithorax [9]. Upon arrival to the trauma center, a thoracostomy tube should be placed. Evacuation of intrapleural air or blood allows for lung re-expansion, facilitates appropriate oxygenation and ventilation, and decreases the risk of lung injury. Lastly, surveillance of hemothorax will be a factor guiding resuscitation, and findings may prompt an immediate need to proceed to the operating room. Anesthesia for thoracic trauma has its own unique considerations and will be covered in a separate chapter in this text.

## Circulation with Hemorrhage Control

Hemorrhage is responsible for 30–40% of trauma deaths, up to 56% of those occurring prior to arrival at a hospital [10]. In patients that survive to hospitalization, the combination of hypothermia, acidosis, and coagulopathy act as a positive feedback loop that worsens mortality. In an early retrospective review of 71 patients with injury severity score > 25 and truncal trauma, 100% of patients with a core body temperature below 32 °C died. In comparison, mortality rates for patients with core temperatures <33 °C and <34 °C were 69% and 40% respectively. Patients whose body temperature remained 34 °C or higher had a mortality rate of 7% [11]. Hypothermia has deleterious effects on the cardiovascular system, enzymatic reactions, and the coagulation cascade. During the primary assessment, a patient should receive two large-bore (16G or larger) intravenous catheters and resuscitation begun with a warmed crystalloid solution. Further discussion of fluid resuscitation occurs later in this chapter. Pressure should be applied to visible bleeding. Non-visible bleeding can occur in the chest, abdomen, and pelvis, and must be detected utilizing physical examination or imaging modalities. Long bone fractures can also account for significant hemorrhage. Table 69.1 provides essential information regarding classification of Hemorrhage.

There is a high incidence of injury to the spleen and liver in abdominal trauma, which can be diagnosed utilizing abdominal imaging. Although the Focused Assessment with Sonography for Trauma [FAST] exam is widely utilized to evaluate blunt abdominal injuries, it has been shown repeatedly to under diagnose intra-abdominal injuries, with variable sensitivities (42–99.8%) being reported [12–17]. Furthermore, a prospective observational study of 547 trauma patients at a level 1 trauma center revealed that a secondary ultrasound examination performed between 30 min and 24 h after arrival increased the sensitivity of detection of abdominal injury from 31.1% on initial assessment to 72.1% on second look [18]. Serial exams are recommended to detect intraperitoneal fluid accumulation that is suspicious for intra-abdominal traumatic injury. In stable patients, computed tomography (CT) is indicated for definitive diagnosis [14].

In pelvic injuries, damage control using an abdominal binder remains the initial treatment. Consultation with an interventional radiologist determines need for angiography with possible embolization of bleeding vessels. Immobilization of known extremity fractures with frequent pulse checks precedes operative management. Hemorrhagic shock is the most common cause of shock in trauma, and can be the result of internal hemorrhage. The patient's initial response to fluid resuscitation, paired with diagnostic findings, guides the decision to proceed to surgical intervention.

## Disability/Neurologic Assessment

Initial neurologic assessment utilizing a mnemonic "AVPU" is discussed as part of the primary survey in ATLS. "AVPU" stands for Alert, Verbal, Painful, Unresponsive, and denotes different levels of consciousness. Use of this mnemonic is swift, but not objective. The Glasgow Coma Scale (GCS, Table 69.2) is an objective neurological scale utilized to record and trend level of consciousness in trauma victims. A baseline neurologic status is critical such that developing changes can be immediately recognized and evaluated. Calculation of the GCS involves a three-component scoring system, adding the best score present for eye opening, verbal response, and motor response. A GCS < 8 in a trauma patient likely indicates need for airway intervention to prevent untoward outcomes such as

**Table 69.1** Classification of hemorrhage

| Estimated blood loss[a] based on patient's initial presentation | | | | |
|---|---|---|---|---|
| | Class I | Class II | Class III | Class IV |
| Blood loss (mL) | Up to 750 | 750–1500 | 1500–2000 | >2000 |
| Blood loss (% of blood volume) | Up to 15% | 15–30% | 30–40% | >40% |
| Pulse rate (BPM) | <100 | 100–120 | 120–140 | >140 |
| Systolic blood pressure | Normal | Normal | Decreased | Decreased |
| Pulse pressure (mmHg) | Normal or increased | Decreased | Decreased | Decreased |
| Respiratory rate | 14–20 | 20–30 | 30–40 | >35 |
| Urine output (mL/h) | >30 | 20–30 | 5–15 | Negligible |
| CNS/mental status | Slightly anxious | Mildly anxious | Anxious, confused | Confused, lethargic |
| Initial fluid replacement | Crystalloid | Crystalloid | Crystalloid and blood | Crystalloid and blood |

[a]For a 70-kg man

**Table 69.2** Glasgow Coma Scale

| Score | Eye | Verbal | Motor |
|---|---|---|---|
| 1 | Does not open eyes | Does not make sounds | No movement |
| 2 | Opens eyes to painful stimuli | Incomprehensible sounds | Decerebrate [Extension to painful stimuli] |
| 3 | Open eyes to voice | Incoherent words | Decorticate [Flexion to painful stimuli] |
| 4 | Spontaneously opens eyes | Confused or disoriented speech | Flexion/Withdrawal to painful stimuli |
| 5 | Not applicable | Oriented, normal conversation | Localizes to painful stimuli |
| 6 | Not applicable | Not applicable | Obeys motor commands |

aspiration, hypoxia, and hypercarbia. However, a decreased GCS score does not mandate intubation in all trauma patients, specifically those intoxicated with drugs or alcohol [19]. The GCS is modified with the letter "C" for "closed" if the eyes are swollen shut, damaged, or not present. It can also be modified with a "T" for "tube" if an endotracheal or tracheostomy tube are present. GCS scoring is less applicable to children because many are too young to be expected to generate an appropriate verbal response.

Patients with a score less than 8–9 have an impaired level of consciousness. These patients have increased anesthetic risk secondary to prior loss of airway reflexes, depressed level of consciousness, intracranial injury, and an inability to give a medical history. Severely injured patients have the potential for altered sensitivity or reaction to anesthetic agents depending on injury complex. Another factor that increases the risk of death from trauma, which is commonly found in trauma patients, is substance abuse. Approximately 40% of motor vehicle crash deaths involve alcohol, and alcohol is responsible for approximately half of all trauma deaths and nonfatal injuries in the United States [20].

## Exposure/Environmental Control

The final component to the primary survey involves full exposure of the patient and subsequent control of environmental factors. A patient's clothing should be removed or cut away, with the goal to reveal further injuries that may otherwise be unrecognized. At this point in the primary survey, a logroll is generally performed to assess for spine injury. Warm blankets or a warming device is swiftly applied to the patient to mitigate heat loss leading to hypothermia, and the temperature of the trauma bay (and operating room) should be raised to slow the onset of hypothermia.

## Secondary and Tertiary Survey

If the patient is stable, ATLS proceeds with a secondary and tertiary survey. The secondary survey is a systematic head-to-toe examination of the patient. A complete history is also taken at this point in the algorithm. Radiographs and/or computed tomography, as relevant, are obtained. If the patient becomes unstable, the primary survey is restarted to guide resuscitation and elucidate any life-threatening injuries that were missed on a prior survey. The tertiary survey is simply a serial reexamination to find missed injuries and to generate a complete injury complex.

## The Operating Room

### Introduction

At a level 1 trauma center, an operating room is always prepared and available for emergency surgery. Rapid information gathering and patient assessment occurs upon patient arrival. The great majority of trauma surgery is performed under general anesthesia, which necessitates rapid sequence induction and intubation if an airway is not already in place. Special considerations for airway management are discussed in the airway assessment section. Many trauma patients present in hypovolemic shock with superimposed organ dysfunction; care must be taken to mitigate changes in hemodynamics, to provide guided and rapid resuscitation and to prevent and treat trauma-induced coagulopathy. These decisions and management impact patient survival.

## Pre-arrival Preparation

A designated trauma operating room should be prepared with a comprehensive set of tools and medications necessary to safely resuscitate and anesthetize the whole spectrum of trauma patients. In addition to standard American Society of Anesthesiologists monitors, invasive monitors should be available including arterial and central venous access. Intravenous (IV) line kits are recommended to provide fast vascular access. A "dry" setup for fluid warming devices is appropriate. A rapid transfusion device must be checked and available in the room. An arterial line, pressure bag, and transducer should be primed and zeroed. Emergency resuscitation drugs must be available in all trauma operating rooms. Point of care blood gas analysis should be immediately available to the anesthesia team. If the hospital provides for uncrossmatched blood in an OR refrigerator, availability and expiration should be confirmed each shift. If possible to obtain, the patient's gender provides vital information so that appropriate uncrossmatched blood can be secured from the blood bank: O-positive for males or O-negative for females of childbearing age.

## Arrival in the Operating Room

In conscious patients, a quick screen for medication allergies, medical history, surgical history, history of anesthetic complications, oral intake status, and home medications is performed. The trauma team should communicate details of the trauma mechanism and injury complex, along with the surgical plan. Preoxygenation should be started immediately while standard ASA monitors are applied.

## Induction of Anesthesia and Airway Management

Induction of anesthesia in the trauma patient must account for patient instability and anticipated changes in hemodynamics; trauma patients may present as exquisitely sensitive to many anesthetics due to vasodilatory and cardiac depressive effects. Young, stable patients may not require significant changes to rapid sequence induction and intubation, whereas patients that present in *extremis* may require little to no anesthetic to optimize intubating conditions due to depressed level of consciousness or lack of muscle tone. Preoxygenation is critical in the trauma population, as overall oxygen consumption is increased due to the patient's sympathetic drive, and shock states result in decreased oxygen delivery to tissues. Rapid sequence induction is required. Since its introduction by Sellick in 1961 [21], the application of cricoid pressure has been accepted as the standard of care as an attempt to prevent regurgitation of gastric contents in individuals at a high risk of aspiration. However, evidence is lacking regarding its efficacy, and a study of 52 trials evaluating cricoid pressure revealed an absence of quality evidence for or against the practice [22]. A "defasciculating" dose of nondepolarizing neuromuscular blocking agent (0.03 mg/kg for rocuronium) may be utilized for pre-curarization. This may decrease fasciculations, myalgias, and catecholamine release related to succinylcholine administration. Patient factors such as closed head injury or known hyperkalemia may preclude use of succinylcholine. In these settings rocuronium can also be used to facilitate rapid sequence intubation. A retrospective cohort study examining brain-injured patients undergoing RSI in the emergency department did not demonstrate a significant increase in mortality when succinylcholine was utilized instead of rocuronium in patients with low severity of head injury. However, in patients that fell into a high-severity group [severe or critical head injury], a significant increase in mortality occurred when succinylcholine was used [23]. Propofol induction in trauma patients is appropriate but must be used with caution. Propofol is of limited use in patients with conditions worsened by limited venous preload (hemorrhagic shock, cardiac tamponade). Etomidate is an alternative induction agent and prevents further cardiac depression in unstable patients. Ketamine preserves spontaneous ventilation, has sympathomimetic hemodynamic effects, and is a potent analgesic. It is therefore often an ideal induction agent in the trauma patient.

## Maintenance of Anesthesia

Volatile anesthetics remain the foundation of anesthetic maintenance in trauma. As with any anesthetic, analgesics may be titrated to effect if the patient can tolerate blunting of their sympathetic response to pain. Minimum alveolar concentration (MAC) is decreased in trauma patients by as much as 25% [24]. In unstable patients, neuromuscular blockade is monitored and re-dosed vigilantly, because the tolerated volatile anesthetic is often inadequate to prevent movement in the patient. Due to their inability to tolerate even moderate anesthetic doses, trauma patients experience a higher incidence of intraoperative recall [25]. If concern for inadequate anesthetic depth arises, amnestic agents, such as benzodiazepines or intravenous scopolamine, may be considered. Furthermore, the anesthesiologist may choose to utilize frontal EEG monitoring in an attempt to guide anesthetic depth.

## Resuscitation

Regaining homeostasis through resuscitation as the trauma team works to control hemorrhage or repair injury is a key component of the trauma anesthetic. Blood loss yields hypotension, hypoperfusion, and ultimately cellular ischemia. It is paramount to address acute hemorrhage and hemorrhagic shock before organ failure becomes irreversible. Even after resuscitation, reperfusion injury can occur and lead to worsened coagulopathy or end-organ dysfunction. All efforts to temporize or treat a patient in hemorrhagic shock begin with recognition. The American College of Surgeons ATLS Classification of Hemorrhage Severity notes that up to 30% of a patient's circulating blood volume may be lost before a drop in systolic blood pressure occurs [26].

Replacement of circulating volume begins with a temporizing crystalloid solution followed by blood product administration. Volume expansion with crystalloid increases venous return and subsequently cardiac output. The clinical evidence currently available on resuscitation with colloids does not support their use in trauma patients. Specific concerns with various colloid solutions include: increased mortality in patients with traumatic brain injury, worsening coagulopathy, higher cost of intervention, and inability to show volume or blood product sparing when colloids are used [27]. At this time, the use of colloid—whether albumin or Hydroxyethyl starch—is not recommended for trauma resuscitation [28].

Class III hemorrhage indicates that the patient needs blood products. Aggressive fluid resuscitation with crystalloid solution has been shown to be potentially detrimental if crystalloid is rapidly administered to a patient prior to control of bleeding. Over-resuscitation with crystalloid results in dilutional thrombocytopenia and worsening coagulopathy. As crystalloid is administered out of proportion to blood products, blood pressure may increase; however, when blood pressure elevates prior to source control, this yields more blood loss and jeopardizes endogenous hemostasis by compromising soft clot [29]. Aggressive crystalloid administration is associated with shorter survival [30].

The goal of trauma resuscitation is to ensure appropriate tissue oxygen delivery, replace needed clotting factors, and replete electrolytes. The initial phase of hypovolemia directly results from acute bleeding. Although several studies have looked at timing of fluid resuscitation in trauma patients with uncontrolled hemorrhage, withholding resuscitation until operative management remains controversial. Permissive hypotension has been shown to increase mortality in patients with traumatic brain injury [31]. Maintenance of normotension in the preoperative setting may be the safest approach. A previous prospective randomized controlled trial examining hypotensive resuscitation with a MAP goal of 50 mmHg was ended early, due to the Inability to demonstrate reduced 30-day mortality or transfusion requirements [32].

The complexities of blood banking and storage have made whole-blood unavailable for transfusion at this time. Particular care is taken in trauma patients to replace individual factors in appropriate ratios. Trauma resuscitation studies note a significant survival advantage if blood products are administered in a ratio that mimics whole blood, specifically when fresh frozen plasma (FFP) and platelets are administered early [33]. Thus, many trauma centers have adopted massive transfusion protocols (MTP) that dictate how products are administered during resuscitation efforts. Historically, massive transfusion has been defined as the transfusion of ten units of packed red blood cells (pRBC) in a 24-h period. These protocols allow providers, the blood bank, and hospital resources to singularly be directed toward the same goal. It is well recognized today that massive transfusion cannot only include pRBCs and protocols are moving to include all blood components. There is, however, still question about the ideal transfusion ratio. *The Prospective, Observational, Multicenter, Major Trauma Transfusion* (PROMMTT) Study, published in 2013, demonstrated that higher early ratios of plasma and platelets to pRBCs decreased 6 h mortality. Patients resuscitated using ratios <1:2 were three times more likely to die during the first 6 h of resuscitation when hemorrhagic shock predominates trauma fatality [34]. Given these results, The Pragmatic Randomized Optimal Platelet and Plasma Ratios (PROPPR) Trial examined 680 severely injured trauma patients (11,185 screened) at 12 level 1 trauma centers in North America to compare a transfusion ratio of 1:1:1 plasma, platelets, and red blood cells to a 1:1:2 ratio. The study showed no difference in 24-h or 30-day mortality between groups, however, there was a statistically significant decrease in death due to exsanguination in the 1:1:1 group (9.2%) versus the 1:1:2 group (14.6%) at the 24-h interval [35].

Antifibrinolytic therapy is also a growing part of trauma resuscitation and massive transfusion. In the 2010 'Clinical Randomization of an Antifibrinolytic in Significant Hemorrhage-2 (CRASH2) Trial,' early administration of transexamic acid (within 3 h of injury), reduced all-cause mortality, as well as risk of death specifically due to bleeding in adult trauma patients [36]. At the 4-week interval, TXA was associated with a 1.5% absolute reduction in mortality when compared to placebo. Table 69.3 outlines recent literature examining trialed interventions to decrease blood product administration, morbidity and mortality during resuscitation efforts.

In addition to resuscitation and antifibrinolytic therapy, aggressive patient temperature management should be employed in the trauma OR for the reasons mentioned previously in this chapter. Strategies utilized to combat hypothermia include: elevated ambient OR temperature, forced air warming devices, heating elements on rapid transfusion devices, fluid warmers on intravenous lines, and lowest allowable fresh gas flows for a specific volatile anesthetic agent.

## Vasopressors

The role of vasopressors remains controversial in trauma resuscitation. The current literature has insufficient clinical evidence to conclusively show harm or benefit when vasopressors are used *intermittently* in trauma [45]. Although no clinical studies have yet validated any vasopressor support for the management of hemorrhagic shock [45], the VITRIS (Vasopressin in Traumatic Hemorrhagic Shock Study) Trial—a multicenter randomized placebo-controlled trial assessing vasopressin versus placebo in refractory traumatic hemorrhagic shock patients—has been completed and is being analyzed. This may provide some insight into the use of vasopressin specifically. When given judiciously in association with

**Table 69.3** Resuscitation interventions trialed in trauma patients

| Study name | Year | Type of study | Primary result |
|---|---|---|---|
| Immediate versus delayed fluid resuscitation for hypotensive patients with penetrating torso injuries [29] | 1994 | Prospective RCT, single hospital, 598 adults with penetrating torso injuries, hypotensive at presentation evaluating immediate vs. delayed resuscitation. | Delayed resuscitation (until patient had operative intervention for their injuries) results in increased survival. |
| SAFE [37], SAFE-TBI [38], and SAFE-TBI II [39] | 2004, 2007, 2013 | Multicenter, double blind, parallel group, RCT. 6997 ICU patients, including trauma and TBI subsets examining albumin to saline resuscitation in ICU. | **SAFE**: No difference in all-cause mortality at 28 d. Subgroup analysis demonstrated albumin leads to worse outcomes in TBI. **SAFE-TBI**: significant increase in mortality at 24 months in albumin group. **SAFE-TBI II**: (post-hoc analysis) Albumin may lead to elevated ICP and reduced CPP. |
| First report on safety and efficacy of hetastarch solution for initial fluid resuscitation at a level 1 trauma center [40] | 2008 | At surgeon discretion (not randomized), hetastarch administered as single bolus during initial fluid resuscitation. Care after bolus otherwise identical. 1714 enrollees with blunt or penetrating trauma. | Multivariate analysis reveals no significant difference in mortality between groups. Lower overall mortality in penetrating subgroup that received hetastarch however, higher rates of ICU admission, blood product administration, ARDS, and sepsis in hetastarch cohort. |
| CRASH-2 [36] | 2010 | Multicenter RCT. 20,207 trauma patients, 274 hospitals, 40 countries evaluating use of TXA vs. placebo. | TXA, when administered within 3 h of trauma, reduces all cause-mortality, and death due to bleeding. |
| Association of 6% hetastarch resuscitation with adverse outcomes in critically ill trauma patients [41] | 2011 | Retrospective review of 2225 adult, severely injured trauma patients, admitted to ICU. Evaluated used of hetastarch as a component of resuscitation | Hetastarch group: higher in-hospital mortality, increased total fluid requirement, increased blood product transfusion, AKI and mortality. |
| MATTERs [42] | 2012 | Retrospective, observational trial of 896 combat trauma patients in Afghanistan | TXA, when given to patients receiving ≥1unit reduces mortality. In MTP resuscitation, TXA is associated with increased survival and decreased coagulopathy. |
| Effect of hetastarch bolus in trauma patients requiring emergency surgery [43] | 2012 | Retrospective, cohort, observational study of 281 patients with blunt or penetrating trauma. | Resuscitated with standard of care vs. standard of care plus hetastarch bolus. Use of hetastarch leads to higher rates of anemia, thrombocytopenia, transfusion. No mortality difference observed. |
| PROMMTT [44] | 2013 | Prospective, multicenter, observational cohort study at 10 level I trauma centers. Eligible if age > 16 and received ≥1uPRBC in first 6 h of admission. 1245 patients. | Early administration of high ratio FFP and platelets to pRBCs decrease in-hospital mortality in the first 6 h in patients with substantial bleeding. Ratios <1:2 are associated with 3× higher mortality in first 6 h. Low plasma ratio was associated with higher risk of death at 24 h. Transfusion ratios do not impact 30 d mortality in those that survive to 24 h. |
| PROPPR [35] | 2015 | Phase 3, multisite RCT of 680 severely-injured trauma patients requiring MT. 12 level I trauma centers in North America, followed up at 24 h and 30 d | No difference in mortality at 24 h or 30 d between a 1:1:1 and 1:1:2 administration of plasma, platelets, and red blood cells in patients who present in hemorrhagic shock requiring MT. Decreased mortality due to exsanguination at 24 h in the 1:1:1 group. |

*RCT* randomized controlled trial, *TBI* traumatic brain injury, *ICU* intensive care unit, *TXA* tranexamic acid, *AKI* acute kidney injury, *ARDS* adult respiratory distress syndrome, *pRBC* packed red blood cells, *MTP* massive transfusion, *d* day, *h* hour fluids, vasopressors *may* offer advantages in trauma patients to improve end-organ perfusion. At this time, routine use of vasopressors should likely be held until surgical hemostasis and appropriate resuscitation has been achieved.

## Laboratory Monitoring

On arrival to the OR, initial labs should be sent including arterial blood gas, complete blood count, complete metabolic panel, coagulation panel, and type and screen. Placement of invasive arterial access will allow for frequent laboratory sampling and hemodynamic monitoring, and should be considered based on projected blood loss, anticipated or witnessed hemodynamic instability. Point of care testing and blood gas analysis in the OR allows the anesthesiologist to follow acid base disturbances, electrolytes, hyper- and hypoglycemia, lactic acid levels, and base deficit measurements to evaluate efficacy of resuscitation. Hematocrit can also be assessed with point of care testing; however, the results may be inaccurate in the rapidly bleeding patient. Special attention should be given to calcium repletion during rapid blood transfusion secondary to citrate chelation. Citrate is the anticoagulant utilized in stored blood products. Small quantities are rapidly metabolized by the liver however, massive transfusion results in plasma citrate levels that outpace hepatic metabolism. Subsequently, citrate binds both calcium and magnesium and can cause cardiac dysrhythmias, vasoplegia and hypotension, negative inotropy, and hypocoagulability [Calcium is Factor IV in the coagulation cascade].

Increasingly, point of care testing of coagulation with thromboelastography is being evaluated and utilized in the trauma operating room. At present, the most recent Cochrane Review (2016) assessing efficacy of thromboelastography (TEG and ROTEM) in guiding use of blood products noted a trend to reduce the need for blood product transfusion. However, the quality of the evidence is "low," with a "high risk of bias," and not directly applicable to trauma, as the majority of the trials were performed in cardiac surgical patients [46].

The last laboratory markers worth noting are lactate level and base deficit (BD). Lactate levels in trauma patients are a direct measure of anaerobic metabolism, whereas base deficit is calculated and may be affected by other factors such as fluctuations in hemoglobin or $CO_2$ (which may change significantly during a trauma resuscitation), administration of chloride-containing solutions, ketoacidosis, or even renal dysfunction. Both lab values are frequently available via in-OR point of care testing and while elevations in either can predict overall mortality, the initial lactate value has been demonstrated to better predict in-hospital mortality when compared to initial BD [47, 48].

## Burns and Head Injury

It is the job of the anesthesiologist to begin fluid resuscitation of burn patients, and to manage elevated intracranial pressure in the operating room. Separate chapters in this text entitled "Anesthesia for Burns" and "Perioperative Management of Adult Patients with Severe Head Injury" are devoted to these frequently encountered sequelae of trauma. Ultimately, traumatic brain injury is the most common cause of death by injury in the United States, even more so than hemorrhage.

## Post-operative Care

Although initial resuscitation efforts occur in the OR and hemorrhage and injury control is surgically achieved, postoperative care is a continuum of original care principles. Treatment of hypothermia, coagulopathy and hypovolemia are key components of trauma management in the intensive care unit. End-organ perfusion may continue to be at risk for several hours despite surgical correction of life-threatening injuries. Further radiographic examination often immediately follows operative management of life-threatening injuries. After arrival in the ICU or PACU, full report should be given to the receiving team including what is known about the patient and their mechanism of trauma, existing vascular access, prior airway management, fluid status, intraoperative events, and any other pertinent patient-specific factors that will aid in resuscitation and recovery. Thorough—and even protocolized—handoffs have been shown to reduce medical errors and subsequently improve patient outcomes [49, 50].

## References

1. Centers for Disease Control and Prevention, National Center for Injury Prevention and Control. Web-based Injury Statistics Query and Reporting System (WISQARS). http://www.cdc.gov/injury/wisqars. Accessed 12 Dec 2016.
2. Smith JS Jr, Martin LF, Young WW, Macioce DP. Do trauma centers improve outcome over non-trauma centers: the evaluation of regional trauma care using discharge abstract data and patient management categories. J Trauma. 1990;30(12):1533–8.
3. American College of Surgeons. About Advanced Trauma Life Support. https://www.facs.org/quality-programs/trauma/atls/about. Accessed 12 Dec 2016.
4. Ottosson A. Aspiration and obstructed airways as the cause of death in 158 consecutive traffic fatalities. J Trauma. 1985;25(6):538–40.
5. Yates DW. Airway patency in fatal accidents. Br Med J. 1977;2:1249–51.
6. McNicholl BP. The golden hour and prehospital trauma care. Injury. 1994;25(4):251–4.
7. Milby AH, Halpern CH, Guo W, Stein SC. Prevalence of cervical spinal injury in trauma. Neurosurg Focus. 2008;25(5):E10. https://doi.org/10.3171/FOC.2008.25.11.E10.
8. Dries DJ, Endorf FW. Inhalation injury: epidemiology, pathology, treatment strategies. Scand J Trauma Resusc Emerg Med. 2013;21:31.
9. Waydhas C, Sauerland S. Pre-hospital pleural decompression and chest tube placement after blunt trauma: a systematic review. Resuscitation. 2007;72(1):11–25.
10. Kauvar DS, Lefering R, Wade CE. Impact of hemorrhage on trauma outcome: an overview of epidemiology, clinical presentations, and therapeutic considerations. J Trauma. 2006 Jun;60(6 Suppl):S3–11.
11. Jurkovich GJ, Greiser WB, Luterman A, Curreri PW. Hypothermia in trauma victims: an ominous predictor of survival. J Trauma. 1987;27(9):1019–24.
12. Kornezos I, Chatziioannou A, Kokkonouzis I, et al. Eur Radiol. 2010;20:234. https://doi.org/10.1007/s00330-009-1516-1.
13. Kimura A, Otsuka T. Emergency center ultrasonography in the evaluation of hemoperitoneum: a prospective study. J Trauma. 1991;31(1):20–3.
14. Miller MT, Pasquale MD, Bromberg WJ, Wasser TE, Cox J. Not so FAST. J Trauma. 2003;54(1):52–9. discussion 59–60
15. Jehle D, Guarino J, Karamanoukian H. Emergency department ultrasound in the evaluation of blunt abdominal trauma. Am J Emerg Med. 1993;11(4):342–6.
16. Lee BC, Ormsby EL, McGahan JP, et al. The utility of sonography for the triage of blunt abdominal trauma patients to exploratory laparotomy. AJR Am J Roentgenol. 2007;188:415–21.
17. McKenney KL, Nunez DB, McKenney MG, Asher J, Zelnick K, Shipshak D. Sonography as the primary screening technique for blunt abdominal trauma: experience with 899 patients. AJR Am J Roentgenol. 1998;170:979–85.
18. Blackbourne LH, Soffer D, McKenney M, Amortegui J, Schulman CI, Crookes B, et al. Secondary ultrasound examination increases the sensitivity of the FAST exam in blunt trauma. J Trauma. 2004;57(5):934–8.
19. Duncan R, Thakore S. Decreased Glasgow Coma Scale score does not mandate endotracheal intubation in the emergency department. J Emerg Med. 2009;37(4):451–5. https://doi.org/10.1016/j.jemermed.2008.11.026. Epub 2009 Mar 9
20. Rivara FP, Jurkovich GJ, Gurney JG, Seguin D, Fligner CL, Ries R, et al. The magnitude of acute and chronic alcohol abuse in trauma patients. Arch Surg. 1993;128(8):907–12. discussion 912–3
21. Sellick BA. Cricoid pressure to control regurgitation of stomach contents during induction of anaesthesia. Lancet. 1961;2(7199):404–6.
22. Nilipovitz DT, Crosby ET. No evidence for decreased incidence of aspiration after rapid sequence induction. Can J Anaesth. 2007;54(9):748–64.
23. Patanwala AE, Erstad BL, Roe DJ, Sakles JC. Succinylcholine is associated with increased mortality when used for rapid sequence intubation of severely brain injured patients in the emergency department. Pharmacotherapy. 2016;36(1):57–63. https://doi.org/10.1002/phar.1683.
24. Varon AJ, Smith CE. Essentials of trauma anesthesia. Cambridge: Cambridge University Press; 2012. pg 87
25. Domino KB, Posner KL, Caplan RA, Cheney FW. Awareness during anesthesia: a closed claims analysis. Anesthesiology. 1999;90(4):1053–61.
26. American College of Surgeons Committee on Trauma. Ch 3: Shock. In: Advanced trauma life support: student course manual. 9th ed. Chicago, IL: American College of Surgeons; 2012. p. 62–81.
27. Jabaley C, Dudaryk R. Fluid resuscitation for trauma patients: crystalloids versus colloids. Curr Anesthesiol Rep. 2014;4:216. https://doi.org/10.1007/s40140-014-0067-4.
28. Perel P, Roberts I, Ker K. Colloids versus crystalloids for fluid resuscitation in critically ill patients. Cochrane Database Syst Rev. 2007;4:CD000567.
29. Bickell WH, Wall MJ Jr, Pepe PE, Martin RR, Ginger VF, Allen MK, Mattox KL. Immediate versus delayed fluid resuscitation for hypotensive patients

with penetrating torso injuries. N Engl J Med. 1994;331(17):1105–9.
30. Solomonov E, Hirsh M, Yahiya A, Krausz MM. The effect of vigorous fluid resuscitation in uncontrolled hemorrhagic shock after massive splenic injury. Crit Care Med. 2000;28(3):749–54.
31. Kochanek PM, Carney N, Adelson PD, Ashwal S, Bell MJ, Bratton S, et al. Guidelines for the acute medical management of severe traumatic brain injury in infants, children, and adolescents – Second edition. Pediatr Crit Care Med. 2012;13(Suppl 1):S1–82.
32. Carick MM, Morrison CA, Tapia NM, Leonard J, Suliburk JW, Norman MA, et al. Intraoperative hypotensive resuscitation for patients undergoing laparotomy or thoracotomy for trauma: early termination of a randomized prospective clinical trial. J Trauma Acute Care Surg. 2016;80(6):886–96. https://doi.org/10.1097/TA.0000000000001044.
33. Zink KA, Sambasivan CN, Holcomb JB, Chisholm G, Schreiber MA. A high ratio of plasma and platelets to packed red blood cells in the first 6 hours of massive transfusion improves outcomes in a large multicenter study. Am J Surg. 2009;197(5):565–70; discussion 570
34. Holcomb JB, del Junco Deborah J, Fox EE, for the PROMMTT Study Group. The Prospective, Observational, Multicenter, Major Trauma Transfusion (PROMMTT) Study. JAMA Surg. 2013;148(2):127–136.
35. Holcomb JB, Tilley BC, Baraniuk S, Fox EE, Wade CE, Podbielski JM, et al. Transfusion of plasma, platelets, and red blood cells in a 1:1:1 vs a 1:1:2 ratio and mortality in patients with severe trauma: the PROPPR randomized clinical trial. JAMA. 2015;313(5):471–82. https://doi.org/10.1001/jama.2015.12.
36. Roberts I, Shakur H, Coats T, Hunt B, Balogun E, Barnetson L, Cook L, et al. The CRASH-2 trial: a randomised controlled trial and economic evaluation of the effects of tranexamic acid on death, vascular occlusive events and transfusion requirement in bleeding trauma patients. Health Technol Assess. 2013;17(10):1–79. https://doi.org/10.3310/hta17100.
37. Finfer S, Bellomo R, Boyce N, French J, Myburgh J, Norton R, et al. A comparison of albumin and saline for fluid resuscitation in the intensive care unit. N Engl J Med. 2004;350(22):2247–56.
38. Myburgh J, Cooper DJ, Finfer S, Bellomo R, Norton R, Bishop N, et al. Saline or albumin for fluid resuscitation in patients with traumatic brain injury. N Engl J Med. 2007;357(9):874–84.
39. Cooper D, Myburgh J, Heritier S, Finfer S, Bellomo R, Billot L, et al. Albumin resuscitation for traumatic brain injury: is intracranial hypertension the cause of increased mortality? J Neurotrauma. 2013;30(7):512–8.
40. Ogilvie MP, Pereira BM, McKenny MG, McMahon PJ, Manning RJ, Namais N, et al. First report on safety and efficacy of hetastarch solution for initial fluid resuscitation at a Level 1 trauma center. J Am Coll Surg. 2010;210(5):870–80.
41. Lissauer ME, Chi A, Kramer ME, Scalea TM, Johnson SB. Association of 6% hetastarch resuscitation with adverse outcomes in critically ill trauma patients. Am J Surg. 2011;202(1):53–8.
42. Morrison JJ, Dubose JJ, Rasmussen TE, Midwinter MJ. Military Application of Tranexamic Acid in Trauma Emergency Resuscitation (MATTERs) Study. Arch Surg. 2012;147(2):113–9. https://doi.org/10.1001/archsurg.2011.287. Epub 2011 Oct 17
43. Ryan ML, Ogilvie MP, Pereira BM, Gomez-Rodriguz JC, Livingstone AS, Proctor KG. Effect of hetastarch bolus in trauma patients requiring emergency surgery. J Spec Oper Med. 2012;12(3):57–67.
44. Holcomb JB, del Junco Deborah J, Fox EE, for the PROMMTT Study Group. The prospective, observational, multicenter, major trauma transfusion (PROMMTT) study. JAMA Surg. 2013;148(2):127–36.
45. Beloncle F, Meziani F, Lerolle N, Radermacher P, Asfar P. Does vasopressor therapy have an indication in hemorrhagic shock? Ann Intensive Care. 2013;3:13. https://doi.org/10.1186/2110-5820-3-13.
46. Wikkelsø A, Wetterslev J, Møller AM, Afshari A. Thromboelastography (TEG) or thromboelastometry (ROTEM) to monitor haemostatic treatment versus usual care in adults or children with bleeding. Cochrane Database Syst Rev. 2016(8). Art. No.: CD007871. DOI:10.1002/14651858.CD007871.pub3.
47. Gale SC, Kocik JF, Creath R, Crystal JS, Dombrovskiy VY. A comparison of initial lactate and initial base deficit as predictors of mortality after severe blunt trauma. J Surg Res. 2016;205(2):446–55. https://doi.org/10.1016/j.jss.2016.06.103. Epub 2016 Jul 5.
48. Raux M, Le Manach Y, Gauss T, Baumgarten R, Hamada S, Harrois A, et al. Comparison of the prognostic significance of initial blood lactate and base deficit in trauma patients. Anesthesiology. 2017;126(3):522–33. https://doi.org/10.1097/ALN.0000000000001490.
49. Starmer AJ, Spector ND, Srivastava R, West DC, Rosenbluth G, Allen AD, et al. Changes in medical errors after implementation of a handoff program. N Engl J Med. 2014;371:1803–12. https://doi.org/10.1056/NEJMsa1405556.
50. Salzwedel C, Mai V, Punke MA, Kluge S, Reuter DA. The effect of a checklist on the quality of patient handover from the operating room to the intensive care unit: a randomized controlled trial. J Crit Care. 2016;32:170–4. https://doi.org/10.1016/j.jcrc.2015.12.016. Epub 2015 Dec 29

# Anesthesia for Pheochromocytoma and Glomus Jugulare

Courtney C. Elder and Kavitha A. Mathew

## Introduction

Patients commonly present for surgery with poorly controlled or refractory hypertension, however those with adrenal neuroendocrine pathology require additional anesthetic consideration throughout the perioperative period. Resection of pheochromocytomas (PCC) and paragangliomas (PGL) is associated with increased perioperative risk due to hypertensive and hypotensive crises and adverse cardiac events. These patients also have an increased risk of mortality due to the secretion of vasoactive catecholamines.

Historically, mortality rates in the 1950s for PCC resection were as high as 20–45%. They have since declined significantly in the past few decades to <3% [1]. The lower rates of morbidity and mortality associated with PCC and PGL resection today are frequently attributed to patient identification, preoperative pharmacologic optimization, the availability of continuous arterial blood pressure monitoring, short-acting vasoactive agents in the intraoperative setting, and improvements in surgical techniques. Although perioperative management guidelines have been established, no clear evidence-based consensus has been reached due to lack of prospective data in the field.

## Definition and Prevalence of Pheochromocytomas and Paragangliomas

Pheochromocytomas are neuroendocrine tumors that originate from neuroectodermal chromaffin tissue in the adrenal medulla. Paraganglionomas in comparison, arise from chromaffin tissue outside of the adrenal gland and account for approximately 20% of all neuroendocrine tumors. These tumors are referred to as paragangliomas (PGL) due to their frequent location along paravertebral sympathetic ganglia in the abdomen, pelvis and thorax [2]. While these highly vascular lesions can be hormonally silent, both PCCs and PGLs are capable of secreting supraphysiologic levels of catecholamines into the systemic circulation leading to a global increase in sympathetic tone.

Pheochromocytomas are exceedingly rare and account for less than 0.1% of patients with diagnosed hypertension [3, 4]. The incidence of tumor is approximately 2–8 per one million people [5], and only 5% of incidental adrenal masses found on imaging represent actual pheochromocytomas [6].

Pheochromocytomas and paragangliomas occur sporadically in the population, however approximately 25% of these tumors arise in the setting of inherited germ line mutations [5, 7].

C. C. Elder, M.D. · K. A. Mathew, M.D., M.P.H. (✉)
Emory University School of Medicine,
Atlanta, GA, USA
e-mail: ccron@emory.edu; kmathew@emory.edu

**Table 70.1** Genetic mutations associated with PCC/PGL [5, 7]

| Cancer syndrome | Genetic mutation | Tumor location | Inheritance pattern |
| --- | --- | --- | --- |
| Multiple Endocrine Neoplasia (MEN), Type 2A and 2B | RET proto-oncogene (germline) | Adrenal-bilateral | Autosomal dominant |
| Von Hippel-Lindau disease (VHL), Types 2A, 2B, and 2C | VHL tumor suppressor gene | Adrenal-bilateral | Autosomal dominant |
| Neurofibromatosis Type 1 (NF1) | NF1 gene | Adrenal | Autosomal dominant |
| PCC-PGL Syndrome (PGL-1) | SDHD gene | Head and neck, extra-adrenal | Maternal genomic imprinting |
| PCC-PGL 2 | Unknown | | Unknown |
| PCC-PGL 3 | SDHC gene | Head and Neck | |
| PCC-PGL 4 | SDHB gene | Extra-adrenal | Autosomal dominant |

*SDH* succinate dehydrogenase gene family

The most common associated mutations include Multiple Endocrine Neoplasia Type II, Von Hippel-Lindau disease, and Neurofibromatosis Type 1. Familial pheochromocytomas are more likely to be multifocal or bilaterally affect the adrenal glands (Table 70.1). Pheochromocytomas and paragangliomas have the potential for malignant spread. These tumors metastasize 10–15% of the time, but currently there is no way to distinguish tumors with malignant potential. Typical metastatic pathway is via venous and lymphatic channels to the lungs, liver and bone [3].

**Table 70.2** Frequency of signs and symptoms of pheochromocytoma. Adapted from [5]

| Signs and symptoms of pheochromocytoma | % of Patients |
| --- | --- |
| Headache | 60–90 |
| Palpitations | 50–70 |
| Sweating | 55–75 |
| Pallor | 40–45 |
| Nausea | 20–40 |
| Flushing | 10–20 |
| Weight loss | 20–40 |
| Fatigue | 25–40 |
| Psychiatric symptoms (anxiety, panic) | 20–40 |
| Hypertension | 80–90 |
| Incidentaloma | 5–10 |

## Clinical Presentation

Patients with secretory pheochromocytomas present with signs and symptoms of catecholamine excess (Table 70.2). Increased peripheral vascular resistance leading to elevated arterial blood pressure occurs due to widespread peripheral alpha-adrenergic stimulation. Patients may also endorse palpitations, tachycardia, and tremor associated with increased beta$_1$ adrenergic receptor activity. Other common presenting symptoms include headache, excessive sweating, postural hypotension, and glucose intolerance [3, 6].

Many of the symptoms associated with pheochromocytomas transpire in a paroxysmal fashion. Symptoms may also manifest incidentally during an abdominal exam. Cases reports additionally outline patients who have been diagnosed with PCC/PGL when profound hemodynamic crisis occurred on induction of general anesthesia for an unrelated procedure. The long-term sequelae of hyperadrenergic activity in this patient population includes end-organ effects such as myocardial infarction, cerebral hemorrhage, renal failure and hypertensive cardiomyopathy with left ventricular failure.

Many patients will present for preoperative evaluation prior to pheochromocytoma resection with a comprehensive endocrine workup. Anesthesiologists should include pheochromocytoma on their differential diagnosis in patients presenting for other surgical procedures with suggestive symptomology (Table 70.2). A higher index of suspicion should arise for patients with unaddressed adrenal masses on imaging, positive family history of pheochromocytoma or associated familial cancer syndrome, and reports of dysrhythmias or hemodynamic volatility with prior anesthetics.

**Fig. 70.1** Differential diagnosis for pheochromocytoma [7]

- Adrenal medullary hyperplasia
- Thyrotoxicosis
- Adrenal adenoma/cyst
- Adrenal metastasis
- Cocaine, amphetamine intoxication
- Alcohol, BZD, clonidine withdrawal
- Serotonin syndrome
- Pre-eclampsia
- Renal artery disease
- Subarachnoid hemorrhage
- MAOI-tyramine hypertensive crisis
- Anxiety/panic attacks
- Migraine/cluster headaches
- Autonomic epilepsy
- Angina pectoris, myocardial infarction
- Baroreceptor failure
- Paroxysmal tachycardias, POT syndrome
- Acute intermittent porphyria
- Hyperadrenergic hypertension
- Neuroblastoma

The differential diagnosis for pheochromocytoma is wide depending on the patient's presenting symptomology. Possible causes of similar symptomatology range widely and include other endocrine syndromes, neurologic pathology, and adverse pharmacologic interactions or medication overdose (Fig. 70.1). One of the most common conditions to mimic the physiologic effects of a pheochromocytoma is hyperadrenergic hypertension. This condition represents a state of centrally-mediated adrenergic excess that presents with hypertension, tachycardia, sweating, anxiety and increased cardiac output [7]. While both conditions present with increased circulating catecholamines, hyperadrenergic hypertension can be differentiated from a pheochromocytoma by the clonidine suppression test. Administration of clonidine will suppress central sympathetic outflow, but will not impact plasma catecholamine levels originating from a PCC/PGL tumor.

## Diagnosis

The diagnosis of a suspected PCC/PGL is established by biochemical tests measuring the plasma or urine levels of catecholamines and their metabolic byproducts. Recent guidelines developed by the Society for Endocrinology recommend initial screening with measurement of plasma free or urinary fractionated metanephrines. Compared to levels of individual catecholamines and vanillylmandelic acid (VMA), plasma free and urine metanephrines have well-established superior diagnostic sensitivity [6]. Although assessment of urinary and plasma metanephrines are considered gold-standard, it has been suggested that the clinical triad of hypertension, headache and excessive sweating is more sensitive and specific than any single biochemical test for pheochromocytoma [3].

After biochemical evidence of excess catecholamine secretion has been demonstrated, imaging should be obtained via CT, MRI or $^{123}$I-MIBG SPECT to determine the location of the tumor. It may also be appropriate for the patient to undergo genetic testing for hereditary types of PCC/PGL, particularly if the family history is suspicious for disease. This decision will likely be deferred to endocrinology specialists.

## Pathophysiology

Adrenal medullary chromaffin cells and peripheral sympathetic nerves synthesize, store and secrete epinephrine and norepinephrine. Production of catecholamines is localized to these tissues due to the tissue-specific expression of specific synthetic enzymes. The precursor amino acid tyrosine is initially converted to dopamine from L-DOPA, which is then hydroxylated by dopamine-b-hydroxylase (DBH) to form norepinephrine in chromaffin tissue. Norepinephrine is subsequently converted to epinephrine by the enzyme phenylethanolamine N-methyltransferase (PNMT) (Fig. 70.2). Dopamine secreting PCC/PGL are rare due to enzymatic conversion to norepinephrine, and occur more frequently as extra-adrenal paragangliomas. Adrenal PCCs tend to produce and store large amounts of epinephrine due to high local expression of PMNT, while extra-adrenal paragangliomas predominantly secrete norepinephrine [2].

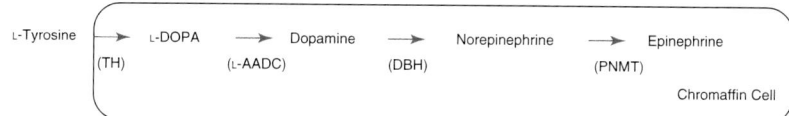

**Fig. 70.2** Catecholamine synthesis pathway

The release of norepinephrine and epinephrine into the systemic circulation causes global stimulation of adrenergic receptors. Alpha$_1$ adrenergic receptor stimulation causes increased peripheral vasoconstriction leading to elevated peripheral vascular resistance and arterial blood pressure. Alpha-receptor stimulation also increases hepatic glycogenolysis and gluconeogenesis, and inhibits pancreatic insulin release and peripheral uptake of glucose; this may cause clinically significant hyperglycemia during paroxysms of catecholamine release.

Beta$_1$ adrenergic stimulation is responsible for increased cardiac chronotropy, dromotropy and inotropy, as well as increased renin secretion. These effects contribute to increased heart rate and cardiac work in the setting of increased alpha-mediated afterload. Beta$_2$ receptor effects can lead to vasodilation and postural hypotension. Patients with pheochromocytoma are traditionally thought to present with baseline hypovolemia due to decreased plasma volume. Although volume contraction in these patients and the value of preoperative salt and fluid loading has been questioned in the existing pheochromocytoma literature [9], current guidelines continue to support preoperative fluid administration for blood volume expansion prior to surgery [6].

## Pharmacology

Pharmacologic agents utilized during the preoperative period predominantly target alpha receptor-mediated hypertension followed by control of beta receptor-mediated symptoms such as tachycardia, ectopy and dysrhythmias. Other agents such as calcium channel blockers, magnesium and tyrosine analogs are also employed.

Alpha-antagonists (selective and non-selective for the alpha$_1$ receptor) are considered first-line agents in the preoperative treatment of functional pheochromocytomas and paragangliomas. Non-selective alpha-antagonists include agents such as oral phenoxybenzamine (PBZ) or intravenous (IV) or intramuscular (IM) phentolamine. Phenoxybenzamine has a relatively long half-life of 24 h. Phentolamine is shorter-acting as an intravenous preparation and may be more useful in the acute inpatient setting. While PBZ effectively decreases arterial blood pressure, side effects can include reflex tachycardia and orthostatic hypotension [1]. Importantly, PBZ is a noncompetitive antagonist, preventing catecholamine surges from out-competing the drug at the receptor site. A primary concern with PBZ is the incidence of postoperative hypotension following pheochromocytoma resection due to prolonged alpha-blocking effects in the absence of supraphysiologic catecholamine levels.

Selective alpha$_1$-antagonists include doxazosin, prazosin, and terazosin, all more commonly known for their application in prostatic hypertrophy. These agents are competitive inhibitors at the alpha$_1$-receptor, and all but doxazosin have short half-lives compared to PBZ. These agents cause less reflex tachycardia and potentially, result in decreased postoperative hypotension. Both non-selective and selective alpha-blockade can lead to orthostatic hypotension because baroreceptor-mediated vasoconstriction is effectively blocked in these patients. This side effect has been utilized as a metric for adequacy of alpha blockade prior to surgery. In addition to anti-hypertensive effects, alpha-antagonists may also help to restore intravascular volume by promoting vasodilation.

Other agents that are used in the preoperative management of PCCs and PGLs are often employed as adjunctive therapy alongside alpha blockade. Beta-blockers can be added to the preoperative regimen to prevent or treat arrhythmias and control reflex tachycardia after the initiation of alpha-blockade [6]. The sequence of adequate alpha-blockade prior to beta blockade is a crucial consideration in the management of these patients. Beta-blockers can precipitate a hypertensive crisis when used as monotherapy due to unopposed alpha stimulation. Additionally, the sudden increase in afterload from unopposed alpha-mediated vasoconstriction with concomitant depression of cardiac function can give rise to acute decompensated heart failure and death. For this reason, beta-blockers are contraindicated in pheochromocytoma hypertension management until alpha-blockade has been successfully established.

Calcium channel blockers can be utilized as monotherapy or as adjunctive treatment for PCC-induced hypertension [8]. These agents cause minimal orthostatic hypotension, prevent coronary vasospasm and may be best tolerated in normotensive patients with paroxysmal hypertension [1, 6, 8]. Metyrosine (methyl-tyrosine) is a tyrosine analog that inhibits the enzyme tyrosine hydroxylase in the catecholamine synthesis pathway. This agent decreases catecholamine production by preventing the formation of precursor molecules. It can be used preoperatively as an adjunct to alpha-blockade if hypertension is not adequately controlled. Metyrosine is often utilized in cases of metastatic or un-resectable disease; it has not been shown to confer differences in surgical outcomes [1].

## Preoperative Evaluation, Management and Optimization

While surgical resection is the only definitive cure for pheochromocytoma, induction of general anesthesia and surgical manipulation carry the risk of hemodynamic instability, cardiac arrhythmias, myocardial infarction, stroke and death. Although mortality rates today currently approach 0% for elective resection, patients with pheochromocytoma have a 14-fold higher rate of cardiovascular morbidity during the perioperative period than those with essential hypertension [9], emphasizing the importance of careful preoperative evaluation and optimization.

In order to reduce intraoperative hemodynamic instability and ultimately postoperative morbidity and mortality, preoperative management of pheochromocytoma has conventionally focused on optimization of blood pressure and volume status prior to surgical resection. Current Endocrine Society Practice Guidelines endorse the use of alpha-antagonists as first line agents for blood pressure control in the preoperative period. These recommendations suggest a 7 to 14-day regimen for all patients with functional PCCs and PGLs prior to surgery, and implementation of a high-sodium diet with increased fluid intake for volume expansion. No randomized control trials have been completed to date on the efficacy of this regimen for reducing perioperative complications; these recommendations are based largely on retrospective studies that yield heterogeneous results.

Preoperative alpha-blockade can be achieved with either selective or nonselective alpha antagonists; neither class has demonstrated clinically significant superiority over the other [1, 7]. There is currently no consensus on the thresholds that indicate the adequacy of adrenergic blockade. Endocrine Society guidelines define optimization as blood pressure less than 130/80 while seated, a systolic blood pressure greater than 90 while standing, and heart rate between 60 and 70 bpm [6]. Other proposed parameters include no blood pressures greater than 160/90 within 24–48 h of surgery, no postural hypotension less than 80/45, no ST-T wave change on electrocardiogram one week prior to surgery, and no more than five premature ventricular contractions per minute [1, 3]. Depending on the agents used for preoperative blood pressure management, discontinuation of these agents prior to surgery should be guided by the half-life of each antihypertensive medication. Longer acting agents should be discontinued immediately prior to surgery to avoid persistent hypotension intra-operatively and in the postoperative period.

Several studies suggest that neither preoperative normalization of blood pressure nor preoperative hypertension is predictive of intraoperative hemodynamic instability or postoperative morbidity for pheochromocytoma resection [1, 4, 8,

9]. Significant hemodynamic volatility can occur despite pharmacologic optimization prior to surgery or in the setting of normal preoperative catecholamine levels [1, 10]. Additionally, it is arguable whether normotensive patients require alpha-blockade in the absence of symptoms; however, experts suggest that the benefits of potentially improved intraoperative hemodynamics outweigh the risk of alpha-blockade [6]. Patients with evidence of ischemic heart disease or hypertensive organ dysfunction should achieve normalization of blood pressure prior to surgical resection, as these conditions are associated with increased morbidity and mortality [8, 9].

Patients should be assessed for signs of hypovolemia prior to undergoing pheochromocytoma resection. Because preoperative orthostatic hypotension may be desirable as a marker of adequate alpha blockade, it may not accurately reflect preoperative volume status. Laboratory measurement of hemoglobin to assess for hemoconcentration, and blood urea nitrogen (BUN) and creatinine (Cr) to assess for pre-renal azotemia, provide objective findings to guide preoperative fluid management. Volume resuscitation in the preoperative period should be performed at the discretion of the provider; no randomized controlled trials have been performed to support this practice. According to retrospective data, fluid loading may limit postural and postoperative hypotension, but does not appear to impact outcomes.

In addition to preoperative optimization of blood pressure and volume status, patients should be monitored for fluctuations in blood glucose levels in the perioperative period. Hyperglycemia may occur due to elevated levels of circulating catecholamines, however preoperative adrenergic blockade may result in clinically significant hypoglycemia prior to surgery.

## Intraoperative Management/Surgical Technique

The relatively low morbidity and mortality rates for elective pheochromocytoma and paraganglioma resection over the past several decades can likely be attributed in part to the regular use of invasive hemodynamic monitoring and the availability of short-acting vasoactive drugs [8, 9]. These tools allow for minimization of the hemodynamic volatility associated with intraoperative catecholamine surges. Catecholamine release is frequently stimulated by induction of anesthesia, endotracheal intubation and direct tumor manipulation. It can also be triggered by patient positioning, light sedation, changes in intra-abdominal pressure with positive pressure ventilation or with creation of pneumoperitoneum. It is appropriate to place an invasive arterial line and establish adequate intravenous access prior to induction of general anesthesia in anticipation of the hemodynamic perturbation. The placement of a central venous catheter can be considered in individual patients depending on the anticipated need for central administration of vaso/venodilators, pressors and inotropes.

Induction of anesthesia and direct laryngoscopy should occur under deep anesthesia; topicalization of airway structures can also be considered to further decrease stimulation. The use of neuromuscular blockade is common, however succinylcholine is often avoided due to the increase in intra-abdominal pressure caused by widespread fasciculation with muscle depolarization. Agents that can potentially stimulate catecholamine release should be avoided, such as ketamine, ephedrine, and pancuronium. Likewise, drugs that stimulate a histaminergic response such as atracurium and morphine sulfate should not be used in this patient population. Care should be taken with use of anticholinergic agents due to loss of vagal tone.

Multiple pharmacologic approaches have been successfully used for management of intraoperative hypertension. Nitroprusside is a rapid-acting vasodilator that decreases both preload and afterload, but can cause a coronary steal phenomenon in patients with underlying CAD. Nitroglycerin acts primarily as a venodilator, but in higher doses can also produce arteriolar dilation. Dihydropyridine calcium channel blockers such as nicardipine provide short-acting arteriolar dilation, resulting in reduced afterload and improved left ventricular function.

Conversely, magnesium sulfate has not been shown to consistently produce adequate control of hypertension in pheochromocytoma [9]. The use of neuraxial techniques as primary or adjunctive anesthetics also do not provide sufficient sympathetic blockade to protect against pheochromocytoma catecholamine release.

Intraoperative hypotension encountered during pheochromocytoma resection is often seen following ligation of the tumor venous blood supply. Hypotension is likely multifactorial due to acute loss of chronic sympathetic tone, underlying hypovolemia, and persistent preoperative alpha blockade. Blood pressure normalizes in many patients following tumor removal if adequate fluid resuscitation has been achieved, however some patients may present with vasoplegic shock requiring additional adrenergic therapy, such as phenylephrine, dopamine, norepinephrine or epinephrine.

The surgical approach to pheochromocytoma and paraganglioma resection plays an important role in the outcomes of these patients. Prior to the 1990s, a majority of pheochromocytomas were resected with an open thoraco-abdominal approach or midline abdominal incision [9]. Minimally invasive laparoscopic removal of these tumors became more commonplace in the mid to late 1990s and is now considered the preferred method for tumors less than 6 cm [6]. Open procedures are reserved for large or invasive tumors to ensure complete resection with negative margins and to prevent tumor rupture [6]. Open resection continues to be more common for paragangliomas as these lesions are more frequently malignant and can be more difficult to access laparoscopically.

Occasionally, patients undergoing routine surgery for other medical conditions are found to have previously undetected pheochromocytomas. The perioperative mortality for these patients has been estimated at approximately 8% [10]. In patients with severe intraoperative hypertensive crises on induction of general anesthesia and with surgical manipulation of abdominal structures, a high index of suspicion for possible catecholamine-secreting tumors should prompt the use of intravenous alpha-blockers and nitrates to reduce hemodynamic volatility and cardiovascular morbidity.

## Postoperative Management and Complications

In the postoperative period following pheochromocytoma or paraganglioma resection, patients should undergo 24–48 h of hemodynamic monitoring. Postoperative hypotension is not uncommon following resection due to an abrupt decrease in circulating catecholamine levels with tumor removal. Residual vasoplegia may also be a consequence of persistent alpha-blockade or metyrosine activity due to the long half-lives of these agents. Postoperative hypotension is ideally treated with volume resuscitation, but may require the addition of vasopressor infusions [3, 7, 9]. Hypotension should resolve within several hours following resection of the lesion.

Patients may present in the postoperative period with residual hypertension. Elevated blood pressure in this setting could be indicative of residual or occult tumor. The differential diagnosis should also include uncontrolled pain, volume overload, autonomic instability and underlying essential hypertension. Therapy should be directed to control symptoms in the immediate postoperative period. Patients should not undergo further biochemical testing for residual tumor for at least 5–7 days to avoid confounding by surgery-induced catecholamine stimulation.

Blood glucose monitoring should continue for at least 24 h after surgery due to the concern for rebound hypoglycemia in the absence of chronic adrenergic activity.

## Directions in Research

A recent focus in pheochromocytoma research has been the preoperative use of selective versus non-selective alpha blockade. The existing body of literature on this topic is based on retrospective cohort data with varied results. Most of this data has demonstrated no superiority of one agent over the other [1, 6]. A lack of consensus definitions for hemodynamic instability and preoperative optimization confer heterogeneity to these studies, and many are confounded by variability in parameters such as surgical technique, preoperative regimens, and tumor size. A prospective, randomized controlled trial comparing non-selective phenoxybenzamine and selective doxazosin is currently underway and is set to complete data collection in 2017 (PRESCRIPT, clinicaltrials.gov).

| Plan/preparation/adverse events | Reasoning/management |
| --- | --- |
| If anticipate need for central administration of vasopressors and inotropes, consider preoperative or post-induction placement of central venous access catheter. | Hemodynamic instability is a common manifestation of pheochromocytoma, and patients with underlying cardiac dysfunction or coronary disease may require central infusion of vasoactive agents to avoid cardiovascular morbidity and mortality. |
| Preprocedural evaluation<br>  Adequacy of blood pressure control<br>  Postural hypotension<br>  Volume status<br>  Signs/symptoms of CAD, CHF<br>  Hyperglycemia | Preoperative optimization of blood pressure and volume status may decrease intraoperative hemodynamic instability. Postural/orthostatic hypotension suggests adequate alpha blockade. Patients may require intravascular volume repletion prior to procedure. |
| Position—typically lateral decubitus with kidney rest and table flexion | Anticipate possible catecholamine release with positioning. |
| IV access—large bore peripheral IV and arterial line | Consider accessibility of upper versus dependent arm in the lateral decubitus position. |
| Analgesia-<br>  Laparoscopic approach- bolus dosing of opioid narcotics<br>  Open approach- consider adjunct epidural analgesia | Decreased opioid requirements with laparoscopic approach. Epidural analgesia does not blunt sympathetic stimulation from pathologic catecholamine excess, so should be utilized primarily for postoperative pain control as indicated. |
| GA with ETT | Need for secure airway. Use of NMB and deep anesthetic can prevent detrimental sympathetic stimulation and catecholamine release. Sufficient depth of anesthesia should be achieved prior to manipulation of the airway. |
| Procedural adverse events<br>  Hyper/hypotension<br>  Dysrhythmias<br>  Intraoperative MI<br>  Hypovolemia<br>  Bleeding | As indicated |
| Postoperative and Post-Discharge Considerations<br>  Hyper/hypotension<br>  Cardiac arrhythmias<br>  Hyper/hypoglycemia | As indicated |

# References

1. Challis BG, Casey RT, Simpson HL, Gurnell M. Is there an optimal preoperative management strategy for phaeochromocytoma/paraganglioma? Clin Endocrinol. 2017;86:163–7. https://doi.org/10.1111/cen.13252.
2. Pacak K, Timmers HJ, Eisenhofer G. Pheochromocytoma. In: Jameson JL, De Groot LJ, de Kretser DM, Guidice LC, Grossman AB, Melmed S, et al., editors. Endocrinology: adult and pediatric. 7th ed. Philadelphia: Elsevier; 2016. p. 1902–30.
3. Fleisher LA, Mythen M. Anesthetic implications of concurrent diseases. In: Miller's anesthesia. 8th ed. Philadelphia: Elsevier; 2015. p. 1156–225.
4. Randle RW, Balentine CJ, Pitt SC, Schneider DF, Sippel RS. Selective versus nonselective α-blockade prior to laparoscopic adrenalectomy for pheochromocytoma. Ann Surg Oncol. 2017;24:244–50. https://doi.org/10.1245/s10434-016-5514-7.

5. Petri BJ, van Eijck CH, de Herder WW, Wagner A, de Krijer RR. Phaeochromocytomas and sympathetic paragangliomas. Br J Surg. 2009;96:1381–92. https://doi.org/10.1002/bjs.6821.
6. Lenders JW, Duh QY, Eisenhofer G, Gimenez-Roqueplo AP, Grebe SK, Murad MH, et al. Pheochromocytoma and paraganglioma: an Endocrine Society clinical practice guideline. J Clin Endocrinol Metab. 2014;99:1915–42. https://doi.org/10.1210/jc.2014-1498.
7. Weingarten TN, Weich TL, Moore TL, Walters GF, Whipple JL, Cavalcante A, et al. Preoperative levels of catecholamines and metanephrines and intraoperative hemodynamics of patients undergoing pheochromocytoma and paraganglioma resection. Urology. 2017;100:131–8. https://doi.org/10.1016/j.urology.2016.10.012.
8. Brunaud L, Nguyen-Thi PL, Miralle E, Rafaelli M, Vriens M, Theveniaud PE, et al. Predictive factors for postoperative morbidity after laparoscopic adrenalectomy for pheochromocytoma: a multicenter retrospective analysis in 225 patients. Surg Endosc. 2016;30:1051–9. https://doi.org/10.1007/s00464-015-4294-7.
9. Lentschener C, Gaujoux S, Tesniere A, Dousset B. Point of controversy: perioperative care of patients undergoing pheochromocytoma removal- time for a reappraisal? Eur J Endocrinol. 2011;165:365–73. https://doi.org/10.1530/EJE-11-0162.
10. Hariskov S, Schumann R. Intraoperative management of patients with incidental catecholamine producing tumors: a literature review and analysis. J Anaesthesiol Clin Pharamcol. 2013;29:41–6. https://doi.org/10.4103/0970-9185.105793.

# Anesthesia for TIPS

Ricky Matkins and W. Thomas Daniel III

## Introduction

Chronic liver disease is the leading cause of portal hypertension in the United States. Portal hypertension is defined as an increase in the hepatic pressure venous gradient (HPVG), often resulting in sequelae of morbid medical conditions including ascites, thrombocytopenia, esophageal varices and spontaneous bacterial peritonitis [1]. The HPVG pressure gradient is measured via catheterization of the hepatic vein and represents the pressure difference between the portal vein and inferior vena cava (IVC) [2]. A pressure gradient >5 millimeters of mercury (mmHg) meets the diagnostic criteria for portal hypertension however, clinical symptoms and disease typically present at pressures ≥10 mmHg [3]. Of great concern and importance in those patients diagnosed with portal hypertension is the presence or development of gastroesophageal (GE) varices. At the time of diagnosis, GE varices will be present in over half of patients with portal hypertension [1]. Those without varices are at risk of developing this comorbid complication at a rate of 5–9% per year [4]. Varices can become a devastating medical emergency with a 6-week mortality of 15% once ruptured [1].

R. Matkins, M.D. (✉) · W. T. Daniel III, M.D.
Emory University Hospital, Emory University School of Medicine, Atlanta, GA, USA
e-mail: rmatkin@emory.edu;
thomas.daniel.iii@emory.edu

## Pathophysiology and Anatomy

Portal hypertension most commonly develops in the setting of liver disease but can occur in the setting of portal vein thrombosis without underlying liver dysfunction [4]. Liver injury leads to fibrosis formation resulting in resistance to blood flow within the intrahepatic portal veins. Cirrhosis also causes additional architectural changes in the liver such as angiogenesis and sinusoidal remodeling which further increase vascular resistance. The end product is a reduction in portal blood flow due to the increased pressure gradient ultimately causing increased portal pressure, splanchnic vasodilation and the development of portal-collateral blood flow channels [1]. As the collateral flow surges through less resistant vessels, native portal flow declines leading to the vasoconstriction of the hepatic system. This further worsens portal hypertension and creates a continuous cycle where collateral flow surges at the expense of portal flow, further exacerbating the disease [1].

TIPS is often performed for acute variceal bleeding and refractory ascites [1]. It is minimally invasive, utilizing fluoroscopy guidance to place a catheter in the hepatic vein. Access to the vein is gained using a guidewire thread through the superior vena cava (SVC) via internal jugular access. The guidewire is then directed into the inferior vena cava (IVC) and finally into the hepatic vein. A needle is advanced through the liver parenchyma into the centralized portal vein and a tract is opened using an angioplasty balloon. Finally, a stent is deployed into the channel to create a direct shunt from the portal vein to the hepatic vein to facilitate blood flow through a low resistance pathway within the liver. Portal pressures are thus improved, and the sequelae of portal hypertension better managed [1].

## Indications and Contraindications

The primary indications for TIPS are the prevention of variceal hemorrhage and management of refractory ascites. Although there is less evidence to support TIPS in other settings, it has also been used to successfully control acute variceal bleeding, treat portal hypertensive gastropathy and augment medical treatment of hepatorenal syndrome [5]. TIPS has been demonstrated to control variceal bleeding in 93.6% of patients who fail medical therapy with only a 12.4% re-bleed rate. However, 6-week mortality in this subset of patients was 35.8% following TIPS [6]. The procedure has also been indicated for the prevention of variceal re-bleeding because it has been demonstrated to decrease the >50% risk of repeated hemorrhage in patients with varices [7, 8].

TIPS is also performed in patients with ascites refractory to medical treatment. The subgroup of patients are unresponsive to sodium restriction and high doses of diuretics, or are intolerant to the doses of diuretic therapy needed to control their disease, may demonstrate disease response following TIPS [9]. For patients frequently needing large volume paracentesis, TIPS patients experienced a 62% decrease in the need for paracentesis, as compared to only 23.6% in group using optimal medication management alone [10–14].

Hepatorenal syndrome (HRS) may be treated with TIPS but it is an indication still under investigation. In a small series of studies, both Type 1 and Type 2 HRS patients demonstrated improvement in glomerular filtration rate, renal plasma flow and improvements in creatinine clearance and aldosterone levels [15–17].

## Preoperative Evaluation

There are several important contraindications to consider when evaluating a patient for TIPS. Given that there are known predictors for poor outcomes following the procedure, the decision to offer TIPS to a patient is often jointly made by hepatology, interventional radiology and anesthesiology teams. Absolute and relative contraindications to TIPS are listed in Table 71.1 [5]. The experience of the interventional team is often factored into the decision to proceed in patients with a relative contraindication. If significant patient coagulopathy prevents TIPS, careful correction may allow a window in which the procedure can be performed. Finally, in the setting of disease palliation, relative contraindications may be overshadowed by a careful assessment of the risk to benefit ratio [5].

Preoperative evaluations, when possible, ensure best care is provided to the patient. Often, these patients are concomitantly being evaluated and medically optimized for liver transplant and have already undergone an extensive medical assessment. For those patients without previous encompassing work-up, a systems approach should be initiated to determine needed preoperative testing.

## Cardiovascular

Due to the overproduction of nitric oxide (NO) in cirrhosis, patients have low systemic vascular

**Table 71.1** Contraindications to TIPS placement

| Absolute | Relative |
|---|---|
| Congestive heart failure | Portal vein thrombus |
| Multiple hepatic cysts | Coagulopathy (severe, INR >5) |
| Uncontrolled infection | Platelets <20,000/cm$^3$ |
| Biliary obstruction, unrelieved | Hepatoma |
| Severe pulmonary hypertension (mean pulmonary artery pressure >45 mmHg) | Moderate pulmonary hypertension |
| Primary prevention of variceal bleeding | |

resistance (SVR) and compensatory high cardiac output. In the setting of variceal formation, large volumes of blood are delivered back to the heart, increasing cardiac preload. However, a rise in preload in cirrhosis does not routinely result in the expected increase in cardiac output [18]; this state is frequently described as "cirrhotic cardiomyopathy," and is characterized by an abnormal Starling Curve. Additionally, these patients are at risk to develop a prolonged QT interval and should be evaluated with preoperative electrocardiogram [18]. When possible, transthoracic echocardiogram should be considered to evaluate cardiac function and volume status.

## Pulmonary

Compression of the diaphragm by ascites, and of the lungs by pleural effusions, can result in atelectasis which will limit oxygenation and ventilation [18]. In subjects with tense ascites, lung function was evaluated with pulmonary function tests both before and after large volume paracentesis (LVP). Functional reserve capacity (FRC), forced expiratory volume in 1 s (FEV1) and expiratory reserve volume (ERV) all demonstrate significant improvement after LVP [19]. As expected, lung mechanics improved with the drop in transdiaphragmatic pressure allowing more normal tidal breathing [19].

Just as varices form in other areas of the body, similar intravascular pulmonary vasodilations can form within the lungs leading to hepatopulmonary syndrome [20–23]. Venous blood within the lungs passes through intravascular pulmonary vasodilations (IVPD) instead of pulmonary capillaries. As a result, the red cells in these channels bypass gas exchange resulting in hypoxemia and an increased Alveolar-arterial gradient [18].

Portopulmonary hypertension (POPH) is diagnosed in 5–10 % of patients with ESLD [22, 24]. The pathophysiology of POPH is similar to idiopathic pulmonary hypertension. Pulmonary vascular obstruction develops as a result of endothelial proliferation, periarteriolar smooth muscle cell proliferation, and the increasing presence of endothelin. The increasing obstruction to flow contributes to platelet aggregation and in situ thrombosis, worsening vascular resistance in pulmonary arterial beds. Of note, POPH development does not correlate with severity of liver disease [22]. POPH is defined as mean pulmonary artery pressure (mPAP) > 25 mmHg at rest, pulmonary vascular resistance (PVR) > 240 dynes s cm$^{-5}$ and pulmonary artery occlusion pressure (PaOP) less than 15 mmHg. Evaluating and diagnosing POPH in potential TIPS patients is critical; in those with severe POPH, the increased cardiac preload delivered through the hepatic shunt created by TIPS often leads to immediate right ventricular failure [18]. Patients with a mPAP over 45 mmHg are not considered candidates for TIPS (nor liver transplant). Those with elevated mPAP, but less than 45 mmHg, are considered on an individual basis to determine if TIPS is a safe treatment option [5].

## Neurologic

Any patient scheduled for TIPS should have a detailed neurologic examination. Often, these patients suffer from encephalopathy due to decreased metabolism of nitrogenous waste produced by intestinal flora. Post-TIPS, encephalopathy may worsen. The accumulation of ammonia and other toxins normally metabolized by the liver are suddenly redistributed around the fibrotic liver and directed back into systemic circulation [20]. The main contributor to neurologic decline in hepatic encephalopathy is thought to be elevated ammonia levels and as such, mental status changes or delay in arousal may improve by lowering systemic ammonia levels [20].

## Coagulation

Although minimally invasive, patients undergoing TIPS should be thoroughly evaluated for coagulopathy. Multiple potential bleeding sites and risks have been reported during TIPS: capsular tears, portal vein disruption and hepatic vein tears [18, 25]. Factors II, VII, IX and X are normally synthesized by the liver and in TIPS patients with cirrhosis, the ability to form clot is decreased. Platelet trapping due to splenic sequestration can lead to thrombocytopenia [18]. As liver function decreases, less thrombopoetin is produced which additionally contributes to thrombocytopenia [18]. Although coagulopathic by standard coagulation tests (prothrombin time, partial thromboplastin time and international normalized ratio), the degree of lab abnormality does not predict the risk of bleeding for a procedure. Furthermore, the balance between coagulopathy and thrombus formation cannot be appreciated by standard lab testing. Use of thromboelastogram is warranted in these patients to determine the coagulation status of the patient at the time of the procedure and to guide resuscitation if needed.

## Renal

Renal disease is prevalent in this patient population. A complex relationship exists between the liver and kidneys with the potential for the development of hepatorenal syndrome. As portal pressure increases from the cirrhotic liver, splanchnic blood pooling occurs and creates relative hypovolemia and renal hypoperfusion [25]. The syndrome can lead to renal failure and in more extreme cases, the need for dialysis. Pre-operative laboratory evaluation of serum creatinine and the glomerular filtration rate determines kidney function, and is warranted as it may impact fluid and medication management.

## Preparation

TIPS can be done in the operating room with a fluoroscopic C-arm or in the interventional radiology suite. If performed in an interventional suite away from the operating room, all resources needed must be available to provide an anesthetic. This includes the ability to place invasive monitors and large bore intravenous access, provide for large volume resuscitation, and administer vasopressor and inotrope therapy if needed.

Supine positioning with the patient's head turned to the left provides access to the right internal jugular vein [26]. Both arms are tucked at patient's side. Following the induction of anesthesia, access to the airway is limited, so placement of an endotracheal tube is recommended. An adequate length breathing circuit is recommended to ensure that the distance between the anesthesia machine and patient is safely managed without placing strain on the airway.

In addition to the American Society of Anesthesiologists standard monitors, an arterial line is inserted to monitor acute changes in hemodynamics and provide easy access for arterial blood gas sampling and coagulation testing. An additional transducer needs to be available to the interventional radiologists to measure HPVG during the procedure. In addition to the arterial line, intravenous access should minimally include two large bore intravenous (IV) catheters, 16 gauge or larger. In some cases, the patient will have an existing right internal jugular central line. In these cases, the central line can be used for induction but other access will need to be obtained, as this will be the procedural site. A Foley catheter is placed to monitor urine output but, in the setting of cirrhosis, portal hypertension and possible HRS or relative hypovolemia, urine output is not a reliable marker of volume status. Blood products need to be ordered and readily available based on the patient's lab results. Glucose-containing solutions may be required due to impaired gluconeogenesis.

## Intraoperative Management

### Type of Anesthesia

TIPS is performed in both elective and emergent settings. Emergently, the TIPS procedure is best performed under general anesthesia. The most frequent emergent indication is control of acute variceal bleeding, which places patients at high risk of compromised airway, aspiration, hemodynamic instability, and hepatic encephalopathy. Electively, TIPS can be performed under monitored anesthesia care (MAC) with local anesthesia. The choice between MAC or general anesthesia will depend on patient factors and local practice. There is little literature comparing different methods, so the advantages and disadvantages of each must be considered for each individual case [27]. Major procedural complications during TIPS are rare and expected in approximately 3% of cases; fatal complications are less frequent but still occur in 2% of patients (range, 0.6–4.3%). Depending on the volume of TIPS performed at the center annually, the familiarity of the anesthesiologist with the procedure, the availability of resuscitation equipment and the capability of the team (proceduralist, anesthesiologist, nursing) to manage a sedated patient, the decision to use MAC versus general can be hospital specific. Particularly in situations where the patient is acutely ill or the team is less equipped to manage an emergency, one could argue if a complication were to occur, the anesthesiologist could respond and treat the patient more effectively under general anesthesia.

General endotracheal anesthesia is usually preferred in most institutions performing TIPS. If induction is performed in the interventional suite, the procedural table is most often a fixed surface without the ability to elevate the head of the bed. Many patients with significant ascites will not tolerate being supine and induction on a patient stretcher with head up is a safe option. The patient is then transferred to the interventional suite table. A rapid sequence induction is necessary in patients with abdominal distention or recent variceal bleed [28]. General anesthesia with endotracheal intubation allows for optimal patient comfort, careful cardiorespiratory monitoring, a secure airway, and lack of patient movement.

When performed under MAC, the anesthesiologist needs to be comfortable managing an airway that is minimally accessible during the procedure. MAC may allow for minimal hemodynamic perturbations compared even to controlled induction of general anesthesia. Patients with significant ascites or recent variceal bleeds are at high risk of aspiration; the authors recommend obtaining a secure airway with an endotracheal tube in these patients. If airway obstruction occurs due to sedation or hematoma formation following cannulation of the internal jugular vein, it needs to be quickly recognized and a preemptive management plan should be discussed with the procedural team. Additionally, balloon dilation of the intrahepatic tract can be particularly painful and MAC may not provide sufficient pain relief without risking airway compromise [28]. Regardless of the anesthetic choice, the anesthesiologist is vital in providing perioperative care for these complicated patients [29].

## Anesthetics and Medications

Optimal anesthetic drugs for patients with ESLD is not defined [30]. Sensitivity to sedatives is increased and caution should be used in the administration of benzodiazepines, propofol and narcotics. The cardiorespiratory effects of induction drugs are unpredictable because cirrhosis alters normal pharmacokinetics, including volume of distribution, hepatic extraction and metabolism, renal excretion and levels of serum proteins including albumin. Consideration of these factors is crucial, and pre-anesthetic planning needs to ensure adequate hepatic perfusion. Decreased liver blood flow contributes to hepatocellular injury and can result in further decompensation. Hepatic arterial flow is the main determinant perfusion to the liver; keeping mean arterial pressure normal by titrating anesthetic agents to effect and using pressors as needed is the safest approach to managing TIPS patients [31].

Intravascular volume maintenance is critical in patients with ESLD and may avert worsening hepatorenal syndrome. Cirrhotic patients suffer from a vasoplegic-like state characterized by a high cardiac output and low systemic vascular resistance and are often reliant on intravascular volume to maintain cardiac output and blood pressure. These patients may be poorly responsive to alpha-agonists compared to patients without liver disease [32]. Rising doses of phenylephrine result in increased hepatosplanchnic vasoconstriction [33] with minimal rises in blood pressure. Norepinephrine is the first line of vasopressor in these patients.

Vasopressin is considered as a second line agent to increase SVR in cirrhotic patients [34] and may be a first line agent in those with increased pulmonary pressures as it has been demonstrated in animal models to result in a 45% decrease in the PVR/SVR ratio compared to phenylephrine [35]. Patients with bleeding varices will also benefit from vasopressin because it reduces portal blood flow and in combination with procedural intervention, has been demonstrated to decrease the need for blood transfusion [36].

Although infrequently clinically significant, severe liver disease lowers circulating levels of pseudocholinesterase which can prolong the duration of succinylcholine [30]. Due to the increased volume of distribution, larger doses of vecuronium/rocuronium are often needed. However, because the elimination phase in severe liver disease is prolonged, subsequent doses are reduced. Cisatracurium is a suitable for neuromuscular blockade because it does not rely on hepatic excretion. In all cases, it is advisable to monitor neuromuscular function [37].

Maintenance of anesthesia can be accomplished with inhalational or intravenous agents. All volatile anesthetics reduce cardiac output and mean arterial pressure and thereby reduce liver blood flow that could result in exaggerated postoperative liver dysfunction. It is therefore prudent to limit the dose of volatile anesthetics. Isoflurane, sevoflurane, and desflurane undergo minimal hepatic metabolism. Maintenance of anesthesia with intravenous agents is appropriate but a prolonged duration of action is expected because they undergo extensive hepatic metabolism [37].

Elimination of morphine is delayed in cirrhotic patients due to both reduced hepatic blood flow and extraction ratio. In patients with associated renal failure or hepatorenal syndrome, accumulation of the active metabolite morphine-6-glucuronide will occur. Morphine is perhaps best avoided in patients with decompensated liver failure as it may precipitate hepatic encephalopathy. Fentanyl, given in low doses, is suitable for intraoperative use as it does not have an active metabolite and is renally excreted. However, in repeated or large doses, fentanyl will accumulate. Elimination of alfentanil is reduced in liver disease, its volume of distribution increased, and protein binding reduced by the lack of alpha-1-acid glycoprotein. Remifentanil is ideally suited to intraoperative use as it is metabolized by tissue and red cell esterases, which unlike plasma esterases, are preserved in patients with severe liver disease. In general, narcotics should be used sparingly as postoperative pain following TIPS is usually minimal and patients are at risk for encephalopathy and post-operative delirium [37].

## Fluids

Fluid replacement to optimize cardiac filling pressures and cardiac output is recommended before vasopressors are started. Although vasopressors may be needed to maintain normal MAP, they can decrease hepatic arterial flow. Goal-directed fluid therapy is guided by systolic pressure variation and pulse pressure variation using the arterial line. Colloids are often chosen over crystalloids in these patients, because of their low oncotic pressure [32]. This is particularly important if LVP is performed concurrently with TIPS.

Following elective TIPS, if there are not contraindications to extubation, the patient is extubated when fully awake and protective laryngeal reflexes are present [18]. Reversal of muscle relaxation with sugammadex has been used in these patients with one case report showing a prolonged time to achieve a TOF ratio > 0.9; this may be explained by the increased volume of distribution common in patients with liver dysfunction [38]. Additionally, in patients with renal impairment (glomerular filtration rate < 30 ml/min) or failure, sugammadex is contraindicated.

## Post-operative Care

Depending on the center and patient, follow-up care may be provided in the post-anesthesia care unit (PACU) or intensive care unit. These patients are at risk of complications that could necessitate ICU admission [39]. Continued routine and arterial blood pressure monitoring is necessary and an assessment completed to evaluate for possible intra and post-operative complications including: bleeding, liver capsule perforation, encephalopathy, hepatic infarction, portal vein thrombus, TIPS dysfunction/thrombosis, accelerated liver failure, contrast induced renal failure, pulmonary edema, congestive heart failure, cardiac arrhythmias, and entry site hematoma [40, 41].

The measures of TIPS success are categorized as technical, hemodynamic, and clinical [42]. The technical success is the physical creation of a patent TIPS between the hepatic vein and a branch of the portal vein and has a 95% success rate. The hemodynamic success is the reduction of portosystemic gradient to the target number, which is typically <12 mmHg, and also has a 95% success rate. The clinical success is resolution of the indication for which the procedure was performed. For variceal bleeding, the success rate is >90% and for ascites, the success rate is broad varying from 55% to 80% with majority of studies reporting approximately 55% [5].

# References

1. Brunner F, Berzigotti A, Bosch J. Prevention and treatment of variceal haemorrhage in 2017. Liver Int. 2017;37(Suppl. 1):104–15.
2. Bosch J, Abraldes JG, Berzigotti A, et al. The clinical use of HVPG measurements in chronic liver disease. Nat Rev Gastroenterol Hepatol. 2009;6:573–82.
3. Ripoll C, Groszmann R, Garcia-Tsao G, et al. Hepatic venous pressure gradient predicts clinical decompensation in patients with compensated cirrhosis. Gastroenterology. 2007;133:481–8.
4. Merli M, Nicolini G, Angeloni S, et al. Incidence and natural history of small esophageal varices in cirrhotic patients. J Hepatol. 2003;38:266–72.
5. Boyer T, Haskal Z. American Association for the Study of Liver Diseases Practice Guidelines: the role of transjugular intrahepatic portosystemic shunt creation in the management of portal hypertension. J Vasc Interv Radiol. 2005;16:615–29.
6. Vangeli M, Patch D, Burroughs AK. Salvage tips for uncontrolled variceal bleeding. J Hepatol. 2003;37:703–4.
7. Sharara A, Rockey D. Gastroesophageal variceal hemorrhage. N Engl J Med. 2001;345:669–81.
8. Chalasani N, Kahi C, Francois F, et al. Improved patient survival after acute variceal bleeding: a Multicenter, Cohort Study. Am J Gastroenterol. 2003;98:653–9.
9. Runyon B. Management of adult patients with ascites due to cirrhosis. Hepatology. 2004;39:841–56.
10. Sanyal A, Genning C, Reddy K, et al., NASTRA group. The North American Study for the treatment of refractory ascites. Gastroenterology. 2003;124:634–41.
11. Lebrec D, Giuily N, Hadengue A, Vilgrain V, Moreau R, Poynard T, et al. Transjugular intrahepatic portosystemic shunts: comparison with paracentesis in patients with cirrhosis and refractory ascites: a randomized trial. J Hepatol. 1996;25:135–44.
12. Rossle M, Ochs A, Gullberg V, Siegerstetter V, Holl J, Deibert P, et al. A comparison of paracentesis and transjugular intrahepatic portosystemic shunting in patients with ascites. N Engl J Med. 2000;342:1701–7.
13. Gines P, Uriz J, Calaborra B, et al. Transjugular intrahepatic portosystemic shunting versus paracentesis plus albumin for refractory ascites in cirrhosis. Gastroeterology. 2002;123:1839–47.
14. Salerno F, Merli M, Riggio O, Cazzaniga M, Valeriano V, Pozzi M, et al. Randomized Controlled Study of TIPS versus paracentesis plus albumin in cirrhosis with severe ascites. Hepatology. 2004;40:629–35.
15. Brensing K, Textor J, Perz J, et al. Long term outcome after transjugular intrahepatic portosytemic stentshunt in non-transplant cirrhotics with hepatorenal syndrome: a phase II study. Gut. 2000;47:288–95.
16. Wong F, Sniderman K, Liu P, et al. Transjugular stent shunt: effects on hemodynamics and sodium homeostasis in cirrhosis and refractory ascites. Ann Intern Med. 1995;122:816–22.
17. Guevara M, Gines P, Bandi J, et al. Transjugular intrahepatic portosystemic shunt in hepatorenal syndrome: effects on renal function and vasoactive systems. Hepatology. 1998;28:416–22.
18. Scher C. Anesthesia for transjugular intrahepatic portosystemic shunt. Int Anesthesiol Clin. 2009;47:21–8.
19. Duranti R, Laffi G, Misuri G, et al. Respiratory mechanics in patients with tense cirrhotic ascites. Eur Respir J. 1997;10:1622–30.
20. Monfort P, Cauli O, Montoliu C, et al. Mechanisms of cognitive alterations in hyperammonemia and hepatic encephalopathy: therapeutical implications. Neurochem Int. 2009;55:106–12.
21. Schenk P, Fuhrmann V, Madl C, et al. Hepatopulmonary syndrome: prevalence and predictive value of various cut offs for arterial oxygenation and their clinical consequences. Gut. 2002;51:853–9.
22. Dalal A. Anesthesia for liver transplantation. Transplant Rev. 2016;30:51–60.
23. Swanson K, Wiesner R, Nyberg S, et al. Survival in portopulmonary hypertension: Mayo Clinic experience categorized by treatment subgroups. Am J Transplant. 2008;8:2445–53.
24. Krowka MJ, Swanson KL, Frantz RP, et al. Portopulmonary hypertension: results from a 10-year screening algorithm. Hepatology. 2006;44:1502–10.
25. Krug S, Seyfarth H, Hagendorff A, et al. Inhaled iloprost for hepatopulmonary syndrome: improvements

of hypoxemia. Eur J Gastroenterol Hepatol. 2007;19:1140–3.
26. Peck-Radosavljevic M. Review article: coagulation disorders in chronic liver disease. Ailment Pharmacol Ther. 2007;26(suppl 1):21–8.
27. Chana A, James M, Veale P. Anesthesia for transjugular intrahepatic portosystemic shunt insertion. BJA Educ. 2016;16:405–9.
28. Moreau R, Lebrec D. Acute kidney injury: new concepts. Hepatorenal syndrome: the role of vasopressors. Nephron Physiol. 2008;109:73–9.
29. Andrea DG, Andrea C, Rocco C, Antonio R, Elena R, Ernestine M, Giuliana F, Manlio P. Transjugular intrahepatic portosystemic shunt (TIPS): the anesthesiological point of view after 150 procedures managed under total intravenous anesthesia. J Clin Monit Comput. 2009;23:341–6.
30. Roberta H, Katherine M. Stoelting's Anesthesia and co-existing disease. 2008; p. 259–78.
31. Fun-Sun Y, Robert P, Rae A. Yao and Artusio's Anesthesiology. 2003; p. 485–509.
32. Thierry G, Francois D, Didier L, Jean-Louis V, Richard M. J Hepatol. 2009;50:2022–33.
33. Berend M. Should norepinephrine, rather than phenylephrine, be considered the primary vasopressor in anesthetic practice? Anesth Analg. 2016;122:1707–14.
34. Dennis D, et al. Canadian. J Emerg Med. 2015;17(S1):1–16.
35. Sarkar J, Golden PJ, Kajiura LN, Murata LM, CFT U. Vasopressin decreases pulmonary to systemic vascular resistance ratio in a porcine model of severe hemorrhagic shock. Shock. 2015;43(5):475–82.
36. Sun G, Wang J, Teng F, Lu Y, Li Y, Wen A. The effect of acute variceal bleeding interventions on reducing the requirement of blood transfusions in cirrhotic patients: a systematic review. Int J Clin Exp Med. 2016;9(3):6166–77.
37. Rakesh V, Larry MN, Imogen S. Contin Educ Anaesth Crit Care Pain. 2010;10:15–9.
38. Fagiuoli S, Bruno R, Venon W, Schepis F, Vizzutti F, Toniutto P, Senzolo M, Caraceni P, Salerno F, Angeli P, Cioni R, Vitale A, Grosso M, DeGasperi A, D'Amico G, Marzano A. Consensus Conference on TIPS management: techniques, indications, and contraindications. Dig Liver Dis. 2017;49(2):121–37.
39. Ginès P, Fernández J, Durand F, Saliba F. Management of critically-ill cirrhotic patients. J Hepatol. 2012;56(Suppl 1):S13–24.
40. Batistaki C, Matsota P, Kalimeris K, Brountzos E, Kostopanagiotou G. Sugammadex antagonizing rocuronium in three patients with liver dysfunction undergoing transjugular intrahepatic portosystemic shunt. Anaesth Intensive Care. 2012;40(3):556–71.
41. Dariushnia S, Haskal Z, Midia M, Martin L, Walker T, Kalva S, Clark T, Ganguli S, Krishnamurthy V, Saiter C, Nikilic B. Quality improvement guidelines for transjugular intrahepatic portosystemic shunts. J Vasc Interv Radiol. 2016;27:1–7.
42. Jaffe, R. Anesthesiologists manual of surgical procedures. 5th ed. Philadelphia, PA: Wolters Kluwer; 2014. p. 1507–12.

# Anesthesia for Liver Transplantation

**Philip L. Kalarickal and Daniel J. Viox**

## Introduction

Liver transplantation is the definitive treatment option for patients with fulminant liver failure, hepatocellular carcinoma (HCC), and end-stage liver disease (ESLD) when the limits of medical therapy have been reached. ESLD affects the majority of the body's organ systems, making liver transplantation amongst the most challenging surgeries for the anesthesiologist to manage. A summary of anesthetic considerations during liver transplantation surgery is provided in Table 72.1.

Pioneering transplant surgeon Dr. Thomas E. Starzl of the University of Colorado School of Medicine attempted the first human liver transplant in 1963, and performed the first successful (survival greater than 1 year after transplantation) human liver transplant in 1967 [1–3]. Over the past 50 years, numerous improvements in liver preservation and allocation, surgical and anesthetic techniques, and immunosuppression have improved morbidity and mortality. Approximately 7800 liver transplants were performed in the United States in 2016. The most recent data examining American transplant centers indicate greater than 90% 1-year survival and greater than 75% survival at 5 years post transplantation [4]. Despite these advances, there remains a scarcity of donor organs, and more than 14,000 candidates remain on the waiting list for liver transplant in the United States [4].

In 2002, the United Network for Organ Sharing (UNOS) established the Model for End-stage Liver Disease (MELD) score to prioritize transplant allocation. The score is calculated as a weighted average of the natural logarithms of International Normalized Ratio (INR), serum bilirubin, and serum creatinine, as the primary determinant of priority for liver allocation in the United States [5, 6]. In January 2016, this scoring system was modified by UNOS to incorporate the patient's serum sodium concentrations [7]. This modified score is called the MELD-Na. MELD-Na has been demonstrated to be a more accurate predictor of waitlist mortality than MELD score alone [8]. The MELD score was originally developed to estimate 90-day mortality after transjugular intrahepatic portosystemic shunt (TIPS) placement [9]. Subsequent evaluations of the score reveal that survival benefit increases with increasing MELD score, and that at lower MELD scores, recipient mortality risk during the first post-transplantation year is higher than for candidates who remain on the waiting list. Exception points are awarded to patients with HCC because although their liver function often remains relatively normal, transplant provides cancer cure [10–12].

P. L. Kalarickal, M.D., M.P.H. (✉) · D. J. Viox, M.D.
Emory University School of Medicine,
Atlanta, GA, USA
e-mail: pkalari@emory.edu; dan.viox@emory.edu

**Table 72.1** Summary of anesthesia considerations in patients undergoing liver transplantation

| Plan/preparation/adverse events | Reasoning/management |
|---|---|
| Preoperative evaluation (see Table 72.2) | Room-air ABG, contrast-enhanced TTE, CXR, PFTs, CT chest<br>ECG, TTE, ± noninvasive stress testing<br>CBC, PT, PTT, INR, fibrinogen, d-dimer<br>Serum BUN, serum Cr, BMP |
| Position | Supine |
| Access | ≥1 14- or 16-gauge IV—Rapid fluid and blood product administration<br>Arterial line—Anticipation of hemodynamic instability, frequent blood sampling, vasoactive drug administration<br>Central venous catheter—CVP and PAP transduction, rapid fluid and blood product administration, vasoactive drug administration |
| GETA | |
|   IV induction | Even if metabolism and/or excretion are hepatic, duration of action determined by redistribution |
|   RSI | Increased risk for regurgitation and aspiration |
|   Maintenance | Isoflurane or sevoflurane preferred given no significant decrease in hepatic blood flow or $O_2$ delivery |
| Procedural adverse events | |
|   Aspiration | RSI as above |
|   Coagulopathy | Transfuse blood products to approximate goals of INR < 3.5, platelets > 20, and fibrinogen > 100 and clinical coagulation status |
|   Hemorrhage | Transfuse pRBCs to goal of hematocrit > 25 |
| | Rapid infuser should be available |
|   Hypotension | Relative hypovolemia during dissection phase, euvolemia after; titrate vasopressors to effect |
|   Hyperkalemic cardiac arrest | Apply defibrillation pads before induction; send ABGs q20–30 min during anhepatic phase; administer $Ca^{2+}$, dextrose, and insulin as indicated |
|   Postreperfusion syndrome | Titrate inotropes and vasopressors to effect |
| Postoperative and post-discharge considerations | |
|   Extubation | May consider if hemodynamically stable and no significant transfusion requirements |

# Applied Anatomy and Physiology of Liver Transplantation

Liver transplantation is divided into three phases: the dissection, anhepatic, and neohepatic phases. Each phase is characterized by different anesthetic goals, and knowledge of surgical technique critically determines hemodynamic aims and resuscitation efforts.

## Dissection Phase

With the patient anesthetized and in the supine position, a bilateral subcostal incision with midline extension cephalad to the xiphoid process (Calne or "Mercedes-Benz" incision) is made. The abdomen is manually explored for evidence of metastatic HCC, other extra-hepatic malignancy, infection, or other contraindication to liver transplantation. Assuming that there are no unexpected findings that act as a contraindication to transplant, the liver is mobilized by dissection of the falciform, round, left and right triangular, and gastrohepatic ligaments in addition to ligation of any varices and/or adhesions. The porta hepatis is dissected, and the hepatic artery, common bile duct, and portal vein successively ligated. In the setting of severe portal hypertension, a temporary portacaval shunt can be created prior to portal vein ligation to help decompress varices and control variceal hemorrhage. The final steps of the dissection phase depend on the chosen technique of anastomosis—standard or piggyback—but end with recipient hepatectomy [13, 14]. During the dissection, significant coagulopathy and surgical bleeding require active management.

## Anhepatic Phase

The standard transplant technique employs a bicaval anastomosis, in which the recipient infrahepatic and suprahepatic vena cava are ligated and anastomosed to the corresponding segments of the donor vena cava in the reverse order. This technique is illustrated in (Fig. 72.1) and is associated with a shorter dissection phase, but has the disadvantage of significantly decreasing systemic venous return from the lower extremities and kidneys because the vena cava is completely clamped in the infra- and supra-hepatic positions. The decreased venous return can be offset by veno-venous bypass (VVB); this removes blood from cannulae in the femoral and portal veins and returns it to the central circulation via a cannula in the axillary or internal jugular vein. However, veno-venous bypass has its own set of risks, including vascular injury, hemomediastinum, and air or thromboembolism [13, 14].

The piggyback technique preserves the recipient vena cava and involves anastomosing the donor suprahepatic vena cava to a cuff created from the three, main recipient hepatic veins. The donor infrahepatic vena cava is ligated. This technique is illustrated in (Fig. 72.2). To access the main hepatic veins, numerous short hepatic veins connecting the caudate lobe of the liver to the vena cava must first be ligated. The liver is then lifted and rotated off of the vena cava to increase exposure. This maneuver may partially occlude the inferior vena cava and temporarily decrease blood pressure, however the ultimate result is maintenance of systemic venous return during the anhepatic phase [13, 14].

With either technique, the donor suprahepatic vena cava is anastomosed first. Immediately before the donor infrahepatic vena cava is anastomosed (standard technique) or ligated (piggyback technique), the cold storage solution and air within the donor liver are flushed to minimize the respective risks of hyperkalemia and air embolism that occur with reperfusion. Donor infrahepatic vena cava anastomosis/ligation is followed by portal vein anastomosis, at which point venous blood flow is carefully reestablished, and the donor liver re-perfused [13, 14].

## Neohepatic Phase

Reperfusion frequently leads to a postreperfusion syndrome (PRS), which can result in severe hemodynamic disturbance. PRS is defined as a decrease in mean arterial pressure (MAP) or heart rate (HR) of greater than 30% from baseline and may result in asystole and/or hemodynamically significant dysrhythmias. PRS incidence varies greatly in the literature from 12 to 77% [15]. Reperfusion of the liver results in a sudden load of cold, acidotic, hyperkalemic blood and preservative solution being released from the liver graft. If VVB is not used, venous blood from the portal system will also be released having been without oxygen since

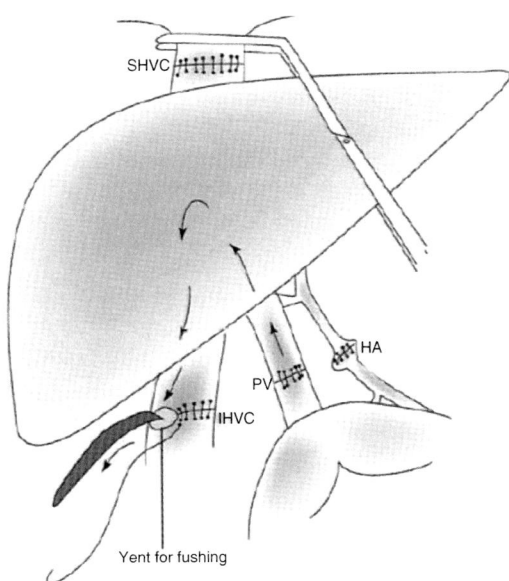

**Fig. 72.1** The standard bicaval technique of liver transplantation. Initial anastomoses include the suprahepatic vena cava (SHVC), infrahepatic vena cava (IHVC), and portal vein (PV). The hepatic artery (HA) and bile duct are anastomosed after reperfusion and hemostasis. Modified from: Atlas of Organ Transplantation, Humar, Matas and Payned eds, 2009

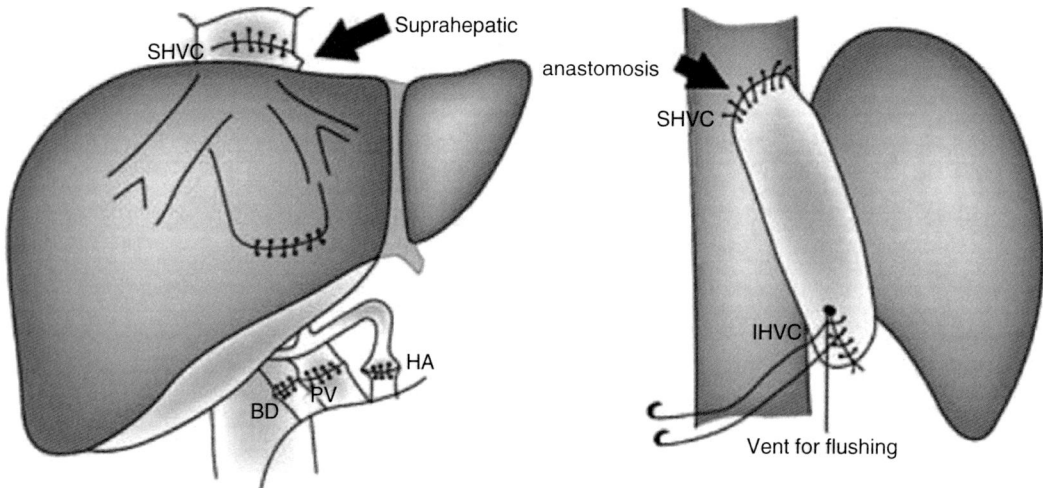

**Fig. 72.2** The piggyback technique of liver transplantation. The donor suprahepatic vena cava (SHVC) is sewn to the confluence of hepatic veins returning blood to the recipient vena cava. The donor infrahepatic vena cava (IHVC) is ligated. Additionally, the portal vein (PV) is anastomosed prior to reperfusion. After reperfusion, the hepatic artery (HA) and bile duct (BD) are anastomosed. Modified from: Atlas of Organ Transplantation, Humar, Matas and Payned eds, 2009

time of clamp placement. As the byproducts of the liver graft, and products of anaerobic metabolism from the portal circulation, are delivered to the heart and lungs. The result is an increase in pulmonary vascular resistance (PVR), which can result in right heart dysfunction and cardiac arrest, particularly in patients with portopulmonary hypertension (POPH). Additionally, right heart dysfunction can prevent left heart filling and lead to notably decreased cardiac output. Often, significant vasopressor and inotrope infusions are necessary to maintain adequate systemic and coronary perfusion pressure. After the patient has been stabilized, hepatic artery anastomosis, cholecystectomy, and common bile duct reconstruction are the last steps before verification of hemostasis and closure [13, 14].

## Preoperative Evaluation

Fulminant liver failure and end-stage liver disease affect multiple organ systems. Clinical manifestations are summarized by organ system in Table 72.2 and described in detail below.

## Neurologic

The primary neurologic manifestation of cirrhosis and end-stage liver disease is encephalopathy, due to decreased metabolism of nitrogenous waste produced by intestinal flora. Hepatic encephalopathy is a diagnosis of exclusion, and other possible etiologies of delirium should first be ruled out. If time and circumstance allow, preoperative treatment of hepatic encephalopathy includes optimizing the patient's other comorbidities, titrating lactulose to three bowel movements per day, and administering oral antibiotics like rifaximin [16]. In fulminant liver failure, cerebral edema may increase intracranial pressure, increasing the risk of brainstem herniation. Placement of an intracranial transducer and drain has been advocated at times as means monitor intracranial pressure and drain cerebral spinal fluid. It's safety in the setting of coagulopathy has not been established and outcome improvements thus far have not been demonstrated [17]. Treatment of increased intracranial pressure may include elevation of the head, hyperventilation, hypertonic saline infusion, and osmotic diuretics such as mannitol.

**Table 72.2** Clinical manifestations of end-stage liver disease

| Organ system | Clinical manifestations |
|---|---|
| Neurological | • Hepatic encephalopathy (due to decreased metabolism of nitrogenous waste)<br>• Elevated intracranial pressure (fulminant liver failure) |
| Respiratory | • Decreased functional residual capacity<br>• Restrictive ventilatory defects<br>• Primary respiratory alkalosis<br>• Hepatopulmonary syndrome (liver disease, hypoxemia, and shunting due to intrapulmonary vasodilation) |
| Cardiovascular | • Hyperdynamic circulation (due to low blood pressure, low systemic vascular resistance, and high cardiac output)<br>• Hypervolemia<br>• Cirrhotic cardiomyopathy<br>• Coronary artery disease<br>• Portopulmonary hypertension |
| Hematologic | • Anemia<br>• Thrombocytopenia<br>• Complex coagulopathy (due to decreased synthesis of coagulation factors and proteins C and S) |
| Renal | • Intravascular volume depletion (due to low plasma oncotic pressure)<br>• Chronic renal failure (due to intravascular volume depletion)<br>• Electrolyte imbalances (e.g., hyponatremia, hypo- or hyperkalemia)<br>• Hepatorenal syndrome |
| Hepatic | • Decreased synthetic function<br>• Hypoalbuminemia, ascites, and peripheral edema<br>• Lactic acidosis |
| Gastrointestinal | • Increased risk of aspiration<br>• Ascites<br>• Esophageal and gastric varices<br>• GI bleeding |

## Respiratory

Respiratory manifestations of liver disease include decreased functional residual capacity and restrictive ventilatory defects secondary to ascites and pleural effusions (hepatic hydrothorax). Patients may also experience hypoxemia, primary respiratory alkalosis, and hepatopulmonary syndrome (HPS). HPS is defined as the triad of liver disease, $PAO_2$–$paO_2$ gradient >15 mmHg, and pulmonary arteriovenous shunting. Characteristic clinical manifestations include platypnea and orthodeoxia, which result from increased right-to-left shunting of deoxygenated blood through dependent pulmonary vascular dilatations. Preoperative evaluation for HPS should include a room-air arterial blood gas (ABG) and contrast-enhanced transthoracic echocardiogram (to evaluate for the presence of bubbles in the left atrium after five heart beats). A chest radiograph, pulmonary functions tests, and chest computed tomography (CT) should be performed to rule out other causes of hypoxemia [6].

## Cardiovascular

Patients with cirrhosis have low systemic vascular resistance (SVR) and high cardiac output due to splanchnic arterial vasodilation. Patients are often hypervolemic and suffer from coexisting cirrhotic cardiomyopathy, coronary artery disease (CAD), and/or POPH. Cirrhotic cardiomyopathy is characterized by electrophysiologic abnormalities, systolic and diastolic dysfunction, and an impaired contractile response to stress due to downregulation of β-adrenergic receptors. While electrocardiogram (ECG) findings consistent with cirrhotic cardiomyopathy (QT interval prolongation, e.g.), TTE may not reveal classic findings of the disease if systolic dysfunction is compensated due to low SVR state.

As cirrhotic patients age, the risk and surgical impact of CAD grows. Although, historically, cirrhosis has been considered "protective" with regards to incidence coronary atherosclerosis, more recent evidence suggests that this may not be the case [18, 19]. Additionally, as the demographics of potential liver transplant recipients shift more towards the elderly, the incidence and severity of CAD may increase. The controversy surrounding incidence and evaluation are covered in greater detail elsewhere [20]. Current best practice in evaluation for CAD in liver transplant candidates includes ECG and TTE. Screening for CAD may also include noninvasive stress testing in patients greater than 60-years-old or with a history of diabetes, hyperlipidemia, hypertension, or tobacco abuse [20–22].

The diagnostic criteria for POPH include mean pulmonary artery pressure (mPAP) > 25 mmHg at rest, pulmonary vascular resistance (PVR) > 240 dynes, and pulmonary artery occlusion pressure (PAoP) < 15 mmHg in the presence of known portal hypertension. The disease affects approximately 5–6% of patients evaluated for liver transplantation, and it portends worse survival at both two (67% vs. 85%) and 5 years (40% vs. 64%) versus isolated idiopathic or familial pulmonary arterial hypertension [23]. POPH may precipitate acute right ventricular failure in the setting of the increased cardiac output, volume, and pulmonary artery pressures that occur with PRS and as such, has been associated with significant intraoperative mortality. Older studies demonstrate up to 50% mortality with mean pulmonary arterial pressure (mPAP) 35–49 mmHg and 100% mortality with mPAP 50 mmHg or greater [24]. All patients presenting for liver transplantation evaluation should have a screening TTE with determination of right ventricular systolic pressure (RVSP) from the tricuspid regurgitant jet. Patients with RVSP ≥ 50 mmHg should be referred for right heart catheterization. Patients with evidence of POPH should be evaluated for initiation of pulmonary vasodilator therapy to reduce the perioperative risk of cardiovascular event. Treatment advances for POPH have resulted in improved outcomes for patients [25] and for patients those patients whose disease demonstrates reversibility, proceeding with transplantation can be safe.

## Hematologic

Anemia, thrombocytopenia, and coagulopathy are common hematologic manifestations of cirrhosis and ESLD. Anemia is frequently due to gastrointestinal blood loss and/or malabsorption of folic acid and vitamin B12. Thrombocytopenia is similarly multifactorial in etiology and may be due to decreased production of thrombopoietin and/or splenic sequestration. Coagulopathy is primarily mediated by decreased hepatic synthesis of coagulation factors and anticoagulation proteins C and S. In practice, the coagulopathy is complex as these patients may be clinically coagulopathic, or may be predisposed to pathologic thrombus formation (portal vein thrombus, e.g.). Preoperative evaluation of hematologic manifestations should include a complete blood count and clotting tests (prothromin time, activated prothrombin time and international normalized ration, fibrinogen, and d-dimer). Due to these factors, as well as portal hypertension, ESLD patients are at significant risk of massive and rapid blood loss during liver transplantation. Red blood cell and plasma transfusion products must be readily available as the patient enters the operating room.

## Renal

Low plasma oncotic pressure due to hypoalbuminemia may cause intravascular volume depletion despite a state of increased total body water. This intravascular volume depletion decreases glomerular filtration rate (GFR), and in susceptible patients, leads to acute or chronic renal failure. Electrolyte abnormalities are common, especially hypervolemic hyponatremia and hypokalemia. Hepatorenal syndrome is an especially ominous complication of both fulminant and chronic liver failure and is the result of splanchnic arterial vasodilation, followed by renal arterial vasoconstriction and ultimately renal failure. Preoperative evaluation of renal function should include serum BUN, serum creatinine, and a basic metabolic panel. Depending on the severity of renal failure, preoperative hemodialysis (HD) or intraoperative continuous renal replacement therapy (CRRT) may be indicated.

## Hepatic

Fulminant acute liver failure and cirrhotic ESLD disrupt both the synthetic and metabolic functions of the liver. INR is typically used to track synthetic function of the liver. While increases in INR do correlate with coagulopathy, the relationship is not linear. Procoagulant therapy should be guided by clinical coagulopathy and not laboratory values alone.

In addition to decreased synthesis of procoagulation factors and anticoagulation proteins C and S, there is decreased synthesis of albumin. This results in low plasma oncotic pressure, ascites and peripheral edema. Decreased metabolism of lactic acid may result in lactic acidosis, which may be profound during the anhepatic phase of liver transplantation.

## Gastrointestinal

ESLD patients are at risk for regurgitation and aspiration due to increased abdominal pressure from ascites and altered mental status from hepatic encephalopathy. Additionally, due to their portal hypertension, these patients often have esophageal and gastric varices. Concomitant coagulopathy puts these patients at increased risk of GI bleeding when the esophagus is instrumented with naso- or oro-gastric tubes or transesophageal echocardiogram (TEE) probe. Risk/benefit analysis should be undertaken prior to these procedures.

## Intraoperative Anesthetic Considerations

### Pre-incision

Given the uncertain volume status and low SVR states of end-stage cirrhosis, an arterial catheter should be considered prior to induction of anesthesia, particularly in unstable patients or those in fulminant failure. In the setting of ascites and deceased lung compliance, consideration should be given to a rapid sequence intubation. Establishment of general endotracheal anesthesia followed by maintenance with a volatile agent and narcotic. Paralysis should be maintained with an aminosteroid or a tetrahydroisoquinoline derivative neuromuscular blocker. Although propofol and most other intravenous induction agents are metabolized and/or excreted by the liver, their duration of action is primarily determined by redistribution, rendering them safe to use for induction. Higher doses of neuromuscular blockers may be required to achieve optimal intubating conditions due to the enlarged extracellular fluid compartment resulting in an increased volume of distribution. After intubation, an arterial line should be placed if not done before induction. Additional vascular access should be secured, including at least one 14- or 16-gauge IV, and a large central venous catheter with multi-lumen access. A rapid infuser needs to be available, and defibrillation pads should be applied early in anticipation of possible cardiac arrest upon reperfusion. Given the importance of assessing cardiac performance, consideration should be given to placement of a pulmonary artery catheter or TEE probe unless contraindicated. Packed red blood cells (pRBCs) and fresh frozen plasma (FFP) should be available in the operating room due to the high risk of significant bleeding (coagulopathic and surgical), At the authors' institution, liver transplantation is started with 10 units of pRBC and 10 units of FFP in the operating room prior to incision. Additional pRBCs, FFP, cryoprecipitate, and platelets are ordered and administered based on laboratory values and clinical coagulopathy. Common laboratory investigations intraoperatively include blood gases, platelet counts, PT, PTT, INR, and thromboelastography.

### Dissection Phase

After incision is made, the peritoneal cavity should be assessed for the presence of ascites. If more than 5 L of ascites is drained and/or there is evidence of intravascular volume depletion, consideration should be given to replacement of fluid losses with albumin; overall volume status goal during dissection is however, relative hypovolemia as a means to reduce blood loss. The decision for transfusion of blood products is based primarily on clinical assessment of volume status and coagulopathy. Good communication regarding on-going bleeding and coagulopathy between surgical and anesthetic teams is of critical importance. Although no specific guidelines exist, at the authors' institution, blood products are transfused based on the clinical impression of coagulopathy and on-going bleeding to approximate goals of hematocrit >25%, INR <3.0, platelets >20,000–30,000/mL and fibrinogen > 100 mg/dL. Crystalloid should be minimized in the setting of low plasma oncotic pressure, although this practice is mostly empiric, not evidence based. Patients may become hypotensive due to further decreases in SVR from inhalational anesthetics and/or fluid shifts. If a vasopressor is needed to maintain MAP goals, norepinephrine is typically first-line, followed by vasopressin. Patients with end-stage liver disease may demonstrate resistance to α-adrenergic agonists like phenylephrine, limiting their usefulness [22].

## Anhepatic Phase

The primary goal of the anhepatic phase is to optimize the patient for reperfusion. During this phase, ABGs are sent every 20–30 min, and dextrose and insulin should be co-administered as necessary to achieve a goal potassium concentration < 4 mEq/L. In the presence of acidosis or a base deficit, sodium bicarbonate may also be administered. Calcium chloride or calcium gluconate are administered for the dual purposes of repletion of calcium chelated by citrated blood products and cardiac membrane stabilization prior to reperfusion. Special attention should be paid to the volume status, with the goal of adequate intravascular volume to re-perfuse the donor liver [21].

## Neohepatic Phase

Given the relatively high concentration of potassium in the cold storage solution in the donor liver, the surgical team may flush the new liver with blood into the surgical field before unclamping the portal vein. The flush decreases the risk of hyperkalemia and cardiac arrest by washing the preservation solution from the donor liver. The University of Wisconsin liver preservation solution, with a potassium concentration of 120 mmol/L, is a significant donor-related mechanism of hyperkalemia following reperfusion. ECG changes, especially peaked T waves, may accompany reperfusion and necessitate immediate treatment of hyperkalemia. Replacing the portal clamping may also be exercised to prevent progression to hyperkalemic cardiac arrest. Additionally, significant bradycardia may result within the first 5 min as the cold storage solution stuns the right heart. Cytokine release syndrome may follow 12–15 min after reperfusion and should be treated aggressively with vasopressors and inotropic agents. PRS may last for several hours with a low SVR state. Additionally, this is typically a period of increased coagulopathy due to a combination of surgical loss, depletion of pre-existing recipient procoagulant factors, and lack of new factors being formed by the reperfused donor organ. As synthetic function resumes, the coagulopathy will also improve, but this process may take several hours. Significant transfusion of blood products is often required until function in the donor graft returns. Extreme cases of coagulopathy and blood loss may require extreme measures such as recombinant Factor VII administration.

After hemostasis of the large vascular anastomoses, immunosuppression is typically given. Intraoperative immunosuppression is institution-specific but often includes steroids, specifically methylprednisolone.

The final portion of the case includes the last vascular anastomosis—the hepatic artery. Cholecystectomy and bile duct anastomosis follow. Assuming adequate hemostasis, the patient's abdomen is closed, and the patient can be transported to the ICU for monitoring and continued management. At large liver transplant centers, more patients are being considered for early extubation. If the patient is hemodynamically stable and transfusion requirements were not significant, extubation in the OR can be successfully performed.

## Summary

Patients with ESLD have significant manifestations of their cirrhosis that impacts every major organ system. Liver transplantation surgery, despite significant advancements, still involves significant blood loss and hemodynamic derangements. It is critical for the Anesthesiologist caring for these patients to be very familiar and experienced in managing these aspects of liver transplantation.

## References

1. Starzl TE, Marchioro TL, Vonkaulla KN, Hermann G, Brittain RS, Waddell WR. Homotransplantation of the liver in humans. Surg Gynecol Obstet. 1963;117:659–76.
2. Starzl TE, Groth CG, Brettschneider L, Penn I, Fulginiti VA, Moon JB, Blanchard H, Martin AJ Jr, Porter KA. Orthotopic homotransplantation of the human liver. Ann Surg. 1968;168(3):392–415.
3. Starzl TE, Brettschneider L, Penn I, Bell P, Groth CG, Blanchard H, Kashiwagi N, Putnam CW. Orthotopic liver transplantation in man. Transplant Proc. 1969;1(1):216–22.
4. Based on OPTN data as of March 23, 2017. https://optn.transplant.hrsa.gov/data/citing-data/.
5. Malik SM, Ahmad J. Preoperative risk assessment for patients with liver disease. Med Clin North Am. 2009 Jul;93(4):917–29.
6. Martin P, DiMartini A, Feng S, Brown R Jr, Fallon M. Evaluation for liver transplantation in adults: 2013 practice guideline by the American Association for the Study of Liver Diseases and the American Society of Transplantation. Hepatology. 2014;59(3):1144–65.
7. Changes to OPTN bylaws and policies from actions at the OPTN/UNOS Executive Committee meetings July 2015–November 2015. https://optn.transplant.hrsa.gov/media/1575/policynotice_20151101.pdf. Accessed 9 May 2017.
8. Kim WR, Biggins SW, Kremers WK, et al. Hyponatremia and mortality among patients on the liver-transplant waiting list. N Engl J Med. 2008;359(10):1018–26.
9. Kamath PS, Wiesner RH, Malinchoc M, Kremers W, Therneau TM, Kosberg CL, D'Amico G, Dickson ER, Kim WR. A model to predict survival in patients with end-stage liver disease. Hepatology. 2001;33(2):464–70.
10. Gleisner AL, Muñoz A, Brandao A, et al. Survival benefit of liver transplantation and the effect of underlying liver disease. Surgery. 2010;147:392–404.
11. Schaubel DE, Guidinger MK, Biggins SW, et al. Survival benefit-based deceased-donor liver allocation. Am J Transplant. 2009;9:970–81.
12. Merion RM, Schaubel DE, Dykstra DM, et al. The survival benefit of liver transplantation. Am J Transplant. 2005;5:307–13.
13. Lladó L, Figueras J. Techniques of orthotopic liver transplantation. HPB. 2004;6(2):69–75.
14. Gallo AE, Melcher ML, Desai DM, Esquivel CO, Angelotti T, Lemmens HJM. Chapter 7.12. Liver/kidney/pancreas transplantation. In: Jaffe RA, Schmiesing CA, Golianu B, editors. Anesthesiologist's manual of surgical procedures. 5th ed. Philadelphia: Wolters Kluwer Health; 2014.
15. Siniscalchi A, et al. Post reperfusion syndrome during liver transplantation: from pathophysiology to therapy and preventive strategies. World J. Gastroenterol.. 2016;22(4):1551–69.
16. Muilenburg DJ, Singh A, Torzilli G, Khatri VP. Surgery in the patient with liver disease. Anesthesiol Clin. 2009;27(4):721–37.
17. Karvellas CJ, Fix OK, Battenhouse H, Durkalski V, Sanders C, Lee WM, et al. Outcomes and complications of intracranial pressure monitoring in acute liver failure: a retrospective cohort study. Crit Care Med. 2014;42(5):11571157s.
18. Carey WD, Dumot JA, Pimentel RR, et al. The prevalence of coronary artery disease in liver transplant candidates over age 50. Transplantation. 1995;59:859–64.
19. Tiukinhoy-Laing SD, Rossi JS, Bayram M, et al. Cardiac hemodynamic and coronary angiographic characteristics of patients being evaluated for liver transplantation. Am J Cardiol. 2006;98:178–81.
20. Steadman RH, Wray CL. Cardiovascular assessment of the liver transplant candidate. Int Anesthesiol Clin. 2017;55:42–66.
21. Findlay JY. Patient selection and preoperative evaluation for transplant surgery. Anesthesiol Clin. 2013;31(4):689–704.
22. Hannaman MJ, Hevesi ZG. Anesthesia care for liver transplantation. Transplant Rev. 2011;25(1):36–43.
23. DuBrock HM, Channick RN, Krowka MJ. What's new in the treatment of portopulmonary hypertension? Expert Rev Gastroenterol Hepatol. 2015;9(7):983–92.
24. Krowka MJ, Plevak DJ, Findlay JY, Rosen CB, Wiesner RH, Krom RAF. Pulmonary hemodynamics and perioperative cardiopulmonary-related mortality in patients with portopulmonary hypertension undergoing liver transplantation. Liver Transpl. 2000;6:443–50.
25. DeMartino ES, Cartin-Ceba R, Findlay JY, Heimbach JK, Krowka MJ. Frequency and outcomes of patients with increased mean pulmonary artery pressure at the time of liver transplantation. Transplantation. 2017;101(1):101–6.

# Anesthesia for Kidney Transplantation

## 73

Ellen Cho and Gaurav P. Patel

## Introduction

Historically, the majority of transplanted kidneys were recovered from deceased donors following brain or cardiac death. However, in recent years there has been an exponential increase in the number of living donors, increasing the pool of available organs for renal transplantation (Fig. 73.1). Compared to deceased donor recipients, those patients receiving living donor organs have better allograft and surgical outcomes [1–4]. Anesthesiologists now care for kidney recipients undergoing planned living directed donor transplants as well as more urgent surgery for those receiving a kidney from a deceased donor. This chapter outlines the surgical technique for renal transplantation as well as the unique patient and anesthetic considerations for both living and deceased donor renal transplants.

## Surgical Considerations and Technique

Following procurement, the donated kidney is prepared with various degrees of dissection that depend on donor anatomy as well as if the kidney

E. Cho, M.D. · G. P. Patel, M.D. (✉)
Emory University School of Medicine,
Atlanta, GA, USA
e-mail: ellen.cho@emory.edu; gppatel@emory.edu

was obtained from a deceased or living donor. Kidney preparation is a meticulous process, and requires surgeon attention and care to ensure optimal outcomes in the recipient. This however, must be balanced with the need to limit organ ischemia. The warm ischemic phase begins when blood flow to the kidney is interrupted during the procurement period and may coincide with renal artery cross-clamp or, in donation after cardiac death (DCD), may commence at the time that the kidney is no longer receiving sufficient blood flow in the donor. Cold ischemia starts when the donor kidney is placed in the hypothermic preservative solution prior to its implantation into the recipient. For deceased donor kidneys, the core temperature is reduced below 4 °C during the cold ischemic phase to minimize inherent metabolism and decrease enzyme activity [5]. The kidney is also flushed with a preservative solution to maintain the organ's viability while it is being transported to the recipient. Despite a significant decrease in enzymatic activity, there is still an appreciable buildup of byproducts such as lactic acid, which can have important physiologic effects on the recipient's homeostasis during the reperfusion period of the transplant surgery. Although cold ischemic time varies amongst organs and individual transplant centers, typically an acceptable time before transplantation is 24 h, with the goal being to re-perfuse the donated kidney as is immediately feasible. The cold ischemia time in a living donor kidney is typically restricted to 20–30 min.

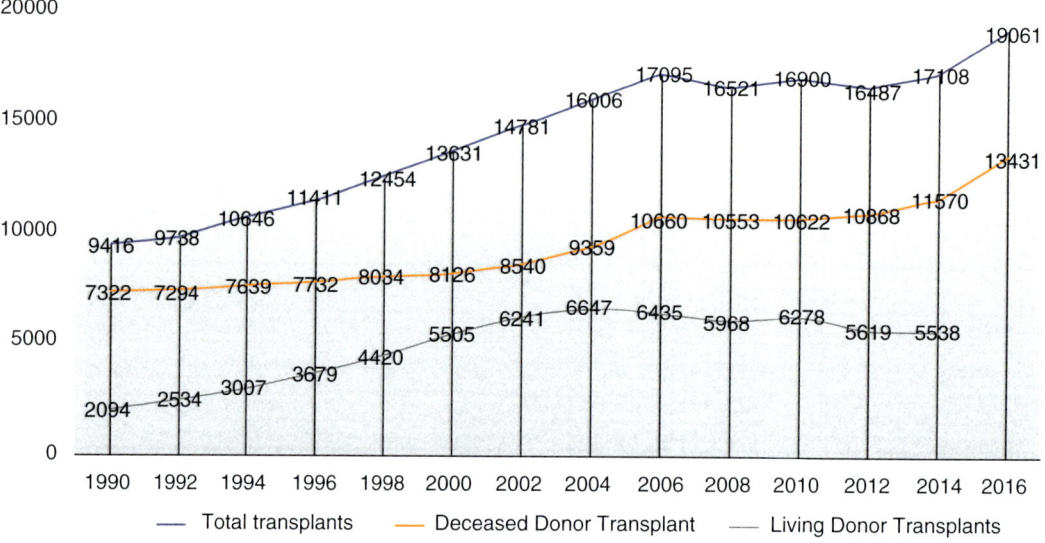

**Fig. 73.1** Kidney transplant by donor type 1990–2016. Organ procurement and transplantation network 2017 [3]

Several surgical approaches to renal transplantation have been described. Currently, the most common is the Gibson incision in the lower abdominal quadrant. Historically, the donated kidney was placed in the contralateral recipient side. Today, surgeons use either side of the recipient's pelvis however, a number of factors are considered when planning kidney placement in the pelvis. In most patients, the left external iliac vessels are shorter than those on the right, which may impact surgical decision-making [6]. In addition, previous surgical sites and location of peritoneal dialysis catheters influence operative side. Through a curvilinear incision, the retroperitoneal space is dissected to expose the bladder and necessary vasculature. In complex cases or in patients who have undergone previous transplants, a larger transabdominal incision may be necessary.

After dissection and exposure, vascular anastomoses are performed. Although the venous anastomosis is traditionally performed first, this can vary depending on surgeon preference as well as donor and recipient anatomic variation. Most commonly, the donor renal vein is anastomosed to the recipient external iliac vein in an end-to-side fashion. Subsequently, the donor renal artery is juxtaposed to the recipient external iliac artery to create the arterial anastomosis. This may be accomplished via an end-to-side or end-to-end fashion. In situations of anatomic variance or previous transplant surgery, it may be necessary to anastomose the donor renal artery to the common iliac artery, aorta or hypogastric artery [7].

Once vascular anastomoses are complete, the vessel cross clamps are removed, resulting in reperfusion of the new kidney. At this point, significant bleeding is identified and corrected, and reconstruction begins on the urinary tract. The donor ureter is directly attached to the recipient bladder—a ureteroneocystostomy. The donor ureter may occasionally need to be anastomosed directly into the native recipient ureter. In these cases, many surgeons will leave an indwelling stent because it is well tolerated by the recipient and may minimize postoperative urinary complications [8].

Performance of the newly transplanted kidney depends significantly on ischemic time. Living donor kidneys are expected to produce urine quickly while deceased donor kidneys may take longer to become fully functional. It is not uncommon for recipients of deceased donor kidneys to require dialysis in the immediate postoperative period while waiting for the donor kidney to function appropriately. Some of the more commonly seen complications of renal transplant surgery include bladder dysfunction, delayed graft function, urinary obstruction, bleeding, hematoma formation and arterial stenosis. It is also possible to have complications related to medication administration, specifically calcineurin inhibitors which are frequently used in immunosuppression regimens.

## Anesthetic Considerations

### Preoperative Management

A detailed pre-operative assessment prior to renal transplantation is required (see Table 73.1). Comorbidities are assessed to determine if the patient is medically optimized to tolerate an anesthetic and the stress of surgery. In most centers, the transplant recipient undergoes significant pre-operative workup and must be deemed an operative candidate by a selection committee.

### Cardiac

Risks for ESRD are also often the same factors that contribute to ischemic heart disease and heart failure. Patients with ESRD due to diabetes are evaluated for concurrent coronary artery disease and peripheral vascular disease. Uncontrolled hypertension is the second leading cause of ESRD in the Unites Stated [9]; progressive renal disease also worsens hypertension in a circular relationship making blood pressure more difficult to control. These patients are often on multiple antihypertensive agents and are at risk to develop ischemic heart disease, heart failure and atrial fibrillation. A 12 lead electrocardiogram (ECG) is obtained to assess for dysrhythmias; and although poorly sensitive in the absence of active symptoms, it may reveal underlying coronary artery disease. Screening the patient's metabolic equivalents (METS) allow assessment of cardiac fitness. Stress testing for those with less than four METS is done in accordance with the evidence-based guidelines put forth by the American Heart Association and The American College of Cardiology [10]. Additionally, given the high incidence of cardiac dysfunction, a transthoracic echocardiogram (TTE) may also be useful to assess structural changes, systolic function, the presence of diastolic dysfunction, common in patients with long standing hypertension [11]. Most centers routinely obtain a TTE and EKG every year for candidates on the transplant waiting list [11, 12].

**Table 73.1** Preoperative considerations

| Organ system | Specific considerations | Tests/workup |
|---|---|---|
| Cardiovascular | Increased risk of CAD<br>Pericarditis/pericardial effusion<br>Volume status (CHF)<br>Presence of dysrhythmias | EKG<br>TTE<br>CXR<br>Stress testing (as indicated by history and physical) |
| Respiratory | Pleural effusions/pleuritic<br>Coexisting COPD/asthma/reactive airway disease | CXR<br>PFTs (rarely indicated) |
| Renal | Pre or post dialysis<br>Dialysis access<br>Electrolyte and acid/base status (presence of hyperkalemia, metabolic acidosis) | Creatinine clearance<br>BUN/Creatinine<br>Electrolytes |
| Hematology | Chronic anemia<br>Presence of coagulopathy<br>Thrombocytopenia/platelet dysfunction | CBC<br>PT/PTT/INR |
| Endocrine | Glycemic control | Glucose level, HgbA1C |

## Pulmonary

Pulmonary disease may develop independently of ESRD or as direct sequelae of renal failure. Volume overload may manifest as pulmonary edema or congestive heart failure. Additionally, patients with ESRD are prone to the development of pleural effusions that prohibit optimal intraoperative oxygenation and ventilation [11]. Smoking has been demonstrated to correlate with the progression of chronic kidney disease [13] and carries a hazard ration for the development of ESRD of 2.4 in men and 2.9 in women [14]. A concomitant diagnosis of emphysema or chronic obstructive pulmonary disease is common in patients with ESRD presenting for transplant evaluation. A baseline chest radiograph is not recommended unless patients demonstrate acute worsening of their condition, signs of infection such as fever or increasingly productive cough, or complain of new or atypical symptoms. An assessment of room air saturation will provide a simple evaluation of the Alveolar-arterial gradient; if concerning, an arterial blood gas sample may be useful [15]. Pulmonary function testing (PFT) may provide further information if significant respiratory disease is suspected, however will not necessarily alter anesthetic or surgical management [7, 12, 15].

## Renal

Fluid management is evaluated as part of the transplant work-up, however current volume status must be clinically assessed prior to proceeding to the operating room for surgery. Those with non-functioning kidneys, even if well managed and adherent to frequent hemodialysis (HD), are prone to volume overload. If possible, those on scheduled HD need to have their session appropriately timed before surgery. Pre-operative HD prevents volume overload and aids in achieving electrolyte imbalance (with special attention to potassium levels). Routine pre-operative use of HD in all patients (even those who exhibit a normal fluid and electrolyte status) is debatable. Several studies show conflicting data correlating preoperative HD to best outcomes [11]. Dialysis should strongly be considered prior to transplant in patients whose serum potassium levels are greater than 6.0 milliequivalents per liter (mEq/L) because potassium is released during graft reperfusion can result in malignant dysrhythmias or in severe circumstances, hyperkalemic cardiac arrest [16].

## Hematologic

A complete blood count (CBC) and coagulation studies should be ordered prior to surgery. A large portion of ESRD patients have chronic anemia secondary to low levels of erythropoietin production. Pre-operative correction is rarely necessary unless the anemia is severe and symptomatic. Thrombocytopenia may accompany renal disease and is theorized to be related to a number of factors including platelet consumption during dialysis (with compensatory release of platelets from the bone marrow) [17], constant heparin exposure during HD [18], increased consumption and decreased production, Platelet function is also poor secondary to uremia. Those undergoing routine hemodialysis demonstrate improvement in platelet function, but their bleeding time is still often prolonged [19]. Prothrombin time (PT/INR) and partial thromboplastin time (PTT) should be measured and evaluated in conjunction with other data [15]. Even when normal, bleeding is more commonly seen in ESRD than in normal kidney function. Platelet transfusions, cryoprecipitate, desmopressin and conjugated estrogens have all demonstrated roles in treatment of ESRD patients during procedural or operating room bleeding [20].

## Endocrine

Diabetes mellitus (DM) is one of the most common causes of ESRD. Cardiovascular disease frequently exists in patients with DM, and appropriate testing to evaluate cardiac function is necessary. Adequate glycemic control is crucial as it is related to perioperative mortality with current recommendations in place to maintain perioperative glucose levels <180 mg/dL [21]. Patients with DM are also at risk of diabetic gastroparesis, suggesting that intraoperative management include a rapid sequence intubation. Additionally, for those with diabetic neuropathy, pre-operative documentation should include baseline sensory deficits with vigilant attention to intraoperative positioning [22].

## Urgent Versus Emergent?

The cadaveric kidney is often viable for 24+ h; thus, if a change in patient condition is recognized in the immediate preoperative period, the case may occasionally need to be delayed to provide urgent medical care. Discussion with the surgeon regarding graft viability is important. Given the donor kidney's ischemic time limitations, it is debatable if this is considered an elective or urgent procedure.

## Intraoperative Concerns and Management

### Anesthetic Technique

The vast majority of centers in the United States perform kidney transplantation under general endotracheal anesthesia. There are reports and studies of the surgery being completed using spinal or epidural anesthesia [11], however this is relatively uncommon.

Patients with ESRD often have low serum protein levels. This will affect medications that are highly protein bound in circulation; low serum albumin levels lead to an increased fraction of free (unbound) drug. Oppositely, the increased volume of distribution often increased the drug dose needed to achieve effect. Careful titration of anesthetics is merited in renal failure because the pharmaco-kinetics and dynamics of anesthetic agents is less predictable.

Propofol and etomidate are commonly used induction agents in kidney transplantation. The use of etomidate has been documented to lead to adrenal insufficiency however, it has been debated if this is of clinical significance in renal transplant patients who will receive steroids and other medications to achieve a state of profound immunosuppression following transplantation [23]. If rapid sequence induction is used, a serum potassium concentration prior to induction of less than 5.0–5.5 mEq/L is considered safe for the use of succinylcholine [15]. Close monitoring of the electrocardiogram during induction is prudent, and any changes, particularly peaked t waves, prompt treatment to correct hyperkalemia [11, 12].

Anesthesia during renal transplantation is maintained using a balanced technique. Inhalational anesthetics or total intravenous anesthesia are both appropriate. Although there is theoretical debate regarding the use of sevoflurane and possible nephrotoxicity in rat models due to compound A, this has not been replicated in humans. Sevoflurane, isoflurane, or desflurane are safe volatile agents for the procedure [12].

Neuromuscular blockade is recommended to optimize surgical conditions. Any movement, especially during anastomosis can be devastating. Cisatracurium or rocuronium can be used however, cisatracurium is often preferred due to its renal-independent metabolism by Hoffman degradation. Prolonged neuromuscular blockade can occur with the use of the latter of the two drugs, and care must be taken upon re-dosing. Reversal agents are administered based on careful monitoring of neuromuscular blockade, and a train-of-four (TOF) ratio > 0.9 is recommended prior to extubation [12, 16]. Reversal is accomplished using a combination of neostigmine and glycopyrrolate. Sugammadex is not currently FDA approved for use in patients with severe renal disease [12].

Several medications utilize the renal system as a predominant method of excretion or metabolism. Morphine-6-glucoronide is an active metabolite of morphine and can lead to increased respiratory depression in renal insufficiency; therefore, use of morphine in this patient population is minimized or avoided. Normoperidine is a byproduct of meperidine metabolism and can result in seizure activity in patients with renal insufficiency. Fentanyl and hydromorphone are safe and the most commonly used medications for pain control as part of a balanced anesthetic [15]. Avoidance of other nephrotoxic agents, such as aminoglycosides and non-steroidal anti-inflammatory, minimizes risk to the transplanted kidney.

Extubation following kidney transplant is common, but depends on patient specific and surgical factors. If extubation is planned, it important to ensure that appropriate depth of anesthesia and relaxation are maintained during fascial closure. Coughing and bucking during surgery or emergence, must be avoided because it places stress on the transplanted kidney and interruption of anastomoses [24]. There are several case reports in the literature of bucking leading to ischemia in the newly transplanted kidney [12, 15, 24–26].

## Monitoring and Access

Standard American Society of Anesthesiologists (ASA) monitors are used for all patients. An arterial line may be inserted, and should be considered in patients with poorly controlled hypertension, brittle diabetes, significant pulmonary disease, or those with suspected fluid overload, electrolyte or acid/base imbalance without time for pre-operative HD. Although most renal recipients are accepted based on an absence of severe ischemic heart disease, an arterial line is recommended in patients with significant valve dysfunction, recent exacerbations in heart failure or those with a recent history of unstable dysrhythmias. Central venous pressure monitoring, while historically common, is no longer a standard practice. The majority of major transplant centers have moved away from placing central venous lines in all renal transplant patients. Current literature suggests less than 30% of patients undergo placement of central venous lines [11, 24].

Peripheral access can be challenging in this patient population. Often, one upper extremity is the site of an arteriovenous (AV) fistula or graft; peripheral access may be limited to the opposite upper extremity. Large bore access is ideal with placement of an 18-gauge peripheral line or larger. A second large peripheral line additionally facilitates medication infusions, resuscitation and fluid administration. If large bore access cannot be obtained, a central line should be placed in the internal jugular vein. A subclavian catheter may be considered but care should be taken if placed on the same side as an AV fistula or graft; Arterialization of the subclavian vein may be present [24] and properly identifying catheter location can be more difficult due to pulsatility and increased oxygenation in the subclavian vein. Femoral vein access can be obtained if other sites are unsuccessful; however, due to risk of infection associated with femoral central access, caution should be exercised in transplant patients particularly due to the initiation of postoperative immunosuppression [24]. Strict aseptic technique should be maintained for central line placement.

## Fluid Management

Fluid management requires particular attention in the operating room and needs to be optimized to promote perfusion of the newly transplanted kidney [11]. Patients may arrive in extremes of baseline volume status; those who missed HD due to timing of transplant, are volume overloaded. Postdialysis patients presenting immediately for surgery are often be volume deplete. Typically, volume loading in the operating room is encouraged however, it has been debated to what degree, mild to significant, hypervolemia is beneficial is to a newly transplanted kidney [15]. Appropriate fluid goals are now frequently based on specific transplant center practice. The primary aim of volume administration is perfusion of the new graft [12]. Avoidance of hypovolemia is widely accepted as a key to the success of these practice specific algorithms to prevent renal ischemia and acute tubular necrosis. Previously, normal saline was the crystalloid of choice in renal transplant surgery with the intended goal of avoiding hyperkalemia however, recent studies, demonstrate that the use of normal saline may lead to potassium concentration compared to lactated ringers [11, 15]. Furthermore, the use of normal saline results in acidosis when administered in large volumes, which may potentially worsen existing hyperkalemia. Currently, balanced solutions such as plasmalyte or normosol are recommended [11, 15].

## Medication Management

Heparin is given during renal transplantation immediately prior to clamp placement on the renal vessels. Typical doses are 2000–5000 IU. Dose and timing should be confirmed with the surgeon.

Although transplant center dependent, medications such as furosemide and mannitol have been suggested to facilitate renal blood flow and urine production, so are often administered in the operating room. Historically, by blocking the Na/K channels in the Loop of Henle, furosemide was given to improve urine output in the newly transplanted kidney. It is unclear however, if loop diuretics improve outcomes or long-term graft survival [27]. Mannitol is widely used in kidney transplantation prior to reperfusion of the vascular anastomosis. Theoretically, mannitol increases tubular flow rate and may increase the release of vasodilatory prostaglandins [28]. To date, it is the only agent shown to decrease immediate acute kidney injury [12]. Long-term renal function does not appear to be impacted by mannitol use [29]. Despite this, current data regarding the use of either of these agents remains controversial. There also may be a difference in the need/use of diuretics when comparing deceased donor versus living donor kidney transplants. Living donor kidneys may not require diuretic agents because the baseline incidence of delayed graft function is notably decreased compared to cadaveric kidneys [25].

At times during transplantation, despite adequate volume loading, patients may experience episodes of hypotension. This is particularly true with the iliac vessels are unclamped and the graft is reperfused. Vasopressor particularly following establishment of blood flow to the new kidney is controversial. Past teachings in anesthesia emphasized avoidance of pressors because alpha agonist activity decreases renal blood flow with theorized harm to the transplanted organ. Dopamine was originally identified as the preferred inotrope of choice during renal transplantation because it increases renal blood flow and urine output. However, several studies demonstrate a possible negative effect on renal function and it has fallen out of favor [30]. Re-exploring vasopressors with alpha activity, such as norepinephrine or phenylephrine, reveals a lack of negative outcomes with the use of norepinephrine to maintain appropriate blood pressure [11, 15].

Preserving a targeted blood pressure to ensure renal, cardiac, and cerebral perfusion is paramount in the operating room; use of a vasopressor can be considered as needed to help maintain these goals with care that appropriate volume status is also achieved.

Immunosuppressant induction is usually initiated prior to the operating room to decrease the incidence of graft rejection. Induction agents given in the operating room often include high-dose steroids and one of the following agents: thymoglobulin, basiliximab, daclimuzab, or belatacept. Following operating room care and the acute phase of immunosuppression, typical long-term immunosuppressant regimens are comprised of a combination of steroids, calcineurin inhibitors, target of rapamycin (TOR) inhibitors or purine synthesis inhibitors.

## Post-operative Care

Patients are frequently extubated in the operating room, transferred to the Post-Anesthesia Care Unit (PACU), and subsequently to a surgical floor. Urine output is monitored closely to ensure early identification of delayed graft function. Hemodialysis may be necessary in the immediate post-operative period if electrolyte abnormalities are uncontrolled and/or signs of symptomatic fluid overload are present, especially in those with delayed graft function. The use of ultrasound to monitor patent renal vasculature is often performed as soon as possible in the recovery room, particularly if there is concern for delayed graft function or surgical complication. When the ultrasound reveals inappropriate perfusion, often the patient is taken back to the operating room.

Cardiovascular complications are amongst the most common following renal transplant. Close monitoring in high-risk patients and immediate work-up for those with suspicious changes in EKG or complaints of cardiopulmonary symptoms is merited.

Other PACU concerns include bleeding, hemorrhage and adverse reactions to immunosuppressants. These factors, in addition to standard postoperative anesthetic concerns, should be addressed prior to discharge from the PACU to the floor.

## Special Considerations

In circumstances when a single donor kidney is deemed insufficient to supply a recipient with adequate renal function, both kidneys may be transplanted. For example, pediatric donor kidneys may be resected en bloc and transplanted together in an adult recipient. Similarly, dual kidneys from an adult donor may be used in a single recipient if the kidneys are deemed to have unlikely success rates if transplanted alone.

Renal transplantation also frequently occurs in conjunction with other organs such as the pancreas and liver. Pancreas transplants are performed to treat insulin-dependent type 1 diabetes mellitus, and are combined with renal transplantation for patients who have chronic kidney disease (CKD) or ESRD secondary to diabetic nephropathy. These cases are usually performed through one abdominal, midline incision as opposed to the traditional lower quadrant incision used for renal transplants. Appropriate access includes at least two large bore peripheral intravenous lines for volume resuscitation and medication administration. Depending on the recipient's comorbidities, it may be reasonable to consider an arterial line and central venous access as well. Intraoperatively, serum glucose is monitored diligently and controlled with a variable rate insulin infusion if necessary. Serum glucose levels need to be continuously monitored postoperatively with careful attention to the development of hypoglycemia as soon as the newly transplanted pancreas begins to function.

Combined liver-kidney transplantation is being performed more frequently in patients with cirrhosis and associated refractory hepatorenal disease or parenchymal diseases related to chronic hepatitis B or C infection. Patients with hepatorenal syndrome deserve special consideration prior to kidney transplantation due to the potential for disease resolution following liver transplant alone [26]. Most commonly, the liver will be transplanted first through a subcostal abdominal incision with the kidney subsequently transplanted through a separate lower quadrant incision. This is to ensure that hemostasis is satisfactory after hepatic reperfusion before proceeding with renal transplantation. These patients are severely morbid with multiple medical comorbidities. The liver transplantation portion of the operation largely dictates anesthetic care in these cases. See chapter on liver transplantation.

## References

1. Transplant trends | UNOS [Internet]. Unos.org. 2017 [cited 30 January 2017]. https://www.unos.org/data/transplant-trends/#transplants_by_organ_type+year+2016.
2. OPTN/SRTR 2015 Annual Data Report. Organ Procurement and Transplantation Network (OPTN) and Scientific Registry of Transplant Recipients (SRTR). 2016.
3. Organ Procurement and Transplantation Network. National Data, Donors Recovered in the United States by Donor Type 2017. https://optn.transplant.hrsa.gov/data/view-data-reports/national-data/#. Accessed 30 May 2017.
4. Meier-Kriesche H, Kaplan B. Waiting time on dialysis as the strongest modifiable risk factor for renal transplant outcomes: a paired donor kidney analysis. Transplantation. 2002;74(10):1377–81.
5. Southard J, Belzer F. Organ preservation. Annu Rev Med. 1995;46:235–47.
6. Flechner S. Renal Transplantation. In: McAninch J, Lue T, ed. by. Smith and Tanagho's General Urology [Internet]. 18th Ed New York: McGraw-Hill; 2013 [cited 30 January 2017]. http://accesssurgery.mhmedical.com.proxy.library.emory.edu/content.aspx?bookid=508&sectionid=41088113.
7. Danovitch G. Handbook of kidney transplantation. 5th ed. Philadelphia: Lippincott, Williams & Wilkins; 2009.
8. Mangus R, Haag B. Stented versus nonstented extravesical ureteroneocystostomy in renal transplantation: a meta-analysis. Am J Transplant. 2004;4:1889–96.
9. Botdorf J, Chaundhary K, Whaley-Connell A. Hpertension in cardiovascular and kidney disease. Cardioremal Med. 2011;1:183–92.
10. Fleisher L, Fleischmann K, Auerbach A, Branson S, Beckman J, Bozkurt B, et al. 2014 ACC/AHA guideline on perioperative cardiovascular evaluation and management of patients undergoing noncardiac surgery. J Am Coll Cardiol. 2014;64(22):e77–e137.
11. Schmid S, Jungwirth B. Anaesthesia for renal transplant surgery: an update. Eur J Anaesthesiol. 2012;29:552–8.

12. Lemmens H. Kidney transplantation: recent developments and recommendations for anesthetic management. Anesthesiol Clin North Am. 2004;22(4):651–62.
13. Bleyer AJ, Shemanski LR, Burke GL, Hansen KJ, Appel RG. Tobacco, hypertension, and vascular disease: risk factors for renal functional decline in an older population. Kidney Int. 2000;57:2072–9.
14. Haroun MK, Jaar BG, Hoffman SC, Comstock GW, Klag MJ, Coresh J. Risk factors for chronic kidney disease: a prospective study of 23,534 men and women in Washington County, Maryland. J Am Soc Nephrol. 2003;14:2934–41.
15. Martinez B, et al. Anesthesia for kidney transplantation—a review. J Anesth Clin Res. 2013;4:1.
16. Jaffe RA, Schmiesing C, Golianu B. Anesthesiologist's manual of surgical procedures. 4th ed. Philadelphia: Lippincott Williams & Wilkins; 2009.
17. Bat T, Bat BE, El-Moghraby A, Samir P, Xingmin F, Dunbar CE, Sarac E. Thrombopoietic status of patients on haemodialysis. Br J Haematol. 2016;172(6): 954–7.
18. Malhotra V, Sudheendra V, Diwan S. Miller's anesthesia. In: Anesthesia and the renal and genitourinary systems. 6th ed. Philadelphia: Churchill Livingstone; 2005. p. 2181–7.
19. Dorgalaleh A, Mahmudi M, Tabibian S, et al. Anemia and thrombocytopenia in acute and chronic renal failure. Int J Hematol Oncol Stem Cell Res. 2013;7(4):34–9.
20. Hedges SJ, Dehoney SB, Hooper JS, Amanzadeh J, Busti AJ. Evidence-based treatment recommendations for uremic bleeding. Nat Clin Pract Nephrol. 2007;3(3):138–53.
21. Moghissi ES, Korytkowski MT, DiNardo M, et al. American Association of Clinical Endocrinologists and American Diabetes Association consensus statement on inpatient glycemic control. Endocr Pract. 2009;15(4):353–69.
22. Norio K, Makisalo H, Isoniemi H, Grop PH, Pere P. Are diabetic patients in danger at renal transplantation? An invasive perioperative study. Eur J Anaesthesiol. 2000;17:729–36.
23. Baxi V, Jain A, Dasgupta D. Anaesthesia for renal transplantation: an update. Indian J Anaesth. 2009;53(2):139–47.
24. Barash PG, Cullen BF, Stoelting RK. Clinical anesthesia. 6th ed. Philadelphia: Lippincott; 2009.
25. Rabey P. Anesthesia for renal transplantation. Br J Anaesth. 2001;1:24–7.
26. David C, Gonwa T, Wilkinson A. Identification of patients best suited for combined liver-kidney transplantation: part II. Liver Transpl. 2002;8:193–211.
27. Lachance SL, Barry JM. Effect of furosemide on dialysis requirement following cadaveric kidney transplantation. J Urol. 1985;133:950–1.
28. Johnston PA, Bernard DB, Perrin NS, Levinsky NG. Prostaglandins mediate the vasodilatory effect of mannitol in the hypoperfused rat kidney. J Clin Invest. 1981;68:127–33.
29. Weimar W, Geerlings W, Bijnen AB, et al. A controlled study on the effect of mannitol on immediate renal function after cadaver donor kidney transplantation. Transplantation. 1983;35:99–101.
30. Kellum J, Decker J. Use of dopamine in acute renal failure: a meta-analysis. Crit Care Med. 2001;29:1526–31.

# Part VII

# Others

# Anesthesia Issues in Patients with Obstructive Sleep Apnea

Amélie Dallaire and Mandeep Singh

## Introduction

Obstructive sleep apnea (OSA) is a serious and common sleep disorder. OSA is characterized by repetitive cessation of breathing lasting 10 s or more resulting in varying severity of hypoxemia and/or hypercapnia. Exaggerated reduction in pharyngeal muscle tone leads to partial or complete closure of the pharynx, accompanied with hypoventilation, desaturation and frequent arousals [1]. Clinically, OSA results in daytime symptoms attributable to impaired sleep, such as sleepiness, fatigue, poor concentration, memory loss, cognitive and behavioral dysfunctions [2].

A. Dallaire, M.D., F.R.C.P.C.
Department of Anesthesiology and Pain Medicine, Toronto Western Hospital, University Health Network, University of Toronto, Toronto, ON, Canada
e-mail: amelie.dallaire.1@ulaval.ca

M. Singh, M.D., M.Sc. (✉)
Department of Anesthesiology and Pain Medicine, Toronto Western Hospital, University Health Network, University of Toronto, Toronto, ON, Canada

Department of Anesthesiology and Pain Management, Women's College Hospital, Toronto, ON, Canada

Toronto Sleep and Pulmonary Centre, Toronto, Canada
e-mail: mandeep.singh@uhn.ca

## Pathophysiology of Airway Collapse in OSA

The upper airway (UA) is a complex structure able to change and adapt its shape in order to fulfill its different functions, such as breathing, speaking and swallowing. UA collapsibility and patency are dependent on a continuous balance between collapsing and expanding forces. During wakefulness, the UA patency is achieved by increased dilatator muscle tone, especially the genioglossus muscle that pulls the tongue forward [3, 4]. The UA of patients with OSA is narrower and more prone to collapse [5]. During sleep, a complex interaction of factors such as, loss of UA dilating muscle tone, impaired response to mechanoreceptors sensing intrapharyngeal pressure and an increased arousal threshold [3, 4], can all predispose to increased propensity for UA collapse in OSA patients. Additionally, overnight rostral fluid shift from the legs to neck may lead to even more UA narrowing in some patients [6]. Arousal from sleep helps to restore airway patency, however at the expense of poor-quality sleep.

The UA collapse and obstructive events tend to occur more frequently under general anesthesia. In addition, decreased upper airway dilator muscle tone and abolition of protective arousal response predisposes to prolonged and more severe oxygen desaturation. Worsening of OSA persists during the postoperative period. Compared to the preoperative baseline, complete or partial obstruction episodes significantly increase during the first postoperative night, with peak increase occurring on the third night [7, 8].

## OSA and Comorbid Conditions

The patient with OSA who presents to the operating room may have multiple comorbid conditions. OSA is associated with obesity, metabolic syndrome, insulin resistance, gastroesophageal reflux and long-term cardiovascular morbidity including myocardial ischemia, heart failure arrhythmias and cerebrovascular disease. Craniofacial deformities (e.g. macroglossia, small chin, mid-facial hypoplasia), endocrine disorders (e.g. hypothyroidism, Cushing disease), demographic (male sex, age > 50 years old) and life style factors (e.g. smoking, alcohol consumption) represent risk factors closely associated with OSA [9]. These comorbidities may require further optimization and risk stratification before surgery.

## Clinical Diagnosis Criteria

Classically the gold-standard for diagnosing OSA is an overnight polysomnography. This study determines the number of abnormal respiratory events (partial obstruction or complete cessation) per hour of sleep. Based on the American Academy of Sleep Medicine (AASM) recommendations, apneas and hypopneas are defined as a reduction in airflow from intranasal pressure of at least 90%, or between 50 and 90%, respectively for at least 10 s accompanied by either a 3–4% drop in oxygen saturation or an EEG arousal [10, 11].

The Apnea-Hypopnea Index (AHI) corresponds to the average number of abnormal breathing events per hour of sleep. AHI is used by the AASM to describe the severity of OSA. Mild OSA is defined as AHI between 5 and 15 events/h, moderate OSA as AHI between 15 and 30 events/h, and severe OSA as AHI greater than 30 events/h [10, 11]. The clinical diagnosis of OSA requires either an AHI of 15 or more, or AHI greater than or equal to 5, with symptoms such as excessive daytime sleepiness, unintentional sleep during wakefulness, unrefreshing sleep, loud snoring reported by a partner, or observed obstruction during sleep [12, 13].

Polysomnography is a laboratory based sleep study registered and analyzed by a technologist using standard criteria. Cost and requirement of technical expertise may limit accessibility of this test. Home sleep testing and nocturnal oximetry may be a reliable alternative to standard polysomnography for the diagnosis of OSA in certain subsets of patients like high-risk surgical patients [12, 14, 15]. Testing with portable devices may be considered when there is high probability of moderate to severe OSA without other substantial comorbidities [14], and proper standards for conducting the test and interpreting the results are met [12].

## Prevalence of OSA

In the general population, the prevalence of moderate to severe OSA (AHI $\geq$ 15 events/h) is 13% among men and 6% among women [16]. The estimates are higher with increasing age and body mass index [17]. In obese patients undergoing bariatric surgery, prevalence of OSA increases up to 70% [18]. Between 60 and 90% of surgical patients with moderate to severe OSA remain undiagnosed preoperatively [19].

## OSA and Postoperative Complications

A recent systematic literature review reported that the presence of OSA increases the risk for postoperative adverse events and complications [20]. Patients with a diagnosis of OSA have increased risk of emergent intubation [21–23], non-invasive or mechanical ventilation [21–23], aspiration pneumonia [22], pulmonary embolism [22], delirium [24] and atrial fibrillation [21, 23]. Patients with OSA, compared to non-OSA patients, present a twofold higher risk of postoperative events, such as acute respiratory failure, desaturation and intensive care transfer [25]. Severity of OSA is an important factor in the development of postoperative complications. Patients with severe OSA (AHI > 30) have more than 2.5-fold increase in post-operative respiratory complications [26].

Compared with treated OSA, untreated OSA is associated with more cardiopulmonary complications including unplanned re-intubation and myocardial infarction [27]. Just like untreated patients, OSA patients who remain undiagnosed are at increased risk of postoperative complications [26]. In a study by Mutter et al., patients with undiagnosed OSA were found to have a threefold higher risk of cardiovascular complications, primarily cardiac arrest and shock, compared to diagnosed OSA patients [26]. Given the important adverse consequences associated with OSA, screening for OSA should be included in the preoperative anesthetic evaluation.

## Screening for OSA

Recent guidelines by the Society of Anesthesia and Sleep Medicine (SASM) states that adult patients at risk of OSA should be identified before surgery [28]. Routine screening for asymptomatic patients in general population is not recommended [29]. Routine preoperative screening using polysomnography, the gold-standard diagnostic test, is costly and resource intensive. As a result, a number of simple and economical screening tests have been developed to detect patients at risk of OSA. The STOP-Bang questionnaire [30], P-SAP score [31], Berlin questionnaire [32] and ASA checklist [14] are screening tests that were validated in the surgical population. Among these tests, the STOP-Bang questionnaire is the most validated screening tool for surgical patients [30, 33–36].

The STOP-Bang questionnaire is a concise screening test consisting of eight dichotomous (yes/no) questions related to the clinical features of OSA (**S**noring, **T**iredness, **O**bserved apnea, high blood **P**ressure, **B**MI, **a**ge, **n**eck circumference and male **g**ender) [30]. (Table 74.1) Patients are considered to be at low risk of OSA with a score between 0 and 2, intermediate risk with a score between 3 and 4 and high risk of OSA with a score between 5 and 8 [30, 33, 35, 36]. The questionnaire has demonstrated a high sensitivity

**Table 74.1** STOP-Bang questionnaire

| | | |
|---|---|---|
| Snoring? | Do you **Snore Loudly** (loud enough to be heard through closed doors or your bed-partner elbows you for snoring at night)? | Yes or No |
| Tired? | Do you often feel **tired, fatigued, or sleepy** during the daytime (such as falling asleep during driving)? | Yes or No |
| Observed? | Has anyone **observed** you **stop breathing** or c**hoking/gasping** during your sleep? | Yes or No |
| Pressure? | Do you have or are being treated for **high blood pressure**? | Yes or No |
| Body mass index more than 35 kg/m²? | | Yes or No |
| Age older than 50 year old? | | Yes or No |
| Neck size large? (Measured around Adams apple) For male, is your shirt collar 17 inches or larger? For female, is your shirt collar 16 inches or larger? | | Yes or No |
| Gender = Male? | | Yes or No |

**Scoring Criteria:**
**Low risk of OSA**: Yes to 0–2 questions
**Intermediate risk of OSA**: Yes to 3–4 questions
**High risk of OSA**: Yes to 5–8 questions
 Yes to 2 of 4 STOP questions + individual's gender is male
 Yes to 2 of 4 STOP questions + BMI > 35 kg/m²
Modified from:
Chung F et al. Anesthesiology 2008; 108:812-21, Chung F et al Br J Anaesth 2012; 108:768–75; Chung F et al Obes Surg 2013; 23:2050-57, Chung F et al J Clin Sleep Med Sept 2014

using a cutoff score of ≥3 to predict moderate OSA (AHI > 15) and severe OSA (AHI > 30): 93% and 100% respectively [30]. The corresponding negative predictive values are 90 and 100% [30]. As the STOP-Bang score increases from 0–2 to 7–8, the probability of moderate-to-severe OSA increases from 18 to 60%, and the probability of severe OSA rises from 4 to 38% [33]. A higher score (≥5) on the STOP-Bang questionnaire is more predictive of severe OSA and is associated with higher postoperative complications [36].

Additional criteria may be used to further classify patients scoring for intermediate risk (3 or 4). A STOP score of $\geq 2$ with a BMI $> 35 kg/m^2$ or male or neck circumference $> 43$ cm in males and $> 41$ cm in females would classify that patient as having a high risk for moderate-to-severe OSA [33]. A STOP-Bang score $\geq 3$ + serum $HCO_3 \geq 28$ mmol/L would also classify that patient as being at moderate-to-severe risk for OSA [33].

## Best Preoperative Practices for Surgical Patients with Diagnosed OSA

During preoperative assessment, the severity of OSA should be assessed and OSA diagnosis should be confirmed by reviewing sleep study reports. As per 2016 SASM guidelines, in addition to obtain sleep study results, consideration should be given in obtaining the recommended positive airway pressure (PAP) device setting before surgery [28]. The presence and severity of co-existing major health disorders such as morbid obesity, uncontrolled hypertension, arrhythmias, cerebrovascular disease, heart failure and metabolic syndrome, should be determined [37]. Preoperative overnight oximetry may be used as a useful screening test where mean preoperative overnight saturation $< 93\%$, oxygen desaturation index $> 29$ events/h, overnight duration of oxygen saturation $< 90\%$ for $>7\%$ of total sleep time, have been shown to predict postoperative adverse events [38]. In the presence of resting hypoxemia not attributable to other cardiopulmonary disease, additional problems with ventilation or gas exchange including hypoventilation syndromes, severe pulmonary hypertension or uncontrolled systemic conditions, further investigations and preoperative cardiopulmonary optimization are required [28].

According to the 2016 SASM guidelines, in the presence of optimized comorbid conditions, patients with untreated or partially treated OSA may undergo surgery as long as strategies for mitigation of postoperative complications are implemented [28]. (Table 74.2) A growing body of literature suggests that CPAP therapy in the perioperative period may play a role in reducing postoperative complications by improving

**Table 74.2** Anesthetic considerations and perioperative management of obstructive sleep apnea in adults

| | |
|---|---|
| Pre-operative management | • Identify patients at risk of OSA by using a screening tool<br>• Confirm OSA severity (mild, moderate or severe) by reviewing sleep study results<br>• Assess treatment effectiveness (treated, partially treated, or non-compliant) and review current settings, such as the optimal PAP to abolish OSA<br>• Initiate discussion early on to include opioid sparing techniques such as a regional anesthetic, and multi-modal analgesia options As per SASM guidelines [28], may consider delaying surgery to optimize cardio-respiratory status and refer to sleep medicine if:<br>• Obesity-hypoventilation syndrome ($HCO_3 \geq 28$ mmol/L)<br>• Severe pulmonary hypertension<br>• Resting hypoxemia in the absence of other cardiopulmonary cause<br>• Associated significant or uncontrolled systemic disease |
| Intra-operative risk mitigation strategies | • Favor local or regional anesthesia<br>• Avoid sedating medication in an unmonitored environment<br>• Capnography or minute ventilation monitoring during sedation<br>• Consider intubation for procedures requiring deep sedation<br>If general anesthesia required:<br>• Head elevated laryngoscopy position if obesity<br>• Use short acting agents (remifentanyl, propofol, desflurane)<br>• Consider short acting agents (succinylcholine), and adequate reversal of neuromuscular blockade by using neuromuscular transmission monitoring<br>• Use lung recruitment strategies, and apply positive end-expiratory pressure (PEEP)<br>• Minimize use of opioids analgesics<br>• Non-supine posture for extubation and recovery |

| | |
|---|---|
| Table 74.2 (continued) | |
| Post-operative management | • Continue PAP therapy at previously prescribed settings during periods of sleep<br>• Minimize use of opioids analgesics and favor multi-modal analgesia<br>• Extended observation period in PACU<br>  – Post-operative respiratory monitoring (oximetry and ventilation) required if PACU respiratory events[a] or unable to use PAP<br>• Ambulatory surgery possible if:<br>  – Optimized OSA status and comorbid conditions<br>  – Pain manageable with opioid sparing techniques<br>  – Able to use PAP therapy at home |

*OSA* obstructive sleep apnea, *PAP* positive airway pressure, *PACU* post-anesthesia care unit

[a]Oxygen saturation < 90% (3 episodes), bradypnea <8 breaths/min (3 episodes), apnea ≥ 10 s (1 episode), pain sedation mismatch [49]

Adapted from:

Chung, F. et al. Society of Anesthesia and Sleep Medicine Guidelines on Preoperative Screening and Assessment of Adult Patients with Obstructive Sleep Apnea. *Anesth. Analg.* **123**, 452–473 (2016)

Gali, B., Whalen, F. X., Schroeder, D. R., Gay, P. C. & Plevak, D. J. Identification of patients at risk for postoperative respiratory complications using a preoperative obstructive sleep apnea screening tool and postanesthesia care assessment. *Anesthesiology* **110**, 869–877 (2009)

Seet, E. & Chung, F. La prise en charge de l'apnée du sommeil chez l'adulte: Algorithmes fonctionnels en période périopératoire. *Can. J. Anesth.* **57**, 849–864 (2010)

Joshi, G. P., Ankichetty, S. P., Gan, T. J. & Chung, F Society for ambulatory anesthesia consensus statement on preoperative selection of adult patients with obstructive sleep apnea scheduled for ambulatory surgery. *Anesth. Analg.* **115**, 1060–1068 (2012)

oxygenation and preventing worsening of OSA [26, 27]. Current guidelines recommend that surgical patients with moderate to severe OSA compliant with PAP therapy should bring their device to the hospital and continue its use during their hospitalization [28]. The previous prescribed settings can be used during periods of sleep. Sometimes postoperative adjustment may be needed. Mild OSA is not an independent risk factor for higher mortality in general population [39]. Therefore, patients with mild OSA may not be at higher risk of undergoing surgery and anesthesia and the requirements for PAP therapy and postoperative monitoring may not be that strictly enforced.

## Best Preoperative Practices for Surgical Patients with High Probability of OSA

In patients suspected of OSA, a focused history should be taken with emphasis on pertinent symptoms and signs of OSA. History of loud snoring and observed apneic episodes while asleep can be obtained from the bed partner. Major comorbidities should be looked for just like a patient with known OSA (see above).

In emergency situations, the patient should proceed for surgery with OSA specific risk mitigation strategies (see below). For elective non-urgent surgery, current SASM guidelines state that insufficient evidence exists to support cancelling or delaying surgery to formally diagnose OSA in those patients identified as being at high risk of OSA preoperatively, unless there is evidence of uncontrolled systemic disease or additional problems with ventilation or gas exchange [28]. Additional evaluation for preoperative cardiopulmonary optimization should be considered in patients who have a high probability of having OSA and have uncontrolled systemic conditions or additional problems with ventilation or gas exchange such as: hypoventilation syndromes, severe pulmonary hypertension, and resting hypoxemia in the absence of other cardiopulmonary disease [28]. In these cases, surgery should be delayed and a sleep medicine referral should be considered for preoperative cardiopulmonary optimization and initiation of treatment. Any discussion about delaying surgery should be taken with careful discussion of risks and benefits, and involving the surgical team in the decision. Otherwise, patients with suspected OSA should be assumed to have moderate-to-severe OSA and strategies to reduce postoperative complications be adopted in the perioperative period (Table 74.2). Since OSA carries significant comorbidities risks, screen-positive patients should be advised to notify their primary care provider that they were found to have a high probability of having OSA, thus allowing for appropriate referral for further evaluation.

## Peri-operative Considerations and Risk-Mitigation Strategies

OSA patients present many challenges to the anesthesiologist (Table 74.2). First, the anesthesiologist may have to manage different comorbidities such as obesity, hypertension, atrial fibrillation, heart failure, cerebrovascular disease and obesity hypoventilation syndrome. Moreover, OSA may induce physiologic changes like arterial hypoxemia, polycythemia, hypercapnia and pulmonary hypertension. In the presence of pulmonary hypertension, care should be taken to prevent elevation of pulmonary artery pressure by avoiding hypercarbia, hypoxemia, hypothermia and acidosis.

In addition, OSA patients present a higher risk of difficult mask ventilation, difficult laryngoscopy and intubation [40, 41]. Guidance from the ASA guidelines for the management of the difficult airway is useful and advance airway equipment may be required at the time of airway management [42]. Adequate preoxygenation should be made with the patient positioned on an elevation pillow or ramp with the head in the sniffing position. Measures to decrease the risk of aspiration such as preoperative proton-pump inhibitors, antacid and modified rapid sequence induction with cricoid pressure should be considered. Extubation should be performed in an upright or reverse trendelenberg position in an awake patient, with complete reversal of neuromuscular blockade who is able to obey commands and maintain a patent airway [46].

OSA patients have increased sensitivity to respiratory depressants. Therefore, short-acting agents such as propofol, remifentanyl and desflurane should be used whereas long-acting agents should be minimized. Increased sensitivity to opioids analgesic administration can result in respiratory depression [43]. Opioid sparing techniques wherever possible using regional anesthesia should be considered. Multimodal analgesia using non-sedating and opioid-sparing agents (nonsteroidal anti-inflammatory, acetaminophen, partial opioid analgesics, anticonvulsivant, corticosteroids, N-methyl-d-aspartate receptor antagonist [44], $\alpha_2$-agonist [45]) should be considered. Local or regional anesthesia are beneficial techniques for OSA patients since they reduce opioids requirement and avoid airway manipulation. Sedation must be given in a monitored setting. Patients previously on PAP therapy at home may continue using their PAP device during procedures under mild to moderate sedation, if necessary. A secured airway is prefered to an unprotected one for procedures requiring deep sedation [47].

## Post-operative Management of OSA Patients

The attending anesthesiologist is responsible to decide whether or not the patient is suitable for ambulatory surgery. If hospitalization is required, evaluation and plans for adequate postoperative monitoring should be made. Therefore, postoperative disposition of these patients depends on type of surgery, OSA severity and treatment, as well as postoperative parenteral opioid requirement.

All patients with known or suspected OSA who have received a general anesthesia should have an extended stay in the post-anesthesia care unit (PACU) with at least continous oximetry, with or without minute ventilation monitoring [48, 49]. The optimal length of the observation period has not been determined. It is reasonable to observe a suspected or documented OSA patient in PACU for an additional 60 min after the modified Aldrete criteria for discharge has been met [48]. During this observation period, occurrence of recurrent respiratory events (episodes of apnea for 10 s or more, bradypnea fewer than 8 breaths per minute, pain-sedation mismatch, repeat oxygen desaturation to less than 90%) should be recorded [50]. The occurrence of one or many PACU respiratory events mandates continous post-operative monitoring. Decision regarding the final patient's disposition (intensive care unit, step-down unit, or surgical ward with continous oximetry) should be made by the attending anesthesiologist. Empiric PAP therapy may be required to abolish recurrent obstructive events associated with significant hypoxemia [51]. For patients who decline PAP therapy due to poor tolerance, close monitoring, positional therapy and oxygen supplementation should be provided.

Concerning ambulatory anesthesia, it is agreed that OSA patients can be safely discharged home when local or regional anesthesia is administered. When a general anesthesia is planned, postoperative opioids requirement, PAP compliance and comorbidities should be assessed in the preoperative period to determine if the patient is suitable for ambulatory surgery. According to the Society for Ambulatory Anesthesia Consensus Statement, patients with a known diagnosis of OSA and optimized comorbid conditions can be considered for ambulatory surgery if they are able to use a CPAP device in the postoperative period and if postoperative pain relief can be provided predominantly with non-opioid analgesic techniques [51]. Plans for an overnight stay with adequate monitoring should be made for OSA patients not suitable for ambulatory surgery. The facility treating OSA patients as outpatients should possess the necessary equipment for continuous postoperative oximetry monitoring and overnight stay in case of any significant respiratory events in PACU. Otherwise, transfer agreements with an in-patient facility should be in place.

### Conclusion

OSA patients are associated with significant comorbidities, serious postoperative consequences and increased cost and resource utilization. Screening for OSA should be incorporated in the preoperative clinics for risk-stratification. To enhance patient safety and ensure the best possible outcomes, institutions should develop protocols for patients with known or suspected OSA regarding preoperative screening strategies, PACU observation, postoperative analgesic regimens and postoperative monitoring.

## References

1. Isono MDS. Obstructive sleep apnea of obese adults pathophysiology and perioperative airway management. Anesthesiology. 2009;110:908–21.
2. Beebe D, Gozal D. Obstructive sleep apnea and the prefrontal cortex: towards a comprehensive model linking nocturnal upper airway obstruction to daytime cognitive and behavioral deficits. J Sleep Res. 2002;11:1–16.
3. Eckert DJ, White DP, Jordan AS, Malhotra A, Wellman A. Defining phenotypic causes of obstructive sleep apnea: identification of novel therapeutic targets. Am J Respir Crit Care Med. 2013;188:996–1004.
4. Subramani Y, et al. Understanding phenotypes of obstructive sleep apnea. Anesth Analg. 2016;124:1.
5. Isono S, et al. Anatomy of pharynx in patients with obstructive sleep apnea and in normal subjects. J Appl Physiol. 1997;82(4):1319–26.
6. Lam T, Singh M, Yadollahi A, Chung F. Is perioperative fluid and salt balance a contributing factor in postoperative worsening of obstructive sleep apnea? Anesth Analg. 2016;122:1335–9.
7. Chung F, Liao P, Yegneswaran B, Shapiro CM, Kang W. Postoperative changes in sleep-disordered breathing and sleep architecture in patients with obstructive sleep apnea. Anesthesiol. 2014;120(2):287–98.
8. Chung F, Liao P, Elsaid H, Shapiro CM, Kang W. Factors associated with postoperative exacerbation of sleep-disordered breathing. Anesthesiology. 2014;120:299–311.
9. Punjabi NM. The epidemiology of adult obstructive sleep apnea. Proc Am Thorac Soc. 2008;5:136–43.
10. Berry RB, et al. Rules for scoring respiratory events in sleep: update of the 2007 AASM manual for the scoring of sleep and associated events. J Clin Sleep Med. 2012;8:597–619.
11. Iber C, Cheeson A, Quan SF, For the American Academy of Sleep Medicine. The AASM manual for the scoring of sleep and associated events, rules, terminology and techical specifications. 1st ed. Westchester: American Academy of Sleep Medicine; 2007.
12. Fleetham J, et al. Canadian Thoracic Society 2011 guideline update: diagnosis and treatment of sleep disordered breathing. Can Respir J. 2011;18:25–47.
13. American Academy of Sleep Medicine (AASM) 2014. The international classification of sleep disorders – 3rd edition (ICSD-3). www.aasmnet.org. Accessed 30 May 2015.
14. Collop NA, Anderson WM. Clinical guidelines for the use of unattended portable monitors in the diagnosis of obstructive sleep apnea in adult patients. J Clin Sleep Med. 2007;3:737–47.
15. Chung F, et al. Oxygen desaturation index from nocturnal oximetry: a sensitive and specific tool to detect sleep-disordered breathing in surgical patients. Anesth Analg. 2012;114:993–1000.

16. Peppard PE, et al. Increased prevalence of sleep-disordered breathing in adults. Am J Epidemiol. 2013;177:1006–14.
17. Terry Y, et al. The occurrence of sleep-disordered breathing among middle-aged adults. N Engl J Med. 1993;328:1230–5.
18. Frey WC, Pilcher J. Obstructive sleep-related breathing disorders in patients evaluated for bariatric surgery. Obes Surg. 2003;13:676–83.
19. Singh M, et al. Proportion of surgical patients with undiagnosed obstructive sleep apnoea. Br J Anaesth. 2013;110:629–36.
20. Opperer M, et al. Does obstructive sleep apnea influence perioperative outcome? A qualitative systematic review for the Society of Anesthesia and Sleep Medicine Task Force on preoperative preparation of patients with sleep-disordered breathing. Anesth Analg. 2016;122:1321–34.
21. Mokhlesi B, et al. Sleep-disordered breathing and postoperative outcomes after elective surgery: analysis of the nationwide inpatient sample. Chest. 2013;144:903–14.
22. Memtsoudis S, et al. Perioperative pulmonary outcomes in patients with sleep apnea after noncardiac surgery. Anesth Analg. 2011;112:113–21.
23. Mokhlesi B, et al. Sleep-disordered breathing and postoperative outcomes after bariatric surgery: analysis of the nationwide inpatient sample. Obes Surg. 2013;23:1842–51.
24. Flink BJ, et al. Obstructive sleep apnea and incidence of postoperative delirium after elective knee replacement in the nondemented elderly. Anesthesiology. 2012;116:788–96.
25. Kaw R, et al. Meta-analysis of the association between obstructive sleep apnoea and postoperative outcome. Br J Anaesth. 2012;109:897–906.
26. Mutter TC, et al. A matched cohort study of postoperative outcomes in obstructive sleep apnea could preoperative diagnosis and treatment prevent complications? Anesthesiology. 2014;121:707–18.
27. Abdelsattar ZM, Hendren S, Wong SL, Campbell DA, Ramachandran SK. The impact of untreated obstructive sleep apnea on cardiopulmonary complications in general and vascular surgery: a cohort study. Sleep. 2015;38:1205–10.
28. Chung F, et al. Society of Anesthesia and Sleep Medicine guidelines on preoperative screening and assessment of adult patients with obstructive sleep apnea. Anesth Analg. 2016;123:452–73.
29. Bibbins-Domingo K, et al. Screening for obstructive sleep apnea in adults. JAMA. 2017;317:407–33.
30. Chung F, et al. STOP questionnaire. Anesthesiology. 2008;108:812–21.
31. Ramachandran SK, et al. Derivation and validation of a simple perioperative sleep apnea prediction score. Anesth Analg. 2010;110:1007–15.
32. Netzer NC, et al. Prevalence of symptoms and risk of sleep apnea in primary care. Chest. 2003;124:1406–14.
33. Chung F, Abdullah HR, Liao P. STOP-Bang questionnaire a practical approach to screen for obstructive sleep apnea. Chest. 2016;149:631–8.
34. Nagappa M, et al. Validation of the STOP-bang questionnaire as a screening tool for obstructive sleep apnea among different populations: a systematic review and meta-analysis. PLoS One. 2015;10(12):e0143697.
35. Chung F, Yang Y, Brown R, Liao P. Alternative scoring models of STOP-Bang questionnaire improve specificity to detect undiagnosed obstructive sleep apnea. J Clin Sleep Med. 2014;10:951–8.
36. Chung F, et al. High STOP-Bang score indicates a high probability of obstructive sleep apnoea. Br J Anaesth. 2012;108:768–75.
37. Bradley TD, Floras JS. Obstructive sleep apnoea and its cardiovascular consequences. Lancet. 2009;373:82–93.
38. Chung F, Zhou L, Liao P. Parameters from preoperative overnight oximetry predict postoperative adverse events. Minerva Anestesiol. 2014;80:1084–95.
39. Marshall NS, et al. Sleep apnea as an independent risk factor for all-cause mortality: the Busselton Health Study. Sleep. 2008;31:1079–85.
40. Kheterpal S, Martin L, Shanks AM, Tremper KK. Prediction and outcomes of impossible mask ventilation. Anesthesiology. 2009;110:891–7.
41. Siyam MA, Benhamou D. Difficult endotracheal intubation in patients with sleep apnea syndrome. Anesth. Analg. 2002;95:1098–102.
42. Apfelbaum JL, et al. Practice guidelines for management of the difficult airway an updated report by the American Society of Anesthesiologists Task Force on Management of the Difficult Airway. Anesthesiology. 2013;118:251–70.
43. Lam KK, Kunder S, Wong J, Doufas AG, Chung F. Obstructive sleep apnea, pain, and opioids: is the riddle solved? Curr Opin Anaesthesiol. 2016;29:134–40.
44. Eikermann M, et al. Ketamine activates breathing and abolishes the coupling between loss of consciousness and upper airway dilator muscle dysfunction. Anesthesiology. 2012;116:35–46.
45. Ankichetty S, Wong J, Chung F. A systematic review of the effects of sedatives and anesthetics in patients with obstructive sleep apnea. J Anaesthesiol Clin Pharmacol. 2011;27:447–58.
46. American Society of Anesthesiologists Task Force on Perioperative Management of Patients with Obstructive Sleep Apnea. Practice guidelines for the perioperative management of patients with obstructive sleep apnea: an updated report by the American Society of Anesthesiologists Task Force on Perioperative Management of patients with obstructive sleep apnea. Anesthesiology. 2014;120:268–86.
47. Seet E, Chung F. La prise en charge de l'apnée du sommeil chez l'adulte: Algorithmes fonctionnels en période périopératoire. Can J Anesth. 2010;57:849–64.
48. Seet E, Han TL, Chung F. Perioperative clinical pathways to manage sleep-disordered breathing. Sleep Med Clin. 2017;8:105–20.

49. Gali B, Whalen FX, Schroeder DR, Gay PC, Plevak DJ. Identification of patients at risk for postoperative respiratory complications using a preoperative obstructive sleep apnea screening tool and postanesthesia care assessment. Anesthesiology. 2009;110:869–77.
50. Sundar E, Chang J, Smetana GW. Perioperative screening for and management of patients with obstructive sleep apnea. J Clin Outcomes Manag. 2011;18:399–411.
51. Joshi GP, Ankichetty SP, Gan TJ, Chung F. Society for ambulatory anesthesia consensus statement on preoperative selection of adult patients with obstructive sleep apnea scheduled for ambulatory surgery. Anesth Analg. 2012;115:1060–8.

# Anesthesia for Major Orthopedic Surgeries

## George Pan and Bradley Reid

## Introduction

Major orthopedic surgical interventions are commonly performed in the United States, and are amongst the most widespread procedures in the elderly. In patients older than 80 years of age, total hip arthroplasty (THA) increased from 181/100,000—257/100,000 annually between the years 2000–2009. A similar trend was seen with total knee replacement (TKR) with an increase from 300/100,000 to 477/100,000 in a similar time frame [1]. Major joint surgery has both elective and emergent indications and, although in the past these surgeries often required an inpatient hospitalization, the growing number of minimally invasive techniques allows many of these cases to be performed in an outpatient setting.

Patients presenting for joint surgery include a diverse population spanning age ranges from infants to centenarians. Patients range from healthy athletes to the elderly, who are often frail and carry multiple medical comorbidities. As such, there is a diverse range of clinical considerations to address when preparing a patient for major orthopedic surgery. Common indications for pediatric orthopedic surgical interventions include traumatic injuries, cancer, and various congenital malformations. The athletic population often incurs cartilaginous and ligamentous injuries, particularly in the knee and shoulder joint. In the elderly population, joint replacement surgery is the most frequent orthopedic procedure performed in the United States, with an increasing incidence of hip and knee arthroplasty.

The anesthesia provider should also note indications for surgery. Many patients may potentially delay or avoid surgical intervention through more conservative treatment approaches. The METEOR trial published in the New England Journal of Medicine (NEJM) demonstrated no difference in functional outcomes in patients presenting with meniscal tears and concomitant mild to moderate osteoarthritis as versus those who were randomized to surgery PLUS physical therapy versus physical therapy alone [2]. Patients may be debilitated, or suffer from chronic pain or disability, when presenting for joint surgery because they have opted to pursue other well-established treatments prior to considering surgery.

## Regional Versus General Anesthesia

The surgical approach poses unique considerations that must be accounted for in the anesthetic plan. Both general and regional anesthesia (including neuraxial anesthesia) can be used to

G. Pan, M.D. (✉) · B. Reid, M.D.
Department of Anesthesiology and Perioperative Medicine, University of California, Los Angeles, Los Angeles, CA, USA
e-mail: GeorgePan@mednet.ucla.edu; bmreid@mednet.ucla.edu

care for patients undergoing joint surgery. Regional techniques are however, an increasingly accepted practice for most providers. When compared to general anesthesia (GA), patients undergoing major orthopedic surgeries with regional anesthesia (RA) experience less blood loss, a decreased need for transfusions, and lower postoperative pain scores [3]. Additionally, in adult patients, RA is associated with decreased risk of stroke and cardiac risk [4]. Deep venous thrombosis (DVT) and pulmonary embolism (PE) may also be reduced with RA options however, studies that compare with general anesthesia did not account for the use of medical prophylaxis. It remains unclear if thromboembolic events are decreased with RA [4]. The theoretical risk that inadequate muscle relaxation would complicate or lengthen surgical repair when using regional anesthesia instead of general has not been validated.

Pediatric patients should also be considered for regional techniques given their safety profile and potential perioperative benefits [5].

## Anatomy and Physiology of Joint Disease

### Hip

The hip is most frequently surgically approached from a posterior approach but anterior incisions can also be utilized. In THA, the femur is dislocated from the acetabulum with subsequent removal of the femoral head and part of the femoral neck. The acetabulum is then reamed to create a smooth articulation surface. Finally, the prosthetic femoral component is made of metal and sized to fit the patient's anatomy. Revision surgeries involve more scar tissue and tend to take longer to perform because old hardware needs to be removed with specialized equipment.

### Knee

Knee surgery is performed in the supine position such that the surgeon can easily expose the femur, patella and tibia. Following bone exposure, the joint is accessed via arthrotomy and a bone saw is used to create sufficient space to insert the metallic or plastic components onto the knee joint surface. Replacement can involve both sides of the joint or address just the medial or lateral side.

## Pelvic Fracture

Surgical management for pelvic repair is complex, and depends upon the type and extent of the fracture. Involvement of the pubic symphysis or pubic rami, requires an anterior approach with a Pfannenstiel or ilioinguinal incision. A posterior approach is used for sacroiliac joint dislocations and fractures of the ilium or sacrum. Posterior approaches tend to be more extensive incisions and complex surgeries, often increasing the length of the case.

## Preoperative Evaluation and Planning

Orthopedic surgery requires an in-depth evaluation to identify underlying medical conditions and determine their state of control and need for optimization. Patients undergoing major orthopedic surgery are often elderly and may present with a number of significant medical conditions. In a 2014 meta-analysis, it was found that the leading causes of mortality following THA were cardiovascular disease (41.1%), followed by cerebrovascular accidents (23.1%), and pulmonary embolism (11.8%). The risks factors associated with increased mortality included male gender, increasing age, diabetes, liver disease, metastatic cancer, hemiplegia or paraplegia, congestive heart failure, dementia, renal disease, psychosis, cerebrovascular disease, and chronic pulmonary disease. Obesity, however, was not associated with increased mortality. This has been described as the "obesity paradox" and although obesity can lead to the development of the aforementioned conditions, obesity itself appears to protect against mortality in the postoperative period [6]. Risk of adverse events can be calculated on an individual patient basis using the National Surgery Quality Improvement Program (NSQIP) surgical risk calculator [7].

## Airway

Rheumatoid arthritis (RA) is common in patients undergoing orthopedic surgery and presents concerns for airway management. Up to 25% of patients with rheumatoid arthritis have atlantoaxial instability [8]. Care should be taken to ensure safe and proper airway instrumentation. Preoperative assessment can include a history of paraesthesia of the head, neck, arm, or hands [9]. Cervical spine imaging may be helpful in those with symptoms, requesting flexion and extension views of the cervical spine. Additional orthopedic conditions that warrant airway caution include severe cervical osteoarthritis and ankylosing spondylitis.

General airway evaluation for orthopedic surgeries should include a preoperative evaluation of cervical range of motion, mandibular opening, thyromental distance, anatomic alterations of the larynx, presence of a receding chin, hoarseness of voice, and stridor [9]. Tracheal intubation could potentially be more difficult as a result of the aforementioned pathologies.

## Cardiovascular and Pulmonary

Special consideration for cardiovascular fitness should be addressed in patients presenting for major orthopedic surgery. Initial screening for metabolic equivalents (METS) may not truly represent the patient's cardiovascular and respiratory fitness due to their limited mobility. Severe hip and knee pathologic pain often limit walking and other metabolic surrogates used in assessing cardiac and respiratory fitness. If the index of suspicion for active ischemic disease is sufficiently high and/or cardiovascular disease is inadequately managed, further workup or referral should be pursued in congruence to the American College of Cardiology (ACC)/American Heart Association (AHA) clinical practice guidelines [10].

Obese patients are more likely to undergo joint surgery at a younger age [11] thus, considerations for co-morbidities in the obese should be considered in anesthetic planning. Particularly, these patients' pulmonary physiology is complicated by restrictive lung disease, obstructive sleep apnea, and decreased closing and functional reserve capacities. Ventilation strategies under general anesthesia need to take in account reduced chest wall compliance in the morbidly obese, as well as the likeliness of developing atelectasis. The use of sedatives during a regional anesthetic may result in upper airway obstruction and hypoventilation; thoughtful anesthetic planning should consider the risks and benefits of the varied sedatives available.

## Neurologic and Musculoskeletal

Preoperative evaluation should include an assessment of neurologic deficits and musculoskeletal abnormalities, particularly if considering a regional technique where close observation of neurologic function is required postoperatively. According to American Society of Anesthesiology (ASA) Closed Claims project, from 2000 to 2013, 445 claims were made for regional anesthetic complications, the majority being related to neuraxial techniques. Documentation should include the pre-procedural musculoskeletal and neurologic exam along with procedural details which record adherence to appropriate procedural standards. Informed consent should be also documented [12].

Assessment and documentation of neurologic status are particularly important in cases involving hip surgery. Surgical treatment of developmental dysplasia requires lengthening of extremities, increasing the risk of nerve injury fourfold [13]. In revision THA, the risk of nerve damage is increased threefold [14]. Risks for major nerve injury following TKA include severe valgus deformities (>12°), flexion contractures (>10°), prolonged tourniquet times (>120 min), and/or preexisting neuraxial neuropathy [15].

## Hematologic

Blood loss is a distinct possibility in orthopedic surgery, particularly in pelvic and hip procedures. Risks factors for transfusion include low body mass index (BMI) and low preoperative hemoglobin levels, thus, evaluating patient's baseline risk for anemia is merited in these patients [16, 17]. The need for allogeneic blood products should be determined preoperatively and if deemed sufficiently high, a type and screen ordered to ensure rare antibodies can be cross-matched on the day of surgery. Most institutions now employ blood management systems that set standard preoperative orders to ensure safety for 90% of patients undergoing a particular procedure. A practical approach is to order a type and screen for routine TKR, a type and cross for one unit of packed red blood cells (pRBC) for a revision TKR, two units for a standard THA, and three units for a revision THA.

The use of cell salvage should be strongly considered for larger, invasive cases where excessive blood loss is expected. Extensive oncologic surgeries can often lead to greater than 4.5 L of blood loss [18]. As blood loss continues, resuscitation with packed red blood cells should be matched appropriately with fresh frozen plasma and platelets. Active communication with the blood bank should occur as soon as significant intraoperative blood losses begin.

## Chronic Pain and Post-operative Analgesic Planning

An in-depth evaluation of a patient's preoperative pain enables the anesthesia practitioner to tailor their anesthetic plan for both optimal intraoperative safety and postoperative pain management. This includes a thorough assessment of preoperative opioid exposure, detailing the duration and dose of opioid and analgesic therapy. Opioid-dependent patients present unique challenges to the management of perioperative pain. It is important to discuss realistic goals with patients about their current and likely postoperative pain prior to proceeding with a surgical intervention. Regional techniques should be considered to decrease the need for escalating opioid therapy and multimodal analgesia should be employed when appropriate.

Considerations for RA should include the patient's coagulation status, skin lesions/infections, systemic infections, and anatomical abnormalities. Relative contraindications include uncooperative patients, bleeding diathesis, infection, and pre-existing peripheral neuropathy. The dose of local anesthetic needed for an adequate block or continuous catheter needs to be calculated and if above recommended safety guidelines, caution should be exercised prior to proceeding or GA chosen. Published recommendations from the American Society of Regional Anesthesia and Pain Management (ASRA) can guide providers when addressing patients with preexisting spinal stenosis and/or vertebral canal pathologies, preexisting neurologic disease, and inflammatory neuropathies when considering neuraxial techniques [15].

|  | | |
|---|---|---|
| Cardiovascular | Burn shock | Hypermetabolism |
|  | Hypovolemia | Increased cardiac output |
|  | Decreased Cardiac Output | Increased resting heart rate |
|  | Increased systemic vascular resistance (SVR) | Hypertension |
|  | Decreased venous oxygen saturation (SvO$_2$) | Decreased SVR |
|  |  | Increased SvO$_2$ |
|  |  | Altered myocardial contractility |
| Respiratory | Pulmonary edema | ARDS |
|  | Airway edema | Pneumonia |
|  | Inhalation injury | Tracheal Stenosis |
|  |  | Inhalation injury |
| Hematologic | Hemoconcentration | Anemia |
|  | Thrombocytopenia | Thrombocytosis |
|  |  | Coagulopathy |
| Renal | Decreased glomerular filtration rate (GFR) | Increased GFR |
|  | Oliguria | Tubular dysfunction |
|  | Myoglobinuria |  |
| Hepatic | Decreased perfusion | Increased perfusion |
|  |  | Increased drug clearance |
| Neurologic | Increased intracranial pressure | Delirium |
|  | Cerebral Edema | PTSD |
| Other | Generalized edema | Increased core body temperature |
|  | Compartment syndrome | Muscle catabolism |
|  |  | Increased metabolic rate |
|  |  | Insulin resistance |

# Anesthetic Considerations for Intraoperative Care

## Neuraxial Anesthesia

As stated previously, neuraxial techniques such as epidural and spinal anesthesia have been shown to decrease morbidity in joint surgery. While the benefits are outlined above in the preoperative section, risks include nerve injury, local anesthetic systemic toxicity (LAST), bleeding, and infection. When deciding on general anesthesia versus regional approach, combined technique should be considered if best able to provide ideal operative conditions and superior postoperative pain control.

With the advent of new anticoagulant and antiplatelet therapies, staying abreast of the most recent clinical recommendations is paramount, particularly when considering regional techniques in the anesthetic plan. Ascertaining anticoagulant status with attention to specific drug type, dose, duration of therapy, and timing of cessation are paramount before proceeding. Additionally, the anesthesiologist needs to coordinate with the orthopedic surgeon, primary care physician and cardiologist to determine the appropriateness of discontinuing therapy prior to the surgical procedure, An optimal risk/benefit balance between achieving hemostasis versus venous thromboembolism prophylaxis/treatment, management of cardiac stents or anticoagulation for atrial fibrillation must be individually determined for each patient. An exhaustive discussion of the various drugs and perioperative management is not the intent of this chapter however, given the vital need to address these drugs prior to major joint surgery in at-risk patients, this topic cannot be overemphasized [19]. The AHA/ACC 2016 *Guidelines on Duration of Dual Antiplatelet Therapy in Patients with Coronary Artery Disease* advise on length of therapy required following cardiac stenting, and specifically address patients presenting for elective noncardiac surgery [20].

Table 75.1 stratifies the relative risk of bleeding complications associate with procedural pain interventions including the varied regional anesthetic techniques. A list of common anticoagulant/antiplatelet medications and timing of drug discontinuation based on the type of regional anesthesia- neuraxial or peripheral nerve block- is listed in Table 75.2. A more comprehensive explanation and list is provided in the ASRA Guidelines [19]. Drugs not listed within the guidelines are often discontinued in a time frame that allows five half-lives to pass and must account hepatic and renal clearance in those with liver and/or kidney disease.

**Table 75.1** Risk stratification of varied pain (regional) interventions [52]

| High risk | Intermediate risk | Low risk |
| --- | --- | --- |
| SCS trial and implant | Interlaminar ESIs (C, T, L, S) | Peripheral nerve blocks |
| Intrathecal catheter and pump implant | Transforaminal ESIs (C, T, L, S) | Peripheral joints and musculoskeletal vertebral augmentation (vertebroplasty injections |
| Vertebral augmentation (vertebroplasty injections and kyphoplasty) | Facet MBB and RFA (C, T, L) | Trigger point injections including piriformis injection |
| | Paravertebral block (C, T, L) | Sacroiliac joint injection and sacral lateral branch blocks |
| | Intradiscal procedures (C, T, L) | |
| | Sympathetic blocks (stellate, thoracic, splanchnic, celiac, lumbar, hypogastric) | |
| | Peripheral nerve stimulation trial and implant | |
| | Pocket revision and IPG/ITP replacement | |

*SCS* spinal cord stimulator, *C* cervical, *T* thoracic, *L* lumbar, *S* sacral, *MBB* medial branch block, *RFA* radiofrequency ablation, *IPG* implantable pulse generator, *ITP* intrathecal pump

**Table 75.2** Peri-procedural management of anticoagulants and antiplatelet agents according to pain intervention risk [51]

| Generic | Trade name | High risk | Intermediate risk | Low risk | Restart |
|---|---|---|---|---|---|
| Abciximab | ReoPro | 2–5 days | 2–5 days | 2–5 days | 8–12 h |
| Apixaban | Eliquis | 3–5 days | 3–5 days | Shared assessment and risk stratification | 24 h |
| Clopidogrel | Plavix | 7 days | 7 days | No | 12–24 h |
| Coumadin | Warfarin | 5 days, normal INR | 5 days, normal INR | No | 24 h |
| Dabigatran | Pradaxa | 4–5 days 6 days with AKI/CKD | 4–5 days 6 days with AKI/CKD | Shared assessment and risk stratification | 24 h |
| Enoxaparin (prophylactic) | Lovenox | 12 h | 12 h | 12 h | – 4 h after low risk<br>– 12–24 h after medium/high risk pain procedures |
| Enoxaparin (therapeutic) | Lovenox | 24 h | 24 h | 24 h | – 4 h after low risk<br>– 12-24 h after medium/high risk pain procedures |
| Eptifibatide | Integrilin | 8–24 h | 8–24 h | 8–24 h | 8–12 h |
| Fondaparinux | Arixtra | 4 days | 4 days | Shared assessment and risk stratification | 24 h |
| Prasugrel | Effient | 7–10 days | 7–10 days | No | 12–24 h |
| Rivaroxaban | Xarelto | 3 days | 3 days | Shared assessment and risk stratification | 24 h |
| Ticagrelor | Brilinta | 5 days | 5 days | No | 12–24 h |
| Tirofiban | Aggrastat | 8–24 h | 8–24 h | 8–24 h | 8–12 h |

## Peripheral Nerve Blocks

Although peripheral nerve blocks can be used as the primary anesthetic for surgery, they are often additionally utilized for post-operative pain. Pain control increases patient satisfaction, allows for faster mobility and physical therapy and decreases the risks of systemic opioids. Specifically for peripheral nerve blocks, ultrasound-guided anesthesia techniques have expanded and are recommended in the latest ASRA guidelines.

## Hip Surgery

Hip surgery can be performed under neuraxial anesthesia or peripheral nerve block. Often, a combination of lumbar plexus and sciatic nerve block is performed, using a posterior approach with the patient in lateral position. Commonly, a nerve stimulator is utilized to elicit motor response and identify nerve location [21, 22]. A significant advantage of peripheral regional approach over neuraxial technique is the reduced incidence of sympathectomy-induced hypotension. Direct needle trauma to nerve roots has also occurred with this approaches so is a risk that must be addressed when deciding on anesthetic plan. Given its anatomic location of the nerve roots, intrathecal and epidural injection are also potential complications. Following case reports of retroperitoneal and renal capsular bleeds, ASRA recommends that anticoagulants and antiplatelets for these regional blocks be managed similarly to that of a neuraxial technique [19].

## Knee Surgery

Should peripheral nerve blocks be chosen for knee surgery, the most frequently performed include the combination of a femoral and sciatic block. For TKA in particular, a recent meta-analysis looked at acute postoperative pain (during rest and movement), postoperative opioid consumption, and quality of early postoperative rehabilitation. The authors conclude that the combination of femoral and sciatic nerve blocks result in optimal outcomes with respect to these parameters [23]. Medications such as NMDA antagonists, acetaminophen, NSAIDS, and gabapentinoid adjuncts have been demonstrated to help control pain following joint surgery, reduce opioid use and increase rehabilitation parameters [24, 25]. Therefore, combination analgesic therapy is strongly recommended when applicable for major orthopedic surgeries.

## Shoulder Surgery

Regional anesthesia techniques for shoulder surgeries have also proven to be beneficial for both intraoperative and postoperative pain control. This includes a variety of procedures: rotator cuff repair, total shoulder arthroplasty, acromioplasty, humeral fracture surgery, and arthroscopy. While some surgical procedures can be performed successfully under regional technique alone, patient selection is paramount as the proximity of the surgical site and surgical drapes close to/covering a patient's face can induce claustrophobia [26]. The combination of regional and general anesthesia is commonly employed. A variety of regional techniques have been studied and include: intra articular local anesthetic injections, single shot suprascapular nerve block ± axillary nerve block, single shot interscalene block, or interscalene block with continuous local anesthetic infusion.

Post-operative pain scores have been evaluated for patients undergoing arthoscopic shoulder acromioplasty comparing various nerve blocks. Compared to intra-articular local anesthetic injection and single shot suprascapular nerve block, the single shot interscalene block provided greatest analgesia. There was no difference in pain scores between intra-articular local anesthesia and placebo [27]. Following this initial conclusion, multiple papers have emerged supporting the interscalene approach as the block of choice, with the suprascapular nerve block with axillary nerve block acting as an effective alternative [28, 29]. The use of intra-articular local anesthetics is not recommended given the risk of chondrolysis and the lack of postoperative analgesia. When comparing single shot versus continuous interscalene block, continuous infusions offer better pain control, sleep patterns, and decreased opioid usage [30, 31]. Interscalene blocks however, are not without risk. Phrenic nerve blockade occurs in >90% of interscalene blocks and is a concerning hazard in patients at risk for respiratory insufficiency. Therefore, this block is contraindicated in patients with limited pulmonary reserve or patients with severe obstructive/restrictive lung disease, myasthenia gravis, status-post pneumonectomy on the contralateral side, contralateral hemi-diaphragmatic dysfunction, or pre-existing vocal fold paralysis. These contraindications are in addition to local infection, sepsis, coagulopathy, and patient refusal [32]. The risk of pneumothorax, long-term nerve injury, and local anesthetic toxicity remains very low [33].

## Operating Room Preparation

Operating room preparation may vary according to the procedure and patient however, standard ASA monitors and airway equipment need to be available for all cases. Depending upon the relative invasiveness of the procedure and the patient's medical comorbidities, the range of invasive lines and monitors varies. A routine, total knee replacement in an ASA I patient often obviates the need for invasive monitoring while an aggressive oncologic resection in an elderly patient may require arterial monitoring and central venous access for intra- and post-operative anesthesia care. Additional equipment such as urinary catheters, high volume resuscitation equipment, cell salvage, warming devices, and point of care testing should be considered on a case-to-case basis.

## Positioning

The varied procedures addressed in this chapter require specific positions however, as with all patients, pressure point padding and vigilant intraoperative checks are mandated for patient safety.

- Lateral decubitus position provides improved surgical access for most hip procedures and may be preferred by surgeons for visualization and instrumentation. Caution needs to be exercised during initial positioning because the risk of neurovascular injury is increased in this case. An axillary role is placed to decrease brachial plexus injury risk and upper extremity vascular compression.
- Beach chair positioning for shoulder procedures provides easy surgical access to the shoulder, but presents increased risk of venous air emboli with resultant hypotension and possible cerebral ischemia. Most importantly, non-invasive blood pressure readings on the arm or leg will be higher than represents cerebral perfusion. For every 10 cm difference between the blood pressure cuff and external tragus, the mean arterial pressure (MAP) reading should be reduced by approximately 12 mmHg. Cerebral perfusion pressure should be estimated based on the calculated MAP as versus the blood pressure cuff reading. If an arterial line is placed, the transducer should be at the level of the Circle of Willis. There have been case reports of shoulder surgery in the beach chair position in which providers did not account for the discrepancy between blood pressure readings and cerebral/perfusion pressure, resulting in several perioperative cerebrovascular accidents [34]. Moreover, there is an increased incidence of peripheral nerve compression associated with the head holder in beach chair positioning. Should it be indicated, early airway establishment is recommended given the decreased ease of intraoperative airway access in both lateral and upright positioning [35].

## Tranexamic Acid

The regular use of tranexamic acid (TXA) should be considered in hip and knee surgery. TXA is a synthetic antifibrinolytic that competitively inhibits plasminogen. This effectively decreases fibrinolysis with resultant decrease in intraoperative blood loss. The effectiveness and safety profile of TXA in hip and knee surgery have been well studied and documented in a series of randomized, placebo-controlled trials as well as compiled in a meta-analyses [36–40]. The 2015 ASA practice guidelines support the use of prophylactic antifibrinolytic therapy in order to decrease the risk of excessive bleeding [41]. TXA does not significantly increase in the rates of deep vein thrombosis (DVT), pulmonary embolism, or other complications.

## Bone Cement Implantation Syndrome (BCIS)

BCIS is a poorly understood syndrome that primarily occurs when polymethylmethacrylate (PMMA) cementation is used for surgical repair. Bone cement is used to augment the prosthetic joint material to patient bone. BCIS can occur at the time of prosthesis insertion, joint reduction, or deflation of a limb tourniquet [42].

While not completely understood, the pathophysiology of BCIS is theorized to be the result of release of PMMA into circulation. The preparation of PMMA results in an exothermic reaction; the released heat increases intramedullary pressures and can force PMMA to embolize. Early signs include the development of hypoxia and hypotension; ultimately however, the emboli increase pulmonary vascular resistance and can result in right ventricular failure. As the intraventricular septum shifts leftward due to the failing contractility of the right heart, it ultimately alters left ventricular compliance, decreases cardiac output and results in cardiovascular collapse. Proposed mechanisms for the development of increased pulmonary vascular resistance include circulation of PMMA cement monomer, histamine release, complement activation, cannabinoid mediated vasodilation, and medullary component emboli [43]. Treatment is supportive and includes use of pulmonary vasodilators, inotropic therapy, invasive monitors and transesophageal echocardiography (TEE) to optimize medical therapy to support the heart and lungs.

## Fat Embolism Syndrome (FES)

Fat embolism syndrome most often occurs after trauma and usually in patients with long bone fracture. Presentation is typically delayed (1–3 days following injury) and anesthesiologists may not observe signs and symptoms in the operating room. FES results from a release of fat emboli into the pulmonary vasculature, or potentially into the systemic circulation via a patent foramen ovale. A release of inflammatory mediators and vasoactive amines occur with resultant hypotension and spontaneous platelet aggregation. Free fatty acids are formed by the hydrolysis of fat emboli, contributing to multi-organ dysfunction [44]. Clinically, signs and symptoms of FES include hypoxemia, tachycardia, skin petechiae, respiratory failure, adult respiratory distress syndrome (ARDS), and central neurologic dysfunction [45].

Fat emboli occur with fixation of long bone fractures using intraoperative reaming and intramedullary nailing. Cementation of the femoral component during THA can also produce FES. Fat emboli showers can often be seen using TEE in the operating room in patients developing suspicious symptoms [46]. FES rarely occurs in TKR; there are only a handful of case reports in the literature. Treatment of FES is supportive, ensuring adequate oxygenation, and the maintenance of intravascular volume. The use of corticosteroids has been suggested to prevent FES in a recent meta-analysis but the included data was old and generally derived from low-quality studies [47]. The use of steroids, albumin, and heparin has not been shown to be effective and are not recommended.

## Limb Tourniquets

The use of limb tourniquets in certain major orthopedic surgeries is common practice as means to reduce intraoperative blood loss and facilitate better visual conditions for the operative team. However, tourniquet use does introduce clinical risks that merit consideration for anesthetic management. The tourniquet is placed proximal to the operative site and inflated above systemic blood pressure. Inflation should not exceed 100 mgHg over systolic pressure during upper extremity procedures, and 150 mgHg for tourniquets placed on the lower extremity. Limb ischemia can occur above these safety boundaries and rhabdomyolysis has been reported. While the maximum allowable duration of tourniquet time is debatable, current guidelines advise an inflation time no greater than 2 h. If more time is required, a brief deflation of the cuff between 5–10 min is strongly advised. Hemodynamic changes need to be closely monitored with cuff inflation. Tourniquet deflation may result in hypothermic and acidotic blood release into systemic circulation; close monitoring is required during this time and patients should be treated as needed to support their blood pressure and cardiac output.

Despite adequate anesthesia, tourniquet pain can occur. It is described as dull pain in an awake patient and can be accompanied by patient agitation and distress. Changes in hemodynamics also indicate tourniquet pain and may be the only sign in a patient under GA. The most common hemodynamic perturbations include hypertension and tachycardia. Typically, the pain does not resolve until release of the tourniquet.

## Venous Thromboembolism (VTE)

VTE is a significant source of morbidity and mortality for patients undergoing major orthopedic surgery with reported incidence as high as 60% [48]. Prophylaxis of VTE includes early mobilization, adequate fluid resuscitation, mechanical devices, and pharmacologic therapies. The use of neuraxial techniques such as epidural and spinal anesthesia may decrease the incidence and associated mortality of VTE [49]. The incidence of VTE is particularly increased following lower extremity surgery so extreme care in providing both chemical and mechanical prophylaxis is undertaken. The American Association of Orthopedic Surgeons, the American College of Chest Physicians, and the National Institute of Clinical Excellence have published evidence-based guidelines for appropriate VTE prophylaxis across various risk stratifications [50] that include a combination of both mechanical and pharmacologic prophylaxis [51].

## Postoperative Care

A primary consideration for patients undergoing major joint surgery is postoperative pain. As previously mentioned, multi-modal analgesia should be considered in the majority of orthopedic surgical patients. Regional techniques, unless contraindicated, provide superior postoperative pain control in most cases. This expedites return to normal function and participation in physical therapy. Patients with chronic pain, who required opioid therapy preoperatively, should be treated preemptively with an understanding that ideal postoperative pain control does not only apply to the PACU but throughout the entire operative hospitalization. A pain management consultation should be strongly considered in opioid-tolerant patients.

## Summary

Major orthopedic surgeries present a unique challenge to the anesthesia provider. Due to the increasing number of these surgeries, it is imperative for anesthesia providers to become familiar with the procedure, its preoperative considerations and anesthetic options. Risk of clinically significant bleeding, venous thromboembolism, limb ischemia, and patient positioning, combined with a diverse patient population make major orthopedic surgery a distinct perioperative entity. It mandates both short and long term planning for successful perioperative management. When approached thoughtfully, major orthopedic surgery presents a challenging yet rewarding task for the perioperative anesthetic provider.

## References

1. Yoshihara H, Yoneoka D. Trends in the incidence and in-hospital outcomes of elective major orthopaedic surgery in patient eighty years of age and older in the United States from 2000 to 2009. J Bone Joint Surg Am. 2014;96(14):1185–91.
2. Katz JN, et al. Surgery versus physical therapy for meniscal tear and osteoarthritis. N E J M. 2013;2013(368):1675–84.
3. Fischer B. Benefits, risks, and best practice in regional anesthesia. Reg Anesth Pain Med. 2010;35:545–8.
4. Mauermann W, Shilling A, Zuo Z. A comparison of Neuraxial block versus general anesthesia for elective total hip replacement: a meta-analysis. Anesth Analg. 2006;103:1018–25.
5. Polaner D, Taenzer A, Walker B, Bosenberg A, Krane E, Suresh S, Wolf C, Martin L. Pediatric regional anesthesia network (PRAN). Anesth Analg. 2012;115:1353–64.
6. Berstock J, Beswick A, Lenguerrand E, Whitehouse M, Blom A. Mortality after total hip replacement surgery: a systematic review. Bone Joint Res. 2014;3:175–82.
7. Bilimoria K, Liu Y, Paruch J, Zhou L, Kmiecik T, Ko C, Cohen M. Development and evaluation of the universal ACS NSQIP surgical risk calculator: a decision aid and informed consent tool for patients and surgeons. J Am Coll Surg. 2013;217:833–42.
8. Fombon FN, Thompson JP. Anaesthesia for the adult patient with rheumatoid arthritis. Critical Care Pain. 2006;6(6):235–9.
9. Rosenberg AD. Anesthesia for major orthopedic surgery. ASA Refresher Courses Anesthesiol. 1997;25:131–44.
10. Lee AF, et al. 2014 ACC/AHA guideline on perioperative cardiovascular evaluation and management of patients undergoing noncardiac surgery. J Am Coll Cardiol. 2014;64(22):77–137.
11. Skutek M, Wirries N, von Lewinski G. Hip arthroplasty in obese patients: rising prevalence- standard procedures? Orthop Rev. 2016;8(2):6379.
12. Kent C, Posner KL, Lee LA, Domino KB. United States: complications associated with regional anesthesia. In: Finucane B, Tsui B, editors. Complications of regional anesthesia. Cham: Springer; 2017. p. 451–62.
13. Schmalzried TP, Amstutz HC, Dorey FJ. Nerve palsy associated with total hip replacement. Risk factors and prognosis. J Bone Joint Surg Am. 1991;73:1074–80.
14. Schmalzried TP, Noordin S, Amstutz HC. Update on nerve palsy associated with total hip replacement. Clin Orthop Relat Res. 1997;(344):188–206.
15. Neal JM, et al. The second ASRA practice advisory on neurologic complications associated with regional anesthesia and pain medicine: executive summary 2015. Reg Anesth Pain Med. 2015;40(5):401–30.
16. Carling M, Jeppsson A, Eriksson B, Brisby H. Transfusions and blood loss in total hip and knee arthroplasty: a prospective observational study. J Orthop Surg Res. 2015;10:48.
17. Sa-ngasoongsong P, Wongsak S, Kulachote N, Chanplakorn P, Woratanarat P, Kawinwonggowit V. Predicting factors for allogeneic blood transfusion and excessive postoperative blood loss after single low-dosage intra-articular Tranexamic acid application in Total knee replacement. Biomed Res Int. 2017;2017:1–7.
18. Kulkarni A, Gupta A. A retrospective analysis of massive blood transfusion and post-operative complica-

tions in patients undergoing supra-major orthopaedic oncosurgeries. Indian J Anaesth. 2016;60(4):270.
19. Horlocker TT, et al. Regional anesthesia in the patient receiving antithrombotic or thrombolytic therapy: American Society of Regional Anesthesia and Pain Medicine Evidence-Based Guidelines (Third Edition). Reg Anesth Pain Med. 2010;35(1):64–101.
20. Levine GN, et al. 2016 ACC/AHA guideline on duration of dual anti-platelet therapy in patients with coronary artery disease. J Am Col Cardiol. 2016;68(10):1082–115.
21. Kopp SL. Posterior approach to the lumbar plexus. In: Hebl JR, Lennon RL, editors. Mayo Clinic atlas of regional anesthesia and ultrasound-guided nerve blockade. Rochester (MN) and New York: Mayo Clinic Scientific Press and Oxford University Press; 2010.
22. Di Benedetto P, et al. A new posterior approach to the sciatic nerve block: a prospective, randomized comparison with the classic posterior approach. Anesth Analg. 2001;93:1040–4.
23. Terkawi AS, et al. Pain management modalities after total knee arthroplasty a network meta-analysis of 170 randomized controlled trials. Anesthesiology. 2017;126:923–37.
24. Buvanendran A, et al. Perioperative oral Pregabalin reduces chronic pain after total knee arthroplasty: a prospective, randomized, controlled trial. Anesth Analg. 2010;110(1):199–207.
25. Yu-Min H, et al. Perioperative celecoxib administration for pain management after total knee arthroplasty—a randomized, controlled study. BMC Musculoskelet Disord. 2008;9:77. https://doi.org/10.1186/1471-2474-9-77.
26. Sulaiman L. Current concepts in anaesthesia for shoulder surgery. Open Orthop J. 2013;7:323–8.
27. Singelyn F, Lhotel L, Fabre B. Pain relief after arthroscopic shoulder surgery: a comparison of Intraarticular analgesia, Suprascapular nerve block, and Interscalene brachial plexus block. Anesth Analg. 2004;99(2):589–92.
28. Singelyn F, Lhotel L, Fabre B. Pain relief after arthroscopic shoulder surgery: a comparison of Intraarticular analgesia, Suprascapular nerve block, and Interscalene brachial plexus block. Anesth Analg. 2004;99:589–92.
29. Beecroft C, Coventry D. Anaesthesia for shoulder surgery. Critical Care Pain. 2008;8:193–8.
30. Malik T, Mass D, Cohn S. Postoperative analgesia in a prolonged continuous interscalene block versus single-shot block in outpatient arthroscopic rotator cuff repair: a prospective randomized study. Arthroscopy. 2016;32:1544–1550.e1.
31. Fredrickson M, Ball C, Dalgleish A. Analgesic effectiveness of a continuous versus single-injection Interscalene block for minor arthroscopic shoulder surgery. Reg Anesth Pain Med. 2010;35:28–33.
32. Long T, Wass C, Burkle C. Perioperative interscalene blockade: an overview of its history and current clinical use. J Clin Anesth. 2002;14:546–56.
33. Borgeat A, Ekatodramis G, Kalberer F, Benz C. Acute and nonacute complications associated with Interscalene block and shoulder surgery. Anesthesiology. 2001;95:875–80.
34. Pohl A, Cullen D. Cerebral ischemia during shoulder surgery in the upright position: a case series. J Clin Anesth. 2005;17:463–9.
35. Schubert A. Positioning injuries in anesthesia: an update. Adv Anesthesia. 2008;26:31–65.
36. Sukeik M, et al. Systematic review and meta-analysis of the use of tranexamic acid in total hip replacement. J Bone Joint Surg Br. 2010;93(1):39–46.
37. Alshryda S, et al. A systematic review and meta-analysis of the topical administration of tranexamic acid in total hip and knee replacement. Bone Joint J. 2014;96-B(8):1005–15.
38. Gandhi R, et al. Tranexamic acid and the reduction of blood loss in total knee and hip arthroplasty: a meta-analysis. BMC Res Notes. 2013;6(1):184.
39. Wang C, et al. Topical application of tranexamic acid in primary total hip arthroplasty: a systemic review and meta-analysis. Int J Surg. 2015;15:134–9.
40. Moskal JT, Capps SG. Meta-analysis of intravenous Tranexamic acid in primary total hip arthroplasty. Orthopedics. 2016;39(5):e883–92.
41. American Society of Anesthesiologists Task Force on Perioperative Blood Management. Practice guidelines for perioperative blood management. Anesthesiology. 2015;122:241–75.
42. Khanna G, Cernovsky J. Bone cement and the implications for anaesthesia. Critical Care Pain. 2012;12(4):213–6.
43. Donaldson AJ, et al. Bone cement implantation syndrome. Br J Anaesth. 2008;102(1):12–22.
44. Shaikh N. Emergency management of fat embolism syndrome. J Emerg Trauma Shock. 2009;2:29.
45. George J, George R, Dixit R, Gupta R, Gupta N. Fat embolism syndrome. Lung India. 2013;30:47–53.
46. Pitto R, Koessler M, Kuehle J. Comparison of fixation of the femoral component without cement and fixation with use of a bone-vacuum cementing technique for the prevention of fat embolism during total hip arthroplasty. A prospective, randomized clinical trial. J Bone Joint Surg Am. 1999;81:831–43.
47. Bederman SS, et al. Do corticosteroids reduce the risk of fat embolism syndrome in patients with long-bone fractures? A meta-analysis. Can J Surg. 2009;52(5):386–93.
48. Kakkar AK, Rushton-Smith SK. Incidence of venous thromboembolism in orthopedic surgery. In: Llau J, editor. Thromboembolism in orthopedic surgery. London: Springer; 2012. p. 11–7.
49. Warwick D. Prevention of venous thromboembolism in total knee and hip replacement. Circulation. 2012;125:2151–5.
50. Geerts WH, Bergqvist D, Pineo GF, et al. Prevention of venous thromboembolism: American College of Chest Physicians evidence-based clinical practice guidelines (8th edition). Chest. 2008;133(6 Suppl):381S–453S.

51. Horlocker TT, Wedel DJ, Rowlingson JC, et al. Executive summary: regional anesthesia in the patient receiving antithrombotic or thrombolytic therapy: American Society of Regional Anesthesia and Pain Medicine evidence-based guidelines (third edition). Reg Anesth Pain Med. 2010;35(1):102–5.
52. Narouze S, et al. Interventional spine and pain procedures in patients on antiplatelet and anticoagulant medications: guidelines from the American Society of Regional Anesthesia and Pain Medicine, the European Society of Regional Anaesthesia and Pain Therapy, the American Academy of Pain Medicine, the International Neuromodulation Society, the North American Neuromodulation Society, and the World Institute of Pain. Reg Anesth Pain Med. 2015;40(3):182–212.

# Anesthesia for Urological Procedures

Hussam Ghabra and Susan A. Smith

## Introduction

Adult urologic surgery involves pathology of the genitourinary system including procedures involving the kidney, ureters, bladder, prostate and urethra. Typically, these types of surgery fall into one of two groups: endourologic and major abdominal procedures. Patients presenting for urologic surgery are often elderly with multiple medical comorbidities; a pre-operative evaluation is critical to address conditions that require optimization, to assess the appropriateness of the patient for an ambulatory surgery environment, and determine the risk, monitors and anesthetic considerations for each procedure. This chapter discusses the frequent anesthetic challenges associated with the most common urologic procedures.

## Pre-operative Evaluation

The increasing number of patients over the age of 65 in the United States has amplified the demand for numerous healthcare services, including the need for outpatient surgery [1]. Due to the large proportion of patients of elderly patients undergoing urological procedures, an evaluation of medical comorbidities is required. Optimization of concomitant diseases is challenging and requires close attention when preparing patients for surgery [2]. Particularly in the elderly, a frailty evaluation offers an additional risk assessment in those presenting for surgery. Numerous studies demonstrate that frail patients have a greater incidence of postoperative complications than non-frail patients [3, 4]. Furthermore, recent publications propose that age, in the absence of frailty, is not an independent risk factor for postoperative surgical complications [5].

Common cardiovascular conditions in urologic patients include coronary artery disease, congestive heart failure, valvular heart disease, systemic hypertension, dysrhythmias, heart block, and peripheral vascular disease. Therefore, a detailed clinical evaluation determining cardiovascular risk is required. The evidence regarding routine use of preoperative electrocardiogram (ECG) demonstrates necessity in only a select group of patients [6]. Additionally, for patients who do have an abnormal ECG, only a small number require preoperative intervention and change in medical management based the results. As a result, the American Society of Anesthesiologists Task Force report on preanesthesia evaluation recommends against routine preoperative ECG [7]. Instead, the task force recommends selective preoperative testing based on history, physical examination, and the type of surgery.

H. Ghabra, M.D. · S. A. Smith, M.D. (✉)
Department of Anesthesiology, Oschner Medical Center, New Orleans, LA, USA
e-mail: hussam.ghabra@ochsner.org; susan.smith@ochsner.org

The American College of Cardiology (ACC) and the American Heart Association (AHA) Guidelines on Preoperative Electrocardiogram [8]:

1. ECG is recommended for patients with history of ischemic heart disease, history of congestive heart failure, history of cerebrovascular disease, diabetes, renal insufficiency, or peripheral vascular disease who will undergo high or intermediate-risk surgery.
2. ECG is reasonable for patients with no risk factors who will undergo high-risk surgery.
3. ECG is not indicated for asymptomatic patients who will undergo low-risk surgery.

The 2014 AHA/ACC *Preoperative Cardiovascular Guidelines for Noncardiac Surgery* provide evidence-based recommendations for cardiac stress testing prior to surgery [8]. Given the varied risk profiles of the different urologic surgeries, patients need to be evaluated for their individual revised cardiac risk index (RCRI), as well as in context for the upcoming surgery. Most endourological procedures are considered low risk. Major urologic procedures (nephrectomy and cystectomy) are considered intermediate risk. However, in the absence of other concerns as detailed in the AHA/ACC Guidelines, ischemic evaluations have not shown to decrease perioperative cardiac events and thus, improve patient outcomes [7, 8].

Due to the extensive smoking history common in urologic patients, one of the most common pulmonary comorbidities is chronic obstructive pulmonary disease (COPD). Smokers are three times more likely to develop bladder cancer than non-smokers [9] and smoking increases the risk of renal cancer by 50% [10]. Yet, the value of preoperative chest radiograph (CXR) is limited. If clinical history and exam indicate a recent change in disease, new-onset symptoms, or unstable cardiopulmonary disease, a CXR may provide valuable information when intervention is needed prior to surgery [7].

Other common comorbidities in patients presenting for urologic surgery include diabetes, joint disease and cognitive and hearing impairment [11]. Evaluating baseline glycemic control, determining use of oral agent versus insulin therapy, and measuring blood glucose levels on the day of surgery aid in management of hyperglycemia in the perioperative period.

Preoperative laboratory testing is considered based on established guidelines [5] and may include a complete blood count, and comprehensive or basic metabolic panel or basic metabolic panel, including renal function tests (baseline serum creatinine and glomerular filtration rate (GFR)). Patients undergoing surgery in the urologic system may have transient changes in renal functions due to their underlying disease or, suffer from chronic kidney disease or end-stage renal disease. If concern for renal function is merited given the current pathophysiology or other medical comorbidities, renal function testing is imperative. Anesthetic medications metabolized by the kidney should be minimized or avoided in patients with decreasing renal function or acute kidney injury. Perioperative assessment also includes determining the patient's volume status and/or risk of electrolyte imbalance. A type and screen/cross should be ordered in certain patients; this is addressed in the separate procedure types and should be added to preoperative labs if needed.

Most urologic procedures are endourologic and can be performed as outpatient surgery. This is advantageous to elderly patients because they are less adaptable to the environmental changes that accompany inpatient surgery. Of added benefit, outpatient surgery reduces hospital and patient cost. Careful outpatient selection optimizes patient safety and efficiently employs available resources. In 2013, a large retrospective study using the National Surgical Quality Improvement Program's data examined 250,000 patients undergoing a wide variety of outpatient surgeries [12]. The incidence of morbidity and mortality for patients undergoing cystoscopy was 1–3%. Risk factors for poor outcome include obesity, chronic obstructive pulmonary disease, history of transient ischemic attack/stroke, hypertension, previous cardiac surgical intervention, and prolonged operative time [13].

## Endourological Procedures

Endourology procedures are those that allow visualization and intervention in the urinary tract without considerable incisions. Endoscopes are generally inserted into the urethra and used to perform procedures on the prostate, bladder, ureters and potentially the kidneys. Although these procedures are considered less invasive than more major urologic procedures, they constitute a large portion of urologic practice and can be associated with significant morbidity. Some of the most common endourologic procedures encountered by the anesthesiologist include: cystoscopy and ureteroscopy performed for urologic cancer surveillance, ureteral stent placement and stone retrieval for nephrolithiasis and transurethral resection of the prostate (TURP) for benign prostatic hypertrophy (BPH).

An important consideration for all endourologic procedures is the use of the lithotomy position. It is the most common position used for these surgeries, and causes notable physiologic changes in the body. (Table 76.1). Use of the lithotomy position is associated with pressure ulcers, peripheral nerve injury and compartment syndrome.

The most important risk factor for nerve injury is the duration of the operation [15, 16]. Operative time exceeding 2–3 h is associated with an increase in the incidence of peripheral nerve injury. Furthermore, incorrect lithotomy, exaggerated lithotomy position, and pressure applied by surgical providers during the operation can increase the risk of nerve injury [15]. The most commonly affected nerves include the lateral femoral cutaneous, obturator, sciatic, and peroneal nerves. Most nerve injuries post-lithotomy are reversible [15, 16]; however, irreversible nerve injuries are associated with significant morbidity [15]. Paresthesia is usually the first reported symptom postoperatively [16]. The American Society of Anesthesiologists Task Force has recommended the avoidance of hamstring muscle group stretching and limiting hip flexion to decrease the risk of sciatic nerve injury [17]. Further recommendations include preventing prolonged pressure on the peroneal nerve at the fibular head and use of padding to prevent nerve pressure against the hard surface of the lithotomy boot [18].

Lithotomy position increases intracompartmental pressure in the lower leg. The pressure escalates when the leg prop device places pressure behind the calf instead of supporting the ankle [19]. Due to the dense fascia in the lower leg, increases in pressure are poorly tolerated in the muscle bed. Should pressure escalate sufficiently to impede blood flow, compartment syndrome can develop. This is a rare but devastating complication and may result in permanent disability if not diagnosed and treated promptly [20]. Despite close supervision of the patient and positioning by a senior surgeon, compartment syndrome has been reported. It most frequently occurs in cases with an operative time greater than 4 h [20, 21]. Trendelenburg position in combination with lithotomy is also an identified risk. The use of intermittent pneumatic external compression devices has been shown to lower the intracompartmental pressure, which may reducing the risk for compartment syndrome [19]. The treatment for the acute development of compartment syndrome is surgical decompression by a fasciotomy.

**Table 76.1** Physiologic changes associated with lithotomy position [14]

| Physiological change | Effect |
| --- | --- |
| Decreased functional residual capacity | Atelectasis and hypoxia |
| Increase in blood in the central circulation (leg elevation with possible Trendelenburg) | Worsening of heart failure, increase in mean arterial pressure, and increase in cardiac output |
| Decrease in venous return (rapid leg lowering) | Hypotension |

## Transurethral Resection of the Prostate (TURP)

### Indication and Procedure

Transurethral resection of the prostate (TURP) and is a common procedure used to treat benign prostatic hypertrophy (BPH) with or without urinary retention. BPH is characterized by proliferation of smooth and epithelial cells in the transition zone of the prostate gland and can significantly increase the size of the gland. Because the gland surrounds the urethra, BPH can effectively constrict the lumen of the urethra resulting in obstructive urinary symptoms [22]. The population of patients undergoing TURP continues to be largely geriatric. The average age of a patient presenting for TURP is 69 years old, with over half of TURP patients being 75 years of older [23]. In recent years, other pathologic factors such as sleep disturbance, hypertension, diabetes, and hyperlipidemia have been identified to further contribute to the development of urinary symptoms [23–25] and these are common co-morbidities in TURP patients. Although TURP remains the definitive treatment for BPH, there has been a consistent decline in the number of TURPs being performed annually because medical therapy (5-alpha reductase inhibitors and alpha-adrenergic blockers) has proven to be an effective treatment alternative.

## Intraoperative Management

Choice of anesthetic for TURP includes both general and neuraxial anesthesia. Neuraxial anesthesia is appropriate and may include spinal, epidural or combined spinal epidural (CSE). Consideration for neuraxial anesthesia must take into account a patient's anticoagulation regimen and the American Society of Regional Anesthesia and Pain Medicine (ASRA) Guidelines should be followed [26]. To date, evidence does not demonstrate general anesthesia or neuraxial techniques to be superior for TURP [27]. There are advantages and disadvantages to each of these techniques, thus the patient's individual risk factors should be taken into consideration when deciding which technique is optimal for each patient. A significant advantage of neuraxial technique is that the patient remains awake in the operating room. Detection of TURP syndrome is highly sensitive in this situation because immediate neurologic exam is possible. Symptoms of TURP syndrome are often masked under a general anesthetic. Karamaz et al., demonstrated that in elderly patients, a low dose (4 mg) bupivacaine spinal (with 25mcg fentanyl) provides adequate sensory block for TURP, but with shorter prolonged motor blockade, less shivering and a lower incidence of hypotension than more traditional dosing (7.5 mg bupivacaine) [28]. If using a neuraxial approach, a T10-T11 sensory level is required. However, despite sufficient sensory level, the patient's obturator reflex remains intact. Although stimulation of the obturator nerve is more commonly seen in procedures involving the bladder, involuntary movement during TURP can complicate the procedure. Additionally, neuraxial anesthesia does appear to decrease initial postoperative pain however, relief did not extend more than 8–12 h following the procedure [29].

Patients with chronic cough are not ideal candidates for a neuraxial block because despite adequate anesthesia and analgesia. Frequent movements generated in a coughing patient make the procedure difficult to perform. Additionally, those with musculoskeletal comorbidities that prevent comfortable supine or lithotomy positioning may not tolerate a neuraxial anesthetic. A general anesthetic with muscle paralysis eliminates the obturator reflex.

Complications associated with TURP include TURP syndrome, bladder perforation, coagulopathy, bleeding and septicemia. Of these, TURP syndrome is the most unique, and warrants consideration in patients undergoing the procedure, particularly if the procedure is long and significant irrigation fluid is used (Table 76.2). It is reported that mild-moderate TURP syndrome occurs in 1–8% of patients; the mortality of severe TURP syndrome may be upwards of 25% [30]. During a TURP, the well-developed vascular bed of the prostate is opened and exposed to the irrigation solution used during the procedure. This presents the opportunity for the solution to be readily absorbed into the systemic circulation. Based on the irrigant solution and the volume absorbed, the patient may experience a variety of deleterious effects that define TURP syndrome. The state is largely characterized by volume overload with hypo-osmotic fluids [31–33].

Table 76.2 Signs and symptoms of TURP syndrome

| Neurologic symptoms | Cardiovascular and pulmonary symptoms | Other symptoms |
|---|---|---|
| Restlessness | Hypertension and tachycardia | Hyponatremia |
| Headache/confusion | Tachypnea | Hyperglycemia |
| Visual disturbances | Hypoxia | Acute renal failure |
| Nausea | Flash pulmonary edema | |
| Seizure | Hypotension and Bradycardia | |
| Obtundation | | |

## Lithotripsy

### Indication and Procedure

Prior management of urolithiasis (stones in the ureteral tract) often included open surgical procedures. Over the past 15 years however, dramatic changes in surgical treatment have become available and less invasive options are now the preferred procedural approach. Stones located in the bladder, and lower part of the ureters, are amenable to treatment with extraction by cystoscopy, placement of a stent or intracorpoareal lithotripsy. Stones in the upper regions of the ureters or in the kidney are treated with extracorporeal lithotripsy [30].

Urolithiasis can result in a variety of clinical manifestations based upon location of the stone. Patients with nephrolithiasis (kidney stones) most commonly present with renal colic but some can present with painless hematuria [29]. Unfortunately for those who present with a kidney stone, there is a 50% recurrence rate [29]. Thus, they may require multiple interventions over their lifetime, the most common treatment choice being shock wave lithotripsy (SWL). Lithotripsy uses ultrasound shock waves (pressure pulses) targeted at the stone(s) to break it down into small pieces that can more easily traverse the urinary tract. Early use of SWL required the patient to be immersed in water to conduct the waves however; more modern equipment has eliminated the water bath making the procedure amenable to outpatient surgical centers.

### Intraoperative Management

Monitored anesthesia care (MAC) may be appropriate for some patients undergoing ESWL. More frequently however, a regional or general anesthetic is required or requested based on individual patient factors. Factors that determine the need for a general versus neuraxial anesthetic are determined by patient comorbidities or request. To date, there is no definitive evidence demonstrating that either type of anesthetic is superior for lithotripsy. In 2014, a prospective randomized controlled trial examined the incidence of postoperative cognitive dysfunction following general versus spinal anesthesia for patients undergoing lithotripsy. Compared to earlier studies, a unique aspect of this investigation was that no sedatives or opiates were administered to the spinal anesthetic group. Results showed no significant difference in postoperative cognitive dysfunction 7 days after surgery between the groups [34]. If regional anesthesia is utilized, a T6 sensory level is needed to ensure the potential field of the shock wave is covered.

Patients with cardiac implantable electronic devices (CIEDs) require special consideration. Shock waves produced by the lithotripsy unit can damage a CIED, particularly if the shock is directed in proximity to the CIED generator. Electromagnetic interference (EMI) may occur because the forces generated by lithotripsy cause inappropriate sensing of arrhythmias. If inappropriate shocks are of considerate concern, the tachyarrythmia detection function of the defibrillator should be deactivated. Pressure pulses during SWL are delivered in two ways: synchronized with the patient's R waves as detected by internal EKG or non-synchronized such that they are delivered at a specific rate. If the lithotripsy equipment is programmed to synchronize with ventricular contractions, atrial pacing pulses by the implanted device can trigger the pressure pulse prematurely. If deemed appropriate by electrophysiology, treatment may warrant atrial pacing be turned off [35]. As per the American Society of Anesthesiologists (ASA) guidelines, preoperative evaluation of the patient should include this planning and require information from the CIED manufacturer if needed.

## Prostatectomy

### Indication and Procedure

Cancer of the prostate gland constitutes the second most common cancer in men. The American Cancer Society predicts that in 2017, 161,360 new cases will be diagnosed and 26,730 deaths will occurred as a result of prostate cancer in the United States [36]. The field of urological oncology has undergone remarkable change with the advent of robotic surgery. Robotics were first reported as an adjunct to surgery in 1985, and trialed in urology in 1989 [37]. In 2000, the Di Vinci robot was approved by the Food and Drug Administration for use and since that time, robotic prostatectomy has been become the most popular surgical technique for removal of the prostate in the United States [37]. Studies comparing open versus laparoscopic versus robotic prostatectomy specifically hypothesize superiority of one over the others. Outcomes most commonly examined include the incidence of incontinence, erectile dysfunction and presence of positive surgical margins. A large multinational retrospective study compared open versus laparoscopic versus robotic radical prostatectomies and found positive surgical margins present at a rate of 22.8%, 16.3% and 13.8% respectively [38]. No differences were identified in incontinence or erectile dysfunction up to 12 weeks post operatively comparing open versus robotic-assisted laparoscopic prostatectomy [39].

Preoperative evaluation of these patients should be geared to optimize medical comorbidities and minimize surgical stress. This topic is addressed in the preoperative section and additionally, in the Enhanced Recovery After Surgery (ERAS) discussion.

### Intraoperative Management

Largely, patients undergoing prostatectomy require general anesthesia with a secured airway, two peripheral intravenous lines and standard ASA monitors. If patient comorbidities (particularly active cardiopulmonary conditions) merit the need for invasive monitoring, arterial or central access requires early consideration. Positioning for robotic prostatectomy requires the patient's arms to be tucked, and the bed to be moved into optimal location for the robot. Once appropriately positioned in the room in relation to the robot, the bed is placed in steep Trendelenberg. Loss of access to the patient after positioning, prepping and draping makes line placement during the procedure difficult, if not impossible. Experience of the surgeon has been shown to be associated with not only the duration of the procedure, but also with patient outcomes [36]. Thus, optimal anesthetic planning and monitoring needs to account for surgeon familiarity and volume.

Positioning patients for robotic procedures is considerably more complicated than traditional open procedures. Like other urologic procedures where lithotomy position is used, care must be taken to protect peripheral nerves and understand the physiologic changes associated with this position. Steep Trendelenburg is necessary to displace the pelvic viscera from the surgeon's surgical field. Special consideration should be given to pad all pressure points and ensure that the patient is secured to the table. The use of nonslip padding prevents patient migration. The calves should be free of contact with the lower portion of the OR table and the lateral portion of the calf and knee should be well padded and supported to protect from peroneal nerve injury. The arms and hands should be adequately padded, with the palms facing the legs and all intravenous and arterial lines should be confirmed patent after positioning [40]. The head and face should be free of any instruments and protective goggles over the eyes may prevent corneal/eye injury. Braces on the operating room table placing pressure on the top of the shoulder (to stabilize the patient on the operating room table) should be used with caution due to their association with brachial plexus injuries [41].

After the patient is prepped and draped, the anesthesia provider will have minimal access to the patient. Contact with the patient's head and airway is maintained and should be checked regularly. The surgeon's assistant establishes port placement because the surgeon is positioned in a console, away from the table, using a telescoping monitor to drive the robotic arms. Generation of pneumoperitoneum augments visualization of the surgical field but simultaneously produces a number of cardiovascular changes that are exacerbated in the Trendelenburg position. As the patient's head falls well below the heart, an increase in intrathoracic pressure results in decreased venous return and increased pulmonary vascular resistance [42, 43]. Further, the development of the pneumoperitoneum, increases vascular resistance in the intraabdominal organs and may cause a subsequent rise in arterial blood pressure [42, 43]. For patients with preexisting cardiovascular disease, these physiologic changes place strain on the left ventricle and cardiac output falls.

Patients with moderate to severe pulmonary hypertension may not tolerate the additional increase in pulmonary vascular resistance, particularly those with compromised right ventricular function. Patients with pulmonary disease, including advanced COPD, may not be ideal candidates for robotic prostatectomy because the added airway pressures often limit ventilation resulting in notable hypercarbia. The morbidly obese also pose unique challenges due to the added weight on the diaphragm and chest wall. Their baseline restrictive lung disease worsens in both the Trendelenburg position and with pneumoperitoneum, the airway and driving pressures needed to successfully oxygenate and ventilate during the procedure may exceed safe limits. Lung-protective ventilation is recommended setting tidal volume at 6–8 mL/kg ideal body weight and positive end expiratory pressure (PEEP) at 5–10 cm of water pressure [44]. There is insufficient data at this time to recommend which patients should have an open versus robotic prostatectomy; the anesthesiologist's discretion and open communication with the surgeon is recommended for patients considered too high risk to tolerate the positioning and pneumoperitoneum needed in the robotic approach.

Several complications have been recognized in these patients, most due to the extreme intraoperative positioning. Edema develops around the head and eyes and can potentially result in transient visual disturbances. Edema can also compromise the patient's airway. Checking for an endotracheal tube leak test at the end of the surgery should be used to guide extubation. If the leak test is positive, placing the head of the patient's bed at 30 degrees is recommended until they pass the leak test and can be safely extubated.

Multimodal pain management with the aim of minimizing narcotics use has been demonstrated to be effective in ERAS models. More can be found regarding this topic in the ERAS section.

## Nephrectomy

### Indication and Procedure

Elderly patients are most affected by renal cancer, the average age at diagnosis being 64 years old [45]. In 2017, the American Cancer Society expects 64,000 new diagnoses of the disease [45]. The most common kidney cancer is renal cell carcinoma (RCC). Surgical treatment for RCC includes partial or radical nephrectomy. For small, localized cancers, long-term morbidity improves when patients are treated with partial nephrectomy. Renal function is better preserved in these patients; furthermore, other systemic conditions, such as cardiovascular disease, malnutrition, anemia and neuropathy also demonstrate improved long-term control [46]. These findings are consistent with the landmark study in 2008 by Go et al., that demonstrate reduced glomerular filtration rate (GFR) is associated with an increased risk of hospitalization and death [47]. When kidney function can be maintained with appropriate selection of patient and disease for partial nephrectomy, there does appear to be a survival and wellness advantage.

Of note, a partial nephrectomy is technically more complicated than radical nephrectomy, especially with the continuing evolution of the minimally invasive approach. The risk of intraoperative and postoperative bleeding is higher in partial nephrectomy given the vascularity of the organ parenchyma.

Cigarette smoking is an established risk factor for patients with renal cancer. Therefore it stands to reason that many of these patients have comorbidities associated with long-term cigarette smoking such as cardiovascular disease and chronic obstructive pulmonary disease (COPD). Further, impaired renal function is a common finding in these patients as well. See the preoperative section for further discussion on patient optimization prior to surgery.

## Intraoperative Management

All patients undergoing nephrectomy need a type and screen prior to surgery. The decision to cross-match blood can be decided on an individual case basis but, conditions and surgical factors that merit consideration for a type and cross include preoperative anemia, history of multiple abdominal surgeries, and large tumors involving vascular structures. A discussion with the surgeon is also imperative to fully discern surgical concerns and considerations with regards to bleeding risk. General endotracheal anesthesia is used for these patients with standard ASA monitors. Large bore intravenous (IV) access is routinely obtained; invasive monitors are generally reserved for those patients with symptomatic or severe cardiopulmonary disease. The exception to this is for patients with tumor thrombus that might require an inferior vena cava thrombectomy with nephrectomy (see chapter on *IVC Thrombectomy*).

A flank incision is the most common surgical approach for patients undergoing nephrectomy. This requires lateral decubitus position with the kidney bar raised just beyond the iliac crest. Yokoyama et al., evaluated blood pressure in the lateral decubitus position during nephrectomy. Results demonstrate that insignificant hemodynamic changes occur with placement in lateral decubitus position, however a significant reduction in blood pressure was appreciated when the kidney bar was raised [48]. Special positioning consideration needs to be made to prevent peripheral nerve injuries. A pillow is typically placed between the patient's lower leg (flexed at the knee) and the upper leg. The upper leg is straight and in alignment with the spine. The dependent arm rests on the operating room table and padding is used to support the arm in neutral position to the shoulder and particularly to protect the ulnar nerve near the elbow. The arm ipsilateral to the surgical side (independent or up arm) is maintained on padding, pillows or within an arm support device that keeps the arm neutral to the shoulder. The elbow is bent in a cephalad position with palm down to prevent nerve stretch or compression [49]. An axillary roll is placed with 2–3 fingerbreadths between the roll and axilla and extended to the area beneath the scapula. This relieves pressure on neurovascular structure to prevent brachial plexus injury and maintain blood flow to the dependent arm. Avoid direct pressure on the ear and eye close to the operating room table. A neutral cervical spine is imperative to prevent neck injuries.

A nephrectomy is a major intraabdominal procedure and fluid management requires constant and thoughtful evaluation throughout operating room and post anesthesia care. Goal-directed fluid therapy (GDFT) is recommended in nephrectomy patients and a number of non-invasive monitors are available to guide fluid administration. The International Fluid Optimization Group published a number of recommendations in 2015 to consolidate the large amount of information that exists regarding GDFT. The highlights are as follows [50]:

1. A consistent technique should be measured in the operating room both before and after fluid therapies are given. Common techniques are systolic pressure variation (SPV), pulse pressure variation (PPV), stroke volume variation (SVV), and plethysmographic waveform variation (PWV).

2. Transesophageal echocardiography can be useful in evaluation of patient's response to

fluid therapy. It should be emphasized that using dynamic and not static measurements are appropriate to use for guidance.
3. Common techniques such as systolic pressure variation (SPV), pulse pressure variation (PPV), stroke volume variation (SVV), and plethysmographic waveform variation (PWV) have been validated in multiple studies with various types of patients including major abdominal, neurosurgery, vascular and cardiac. Each technique requires understanding by providers when fluid therapy is given.

Pain management is as described and discussed in the ERAS portion of this chapter with emphasis on multimodal techniques and consideration for neuraxial techniques.

## Cystectomy

### Indication and Procedure

Bladder cancer represents 5% of all new cancers diagnosed, with an estimated 80,000 new diagnoses being expected this year [51]. Men are 3–4 times more likely to be diagnosed than women, and at an average age of 73 years old [51]. Similar to renal cancer, cigarette smoking is a known risk factor for bladder cancer and many carry the concomitant diagnoses of cardiovascular and chronic obstructive pulmonary disease. The typical patient receiving a cystectomy is elderly with multiple comorbidities.

Radical cystectomy involves surgical removal of the bladder and may result in blood loss and need for transfusion. General endotracheal anesthesia is universally accepted as the anesthetic of choice. In addition to standard ASA monitors, an arterial line is recommended for hemodynamic monitoring, blood gas sampling and pulse pressure variation to guide resuscitation. Central access is frequently placed for potential vasopressor administration and rapid resuscitation if needed. Two to four red blood cell units should be cross-matched and easily available for the procedure. Volume assessment can be difficult because of large volume intraoperative fluid shifts; also, unique to cystectomy, urine output cannot be measured because it falls into the surgical field. GDFT is recommended and should be directed by PPV/SPV/SVV assessment, blood gas monitoring, and strict and frequent blood loss measurement.

## Enhanced Recovery After Major Urological Procedures

Enhanced recovery after surgery (ERAS) has gained a great deal of attention given the vast amount of evidence showing improvements in surgical outcomes. Many surgical specialties have adapted use around the world and continue to perfect protocols. Major components of these protocols are outlined in Table 76.3.

Each of these components has been used in isolation in various settings for many years. However, using all components together in continuity with consistent adherence amongst multiple disciplines, has led to improvement in postoperative outcomes [52]. Using an ERAS protocol, Shah and Abaza followed 30 consecutive patients undergoing robotic cystectomy and decreased length of stay (LOS) to 3.3 days (as versus typical LOS 5–7 days) [54]. Chang et al., reviewed 304 patients undergoing open radical cystectomy using an ERAS protocol and reported a major complication rate of 4.9% and mortality of 0.3% [55]. Compared to previous reports by Frazier et al., patients undergoing radical cystectomy using a non-ERAS pathway have an overall 30-day complication rate of 32% and mortality rate of 2.5% [56]. Other studies have shown similar improvement in outcomes and reduction in complications [57]. Despite the preponderance of evidence showing the positive outcomes of ERAS, a recent survey by Kukreja et al., showed that 64% of radical cystectomy providers follow an ERAS protocol and of those who do use an ERAS algorithm, only 20% complied with all interventions [62]. Therefore, it should be noted that although different institutions may report use of an ERAS protocol, it likely varies in method.

Designing an anesthetic to minimize narcotics is an integral component of ERAS pathway. In

**Table 76.3** Major components of enhanced recovery after surgery (ERAS) [52–61]

| Recommendations | Reasoning for recommendation |
|---|---|
| Provide preoperative patient counseling regarding surgical course | Set recovery expectations about what is/is not normal for the surgical course. Adjust the patient's understanding of expected level of postoperative pain. Improve patient satisfaction |
| Identify patient specific factors to reduce risk and counsel regarding modification (improve pre-operative nutrition, recommend smoking cessation, encourage activity/exercise, e.g.) | Optimize preoperative condition to minimize postoperative morbidity and mortality |
| Omission of preoperative bowel preparation | Decrease the risk of volume depletion and the metabolic and electrolyte deficiencies associated with bowel prep solution and administration. The bowel prep may be associated with fecal leakage (not prevent fecal contamination/leak) |
| Omission of prolonged fasting (withhold solids for 6 h and fluids for 2 h) | Prolonged fasting may increase hyperglycemia and insulin resistance. Hyperglycemia is associated with delayed wound healing, infection, acute kidney injury and increased length of hospital stay |
| Carbohydrate loading prior to surgery | Decrease the body's stress state, facilitate normal insulin release and peripheral glucose uptake. Promote anabolic metabolism, allowing the body to create new cells and possibly heal tissues more quickly |
| Use of Alvimopan | l-opioid receptor antagonist; reduces postoperative ileus |
| Protocol driven intraoperative anesthetic management (goal-directed fluid therapy, multimodal treatment of nausea/vomiting and pain) | Possibly decrease length of stay. Improve post-operative pain control. Reduce surgical stress. Decrease complications associated with nausea and vomiting (allows earlier food intake, prevents retching against new incision lines, increases patient satisfaction) |
| Minimally invasive surgical approach | Improves patient satisfaction. Reduce length of stay. Reduce postoperative pain |
| Minimal use of nasogastric tubes(NGT) | May decrease the risk of fever, atelectasis and pneumonia. Also, allows for earlier food intake |
| Early feeding | Preservation of metabolic homeostasis. May protect against insulin resistance. Likely promotes anabolic metabolism with preservation of the body's protein stores |
| Early ambulation | Reduce post-operative deconditioning. Enable quicker return of bowel function. Reduce postoperative pulmonary complications and deep venous thrombosis |

February 2016, the American Pain Society published clinical practice guidelines for the management of postoperative pain [58]. For open laparotomy, which would be most consistent with major open urologic procedures, systemic non-opioid treatments include non-steroidal anti-inflammatory agents, acetaminophen, gabapentin, and intravenous ketamine and lidocaine infusions [58]. Techniques including a TAP block [61], epidural catheters, and transcutaneous electrical nerve stimulator (TENS) therapy are also recommended. Studies evaluating the use of dexmedetomidine infusions as an anesthetic adjunct, have also demonstrated a reduction in post-operative opioid consumption [59]. Similarly, IV lidocaine infusions may be associated with a reduction in post-operative pain and ileus [60]. However, a recent systematic review emphasized the paucity of safety data that exist for the use of lidocaine in this context [60]. The use of liposomal-bupivicaine (Exparel) TAP blocks for patients undergoing abdominoplasty, demonstrates a reduction in pain and opiate consumption, as well as earlier ambulation [12, 63]. No prospective studies have shown its use major urological procedures and given its substantial costs, this evidence is needed to justify use. Standard bupivacaine is less expensive option and currently, can be used to perform a TAP block as an adjunct to control post-operative pain. Given new analgesic approaches in the setting of more revolutionary surgical techniques, the fields of urology and anesthesiology continue to advance surgical care for an increasingly complex set of patients.

# References

1. Bettelli G. Anaesthesia for the elderly outpatient: preoperative assessment and evaluation, anaesthetic technique and postoperative pain management. Curr Opin Anaesthesiol. 2010;23(6):726–31.
2. Hong JY, Yang SC, Ahn S, Kil HK. Preoperative comorbidities and relationship of comorbidities with postoperative complications in patients undergoing transurethral prostate resection. J Urol. 2011;185(4):1374–8.
3. Makary MA, Segev DL, Pronovost PJ, Syin D, Bandeen-Roche K, Patel P, Takenaga R, Devgan L, Holzmueller CG, Tian J, Fried LP. Frailty as a predictor of surgical outcomes in older patients. J Am Coll Surg. 2010;210(6):901–8. https://doi.org/10.1016/j.jamcollsurg.2010.01.028.
4. Buigues C, Juarros-Folgado P, Fernández-Garrido J, Navarro-Martínez R, Cauli O. Frailty syndrome and pre-operative risk evaluation: a systematic review. Arch Gerontol Geriatr. 2015;61(3):309–21. https://doi.org/10.1016/j.archger.2015.08.002.
5. Michalak MD JR, Lin MD FC, Twiss MD CO. Preoperative evaluation and optimization of the geriatric urologic patient. Urol Pract. 2016. https://doi.org/10.1016/j.urpr.2016.10.00.
6. Fleisher LA. Evidence-based practice of anesthesiology. Philadelphia, PA: Elsevier/Saunders; 2013.
7. Committee on Standards and Practice Parameters, Apfelbaum JL, Connis RT, Nickinovich DG, American Society of Anesthesiologists Task Force on Preanesthesia Evaluation, Pasternak LR, Arens JF, Caplan RA, Connis RT, Fleisher LA, Flowerdew R, Gold BS, Mayhew JF, Nickinovich DG, Rice LJ, Roizen MF, Twersky RS. Practice advisory for preanesthesia evaluation: an updated report by the American Society of Anesthesiologists Task Force on Preanesthesia evaluation. Anesthesiology. 2012;116(3):522–38.
8. Fleisher LA, Beckman JA, Brown KA, Calkins H, Chaikof EL, Fleischmann KE, Freeman WK, Froehlich JB, Kasper EK, Kersten JR, Riegel B, Robb JF, Smith SC Jr, Jacobs AK, Adams CD, Anderson JL, Antman EM, Buller CE, Creager MA, Ettinger SM, Faxon DP, Fuster V, Halperin JL, Hiratzka LF, Hunt SA, Lytle BW, Nishimura R, Ornato JP, Page RL, Riegel B, Tarkington LG, Yancy CW. ACC/AHA 2007 guidelines on perioperative cardiovascular evaluation and care for noncardiac surgery: executive summary: a report of the American College of Cardiology/American Heart Association Task Force on Practice guidelines (writing committee to revise the 2002 guidelines on perioperative cardiovascular evaluation for noncardiac surgery) developed in collaboration with the American Society of Echocardiography, American Society of Nuclear Cardiology, Heart Rhythm Society, Society of Cardiovascular Anesthesiologists, Society for Cardiovascular Angiography and Interventions, Society for Vascular Medicine and Biology, and Society for Vascular Surgery. J Am Coll Cardiol. 2007;50(17):1707–32.
9. The American Cancer Society. https://www.cancer.org/cancer/bladder-cancer/causes-risks-prevention/risk-factors.html. Accessed 29 May 2017.
10. The American Cancer Society. https://www.cancer.org/cancer/kidney-cancer/causes-risks-prevention/risk-factors.html. Accessed 29 May 2017.
11. Longnecker DE, Newman MF, Mackey S, Sandberg WS, Zapol WM. Chapter 21. Anesthesiology. New York: McGraw-Hill Education; 2017.
12. Vyas KS, Rajendran S, Morrison SD, Shakir A, Mardini S, Lemaine V, Nahabedian MY, Baker SB, Rinker BD, Vasconez HC. Systematic review of liposomal bupivacaine (exparel) for postoperative analgesia. Plast Reconstr Surg. 2016;138(4):748e–56e. https://doi.org/10.1097/PRS.0000000000002547.
13. Mathis MR, Naughton NN, Shanks AM, Freundlich RE, Pannucci CJ, Chu Y, Haus J, Morris M, Kheterpal S. Patient selection for day case-eligible surgery: identifying those at high risk for major complications. Anesthesiology. 2013;119(6):1310–21. https://doi.org/10.1097/ALN.0000000000000005.
14. Butterworth JF, Mackey DC, Wasnick JD, Morgan GE, Mikhail MS. Chapter 31. Morgan & Mikhail's Clinical Anesthesiology. New York: McGraw-Hill; 2013.
15. Gumus E, Kendirci M, Horasanli K, Tanriverdi O, Gidemez G, Miroglu C. Neurapraxic complications in operations performed in the lithotomy position. World J Urol. 2002;20(1):68–71.
16. Warner MA, Warner DO, Harper CM, Schroeder DR, Maxson PM. Lower extremity neuropathies associated with lithotomy positions. Anesthesiology. 2000;93(4):938–42.
17. American Society of Anesthesiologists Task Force on Prevention of Perioperative Peripheral Neuropathies. Practice advisory for the prevention of perioperative peripheral neuropathies: an updated report by the American Society of Anesthesiologists Task Force on prevention of perioperative peripheral neuropathies. Anesthesiology. 2011;114(4):741–54.

18. Morgan GE, Mikhail MS, Murray MJ. Anesthesia for genitourinary surgery. In: Clinical anesthesiology. 4th ed. New York: McGraw Hill; 2006. p. 757–72.
19. Pfeffer SD, Halliwill JR, Warner MA. Effects of lithotomy position and external compression on lower leg muscle compartment pressure. Anesthesiology. 2001 Sep;95(3):632–6.
20. Simms MS, Terry TR. Well leg compartment syndrome after pelvic and perineal surgery in the lithotomy position. Postgrad Med J. 2005 Aug;81(958):534–6.
21. Zappa L, Sugarbaker PH. Compartment syndrome of the leg associated with lithotomy position for cytoreductive surgery. J Surg Oncol. 2007;96(7):619–23.
22. Stafford-Smith M, Shaw A, Sandler A, Kuhn C. The renal system and anesthesia for urologic surgery. In: Barish PG, Cullen BF, Stoelting RK, Cahalan MK, Stock MC, Ortega R, editors. Clinical anesthesia. 7th ed. Philadelphia: Wolters Kluwer Health: Lippincott Williams & Wilkins; 2013. p. 1400–39.
23. Parsons JK. Modifiable risk factors for benign prostatic hyperplasia and lower urinary tract symptoms: new approaches to old problems. J Urol. 2007;178(2):395–401; Epub 2007 Jun 11.
24. Chou PS, Chang WC, Chou WP, Liu ME, Lai CL, Liu CK, Ku YC, Tsai SJ, Chou YH, Chang WP. Increased risk of benign prostate hyperplasia in sleep apnea patients: a nationwide population-based study. PLoS One. 2014;9(3):e93081. https://doi.org/10.1371/journal.pone.0093081.
25. Roehrborn CG. Benign prostatic hyperplasia: etiology, pathophysiology, epidemiology, and natural history. In: Wein WJ, editor. Campbell-Walsh urology. 11th ed. Philadelphia: Saunders; 2016. p. 2425–62.
26. Horlocker TT, Wedel DJ, Rowlingson JC, Enneking FK, Kopp SL, Benzon HT, Brown DL, Heit JA, Mulroy MF, Rosenquist RW, Tryba M, Yuan CS. Regional anesthesia in the patient receiving antithrombotic or thrombolytic therapy: American Society of Regional Anesthesia and Pain Medicine Evidence-Based guidelines (Third Edition). Reg Anesth Pain Med. 2010;35(1):64–101.
27. Wasson JH, Bubolz TA, Lu-Yao GL, Walker-Corkery E, Hammond CS, Barry MJ. Transurethral resection of the prostate among medicare beneficiaries: 1984 to 1997. J Urol. 2000;164(4):1212–5.
28. Silbert BS, Evered LA, Scott DA. Incidence of postoperative cognitive dysfunction after general or spinal anaesthesia for extracorporeal shock wave lithotripsy. Br J Anaesth. 2014;113(5):784–91.
29. Tyritzis SI, Stravodimos KG, Vasileiou I, Fotopoulou G, Koritsiadis G, Migdalis V, Michalakis A, Constantinides CA. Spinal versus general anaesthesia in postoperative pain management during transurethral procedures. ISRN Urol. 2011;2011:895874. https://doi.org/10.5402/2011/895874.
30. Hahn RG. Fluid absorption in endoscopic surgery. Br J Anaesth. 2006;96:8–20.
31. Gravenstein D. Transurethral resection of the prostate (TURP) syndrome: a review of the pathophysiology and management. Anesth Analg. 1997;84(2):438–46.
32. Hawary A, Mukhtar K, Sinclair A, Pearce I. Transurethral resection of the prostate syndrome: almost gone but not forgotten. J Endourol. 2009;23(12):2013–20. https://doi.org/10.1089/end.2009.0129.
33. Aidan M. O'Donnell, , Irwin T.H. Foo. Anaesthesia for transurethral resection of the prostate. Contin Educ Anaesth Crit Care Pain (2009) 9(3):92–96. doi:https://doi.org/10.1093/bjaceaccp/mkp012
34. A K, Kaya S, Turhanoglu S, Ozyilmaz MA. Low-dose bupivacaine-fentanyl spinal anaesthesia for transurethral prostatectomy. Anaesthesia. 2003;58(6):526–30.
35. American Society of Anesthesiologists. Practice advisory for the perioperative management of patients with cardiac implantable electronic devices: pacemakers and implantable cardioverter-defibrillators: an updated report by the American Society of Anesthesiologists Task Force on Perioperative Management of Patients with Cardiac Implantable Electronic Devices. Anesthesiology. 2011;114:247–61.
36. The American Cancer Society. https://www.cancer.org/cancer/prostate-cancer/about/key-statistics.html. Accessed 10 Mar 2017.
37. Thiel DD, Winfield HN. Robotics in urology: past, present, and future. J Endourol. 2008;22(4):825–30.
38. Sooriakumaran P, Srivastava A, Shariat SF, Stricker PD, Ahlering T, Eden CG, Wiklund PN, Sanchez-Salas R, Mottrie A, Lee D, Neal DE, Ghavamian R, Nyirady P, Nilsson A, Carlsson S, Xylinas E, Loidl W, Seitz C, Schramek P, Roehrborn C, Cathelineau X, Skarecky D, Shaw G, Warren A, Delprado WJ, Haynes AM, Steyerberg E, Roobol MJ, Tewari AK. A multinational, multi-institutional study comparing positive surgical margin rates among 22393 open, laparoscopic, and robot-assisted radical prostatectomy patients. Eur Urol. 2014;66(3):450.
39. Yaxley JW, Coughlin GD, Chambers SK. Robot-assisted laparoscopic prostatectomy versus open radical retropubic prostatectomy: early outcomes from a randomized controlled phase 3 study. Lancet. 2016;
40. Danic MJ, Chow M, Alexander G, Bhandari A, Menon M, Brown M. Anesthesia considerations for robotic-assisted laparoscopic prostatectomy: a review of 1,500 cases. J Robot Surg. 2007;1(2):119–23. https://doi.org/10.1007/s11701-007-0024-z.
41. OpenAnesthesia supported by International Anesthesia Research Society. https://www.openanesthesia.org/patient_positioning_and_injury_anesthesia_text/
42. Joris JL, Chiche JD, Canivet JL, Jacquet NJ, Legros JJ, Lamy ML. Hemodynamic changes induced by laparoscopy and their endocrine correlates: effects of clonidine. J Am Coll Cardiol. 1998;32(5):1389–96.
43. Wahba RW, Béïque F, Kleiman SJ. Cardiopulmonary function and laparoscopic cholecystectomy. Can J Anaesth. 1995;42(1):51–6.
44. Güldner A, Kiss T, Serpa Neto A, Hemmes SN, Canet J, Spieth PM, Rocco PR, Schultz MJ, Pelosi P, Gama de Abreu M. Intraoperative protective mechanical ventilation for prevention of postoperative pulmonary complications: a comprehensive review of the role of tidal volume, positive end-expiratory pressure, and lung recruitment maneuvers. Anesthesiology. 2015;123(3):692.

45. The American Cancer Society. https://www.cancer.org/cancer/kidney-cancer/about/key-statistics.html. Accessed 25 Feb 2017.
46. Zini L, Perrotte P, Capitanio U, Jeldres C, Shariat SF, Antebi E, Saad F, Patard JJ, Montorsi F, Karakiewicz PI. Radical versus partial nephrectomy: effect on overall and noncancer mortality. Cancer. 2009;115(7):1465–71. https://doi.org/10.1002/cncr.24035.
47. Go AS, Chertow GM, Fan D, CE MC, Hsu CY. Chronic kidney disease and the risks of death, cardiovascular events, and hospitalization. N Engl J Med. 2004;351(13):1296–305.
48. Yokoyama M, Ueda W, Hirakawa M. Haemodynamic effects of the lateral decubitus position and the kidney rest lateral decubitus position during anaesthesia. Br J Anaesth. 2000;84(6):753–7.
49. Conacher D, Soomro NA, Rix D. Anaesthesia for laparoscopic urological surgery. Br J Anaesth. 2004;93(6):859–64.
50. Navarro LH, Bloomstone JA, Auler JO Jr, Cannesson M, Rocca GD, Gan TJ, Kinsky M, Magder S, Miller TE, Mythen M, Perel A, Reuter DA, Pinsky MR, Kramer GC. Perioperative fluid therapy: a statement from the group. Perioper Med. 2015;4:3. https://doi.org/10.1186/s13741-015-0014-z.
51. American Cancer Society. https://www.cancer.org/cancer/bladder-cancer/about/key-statistics.html. Accessed 10 Mar 2017.
52. Shah AD, Abaza R. Clinical pathway for 3-day stay after robot-assisted cystectomy. J Endourol. 2011;25(8):1253–8. https://doi.org/10.1089/end.2011.0035.
53. Egbert LD, Battit GE, Welch CE, Bartlett MK. Reduction of postoperative pain by encouragement and instruction of patients. A study of doctor-patient rapport. N Engl J Med. 1964;270:825–7.
54. Melnyk M, Casey R, Black P, Koupparis A. Enhanced recovery after surgery (ERAS) protocols: time to change practice? Can Urol Assoc J. 2011;5(5):342–8. https://doi.org/10.5489/cuaj.11002.
55. Chang SS, Cookson MS, Baumgartner RG, Wells N, Smith JA Jr. Analysis of early complications after radical cystectomy: results of a collaborative care pathway. J Urol. 2002;167(5):2012–6.
56. Frazier HA, Robertson JE, Paulson DF. Complications of radical cystectomy and urinary diversion: a retrospective review of 675 cases in 2 decades. J Urol. 1992;148(5):1401–5.
57. Daneshmand S, Ahmadi H, Schuckman AK, Mitra AP, Cai J, Miranda G, Djaladat H. Enhanced recovery protocol after radical cystectomy for bladder cancer. J Urol. 2014;192(1):50–5. https://doi.org/10.1016/j.juro.2014.01.097.
58. Chou R, Gordon DB, de Leon-Casasola OA, Rosenberg JM, Bickler S, Brennan T, Carter T, Cassidy CL, Chittenden EH, Degenhardt E, Griffith S, Manworren R, McCarberg B, Montgomery R, Murphy J, Perkal MF, Suresh S, Sluka K, Strassels S, Thirlby R, Viscusi E, Walco GA, Warner L, Weisman SJ, Wu CL. Management of postoperative pain: a clinical practice guideline from the American Pain Society, the American Society of Regional Anesthesia and Pain Medicine, and the American Society of Anesthesiologists' Committee on Regional Anesthesia, Executive Committee, and Administrative Council. J Pain. 2016;17(2):131–57. https://doi.org/10.1016/j.jpain.2015.12.008.
59. Tufanogullari B, White PF, Peixoto MP, Kianpour D, Lacour T, Griffin J, Skrivanek G, Macaluso A, Shah M, Provost DA. Dexmedetomidine infusion during laparoscopic bariatric surgery: the effect on recovery outcome variables. Anesth Analg. 2008;106(6):1741–8.
60. Weibel S, Jokinen J, Pace NL, Schnabel A, Hollmann MW, Hahnenkamp K, Eberhart LH, Poepping DM, Afshari A, Kranke P. Efficacy and safety of intravenous lidocaine for postoperative analgesia and recovery after surgery: a systematic review with trial sequential analysis. Br J Anaesth. 2016;116(6):770–83. https://doi.org/10.1093/bja/aew101.
61. Qu G, Cui XL, Liu HJ, Ji ZG, Huang YG. Ultrasound-guided transversus abdominis plane block improves postoperative analgesia and early recovery in patients undergoing retroperitoneoscopic urologic surgeries: a randomized controlled double-blinded trial. Chin Med Sci J. 2016;31(3):137–141.59.
62. Baack Kukreja JE, Messing EM, Shah JB. Are we doing "better"? The discrepancy between perception and practice of enhanced recovery after cystectomy principles among urologic oncologists. Urol Oncol. 2016;34(3):120.e17–21. https://doi.org/10.1016/j.urolonc.2015.10.002.
63. Morales R Jr, Mentz H, Newall G, Patronella C, Masters O. Use of abdominal field block injections with liposomal bupivicaine to control postoperative pain after abdominoplasty. Aesthet Surg J. 2013;33(8):1148–53. https://doi.org/10.1177/1090820X13510720.

# Organ Harvesting and the Role of Anesthesiologist

Michael R. Schwartz and Erin W. Pukenas

## Overview

Organ procurement organizations (OPOs) work with hospitals that participate in organ retrieval to facilitate donor organs for allocation and transplant. In 2016, over 33,500 organs were transplanted, an increase of 20% over a 5 year period. However, as of 2017 there were still over 118,000 patients waiting for life-saving transplants.

Increases in knowledge and awareness in organ donation, as well as advances in medicine and technology have not been able to narrow the gap between the supply of organs available and those needed for transplant. According to the Organ Procurement and Transplantation Network [1], although the number of patients needing organ transplants has increased over the 10 year period from 2005–2015, the amount of transplants performed and donors recovered has not met with the demand. In an attempt to keep up with increasing demands for organ transplants, the Joint Commission, along with procurement organizations, have attempted to develop enhanced policies associated with donation after cardiac death (DCD).

M. R. Schwartz, M.D. (✉) · E. W. Pukenas, M.D., F.A.A.P., C.P.P.S.
Department of Anesthesiology, Cooper Medical School of Rowan University/Cooper University Health Care, Camden, NJ, USA
e-mail: schwartz-michael@cooperhealth.edu; pukenas-erin@CooperHealth.edu

The ability to procure and allocate organs is dependent on many factors. Specific medical conditions and blood typing are necessary in all transplants, but each organ-type has specific criteria in determining allocation as seen in Table 77.1.

Factors that put potential organs at risk during organ procurement include hypotension, hypovolemia, hypothermia, diabetes insipidus, blood glucose management and cardiac dysfunction. Therefore it is essential that brain dead donors are still managed appropriately to improve organ conditions for transplant. Anesthesia, as well as critical care providers, should be aware of proper

Table 77.1 Specific factors pertaining to organ-type allocation [1]

| Organ-type | Common maximum preservation times (h) | Factors in organ allocation |
|---|---|---|
| Kidney | 24–36 | Wait time, immune system compatibility, pediatric status, prior living donor, distance from donor hospital, survival benefit |
| Heart | 4–6 | Medical urgency, distance from donor hospital |
| Lung | 4–6 | Distance from donor hospital, waiting time, medical urgency, survival benefit |
| Liver | 8–12 | Medical urgency, distance from donor hospital |
| Pancreas | 12–18 | |

organ procurement management in order to provide optimal transplant management and minimize potential adverse outcomes. In this chapter we will not be discussing organ donation from living donors, but instead focus on donation after brain death and cardiac death.

## Donation After Brain-Death (DBD)

In the United States, brain death criteria may vary from state to state but must include complete and irreversible cessation of both cerebral and brainstem functions. Most guidelines for determining brain death are not evidence-based, and must rely on clinical judgment. Brain death is ultimately a clinical diagnosis, however several test modalities are used to confirm and support the clinical examination. Determination of brain death typically consists of four steps which include clinical evaluation, neurologic exam, ancillary tests and documentation.

Prior to performing a neurological assessment, physicians must determine an irreversible and proximate cause of coma. Other factors that may cause short-term coma must be ruled out, such as pharmaceutical drugs and acute medical pathology. Patients should be normothermic or near normothermic (>36 °C), normocapnic ($PaCO_2$ 35–45 mmHg), euvolemic and normotensive (systolic blood pressure $\geq$ 100 mmHg).

After these prerequisites are achieved, a neurologic exam should be performed to confirm coma, absence of brainstem reflexes, and apnea [2]. Any physician may perform the exam, however usually a neurologist, neurosurgeon or critical care intensivist who specializes and is more familiar with the exam is needed. Some states require two physicians to perform the exam. A patient may be considered brain dead if they are unresponsive to sensory stimuli, and have no brainstem reflexes including ventilatory drive with the apnea test.

After a neurological exam is conducted, imaging studies should be performed to confirm the findings. An electroencephalogram will show a flat tracing. Transcranial doppler will show a lack of circulation to the brain. Finally, traditional cerebral angiography or isotope cerebral scintigraphy may also be used to show a lack of blood-flow throughout the brain.

Once all exams have been performed and brain death has been determined, the time of brain death should be documented. Depending on hospital and state policies, a specific checklist should also be completed and attached to the medical record. Organ procurement agencies must be contacted, but only after brain death has been determined. It is imperative that no physician associated with the organ procurement be a part of brain death determination.

## Donation After Cardiac Death (DCD)

DCD donors and criteria for death are distinct from brain-dead donors. DCD donors do not meet the criteria for brain death as described above. Although they still have electrical activity in the brain, there is usually severe, irreversible, widespread brain dysfunction. Once life-sustaining care is ended they will be declared dead from a cardiopulmonary standpoint [3].

The Joint Commission, in an attempt to increase the number of organs available for allocation, mandated hospitals in 2007 to develop DCD policies. Campbell and Sutherland in 1999 performed a review that showed 10 possible patients who may have been eligible for organ procurement which could have yielded up to 20 kidneys for allocation, an increase in 48% for that institution [4]. Since the mandate, there has been an increase in DCD organs, accounting for 10.6% of all organ transplants in the United States [5]. Chart reviews from the Washington Hospital Center from 1992 to 1994 found that up to 3–6 times more patients were eligible as non-heart-beating cadaver donors (NHBCDs) than compared to brain-dead donors [6]. With the limited number of DBDs in participating hospitals, the addition of NHBCDs may greatly increase the number of potential organs available for donation.

Every hospital that participates in organ procurement should have specific protocols for DCD. Although management of NHBCDs may be similar, anesthesiologists should be familiar with individual institutional protocols to adhere to appropriate management. At times, the anesthesiologist may not be apart of the organ procurement process in NHBCDs as they are terminally extubated prior to arriving to the OR and are then brought in once cardiorespiratory function ceases. However, if lungs are part of the procurement process, then anesthesiologists may be asked to intubate the trachea and provide recruitment maneuvers prior to removal. If this is the case, then lung protective ventilation should be reinstated to prevent acute lung injury, [7] but only after cerebral circulation has been isolated to prevent return of cerebral oxygenation [8, 9].

## Ethics of Organ Procurement

The issue of organ donation can be a very controversial subject. It often requires the ability of physicians to put aside their beliefs of maleficence or "do no harm" and continuing life-saving treatment in order to determine when a subject may be an eligible organ donor. As in the case with NHBCDs, the anesthesiologist may be tasked with disconnecting the patient from life-saving support, which some physicians may find difficult. Again it is important to know individual institutional policies on physician roles during organ procurement.

The ethical concerns relating to brain-death was partially resolved in 1981 when a presidential committee stated the Uniform Determination of Death Act, which states that "An individual who has sustained either (1) irreversible cessation of circulatory and respiratory functions, or (2) irreversible cessation of all functions of the entire brain, including the brainstem, is dead" [10, 11]. This allowed for a more standardized definition that is used the world. However, these are still guidelines and not always universally accepted [12].

Another issue stems from concerns about informing families and the process of beginning organ procurement. It is vital that the concept of organ donation be established as soon as possible, however it should not affect life-sustaining treatments if it goes against the wishes of the patient or family. Family members should be informed about the process and allowed to make a decision based off of pertinent information. Family members often time have a hard time making this delicate decision and often don't fully understand the implication of brain-death and the decision to withdraw care. Finally, it is important that the organ procurement team is not informed, until the decision to proceed with organ donation is decided as not to compromise that decision.

## Cardiovascular System

The main goal of anesthesiologists during organ procurement is to maintain hemodynamic stability to ensure adequate organ perfusion. The challenge is that these patients undergo cardiac dysfunction and hemodynamic instability after brain death. This is usually due to a "catecholamine storm" which occurs shortly after brain death [13]. This "storm" leads to an increase in cardiac output (CO) and sympathetic tone. This sudden increase in sympathetic tone may result in increased heart rate and vasoconstriction. This leads to increase in systemic vascular resistance, which in turn can lead to myocardial injury. After an initial increase in CO, myocardial injury may result in arrhythmias, ventricular dysfunction and decreased CO. This ultimately may lead to further hemodynamic instability and reduce the viability of the organs being procured [14]. One goal to maintain cardiac function, especially if cardiac transplant is desired, is to maintain coronary perfusion pressures [15]. While the autonomic storm is often transient, initial management usually consists of nitroprusside and esmolol to manage hypertension and tachycardia, respectively [16, 17].

Another contributor of hemodynamic instability during organ procurement is hypovolemia, which may be due to fluid shifts, evaporative losses, bleeding and polyuria secondary to diabetes insipidus. Fluid replacement is essential to maintaining perfusion to viable organs, however goals of fluid management is often predicated on what organs are being procured. Whereas kidney transplants may require greater fluid resuscitation, overzealous fluid administration in spleen and lung transplants may be harmful for viability [8]. Initial steps at fluid resuscitation is usually done with infusions of crystalloids. Colloids may have some benefit in intravascular expansion. Transfusion of blood products may be indicated if hypovolemia is thought to be from bleeding. A study by Rosengard et al. showed that colloids may be prefered in lung procurement to prevent fluid overload [18]. The use of hydroxyethyl starch (HES) products has conflicting results. A study by Cittanova et al. showed HES products may impair graft function and should be avoided [19], whereas another study by Blasco et al. using lower molecular weight HES products showed less effect on graft function [20].

After the initial autonomic storm has resolved, the next phase of instability is usually due to loss of sympathetic tone [14]. Once fluid resuscitation is considered adequate, vasopressor or inotropic agents may be necessary to maintain perfusion pressures. Vasopressin appears to be the agent of choice as it works to both restore vascular tone and organ perfusion [16, 21], while also countering the effects of diabetes insipidus from the decrease in ADH that occurs after brain death. Other agents such as phenylephrine, epinephrine, norepinephrine and dopamine have been studied for controlling hemodynamics with no clear evidence of superiority [22–24]. While low-dose dopamine has been shown to improve renal perfusion, long-term graft benefits have not been proven [25]. Regardless of agent chosen, the goal for management is to maintain SBP > 100 mmHg, MAP > 70 mmHg, and HR 60–120 beats per minute [21, 22, 25–29].

## Pulmonary System

The pulmonary system is very susceptible to injury after brain death. Further complicating factors include trauma, infection, aspiration, neurogenic pulmonary edema, pulmonary edema from other causes, acute lung injury/acute respiratory distress syndrome (ALI/ARDS) as well as underlying comorbid conditions. These insults, along with acceptability criteria, limit the availability of transplantable lungs each year.

Patients who have neurologic injury that results in brain death require mechanical ventilation to maintain ventilation and oxygenation to support other organ systems. This increases the risk for ventilator associated pneumonia (VAP) and ventilator-induced lung injury (VILI) along with any other injuries they may have suffered not pertaining to the pulmonary system.

Strategies to increase the viability of lungs for transplant should begin prior to the OR. In the case of intensive care unit (ICU) patients who may be eligible for any type of transplant, studies have shown the benefit of lung-protective ventilation in improving lung transplants. This strategy should be continued into the OR and throughout the period of organ procurement.

Lung-protective ventilation strategies for organ procurement are very similar to the lung-protective strategies seen for ARDS. The main goals are to avoid VILI and pulmonary derecruitment. To avoid these, it is recommended that low tidal volumes (4–8 mL/kg) based on predicted body weight and modest levels of PEEP (8–10 cmH$_2$O) with periodic recruitment maneuvers be used. This, along with limiting high FiO$_2$ and circuit disconnects, can help reduce VILI and improve procurement rates [7, 30].

A European study [7] demonstrated the benefit of lung protective strategy in DBD. Along with low tidal volumes and PEEP administration, CPAP was provided during apnea tests followed by recruitment maneuvers after any circuit disconnections. FiO$_2$ and respiratory rates were adjusted for both groups to maintain PaO$_2$ greater than 90 mmHg and PaCO$_2$ between 40 and 45 mmHg. Ninety-five percent of patients were eligible for lung donation with a lung protective strategy compared to only 54% using conventional ventilation. Also, recipients of these lung transplants had a 6% better survival after 6 months. However, lung protective strategies were not as important in preventing acute kidney injury [31] and their benefit is still not completely clear for improving viability for procuring other organs.

Due to risk of edema and release of inflammatory cytokines with excess fluid administration, a minimal fluid balance should be maintained for lung procurement [28]. This along with lung protective ventilation have been shown to reduce the release of interleukin-6 and tumor necrosis factor when compared to conventional ventilation [7]. Maintaining central venous pressures less than 10 mmHg along with standardized hormone replacement (discussed later in this chapter) have been shown to increase availability of lungs for transplant [24]. Anesthesiologists must balance minimizing fluid administration to improve lung procurement while also maintaining perfusion to other organs.

## Neuromuscular System

As mentioned earlier, despite the presence of brain death, somatic movements mediated by spinal reflexes may occur [26]. This may cause patient movement due to incision or surgical manipulation during organ procurement. Minimal alveolar concentration in one animal study was unaffected by high cervical cord section and suggests that anesthetics prevent motor response via the spinal cord [32]. Anesthesiologists should provide muscle paralysis either through use of volatile anesthetics or specific muscle relaxants to optimize surgical conditions.

The use of volatile anesthetics also blunt the autonomic storm caused by the release of catecholamines that occurs during brainstem ischemia [33]. This can help reduce reperfusion-ischemia injuries in organs [13, 34–39]. Also, despite the lack of higher brain function, volatile anesthetics have been shown to independently act on the spinal cord and their administration may act directly to inhibit spinal reflexes during surgery [40].

## Hematologic System

A major goal of the anesthesiologist is to maintain perfusion and oxygenation to increase viable organs for procurement. Critically ill patients who may be eligible for organ donation often have increased metabolic and oxygen demands, but do not have the ability to increase supply [41]. Packed red blood cells (PRBC) may be used to improve oxygenation during organ procurement. While there is no universal transfusion threshold, most studies indicate maintaining hemoglobin levels above 7 g × dL$^{-1}$ with a target of 9–10 g × dL$^{-1}$ [42, 43]. It is also recommended to target a mixed venous oxygenation saturation of greater than 60% which can be achieved with transfusion of PRBC [22].

Brain death is often complicated by coagulopathy. Degree of coagulopathy is not always indicated, but reports have showed incidences varying widely from less than 10% to over 80% [44]. Brain injury results in release of cytokines which can adversely affect the coagulation pathway and lead to worse outcomes [45, 46]. If coagulopathy is not controlled it may lead to disseminated intravascular coagulation (DIC) and decrease in organ viability [45]. It is recommended that coagulopathy is treated if ongoing bleeding occurs. If clinical bleeding is observed, fresh frozen plasma, platelets, cryoprecipitate or specific clotting factors may be used, but specific lab value goals have not been determined. Antifibrinolytics can be used as well, but studies are conflicting [47–49]. Case reports have shown the use of thromboelastography (TEG) to manage resuscitation efforts in both DBD and DCD patients which allowed for successful procurement of several organs [50]. Further studies may be indicated to determine the use or benefit of TEG for organ procurement.

## Endocrine System

After brain death the majority of potential donors will experience a disruption in their hypothalamic-pituitary axis (HPA). HPA dysfunction can lead to decreases in serum concentrations of either anterior or posterior pituitary hormones [51]. However, usually anterior pituitary function remains after brain death [52]. The major concerns associated with these changes include diabetes insipidus (DI) caused by pituitary infarction, and hyperosmolarity due to hyperglycemia and hypernatremia. Anesthesiologists along with transplant teams should be aware of possible changes in cortisol, T3 and thyroid levels. Several trials have shown increases in organ donation rates and may improve graft and recipient patient survival when corticosteroids, insulin, vasopressin and thyroid hormone are incorporated into organ procurement management [53]. There are many different protocols available for hormone replacement and may vary between institutions.

Corticosteroid administration during organ procurement has been shown to improve donor hemodynamics, oxygenation, organ procurement rates, graft survival, and recipient survival [54]. Protocols for corticosteroid regimens vary and may include cortisol, hydrocortisone or methylprednisolone. One review by Dhar et al. showed that low-dose corticosteroid treatment was as effective as high-dose treatment and showed no difference in cardiopulmonary function, a similar organ transplantation rate, a decreased insulin requirement, and improved glycemic control [55].

Dysfunction in hormone regulation during DBD often leads to hyperglycemia. This may be due to insulin resistance despite the maintenance of pancreatic function after brain death [56]. This may be worsened by epinephrine release, which was mentioned earlier as part of the "catecholamine storm", as well as by corticosteroid administration and infusion of dextrose-containing intravenous solutions. Numerous studies have investigated the benefit of glucose management during organ procurement, however no definitive level for glucose control has been established.

Serum glucose levels greater than 180 mg $\times$ dL$^{-1}$ may lead to protein glycosylation and tissue damage [57]. Persistent levels of hyperglycemia greater than 200 mg $\times$ dL$^{-1}$ may lead to lower rates of viable organs for transplant and decreased renal graft function specifically for kidney transplant [58]. This may be due to increased osmotic diuresis and worsening oxygen supply to demand ratio in the renal medulla which may lead to infarction and damage to kidneys. This has lead to some experts arguing that glucose management should be titrated based on metabolic activity of the donor [57].

Studies on pancreas transplants have shown improved outcomes when maintaining serum glucose levels <200 mg $\times$ dL$^{-1}$ [58]. A study by Blasi-Ibanez et al. on kidney transplants showed that the strongest predictor of serum creatinine and calculated glomerular filtration rate was the average serum glucose of the donor [59]. Also, greater variability in glucose levels was strongly associated with worse graft function. Most experts agree that the serum glucose level should be maintained between 120 and 180 mg $\times$ dL$^{-1}$ [22, 28, 60, 61]. However, critical outcomes of poor glucose management such as stroke and mortality may not be relevant when looking at organ procurement. In order to maintain these levels, it is recommended that insulin infusions be used and titrated throughout procurement.

After brain death, posterior pituitary infarction and dysregulation of HPA may lead to central diabetes insipidus. Central DI is caused by a decrease or complete shutdown in vasopressin, also known as antidiuretic hormone (ADH), production due to a direct insult to the pituitary gland. It differs from nephrogenic DI which is due to normal vasopressin production but impaired regulation at the level of the kidneys. Central DI leads to large amounts of dilute urine and hyperosmolarity due to the lack of ADH. To counteract the lack of ADH, arginine vasopressin (AVP) can be used to decrease urine output and prevent the increase in serum osmolarity. AVP has also been shown to improve systemic blood pressure, cardiac output and serum osmolarity which can lead to an increase in organ recovery rate and graft survival [61].

One cause of hyperosmolarity in DBD is due to hypernatremia. Hypernatremia is defined as a serum concentration of sodium greater than 145 mEq/L and is due a deficit in total body water relative to total body sodium. The hypernatremia in DBD is a hypovolemic hypernatremia caused by the excess quantities of dilute urine lost from decreased ADH. Persistent hypernatremia, especially greater than 155 mEq/L, was shown to increase rate of early graft loss, whereas graft loss was decreased with maintenance of normal osmolarity levels [62]. Initial steps in management of hypernatremia in DBD involve fluid resuscitation and can be achieved by using hypotonic fluids or free water. Hypotonic solutions, such as 0.45% NaCl, may be used as maintenance fluid. In living patients the correction of sodium is usually limited to 0.5–1.0 mEq $\times$ L$^{-1}$ $\times$ h.$^{-1}$ to prevent cerebral edema, however in DBD it is unclear if this correction rate is needed due to the underlying deficit in brain function. Management of hypernatremia can also be guided by the donor's estimated water deficit calculated as follows: Water deficit (L) = 0.6 $\times$ [weight in kg] $\times$ [(current Na$^+$/140) − 1].

Finally, brain-death has an effect on thyroid hormone, and may require thyroid hormone replacement. Thyroid hormone management may improve cardiac function [54] as well as minimize the need for vasopressor support [28]. Triiodothyronine/levothyroxine (T3/T4) replacement is often used for hormone replacement in DBD. Usually an infusion is run during procurement to assist in hemodynamic support [54]. However, some studies indicate thyroid hormone replacement may not improve hemodynamics or decrease myocardial dysfunction [63]. Despite conflicting evidence, multiple hormone replacement regimens, which include methylprednisolone, vasopressin and T3/T4, are often used in DBD and may increase the number of viable transplanted organs and improve early graft function [29, 53, 64].

## Equipment and Monitoring

There are no definitive guidelines on what types of equipment or monitors are needed for organ procurement. However, based on the above clinical management goals, it is recommended that certain modalities are used to guide anesthesiologists in maintaining overall organ viability.

Adequate peripheral and central intravenous (IV) access is imperative during organ procurement. It is recommended that at least two large bore IVs are placed to allow for blood and fluid administration as large fluid shifts and losses may occur during the procedure. Depending on which organs are being recovered, it may be beneficial to have the IVs placed in an upper extremity to prevent issues during surgical clamping. If large peripheral IVs are obtained then smaller central catheters may be appropriate if only being used for drug administration or central venous pressure (CVP) monitoring.

As mentioned earlier, maintaining adequate fluid status during the procedure is very important, and there are numerous monitoring options available. Urinary catheters can be used to track urine output which may be related to kidney perfusion and cardiac output. Urine production may also be affected by diabetes insipidus (DI). If DI is suspected, urinalysis may be collected along with blood samples to monitor electrolytes. It is important to balance the maintenance of intravascular volume with the inherent loss due to DI in order to have adequate volume replacement.

Other ways to track volume status include CVP via central venous access. However, CVP may not be accurate as a continual intravascular monitor during general anesthesia [65]. Often times patients arriving from the ICU may already have pulmonary artery catheters (PACs) placed which were being used for hemodynamic monitoring. These PACs may be continued to be used to guide fluid replacement, determine cardiac output or evaluate mixed venous saturation. A transesophageal echo (TEE) may also be placed intraoperatively to determine heart filling and fluid status as well as cardiac output. For cardiac transplants, the TEE may be beneficial to determine viability of the donor heart prior to procurement. Finally, pulse pressure variation (PPV) which can be calculated from an arterial line waveform, may be used as a surrogate for volume status [66].

Arterial lines are one of the more useful tools for guiding the anesthesiologists during organ procurement. Arterial lines allow for continual blood pressure readings which can allow careful titration of inotropic agents. Frequent laboratory markers can be evaluated which can help guide therapies. Hemoglobin and hematocrit can be sent to determine blood transfusion effectiveness. Frequent blood glucose evaluations can be performed to control glucose homeostasis. Arterial blood gases can help determine acid-base status, as well as ventilation and oxygenation. Trending lactate can help determine perfusion [67]. Electrolytes such as sodium, potassium and calcium which can be effected by fluid administration, DI and blood transfusion can also be monitored. Coagulation status can also be monitored if clinically significant bleeding is present. Blood may also be sent for TEGs, although its use in organ procurement has yet to be fully determined.

## Conclusions

The demand for organ transplantation continues to outpace supply. DCD and NBHCDs have increased the total number of available organs for transplant, and anesthesia care teams should familiarize themselves with institutional policies for this and DBD. Anesthesia providers play an integral role as members of the procurement team through physiologic monitoring and guiding therapies. With precise management of the donor patient, the anesthesia team may contribute to improving outcomes for transplant recipients. While management goals may vary depending on organ type, hemodynamic stability, coagulopathy, oxygenation and ventilation strategies are important parameters to consider for successful organ procurement.

## References

1. http://optn.transplant.hrsa.gov.
2. Wijdicks EFM, Varelas PN, Gronseth GS, et al. Evidence-based guideline update: determining brain death in adults: report of the Quality Standards Subcommittee of the American Academy of Neurology. Neurology. 2010;74:1911–8.
3. Bernat JL, D'lessandro AM, Port FK, et al. Report of a national conference on donation after cardiac death. Am J Transplant. 2006;6:281–91.
4. Campbell GM, Sutherland FR. Non-heart-beating organ donors as a source of kidneys for transplantation: a chart review. CMAJ. 1999;160:1573–6.
5. Klein AS, Messersmith EE, Ratner LE, et al. Organ donation and utilization in the United States, 1999–2008. Am J Transplant. 2010;10(Pt 2):973.
6. Kowalski AE, Light JA, Ritchie WO, Sasaki TM, Callender CO, Gage F. A new approach for increasing the organ supply. Clin Transpl. 1996;10:653–7.
7. Mascia L, Pasero D, Slutsky AS, et al. Effect of a lung protective strategy for organ donors on eligibility and availability of lungs for transplantation: a randomized controlled trial. JAMA. 2010;304:2620–7.
8. Pennefather SH, Bullock RE, Dark JH. The effect of fluid therapy on alveolar arterial oxygen gradient in brain-dead organ donors. Transplantation. 1993;56:1418–21.
9. Martin J, Lutter G, Ihling C, et al. Myocardial viability twenty-four hours after orthotopic heart transplantation from non-heart-beating donors. J Thorac Cardiovasc Surg. 2003;125:1217–28.
10. President's Commission for the Study of Ethical Problems in Medicine and Biomedical and Behavioral Research. Defining death: a report on the medical, legal, and ethical issues in the determination of death. Washington, DC: Government Printing Office; 1981.
11. Barclay WR. Guidelines for the determination of death. JAMA. 1981;246(19):2194. https://doi.org/10.1001/jama.1981.03320190052031.
12. Wijdicks EFM. Brain death worldwide: accepted fact but no global consensus in diagnostic criteria. Neurology. 2002;58:20–5.
13. Avlonitis VS, Wigfield CH, Kirby JA, Dark JH. The hemodynamic mechanisms of lung injury and systemic inflammatory response following brain death in the transplant donor. Am J Transplant. 2005;5(4 Pt 1):684–93.
14. Belzberg H, Shoemaker WC, Wo CC, et al. Hemodynamic and oxygen transport patterns after head trauma and brain death: implications for management of the organ donor. J Trauma. 2007;63:1032–42.
15. Szabo G. Physiologic changes after brain death. J Heart Lung Transplant. 2004;23(9 Suppl):S223–6.
16. Plurad DS, Bricker S, Neville A, Bongard F, Putnam B. Arginine vasopressin significantly increases the rate of successful organ procurement in potential donors. Am J Surg. 2012;204:856–60.
17. Audibert G, Charpentier C, Seguin-Devaux C, et al. Improvement of donor myocardial function after treatment of autonomic storm during brain death. Transplantation. 2006;82:1031–6.
18. Rosengard BR, Feng S, Alfrey EJ, et al. Report of the Crystal City meeting to maximize the use of organs recovered from the cadaver donor. Am J Transplant. 2002;2:701–11.
19. Cittanova ML, Leblanc I, Legendre C, Mouquet C, Riou B, Coriat P. Effect of hydroxyethylstarch in brain-dead kidney donors on renal function in kidney-transplant recipients. Lancet. 1996;348:1620–2.
20. Blasco V, Leone M, Antonini F, Geissler A, Albanese J, Martin C. Comparison of the novel hydroxyethylstarch 130/0.4 and hydroxyethylstarch 200/0.6 in brain-dead donor resuscitation on renal function after transplantation. Br J Anaesth. 2008;100:504–8.
21. Pennefather SH, Bullock RE, Mantle D, Dark JH. Use of low dose arginine vasopressin to support brain-dead organ donors. Transplantation. 1995;59:58–62.
22. Shemie SD, Ross H, Pagliarello J, et al. Organ donor management in Canada: recommendations of the

forum on medical management to optimize donor organ potential. CMAJ. 2006;174:S13–32.
23. Schnuelle P, Lorenz D, Mueller A, Trede M, Van Der Woude FJ. Donor catecholamine use reduces acute allograft rejection and improves graft survival after cadaveric renal transplantation. Kidney Int. 1999;56:738–46.
24. Abdelnour T, Rieke S. Relationship of hormonal resuscitation therapy and central venous pressure on increasing organs for transplant. J Heart Lung Transplant. 2009;28(5):480.
25. Gelb AW, Robertson KM. Anaesthetic management of the brain dead for organ donation. Can J Anaesth. 1990;37:806–12.
26. McKeown DW, Bonser RS, Kellum JA. Management of the heartbeating brain-dead organ donor. Br J Anaesth. 2012;108(Suppl 1):i96–107.
27. Dictus C, Vienenkoetter B, Esmaeilzadeh M, Unterberg A, Ahmadi R. Critical care management of potential organ donors: our current standard. Clin Transpl. 2009;23(Suppl 21):2–9.
28. Wood KE, Becker BN, McCartney JG, D'Alessandro AM, Coursin DB. Care of the potential organ donor. N Engl J Med. 2004;351:2730–9.
29. Rosendale JD, Kauffman HM, McBride MA, et al. Aggressive pharmacological donor management results in more transplanted organs. Transplantation. 2003;75:482–7.
30. Lucangelo U, Del Sorbo L, Boffini M, Ranieri VM. Protective ventilation for lung transplantation. Curr Opin Anaesthesiol. 2012;25(2):170–4.
31. Cortjens B, Royakkers AA, Determann RM, et al. Lung-protective mechanical ventilation does not protect against acute kidney injury in patients without lung injury at onset of mechanical ventilation. J Crit Care. 2011;27(3):261–7.
32. Rampil IJ. Anesthetic potency is not altered after hypothermic spinal cord transection in rats. Anesthesiology. 1994;80:606–10.
33. Yoo KY, Jeong CW, Kim SJ, et al. Sevoflurane concentrations required to block autonomic hyperreflexia during transurethral litholapaxy in patients with complete spinal cord injury. Anesthesiology. 2008;108(5):858–63.
34. De Hert SG, Turani F, Mathur S, Stowe DF. Cardioprotection with volatile anesthetics: mechanisms and clinical implications. Anesth Analg. 2005;100(6):1584–93.
35. Arbour R. Clinical management of the organ donor. AACN Clin Issues. 2005;16(4):551–80.
36. Avlonitis VS, Fisher AJ, Kirby JA, Dark JH. Pulmonary transplantation: the role of brain death in donor lung injury. Transplantation. 2003;75(12):1928–33.
37. Nijboer WN, Schuurs TA, van der Hoeven JA, et al. Effect of brain death on gene expression and tissue activation in human donor kidneys. Transplantation. 2004;78(7):978–86.
38. Kaminska D, Tyran B, Mazanowska O, et al. Cytokine gene expression in kidney allograft biopsies after donor brain death and ischemia-reperfusion injury using in situ reverse-transcription polymerase chain reaction analysis. Transplantation. 2007;84(9):1118–24.
39. Sánchez-Fructuoso AI, Prats D, Marques M, et al. Does donor brain death influence acute vascular rejection in the kidney transplant? Transplantation. 2004;78(1):142–6.
40. Antognini JF, Berg K. Cardiovascular responses to noxious stimuli during isoflurane anesthesia are minimally affected by anesthetic action in the brain. Anesth Analg. 1995;81(4):843–8.
41. Du Pont-Thibodeau G, Harrington K, Lacroix J. Anemia and red blood cell transfusion in critically ill cardiac patients. Ann Intensive Care. 2014;4:16.
42. Van Bakel AB. The cardiac transplant donor: identification, assessment, and management. Am J Med Sci. 1997;314(3):152–63.
43. Zaroff JG, Rosengard BR, Armstrong WF, Babcock WD, D'Alessandro A, Dec GW, Edwards NM, Higgins RS, Jeevanandum V, Kauffman M, Kirklin JK, Large SR, Marelli D, Peterson TS, Ring WS, Robbins RC, Russell SD, Taylor DO, Van Bakel A, Wallwork J, Young JB. Consensus conference report maximizing use of organs recovered from the cadaver donor: cardiac recommendations. Circulation. 2002;106:836–41.
44. Talving P, Benfield R, Hadjizacharia P, Inaba K, Chan LS, Demetriades D. Coagulopathy in severe traumatic brain injury: a prospective study. J Trauma. 2009;66:55–61; discussion 61–2
45. de Oliveira Manoel AL, Neto AC, Veigas PV, Rizoli S. Traumatic brain injury associated coagulopathy. Neurocrit Care. 2014;22(1):34–44. https://doi.org/10.1007/s12028-014-0026-4.
46. Hefty TR, Cotterell LW, Fraser SC, Goodnight SH, Hatch TR. Disseminated intravascular coagulation in cadaveric organ donors: incidence and effect on renal transplantation. Transplantation. 1993;55:442–3.
47. Mannucci PM, Levi M. Prevention and treatment of major blood loss. N Engl J Med. 2007;356:2301–11. https://doi.org/10.1056/NEJMra067742.
48. Brown JE, Olujohungbe A, Chang J, Ryder WD, Morganstern GR, Chopra R, Scarffe JH. All-trans retinoic acid (ATRA) and tranexamic acid as a potentially fatal combination in acute promyelocytic leukaemia. Br J Haematol. 2000;110:1010–2. https://doi.org/10.1046/j.1365-2141.2000.02270-8.x.
49. de la Serna J, Montesinos P, Vellenga E, Rayon C, Parody R, Leon A, Esteve J, Bergua JM, Milone G, Deben G, Rivas C, Gonzalez M, Tormo M, az-Mediavilla J, Gonzalez JD, Negri S, Amutio E, Brunet S, Lowenberg B, Sanz MA. Causes and prognostic factors of remission induction failure in patients with acute promyelocytic leukemia treated with all-trans retinoic acid and idarubicin. Blood. 2008;111:3395–402. https://doi.org/10.1182/blood-2007-07-100669.
50. Walsh M, Thomas SG, Howard JC, Evans E, Guyer K, Medvecz A, et al. Blood component therapy in trauma guided with the utilization of the perfusionist and thromboelastography. J Extra Corpor Technol. 2011;43:162–7.

51. Novitzky D, Cooper DK, Reichart B. Hemodynamic and metabolic responses to hormonal therapy in brain-dead potential organ donors. Transplantation. 1987;43:852–4.
52. Howlett TA, Keogh AM, Perry L, Touzel R, Rees LH. Anterior and posterior pituitary function in brain-stem-dead donors. Transplantation. 1989;47:828–34.
53. Rosendale JD, Chabalewski FL, McBride MA, et al. Increased transplanted organs from the use of a standardized donor management protocol. Am J Transplant. 2002;2:761–8.
54. Novitzky D, Cooper DK, Rosendale JD, Kauffman HM. Hormonal therapy of the brain-dead organ donor: experimental and clinical studies. Transplantation. 2006;82(11):1396–401.
55. Dhar R, Cotton C, Coleman J, et al. Comparison of high- and low-dose corticosteroid regimens for organ donor management. J Crit Care. 2013;28:111.e1–7.
56. Masson F, Thicoipe M, Gin H, De Mascarel A, Angibeau RM, Favarel-Garrigues JF, et al. The endocrine pancreas in brain-dead donors. Transplantation. 1993;56(2):363–7.
57. Nunnally ME, O'Connor MF. Glycemic control for organs: a new approach to a controversial topic. J Cardiothorac Vasc Anesth. 2005;19:689–90.
58. University of Pittsburgh. MOnIToR Study. https://crisma.upmc.com/MonitorStudy/index.asp. Accessed Jan 2015.
59. Blasi-Ibanez A, Hirose R, Feiner J, Freise C, Stock P, Roberts JP, Niemann CU. Predictors associated with terminal renal function in deceased organ donors in the intensive care unit. Anesthesiology. 2009;110:333–41.
60. Sally MB, Ewing T, Crutchfield M, et al. Determining optimal threshold for glucose control in organ donors after neurologic determination of death: a United Network for Organ Sharing Region 5 Donor Management Goals Workgroup prospective analysis. J Trauma Acute Care Surg. 2014;76:62–8; discussion 68–9
61. Malinoski DJ, Patel MS, Daly MC, Oley-Graybill C, Salim A, UNOS Region 5 DMG Workgroup. The impact of meeting donor management goals on the number of organs transplanted per donor: results from the United Network for Organ Sharing Region 5 prospective donor management goals study. Crit Care Med. 2012;40:2773–80.
62. Totsuka E, Dodson F, Urakami A, et al. Influence of high donor serum sodium levels on early postoperative graft function in human liver transplantation: effect of correction of donor hypernatremia. Liver Transpl Surg. 1999;5:421–8.
63. Rech TH, Moraes RB, Crispim D, Czepielewski MA, Leitao CB. Management of the brain-dead organ donor: a systematic review and meta-analysis. Transplantation. 2013;95:966–74.
64. Rosendale JD, Kauffman HM, McBride MA, et al. Hormonal resuscitation yields more transplanted hearts, with improved early function. Transplantation. 2003;75:1336–41.
65. Marik PE, Baram M, Vahid B. Does central venous pressure predict fluid responsiveness? A systematic review of the literature and the tale of seven mares. Chest. 2008;134(1):172–8. https://doi.org/10.1378/chest.07-2331.
66. Michard F. Changes in arterial pressure during mechanical ventilation. Anesthesiology. 2005;103:419–28.
67. Bakkar J, Nijsten M, Jansen T. Clinical use of lactate monitoring in critically ill patients. Ann Intensive Care. 2013;3:12.

# Anesthesia and Burns

Clare R. Herlihy and Cassandra Barry

## Introduction

Approximately 500,000 people seek medical attention annually for burn injuries in the United States. About 10% of those patients are hospitalized for their burns [1]. Although burns continue to be a major source of morbidity and mortality, improvements in care over the last 40 years have significantly reduced this burden. Many of these patients end up in the operating room for care of their burns. On arrival in the operating room, these patients have significant differences in physiology from the typical patient that should be understood by the treating anesthesiologist. Significant concerns in fluid management, airway management, and cardiovascular changes all present challenges in the initial management of burn patients in the emergency department, the intensive care unit, and in the operating room. In addition, pain management and sedation requirements may require further care by an anesthesiologist outside of the operating room. It is important to have an appreciation of the physiology of burn injury to better care for those burn patients and improve outcomes.

C. R. Herlihy, M.D. (✉) · C. Barry, M.B., B.Ch.
University of Cincinnati Medical Center,
Cincinnati, OH, USA
e-mail: herlihcr@ucmail.uc.edu;
barryca@ucmail.uc.edu

## Burn Physiology

Burn injury is categorized by the depth of injury to the dermis and subcutaneous tissues as well as the percent of body surface area involved. Superficial burns (first degree) involve only the epidermis and do not cause significant morbidity or mortality. Partial thickness burns (second degree) involve only dermis and epidermis. Full thickness burns involve all skin layers. Full thickness burns are more likely to lead to scarring. Percent of total body surface area (TBSA) involving at least second degree burns is a strong predictor of degree of morbidity in burn patients [2]. The total body surface area involved can be calculated using the Lund Brower chart. Alternatively, the simple rule of nines can be used [3]. Severe burn injury is categorized as patients with >10% TBSA burn injury in children and >25% TBSA burn injury in adults.

Severe burn injury results in significant tissue destruction and an immediate systemic inflammatory response [4]. The initial injury breaks down the body's natural barrier to infection and alters both fluid and heat regulation. Rapid fluid losses occur due to evaporative loss from the burn surface as well as increased vascular permeability. Patients often can develop significant hypothermia both due to evaporative loss and the loss of homeostatic thermoregulators. The systemic response affects not simply the burned tissue, but tissues throughout the body. Patients can develop pulmonary and cerebral edema from increased permeability, acute respiratory distress syndrome (ARDS), and renal failure from fluid shifts and severe hypovolemia. The systemic response to a burn injury can be predicted in two phases. The initial phase of burn shock (ebb phase) begins immediately and lasts for approximately the first 48 h. After this, a hypermetabolic (flow) phase begins that can last months after the burn injury (Table 78.1) [3]. An understanding of these changes is key to management of these patients throughout their injury course.

## Burn Shock Physiology

Significant burn injury causes a release of inflammatory mediators at the site of the injury. These mediators lead to significant capillary leak. In a small burn this leads to localized edema at the burn site. With larger burns this cascade of inflammation creates systemic capillary leak leading to loss of intravascular fluid and burn shock [5]. The flow of plasma out of the vascular space leads directly to hemoconcentration and requires significant fluid resuscitation to maintain circulating volume. The large volume fluid resuscitation continues to leak into the extravascular space and cause complications associated with edema including respiratory failure and compartment syndrome. Despite adequate resuscitation, patients initially have an elevation in their hematocrit. Without concomitant trauma, these patients rarely require blood product transfusion in their initial presentation.

Many formulae exist to calculate the appropriate volume for fluid resuscitation for burns; the most famous is the Parkland Formula (4 mL × Ideal body weight × %TBSA with ½ given over the first 8 h and the remainder given over the following 16 h) [6]. The Parkland formula tends to overload patients with fluid, leading to increased incidence of compartment syndrome and edema. Other rules have been suggested including the rule of ten's

**Table 78.1** Effect of burns on different organ systems, both resulting from shock and increased metabolism

| | Burn shock | Hypermetabolism |
|---|---|---|
| Cardiovascular | Hypovolemia | Increased cardiac output |
| | Decreased cardiac output | Increased resting heart rate |
| | Increased systemic vascular resistance (SVR) | Hypertension |
| | Decreased venous oxygen saturation ($SvO_2$) | Decreased SVR |
| | | Increased $SvO_2$ |
| | | Altered myocardial contractility |
| Respiratory | Pulmonary edema | ARDS |
| | Airway edema | Pneumonia |
| | Inhalation injury | Tracheal stenosis |
| | | Inhalation injury |
| Hematologic | Hemoconcentration | Anemia |
| | Thrombocytopenia | Thrombocytosis |
| | | Coagulopathy |
| Renal | Decreased glomerular filtration rate (GFR) | Increased GFR |
| | Oliguria | Tubular dysfunction |
| | Myoglobinuria | |
| Hepatic | Decreased perfusion | Increased perfusion |
| | | Increased drug clearance |
| Neurologic | Increased intracranial pressure | Delirium |
| | Cerebral Edema | PTSD |
| Other | Generalized edema | Increased core body temperature |
| | Compartment syndrome | Muscle catabolism |
| | | Increased metabolic rate |
| | | Insulin resistance |

(10 mL/h × %TBSA = hourly rate) [7] or the modified Brooke formula (2 mL × ideal body weight × %TBSA with ½ given over the first 8 h and the remaineder over the following 16 h) [8]. These calculations should be used only to determine an initial rate for fluid resuscitation, more fluid does not necessarily decrease mortality. Resuscitation should then be titrated to physiological endpoints, most commonly urine output. The rate should be adjusted hourly based on the patient's urine output. Algorithms for resuscitation often aim for a goal urine output of 0.3–1 mL/kg per hour [9]. Impaired renal function may prove difficult for titration of fluid resuscitation. Other markers of resuscitation can be used for a more complete picture. In large burns, an arterial line may be placed for close monitoring of hemodynamics. This also allows the use of pulse contour analysis. Stroke volume variation as well as central venous pressure can be followed as a trend to evaluate adequacy of volume resuscitation. Cardiac evaluation can be easily performed with bedside ultrasonography. If evaluation of resuscitation is complicated or confusing, a pulmonary artery catheter may be helpful. In burn patients, it is important to avoid fluid boluses; rather, adjust hourly fluid rate to achieve adequate circulating volume without fluid overload. Initial resuscitation should be done with crystalloid solutions; usually Lactated Ringers or Plasmalyte solution is recommended. Albumin infusion may reduce mortality and incidence of compartment syndrome if patients are exceeding their predicted fluid resuscitation volume [10].

Inadequate volume resuscitation will cause hypovolemic shock and multi-organ dysfunction. Some lab markers that may be useful to trend include lactate and base deficit. Complete blood counts should also be followed monitoring for both anemia and hemoconcentration. Arterial blood gases will be helpful as patients with hypermetabolism may require higher than expected minute ventilation. Over resuscitation can increase morbidity and mortality. Risks are related to volume overload and increased vascular permeability. Complications of over resuscitation include pulmonary edema, respiratory failure, pericardial and pleural effusions, abdominal and limb compartment syndromes, and ileus [6, 11, 12]. Vasopressors may be required to avoid over resuscitation and complications from volume overload. Patients may require escharotomies to prevent compartment syndrome. If there is a concern for abdominal compartment syndrome, bladder pressures should be monitored during the resuscitation phase.

Additionally, in the first 24–48 h, burned patients experience a significant decrease in cardiac output with decreased cardiac contractility. This occurs despite adequate volume resuscitation and is due to direct myocardial depression [13]. Increased pulmonary and systemic vascular resistance contribute to decreased perfusion throughout the body. All of these changes can lead to metabolic acidosis and mixed venous desaturation. Significant fluid shifts in this context lead to renal dysfunction and possibly renal failure. Renal dysfunction can further complicate treatment and possibly lead to over resuscitation, as fluid resuscitation is most often titrated to maintain a goal urine output.

## Hypermetabolism Physiology

After about 48 h, the hypermetabolic phase of the burn injury begins. This flow phase lasts throughout the healing process and can last for months to years after the burn. The cardiac output transitions from low to high with increased stroke volumes [14]. Patients remain tachycardic and later can develop cardiac dysfunction due to this hyperactivity [13]. Systemic vascular resistance decreases and these changes can lead to blood loss. Lungs can be damaged due to continued pulmonary edema or ARDS even in the absence of inhalation injury. Kidneys exhibit increased GFR but decreased tubular function [15]. Hepatic metabolic function can alter drug clearance. Coagulation factor metabolism decreases. Hematopoesis decreases resulting in long lasting anemia. Patients also become immunologically compromised due to poor WBC production.

This phase is also associated with a significant increase in metabolism throughout the body.

Protein breakdown and muscle wasting is a key component of this stage and adequate nutrition is important to minimize long term consequences and enhance healing. Nutrition should be initiated as soon as the patient is stabilized and the initial resuscitation period is over. Glucose and fat metabolism is also altered. Hyperglycemia is common and insulin is often required [16, 17]. Untreated hyperglycemia can contribute to increased infections and mortality.

Several agents have been studied as treatment of hypermetabolism with mixed results. Oxandralone is an anabolic agent that has been studied, and in one RCT this agent has shown to maintain lean body mass and improve hepatic protein synthesis [14]. Propranolol, a beta blocker, has also been studied and has been shown to reduce energy expenditure and accelerate wound healing [18, 19]. There is no consensus on which agents should be used for hypermetabolism treatment, and it is unknown if they reduce morbidity or mortality.

$CO_2$ production increases in this phase of injury and can create acidosis. Conventional ventilation may still result in a respiratory acidosis or an uncorrected metabolic acidosis. At the same time, the patients begin to show signs of inhalation injury, pulmonary edema, and ARDS. Lung protective ventilation with tidal volumes of 6–8 mL/kg should be used to prevent further lung injury and manage ARDS [20]. Occasionally, this is not sufficient to treat this acidosis and some patients may require tidal volumes >8–10 mL/kg IBW to control their acidosis [21]. Alternatively, if patients are having trouble with oxygenation or ventilation, high frequency percussive ventilation can be used to ventilate patients [22].

Table 78.1 highlights effect of burns on different organ systems, both resulting from shock and increased metabolism.

## Inhalation Injury

Inhalation injury is a term used to describe both direct injury to the airway caused by hot gases, steam and chemical injury to the airways and alveoli due to inhaled toxins. This can occur in up to 35% of burn victims. Isolated inhalation injury carries about 10% mortality; however, it will significantly increase mortality from burn injury [23, 24]. Patients with inhalation injury require higher volume fluid resuscitation than anticipated for their %TBSA burn. Airway obstruction is the initial concern in patients who present with possible inhalation injury. Direct burns to the larynx can result in significant injury and poor outcomes if overlooked [25]. Swelling may not occur initially, but can develop during resuscitation. In these patients it is important to secure the airway early because edema can progress rapidly leading to a compromised airway that may be difficult to intubate.

Direct thermal injury to the distal airways can be devastating but occurs rarely unless steam is inhaled. Instead, distal airways are injured by chemical injury from smoke and combustion. The mucociliary clearance is damaged, resulting in decreased clearance from the airways. Oxygenation is impaired due to inactivated surfactant and collapse of alveoli [26]. Inhalation injury is initially suspected in a fire in an enclosed area, and a high level of clinical suspicion is important in those circumstances. Other signs and symptoms include facial burns, singed nasal hairs, stridor, and carbonaceous sputum. Evaluation of the airways with bronchoscopy is the primary method for diagnosing inhalation injury [27, 28]. Treatment for inhalation injury includes N acetyl cysteine, inhaled heparin, bronchodilators, and good pulmonary toilet in addition to supportive therapy [28, 29].

Often patients who are diagnosed with inhalation injury also have exposure to other substances. Carbon monoxide is commonly seen in patients with suspected inhalation injury. A co-oximeter is used to diagnose carbon monoxide poisoning. Carbon monoxide has increased affinity for hemoglobin compared to oxygen. The presence of carbon monoxide shifts the oxyhemoglobin dissociation curve to the left, impairing oxygen delivery to the tissues. Administration of 100% oxygen decreases the half-life of carboxyhemoglobin [30, 31]. Cyanide is another poisonous gas that can produce profound acidosis and unstable hemodynamics along with an altered mental status. Treatment with sodium thiosulfate or hydroxocobalamin is important with suspicion of cyanide poisoning [32, 33].

Patients are at risk for pulmonary edema throughout their hospital course. ARDS and acute lung injury are both concerns given the high volume fluid resuscitation needed and blood transfusions that these patients often require [34]. This contributes to increased mortality in patients, even if they do not present with an inhalation injury.

## Infection

Infections are a major cause of death in burned patients [35]. A major skin function is to provide a barrier to microorganisms, and this is damaged in burn injuries. Mucociliary clearance will be decreased in inhalation injury. Patients are often febrile due to hypermetabolism, but infection should be aggressively searched for and treated. After the initial resuscitation phase, any unnecessary urinary catheters or vascular access devices should be removed. Early burn excision reduces the risk of wound infection.

## Pain Management in Burn Patients

Burn patients experience significant pain from the moment they are injured. Acutely, burn patients require multiple painful procedures to care for their wounds. Additionally, dressing changes both before and after excision can be incredibly painful to patients. Adequate pain control is also an essential part of the patient's ability to participate in successful rehabilitation [36]. Additionally, patients quickly develop tolerance to medications due to their hypermetabolic state. This needs to be consistently addressed throughout their injury course.

Pain in burn patients is a significant issue in the acute phase of injury and can continue to persist through a patient's rehabilitation and for years post injury [37]. Inadequate pain control has been shown to increase the risk of depression and PTSD in burn patients [38, 39]. Achieving adequate pain control in patients is therefore very important to their long term recovery.

Opioids are the cornerstone of management of acute burn pain. Patients with major burns require both background pain control along with intermittent procedural pain control to address pain associated with OR procedures and dressing changes [40]. Most often these patients are placed on continuous opioid therapy that can be titrated; typically, this is achieved through continuous IV infusions or patient-controlled analgesia (PCA) [41]. This allows for adjustments as patients pharmacodynamics change. Opioids should be titrated to effect in burn patients, and opioid requirements are often increased compared to non-burned patients. Methadone is often used as a long acting opioid with NMDA receptor activity to treat background pain [42].

Non opioid analgesia is an important supplement to opioid analgesia. Ketamine is often used in the management of pain in burn patients [43]. It is used as a sedative in procedures, or it can be used in patients with refractory pain as an infusion. Conscious sedation with bolus doses of ketamine can be useful during long and painful dressing changes. Dexmedetomidine is another adjunct that can be very useful in pain management in refractory patients [44, 45]. Maintaining anxiolysis in these patients is important to avoid escalation of pain [46]. Other useful adjuncts include acetaminophen and non-steroidal anti-inflammatory (NSAID) use [39, 47]. These medications help to minimize the requirement for opioid therapy and can be used as sole agents in patients with smaller burns.

In patients who present with large burns, neuropathic pain should be considered due to the direct nerve injury sustained. Alleviating this pain can be very important for long term improvement in pain status. Gabapentin and pregabalin are the primary options for treatment. Antidepressant medications can also be considered for this treatment [40].

Local anesthetics are often used with success in burn patients. Tumescent local anesthetics with or without epinephrine can be injected into donor sites to reduce pain from skin harvesting procedures. Regional anesthesia is an option for many of these patients. This can be used both for the acute burn and for donor site pain. Options for regional anesthesia include peripheral blocks, catheters, and neuraxial blocks [48]. One limitation of this technique is infection risk, so avoiding burned skin for placement of catheters is important. The thigh is often used as a donor site for skin grafts, therefore lateral femoral cutaneous and fascia iliaca nerve blocks are often used for pain at this site [49].

## Practical Management of Burn Patients

Burn patients often require multiple trips to the operating room for escharotomies, burn excision and grafting, reconstructive surgery, and tracheostomies. Prior to bringing a patient with a large burn into the operating room, it is important to begin by preparing the room. Due to the loss of temperature regulation by the skin, these patients can lose heat very quickly. It is the standard to prepare a warm room to minimize heat loss although this can be controversial [50]. It is also important to note the patient's preoperative temperature, as hypermetabolic patients can be hyperthermic at baseline. Decreased body temperature can lead to increased oxygen consumption, increased blood loss, and increased risk of infection [34]. Blood and fluid warmers are important to maintain temperature. Additionally, warming blankets with fluid or blown air can be helpful to maintain temperature. Special care is required in patient positioning in the operating room to avoid damage to the skin or grafts.

Early excision of burn injury and grafting to cover the wound is important to minimize both morbidity and mortality [51, 52]. Often burn patients are in the operating room soon after their injuries, occasionally even while they are still undergoing resuscitation. Because of this, burn patients are often hemodynamically unstable when they are first taken to the operating room and require consistent active management. Burn patients may also have additional traumatic injuries related to the burn event that may require special management. Outside of the operating room burn patients often require sedation for painful procedures [43]. These procedures are often done with sedation managed by the anesthesia team.

## Airway Management

Airway management in these patients can be complicated due to swelling. It is important to have a good airway exam early to prepare for any difficulties. Limited mouth opening due to burns or scarring can complicate airway management. Laryngeal burns are a concern, and if possible, a good look at the larynx is important on intubation for early intervention. Bronchoscopic evaluation for inhalation injury in patients where it is suspected can be beneficial. Patients need to be evaluated also for possible difficult mask ventilation due to facial dressings or wounds [3]. Additionally, securing the airway can be difficult as tape often does not adhere well to burn injuries. Ties can be a concern due to swelling. Securing the airway to the teeth with wire or suture is an option. Stapling tape to the skin is an alternate method to secure the airway. As patients progress through their hospital stay, neck contractures can make airway management increasingly difficult. Laryngeal mask airways (LMA) have been shown to be both safe and effective airway management tools to assist in difficult airways after burns [53]. Fiber optic intubation is occasionally a required technique if the airway appears difficult [3]. If a patient needs to be intubated, consideration for pulmonary toilet and frequent bronchoscopies should be given in choosing an endotracheal tube. Intra-operative ventilation may be difficult due to associated pulmonary edema or ARDS. If the patient has circumferential chest wall burns, this may cause restrictive physiology.

## Fluid Management

Fluid management in the operating room is especially important in burned patients. Patients who are still in their initial resuscitation must continue the resuscitation throughout surgery. Large fluid boluses put patients at risk for fluid overload and compartment syndromes, therefore, it is important to consistently adjust their maintenance rate [12]. Monitoring urine output and vital signs and adjusting fluid rates accordingly is especially important (Goal rate of hourly urine output 0.3–1 mL/kg). In the operating room, this becomes more of a challenge due to insensible fluid losses and blood loss; therefore, consistent vigilance is required.

Excision of burn wounds can cause significant blood loss, which can be incredibly difficult to monitor. The hyperdynamic state of the patient can contribute to increased blood loss. Blood loss during excision has been reported to be 2.6–3.4% of blood volume for every 1%TBSA excised [54]. This can occur very rapidly. Estimating blood loss is difficult as much of the loss cannot be suctioned and sponges contain both blood and irrigation fluid. Significant amounts of blood loss can also collect beneath the patient or in dressings [55]. It is important to be vigilant in monitoring for blood loss. Many techniques have been studied to minimize blood loss in these procedures. Topical thrombin, brisk operative pace, use of tourniquets, injection or topical application of vasoconstrictors have all been attempted [56, 57]. No one method has been shown superior [58]. Often, staged procedures are necessary to avoid hemorrhagic shock in these patients.

Given this predictable blood loss, it is important to be prepared. A type and screen should be performed preoperatively and blood should be available when large blood loss is anticipated. Blood loss should be aggressively treated as it is easy to "get behind" once excision has started. When the patient's predicted blood loss will likely decrease the hematocrit below the patient's transfusion threshold, it can be useful to start blood preoperatively given how rapidly patients can bleed. It is important to avoid over transfusion, as transfusion can be associated with increased risk of infections and mortality [59].

Tumescent crystalloid with a vasoconstrictor can be injected by the surgeon into the subcutaneous tissue to minimize blood loss while excising burned tissue. Occasionally, local anesthetic may be added to the tumescent crystalloid to assist with pain control post-operatively. Significant amounts of this fluid can be injected into tissue, often exceeding 100 mL/kg. This fluid is then gradually absorbed into the vasculature over the following 24–48 h. This can create a delayed fluid overload which must be monitored, especially if patients are returning for subsequent procedures or requiring additional fluid replacement.

## Pharmacologic Management

Succinylcholine use is a concern in burned patients. It is generally safe to use within 48 h of burn injury. After 48 h, an up regulation of extrajunctional acetylcholine receptors put patients at risk for an exaggerated hyperkalemic response after administration of succinylcholine [60]. The severe hyperkalemia can lead to cardiac arrest. Other anesthetic medications are considered safe. There is a decreased sensitivity to non-depolarizing muscle relaxants noted in burned patients [61]. Increased volume of distribution as well as altered plasma proteins may lead to unpredictable drug pharmacokinetics [62]. Drug metabolism may be altered due to hypermetabolism as well as renal or hepatic dysfunction.

## Vascular Access

Intravenous access may be difficult in extensive burn injuries. If possible, vascular access should be obtained from areas of unburned skin to minimize risk of infection. These patients should have at least two large bore IV lines for fluid resuscitation and blood administration. They often require central lines for long term access and vasopressor administration. Securing IVs to burned skin may be difficult as adhesive dressings will not stay in place. A stitch may be used to secure IVs. Central lines should be monitored closely and meticulous care is required to avoid line infections.

## Monitoring

Patients with large burn injury present multiple challenges when it comes to monitoring. Transmission pulse oximetry does not work well through severely burned skin; therefore, alternate unburned sites may need to be considered [63, 64]. Based on the extent of burn injury, EKG electrodes may not stick to the patient. Needle electrodes or an esophageal catheter with an EKG electrode can be useful to obtain EKG monitoring [65]. Core temperature monitoring is essential to maintain body temperature during surgery. Monitoring invasive blood pressure is useful to obtain accurate blood pressure readings depending on the surgical sites. CVP monitoring can be helpful in patients with ongoing resuscitation.

## Nutrition

As detailed above, the hypermetabolic response after burn injury requires significant nutritional support. Burn injured patients may undergo multiple surgical procedures to excise eschar and cover their wounds. Periods of fasting have been shown to cause significant nutritional deficits in these patients, which can lead to poor wound healing and malnutrition [66]. Studies have shown safety in post pyloric feeding through surgery [67]. Parenteral nutrition is occasionally used when enteral feeding is not an option, however, this presents the risk of infection and increased mortality [68, 69].

## Burn Reconstruction

After initial burns are healed, scarring can be a recurrent problem. Many patients will require surgical treatment of their burn scars. Patients with significant burn history often present with very difficult IV access due to scarring and contractures [70]. It can be very useful to have an ultrasound available for IV access. In addition, airway management can be complicated by burn scar contractures to the neck or mouth. Fiber optic intubation or LMA placement can be beneficial in patients with a suspected difficult intubation. Patients with significant previous injuries often still have resistance to nondepolarizing muscle relaxants. They also have higher tolerance with opiate drugs and should be dosed accordingly.

## Reference

1. American Burn Association. Sources: National Hospital Ambulatory Medical Care Survey: 2011 Emergency Department Summary Tables (accessed on January 22, 2015, at http://www.cdc.gov/nchs/ahcd/web_tables.htm#2011). Fire/Smoke Inhalation Deaths:3,275 This total includes 2,745 deaths from residential fires, 310 from vehicle crash fires, and 220 from other sources. One civilian fire death occurs every 2 hours and 41 minutes. The odds of a U.S. resident dying from exposure to fire, flames or smoke is 1 in 1442. Fire and inhalation deaths are combined because deaths from thermal burns in fires cannot always be distinguished from deaths from inhalation of toxins in smoke. 2017. http://www.ameriburn.org/resources_factsheet.php.
2. Tobiasen J, Hiebert JH, Edlich RF. Prediction of burn mortality. Surg Gynecol Obstet. 1982;154(5):711–4.
3. Bittner EA, Shank E, Woodson L, Martyn JA. Acute and perioperative care of the burn-injured patient. Anesthesiology. 2015;122(2):448–64. https://doi.org/10.1097/ALN.0000000000000559.
4. Finnerty CC, Herndon DN, Przkora R, Pereira CT, Oliveira HM, Queiroz DM, et al. Cytokine expression profile over time in severely burned pediatric patients. Shock. 2006;26(1):13–9. https://doi.org/10.1097/01.shk.0000223120.26394.7d.
5. Arturson G, Jonsson CE. Transcapillary transport after thermal injury. Scand J Plast Reconstr Surg. 1979;13(1):29–38.
6. Alvarado R, Chung KK, Cancio LC, Wolf SE. Burn resuscitation. Burns. 2009;35(1):4–14. https://doi.org/10.1016/j.burns.2008.03.008.
7. Chung KK, Salinas J, Renz EM, Alvarado RA, King BT, Barillo DJ, et al. Simple derivation of the initial fluid rate for the resuscitation of severely burned adult combat casualties: in silico validation of the rule of 10. J Trauma. 2010;69(Suppl 1):S49–54. https://doi.org/10.1097/TA.0b013e3181e425f1.
8. Chung KK, Wolf SE, Cancio LC, Alvarado R, Jones JA, McCorcle J, et al. Resuscitation of severely burned military casualties: fluid begets more fluid. J Trauma. 2009;67(2):231–7. https://doi.org/10.1097/TA.0b013e3181ac68cf; discussion 7.
9. Pham TN, Cancio LC, Gibran NS, American Burn Association. American burn association practice guidelines burn shock resuscitation. J Burn Care Res. 2008;29(1):257–66. https://doi.org/10.1097/BCR.0b013e31815f3876.
10. Navickis RJ, Greenhalgh DG, Wilkes MM. Albumin in burn shock resuscitation: a meta-analysis of controlled clinical studies. J Burn Care Res. 2016;37(3):e268–78. https://doi.org/10.1097/BCR.0000000000000201.
11. Klein MB, Hayden D, Elson C, Nathens AB, Gamelli RL, Gibran NS, et al. The association between fluid administration and outcome following major burn: a multicenter study. Ann Surg. 2007;245(4):622–8. https://doi.org/10.1097/01.sla.0000252572.50684.49.

12. Oda J, Yamashita K, Inoue T, Harunari N, Ode Y, Mega K, et al. Resuscitation fluid volume and abdominal compartment syndrome in patients with major burns. Burns. 2006;32(2):151–4. https://doi.org/10.1016/j.burns.2005.08.011.
13. Carleton SC. Cardiac problems associated with burns. Cardiol Clin. 1995;13(2):257–62.
14. Jeschke MG, Finnerty CC, Suman OE, Kulp G, Mlcak RP, Herndon DN. The effect of oxandrolone on the endocrinologic, inflammatory, and hypermetabolic responses during the acute phase postburn. Ann Surg. 2007;246(3):351–60. https://doi.org/10.1097/SLA.0b013e318146980e; discussion 60–2.
15. Chrysopoulo MT, Jeschke MG, Dziewulski P, Barrow RE, Herndon DN. Acute renal dysfunction in severely burned adults. J Trauma. 1999;46(1):141–4.
16. Gore DC, Chinkes D, Heggers J, Herndon DN, Wolf SE, Desai M. Association of hyperglycemia with increased mortality after severe burn injury. J Trauma. 2001;51(3):540–4.
17. Ray JJ, Meizoso JP, Allen CJ, Teisch LF, Yang EY, Foong HY, et al. Admission hyperglycemia predicts infectious complications after burns. J Burn Care Res. 2017;38(2):85–9. https://doi.org/10.1097/BCR.0000000000000381.
18. Ali A, Herndon DN, Mamachen A, Hasan S, Andersen CR, Grogans RJ, et al. Propranolol attenuates hemorrhage and accelerates wound healing in severely burned adults. Crit Care. 2015;19:217. https://doi.org/10.1186/s13054-015-0913-x.
19. Herndon DN, Rodriguez NA, Diaz EC, Hegde S, Jennings K, Mlcak RP, et al. Long-term propranolol use in severely burned pediatric patients: a randomized controlled study. Ann Surg. 2012;256(3):402–11. https://doi.org/10.1097/SLA.0b013e318265427e.
20. Peck MD, Koppelman T. Low-tidal-volume ventilation as a strategy to reduce ventilator-associated injury in ALI and ARDS. J Burn Care Res. 2009;30(1):172–5. https://doi.org/10.1097/BCR.0b013e3181923c32.
21. Sousse LE, Herndon DN, Andersen CR, Ali A, Benjamin NC, Granchi T, et al. High tidal volume decreases adult respiratory distress syndrome, atelectasis, and ventilator days compared with low tidal volume in pediatric burned patients with inhalation injury. J Am Coll Surg. 2015;220(4):570–8. https://doi.org/10.1016/j.jamcollsurg.2014.12.028.
22. Chung KK, Wolf SE, Renz EM, Allan PF, Aden JK, Merrill GA, et al. High-frequency percussive ventilation and low tidal volume ventilation in burns: a randomized controlled trial. Crit Care Med. 2010;38(10):1970–7. https://doi.org/10.1097/CCM.0b013e3181eb9d0b.
23. El-Helbawy RH, Ghareeb FM. Inhalation injury as a prognostic factor for mortality in burn patients. Ann Burns Fire Disasters. 2011;24(2):82–8.
24. Kadri SS, Miller AC, Hohmann S, Bonne S, Nielsen C, Wells C, et al. Risk factors for in-hospital mortality in smoke inhalation-associated acute lung injury: data from 68 United States Hospitals. Chest. 2016;150(6):1260–8. https://doi.org/10.1016/j.chest.2016.06.008.
25. Valdez TA, Desai U, Ruhl CM, Nigri PT. Early laryngeal inhalation injury and its correlation with late sequelae. Laryngoscope. 2006;116(2):283–7. https://doi.org/10.1097/01.mlg.0000197932.09386.0e.
26. Nieman GF, Clark WR, Wax SD, Webb SR. The effect of smoke inhalation on pulmonary surfactant. Ann Surg. 1980;191(2):171–81.
27. Miller K, Chang A. Acute inhalation injury. Emerg Med Clin North Am. 2003;21(2):533–57.
28. Walker PF, Buehner MF, Wood LA, Boyer NL, Driscoll IR, Lundy JB, et al. Diagnosis and management of inhalation injury: an updated review. Crit Care. 2015;19:351. https://doi.org/10.1186/s13054-015-1077-4.
29. Miller AC, Elamin EM, Suffredini AF. Inhaled anticoagulation regimens for the treatment of smoke inhalation-associated acute lung injury: a systematic review. Crit Care Med. 2014;42(2):413–9. https://doi.org/10.1097/CCM.0b013e3182a645e5.
30. Kao LW, Nañagas KA. Carbon monoxide poisoning. Med Clin North Am. 2005;89(6):1161–94. https://doi.org/10.1016/j.mcna.2005.06.007.
31. Varon J, Marik PE, Fromm RE, Gueler A. Carbon monoxide poisoning: a review for clinicians. J Emerg Med. 1999;17(1):87–93.
32. Baud FJ, Barriot P, Toffis V, Riou B, Vicaut E, Lecarpentier Y, et al. Elevated blood cyanide concentrations in victims of smoke inhalation. N Engl J Med. 1991;325(25):1761–6. https://doi.org/10.1056/NEJM199112193252502.
33. Geller RJ, Barthold C, Saiers JA, Hall AH. Pediatric cyanide poisoning: causes, manifestations, management, and unmet needs. Pediatrics. 2006;118(5):2146–58. https://doi.org/10.1542/peds.2006-1251.
34. Oda J, Kasai K, Noborio M, Ueyama M, Yukioka T. Hypothermia during burn surgery and postoperative acute lung injury in extensively burned patients. J Trauma. 2009;66(6):1525–9. https://doi.org/10.1097/TA.0b013e3181a51f35; discussion 9–30.
35. Church D, Elsayed S, Reid O, Winston B, Lindsay R. Burn wound infections. Clin Microbiol Rev. 2006;19(2):403–34. https://doi.org/10.1128/CMR.19.2.403-434.2006.
36. Faucher L, Furukawa K. Practice guidelines for the management of pain. J Burn Care Res. 2006;27(5):659–68. https://doi.org/10.1097/01.BCR.0000238117.41490.00.
37. Duffy JR, Warburg FE, Koelle SF, Werner MU, Nielsen PR. Pain-related psychological distress, self-rated health and significance of neuropathic pain in Danish soldiers injured in Afghanistan. Acta Anaesthesiol Scand. 2015;59(10):1367–76. https://doi.org/10.1111/aas.12579.
38. Sheridan RL, Stoddard FJ, Kazis LE, Lee A, Li NC, Kagan RJ, et al. Long-term posttraumatic stress symptoms vary inversely with early opiate dosing in children recovering from serious burns: effects durable at

39. Pardesi O, Fuzaylov G. Pain management in pediatric burn patients: review of recent literature and future directions. J Burn Care Res. 2016;38(6):335–47. https://doi.org/10.1097/BCR.0000000000000470.
40. Retrouvey H, Shahrokhi S. Pain and the thermally injured patient-a review of current therapies. J Burn Care Res. 2015;36(2):315–23. https://doi.org/10.1097/BCR.0000000000000073.
41. Rovers J, Knighton J, Neligan P, Peters W. Patient-controlled analgesia in burn patients: a critical review of the literature and case report. Hosp Pharm. 1994;29(2):106, 8–11.
42. Williams PI, Sarginson RE, Ratcliffe JM. Use of methadone in the morphine-tolerant burned paediatric patient. Br J Anaesth. 1998;80(1):92–5.
43. Owens VF, Palmieri TL, Comroe CM, Conroy JM, Scavone JA, Greenhalgh DG. Ketamine: a safe and effective agent for painful procedures in the pediatric burn patient. J Burn Care Res. 2006;27(2):211–6. https://doi.org/10.1097/01.BCR.0000204310.67594.A1; discussion 7.
44. Walker J, Maccallum M, Fischer C, Kopcha R, Saylors R, McCall J. Sedation using dexmedetomidine in pediatric burn patients. J Burn Care Res. 2006;27(2):206–10. https://doi.org/10.1097/01.BCR.0000200910.76019.CF.
45. Sheridan R, Stoddard F, Querzoli E. Management of background pain and anxiety in critically burned children requiring protracted mechanical ventilation. J Burn Care Rehabil. 2001;22(2):150–3.
46. Ratcliff SL, Brown A, Rosenberg L, Rosenberg M, Robert RS, Cuervo LJ, et al. The effectiveness of a pain and anxiety protocol to treat the acute pediatric burn patient. Burns. 2006;32(5):554–62. https://doi.org/10.1016/j.burns.2005.12.006.
47. Meyer WJ, Nichols RJ, Cortiella J, Villarreal C, Marvin JA, Blakeney PE, et al. Acetaminophen in the management of background pain in children postburn. J Pain Symptom Manag. 1997;13(1):50–5.
48. Dadure C, Acosta C, Capdevila X. Perioperative pain management of a complex orthopedic surgical procedure with double continuous nerve blocks in a burned child. Anesth Analg. 2004;98(6):1653–5, table of contents.
49. Cuignet O, Pirson J, Boughrouph J, Duville D. The efficacy of continuous fascia iliaca compartment block for pain management in burn patients undergoing skin grafting procedures. Anesth Analg. 2004;98(4):1077–81, table of contents.
50. Rizzo JA, Rowan MP, Driscoll IR, Chan RK, Chung KK. Perioperative temperature management during burn care. J Burn Care Res. 2017;38(1):e277–e83. https://doi.org/10.1097/BCR.0000000000000371.
51. Ong YS, Samuel M, Song C. Meta-analysis of early excision of burns. Burns. 2006;32(2):145–50. https://doi.org/10.1016/j.burns.2005.09.005.
52. Tompkins RG, Remensnyder JP, Burke JF, Tompkins DM, Hilton JF, Schoenfeld DA, et al. Significant 4 years. J Trauma Acute Care Surg. 2014;76(3):828–32. https://doi.org/10.1097/TA.0b013e3182ab111c. reductions in mortality for children with burn injuries through the use of prompt eschar excision. Ann Surg. 1988;208(5):577–85.
53. McCall JE, Fischer CG, Schomaker E, Young JM. Laryngeal mask airway use in children with acute burns: intraoperative airway management. Paediatr Anaesth. 1999;9(6):515–20.
54. Budny PG, Regan PJ, Roberts AH. The estimation of blood loss during burns surgery. Burns. 1993;19(2):134–7.
55. Housinger TA, Lang D, Warden GD. A prospective study of blood loss with excisional therapy in pediatric burn patients. J Trauma. 1993;34(2):262–3.
56. Beausang E, Orr D, Shah M, Dunn KW, Davenport PJ. Subcutaneous adrenaline infiltration in paediatric burn surgery. Br J Plast Surg. 1999;52(6):480–1. https://doi.org/10.1054/bjps.1999.3161.
57. Mitchell RT, Funk D, Spiwak R, Logsetty S. Phenylephrine tumescence in split-thickness skin graft donor sites in surgery for burn injury-a concentration finding study. J Burn Care Res. 2011;32(1):129–34. https://doi.org/10.1097/BCR.0b013e318204b39b.
58. Sterling JP, Heimbach DM. Hemostasis in burn surgery—a review. Burns. 2011;37(4):559–65. https://doi.org/10.1016/j.burns.2010.06.010.
59. Palmieri TL, Caruso DM, Foster KN, Cairns BA, Peck MD, Gamelli RL, et al. Effect of blood transfusion on outcome after major burn injury: a multicenter study. Crit Care Med. 2006;34(6):1602–7. https://doi.org/10.1097/01.CCM.0000217472.97524.0E.
60. Martyn JA, Richtsfeld M. Succinylcholine-induced hyperkalemia in acquired pathologic states: etiologic factors and molecular mechanisms. Anesthesiology. 2006;104(1):158–69.
61. Jaehde U, Sörgel F. Clinical pharmacokinetics in patients with burns. Clin Pharmacokinet. 1995;29(1):15–28. https://doi.org/10.2165/00003088-199529010-00003.
62. Blanchet B, Jullien V, Vinsonneau C, Tod M. Influence of burns on pharmacokinetics and pharmacodynamics of drugs used in the care of burn patients. Clin Pharmacokinet. 2008;47(10):635–54. https://doi.org/10.2165/00003088-200847100-00002.
63. Coté CJ, Daniels AL, Connolly M, Szyfelbein SK, Wickens CD. Tongue oximetry in children with extensive thermal injury: comparison with peripheral oximetry. Can J Anaesth. 1992;39(5 Pt 1):454–7. https://doi.org/10.1007/BF03008709.
64. Pal SK, Kyriacou PA, Kumaran S, Fadheel S, Emamdee R, Langford RM, et al. Evaluation of oesophageal reflectance pulse oximetry in major burns patients. Burns. 2005;31(3):337–41. https://doi.org/10.1016/j.burns.2004.10.025.
65. Reid M, Shaw P, Taylor RH. Oesophageal ECG in a child for burns surgery. Paediatr Anaesth. 1997;7(1):73–6.
66. Pearson KS, From RP, Symreng T, Kealey GP. Continuous enteral feeding and short fasting periods enhance perioperative nutrition in patients with burns. J Burn Care Rehabil. 1992;13(4):477–81.

67. Jenkins ME, Gottschlich MM, Warden GD. Enteral feeding during operative procedures in thermal injuries. J Burn Care Rehabil. 1994;15(2):199–205.
68. Chen Z, Wang S, Yu B, Li A. A comparison study between early enteral nutrition and parenteral nutrition in severe burn patients. Burns. 2007;33(6):708–12. https://doi.org/10.1016/j.burns.2006.10.380.
69. Herndon DN, Barrow RE, Stein M, Linares H, Rutan TC, Rutan R, et al. Increased mortality with intravenous supplemental feeding in severely burned patients. J Burn Care Rehabil. 1989;10(4):309–13.
70. Fuzaylov G, Fidkowski CW. Anesthetic considerations for major burn injury in pediatric patients. Paediatr Anaesth. 2009;19(3):202–11. https://doi.org/10.1111/j.1460-9592.2009.02924.x.

# Anesthesia for Robot Assisted Gynecological Procedures

Eilish M. Galvin and Henri J. D. de Graaff

## Introduction

The use of robots to assist in the performance of surgery has been one of the most important developments in surgery in recent decades. Some would say that robot- assisted surgery as a continuation from minimally invasive laparoscopic surgery is the biggest breakthrough in surgery since the introduction of anesthesia [1]. This has had important implications not only for the surgical technique but also the entire operating room landscape.

Robot-assisted surgery is an extension of laparoscopic procedures which have been performed routinely since the 1980s, and have been shown to effectively reduce complication rates, length of hospital stay and post-operative pain, while showing a better cosmetic result and quicker return to normal daily activities [2]. However, traditional laparoscopic surgery has its drawbacks, such as the 'lack of depth' in the on screen image, which is only 2-dimensional (2D) and the alteration of the interaction between surgeon and patient by the interposition of a technological interface in the form of a display screen. Also the instruments used have a limited range of movement decreasing the precision of the surgeon's movements. Such disadvantages of laparoscopic surgery have to a great extent been solved by the advent of robot-assisted surgery.

The use of robot-assisted surgery across all surgical disciplines is growing rapidly and is currently used in a wide range of surgical procedures from kidney transplantations [3] to oncological surgery [4–6]. The US FDA approved the robot-assisted surgical system for gynecological conditions in 2005, the first robot-assisted radical hysterectomy was in 2006 [7] and currently gynecological together with urological are the most common surgical procedures performed with the Da Vinci® robot [8]. Gynecological procedures for which the robot is currently used are presented in Table 79.1.

**Table 79.1** Gynecological procedures for which the robot is currently used

| |
|---|
| Total and supra-cervical hysterectomy |
| Myomectomy |
| Tubal re-anastomosis |
| Ovarian surgery (cystectomy, oncology) |
| Sacrocolpopexy |
| Cervicectomy |
| Lymphnode dissection |
| Endometriosis resection |
| Ectopic pregnancy |

E. M. Galvin, M.D., F.C.A.R.C.S.I., Ph.D. (✉)
H. J. D. de Graaff, M.D., M.Sc., DESA
Department of Anesthesiology, Erasmus University Medical Center, Rotterdam, The Netherlands

## History of Robot Assisted Surgery

The Zeus® Robotic Surgical System (ZRSS) was a medical robot designed to assist in surgery, originally produced by the American robotics company Computer Motion Inc. (Goleta, California, US). Its predecessor, EASOP, was cleared by the Food and Drug Administration in 1994 to assist surgeons in minimally invasive surgery. The Zeus® itself was cleared by the FDA 7 years later, in 2001. ZEUS had three robotic arms, which were remotely controlled by the surgeon. The first arm, EASOP (Automated Endoscopic System for Optimal Positioning), was a voice-activated endoscope, allowing the surgeon to see inside the patient's body. The other two robotic arms mimicked the surgeon's movements to make precise incisions and extractions [2]. ZEUS® was discontinued in 2003, following the merger of Computer Motion with its rival Intuitive Surgical Inc. (Sunnyvale, California, US); the merged company focused on the developed the Da Vinci® Surgical System.

## The Da Vinci® Robotic Surgical System

The currently used robotic assisted surgical system is called the Da Vinci® Surgical System (Intuitive Surgical, Inc., Sunnyvale, California, US). In 1995 a robotic surgical system called MONA was developed, which had seven degrees of movement due to a joint at the end of the instruments, which was capable of reproducing the surgeon's hand movements, this coupled with a feedback system in 3D vision gave the surgeon the feeling of being immersed in the operative field. The first robot-assisted cholecystectomy was performed in 1997 [9]. The robot-assisted surgical market is rapidly growing, with current market growth predictions estimating a threefold increase in worth from the start to the end of the current decade [10].

The Da Vinci Surgical System comprises three parts connected by a system of electrical cables:

1. control console/ station, where the surgeon seats and performs the surgery (Fig. 79.1)
2. tower/cart which holds the robotic/articulating arms manipulated by the surgeon (one to control the camera and three to manipulate instruments) (Fig. 79.2, arms in folded position)
3. imaging system (high-definition three-dimensional (3D) vision system)

Articulating surgical instruments are mounted on the robotic arms which are introduced into the body through ports. The arms are equipped with a joint at their ends (Endowrist®) that mimics the movements of the wrist and has seven degrees of movement at the tip, with 360° range of motion and 90° of instrument articulation control attached to the robotic arms.

Meticulous surgical dissection is possible and importantly the movement of the instruments is intuitive unlike in traditional laparoscopic surgery where counteractive arm movements were required, meaning the surgeon has to move the equipment outside the patient's body in the opposite direction to achieve the desired movement inside the body [11].

The current Da Vinci® has four robotic arms; arm 1 and 2 are the right and left hand controls, arm 3 is the camera and arm 4 is used as a retractor, which is periodically repositioned and reduces dependency on patient side surgical assistance. These arms lock into place above the surgical field. An assistant at the patient's side is required to exchange instruments, to load sutures and release staples when instructed by the operating surgeon. At the console, two handles or joysticks transmit the surgeon's hand movements to control the instruments and the lens. It works with a device that scales down movements from 1:1 to 5:1, as well as a filtration module to eliminate hand tremors. The console also contains a pedal unit which comprises several pedals used for different types of cautery (unipolar, bipolar, ultrasound), for managing camera movements, and a clutch device for optimal repositioning of the instruments.

The vision system comprises an insufflator, a light source, and a dual camera, and is mounted below a monitor transmitting the image of the surgical field in 2D to other operating room personnel; this is the image which is observed by

**Fig. 79.1** Control console

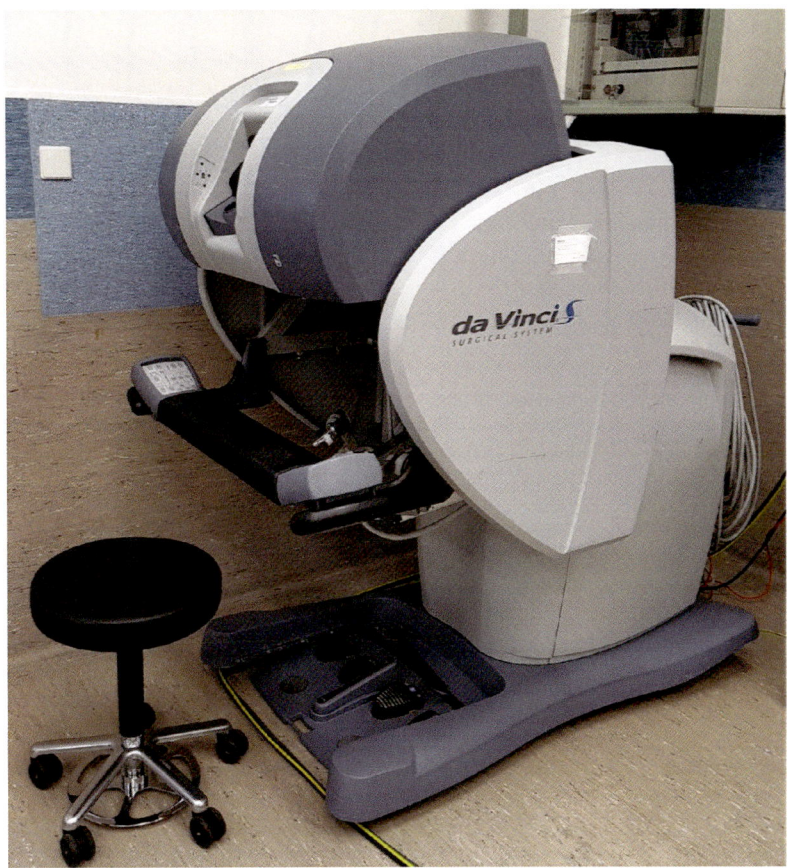

**Fig. 79.2** Tower which holds the robotic/articulating arms

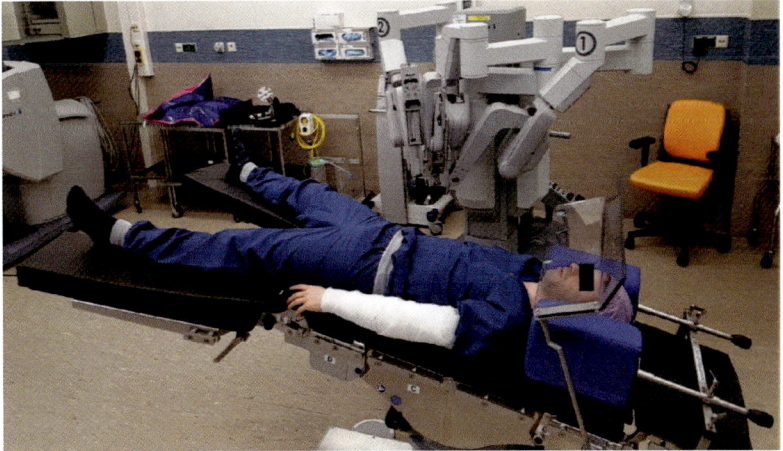

anesthesia personnel. The current version of the Da Vinci® allows a second console to the surgeon console, an innovation that allows a novice surgeon to be coached by a mentor during the procedure and thereby increases safety during the learning curve. For further information on the technological details of the improved imaging and movement using robot-assisted surgery, we refer the reader to an the article by Pugin et al. [2]

## Advantages of Robot-Assisted Surgery

In essence the Da Vinci® system allows a surgeon to operate on a patient from a location remote to the patient, currently beside or in the operating room, but significantly not at the operating table itself. The advantages to the surgical technique are improved accuracy and precision of the actual surgical procedure and a more comfortable, less tiring operating position for the surgeon, which improves the quality of surgical technique. Importantly, in terms of quality of surgical resection, better margin negative rates and improved functional outcomes have been reported [12]. Robot-assisted surgery also has the potential to enable remote surgery, allowing specialized surgical expertise to be delivered to a wider patient population.

## Disadvantages of Robot-Assisted Surgery

The setting up and maintenance of robot assisted surgery is a very significant cost for hospitals; with initial costs of approximately two million dollars, followed by maintenance and update costs, disposable equipment costs, as well as the costs of training staff and allowing for initial longer operating room times during the learning curve phase of such surgery [13]. However, it has been shown that such costs reduce over time mainly due to a shortening of surgical operative time [14].

From an anesthetic view point, there are specific challenges such as spatial restrictions, patient positioning, limited patient access, ventilation, blood pressure management etc. These will be covered in greater detail later in the chapter.

Clearly, with the requirement for so much technical equipment within an operating room, spatial restrictions imposed by the robot relative to the conventional anesthetic area need to be taken into account to ensure safe and effective functioning within the operating room. Indeed, anesthesia itself has increased its footprint within the operating room over recent years, with larger ventilators, more monitoring equipment, greater use of infusion pumps, heating devices and so on. It is essential that the anesthesiologist has a clear plan for the placement of anesthesia equipment to ensure patient safety as well as a comfortable working space.

However, looking forward, as other companies enter the market and develop new robotic surgical systems, it is likely that as demand grows and market competition increases, lower costs and more compact machines will become the norm.

## Pre-operative Assessment

A thorough pre-operative assessment is necessary for robot assisted gynecological operations, because of the considerable challenges during these procedures. This is a consequence of the combination of the following characteristics: pneumoperitoneum, Trendelenburg positioning, lithotomy position and a prolonged operation time.

Frequently, the referring gynecologist will have applied a first patient selection process, based on comorbidities, before considering a patients' eligibility to undergo a robot-assisted operation. However, in the pre-operative assessment a systematic approach to evaluate and optimize the patient's condition where possible is very important.

## Cardiovascular

The cardiac status of each patient must be evaluated according to the current ACC/AHA guideline on perioperative cardiovascular evaluation and management of patients undergoing non cardiac surgery. Robot-assisted gynecological operations are currently regarded as 'elevated risk' operations (risk of >1% of major adverse cardiac event) [15].

Elderly patients frequently use anticoagulants because of a cardiac stent. In deciding whether to temporarily withhold all or some of the anticoagulants, the risk of surgical bleeding should be weighed against the risk of in-stent thrombosis. This remains a topic of discussion; recent reviews show that the duration of dual antiplatelet therapy can be decreased to 3–6 months after percutaneous coronary intervention with drug-eluting stents [16, 17].

The lithotomy position and subsequent pneumoperitoneum increase (left and right) ventricular preload [18], which means an increase in ventricular wall stress and therefore the myocardial oxygen consumption is increased. This can lead to ischemia in patients with coronary artery disease.Alternatively, in patients suffering from heart failure, these changes can lead to acute decompensation. To date, there is no absolute contra-indication or lower limit for the left ventricle ejection fraction for determining a patient eligible for laparoscopic surgery. On the contrary, a recent study concludes that laparoscopy is safe in patients with congestive heart failure, in surgical patients [19].

The management for patients with cardiovascular implantable electronic devices (CIED: ICD/Pacemaker) is not different in robot-assisted operations. Bipolar electrocautery is advised to decrease the likelihood of interaction with the CIED [15].

Consultation by a cardiologist is recommended when (pharmacological) optimization is necessary (i.e.: atrial fibrillation with rapid ventricle response) or further diagnostic evaluation is needed according to the ACC/AHA guideline.

## Pulmonary

During laparoscopy there is an increase in (peak) airway pressures, and a decrease in pulmonary compliance secondary to the increased intra-abdominal pressure (IAP) and due to Trendelenburg positioning [20]. Within minutes after deflation of the pneumoperitoneum, the pressures return to baseline levels. Furthermore, the increased IAP shifts the diaphragm cephalad, resulting in closure of smaller airways leading to atelectasis with a decrease in functional residual capacity. Combined with preferential ventilation of nondependent parts of the lung, the result is a ventilation-perfusion (V/Q) mismatch with a higher degree of intrapulmonary shunting [21]. Even in patients without lung disease the arterial oxygen pressure is significantly decreased during pneumoperitoneum [22].

In patients with severe lung disease, these alterations can be poorly tolerated. Therefore, preoperative pulmonary function testing including arterial blood gas analysis should be performed. For patients with obstructive lung disease, such as COPD or asthma, a consultation with the pulmonologist should be considered for optimization (i.e. corticosteroids and inhaled beta2-sympathomimetic agents) [23].

## Intracranial

Both Trendelenburg positioning and pneumoperitoneum increase the intracranial pressure (ICP) [24–26]. However, the cerebral perfusion pressure remains within the limits of cerebral autoregulation and regional cerebral oxygenation is preserved in patients without intracranial pathology [27]. It has been shown that the proportional relation between $PaCO_2$ and cerebral blood flow remains intact during Trendelenburg positioning and capnoperitoneum: this means that normocapnia should be the target intraoperatively [28].

For patients with intracranial pathology who have a functional shunt, there have been serious concerns about whether creating a pneumoperitoneum is safe and if there should be shunt patency monitoring intraoperatively. Recent literature shows that these patients can undergo laparoscopic operations [29–31], however the use of non-invasive shunt monitoring is still a topic of discussion. Transcranial Doppler monitoring of middle cerebral flow velocity monitoring is suggested by some authors [31], while others recommend routine anesthetic monitoring [29, 30]. We recommend that the anesthesiologist must confirm the functionality of the shunt pre-operative and that these patients should have their surgery performed in hospitals with neurosurgical facilities.

## Intraocular

The intraocular pressure (IOP) is on average 13 mmHg higher at the end of a laparoscopic operation with Trendelenburg positioning. Surgical duration and end-tidal carbon dioxide ($ETCO_2$) measurements are the predictors of this IOP increase [32]. Pneumoperitoneum itself produces only a minimal increase in IOP (up to 3 mmHg) [33]. Prolonged surgery or pre-existing ocular pathology can lead to dangerous intra ocular pressures that risk retinal detachment or periorbital edema [34].

To date, there are no guidelines for monitoring and treating patients with an increased IOP/ glaucoma undergoing surgical procedures while in the Trendelenburg position. In 2016 a case report was published where the authors describe a patient with significant open-angle glaucoma undergoing robotic surgery in whom IOP was monitored (direct measurements were taken by an experienced ophthalmology technician using an applanation tonometer) and successfully treated while maintaining steep Trendelenburg position with acetazolamide and mannitol intravenously during the operation [35]. Therefore a consultation with an ophthalmologist is recommended in patients with (suspected) glaucoma [36]. The anesthesiologist should strive to maintain normocapnia, to prevent a further increase of the IOP.

A recent review based on data from the National Inpatient Sample (NIS) reported that compared with open hysterectomy, the risk of corneal abrasion was increased nearly fourfold with the laparoscopic technique and nearly 6.5-fold with the robotic technique [37]. Several proposed etiologies for perioperative corneal abrasion include exposure, reduced corneal hydration, and chemical or direct mechanical trauma [38]. Corneal or conjunctival edema may also occur from increased central venous pressure and raised intraocular pressure, causing further stress to the eye via direct fluid pressure on the globe or pressure causing the eyes to tend to remain open [38]. Some clinics describe a high incidence of transient postoperative pain in both eyes after robot assisted operations. As a possible cause scleral or corneal edema is proposed [39].

## Renal

The renal function should be determined preoperative by serum creatinine and urea levels, because robot-assisted operations cause a decreased blood flow to the visceral organs. At a pressure of above 10 mmHg, pneumoperitoneum has been shown to produce reduced renal blood flow, renal dysfunction and a transient oliguria [40, 41]. Any decrease in renal function is dependent on preoperative renal function, level of hydration, level of pneumoperitoneum, patient positioning (*reverse* Trendelenburg also worsens renal perfusion), and duration of pneumoperitoneum [42].

## Patient Positioning on the Operating Table: Two Phases

### Phase 1: Patient Positioning for Induction of Anesthesia (Table 79.2)

Prior to positioning of the patient on the operating room table, one must ensure that the appropriate pressure mattress is placed on the table. In our hospital, a specialized mattress with a top layer of memory foam (Premium Sof-Care cushion, Maquet GmBH, Rastatt, Germany) is now routine for robot-assisted surgical procedures. Its use has greatly improved the process of patient positioning from both a time saving and safety perspective. In the past, a vacuum mattress was placed on the operating table from the sacrum to just above the shoulders. Following the removal of air from this mattress, it was shaped to prevent the patient from slipping proximally on the table during Trendelenburg positioning. However, there have been reports and personal communications of alopecia due to pressure effects of the vacuum mattress for prolonged periods of time against the head [43, 44]. As a result, it has been replaced with the aforementioned memory foam mattress.

For induction of anesthesia, the patient lies on the operating table, in a standard supine position, with the head resting on a normal hospital pillow or intubation cushion (Slotted head positioner, Covidien, Mansfield, USA.) which is routinely used in our operating theatres.

**Table 79.2** Patient positioning and protection during robot-assisted gynecological surgery

| Positioning/protection | Reasoning |
|---|---|
| OR mattress with memory foam | Excellent pressure distribution, preventing pressure injuries |
| Disposable surface overlay (foam/paper) | Surface overlay enhances service life of the memory foam |
| IV lines preferably in the lower arms, not near the wrist or elbow joint | The IV lines cannot be inspected during surgery, therefore a location that is the least vulnerable to movement/dislocation should be selected |
| Synthetic cast padding/cotton wool around the arms, extra thick layer around the elbow | Prevention of pressure/nerve injuries, special attention to ulnar groove |
| Legs are moved laterally on movable distal sections of the operating table, so called 'table blades' rather than in classic lithotomy position | The degree of leg elevation is greatly lessened and so also the risk of compartment syndrome |
| Fixation with leg straps | Prevents legs from falling off operating table |
| Positioning of the head on a shoulder supporting head rest with customized metal fixation device | This construction provides good support for the head, neck and shoulders, whilst also preventing the patient from sliding cranially during Trendelenburg positioning |
| Plexiglass shield over the head, making sure that there is space between the plexiglass and the nose of the patient | Prevents surgical equipment/robot arms from compressing the patient's face |
| *Temperature management* | |
| – Oral or nasal pharyngeal temperature probe | Continuous temperature measurement |
| – Forced-air warming blanket | Warm/cool patient as necessary |
| A urinary collection bag is placed hanging from the cranial end of the table | Monitor perioperative urinary output |
| Neuromuscular monitoring device: Train of four monitor, either placed at the hand (ulnar nerve) or at the face (facial nerve) | Monitor level of neuromuscular blockade |

Prior to induction of anesthesia, both arms are placed on arm boards positioned at angles of <90° from the operating table. Standard monitoring equipment is attached to the patient, according to the American society of anesthesia guidelines, 'Standards for basic anesthetic monitoring' [45]. In the past, an arterial line was routinely placed, but gradually as the duration of surgery is shortening, the indication for an arterial line is also lessening. Currently, arterial lines are placed at the discretion of the individual anesthesiologist depending on the overall health status of the patient.

Venous access is obtained and the fluid administration line is lengthened to ensure ease of drug administration during surgery. A second venous line is inserted following induction of anesthesia. One venous line is used for warm fluid administration using a fluid warming device (Hotline Fluid warmer Level 1, Smiths Medical ASD, Inc. Rockland, USA). The other cannula is used for administration of drug infusions. Commonly used infusions are a vasopressor agent, a neuromuscular blocking agent and an opioid infusion. Any bolus dosing of drugs may be administered via the warmed fluid line to avoid inadvertent bolus administration of infusion drugs.

It is standard practice in our operating theatres to perform a 'time out procedure' or surgical safety check list, as recommended by the World Health Organization (WHO) during which special attention is paid to the requirement of careful patient positioning and optimal muscle relaxation during robot-assisted surgery, in addition to the routine questions of importance for all types of surgery [46]. A final check to ensure that all staff are familiar with the process of "undocking' or removing the robotic arms in the event of an emergency also occurs (Table 79.3).

As with anesthesia for all surgical procedures, a variety of anesthetic drug combinations may be used, influenced by patient co-morbidities and likelihood of a difficult intubation. Our preferred technique consists of pre-oxygenation with 100% oxygen, administration of a small bolus of sufentanil or fentanyl, followed by an infusion of

**Table 79.3** Protocol for Emergency undocking of robot during surgery

| | |
|---|---|
| Step 1. Communicate the need to undock to entire theatre team, by clearing stating "EMERGENCY UNDOCK". State reason e.g. cardiac arrest, hemorrhage, equipment malfunction | |
| Step 2. Communicate whether laparoscopic or laparotomy instruments are required | |
| **Member of operation team** | **Role** |
| Robot-assisted operating surgeon | – Place instruments in center of field, ready for removal<br>– Scrub in preparation for surgery |
| Surgical assistant/resident | – Remove instruments/endoscopes from patient<br>– Remove instruments from robot arms<br>– Fold robot arms to resting position<br>– Remove ports if laparotomy<br>– Leave ports in situ if laparoscopy |
| Scrub Nurse | – Remain scrubbed<br>– Prepare instruments for either laparotomy or laparoscopy |
| Circulating nurse | – Move robot tower/cart away from operating table |
| Anesthesiologist | – Return operating table to zero position after surgical instruments removed<br>– Intervene medically as appropriate |
| Anesthetic nurse | – Assist anesthesiologist (call for extra help, contact lab, order blood etc...) |

remifentanil throughout the procedure until approximately 30 min before the end of surgery The advantage of using remifentanil is that patients remain very stable throughout surgery, risk of patient movement is very low and requirement for additional muscle relaxant administration is also reduced. An added benefit is the fast onset and offset time of remifentanil, allowing easy titration during surgery. However, this advantage has to be weighed against the suggested possibility of hyperalgesia and potential opioid tolerance at higher doses in excess of 0.2 µg/kg/min [47]. To avoid this potential risk, our technique utilizes multimodal modes of analgesia with local anesthetic wound infiltration, NMDA receptor antagonists, acetaminophen, non-steroidal anti-inflammatory drugs as well as longer acting opioids towards the end of surgery. During the procedure or in the recovery room, clonidine (1–2 µg/kg) is administered as necessary.

Induction of anesthesia is established with propofol, titrating to loss of consciousness (approximately 1.5–2.5 mg/kg). Subsequently, a muscle relaxant is administered, in the absence of known allergy, our preferred choice is rocuronium. Maintenance of anesthesia is provided with either a propofol infusion (approximately 6–10 mg/kg/h) or an inhalational agent such as Sevoflurane or Isoflurane. To date there is little evidence supporting the use of propofol over inhalational agents for maintenance during robot-assisted surgery, although a study has been published showing less intraocular pressure increase with propofol versus sevoflurane during 30° Trendelenburg position [48]. Further studies are indicated in this area, before any firm conclusion can be made. Another potential advantage of propofol is a lessening of post-operative nausea and vomiting (PONV) [49].

However, in our view, an important advantage for the use of an inhalational agent in such patients is that during robot-assisted surgery, both arms are placed along the patient's side and are not visible to the anesthesiologist. In the event of a propofol line disconnection or displacement of an intravenous cannula into the extravascular space, this would not become apparent until a late stage, risking patient movement, with very serious consequences for the surgical technique and the patient. For this reason, it is standard practice at our center to use an inhalation anesthetic agent for maintenance of anesthesia, with the benefit of continuous measurement of end expiratory inhalational agent concentration.

Anti-emetics are provided depending on patient indication and contra-indications in the form of a low dose of dexamethasone, a 5HT₃ antagonist and a low dose dehydrobenzperidol (0.625 mg) for those with a significant history of PONV. Gynecological robot-assisted operations are associated with a high rate of PONV [50].

An infusion of a neuromuscular blocking agent is administered during the procedure and muscle relaxation is monitored using a train of four device (Tof-Watch ®SX, Organon, Dublin, Ireland). Following intubation of the trachea with a standard cuffed oral endotracheal tube (ETT) and attachment of a cuff manometer, it is important that the ETT is well secured with tape, as the patient is placed in Trendelenburg position during surgery. As a routine, a protective eye gel (Duratears Z (Alcon, Puurs, Belgium) is placed on both eyes followed by taping.

An oral or nasal pharyngeal temperature probe is placed. A gastric tube is passed orally into the stomach to decompress gastric acid and air. As this will be removed at the end of surgery, placement via the nose is not required.

A urinary catheter is placed by the gynecologist under sterile conditions and the urinary collection bag is placed hanging from the cranial end of the table. Due to Trendelenburg positioning, urinary output cannot be reliably measured intraoperatively.

## Phase 2: Patient Positioning for Surgery

Once the induction process of anesthesia is complete, the second phase of patient positioning ahead of the surgical procedure is done. The patient's legs are moved laterally on movable distal sections of the operating table, to allow surgical access (see Fig. 79.2). In the past, the patient's legs were placed in the lithotomy position, raised above the table, however, such a position for several hours with the legs elevated even further during extreme Trendelenburg contributed to the development of compartment syndrome in the lower limbs [51]. With the described leg positioning technique, the degree of leg elevation is greatly lessened and so also the risk of compartment syndrome.

The arms of the patient are placed along the sides of the thorax and abdomen, wrapped in cotton wool/synthetic cast padding (Softban synthetic, BSN Medical GmbH., Hamburg, Germany) (see Fig. 79.2) and secured in position, so that they remain immobile during the procedure. Particular care is taken to ensure that the ulnar nerve is protected and that the IV cannulas and arterial line, if present, are functioning adequately.

Head and shoulder positioning is very important during robot-assisted gynecological procedures. Due to Trendelenburg positioning for long periods, it is essential that the head is carefully positioned on an appropriate cushion and that a system is employed to ensure that the patient does not slip proximally on the operating table. In our hospital, we use a specially designed head, neck and shoulder supporting cushion (Da Vinci Cushion, MediPlac GmbH, Borchen, Germany) that is fixed in place using a metal fixation device (see Fig. 79.3). The soft cushion under the patients head lessens the potential risk of developing localized alopecia.

At this point, it is essential that a careful review of patient positioning is performed. All pressure points need to be checked and additional cotton wool placed where necessary to ensure adequate protection during surgery. Injury to the nerves of both upper and lower limbs have been reported [52]. Once surgery starts, it is very difficult to gain access to the intravenous cannulas and arterial line due to the degree of equipment around the operating table as well as the Trendelenburg positioning, therefore a thorough final check of correct attachment of anesthesia monitoring equipment and venous/arterial line access must be performed before giving the go ahead to commence the surgical procedure.

A warming blanket is now placed over the patient's upper body extending to the level of the xiphisternum and attached to an air blower. A device designed to protect the face of the patient from inadvertent pressure from the robot arms made of plexiglass (local hospital product) (see Fig. 79.3) is then placed over the patient's face, a check that the nose is clear of the plexiglass is performed at regular intervals for the duration of surgery.

Once the anesthesiologist and surgeon are satisfied with patient position, the disinfection

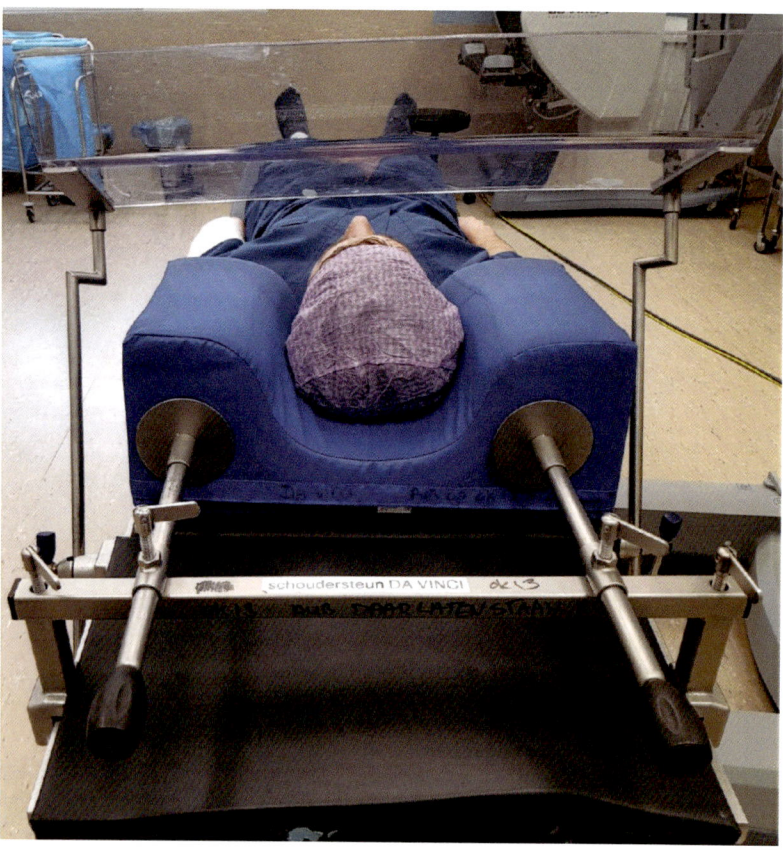

**Fig. 79.3** A specially designed head, neck and shoulder supporting cushion, with a metal fixation device

and surgery can commence. Local anesthetic is injected at the sites of port insertion (ropivicaine 0.75%, 5 ml to each of 4 ports). After the creation of a pneumoperitoneum and port insertions, the patient is placed in Trendelenburg position, with a further check of the head and shoulder position. Unlike during the earlier years of robot-assisted surgery, the amount of Trendelenburg used is no longer extreme; in our hospital a maximum Trendelenburg of 25° is used. Maximum intraperitoneal pressure is limited to 15 mmHg.

## Intra Operative Changes in Physiology

### Hemodynamic

Pneumoperitoneum (IAP limited to 15 mmHg) and Trendelenburg position significantly increase mean arterial pressure and systemic vascular resistance (SVR). However, there are no significant changes in cardiac output or stroke volume [53]. At IAP levels greater than 15 mmHg, venous return decreases as the inferior vena cava and the surrounding collateral vessels are compressed, leading to decreased cardiac output and hypotension [54]. A moderate to low IAP (12 mmHg) is recommended as it limits the decrease in splanchnic perfusion, and consecutive organ dysfunctions will be minimal [40].

Due to the increased SVR, a vasopressor is usually not necessary. Norepinephrine is preferred over phenylephrine, because norepinephrine better maintains the cardiac output and splanchnic perfusion [55]. Special attention is warranted in Trendelenburg position when using invasive blood pressure monitoring that the pressure transducer is positioned at the level of the heart to ensure accurate readings.

In patients with a decreased ventricular function an inotropic agent might be necessary. Both dobutamine and phosphodiesterase type 3 inhibitors (such as enoximone) are possible agents. To date there have not been randomized trials to compare these drugs in patients under general anesthesia.

Maintaining an adequate intravascular volume is important since hypovolemia will exaggerate the decreased venous return during pneumoperitoneum. However, blood loss is significantly lower during robot-assisted gynecological operations as compared to conventional, open procedures [56–58]. Blood loss and urine output should be replaced by crystalloids at first. Furthermore, some authors suggest limiting intravenous fluids to reduce soft-tissue edema of the head and neck from positioning [39]. Bradyarrhythmias, including significant bradycardia, atrioventricular dissociation, nodal rhythm, and asystole can occur. These are the result of vagal stimulation caused by pneumoperitoneum-induced peritoneal stretch, stimulation of the fallopian tube during electrocauterization, or carbon dioxide embolization [59]. Tachyarrhythmias can occur because of increased concentrations of carbon dioxide and catecholamines [21]. The treatment of these arrhythmias is primarily to remove the stimulus (i.e. desufflation of the pneumoperitoneum), rather than pharmacological treatment.

## Ventilation

Pulmonary compliance is decreased during pneumoperitoneum and Trendelenburg positioning, therefore the ventilation strategy is very important. Recent studies prefer pressure controlled ventilation over volume controlled ventilation, because of a lower peak airway pressure, a greater dynamic compliance and a better-preserved ventilation-perfusion matching for the same levels of minute ventilation [60, 61].

A tidal volume of 6–8 ml/kg and a positive end-expiratory pressure of 4–7 $cmH_2O$ are recommended for the prevention of atelectasis, and maximal airway pressure should be kept under 35 $cmH_2O$ [62, 63]. A prolonged inspiratory time has a beneficial effect on both oxygenation as carbon dioxide elimination: instead of the conventional I:E ratio of 1:2, this can be altered to 1:1 or even 2:1 provided there is sufficient time for expiration (no air trapping) [64].

After Trendelenburg positioning and pneumoperitoneum the distance from the vocal cord to the carina is reduced by about 1 cm compared to pre-positioning [65]. Therefore, confirmation of the tracheal tube position is recommended after positioning because the displacement of the tracheal tube may result in endobronchial intubation.

## Emergence from Anesthesia

At the end of surgery, following reversal of pneumoperitoneum and removal of the robotic arms and surgical ports, the operating table is returned to the neutral position. During the initial years of robot-assisted surgery, it was usual to maintain anesthesia for a period of time, up to 2 h after the end of surgery, with the patient in a head up position. The theory was to allow any edema of the head and neck, in particular edema of the airway, to resolve prior to removing the endotracheal tube. Indication for early reintubation as a result of airway edema has been reported [66]. Various recommendations such as performing a leak test have been suggested, although supporting evidence is weak, with low reported positive predictive value and sensitivity scores [67].

Currently, it is no longer standard practice at our institution to mandate a period of head elevation for all robot-assisted surgery patients prior to extubation and instead, a decision is taken on an individual patient basis. Patients who appear to have developed head and facial edema, in particular ocular edema are placed head up and ventilated until the edema is resolved to a satisfactory level.

All patients have the level of residual muscle relaxation measured with a train of four device and where indicated an antagonist such as neostigmine or sugammadex is administered. The ETT is removed as per standard guidelines for extubation and patients remain in the recovery room according to the same rules as for all general anesthesia patients; i.e. stable vital signs including normothermia, awake, pain score ≤4 and no nausea or vomiting.

## Postoperative Analgesia

A standard protocol for postoperative analgesia includes acetaminophen, NSAID (in the absence of contraindications) and a delayed release oral opioid, in addition to an immediate release oral opioid as escape analgesia. In our experience, such a regime maintains satisfactory levels of pain control. Occasionally, when oral opioids are insufficient, a patient controlled analgesia (PCA) device administering an opioid is used. Residual gas can be a prominent cause of post-laparoscopy pain [68].

The role of a transversus abdominis plane (TAP) block after robot-assisted operations is still a subject of discussion: recent randomized controlled trials show conflicting results [69, 70]. Conversion rates for robot-assisted hysterectomy are approximately 5% [71, 72], while for robot-assisted sacrocolpopexy the conversion rate to is less than 1% [73]. Since the post-operative narcotics requirement is significantly higher after open surgery, these patients may receive a PCA device [74]. Epidural analgesia is not routinely used for laparoscopic gynecological procedures [75], because of the good alternative analgesics, combined with the reduced length of hospital stay and enhanced recovery programs [76].

## Intraoperative Emergencies

Intraoperative emergencies are rare during robot-assisted gynecological operations, but when they do happen they represent a major challenge to the anesthesiologist and gynecologist because of the limited access to the patient. These major events lead to the cessation of the surgical procedure and are reason for triggering the 'emergency undocking procedure'. We describe the most life threatening emergencies, followed by an emergency undocking protocol.

## Massive Intraoperative Hemorrhage

Various studies have shown that robot-assisted surgery is associated with less blood loss than either open or traditional laparoscopic techniques [28]. Hemorrhage during robot-assisted surgery is not a common occurrence, however when it does occur there are a number of significant factors which must be taken into account. Due to both the head down positioning and the pneumoperitoneum, a source of bleeding can be masked until a late stage in the surgery. This has been highlighted in the literature, where a case of arterial bleeding during robot-assisted surgery was masked until cessation of abdominal insufflation and return of the patient to the neutral position [77]. The Trendelenburg positioning resulted in adequate blood pressure measurements and the increased intraabdominal pressure likely suppressed the hemorrhage. Massive hemorrhage during robot-assisted surgery triggers the undocking of the robot and usually conversion to an open procedure. Anesthesiologists should be alert to the possibility of operative bleeding right up until the very end of the procedure and any unexpected variations in blood pressure should trigger measurement of a hemoglobin level and clear communication to the operative gynecologist to check for occult bleeding.

## Venous Gas Embolism

Venous gas embolism (VGE) can occur during pneumoperitoneum: direct intravascular gas insufflation, a tear in an abdominal wall or a damaged peritoneum vessel can lead to VGE [21]. It has been reported that up to 100% of the patients undergoing a laparoscopic hysterectomy had intraoperative VGE's (determined by transesophageal echocardiography), although none of these events caused hemodynamic instability or electrocardiogram changes at the time of VGE occurrence [78]. A severe VGE is characterized by a sudden increase of end-tidal $CO_2$, followed by a rapid decrease due to cardiovascular collapse and reduction of pulmonary blood flow. Other signs include tachycardia, hypotension, diminished breath sounds in a specific lung field on auscultation, cyanosis, and a classic cardiac murmur (mill-wheel murmur) [21, 79].

When a VGE is suspected, insufflation of $CO_2$ should be stopped immediately and pneumoperitoneum must be released. Subsequent emergency undocking of the robot must be performed (Table 79.3), while the patient is ventilated with 100% oxygen. After undocking, patients should be turned to the left lateral decubitus with a head-down position. Placement of a central venous line to aspirate the VGE should be considered [21, 39].

## Pneumothorax

Pneumothorax is a known complication of laparoscopic abdominal surgery [80], which can occur when $CO_2$ traverses into the thorax through a tear in the visceral peritoneum or by spontaneous rupture of preexisting emphysematous bulla. The reported incidence of pneumothorax during laparoscopy is 0.01–0.4% [81], however frequently a pneumothorax during laparoscopy is asymptomatic [82]. Symptoms include increased peak airway pressures, decreased oxygen saturation and, in severe cases, significant hypotension and cardiac arrest. The treatment depends on the severity of the situation, from conservative treatment with close observation to chest tube placement [80]. Case reports have been published describing massive subcutaneous emphysema and pneumomediastinum after robotic sacrocolpopexy. Subcutaneous emphysema is recognized by subcutaneous crackles throughout the upper chest and neck, this resolves generally within 1 week after surgery and does not cause airway obstruction [83]. One case report described the symptoms of a pneumomediastinum to include shortness of breath, tachycardia, tachypnea and increased oxygen requirement. Treatment was supportive (while the patient was admitted to the intensive care) and the pneumomediastinum resolved one day after surgery [84].

## Venous Thromboembolism

Patients undergoing major general and gynecological surgery have a risk of 15–40% of developing postoperative venous thromboembolism (VTE) in the absence of thromboprophylaxis [85]. This can lead to very serious consequences: the most severe being a fatal pulmonary embolism, which is known to be the most preventable cause of hospital death [86]. Prevention strategies vary from mechanical prophylaxis (including sequential compression devices and compression hose) to pharmacological prophylaxis with blood thinners such as heparin and low molecular–weight heparin [87].

However, a recent large cohort study compared mechanical prophylaxis (per hospital policy) with combined (mechanical and pharmacologic prophylaxis). The rate of VTE was 0.35% (5/1413), which did not significantly differ among both groups. All women underwent robotic or laparoscopic hysterectomy for endometrial carcinoma or complex hyperplasia with atypia [88]. Indeed, another recent cohort study concluded that women undergoing minimally invasive surgery had a lower venous thromboembolism incidence (0.7%, n = 47) than women undergoing open surgery (2.2%, n = 80) ($P < 0.001$) [89].

In light of the latter studies, the debate is ongoing as to whether mechanical prophylaxis is sufficient for women undergoing minimal invasive (robotic) surgery, since the risk for post operative VTE is significantly lower compared to open surgery.

## Robotic Malfunction

A comprehensive analysis of the adverse events reported to the publicly available MAUDE database (maintained by the U.S. Food and Drug Administration) included data of over 1.75 million robotic procedures performed in the United States across various surgical specialties. During 2007–2013, the estimated rate of deaths has been 5.7 per 100,000 procedures in gynecology, urology, and general surgeries. The rate of injuries and procedure conversions away from robot-assisted, have been 71.5 and 29.2 per 100,000 procedures respectively. Major part of the above-mentioned reports were due to 'device and instrument malfunctions', such as falling of burnt/broken pieces of instruments into the patient, electrical arcing of instruments, unintended operation of instruments, system errors and video/imaging problems [90]. From the anesthesiologist's point of view, we recommend active participation in crew resource management training, frequent performance of the 'emergency undocking' protocol simulation and to report (near) accidents to the appropriate national organization.

## Emergency Undocking Protocol for Da Vinci® Robot

It is essential that there is a clear protocol in place in the event of an emergency situation developing which requires the immediate stopping of robot-assisted surgery, removal of the surgical arms/ports and return of the patient to the supine position for further medical management. All theatre staff should be familiar with the details of such a protocol and the steps should be repeated with the entire team at regular intervals. One possibility is to briefly run through the steps during the 'time out' procedure prior to commencement of surgery. An important part of the undocking procedure is a clear knowledge of individual roles for each member of the theatre team.

Various hospitals have developed their own protocols in keeping with local experience, staffing and in theatre logistics [91]. Indeed simulation has been used to ensure practice of the undocking procedure [92]. A sample protocol is shown in Table 79.3. Of course not all situations in which robotic surgery is stopped are emergencies. In certain situations, for technical reasons or increasing difficulty with lung ventilation, a decision is made to semi electively convert to either an open or laparoscopic procedure. In these non-immediately life-threatening circumstances, undocking of the robotic equipment is also required but not with the same degree of haste, although the steps of the procedure are essentially the same.

## Future of Robot-Assisted Surgery

The future of robot-assisted surgery appears to be exciting. New applications for robot-assisted surgery are published at an increasing rate. It is likely that as equipment improves and surgical teaching and skills progress, that learning curves will shorten and operating times will reduce significantly. New developments such as single port robot-assisted surgery will further improve the quality, leading to improved cosmetic effects and less pain for patients. From an anesthesia point of view, as the robot technology advances and provided that evidence based medicine supports its benefits, it is likely that older and sicker patients will undergo robot-assisted surgery. This will present new challenges for anesthesiologists in terms of ventilation and cardiovascular support. Perhaps most significantly from the point of view of anesthesia, as communication technology further improves allowing high speed, reliable transfer of information, the prospect of surgery being performed by a surgeon based off-site is highly probable, bringing with it new challenges for the anesthesiologist who may no longer have the operating surgeon within arm's length.

## References

1. Ng AT, Tam PC. Current status of robot-assisted surgery. Hong Kong Med J. 2014;20:241–50.
2. Pugin F, Bucher P, Morel P. History of robotic surgery: from AESOP(R) and ZEUS(R) to da Vinci(R). J Visc Surg. 2011;148:e3–8.
3. Territo A, Mottrie A, Abaza R, et al. Robotic kidney transplantation: current status and future perspectives. Minerva Urol Nefrol. 2016;69(1):5–13.
4. Chauvet D, Hans S, Missistrano A, Rebours C, Bakkouri WE, Lot G. Transoral robotic surgery for sellar tumors: first clinical study. J Neurosurg. 2016;127(4):941–8.
5. Zhao Y, Jiao W, Ren X, et al. Left lower lobe sleeve lobectomy for lung cancer using the Da Vinci surgical system. J Cardiothorac Surg. 2016;11:59.
6. Bellia A, Vitale SG, Lagana AS, et al. Feasibility and surgical outcomes of conventional and robot-assisted laparoscopy for early-stage ovarian cancer: a retrospective, multicenter analysis. Arch Gynecol Obstet. 2016;294:615–22.

7. Krill LS, Bristow RE. Robotic surgery: gynecologic oncology. Cancer J. 2013;19:167–76.
8. Lenihan JP Jr. Navigating credentialing, privileging, and learning curves in robotics with an evidence and experienced-based approach. Clin Obstet Gynecol. 2011;54:382–90.
9. Himpens J, Leman G, Cadiere GB. Telesurgical laparoscopic cholecystectomy. Surg Endosc. 1998;12:1091.
10. Medical Robotic Systems Market (Surgical Robots, Non-Invasive Radiosurgery Robotic Systems, Prosthetics and Exoskeletons, Assistive and Rehabilitation Robots, Non-Medical Robotics in Hospitals and Emergency Response Robotic Systems) - Global Industry Analysis, Size, Share, Growth, Trends and Forecast 2012–2018. 2013. http://www.transparencymarketresearch.com/medical-robotic-systems.html. Accessed May 2017.
11. Steenwyk B, Lyerly R 3rd. Advancements in robotic-assisted thoracic surgery. Anesthesiol Clin. 2012;30:699–708.
12. Hu JC, Gu X, Lipsitz SR, et al. Comparative effectiveness of minimally invasive vs open radical prostatectomy. JAMA. 2009;302:1557–64.
13. Lim PC, Kang E, Park DH. Learning curve and surgical outcome for robotic-assisted hysterectomy with lymphadenectomy: case-matched controlled comparison with laparoscopy and laparotomy for treatment of endometrial cancer. J Minim Invasive Gynecol. 2010;17:739–48.
14. Avondstondt AM, Wallenstein M, D'Adamo CR, Ehsanipoor RM. Change in cost after 5 years of experience with robotic-assisted hysterectomy for the treatment of endometrial cancer. J Robot Surg. 2017. https://doi.org/10.1007/s11701-017-0700-6.
15. Fleisher LA, Fleischmann KE, Auerbach AD, et al. 2014 ACC/AHA guideline on perioperative cardiovascular evaluation and management of patients undergoing noncardiac surgery: a report of the American College of Cardiology/American Heart Association Task Force on practice guidelines. J Am Coll Cardiol. 2014;64:e77–137.
16. Montalescot G, Sabatine MS. Oral dual antiplatelet therapy: what have we learnt from recent trials? Eur Heart J. 2016;37:344–52.
17. Evidence Review Committee M, Bittl JA, Baber U, Bradley SM, Wijeysundera DN. Duration of dual antiplatelet therapy: a systematic review for the 2016 ACC/AHA guideline focused update on duration of dual antiplatelet therapy in patients with coronary artery disease: a report of the American College of Cardiology/American Heart Association Task Force on Clinical Practice Guidelines. Circulation. 2016;134:e156–78.
18. Rist M, Hemmerling TM, Rauh R, Siebzehnrubl E, Jacobi KE. Influence of pneumoperitoneum and patient positioning on preload and splanchnic blood volume in laparoscopic surgery of the lower abdomen. J Clin Anesth. 2001;13:244–9.
19. Speicher PJ, Ganapathi AM, Englum BR, Vaslef SN. Laparoscopy is safe among patients with congestive heart failure undergoing general surgery procedures. Surgery. 2014;156:371–8.
20. Rauh R, Hemmerling TM, Rist M, Jacobi KE. Influence of pneumoperitoneum and patient positioning on respiratory system compliance. J Clin Anesth. 2001;13(5):361.
21. Gerges FJ, Kanazi GE, Jabbour-Khoury SI. Anesthesia for laparoscopy: a review. J Clin Anesth. 2006;18:67–78.
22. Salihoglu Z, Demiroluk S, Baca B, Ayan F, Kara H. Effects of pneumoperitoneum and positioning on respiratory mechanics in chronic obstructive pulmonary disease patients during Nissen fundoplication. Surg Laparosc Endosc Percutan Tech. 2008;18:437–40.
23. Silvanus MT, Groeben H, Peters J. Corticosteroids and inhaled salbutamol in patients with reversible airway obstruction markedly decrease the incidence of bronchospasm after tracheal intubation. Anesthesiology. 2004;100:1052–7.
24. Halverson A, Buchanan R, Jacobs L, et al. Evaluation of mechanism of increased intracranial pressure with insufflation. Surg Endosc. 1998;12:266–9.
25. Irgau I, Koyfman Y, Tikellis JI. Elective intraoperative intracranial pressure monitoring during laparoscopic cholecystectomy. Arch Surg. 1995;130:1011–3.
26. Mavrocordatos P, Bissonnette B, Ravussin P. Effects of neck position and head elevation on intracranial pressure in anaesthetized neurosurgical patients: preliminary results. J Neurosurg Anesthesiol. 2000;12:10–4.
27. Kalmar AF, Foubert L, Hendrickx JF, et al. Influence of steep Trendelenburg position and CO(2) pneumoperitoneum on cardiovascular, cerebrovascular, and respiratory homeostasis during robotic prostatectomy. Br J Anaesth. 2010;104:433–9.
28. Park EY, Koo BN, Min KT, Nam SH. The effect of pneumoperitoneum in the steep Trendelenburg position on cerebral oxygenation. Acta Anaesthesiol Scand. 2009;53:895–9.
29. Jackman SV, Weingart JD, Kinsman SL, Docimo SG. Laparoscopic surgery in patients with ventriculoperitoneal shunts: safety and monitoring. J Urol. 2000;164(4):1352.
30. Sankpal R, Chandavarkar A, Chandavarkar M. Safety of laparoscopy in ventriculoperitoneal shunt patients. J Gynecol Endosc Surg. 2011;2:91–3.
31. Staikou C, Tsaroucha A, Mani A, Fassoulaki A. Transcranial Doppler monitoring of middle cerebral flow velocity in a patient with a ventriculoperitoneal shunt undergoing laparoscopy. J Clin Monit Comput. 2012;26:487–9.
32. Awad H, Santilli S, Ohr M, et al. The effects of steep trendelenburg positioning on intraocular pressure during robotic radical prostatectomy. Anesth Analg. 2009;109:473–8.
33. Adisa AO, Onakpoya OH, Adenekan AT, Awe OO. Intraocular pressure changes with positioning during laparoscopy. JSLS. 2016;20(4):e2016.00078.

34. Berger JS, Taghreed A, Dayo L, Paul D. Anesthetic considerations for robot-assisted gynecologic and urology surgery. J Anesthe Clinic Res. 2013;4:8.
35. Lee M, Dallas R, Daniel C, Cotter F. Intraoperative management of increased intraocular pressure in a patient with glaucoma undergoing robotic prostatectomy in the trendelenburg position. A A Case Rep. 2016;6:19–21.
36. Borahay MA, Patel PR, Walsh TM, et al. Intraocular pressure and steep Trendelenburg during minimally invasive gynecologic surgery: is there a risk? J Minim Invasive Gynecol. 2013;20:819–24.
37. Sampat A, Parakati I, Kunnavakkam R, et al. Corneal abrasion in hysterectomy and prostatectomy: role of laparoscopic and robotic assistance. Anesthesiology. 2015;122:994–1001.
38. Roth S, Thisted RA, Erickson JP, Black S, Schreider BD. Eye injuries after nonocular surgery. A study of 60,965 anesthetics from 1988 to 1992. Anesthesiology. 1996;85:1020–7.
39. Awad H, Walker CM, Shaikh M, Dimitrova GT, Abaza R, O'Hara J. Anesthetic considerations for robotic prostatectomy: a review of the literature. J Clin Anesth. 2012;24:494–504.
40. Gutt CN, Oniu T, Mehrabi A, et al. Circulatory and respiratory complications of carbon dioxide insufflation. Dig Surg. 2004;21:95–105.
41. Wiesenthal JD, Fazio LM, Perks AE, et al. Effect of pneumoperitoneum on renal tissue oxygenation and blood flow in a rat model. Urology. 2011;77:1508 e9–15.
42. Demyttenaere S, Feldman LS, Fried GM. Effect of pneumoperitoneum on renal perfusion and function: a systematic review. Surg Endosc. 2007;21:152–60.
43. Bagaria M, Luck AM. Postoperative (pressure) alopecia following sacrocolpopexy. J Robot Surg. 2015;9:149–51.
44. Gollapalli L, Papapetrou P, Gupta D, Fuleihan SF. Post-operative alopecia after robotic surgery in steep Trendelenburg position: a restated observation of pressure alopecia. Middle East J Anaesthesiol. 2013;22:343–5.
45. Standards for Basic Anesthetic Monitoring. 2010. http://www.asahq.org/~/media/Sites/ASAHQ/Files/Public/Resources/standards-guidelines/standards-for-basic-anesthetic-monitoring.pdf. Accessed May 2017.
46. Patient Safety. http://www.who.int/patientsafety/safesurgery/en/. Accessed May 2017.
47. Yu EH, Tran DH, Lam SW, Irwin MG. Remifentanil tolerance and hyperalgesia: short-term gain, long-term pain? Anaesthesia. 2016;71:1347–62.
48. Yoo YC, Shin S, Choi EK, Kim CY, Choi YD, Bai SJ. Increase in intraocular pressure is less with propofol than with sevoflurane during laparoscopic surgery in the steep Trendelenburg position. Can J Anaesth. 2014;61:322–9.
49. Yoo YC, Bai SJ, Lee KY, Shin S, Choi EK, Lee JW. Total intravenous anesthesia with propofol reduces postoperative nausea and vomiting in patients undergoing robot-assisted laparoscopic radical prostatectomy: a prospective randomized trial. Yonsei Med J. 2012;53:1197–202.
50. Turner TB, Habib AS, Broadwater G, et al. Postoperative pain scores and narcotic use in robotic-assisted versus laparoscopic hysterectomy for endometrial cancer staging. J Minim Invasive Gynecol. 2015;22:1004–10.
51. Pridgeon S, Bishop CV, Adshead J. Lower limb compartment syndrome as a complication of robot-assisted radical prostatectomy: the UK experience. BJU Int. 2013;112:485–8.
52. Wen T, Deibert CM, Siringo FS, Spencer BA. Positioning-related complications of minimally invasive radical prostatectomies. J Endourol. 2014;28:660–7.
53. Falabella A, Moore-Jeffries E, Sullivan MJ, Nelson R, Lew M. Cardiac function during steep Trendelenburg position and CO2 pneumoperitoneum for robotic-assisted prostatectomy: a trans-oesophageal Doppler probe study. Int J Med Robot. 2007;3:312–5.
54. Odeberg S, Ljungqvist O, Svenberg T, et al. Haemodynamic effects of pneumoperitoneum and the influence of posture during anaesthesia for laparoscopic surgery. Acta Anaesthesiol Scand. 1994;38:276–83.
55. Mets B. Should norepinephrine, rather than phenylephrine, be considered the primary vasopressor in anesthetic practice? Anesth Analg. 2016;122:1707–14.
56. Ko EM, Muto MG, Berkowitz RS, Feltmate CM. Robotic versus open radical hysterectomy: a comparative study at a single institution. Gynecol Oncol. 2008;111:425–30.
57. Sert BM, Boggess JF, Ahmad S, et al. Robot-assisted versus open radical hysterectomy: a multi-institutional experience for early-stage cervical cancer. Eur J Surg Oncol. 2016;42:513–22.
58. Wallin E, Floter Radestad A, Falconer H. Introduction of robot-assisted radical hysterectomy for early stage cervical cancer: impact on complications, costs and oncologic outcome. Acta Obstet Gynecol Scand. 2017;96:536–42.
59. Sprung J, Abdelmalak B, Schoenwald PK. Recurrent complete heart block in a healthy patient during laparoscopic electrocauterization of the Fallopian tube. Anesthesiology. 1998;88:1401–3.
60. Choi EM, Na S, Choi SH, An J, Rha KH, Oh YJ. Comparison of volume-controlled and pressure-controlled ventilation in steep Trendelenburg position for robot-assisted laparoscopic radical prostatectomy. J Clin Anesth. 2011;23:183–8.
61. Jaju R, Jaju PB, Dubey M, Mohammad S, Bhargava AK. Comparison of volume controlled ventilation and pressure controlled ventilation in patients undergoing robot-assisted pelvic surgeries: an open-label trial. Indian J Anaesth. 2017;61:17–23.
62. Gupta K, Mehta Y, Sarin Jolly A, Khanna S. Anaesthesia for robotic gynaecological surgery. Anaesth Intensive Care. 2012;40:614–21.

63. Lee JR. Anesthetic considerations for robotic surgery. Korean J Anesthesiol. 2014;66:3–11.
64. Kim WH, Hahm TS, Kim JA, et al. Prolonged inspiratory time produces better gas exchange in patients undergoing laparoscopic surgery: a randomised trial. Acta Anaesthesiol Scand. 2013;57:613–22.
65. Chang CH, Lee HK, Nam SH. The displacement of the tracheal tube during robot-assisted radical prostatectomy. Eur J Anaesthesiol. 2010;27:478–80.
66. Phong SV, Koh LK. Anaesthesia for robotic-assisted radical prostatectomy: considerations for laparoscopy in the Trendelenburg position. Anaesth Intensive Care. 2007;35:281–5.
67. Mikaeili H, Yazdchi M, Tarzamni MK, Ansarin K, Ghasemzadeh M. Laryngeal ultrasonography versus cuff leak test in predicting postextubation stridor. J Cardiovasc Thorac Res. 2014;6:25–8.
68. Jackson SA, Laurence AS, Hill JC. Does postlaparoscopy pain relate to residual carbon dioxide? Anaesthesia. 1996;51:485–7.
69. Torup H, Bogeskov M, Hansen EG, et al. Transversus abdominis plane (TAP) block after robot-assisted laparoscopic hysterectomy: a randomised clinical trial. Acta Anaesthesiol Scand. 2015;59:928–35.
70. Hutchins J, Delaney D, Vogel RI, et al. Ultrasound guided subcostal transversus abdominis plane (TAP) infiltration with liposomal bupivacaine for patients undergoing robotic assisted hysterectomy: a prospective randomized controlled study. Gynecol Oncol. 2015;138:609–13.
71. Walters Haygood CL, Fauci JM, Huddleston-Colburn MK, Huh WK, Straughn JM. Outcomes of gynecologic oncology patients undergoing robotic-assisted laparoscopic procedures in a university setting. J Robot Surg. 2014;8:207–11.
72. Gaia G, Holloway RW, Santoro L, Ahmad S, Di Silverio E, Spinillo A. Robotic-assisted hysterectomy for endometrial cancer compared with traditional laparoscopic and laparotomy approaches: a systematic review. Obstet Gynecol. 2010;116:1422–31.
73. Serati M, Bogani G, Sorice P, et al. Robot-assisted sacrocolpopexy for pelvic organ prolapse: a systematic review and meta-analysis of comparative studies. Eur Urol. 2014;66:303–18.
74. Fleming ND, Havrilesky LJ, Valea FA, et al. Analgesic and antiemetic needs following minimally invasive vs open staging for endometrial cancer. Am J Obstet Gynecol. 2011;204:65 e1–6.
75. Baker J, Janda M, Belavy D, Obermair A. Differences in epidural and analgesic use in patients with apparent stage I endometrial cancer treated by open versus laparoscopic surgery: results from the randomised LACE trial. Minim Invasive Surg. 2013;2013(764329)
76. Rawal N. Epidural technique for postoperative pain: gold standard no more? Reg Anesth Pain Med. 2012;37:310–7.
77. Nakano S, Nakahira J, Sawai T, Kadono N, Minami T. Unexpected hemorrhage during robot-assisted laparoscopic prostatectomy: a case report. J Med Case Rep. 2016;10:240.
78. Kim CS, Kim JY, Kwon JY, et al. Venous air embolism during total laparoscopic hysterectomy: comparison to total abdominal hysterectomy. Anesthesiology. 2009;111:50–4.
79. Kaye AD, Vadivelu N, Ahuja N, Mitra S, Silasi D, Urman RD. Anesthetic considerations in robotic-assisted gynecologic surgery. Ochsner J. 2013;13:517–24.
80. Joshi GP. Complications of laparoscopy. Anesthesiol Clin North Am. 2001;19:89–105.
81. Raveendran R, Prabu HN, Ninan S, Darmalingam S. Fast-track management of pneumothorax in laparoscopic surgery. Indian J Anaesth. 2011;55:91–2.
82. Ludemann R, Krysztopik R, Jamieson GG, Watson DI. Pneumothorax during laparoscopy. Surg Endosc. 2003;17:1985–9.
83. Celik H, Cremins A, Jones KA, Harmanli O. Massive subcutaneous emphysema in robotic sacrocolpopexy. JSLS. 2013;17:245–8.
84. Crawford NM, Pathi SD, Corton MM. Pneumomediastinum after robotic sacrocolpopexy. Female Pelvic Med Reconstr Surg. 2014;20:56–8.
85. Geerts WH, Bergqvist D, Pineo GF, et al. Prevention of venous thromboembolism: American College of Chest Physicians Evidence-Based Clinical Practice Guidelines (8th Edition). Chest. 2008;133:381S–453S.
86. Horlander KT, Mannino DM, Leeper KV. Pulmonary embolism mortality in the United States, 1979-1998: an analysis using multiple-cause mortality data. Arch Intern Med. 2003;163:1711–7.
87. Mueller MG, Pilecki MA, Catanzarite T, Jain U, Kim JY, Kenton K. Venous thromboembolism in reconstructive pelvic surgery. Am J Obstet Gynecol. 2014;211, 552 e1:–6.
88. Freeman AH, Barrie A, Lyon L, et al. Venous thromboembolism following minimally invasive surgery among women with endometrial cancer. Gynecol Oncol. 2016;142:267–72.
89. Barber EL, Gehrig PA, Clarke-Pearson DL. Venous thromboembolism in minimally invasive compared with open hysterectomy for endometrial cancer. Obstet Gynecol. 2016;128:121–6.
90. Alemzadeh H, Raman J, Leveson N, Kalbarczyk Z, Iyer RK. Adverse events in robotic surgery: a retrospective study of 14 years of FDA data. PLoS One. 2016;11:e0151470.
91. O'Sullivan OE, O'Sullivan S, Hewitt M, O'Reilly BA. Da Vinci robot emergency undocking protocol. J Robot Surg. 2016;10(3):251.
92. Huser AS, Muller D, Brunkhorst V, et al. Simulated life-threatening emergency during robot-assisted surgery. J Endourol. 2014;28:717–21.

# Anesthesia Issues in Geriatrics

Nalini Kotekar, Anshul Shenkar, and Adarsh A. Hegde

## Introduction

Anesthesia has a pivotal role in any hospital setup and also the ability to influence the outcome for patients with regard to surgery, trauma, intensive care, interventional cardiology, interventional radiology and pain and palliative care. As the specialty of anesthesiology evolves further, the safety index continues to improve and justifiably so because the future generation is going to anaesthetise increasingly older and sicker patients.

The geriatric population is rapidly accelerating world over, from 461 million people over 65 years of age in 2004 to an estimated 2 billion people over 65 years in 2050 [1], which has profound implication for delivering health care and social support system for the elderly. As humans live longer, a substantial percentage of them are potential candidates for major surgery. Around one third of the operations in United States (US) are performed on patients over 65 years of age with 55% of them undergoing at least one surgery. The heterogeneity in geriatric patients is so tremendous that evaluation of this population remains a challenging task with the need to individualise each one of them.

Age related changes in the organ function, physiology, and pharmacology superimposed on pre-existing comorbidities and medications which are inherent in the elderly make the anaesthetic management more complex and complicated as the likelihood of surgeries increase with age.

The severity of the associated disease tends to reduce the functional reserves which can be further detrimental in proportion to the urgency and intricacy of the procedure. Basal organ functions may be sufficient to allow the elderly to meet their resting demands but become inadequate in coping with the stress of anesthesia and surgery. However with advancement in the medical field, it is rare that patients are denied treatment or surgery because of their chronological age. The anaesthesiologist is required to integrate an often extensive medical history with the presenting surgical illness. A sound knowledge of geriatric physiology, pathophysiology and their anaesthetic implications is essential to maximize good outcomes (Table 80.1).

N. Kotekar (✉)
Department of Anesthesiology, Critical Care and Pain Medicine, JSS Medical College, Mysore, India

A. Shenkar, M.B.B.S.
Department of Anesthesiology and Critical Care, A.J. Medical College and Research Centre, Mangalore, India

A. A. Hegde, M.B.B.S.
Department of Anesthesiology, Critical Care and Pain Medicine, JSS Medical College and Hospital, Mysore, India

**Table 80.1** Age related pathophysiological changes

| |
|---|
| 1. Decreased end organ reserve |
| 2. Decreased functional capacity |
| 3. Increased imbalance of homeostatic mechanisms |
| 4. Increased incidence of pathologic processes |

## Physiological Effects of Aging

### Cardiovascular Aging

Cardiovascular disease, predominantly coronary artery disease, hypertension and congestive heart failure rises exponentially with age [1]. The physiological changes that occur in the cardiovascular system with aging results in a lower cardiovascular reserve and also worsens the outcome of disease (Tables 80.1 and 80.2). For example, elderly patients are not only more likely to experience myocardial infarction, they are also more at risk to develop heart failure as a consequence of myocardial infarction than their younger counterparts [2]. Furthermore, elderly patients are also more likely to die from myocardial infarction, develop cardiac arrest, papillary muscle rupture, acquired ventricular septal defect and free wall rupture [2] (Table 80.3).

The age related changes induced within the arteries, veins and myocardium are the same i.e., stiffening, thickening, dilation or enlargement and endothelial or myocardial dysfunction [3].

### Vascular Aging and Stiffening

Aging of the vascular system results in vascular stiffness and a predisposition to atherosclerosis. Vascular stiffness is caused by increased collagen, decreased elastin, glycosylation of proteins,

**Table 80.2** Physiological changes in CVS with aging

| |
|---|
| • Arterial wall thickening, stiffening and decreased compliance |
| • Left ventricular and atrial hypertrophy |
| • Sclerosis of atrial and mitral valves |
| • Decreased beta adrenergic response |
| • Decreased baroreceptor sensitivity |
| • Decreased sinoatrial node automaticity |
| • Diastolic dysfunction |

**Table 80.3** Cardiac pathology in geriatrics

| |
|---|
| • Coronary artery disease |
| • Congestive heart failure |
| • Refractory arrhythmias |
| • Increased blood pressure |
| • Postural hypotension |
| • Valvular heart disease |

free radical damage, calcification and chronic mechanical stress. Atherosclerosis contributes to several age-related diseases such as stroke, coronary artery disease and peripheral vascular disease as a result of arterial occlusion. Age-related arterial endothelial dysfunction promotes atherosclerosis and shifts the endothelium to a more vasoconstricted, pro-coagulant, proliferative and pro-inflammatory state [4, 5] (Fig. 80.1) Atherosclerosis and arteriosclerosis are inflammatory processes. Increased levels of C-reactive proteins, erythrocyte sedimentation rates and an up-regulated range of pro-inflammatory cytokines suggest an increased inflammatory propensity in the elderly. Release of nitric oxide from the endothelial layer has vaso-protective and cardio-protective properties by inhibiting platelet aggregation and inflammatory cell adhesion to endothelial cells. Aging induces an increase in reactive oxygen species within the heart and vasculature which in turn alters the production of nitric oxide, thereby impairing the flow in the microvasculature and increasing chances of organ dysfunction.

Aging also affects the vasculature of small vessels, particularly in the cerebral circulation [6]. Perivascular fibrosis, replacement of vascular smooth muscle cells by fibro-hyaline material and generalized small vessel atrophy is common in the aged. This leads to derangement in microcirculatory controls and predisposes the elderly to ischemic and neurological events. These small vessel changes are also closely related to the development of Alzheimer's, Parkinson's and other neurodegenerative diseases [7, 8].

### Systemic Blood Pressure

A healthy aorta expands during systole and relaxes during diastole; this cyclical repetition propels blood distally, thus maintaining forward flow. In the aged, the stiffer aorta is responsible for higher velocity of pulse wave to travel to the periphery and this reflects back to the aortic root earlier than normal while the ventricle is still in systole and ejecting volume. The early return of reflected wave in elderly during systole results in higher systolic blood pressure [9]. This is in contrast to the healthy aorta in the younger

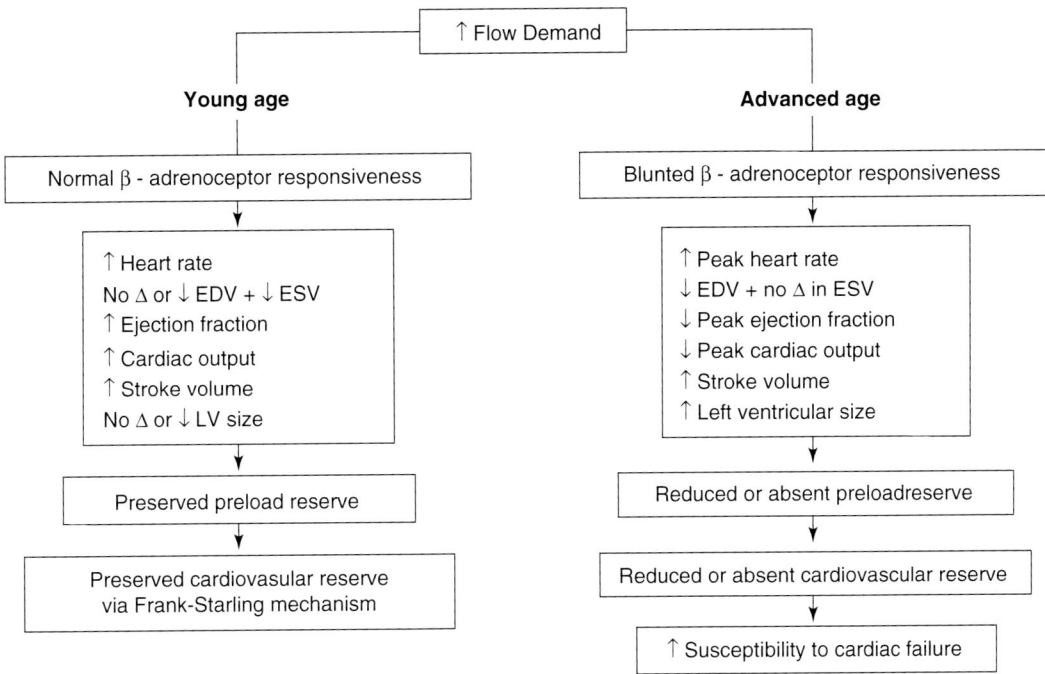

**Fig. 80.1** Age related physiological changes of CVS [Priebe H-J. BJA 2000; 85:763–78]

population, where the slower pulse wave velocity ensures that the reflected wave reaches the heart in early diastole thus augmenting the diastolic pressure. The diastolic augmentation by the reflected pulse wave does not happen in the elderly, thus resulting in lower diastolic pressure. This results in higher afterload and the left ventricle has to generate a higher pressure to overcome the increased resistance, thus resulting in systolic hypertension, increased left ventricular load and hypertrophy.

The altered ventricular-vascular coupling contributes to higher systolic pressure, lower diastolic pressure and wider pulse pressure leading to increased myocardial stress and altered myocardial blood flow (Fig. 80.2). Systolic hypertension and left ventricular hypertrophy increase the myocardial oxygen demand and wall stress combined with a lower diastolic pressure (responsible for the perfusion of the left ventricle) renders the aging heart vulnerable for ischemia [10].

While arterial stiffening leads to increased afterload, venous stiffening impairs the ability of venous system to maintain constant preload to the heart. Reduced compliance of the venous system renders the elderly vulnerable to exaggerated hypotension due to blood loss or peripheral pooling of the blood with general anesthesia or neuraxial block [11].

In a hypertrophic heart with diastolic dysfunction, a delayed relaxation of the left ventricle adversely affects its filling. This is compensated by an increase in the force of left atrial contraction which pushes the blood into the left ventricle. This is termed the *atrial kick* and depends on a sinus rhythm to maintain adequate filling. Any event resulting in tachycardia or arrhythmias including exercise and stress does not increase the cardiac output but could in all probability result in heart failure.

## Diastolic Dysfunction and the Anaesthesiologist

Diastolic dysfunction is caused by the inability of the left ventricle to relax completely. In a significant number of elderly patients with heart failure, the left ventricle ejection fraction may be deceptively normal. As diastole progresses to become increasingly incomplete there is increased impedance to ventricular filling. This abnormal

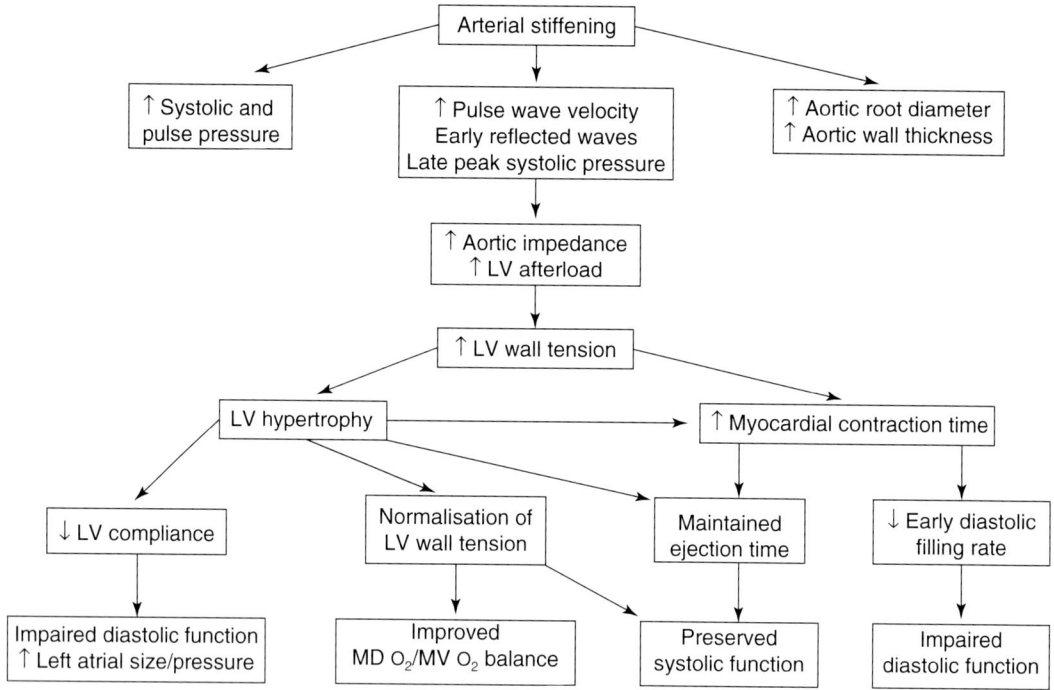

**Fig. 80.2** Effects of changes in vasculature in aging [Priebe H-J. BJA 2000; 85:763–78]

relaxation of the left ventricle results from the normal process of aging, ischemic heart disease, left ventricular hypertrophy, long standing hypertension and aortic stenosis with a normal left ventricular ejection fraction.

Rhythm disturbances in the elderly such as atrial fibrillation, first and second degree heart block and sick sinus syndrome tend to impair relaxation and further reduce diastolic volume.

In patients with atrial fibrillation, loss of atrial kick has a negative influence on emptying of the left atrium and thereby the filling of the left ventricle (LV) and LV stroke volume. Atrial enlargement may predispose patients to atrial fibrillation. Intraoperative events such as hypotension, hypertension, tachycardia, arrhythmias and volume overload should be avoided.

Meticulous evaluation should be aimed at identifying and treating pre-existing hypertension, coronary artery disease, aortic stenosis and irregular cardiac rhythms.

Unexplained hypotension during induction of general anesthesia may indicate diminished cardiac reserve in elderly patients. Onset of action of intravenous drugs may be delayed because of prolonged circulation times and decreased cardiac output.

### Fluid Therapy in the Aged

The United Kingdom National confidential inquiry into preoperative deaths at the extremes of age concluded that errors in fluid management (usually the excess of fluids) were one of the most common causes of avoidable preoperative morbidity and mortality [12]. Their report states that fluid management in the elderly is often suboptimal and it should be considered as important as a drug having pharmacological implications. Hypovolemia and hypervolemia are considered detrimental owing to high incidence of coronary heart disease, diastolic dysfunction, atherosclerosis and stiff ventricles. Organ hypoperfusion or congestive heart failure could prevail on either ends of the spectrum. The physiological response to stress such as hypovolemia may be blunted due to reduced baro-receptor sensitivity and autonomic function. This may be deleterious in patients taking β-blockers or ACE inhibitors.

Goal-directed fluid therapy as an option of fluid management has proved to be beneficial. One of the essential goals of fluid therapy is to achieve adequate cardiac index and stroke volume, depending on the clinical situation by maintaining optimum preload. Fluid status of the patients was earlier determined by using static markers of preload such as central venous pressure and pulmonary artery wedge pressure. These markers are less accurate than the more recent non-invasive dynamic indices like pulse pressure variation (PPV), systolic pressure variation (SPV) and stroke volume variation (SVV) [13].

## Vasopressor Therapy

Beta receptor activity of the myocardium diminishes with age and as a result, responses to commonly used adrenergic drugs are decreased in terms of heart rate and increased contractility of the heart in the event of hypotension, exercise and catecholamine stimulation [13]. Responses to ephedrine and phenylephrine are reduced and higher doses may be required to achieve the desired effect in the event of hypotension after induction of general anesthesia or to overcome the sympatholytic effect of neuraxial blockade. Aging is associated with a reduction in the carotid baroreceptor response to hypotension. Intravenous and inhalational anaesthetics further impair this response and cause depression of cardiac and vascular smooth muscle contractility. Low basal vagal tone could explain the decreased heart rate response to atropine.

## Rhythm Abnormalities

Calcification and fibrosis of the heart increase the incidence of sinus, atrioventricular and ventricular conduction defects. Geriatric patients often suffer from supraventricular and ventricular arrhythmias or conduction blocks that require treatment with anti-arrhythmic drugs or have implantable devices such as permanent pacemakers or cardioverters. Use of anti-muscarinic agents in patients with atrial fibrillation mandates caution, as they may provoke a rapid ventricular rate which would require treatment with beta-blockers, calcium channel blockers or amiodarone [14]. Recommended guidelines should be followed when anaesthetizing patients with implantable devices.

Atrial pacemaker cells decline by 80–90% by 70 years hence causing atrial Fibrillation (AF) to be the most common arrhythmia seen in clinical practice and it worsens with age. AF may result in undesirable consequences such as myocardial ischemia, heart failure, unstable hemodynamics, thromboembolism, stroke and death. Longstanding AF leads to stasis of blood in the atrium causing thrombus formation that may embolize and result in impaired blood circulation. Rate and rhythm should be maintained and atrial clot should be assessed in patients with AF. Perioperative anticoagulation may be considered in long standing AF. Atrial contraction has a vital role in maintaining cardiac output in the elderly, hence it is important to maintain sinus rhythm. If AF is the cause of hemodynamic instability, cardioversion should be a choice prior to anesthesia to control the heart rate to less than 100/min.

## Age Related Valvular Changes

Aortic and mitral valve leaflets undergo thickening with aging. 90% of healthy 80-year olds present with multivalvular regurgitation, which is usually mild, central and presents with leaflets which appear normal [15]. Moderate to severe aortic regurgitation often co-exists in 16% of elderly (Table 80.2). Mitral annular calcification and regurgitation are seen in approximately 50% of females and 36% of males. The valvular disorders have shown an association with coronary events, heart failure, atrial fibrillation, endocarditis, transient ischemic attacks and thrombolic strokes [15]. Significant aortic stenosis predisposes the elderly to coronary events with two to three times increased risk of adverse perioperative cardiac events [16].

## Anaesthetic Management and Cardiovascular Safety in Aged

Arthritis and degenerative diseases may limit exercise capacity and mask poor exertional tolerance due to poor cardiac status. Elderly patients are likely to be on treatment of hypertension, ischemic heart disease and heart failure. These drugs have to be continued during the peri-operative period as sudden cessation of these drugs may be harmful (eg. Beta-blockers). ACE inhibitors should be discontinued on the day of surgery as it may result in fluctuations in peri-operative blood pressure. Anti-platelet agents (eg. clopidogrel) and anti-coagulants (eg. warfarin) need to be discontinued to ensure normal hemostasis.

The aged have decreased tolerance for cardiovascular stress and hemodynamic upheavals, making them more prone for ischemia, arrhythmias and heart failure. Keen attention needs to be paid to maintain the balance between oxygen demand and oxygen supply by avoiding persistent and prolonged changes in systemic blood pressure and heart rate. A safer option is to maintain both within 20% of the normal awake values. Volume overload and rhythm disturbances should be guarded against. Inotropes and drugs that increase heart rate should be avoided. The dose of induction agents should be decreased by 25% and opioid doses may be reduced by 50%. The minimal alveolar concentration (MAC) of induction agents required is 30% lower than younger counterparts. Calcium channel blockers, beta blockers and calcium sensitizing drugs may be beneficial. Ketamine and thiopentone may worsen hemodynamics by reducing contractility.

## Respiratory System and Aging

Most of the respiratory changes occur due to decreased lung elasticity. The chest wall is composed of two elements: the bony and cartilaginous structure of the rib cage and the muscles that move them. Aging diminishes their compliance as a result of calcification and stiffening of the costochondral joints. The typical barrel chest appearance is caused by loss of height and calcification of the vertebral column and rib cage [17]. There is flattening of the diaphragm which becomes mechanically less efficient and functionally impaired by significant loss of muscle mass associated with aging. Age related deterioration of all musculoskeletal structures involves the respiratory muscles and causes weakness and inability to generate adequate inspiratory and expiratory pressures (Table 80.4).

**Table 80.4** Changes in geriatric respiratory system

- Reduced parenchymal tissue
- Increased residual and closing volumes and functional residual capacity
- V/Q mismatch progressively worsens
- Reduced diffusion capacity and increased physiological dead space
- Depressed hypoxic drive
- Decreased protective airway reflexes
- Atrophied muscles
- Decreased cough.
- Decreased maximal breathing capacity

**Table 80.5** Effects of changes in respiratory system

- Decline in functional capacity
- Decrease cough reflex and airway ciliary action
- Frequent airway collapse
- Reduced compliance
- Snoring and sleep apnea
- Higher rates of infection

Poor nutrition and other co-morbidities lead to malnutrition and mal-absorption and have a negative impact on the respiratory function [18]. Loss of lung elastic recoil reduces pulmonary gas exchange, increases work of breathing and allows over-distension of alveoli and collapse of small airways [18, 19] (Table 80.5).

### The Upper Airway

Over the age of 70 years, various factors like loss of muscle supporting the pharyngeal wall, loss of protective laryngeal reflexes, loss of bronchial epithelial cilia and co-morbidities such as chronic obstructive pulmonary disease (COPD), stroke and cognitive decline contribute to impaired cough and swallowing reflexes [20, 21]. The tracheobronchial tree is unable to recognize foreign bodies and there is inadequate generation of cough volume. The inferior cough and swallowing mechanisms provoke a higher risk for tracheo-bronchial aspiration of pharyngeal or gastric contents and therefore increase the risk of aspiration pneumonia [20]. Ventilatory response to hypoxia, hypercapnia and mechanical ventilation is substantially attenuated [22]. With aging peripheral and central chemoreceptor responses diminish along with declining integration of CNS pathways [22].

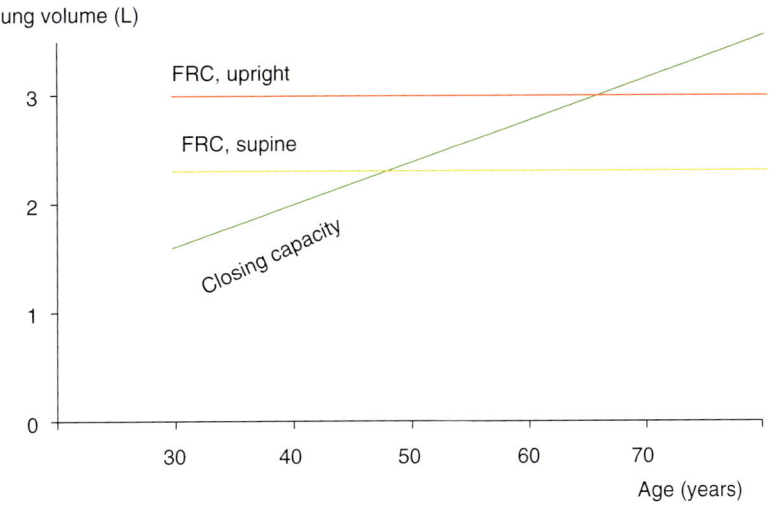

**Fig. 80.3** Changes in respiratory capacity in aged

## Lung Function

Premature airway collapse increases functional residual capacity (FRC), residual volume and closing capacity (CC) resulting in ventilation/perfusion (V/Q) mismatch. CC exceeds FRC at the age of 45 years in the supine position and at the age of 65 years in the sitting position (Fig. 80.3).

V/Q mismatch results in inadequate gas exchange, hypoxemia and increased alveolar-arterial oxygen difference. There is no significant change in arterial pH or $PaCO_2$ with age. With pre-oxygenation, breathing 100% oxygen for 3 minutes or longer will be more beneficial than taking the usual four maximal inspirations of 100% oxygen [23].

## Airway Management

Mask ventilation is difficult in edentulous patients. Continuing the use of dentures in the operating room during induction may facilitate mask ventilation. Arthritis of the temporomandibular joint or glycosylation of the cervical spine may cause difficulty in tracheal intubation.

## Anesthetic Management and Respiratory Pathophysiology in the Aged

The pre-anesthetic evaluation should include the identification of age related respiratory changes and estimation of physiological reserve. COPD and sleep apnea are common in the elderly. A history of smoking, cough, dyspnea and wheezing should be elicited. Smokers should be advised to quit smoking at least 6–8 weeks before surgery to minimize high airway reactivity and risk of bronchospastic airway obstruction, mucus trapping and regional atelectasis. Preoperative optimization with spirometry, bronchodilator therapy, mucolytics, chest physiotherapy and antibiotics is useful.

Neuromuscular disorders such as Parkinson's disease and cerebro-vascular abnormalities as well as cardiac abnormalities have significant impact on the strength of respiratory muscles and can complicate weaning from respiratory support after surgery [24, 25].

A "6 minute walk test" gives an indication of the patient's ability to withstand surgical stress. Arterial blood gases and chest x-ray provide valuable inputs. Pulmonary function testing for Forced Expiratory Volume in 1 s ($FEV_1$) and Forced Vital Capacity (FVC) indicates physiologic reserve. Reversibility with bronchodilators is suggestive of potential for improvement. History of snoring may indicate sleep induced hypoventilation and caution would be needed if benzodiazepines or opioids are used.

## Respiratory Diseases in Elderly

Respiratory disease is a common co-morbidity in the elderly population presenting for surgery, thereby increasing the rate of perioperative morbidity. Age results in a gradual reduction in pulmonary reserve due to structural and functional alterations. The commonly encountered respiratory co-morbidities include COPD, asthma, pneumonia and obstructive sleep apnea. COPD will be discussed in detail here as it is the third leading cause of morbidity in the US and is expected to increase world-wide [26].

## COPD

COPD is a chronic and progressive inflammatory condition affecting central and peripheral airways, lung parenchyma and pulmonary vasculature which results in poorly reversible narrowing of the airways, increased number of mucus-secreting glands and pulmonary vascular changes causing pulmonary hypertension. COPD also results in significant systemic effects [27].

Cigarette smoking is the key noxious inflammatory trigger for the development of COPD with house dust, fumes and smoke from biomass also contributing to the pathophysiology of the disease.

The pathophysiology of COPD is characterised by limitation of expiratory airflow as a result of small airway inflammation (obstructive bronchitis) and parenchymal destruction (emphysema). Small airway inflammation causes obstruction and air trapping resulting in dynamic hyperinflation leading to V/Q mismatch. Emphysema causes destruction of alveolar architecture as a result of elastin breakdown. In the geriatric patient, the chronicity of the disease results in respiratory failure because of V/Q mismatch, decreased gas transfer and alveolar hypoventilation. The extra-pulmonary systemic effects of the disease manifest as cardiovascular and musculoskeletal insufficiencies in the form of hypertension, ischemic heart disease, cardiac arrhythmias and congestive cardiac failure along with muscle mass depletion and weakness respectively. Release of pro-inflammatory cytokines cause muscle weakness and thereby hypoxemia and hypercapnia. Body weight decreases severely, which is an independent marker of poor outcome. The combination of severe COPD and surgery carries poor prognosis with high mortality.

The diagnosis is made by eliciting a history of chronic cough, exertional dyspnea and regular sputum production. In the elderly this should be considered along with the CGA [28] because the risk in elderly patients with COPD is high in terms of well being and functional status, when compared to same aged normal persons. Frequency of exacerbations, forced expiratory volume$_1$ ($FEV_1$) and body mass index(BMI) should be documented.

COPD has to be managed comprehensively with the assessment of severity, reduction of risk factors (cessation of smoking, exposure to irritants), medical management of the disease and prevention of exacerbations.

Pharmacological management is done with inhaled and oral therapy. Short-acting bronchodilators ($\beta$ agonist or muscarinic agonist) are administered for breathlessness and exercise limitation. Long-acting $\beta$ agonists should be substituted if breathlessness persists along with inhaled corticosteroids depending on $FEV_1$ status. Oral corticosteroids, if used for extensive period increases the risk of the patients for osteoporosis, immune-suppression, peptic acid disease, hyperglycemia, impaired wound healing and stress related acute adrenal insufficiency. Oral mucolytics, oxygen therapy, physiotherapy and nutritional supplementation help in optimizing the elderly prior to surgery.

## Choice of Anesthesia in COPD

General anesthesia, endotracheal intubation and intermittent positive pressure ventilation (IPPV) are associated with adverse events in the presence of COPD as these patients are prone to develop laryngospasm, bronchospasm, barotrauma, cardiovascular insufficiencies, hypoxemia and postoperative pulmonary complications. General anesthesia and IPPV carries the risk of air trapping and intrinsic PEEP because the narrow airway traps the inhaled breath prior to exhalation. The raised intra-thoracic pressure caused by IPPV decreases the systemic venous return, which may be transmitted to pulmonary arteries, causing a raised pulmonary vascular resistance leading to right heart strain. The hyper-inflated lungs exert direct pressure on the heart causing cardiovascular instability. Air trapping also may result in volutrauma, hypercapnia and acidosis. Air trapping may be decreased by reducing the I: E ratio (to 1:3–1:5) which allows more time for exhalation but with the concomitant risk of reduced minute volume, hypercapnia, hypoxia or acidosis. Inspiratory flow rate may be increased to combat these problems which may risk the patients for barotrauma. Extubation followed by initiation of non-invasive ventilation may help to reduce work of breathing, re-intubation and air trapping.

Hypoventilation as a result of residual anesthesia may lead to hypercarbia and hypoxia. Pain in the post-operative period may trigger hypoventilation (thoracic or abdominal surgeries) or hyperventilation both of which can have deleterious effects. Epidural or perineural catheters left in-situ is the most appropriate mode of affording safe analgesia.

## Patient Related Factors Responsible for Post-operative Pulmonary Complications (PPC) [29, 30]

Older patients are at a risk of substantial perioperative morbidity and mortality with the additional risk of postoperative pulmonary complications namely pneumonia, atelectasis, bronchospasm, respiratory failure and exacerbation of obstructive lung disease. Hence adequate optimization of the overall health of the aged is a prerogative for an uneventful perioperative period. Smokers, even in the absence of chronic lung disease have a threefold increased risk of PPCs. COPD is the single most important patient related risk factor, accounting for three to fourfold increase in PPCs [31] (Table 80.6).

**Table 80.6** Independent predictors of postoperative pulmonary complications in elderly

| |
|---|
| • Post-operative |
| – Nasogastric intubation |
| – Sputum production |
| • Longer general anesthesia |
| • Surgical procedures |
| • Age |
| • COPD |
| • Smoking |
| • Alcohol abuse |
| • Long term steroid use |
| • Impaired level of consciousness |

Decreased general health status, poor exercise tolerance and serum albumin less than 3.5 g/dl are all implicated in PPCs [32].

Bronchial asthma, if appropriately treated preoperatively, makes the perioperative period relatively safe. Obesity with a BMI in excess of 34 showed 12% incidence of PPCs while those with obstructive sleep apnea (OSA) had complications of 30% as compared to obese patients without OSA (3%) [33].

Risk of PPCs in the elderly are related to procedures. Surgical sites such as thoraco-abdominal surgeries predispose the patients for higher risk. Any procedure lasting more than 3 hours or requires neuromuscular blockade, as well as patients requiring postoperative ventilatory support increases the risk for PPCs [29, 34]. General anesthesia and open surgical procedures are considered to carry a higher risk for PPCs than regional anesthesia and laparoscopic surgeries respectively. Procedures near the diaphragm, surgery over neck vascular and neurosurgery are associated with aspiration risk and therefore increases the risk of mortality. Emergency procedures are considered to be of high risk.

Anesthesia has a significant effect on pulmonary function and results in decreased FRC, reduction in VC, increased closing volume, impaired pulmonary vasoconstriction and impaired mucociliary mechanism. Postoperative hypoventilation secondary to residual anesthetic effects and pain at the incision site contribute to PPCs in the geriatric population [29].

Postoperative strategies which can help reduce the above risk factors include lung expansion maneuvers and adequate pain relief. Both of these methods improve lung expansion, minimize atelectasis and reduce PPCs. Lung expansion can be achieved by using simple deep breathing exercises, incentive spirometry or continuous positive airway pressure (CPAP).

Adequate pain relief strategies in the elderly can prevent PPCs. Multimodal analgesia with central neuraxial analgesia, peripheral nerve blocks, infiltration of incision site with local anesthesia, short acting opioids and anti-inflammatory analgesics will reduce splinting of diaphragm, help in deep breathing and improve lung expansion.

## Gastrointestinal Tract and Liver

Aging of the gastrointestinal tract is not as apparent as that seen in other organs. The esophageal contractions show a decrease in amplitude along with decrease in peristaltic waves which follow the act of swallowing. Gastric emptying takes longer, thus putting the geriatric population at a higher risk for aspiration during the induction of anesthesia and in the postoperative period [35].

There is a decrease of average daily energy intake by up to 30% by the time a person becomes 80 years of age. The decreased intake is probably due to decline in energy expenditure as one ages. Physiological reduction in appetite and energy intake is associated with loss of body weight, a phenomenon which has been termed as "The anorexia of aging" [36].

Gastric acid secretion decreases with age along with a propensity for developing atrophic gastritis which is responsible for decreased secretion of acid and intrinsic factor. Lack of intrinsic factor can lead to vitamin B12 deficiency and pernicious anaemia. Atrophic gastritis may affect calcium bioavailability as a result of decreased dissociation from food complexes. Gastrointestinal bleeding is a frequent presentation in the aged. Upper and lower gastrointestinal bleeding tend to increase with increasing age, longer length of hospital stay and co-morbidities.

The liver undergoes a reduction in volume by 20–40% and there is a decline in hepatic blood flow. Aging does not result in much change in the liver function except for a decline in P450 enzyme system which may result in delayed metabolism of many drugs. Reduced oxidative drug metabolism leads to delayed clearance of drugs that depend on hepatic oxidation for metabolism (Ex. diazepam). Drugs such as lorazepam that depend on glucuronidation for metabolism are degraded similarly in young and old persons. Decreased synthesis of albumin may affect protein binding of drugs. Although serum albumin is purely a marker of nutrition, levels less than 3.5 g/dL are an important predictor of 30-day perioperative morbidity and mortality [37].

The aging liver is more susceptible to oxidative stress and injury, which is why the elderly are more prone for overt liver disease and have higher risk of liver dysfunction and failure following surgical stress.

Hepatic insufficiency may herald poor outcomes after surgery. Preoperative correction of coagulation abnormalities with vitamin K or blood products (eg. Fresh Frozen Plasma and coagulation concentrates) may be required.

## Renal System in the Elderly

The kidneys undergo structural and functional changes with the loss of renal mass, increased numbers of sclerotic glomeruli, a decrease in number of tubules and interstitial fibrosis. The renal blood flow decreases by approximately 50% by the age of 80 years, along with a 45% reduction of glomerular filtration rate(GFR).The lean body mass decreases in the elderly, hence, serum creatinine usually remains unchanged. The kidneys are increasingly susceptible to acute insults, such as perioperative hypotension or hypoxia and are more prone to chronic renal impairment. As renal blood flow is significantly decreased, there is an accompanied decline in responsiveness and auto-regulation of volume status [38].The integrity of biochemical balance of all cells is dependent on the function of the kidneys. Electrolyte homeostasis may be seen as slow responsiveness to sodium changes and diminished ability to adequately dilute or concentrate urine. The transport of other electrolytes and ions across the tubular epithelium may show a global impairment [38].

The renin-angiotensin-aldosterone system (RAAS) is responsible for maintenance of circulating volume and electrolyte balance. This system is altered in the aged even in the absence of hypertension and other cardiovascular diseases because of the decrease in renin levels secondary to glomerulosclerosis. There is a resultant rise in plasma potassium and creatinine levels and close monitoring is essential especially in the elderly with renal impairment in whom angiotensin-converting enzyme inhibitors (ACEIs) or angiotensin receptor blockers (ARBs) may cause further deterioration in renal functions.

The currently available tests to estimate the renal functions do not predict the true functional reserve in the elderly, hence the anesthesiologist needs to exercise caution with respect to drugs such as ACEIs and non-steroidal anti-inflammatory drugs (NSAIDs) along with cautious fluid and electrolyte maintenance. The kidneys have suboptimal ability to conserve body water during states of dehydration along with loss of diluting capacity, which contributes to exacerbation of morbidity due to common clinical conditions such as diarrhea, vomiting, decreased thirst and hypovolemia.

Abnormal serum urea and electrolyte values are not uncommon in elderly, however, normal urea and creatinine values need not indicate a normal renal function. It may result from reduced dietary intake and muscle mass. Only after substantial deterioration of renal functions would the urea and creatinine values become abnormal.

## Endocrine System

Endocrine function shows a decline in terms of decreased tissue responsiveness and diminished hormone secretion from the peripheral glands [39] (Table 80.7). The thyroid hormones, thyroxin (T4) and tri-iodo-thyronine (T3) undergo reduced secretion.

Elderly women have low estrogen levels making them more prone for cardiovascular events, loss of skeletal mass, altered psychological health, vasomotor instability and atrophy of estrogen-responsive tissues [40]. Andropause in elderly males causes the total serum testosterone concentrations to fall.

The hypothalamic–pituitary-adrenal (HPA) axis triggers the secretion of growth hormone (GH) and adrenocorticotropic hormone (ACTH). GH stimulates protein synthesis and inhibits protein breakdown, promotes lipolysis, initiates glycogenolysis in the liver and antagonises the insulin effect by inhibiting glucose uptake and glucose utilization by cells. Following ACTH stimulation, the adrenal cortex secretes cortisol which is responsible for protein breakdown and lipolysis, thus increasing the precursors of gluconeogenesis. Although surgery incites a catabolic hyperglycemic response, the endogenous secretion of insulin may fall in the perioperative period. This may be due to decreased pancreatic beta cell secretion secondary to adrenergic inhibition. This worsens the "insulin resistance", which is seen during surgery. The hormonal changes are insignificant during low-risk procedures and gain significance as the degree of surgical stress increases [41]. Endocrine responses to elective surgical procedures are intact in older patients in terms of plasma cortisol levels and urinary excretion of adrenaline, nor-adrenaline and 17-hydroxy-corticosteroid, thereby explaining the intact endocrine response to surgical stress. The proportionate increase in the energy expenditure is independent of the age of the patient [42].

### Diabetes Mellitus

The elderly have deterioration of glucose metabolism which makes them prone to inadequate glycemic control in the perioperative period. Increased body fat and decreased lean body mass results in insulin resistance in addition to decreased production of insulin by beta cells.

Diabetes causes exacerbations in age-related physiological changes including decline in physiological reserve in major organs. The geriatric diabetics are more at risk of atherosclerotic related comorbidities. In the US, diabetes contributes significantly to the development of renal failure and dialysis in the elderly. Diabetic retinopathy causes a significant number of elderly persons to suffer from loss of vision, disability and depression. Hyperglycemic hyperosmolar nonketotic coma is a severe complication of diabetes in elderly [40].

In the perioperative settings, inadequate control of blood glucose can result in hyperglycemia,

**Table 80.7** Endocrinal changes in aged

| |
|---|
| • Impaired glucose homeostasis |
| • Reduced response to thyroid hormone, hypothyroidism |
| • Increased ADH, reduced renin and aldosterone |
| • Reduced testosterone production, impotency |
| • Vitamin-D homeostasis impairment, osteopenia |

acidemia, hyperosmolar crisis and ketosis, accompanied with severe fluid and electrolyte imbalances or even hypoglycemia.

Perioperative care of the diabetic elderly should ensure normal metabolism so as to ensure that the patient is not subjected to excessive hyperglycemia, hypoglycemia, lipolysis, ketogenesis, protein catabolism and dyselectrolytemia. This goal is best achieved by providing adequate insulin to counterbalance the catabolic response to surgery and anesthesia. There is an increased requirement of carbohydrate in the perioperative period as a result of stress. The endogenous insulin becomes less effective than usual as a result of counter regulatory hormones. As the patients are starved preoperatively, there is lack of carbohydrates as well as suboptimal disposal of existing carbohydrates as insulin is generally avoided before surgery. The omission of carbohydrates and insulin can be detrimental in the diabetic elderly patient. Hence sufficient glucose needs to be provided in order to meet the increased requirements of surgical stress in addition to basal caloric requirements along with an insulin regimen to match. One unit of insulin decreases blood glucose by 25–30 mg/dl in a 70–80 kg person and 10 g glucose raises it by 35–40 mg/dl [43]. Geriatric medications can include diuretics, sympathomimetics, oestrogen, glucocorticoids, phenytoin and tricyclic antidepressants. These can adversely affect glucose metabolism, exacerbating glucose intolerance. Stressful situations such as myocardial infarction, infections, surgery and burns can worsen glucose intolerance and precipitate fasting hyperglycemia [44].

## Age and Central Nervous System

Beyond the age of 60 years, there is a loss of 2–3 g of brain weight every year, thereby causing significant decrease in the brain mass and weight. The neuronal function shows a decline with decreased neuronal size and synapses. Dendritic architecture undergoes significant change. There is decreased synthesis of neurotransmitters, increased fibrosis of peripheral sympathetic neurons and impaired responses of cardiovascular reflexes. Neurofibrillary tangles and senile plaques are seen more extensively in Alzheimer's disease.

Degeneration of peripheral nerve cells decreases conduction velocity and results in atrophy of skeletal muscles, hence the decrease in local anaesthetic requirement.

A decrease of 10–20% of global cerebral blood flow is seen due to decreased brain mass, but the cerebral blood flow per unit of weight remains normal. Vertibro-basilar insufficiency is seen frequently and can be evaluated by assessing the effect of extension and rotation of the head on higher mental functions.

About 40% of elderly people suffer from sleep related problems, which may be associated with sleep apnea, dysomnias and nocturnal myoclonus.

Meaningful communication during the history and physical exam may not be possible because of hearing and vision impairments and anesthesiologist may need to dedicate more time and patience to elicit pertinent information.

Cognitive function is found to be reduced in terms of perception, memory, information processing, problem solving and reaction time. Cognitive function is important in order to select, store and retrieve information to allow adequate response. The elderly tend to suffer from memory loss with loss of immediate or recent memory being more affected than the long term, crystallized memory of the past.

Neurological disorders are more common as one ages, leading to loss of functional independence and financial burden which affects society as a whole. The burden to the society is in the form of loss of mobility, stability, impairment of intellect in addition to incontinence and iatrogenic disorders. All of the above constitute the five undesirable 'I's of Geriatrics (Table 80.8).

**Table 80.8** Five Is of geriatrics

| |
|---|
| • Intellectual impairment |
| • Immobility |
| • Instability |
| • Incontinence |
| • Iatrogenic disorders |

## Nutritional Status

Nearly a quarter of the aged are vulnerable to malnutrition, probably due to unavailability of wholesome food, decreased appetite, co-morbidities, polymedications, metabolic causes and psychosocial issues [45]. Muscle mass decreases as well as physical activity resulting in a fall in total energy expenditure with increasing age. Energy requirements decrease with aging; however these requirement increases during periods of stress related to surgery or infection.

Preoperative albumin levels have been used as a nutrition marker to predict postoperative outcomes. Age, low albumin, weight loss of ≥10%, poor functional status are considered as risk factors for postoperative respiratory failures [46, 47] and poor postoperative outcomes.

The hepatic protein, pre-albumin is also a reflection of nutritional status. Pre-albumin is a better predictor of malnutrition owing to the shorter half-life (2 days) compared to 20 days of albumin, thereby making it a better predictor of short term changes pertaining to nutritional status. Pre-albumin is independent of hydration status; hence, in patients with fluid fluctuation such as patients on dialysis and congestive cardiac failure, it is a more dependable marker of nourishment than albumin. A pre-albumin level less than 10 mg/dL is a predictor of increased morbidity and mortality. Deficiencies of minerals and vitamins are also known to impact outcomes; hence replacement of iron, vitamin B12 and folate could reduce adverse outcomes. Frailty and sarcopenia could result from deficiency of vitamin D and worsen outcomes. Promotion of preoperative nutrition with the help of nutritional supplementation and pharmaco-nutrients may improve surgical outcome [48].

Nutritional assessment in the elderly should be a routine preoperative assessment. Nutritional indices usually incorporate BMI and weight loss of greater than 5% in 3 months. Commonly used screening tests are the Malnutrition Universal Screening Tool (MUST) and the Mini-Nutritional Assessment [49].

## Hydration

Dehydration is common in the aged because of multiple reasons such as: inability to recognize thirst, decreased urine concentrating ability resulting in frequent urination and fluid loss, use of diuretics or laxatives and presence of fever or infections. Adequate hydration could be ensured by following the current fasting guidelines which allows clear fluids to be consumed upto 2 hours prior to surgery.

Elderly patients can present with hypovolemia even in the absence of shock or bleeding. The aged heart depends on increased ventricular filling (Frank-Starling Law) and stroke volume to maintain adequate cardiac output because of decreased beta responsiveness and inability to increase the heart rate on demand. General anesthesia and central neuraxial blockade cause decline in sympathetic activity which may result in profound hypotension. The correction of this hypotension with rapid fluid loading may trigger pulmonary oedema and cardiac failure, hence early initiation of vasopressors is desirable. Trans-oesophageal echocardiography and continuous arterial pressure monitoring may assist in goal directed fluid therapy in geriatrics.

## Geriatric Related Syndromes

Surgical stress in the elderly is known to evoke imbalances in the physiological haemostasis, as seen by endocrine and hemodynamic alterations. The gravity of the stress response depends on patient-related comorbidities as well as anaesthetic and surgical insults. The prevalence of comorbidities increases with age along with multiplicity of comorbidities, all of which result in poor postoperative functional outcome. The routine preoperative assessment which grades the risk based on The American Society of Anaesthesiologists (ASA) risk stratification is now considered inadequate in the geriatric patient. The consideration of under-estimated geriatric-specific syndromes, such as frailty, restricted mobility, functional and cognitive status and malnutrition constitutes the comprehensive geriatric assessment scale (CGA). This scale helps in determining the efficiency of compensatory mechanisms necessary for combating perioperative stress in elderly.

## Frailty

Cardiorespiratory reserve has always been emphasized as the main determinant of functional capacity. Frailty reflects the diminished physiologic reserve across multiple organ systems. Studies in various surgical populations have identified frailty as an independent risk factor for major morbidity, mortality, increased length of hospital stay and institutional discharge [50]. Two categories of frailty have been described. The physical category of frailty should comprise three or more of the following: unexplained weight loss of over 10 lbs. in past 1 year, easy fatigability, muscular weakness, slow paced walking, and low physical activity [51]. The multi-domain category of frailty incudes additional factors such as cognition, mood abnormalities, sensory decline, suboptimal social conditions and support system, comorbid conditions and disability.

Frailty status, when combined with other preoperative assessment tools including ASA physical status, improves the predictability of peri-operative morbidity and mortality. The parameters used for assessing frailty measure both performance and non-performance based functions, provides insight into the postoperative outcomes and also identifies potentially modifiable factors to be optimised preoperatively.

## Sarcopenia in the Aged

The key component of disability in frail elderly patients is the progressive loss of skeletal muscle mass, strength and power [52]. The CNS, endocrine and immune system collectively co-ordinates the muscle homeostasis by sequential formation of new muscle tissue, hypertrophy and protein loss in young adult. The low physical activity and malnutrition is closely related to sarcopenia in the elderly. Pro-inflammatory cytokines including IL-6 and TNF-α enhance muscle breakdown to produce amino-acids for energy production. Frailty may result in an excess of inflammatory responses causing further debility with decline in muscle mass, strength and functional status. Sarcopenia in the elderly population contributes to risk of falls, long term dependency, disability and death.

## Functional Status

Functional status (FS) is known to be a reliable indicator of outcomes following surgery in the elderly and is quantified by using a questionnaire. It is defined as the sum of behaviours that are needed to maintain daily activities, including social and cognitive functions [53]. It assesses the patient's ability to actively mobilize and attend to basic(BADL) [54] and instrumental (IADL) [55] activities of daily life. The score is determined by adding up the number of activities the patient can perform, thereby determining the patient's degree of independence. Poor exercise tolerance, defined as the inability to walk beyond two blocks or climb two flights of stairs without any symptoms, was indicative of increased length of hospital stay. This in combination with older age, single status, living alone, more than five medications, anesthesia duration over 4 hours, orthopaedic surgery and serious postoperative complications form part of the questionnaire [46].

A rough evaluation of FS can be done by observing the patients when they enter the consultation room, asking them to sit, get up from the chair, walk around, and sit down again, while calculating the time required (6 minute walk test).

Functional dependence also contributes to postoperative surgical site infection apart from being a predictor for postoperative pulmonary complications. Assessment of functional status provides an easily available predictive tool which can be invaluable for the surgeons, patients and their families [56].

## Cognitive Assessment

Preoperative cognitive dysfunction is a major predictor for perioperative delirium. Anesthesia and surgery are forever locked together as agents of any cognitive change after surgical interventions and the concept of postoperative disturbance in cognition is referred to as postoperative cognitive dysfunction (POCD). The term is, however, used variably, and it is imperative to distinguish among three types of cognitive deterioration after surgery.

1. Delirium is an acute disturbance in consciousness and cognition characterized by signs of disorientation, attention deficits and clouding of consciousness which develops over a short period of time with degree of severity ranging from mild to very severe [57]. Delirium may be precipitated by peri-operative hypoxia, anti-cholinergic medication, infections, opiates, sedatives and abnormalities of glucose, calcium and sodium.
2. Short term cognitive disturbances may be apparent the day after surgery. This is a frequent observation. This condition is transitory and may not be long lasting.
3. POCD is a more subtle and prolonged change in cognition, with clinical manifestations similar to those seen in neurodegenerative disorders, and is diagnosed as a "more than expected" postoperative deterioration in cognitive domains, including short term memory (reduced ability to learn or recall information), mood, consciousness and circadian rhythm [58].

Etiopathogenesis of POCD is believed to be an anesthesia related neurotoxicity which results in apoptosis of neuroglial cells and worsening of beta amyloid oligomerization and deposition, a process associated with Alzheimer's disease and cognitive dysfunction [59]. Inflammation and activation of the immune system are associated with cognitive decline. Surgical patients exhibit elevations of pro-inflammatory cytokines especially during major procedures such as cardiac and orthopaedic surgeries which expose patients to excessive trauma, blood loss and extensive tissue injury.

Major surgery causes an endocrine response with release of hypothalamic-pituitary-adrenal axis (HPA) and sympathetic nervous system hormones [60]. Hypercortisolaemeia has been well known for some time to impair cognitive function.

Microembolization caused by air introduced into the venous circulation, during cardiopulmonary bypass has been implicated for causing POCD. Genetic propensity, for POCD after non-cardiac surgery, in certain individuals has been suggested [61].

POCD is a multifactorial disease with many factors contributing to its development. Possible risk factors are: increasing age, lower educational level, higher ASA physical status, pre-existing cognitive impairment, history of cerebrovascular impairment, major surgery, cardiac surgery, longer duration of surgery and anesthesia, intraoperative cerebral desaturation and postoperative infection.

The adage "prevention is better than cure" is very salient with regard to POCD because evidence of successful treatment is still elusive. A multicomponent intervention strategy has been suggested for effective prevention of POCD [30]. It includes prevention of hypoxia, dyselectrytemia and polypharmacy as well as proper dosing and allowing the elderly to recover postoperatively in a familiar atmosphere preferably in the presence of family. The recovery area should be quiet, well-lit and have compassionate caregivers. Adequate pain relief, early mobilization and maintenance of good hydration are of paramount importance. Patients and family members need to be counselled and reassured.

## Assessment of Cognitive Abilities

Multiple methods can be used to assess patient's cognitive abilities preoperatively and postoperatively. The Mini Mental State Examination (MMSE) includes simple questions to allow clinicians to rapidly assess multiple cognitive domains including cognition, short term and long term memory, visual-motor skills, language, comprehensibility and executive skills [62, 63].

Neuropsychological test batteries are subject to large variability. The International Study on Post Operative Cognitive Dysfunction (ISPOCD) study results revealed that the letter digit coding, Stroop color interference and visual verbal learning tests had a high correlation with both age and IQ [64, 65].

With the increasing trend of the aged population presenting for surgery, only now are we beginning to graze the surface of its proclivity, etiopathogenesis and diagnosis. Novel therapeutic interventions with alterations in the delivery of current regimens may help prevent devastating consequence of POCD in the elderly [66].

## Mood/Depression

Depression is highly prevalent among elderly patients in the pre-operative period which diminishes after surgery. Patients with preoperative anxiety and depression showed unfavourable postoperative outcomes [67], such as, longer length of stay (LOS) and a higher requirement of skilled nursing after discharge from hospital. Depression has been found to be an important predictor of 6 month mortality, similar to chronic obstructive pulmonary disease, hypertension, stroke, Parkinson's disease, age, dementia and elevated serum creatinine levels [68].

A higher incidence of depression is documented when deliberate screening is undertaken rather than detecting it from prior history. Preoperative assessment for geriatric patients would benefit more from inclusion of a simple depression questionnaire, eg. the geriatric questionnaire scale [69] which stratifies the patients into normal, mild and severe depressives. Depression may be a precursor to further complications, and be implicated with the elderly getting discharged to a place other than his home or even mortality.

## Pharmacokinetics and Pharmacodynamics in the Elderly

Altered physiology in the aged has an impact on the pharmacokinetics and pharmacodynamics of anaesthetics, thereby affecting the metabolism, sensitivity, drug-body interaction and elimination of each drug. Pharmacokinetics refers to the fate of the drug or what the body does to the drug while pharmacodynamics refers to how the drug affects the body.

## Body Compartments and Drug Distribution

Age impacts the body composition by causing an increased percentage of body fat, decreased lean body mass and decreased total body water. Most anaesthetic drugs are lipid soluble. Due to increased body fat and availability of lipid storage sites, there is accumulation of drugs in fat reservoirs and protracted elution of drugs thereafter. This result in greater plasma concentration of the drugs contributing to prolonged anaesthetic effects and longer periods required for their elimination. Decreased muscle mass and body water reduces the distribution volume for water soluble drugs, causing higher plasma concentrations of the active drug form.

Drugs are not distributed uniformly throughout the body. The speed with which a drug reaches a particular tissue is largely dependent on its blood flow. Similar tissue types are grouped together into various 'compartments' depending on their blood supply. Each compartment serves as a reservoir for the drug depending on its size and affinity for the drug. The three compartment model, shown in Fig. 80.4 depicts the vessel rich, intermediate and vessel poor tissues with a central compartment(blood), through which drugs must pass during uptake or elimination [70].

On entering the blood stream, a percentage of the drug binds to the plasma proteins, and the rest remain 'free' or 'unbound'. The physical characteristics of the drug such as lipid solubility and protein binding capacity will decide the degree of protein binding. The drug gets carried to the right side of the heart and through the pulmonary circulation to the left side of the heart into the systemic circulation.

About 70% of the cardiac output supplies the brain, liver and kidneys (vessel rich organs) thus a high proportion of the initial bolus is delivered to cerebral circulation. The drug diffuses along a concentration gradient from the blood into the brain. The rapidity with which this transfer occurs depends on the arterial concentration of the unbound free drugs, lipid solubility of the drug and degree of ionization. The quickest

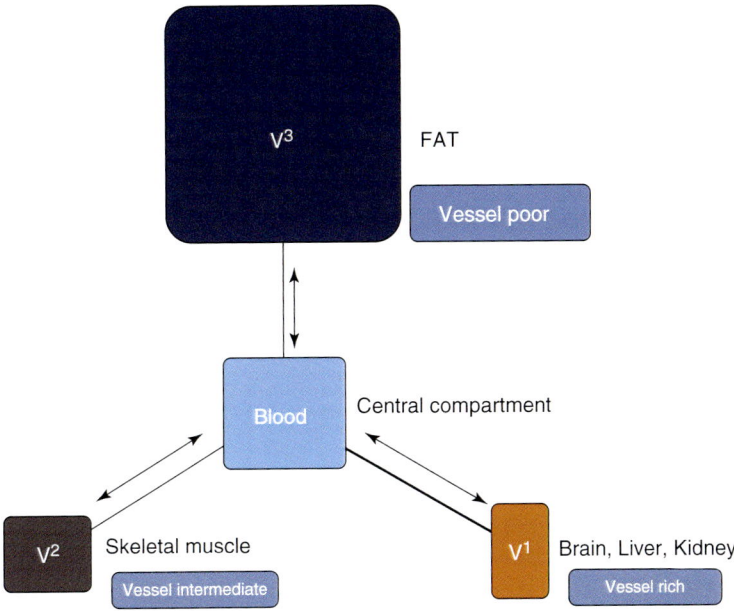

**Fig. 80.4** Illustration of a three compartment model for a lipid-soluble drug. Tank size indicates the capacity of the drug reservoir

molecules to cross the blood-brain barrier are the ones which are unbound, lipid soluble and unionised. On penetrating the CNS tissue, the drug exerts its effects.

Following the initial flooding of the CNS and vessel rich tissues with non ionised molecules, the drug starts to diffuse into other tissues which do not have rich blood supply. The drug moves down the concentration gradient from CNS to the area of secondary tissue uptake, predominantly the skeletal muscle. This initial redistribution of the drug into other tissues leads to the rapid wake up after a single induction dose. Fat (the vessel poor tissue) has poor blood supply and following repeated doses or infusion, the drug equilibrates with adipose tissue to form a drug reservoir often causing prolonged action of the drug.

In the elderly, with reduced cardiac output, the body compensates by diverting higher proportion of the cardiac output to the cerebral circulation. Since a greater proportion of injected drugs will enter the CNS, the dose of induction agents must be reduced. In addition, with reduced cardiac output, the time taken for the drug to reach the brain and exert its effect is prolonged. Thus slow titration of reduced dose of the drug is mandatory for the safe induction in the aged [71].

### Protein Binding

Anaesthetic drugs tend to bind to plasma proteins, rendering them unable to cross membranes to produce the desired drug effect. Acidic drugs bind to albumin. The concentration of albumin in the aged decreases, resulting in an increase in the unbound fraction of acidic anaesthetics such as benzodiazepines, barbituarates and opioids. Decreased protein binding increases the amount of drug available for interaction with target receptors thereby causing an increase in the depth and duration of anaesthetic action. Some chronic diseases such as cardiac and renal failure are also associated with decreased albumin levels and altered quantity of available protein [72]. The levels of α1-acid glycoprotein, which binds to basic drugs, (Eg. local anaesthetics and muscle relaxants) does not change or increase, thereby decreasing their action.

### Biotransformation of Drugs

Metabolism of anaesthetic drugs depends on the enzyme reactions that occur in the liver. Phase 1 reactions result in oxidation, reduction and hydrolytic reactions. The cytochrome P450 enzyme system of phase 1 reactions is responsible for metabolism of anaesthetic drugs. i.e., inhalational agents [73]. Phase 1 reactions generally result in loss of pharmacological activity and phase 2 reactions make compounds more water soluble and increase the excretion into urine or bile.

The mass of the liver, hepatic blood flow and intrinsic hepatic capacity is reduced in the elderly leading to decreased metabolism and drug clearance. This causes a prolonged duration of action of anesthetics and the need to reduce the dosages of drugs.

Loss of renal parenchymal tissue and decline in glomerular filtration rate interferes with elimination of anaesthetics which are dependent on renal excretion. Comorbid conditions like hypertension and coronary artery disease may worsen kidney function. Reduced elimination leads to accumulation of the drugs, leading to toxicity.

## Inhalational Anaesthetics

Pharmacodynamics of all inhaled anaesthetics are altered by age (Table 80.9). The MAC of volatile anaesthetics decreases with age [74]. The MAC decreases by 4% per decade after the age of 40.

A decrease of 4% in MAC and also similarly in MAC awake, for each decade of aging results in increased potency by approximately 6% for each decade. The increase in potency might be due to age- related changes in neurotransmitters and target receptors. A higher volume of distribution and low hepatic function is also a cause of delay in recovery following induction and maintenance with volatile anaesthetics. A reduction in dose is advised as cerebral electrical activity suppression may be achieved with lower concentrations.

Halothane is a lipid soluble volatile anaesthetic agent with a rapid rate of induction and higher risk of adverse events in the elderly when compared to less lipid soluble agents [75]. Isoflurane is less lipid soluble and can be titrated for a more stable induction in the elderly.

**Table 80.9** Dose adjustments of drugs in elderly

| Drug | Usual adult doses | Suggested adjustment in elderly |
|---|---|---|
| Induction agents | | |
| Propofol | Bolus 2–2.5 mg/kg, infusion dose 100–250 mcg/kg/min | 40–50% dose reduction, 30% dose reduction in infusion dose |
| Thiopentone | 4–5 mg/kg | 50–67% reduction in dosage |
| Etomidate | 0.3–0.4 mg/kg | 0.2 mg/kg |
| Ketamine | 2 mg/kg | No available literature |
| Midazolam | | 50% dose reduction |
| Inhalational agents | | |
| Isoflurane | 1.17 MAC | The MAC decreases by 4% per decade of age more than 40 years. Potency increases by 6% for every decade after 40 years |
| Sevoflurane | 1.8 MAC | |
| Desflurane | 6.6 MAC | |
| Halothane | 0.8 MAC | |
| Opioids | | |
| Morphine | 0.1–0.2 mg/kg intraoperatively | 50% dose reduction |
| Fentanyl | 1–2 mcg/kg for short term analgesia | 50% dose reduction |
| Alfentanyl | 5–25 mcg/kg for short term analgesia | 50% dose reduction |
| Remifentanyl | 0.5–1 mcg/kg Infusion 0.2–0.5 mcg/kg/min | 50% dose reduction-bolus 33% reduction-infusion |
| Neuromuscular blockers | | |
| Vecuronium | 0.1–0.15 mg/kg | 30% dose reduction |
| Rocuronium | 0.6 mg/kg | |

Halothane and isoflurane in combination with nitrous oxide have the property to impair peripheral blood flow in the older age group of patients. Sevoflurane also has less solubility and can provide a relatively controlled induction. Desflurane has a very low blood- gas solubility which provides the elderly with very rapid induction and emergence, even better when compared to sevoflurane.

The reduced cerebral blood flow, cell density and cerebral oxygen consumption appears to be the reason for decreased anaesthetic requirement in elderly. Xenon, an inert gas might prove to be a an ideal inhalational agent in future in the aged because its anaesthetic properties have the advantage of fast emergence from anesthesia without undergoing any metabolism in the body apart from affording cardiovascular and hemodynamic stability [75]. With respect to overall inhalational anaesthetics, the principal pharmacodynamical change associated with aging would be reduced anaesthetic requirement, represented by a lower MAC.

"Triple Low", a condition associated with low BiSpectral Index (<45), low mean arterial pressure(<75 mmHg) and low end tidal volatile anesthetic concentration in MAC equivalent(<0.7) is an ominous combination which may identify patients who are specially sensitive to anesthesia, and probably, at risk of brain hypoperfusion and high post-operative mortality rates [76].

## Intravenous Anaesthetics

The age related decrease of the dose required to produce a particular drug effect is due to changes in the volume of distribution and intercompartmental clearance. The reduced volume of distribution in the geriatric age group causes higher concentrations of thiopentone in plasma, since the effects of a single bolus of the drug is terminated by redistribution rather than metabolism in the liver. Due to low intercompartmental clearance, more thiopentone is available for distribution into the brain, thereby producing a profound effect. Thereafter if repeated doses of thiopentone are given, the elimination depends on the hepatic enzymes and plasma protein binding [75]. Thiopentone when compared to propofol affords faster onset and better hemodynamic stability. Dose requirement of thiopentone reduces to 50–67% in the elderly when compared to adults. A reduction in doses of propofol by 40–50% would be reasonable due to decreased clearance and increased sensitivity to drug in the elderly. With increasing age, the dose of etomidate needs to be reduced by 50%. The incidence of apnea and respiratory depression is less in patients receiving etomidate than those induced with thiopentone [77].

The pharmacokinetics and pharmacodynamics of benzodiazepines are impaired by increased age. Reduced hepatic perfusion and clearance in the elderly may lead to accumulation of the more potent hydroxylated metabolite of diazepam i.e., desmethyldiazepam resulting in prolonged clinical effects [78]. Midazolam requirement is reduced by 25–75% because of decreased enzyme activity and hepatic perfusion. Benzodiazepines need to be administered in reduced doses in the aged as they are more vulnerable to the central depressant actions. Flumazenil, the benzodiazepine receptor antagonist, can be used to reverse the untoward effects of benzodiazepines. The absorption, distribution and bio-availability of flumazenil in the elderly is comparable to that in the younger patients.

Opioid pharmacokinetics in the elderly are altered because of changes in the distribution volumes and decreased liver and renal blood flows. The elderly are very sensitive to the effects of the opioids via all the routes of administration and develop exaggerated physiological responses which mandate dose reductions.

Morphine in the elderly causes prolonged effects because it's clearance is decreased by 50% and half-life is prolonged by 50% when compared to that in young adults. The active metabolite of morphine is morphine-6-glucuronide which is dependent on renal excretion for clearance. Respiratory depression and immune suppression are the undesired side effects of morphine. Dose reduction of morphine is advocated [79].

Fentanyl has an elimination half-life of 925 min in the elderly when compared to 250 min in young adults. The dose requirement for fentanyl and alfentanyl decreases by 50% in the aged. Age does not significantly affect the pharmacokinetics of both these drugs, however, altered pharmacodynamics make them twice as potent in the elderly when compared to younger patients [79]. Sufentanyl also requires dose reduction by 50% in the aged due to increased brain sensitivity to opioids due to change in the number of opiate receptors or opiate receptor binding [80].

Remifentanyl, an ultra-short acting opioid exhibits altered pharmacokinetics and pharmacodynamics in the elderly. Dose reduction of 50% is recommended and infusion rates should be adjusted accordingly, because profound hemodynamic, central nervous system and respiratory system depression may result in delayed recovery [81].

Tramadol is a centrally acting synthetic analgesic which binds to the µ-opioid receptor and inhibits noradrenaline and serotonin re-uptake. A longer half-life of tramadol is seen after the age of 75 years and a reduction in dose is advisable. There is less risk of respiratory depression on one hand and propensity of causing post-operative delirium on the other, in the elderly population [82].

Meperidine (Pethidine) is known to cause profound clinical effects in the elderly because of the accumulation of it's active metabolite, normeperidine, due to decreased renal function which causes central nervous system toxicity. Decreased protein binding causes increase in free fraction of the drug which adds to the toxic effects [83].

## Neuromuscular Blocking Drugs

Age causes increased drug concentration in the blood as a result of reduced volume of distribution, clearance and altered pharmacokinetics. The aminosteroid group of non-depolarizing neuromuscular agents (pancuronium, vecuronium, rocuronium) depend on hepatic and renal function and blood flow for their elimination. Pancuronium bromide is not preferred in geriatrics because of higher incidences of tachycardia, hypertension and residual neuromuscular block. Vecuronium bromide, in the presence of age related decreased hepatic and renal blood flow, causes prolonged effect and decreased elimination. Drug dose should be reduced by 30% of that of younger adults. Rocuronium also displays prolonged action due to age related pharmacokinetics.

The benzylisoquinolone group of muscle relaxants (atracurium and cis-atracurium) undergo elimination by Hoffmann degradation with less variability in the effect of action in the elderly when compared to the aminosteroid group of relaxants. The depolarising neuromuscular blocking agent succinylcholine may result in prolonged action because of reduced level of pseudocholinesterase levels in frail geriatric patients.

Administration of neuromuscular blockers should be dosed keeping in mind that the elderly have decreased muscle blood flow and an altered number of acetyl choline receptors due to reduced physical activity and hence a delay in recovery and prolonged duration of action may result [72].

Age-appropriate dosing, monitoring and reversal strategies are required in the elderly to avoid delayed recovery and the risk of post-operative residual neuro-muscular block (PRNB). Age-related reductions in renal and hepatic function, cardiac output, muscle mass and ability to regulate temperature are present in older patient, thereby subjecting them to a higher incidence of adverse respiratory events [84]. Pre-existing decrease in vital capacity, maximum voluntary ventilation and total lung capacity are seen in elderly whereas closing volume is increased. PRNB is an important risk factor for pharyngeal dysfunction, upper airway obstruction, reduced upper oesophageal sphincter tone and an increased risk of aspiration. It predisposes the aged to a high risk of respiratory muscle weakness and subsequent hypoxemic events and pulmonary complications in the PACU. Hence the use of quantitative monitoring and sugammadex is beneficial in ensuring full recovery of neuromuscular function in the elderly surgical patient [85].

## Local Anaesthetics

Age related alterations in pharmacokinetics in the elderly result in higher blood concentration and longer half-lives of local anaesthetics. The elderly are prone to high sensitivity to local anesthetics in the form of persistent numbness, nerve palsies, increased block duration and level and increased degree of hypotension and bradycardia with equivalent doses when compared to young adults. These effects may be due to structural and functional changes in central and peripheral nervous systems. Dose reduction is advisable to avoid age related increase in duration and intensity of blockade. Biotransformation of local anaesthetics is dependent on hydrolysis by pseudocholinesterases or enzymatic degradation in liver. Compromised hepatic blood flow and enzyme levels due to age results in higher blood concentrations and longer half-lives of the drugs. Thoracic epidural with local anaesthetics reduces MAC and MAC awake by as much as by 50%, thereby reducing the concentration of inhalational anaesthetics required during combined epidural- GA for prolonged surgeries. Lidocaine, bupivacaine, levo-bupivacaine and ropivaciane are the commonly used local anaesthetics.

## Anticoagulants in the Elderly

The elderly have a higher prevalence of medical conditions with predisposition for thromboembolic complications, hence increasing the requirement of antithrombotic therapy [86]. The American College Of Cardiology/American Heart Association (ACC/AHA) guidelines can be utilized in addition to patient history and exercise tolerance to assess cardiac risk for patients undergoing non cardiac surgery. In the case of patients who have existing stents, the type and location have to be ascertained. Patients with drug eluting stents placed within the past year prior to their surgery are not candidates for elective surgery because of the risk of thrombosis from the discontinuation of antiplatelet agents in the perioperative period. A patient who is likely to undergo a surgery might be in need for a stent placement, in which case, the appropriate timing and type of intervention should be discussed with the cardiologist.

Antiplatelet medication like clopidogrel and ticlopidine should be discontinued 7 days prior to surgery, however low dose aspirin should be continued throughout the perioperative period.

## Indications for Anticoagulation

The incidence of venous thromboembolism (VTE) increases as a person ages [87] with higher prevalence of deep vein thrombosis (DVT) and pulmonary embolism (PE) in elderly patients above 70 years compared to younger patients. This could be attributed to higher prevalence of comorbidities such as malignancy or heart failure in the aged.

Anticoagulant therapy in VTE prevents extension of thrombus, recurrence of VTE and post-thrombotic syndrome. Subcutaneous Low Molecular Weight Heparin (LMWH), synthetic anti-factor Xa pentasaccharide (fondaparinux) or unfractionated heparin (UFH) are the therapy options in case of severe renal insufficiency, followed by an oral vitamin K Antagonist (VKA).

Parenteral anticoagulants treatment is accompanied with vitamin K antagonists for treating VTE. The parenteral agent can be stopped after 5 days, provided the INR is ≥2.0 for at least 24 hours [88].

## Atrial Fibrillation

The prevalence of atrial fibrillation (AF) increases significantly with age, in around 10% of people above 80 years of age [87]. Atrial fibrillation is implicated in 15% of ischemic strokes in the US. Long term anticoagulation is required in these patients and oral vitamin K anti-coagulants are recommended. Warfarin is a commonly used molecule and is considered more efficient than aspirin in elderly patients with AF in stroke prevention, provided there are no contra-indications.

## Valvular Heart Disease

Prosthetic heart valves pose a high risk of systemic embolism and are an indication for long term anti-coagulation. The latest recommendations according to ACCP guidelines recommend anticoagulation with a VKA for all mechanical valves. The target INR is 2.5–3.5 for different valves. Low dose aspirin (50–100 mg/day) is recommended in the presence of additional risk factors such as AF, hyper-coagulable state, low ejection fraction and left atrial enlargement [89].

## Pharmacology of VKA in the Elderly

The vitamin K antagonist warfarin belongs to the coumarin group and is used worldwide. It is absorbed rapidly from the gastrointestinal tract after oral administration. Its anticoagulant effect is caused by interfering with vitamin K metabolism thus impairing the hemostatic properties of factors II, VII, IX, X. Warfarin is predominantly plasma protein bound and is metabolised by the liver cytochrome CYP2C9 [90]. As a result of polypharmacy in the elderly they are at risk of drug interactions when on warfarin therapy. Aging results in decline in synthesis of clotting factors in patients with hepatic disease and less intake of vitamin K in the diet. Drug interactions with NSAIDs or aspirin may interfere with the pharmacodynamics of warfarin. Hence maintaining safe anticoagulation with VKA is imperative in view of increased response to warfarin in the elderly. INR should be closely monitored in order to avoid anticoagulation associated bleeding complications (Fig. 80.5).

## Newer Anticoagulation Agents

These therapeutic agents target specific steps in the coagulation cascade. They target factor Xa and factor IIa (Thrombin). Factor Xa initiates the common pathway of coagulation and thrombin has a pivotal role in converting fibrinogen to fibrin, and activating coagulation factors (V, VII, XI, XIII) and platelets.

1. Indirect Xa inhibitors—fondaparinux, idraparinux
2. Direct Xa inhibitors—apixaban, rivaroxaban
3. Direct thrombin inhibitors—hirudin, argatroban

Elderly people are at high thromboembolic risk on one hand and also at high risk of haemorrhage on the other hand. Analysing the benefit-risk ratio of anticoagulation is a highly challenging issue in the elderly in order to afford maximum safety.

## Special Considerations in Geriatric Patients on Anticoagulants

Anticoagulants in the elderly are associated with the inherent bleeding risk. Age related decrease in renal function has to be considered in patients treated with LMWHs and fondaparinux, as these depend on the kidneys for excretion. Assessment of kidney function is important when prescribing anti-coagulants in the elderly, because even minimal decreases in creatinine clearance can result in accumulation of LMWHs.

Comorbidities such as hypertension, cerebrovascular disease, ischemic stroke, diabetes, heart disease, renal in-sufficiency, hepatic disease and alcoholism have been incriminated in the increased risk of bleeding in patients on VKA therapy. This has to be considered while estimating risk-benefit ratio of oral anticoagulation [91].

Geriatric patients with a history of "frequent falls", "history of falls", "multiple falls" or "tendency of falls" and who are also on VKA show an increased risk of intracranial haemorrhage (ICH). Prescription of warfarin has not been found to affect the incidence rate of ICH. Anti-coagulation affords benefit for patients in AF (with additional risk of stroke) even though they are at high risk for falls [92].

## Preoperative Assessment of Functional Reserve in Elderly

Preoperative evaluation is a crucial and significant part in assessing and reducing post-operative complications in the elderly. It is useful in identifying the risks associated with specific complications and to have a management plan that minimizes those risks. Although age is a big risk factor for elderly patients undergoing a surgery, each patient should be assessed individually focussing on the problems associated and his/her physiologic status (Table 80.11).

Metabolic equivalents and ASA physical status are the commonly used tools for quantifying functional reserve.

| \multicolumn{3}{l}{**MANAGING ORAL ANTICOAGULATION in the ELDERLY**} | |
|---|---|---|
| Initiation of Therapy | ■ Obtain baseline INR (and APTT if on heparin).<br>■ Determine if drug interactions with warfarin are present.<br>■ Initial dosage should be an estimate of the average daily dosage of warfarin, usually less then 5 mg daily in the elderly due to increased pharmacodynamic activity.<br>■ Discontinue heparin, if being administered concurrently, after the INR has been in the therapeutic range for at least two measurements taken ≥ 24 hours apart. | |
| Monitoring of Therapy | ■ Monitor INR daily until stable; a therapeutic INR is usually achieved in 5 to 7 days.<br>■ The INR can be monitored 2-3 times weekly for 1-2 weeks, then weekly for one month, and monthly thereafter. More frequent monitoring is required in some patients, particularly during changes in medications, particularly antibiotics, and changes in diet. | |
| Managing High INR Values | INR 3.0 - 5.0<br>No significant bleeding | ■ Withhold one dose or lower the dose<br>■ Resume therapy when INR in desired range |
| | INR 5.0 - 9.0<br>No significant bleeding | ■ Withhold 1-2 doses, resume when INR in desired range<br>■ Consider Vitamin K1 (1-2.5 mg p.o.). especially if increased bleeding risk<br>■ If urgent correction required, give Vitamin K1 (2-4 mg p.o); if INR remains high give additional Vitamin K1 (1-2 mg p.o)<br>*Grade 2G evidence as compared with no treatment* |
| | INR > 9.0<br>No significant bleeding | ■ Withhold warfarin; give Vitamin K1 (3-5 mg p.o)<br>■ Closely monitor INR; if not substantially reduced in 24-48 hrs., may require additional Vitamin K1. |
| | Significant bleeding | ■ Discontinue warfarin<br>■ Administer Vitamin K1 (10 mg slow IV infusion); supplemented with fresh plasma or prothrombin complex concentrate, depending on urgency; Vitamin K1 injections can be repeated every 12 hours. (*grade 2C*) |
| Managing oral anticoagulation During invasive procedures | Low risk for thromboembolism<br>■ No VTE > 3 mos.<br>■ AF without history of stroke<br>■ Bileaflet mechanical valve in the aortic position | ■ Stop warfarin about 4 days prior to procedure<br>■ Consider short term LMWH or LDUH when INR is reduced if procedure increases risk for thrombosis<br>■ Resume warfarin following |
| | Intermediate risk for Thromboembolism | ■ Stop warfarin about 4 days prior to procedure and allow INR to return to normal range<br>■ Administer LMWH or LDUH (5000 IU SC) about 2 days prior to procedure; and following the procedure<br>■ Resume warfarin and discontinue LDUH when INR is therapeutic for ≥ 48 hours |
| | High risk for thromboembolism<br>■ VTE in < 3 months<br>■ History of VTE<br>■ Mechanical cardiac valve in mitral position<br>■ Old model cardiac valve (ball/cage) | ■ Stop warfarin about 4 days prior to procedure and allow INR to fall to normal range<br>■ Administer full dose heparin (SC or IV) as INR falls, and discontinue about 5 hours prior to procedure; or alternately administer LMWH untill 12 to 24 hours prior to the procedure<br>■ Resume heparin or LMWH and warfarin after procedure and discontinue LDUH when INR is therapeutic for ≥ 48 hours |

**Fig. 80.5** The American Geriatrics Society guidelines for managing oral anticoagulation in the elderly

### ORAL ANTICOAGULANT GUIDELINES FOR THE CARE OF OLDER ADULTS*

#### VENOUS THROMBOEMBOLISM

| DISORDER | INR Gial, range | CLINICAL COMMENTS |
|---|---|---|
| Surgical prophylaxis for High Risk Patients | 2.5 (2.0-3.0) | In older adults (> 60 years), undergoing general, gynecologic, urologic surgery, perioperative prophylaxis with LDUH, LMWH, IPC device, ES, is preferred over oral warfarin (grade 1A-C). For major orthopedic surgery, THR, TKR, hip fracture surgery, LMWH is preferred, but adjusted dose oral warfarin may be used alternatively to LMWH, adjusted dose heparin, (grade 1A), or IPC device (grade 1B). Anticoagulants are given preoperatively or immediately postoperatively, and continued at least 7-10 days postoperatively. |
| Deep Venous Thrombosis (DVT) or Pulmonary Embolism (PE) | 2.5 (2.0-3.0) | Oral warfarin should be initiated with LMWH on day 1; discontinue LMWH after ≥ 4 to 5 days of combined therapy when INR is >2.0.<br>Duration:<br>■ ≥ 6 to 12 weeks for symptomatic isolated calf thrombosis (grade 1A)<br>■ ≥ 3 months for first episode with reversible or time-limited risk factor (grade 1A)<br>■ ≥ 6 months for idiopathic first episode (grade 1A)<br>■ ≥ 12 months for recurrent idiopathic or continuing risk factor (grade 1C) Therapy should be individualized; for many patients, lifelong therapy is indicated.<br>Time-limited risk factors include surgery, trauma, immobilization, estrogen use. Continuing risk factors include cancer, antithrombin deficiency, anticardiolipin antibody syndrome. IVC filters recommended for placement with proximal vein thrombosis or PE or with high risk for these conditions when anticoagulant therapy is contraindicated or has resulted in a complication (grade 1C+) or with recurrent VTE despite adequate anticoagulation, with chronic recurrent embolism and pulmonary hypertension, and with surgical pulmonary embolectomy, (grade 1C) with continued warfarin. |

#### PREVENTION OF SYSTEMIC EMBOLISM

| | | |
|---|---|---|
| Atrial fibrillation (AF) | 2.5 (2.0-3.0) | For patients with any high risk factor or more than one moderate risk factor, warfarin is recommended. For patients with one moderate risk factor, aspirin 325 mg/d or warfarin is recommended. High risk factors include age ≥ 75; previous TIA, SE, or stroke; poor LV systolic function, hypertension, rheumatic mitral valve disease; or prosthetic heart valve (grade 1A). Moderate risk factors include age 65-75, diabetes mellitus, CAD, with preserved LV function, (grade 1A) |
| Cardioversion Atrial Fibrillation or Atrial Flutter | 2.5 (2.0-3.0) | Patients with AF for < 48 hours should be offered anticoagulation during the pericardioversion period (grade 2C). If > 48 hrs or indeterminate, anticoagulate as below; Duration: 3 weeks prior and ≥ 4 weeks after procedure (grade 1C+); or alternatively, if < 48 hrs and TEE is negative for thrombus, anticoagulation until NSR is maintained ≥ 4 weeks (grade 1C). |
| Acute Myocardial Infarction | | Anticoagulate for ≤ 3 months in patients who may or may not have received thrombolytic and are at high risk for systemic embolism or VTE (anterior Q-wave infarction, severe LV dysfunction, congestive heart failure, history of SE or PE, 2D-echo evidence of mural thrombus. (grade 2A) or AF [grade 1A]), indefinitely with AF |
| Rheumatic Mitral Valve Disease (MS, MR) | 2.5 (2.0-3.0) | Indefinite treatment with history of SE or AF (grade 1C+). Consideration of long-term warfarin therapy based on risk factors for SE (LA size, patient's age, hemodynamic severity) (grade 2C). Oral anticoagulation for mitral valve prolapse recommended when a documented SE or recurrent TIA has occurred despite aspirin (grade 1C) |
| Aortic Valve and Aortic Arch Disorders | | Oral warfarin is only recommended for mobile aortic atheroma and aortic plaque > 4 mm by TEE (grade 2C) |
| Prothetic Heart Valves; Any bileaflet or tilting disk in aortic position | 2.5 (2.0-3.0) (grade 1A) | St. Jude Medical (grade 1A) or CarboMedics bileaflet, or Medtronic-Hall tilting disk (grade 1C); left atrium normal size, NSR |
| Prosthetic Heart Valves: Tilting disk valve or bileaflet mechanical valve in mitral position | 3.0 (2.5-3.5) | Alternatively, INR 2.5 (2.0 - 3.0) and aspirin therapy (80-100 mg/d) (grade 2C) |
| Prosthetic Heart Valves: Any mechanical aortic with AF | 3.0 (2.5-3.5) | Alternatively, INR 2.5 (2.0 - 3.0) and aspirin therapy (80-100 mg/d) (grade 2C) |
| Prosthetic Heart Valves: Caged ball or caged disk valve | 3.0 (2.5-3.5) | Alternatively, INR 2.5 (2.0 - 3.0) and aspirin therapy (80-100 mg/d) (grade 2C) |
| Prosthetic Heart Valves; Additional risk factors or Systemic embolism despite adequate therapy with oral anticoagulants | 3.0 (2.5-3.5) | INR 2.5 (2.0 - 3.0) and aspirin therapy (80-100 mg/d) (grade 1C+) |

Abbreviations:

| | | | | | |
|---|---|---|---|---|---|
| AF | Atrial fibrillation | LMWH | Low molecular weight heparin | SE | Systemic Embolism |
| CAD | Coronary artery disease | LA | Left Atrial | TEE | Transesophageal echocardiogram |
| ES | Elastic Stockings | LV | Left ventricular | TIA | Transient ischemic attack |
| IPC | Intermittent Pneumatic Compression | NSR | Normal sinus rhythm | THR | Total hip replacement |
| LDUH | Low dose unfractionated heparin | PE | Pulmonary embolism | TKR | Total knee replacement |

*Modified from Chest 2001;119/1(Suppl.) by Laurie G. Jacobs, MD for the Clinical Practice Committee of the American geriatrics Society. For further information, visit the AGS web-site (www.americangeriatrics.org)
This pocket card has been reviewed and approved by the Society of Geriatric Cardiology
The development of this pocket card was supported by an unrestricted educational grant from Bristol-Meyers Squibb.

**Fig. 80.5** (continued)

## Metabolic equivalents (METs)

Metabolic equivalents is based on the calculation of the basal oxygen requirements, at rest, of a 40 year old male weighing 70 kg (about 3.5 ml/kg/min) and then gradually stepping up his workload and simultaneously recording the increase in oxygen uptake.

The aged patients with restricted cardiorespiratory reserve have limited capacity to increase their cardiac output and oxygen delivery so as to compensate for the oxygen debt in the postoperative period. This functional limitation is calculated in terms of METs that they can achieve, which gives an insight into the ability of the elderly to meet the increased post-operative oxygen demand secondary to surgical stress. Systemic Inflammatory Response Syndrome (SIRS) secondary to surgery increases oxygen requirement from an average of 110 ml/min/m$^2$ at rest to an average of 170 ml/min/m². The failure to cope may be a predictor of organ failure and death. METs is difficult to assess in patients with arthritis, blindness or stroke. Exercise testing for ischemia remains a reliable measure but in cases of mobility restriction, an inotrope-induced stress test is a viable option. If available, dipyridamole-thallium scanning, trans-oesophageal ECHO or Holter monitoring may be of benefit.

The **ASA Physical Status Classification** aims at identifying dysfunction of organ systems and severity of functional impairment thereby predicting morbidity and mortality in patients undergoing surgery. This assessment lacks specificity and precision. It does not grade the risk with respect to patient's age, type of surgery, physical and mental status, all of which have an impact in geriatric anesthesia.

**Table 80.10** Risk factors for increased morbidity and mortality

| |
|---|
| • ASA Physical risk status—Class 3 and 4 |
| • Severe coexisting systemic disease |
| • Functional Status—less than 1–4 METs |
| • Serum Albumin <3.5 g/dL |
| • Anaemia with Hb <8 g/dL |
| • Unable to do daily activities before surgery |

patient was admitted, whereas the recent development has given rise to the current methodology known as Comprehensive Geriatric Assessment (CGA) [93]. The CGA includes multiple geriatric related domains to predict post-operative outcomes so as to identify the older patients at risk and help devise appropriate and realistic perioperative care plans (Table 80.10) (Fig. 80.6).

## POSSUM (Physiological and Operative Severity Score for the enUmeration of Mortality and Morbidity)

This assessment includes physiological and operative variables to assess the risk of morbidity and mortality in surgical patients. Age is a component of the physiological portion and increasing age is accorded higher scores. The operative score includes variables such as operative magnitude, predicted blood loss and whether the surgery is elective or emergency.

## Comprehensive Geriatric Assessment (CGA)

As one ages, multiple organ systems undergo physiological changes, and the cumulative effects of the sum of these changes involve more than one set of measurements. In the current scenario, a new approach to geriatric assessment has taken shape, evaluating comorbidities, nutritional and mental status, living circumstances, polypharmacy and collateral support systems. The traditional mono-dimensional assessment concentrated more on the illness per se for which the

## Preoperative Assessment in the Elderly for Emergency Procedures

The elderly presenting for emergency procedures have to be accepted for emergency anesthesia even if they were to be unfit for elective procedures. These patients may present with trauma, involving fractured limbs and facial or neurotrauma. Abdominal emergencies in geriatrics often present as bowel perforations, appendicitis, cholecystitis, mesenteric ischemia, occlusive syndromes involving hernias or colon, cancers and peritonitis. These patients often present in suboptimal conditions due to the late discovery of their conditions, fluid depleted states, metabolic derangements, pain and suboptimally managed chronic ailments. Such patients would present with confused mental status and incomplete medical history.

Depending on the emergent situation, optimal preoperative assessment is mandatory and optimisation of co-existing medical conditions should be simultaneously aimed at. Delaying orthopaedic corrections of lower limbs have shown to result in increased risk of death in the elderly. A meticulous general physical examination with basic investigations such as ECG and Echocardiography (if possible, to determine cardiac status) and blood

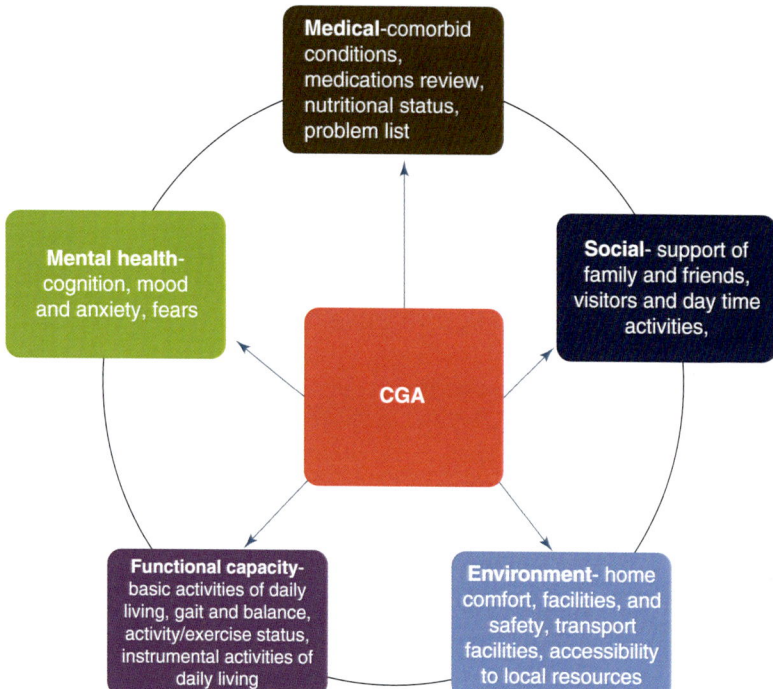

**Fig. 80.6** Components of comprehensive geriatric assessment

chemistry should be undertaken. These patients often present with history of anti-coagulant or anti-platelet medications which have anaesthetic and surgical implications.

## Informed Consent

An essential requirement to give an informed consent is the ability of a person to understand the type of procedure and the risk and benefits associated with it. More often than not, the elderly patient may not be fully aware of the severity of the illness or the degree of complications that is associated with the planned surgery. In such instances family members or the legal guardians should be informed about the surgical interventions and the likely complications. It is advisable to involve a close relative in obtaining the consent. Patient's mental and cognitive status must be documented for legal purposes.

## History and Nutritional Assessment

A complete medical and surgical history will prove to be useful in assessment of the patient. Likewise the list of all the medications that the patient has been taking prior to the surgery may help in assessing the severity of the comorbidity. Malnutrition is common in the elderly. A BMI of less than 20 kg/m$^2$ might pose a problem as it can lead to delayed wound healing. Albumin levels of less than 3.5 g/dL in hospitalized elderly highly predict the subsequent mortality and morbidity. A cholesterol level of less than 160 mg/dL in a frail elderly person is also a marker for increased mortality. Supplementing with nutritional supplements preoperatively in forms of high energy foods, protein diet and vitamins should be considered.

## Best Practices for Communication with Older Adults

1. Assessment should be made face to face to allow the patients to see lip movements when speaking, especially with hearing impaired
2. Clear, slow voice tone but louder than usual
3. Leading question to the companion or caregiver to understand the condition better
4. Allow sufficient time for the patient to respond.
5. Use common and layman terms avoiding medical terminologies
6. In patients with cognitive impairment, responses should be verified with the caregivers.

## Physical Examination

Hydration and nutrition can be assessed by examination of skin, oral mucosa and tongue. Thin and fragile skin can give valuable inputs of a poorly maintained collagen matrix and a risk of potential damage to ligaments and joint subluxation. Bruised skin is an indication of intra-operative tendencies of increased bleeding. These patients are prone to developing pressure sores as a result of minute trauma during shifting. Subcutaneous fat is limited, so is muscle mass, thereby subjecting the aged to the risk of hypothermia. Fragility of skin may make inserting of i.v. lines difficult and fluids administered under pressure may cause rupture of fragile vessel walls leading to fluid extravasation.

The aged have osteoporotic bones and lax ligaments making positioning for central neuraxial blockade difficult. Fractures and joint dislocations under anesthesia should be carefully avoided and pressure points well padded.

A detailed examination of blood pressure, pulse irregularities and systemic examination should be included and can prove useful with respect to intra-op management. Pre-operative dementia is an important predictor of poor surgical outcome. A detailed systemic examination should be conducted to identify physiologic deficits and comorbid conditions that may increase the chances of post-operative complications.

## Pre-operative Investigations

Various objective parameters can be used to determine the health status of elderly objectively. Investigations serve as baseline data for comparing the status of the patient post-operatively and also to identify complications (Table 80.11). These include

- Complete blood count
- Renal function tests (deteriorate gradually with age)
- Blood glucose and cholesterol levels.
- Albumin level and coagulation profile
- Serum Electrolytes
- ECG/Echocardiography
- Chest radiograph and pulmonary function tests for assessing lungs

**Table 80.11** Checklist for effective pre-anaesthetic evaluation

- Functional status and nutritional evaluation
- Procedural risk estimation
- Optimize medical conditions
- Medical history and physical examination
- Relevant investigations

## Choice of Anesthesia Technique

Clear answers to the choice of anesthesia technique (whether regional or GA) in the elderly is still elusive because very few anaesthetic agents which are in current use have been evaluated in the elderly, and usually not in large enough studies to arrive at a definite conclusion.

Regional anaesthesia (RA) offers the inherent element of safety as it allows for the preservation of the mental functions. In the elderly population, cognitive dysfunction is an incapacitating entity which occurs in a significant number of elderly following surgery. Several studies done have not found any conclusive evidence that occurrence of postoperative cognitive dysfunction is more in GA than regional anesthesia [66].

However RA offers several benefits in terms of decreased adverse cardiac and respiratory outcomes. Intense analgesia and excellent operative relaxation reduces surgical stress response especially in debilitated elderly patients. Physiology of aging has adverse effects on the pulmonary gas exchange which can cause severe V/Q mismatch especially in elderly pulmonary cripples subjected to GA. Regional techniques, in the form of central neuraxial blockade and regional nerve blocks may help preserve pulmonary functions. RA along with sedation has now almost monopolized contemporary anesthesia practice. Postoperative pain relief afforded by a combination of local anaesthetics and opioids as a part of central neuraxial blockade is far superior to intravenous patient controlled analgesia (PCA). The latter is known to cause undesirable opioid related respiratory depression, post-operative nausea and vomiting and chest wall rigidity. In major abdominal surgeries where epidural catheterisation is supplementary to GA, the requirement of polypharmacy is substantially reduced and postoperative analgesia is excellent.

Regional anesthesia might be technically challenging in the geriatric patients, in terms of positioning because of rigidity, arthritis, calcification and osteoporotic bones, resulting in difficult or unsuccessful regional blocks or central neuraxial blockade. The use of large gauge spinal needles is acceptable because the incidence of post dural puncture headache (PDPH) is less in elderly. Ultrasound guided nerve blocks have become popular as it offers the advantage of blocking selective nerves with minimum drug volume when compared to traditional landmark techniques which use larger volumes of local anaesthetics.

Regional blocks may be extended into the postoperative period with the insertion of perineural catheters and this is equally beneficial during physiotherapy, should it be required [94].

Central neuraxial blockade has the disadvantage of causing hypotension and bradycardia as a result of sympatho-adrenal suppression. Routine pre-hydration in frail elderly may lead to volume load and result in congestive heart failure and pulmonary edema.

GA is a technically simpler option provided the airway related problems can be circumvented and is usually preferred in emergency situations when the patients are hypovolemic or dehydrated. However the risk of polypharmacy and postoperative pulmonary complications in GA are pertinent issues of this technique [95].

The issues that negatively affect the safety profile of GA in the elderly are that pertaining to the physiology and comorbidity. There is a greater incidence of the following events: cardiovascular (MI, CHF, arrhythmias); respiratory (respiratory insufficiency, hypoxemia, PPC, difficult weaning from ventilatory support); gastrointestinal (ileus, anastomotic disruptions) [96]; neurologic (delirium, confusion, POCD); airway difficulty(edentulous, neck stiffness) and urologic (retention). These are further magnified with increased surgical duration, in emergency surgeries and increasing age.

## Conclusion

It is beyond doubt that the fastest growing population globally is the geriatric population (>65 years). With the number of 'old olds' (75–84 years) and 'oldest' (over 85 years) slated to rise exponentially as a result of advances in health care, we will be required to better understand these patients so as to provide them with safe anesthetic care. Rather than making their later years a period of dependency and debility, we should strive to convert this phase of life into one of independence and productivity. The unpredictable responses of the aged have to be managed with higher levels of care and vigilance to ensure safer outcomes. Updated knowledge of the pathophysiology of aged organ system, metabolism, pharmacokinetics and pharmacodynamics of anaesthetic drugs will go a long way in individualizing and managing geriatric patients.

## References

1. Christensen K, Doblhammer G, Rao R, Vaupel JW. Aging populations: the challenges ahead. Lancet. 2009;374:1196–208.
2. Sabate S, Canet J, Gomar C, Castillo J, Villalonga A. ANESCAT Investigators. Cross sectional survey of anaesthetic practices in Catalonia, Spain. Ann Fr Anesth Reanim. 2008;27(5):371–83.
3. Akhtar S, Alec Rooke G. Cardiovascular ageing; Chapter 6. In: Dodds C, Kumar C, Veering B, editors. Oxford textbook of anesthesia for the elderly patient. Oxford: Oxford University Press; 2014. p. 41–9.
4. Stassijns G, Lysens R, Decramer M. Peripheral and respiratory muscles in chronic heart failure. Eur Respir J. 1996;9(10):2161–7.
5. Crapo RO. The ageing lung. In: Mahler DA, editor. Pulmonary disease in the elderly patient, vol. 63. New York: Marcel Dekker; 1993. p. 1–21.
6. Griffith KA, Sherrill DL, Siegel EM, Manolio TA, Bonekat HW, Enright PL. Predictors of loss of lung function in the elderly: the Cardiovascular Health study. Am J Respir Crit Care Med. 2001;163(1):61–8.
7. Wahba WM. Influence of ageing on lung function – clinical significance of changes from age twenty. Anaesth Analg. 1983;62(8):764–76.
8. Smith TC. Respiratory effects of aging. Semin Anesth. 1986;5(1):14–22.
9. Vait Kevicius PV, Fleg JL, Engel JH, et al. Effects of age and aerobic capacity on arterial stiffness in healthy adults. Circulation. 1993;88:1456–62.

10. Karlekar A, Sarkar D. Cardiovascular system and the elderly surgical patient: changes and implications. In: Kumra VP, editor. Applied geriatric anesthesia. 1st ed. New Delhi: Jaypee Brothers; 2008. p. 57–85.
11. Rooke GA, Robinson BJ. Cardiovascular and autonomic nervous system aging. Probl Anesth. 1997;9:482–97.
12. Powell-Tuck J, Gosling P, Lobo D, et al. British consensus guidelines on intravenous fluid therapy for adult surgical patient. 2008. https://www.ics.ac.uk/ICS/guidelines-and-standards.aspx.
13. Rooke GA. Cardiovascular aging and anaesthetic implications. J Cardiothorac Vasc Anesth. 2003;17:512–23. Pub Med: 12968244
14. Barnett SR. Polypharmacy and perioperative medications in the elderly. Anesthesiol Clin. 2009;27(3):377–89.
15. Aronow WS. Heart disease and aging. Med Clin North Am. 2006;90(5):849–62.
16. Kertai MD, Bountioukos M, Boersma E, et al. Aortic stenosis: an underestimated risk factor for perioperative complications in patients undergoing non cardiac surgery. Am J Med. 2004;116(1):8–13.
17. Canet J, Sanchis J. Respiratory ageing. Chapter 7. In: Oxford textbook of anesthesia for the elderly patient. Oxford: Oxford University Press; 2014. p. 53–8.
18. Zaugg M, Lucchinetti E. Respiratory function in the elderly. Anesthesiol Clin North Am. 2000;18(1):47–58.
19. Enright P, Kronmal R, Manolio T, Schenker MB, Hyatt RE. Respiratory muscle strength in the elderly: correlates and reference values. Am J Respir Crit Care Med. 1994;149(3 pt1):430–8.
20. Marik PE, Kaplan D. Aspiration pneumonia and dysphagia in the elderly. Chest. 2003;124(1):328–36.
21. White DP, Lombard RM, Cadieux RJ, Zwillich CW. Pharyngeal resistance in normal human: influence of gender, age and obesity. J Appl Physiol. 1985;58(2):365–71.
22. Krumpe PE, Knudson RG, Parsons G, Reiserk. The aging respiratory system. Clin Geriatr Med. 1985;1(1):143–75.
23. Valentine SJ, Marjot R, Monk CR. Pre-oxygention in the elderly: a comparison of the four-maximal-breath and three minute ventilation techniques. Anesth Analg. 1990;71(5):516–9.
24. Brown L. Respiratory dysfunction in Parkinson's disease. Clin Chest Med. 1994;15(4):715–27.
25. Vingerhoets F, Bogousslavsky J. Respiratory dysfunction in stroke. Clin Chest Med. 1994;15(4):729–37.
26. World Health Organization. Global surveillance, prevention and control of chronic respiratory disease. A comprehensive approach. Genera: WHO Publication; 2007.
27. Lumb A, Bier Camp C. Chronic obstructive pulmonary disease and anesthesia. Contin Educ Anaesth Crit Care Pain. 2014;14(1):1–5.
28. Antonelli-Incalzi R, Pedone C, Pahor M. Multidimensional assessment and treatment of the elderly with COPD. Eur Respir Mongr. 2009;43:35–55.
29. Trayner E, Celli BR. Postoperative medical complications. Med Clin North Am. 2001;85(5):1129–39.
30. Kumra VP. Preoperative assessment and preparation. In: Applied geriatric anesthesia. 1st ed. New Delhi: Jaypee Brothers; 2008. p. 20–46.
31. Tarhan S, Moffitt ET, et al. Role of anesthesia and surgery with chronic bronchitis and COPD. Surgery. 1973;74:720–6.
32. Arozullah AM, Daley J, et al. Multifactorial risk index for predicting postoperative respiratory failure in men after major non-cardiac surgery. Ann Surg. 2000;232:42–53.
33. Gupta RM, Parizi J, et al. Postoperative complications in patients with OSA syndrome undergoing hip and knee replacement. Mayo Clin Proc. 76:897.
34. Beliveau MM, Multach M. Perioperative care for the elderly patients. Med Clin North Am. 2003;87(1):273–89.
35. Russell RM. Changes in gastrointestinal function attributed to ageing. Am J Clin Nutr. 1992;55:1230S–7S. Pubmed;15-90257
36. Morley JE. Anorexia of ageing: physiologic and pathogenic. Am J Clin Nutr. 1997;66(4):760–73.
37. Gibbs J, Cull W, Henderson W, Daley J, Hur K, Khuri SF. Peri-operative serum albumin levels as a predictor of mortality and morbidity: results from national VA surgical risk study. Arch Surg. 1999;134(1):36–42.
38. Martin JE, Sheaff MT. Renal ageing. J Pathol. 2007;211:198–205. Pubmed: 17200944
39. Chahal HS, Drake WM. The endocrine system and ageing. J Pathol. 2007;211:173–80. Pubmed: 17200939
40. Lamberts SW, van den Beld AW, van der Lely AJ. The endocrinology of ageing. Science. 1997;278:419–24. Pubmed: 9334293
41. Burton D. Endocrine and metabolic response to surgery. Contin Educ Anaesth Crit Care Pain. 2004;4(5):144–7.
42. Kim S, Brooks AK, Groban L. Perioperative assessment of the older surgical patient: honing in on geriatric syndromes. Clin Interv Ageing. Dovepress. http://dx.doi.org/https://doi.org/10.2147/CIA.S75285.
43. Kumar R, Kumra VP. Diabetes mellitus in geriatric patients. In: Applied geriatric anesthesia. 1st ed. New Delhi: Jaypee Brothers; 2008. p. 158–83.
44. Blaum CS, Halter JB. Treatment of older adults with diabetes. In: Kahn CR, Weir GC, King GL, Jacobson AM, Moses AC, Smith RJ, editors. Joslin's Diabetes Mellitus. 14th ed. Philadelphia: Lippincott Williams and Wilkins; 2005. p. 737–46.
45. Kaiser MJ, Bauer JM, Ramsch C, et al. Mini Nutritional Assessment International Group. Frequency of malnutrition in older adults: a multinational perspective using the mini nutritional assessment. J Am Geriatr Soc. 2010;58(9):1734–8.
46. Arozullah AM, Daley J, Henderson WG, Khuri SF. Multifactorial risk index for predicting postoperative respiratory failure in men after major non cardiac surgery. The National Veterans Administration

47. VanStijn MFM, Korkic-Halilovic I, MSM B, VanderPloeg T, PAM VL, APJ H. Preoperative nutrition status and postoperative outcome in elderly general surgery patients: a systematic review. JPEN J Parenter Enteral Nutr. 2013;37(1):37–43.
48. Osland EJ, Memon MA. Are we jumping the gun with pharmaconutrition (immunonutrition) in gastrointestinal oncological surgery? World J Gastrointest Oncol. 2011;3(9):128–30.
49. Guigoz Y, Lauque S, Vellas BJ. Identifying the elderly at risk for malnutrition. The mini-nutritional assessment. Clin Geriatr Med. 2002;18:737–57.
50. Guidelines for pre-operative cardiac risk assessment and perioperative cardiac management in Non-cardiac Surgery of the European Society of Cardiology (ESC) and endorsed by the European Society Anaesthesiology (ESE). Eur J Anesthesial. 2010;27:92–137.
51. Fried LP, Tangen CM, Walston J, et al. Cardiovascular Health Study Collaborative Research Group. Frailty in older adults: evidence for a phenotype. J Gerontol A Biol Sci Med Sci. 2001;56(3):M146–56.
52. Cruz-Jentoft AJ, Baeyens JP, Bauer JM, Boirie Y, Cederholm T, Landi F, et al. Sarcopenia: European Consesus on definition and diagnosis: Report of the European Working Group on Sarcopenia in the older people. Age Ageing. 2010;39(4):412–23. Pubmed:20392703
53. Mocchegiani E, Corsonello A, Lattanzio F. Frailty, ageing and inflammation: reality and perspectives. Biogerontology. 2010;11:523–5.
54. McCusker J, Bellavalce F, Cardin S, Belzile E. Validity of an activities of daily life questionnaire among older patients in the emergency department. J Clin Epidemiol. 1999;52:1023–30.
55. Lawton MP, Brody EM. Self maintaining and instrumental activities of daily living. Gerontologist. 1969;9:179–86.
56. Dodds C, Kumar MC, Servin F. Anesthesia for the elderly patient. Oxford Anesthesia Library. 2016; Chapter 12, p. 107–12.
57. Grape S, Ravussin P, Rossi A, Kern C, Steiner LA. Postoperative cognitive dysfunction. Trends Anesth Crit Care. 2012;2:98–103.
58. Caza N, Taha R, Qi Y, Blaise G. The effects of surgery and anesthesia on memory and cognition. Prog Brain Res. 2008;169:409–22.
59. Baranov D, Bickler PE, Crosby GJ, Culley DJ, Eckenhoff MF, Eckenoff RG, et al. Consensus statement: first international workshop on anaesthetics and Alzheimer's disease. Anesth Analg. 2009;108(5):1627–30.
60. Newcomer JW, Craft S, Hershey T, Askins K, Bardgett ME. Glucocortocoids-induced impairment in declarative memory performance in adult humans. J Neurosci. 1994;14:2047–53.
61. Abildstorm H, Christiansen M, Siersma VD, Rasmussen LS, ISPOCD2 Investigators. Apoprotein E genotype and cognitive dysfunction after non-cardiac surgery. Anaesthesiology. 2004;101:855–61.
62. Folstein MF, Folstein SE, McHugh PR. "Mini Mental State" a practical method for grading the cognitive state of patients for the clinician. J Psychiatr Res. 1975;12:189–98.
63. Robinson TN, Wu DS, Pointer LF, Dunn CL, Moss M. Preoperative Cognition Dysfunction is related to adverse postoperative outcomes in the elderly. J Am Coll Surg. 2012;215(1):12–7.
64. Moller JT, Cluitmans P, Rasmussen LS, Houx P, Rasmussen H, Canet J, et al. Long term postoperative cognitive dysfunction in the elderly. ISPOCD1 study. ISPOCD investigators. International study of postoperative dysfunction. Lancet. 1998;351:857–61.
65. Dijkstra JB, Houx PJ, Jolles J. Cognition after major surgery in the elderly: test performance and complaints. Br J Anaesth. 1999;82:867–74.
66. Kotekar N, Kuruvilla CS, Murthy V. Post-operative cognitive dysfunction in the elderly: a prospective clinical study. Indian J Anaesth. 2014;58:263–8.
67. Duivenvoorden T, Vissers MM, Verhaar JA, Busschbach J, Gosens T, Bloem R, et al. Anxiety and depressive symptoms before and after total hip and knee arthroplasty: a prospective multicentre study. Osteoarthr Cartil. 2013;21(12):1834–40.
68. Blumenthal JA, Blumenthal J, Lett HS, Babyak MA, White W, Smith P, et al. NORG investigators. Depression as a risk factor for mortality after coronary artery bypass surgery. Lancet. 2003;362(9384):604–9.
69. Yesavage JA, Brink TL, Rose TL, et al. Development and validation of a geriatric depression screening scale: a preliminary report. J Psychiatr Res. 1983;17:37–49.
70. Roberts F, Freshwater-Turner D. Pharmacokinetics and anesthesia. Update Anesthesia. 2008;24(2):82–5.
71. Lupton T, Pratt O. Intravenous drugs used for the induction of anaesthesia. Update Anaesthesia. 2008;24(2):91–101.
72. Christmann IY, Cok O. Drug mechanisms in the elderly. Chapter 3. In: Oxford textbook of anaesthesia for the elderly patient. 1st ed. Oxford: Oxford University Press; 2014. p. 13–25.
73. Kharash ED, Thummel KE. Identification of cytochrome P4502E1 as the predominant enzyme catalysing human liver microsomal deflourination of sevoflurane, isoflurane and methoxyflurane. Anaesthesiology. 1993;79(4):795–807.
74. Eger EI. Age, minimum alveolar anaesthetic concentration and minimum alveolar anaesthetic concentration- awake. Anesth Analg. 2001;93(4):947–53.
75. Hall JE, Oldham T, Stewart JI, Harmer M. Comparison between halothane and sevoflurane for adult vital capacity induction. Br J Anaesth. 1997;79(3):285–8.
76. Saager L, Greenwald SD, Kelley SD, Schubert A, Sessler DI. Vasopressor may reduce mortality associated with a "triple low" of blood pressure, BIS and MAC. 2009. A.354.
77. Sadean MR, Glass PSA. Pharmacokinetics in the elderly. Best Pract Res Clin Anaesthiol. 2003;17(2): 191–205.

78. Ochs H, Greenblatt D, Divoll M, Abernethy D, Feyerabend H, Dengler H. Diazepam kinetics in relation to age and sex. Pharmacology. 1981;23(1):24–30.
79. Pergolizzi J, Böger R, Budd K, Dahan A, Erdine S, Hans G, et al. Opioids and the management of chronic severe pain in the elderly: consensus statement of an International Expert Panel with focus on the six clinically most often used World Health Organization step III opioids (buprenorphine, fentanyl, hydromorphone, methadone, morphine, oxycodone). Pain Pract. 2008;8(4):287–313.
80. Helmers JH, van Leeuwen L, Zuurmond WW. Sufentanyl pharmacokinetics in young adult and elderly surgical patients. Eur J Anaesthiol. 1994;11(3):181–5.
81. Kruijt Spanjer MR, Bakker N, Absalom AR. Pharmacology in the elderly and newer anaesthesia drugs. Best Pract Res Clin Anaesthesiol. 2011;25(3):355–65.
82. Brouquet A, Cudennec T, Benoist S, et al. Impaired mobility, ASA status and administration of tramadol are risk factors for postoperative delirium in patients aged 75 years or more after major abdominal surgery. Ann Surg. 2010;251(4):759–65.
83. Fosnight SM, Holder CM, Allen K, Hazelett S. A strategy to decrease the use of risky drugs in the elderly. Cleve Clin J Med. 2004;71(7):561–8.
84. Cope TM, Hunter JM. Selecting neuromuscular-blocking drugs for elderly patients. Drugs Aging. 2003;20(2):125–40.
85. Murphy G, Szokol J, Avram M, Greenberg S, Shear T, Vender J, et al. Residual neuromuscular block in the elderly. Anesthesiology. 2015;123(6):1322–36.
86. Ebadi HR, LeGal G, Righini M. Use of anticoagulant in elderly patients: practical recommendations. Clin Interv Aging. 2009;4:165–77.
87. Go AS, Hylek EM, Phillips KA, et al. Prevalence of diagnosed atrial fibrillation in adults: national implications for rhythm management and stroke prevention: the AnTicoagulation and Risk factors in Atrial fibrillation (ATRIA) Study. JAMA. 2001;285(18):2370–5.
88. Kearon C, Kahn SR, Agnelli G, Goldhaber S, Raskob GE, Comerota AJ. Antithrombotic therapy for venous thromboembolic disease: American College of Chest Physicians Evidence-Based Clinical Practice Guidelines (8th edition). Chest. 2008;133(6 Suppl):454S–545S.
89. Salem DN, O'Gara PT, Madias C, Pauker SG. Valvular and structural heart disease: American College of Chest Physicians Evidence-Based Clinical Practice Guidelines (8th edition). Chest. 2008;133(6 Suppl):593S–629S.
90. Jacobs LG. Warfarin pharmacology, clinical management, and evaluation of hemorrhagic risk for the elderly. Cardiol Clin. 2008;26(2):157–67.
91. Schulman S, Beyth RJ, Kearon C, Levine MN. Hemorrhagic complications of anti coagulant and thrombolytic treatment: American College of Chest Physicians Evidence Based Clinical Practice Guidelines (8th Edition). Chest. 2008;133(6 suppl):257S–98S.
92. Gage BF, Birman-Deych E, Kerzner R, Radford MJ, Nilasena DS, Rich MW. Incidence of intracranial hemorrhage in patients with atrial fibrillation who are prone to fall. Am J Med. 2005;118(6):612–7.
93. Inonye SK, Peduzzi PN, Robinson JT. Importance of functional measures in predicting mortality among older hospitalized patients. JAMA. 1998;279:1187–93.
94. Carli F, Halliday D. Continuous epidural blockade arrest the postoperative decrease in muscle protein fractional synthetic rate in surgical patients. Anesthesiology. 1997;86(5):1033–40.
95. Roy R. Choosing general versus regional anesthesia for the elderly. Anesthesiol Clin North Am. 2000;18(1):91–104.
96. Watters JM, Clancey SM, Meulton SB, Briere KM, Zhu JM. Impaired recovery of strength in older patients after major abdominal surgery. Ann Surg. 1993;218(3):380–90.

# Anesthesia for Weight Reduction Surgery

Angelo Andonakakis and Kathleen Kwiatt

## Obesity Prevalence
- 200 million, or 66% of the adult population in the United States are classified as overweight or obese.
- It is the most common nutritional disorder in the U.S.

## Obesity Statistics
- It is estimated 26 million people in the U.S. have a Body Mass Index (BMI) greater than 35 kg/m² and 15 million have a BMI of 40 kg/m² or greater.
- The World Health Organization (WHO) is predicting by 2025 the number of severely overweight adults will double.
- WHO reports obesity accounts for 400,000 deaths annually, second only to tobacco-related disease worldwide.

## Definition
- *Obesity*—Weight greater than 20% above ideal body weight.
- *Morbid Obesity*—Body weight two times the predicted ideal body weight, or greater than 100 pounds above ideal body weight.

Illustrations by Angelo Andonakakis D.O.

A. Andonakakis, D.O. (✉) · K. Kwiatt, D.O.
Department of Anesthesiology, Cooper University Hospital, Camden, NJ, USA
e-mail: Kwiatt-Kathleen@cooperhealth.edu

- *Waist Circumference*—Circumference greater than 102 cm or 40″ in men, and 88 cm or 35″ in women predispose to certain diseases and conditions.
- *Body Mass Index: BMI*

$$\text{BMI} = \frac{\text{weight in kilograms}}{\text{height in meters squared}}$$

- Has been adopted as the most useful index for evaluating obesity.
- Values greater than 28 for males and 27 for females represent 20% above ideal body weight.
- BMI of 40 or greater represents morbid obesity

## Who Is a Good Candidate for Surgery?
- According to the National Institute of Health (1991), anyone greater than BMI of 40, or BMI of 35–40 with associated comorbidities of hypertension, heart disease, sleep apnea, or diabetes.
- Age plays an important role in the patient selection process.
- Several studies show increased mortality and complications with increased age:
  - Flum = 65 (JAMA. 2000;294(15):1903–1908)
  - MBSC =50-OR 1.38 (Ann Surg. 2011;254:633–640)
  - DeMaria = 45-OR 1.64 (SOARD. 2007;3:134–140)
  - Sanni et al. "Post op complications increase by 2% per year of age" (Sanni et al. Surg Endosc. 2014;28(12):3302–3309)

## Greater BMI Poses Increasing Risks of Surgical Complications

- DeMaria and Livingston; BMI >50
- Gupta (J Am Coll Surg. 2011 Mar;212(3):301–309) BMI >60
- Flum—BMI >70

## Data-Driven Quality Improvement Through Risk Stratification Studies

- DeMaria EJ, Murr M, Byrne TK, et al. Validation of the obesity mortality risk score in a multicenter study proves it stratifies mortality risk in patients undergoing gastric bypass for morbid obesity. Ann Surg. 2007;246:578–582
- Thomas H. Agrawal S. Systematic review of obesity surgery mortality risk score—preoperative risk stratification in bariatric surgery. Obes Surg. 2012;22:1135–1140
- Sarela AI, Dexter SP, McMahon MJ. Use of the obesity surgery mortality risk score to predict complications of laparoscopic bariatric surgery. Obes Surg. 2011;21:1698–1703.
- Variables in the patient selection process posing increased risk stratification include: male gender, hypertension, BMI >50, increased risk of pulmonary embolism and age greater than 45.
- Risk stratification values are based on points awarded for each:
  - 0–1 = low
  - 2–3 = intermediate
  - 4–5 = high (DeMaria et al.)

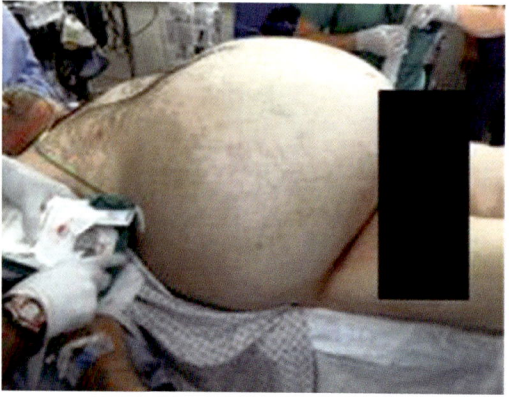

**Fig. 81.1** High risk stratification: male, age >45, BMI >50

## Psychological Considerations and Mobility

- Active drug use, Schizophrenia, low intellectual capacity, untreated depression, psychosis, bipolar disorder and inappropriate expectations or understanding of the surgery may delay or deny the surgical process (Walfish S, Vance D, Fabricatore AN. Psychological evaluation of bariatric surgery applicants: procedures and reasons for delay or denial of surgery. Obes Surg. 2007;17:1578–1783)
- Psychosocial issues may be discussed prior to procedure, such as ability to stay strict with specified diet, willingness to follow through with goals and objectives and available peer or family support.
- Both patient mobility and psychological status play a role in patient selection process, via data-driven quality improvement.

## Medical Conditions Statistically Associated with Obesity Include:

- Hypertension, Diabetes, Coronary Artery Disease, Cardiac Failure, Lipid abnormalities, Pancreatitis, Metabolic abnormalities, Cholelithiasis, Obstructive Sleep Apnea, Esophageal reflux, Non Alcoholic Steatohepatitis and Osteoarthritis may all be implicated in obesity and morbid obesity states.

## Physiologic Abnormalities Associated with Obesity

### Metabolic

- Metabolic or metabolic syndrome, which includes a host of indicators; such as increases waist circumference, elevated triglycerides, reduction in HDL, HTN, and elevations in fasting glucose.

### Pulmonary

- Hypoxemia is secondary to increased tissue mass requiring increased energy consumption, and oxygen utilization. There is increased work of breathing along with changes in lung

# 81 Anesthesia for Weight Reduction Surgery

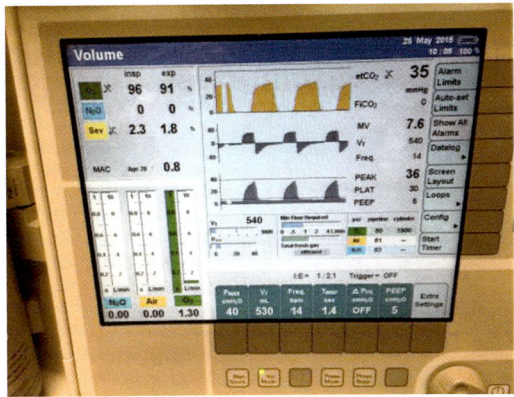

**Fig. 81.2** Classic respiratory pattern observed in obese patients: increased peak pressures, obstructive pattern, and absence of plateau

volumes resulting in closure of small airways. V/Q mismatch may be present.
- *Functional residual capacity*, *vital capacity*, *total lung capacity*, *ERV*, and *inspiratory capacity* are **reduced** as a result of lower respiratory compliance.
- PaCO2 and the ventilatory response to CO2 is unchanged.
- Obese patients typically breathe rapidly and shallowly, as this pattern results in the least oxygen cost of breathing.

## Obstructive Sleep Apnea, (OSA)
- Characterized with intermittent closure or narrowing of the upper airway during sleep, excess episodes of apnea, in spite of respiratory effort, resulting in complete or partial airway obstruction.
- As many as 80–95% of individuals are undiagnosed, and approximately 18 million Americans have this disorder.
- Hypopnea is defined as 50% reduction in airflow for 10 s, for 15 or more times per hour of sleep, associated with snoring and a 4% drop in oxygen saturation.
- Apnea is considered obstructive if there is cessation of airflow at the nose or mouth for more than 10 s, despite of respiratory effort.
- American Academy of Sleep Medicine distinguishes grades of OSA, via an apnea-hypopnea index (AHI); relating to number apneic episodes per hour of sleep.
- *Mild*: 5–15, *moderate*: 15–30, and *severe*: greater than 30 episodes of abnormal respiratory events.

## Obesity Hypoventilation Syndrome (Pickwickian Syndrome)
- Occurs in 8% of obese patients and episodic day time somnolence may be present.
- **There is an elevation in PaCO2** resulting in respiratory acidosis.
- Arterial hypoxemia, Polycythemia and Pulmonary hypertension may result in right heart failure.
- Obstructive sleep apnea is closely associated with this disorder, although it may be present without it.
- These patients are exquisitely sensitive to opioids and sedatives, and caution is recommended when MAC sedation is the anesthetic plan.
- These people must be done with a good local and minimal sedation.
- Distinct characteristics of this syndrome setting it apart from obesity and OSA are:
- $PaCO_2$ greater than 45 during wakefulness
- $PaO_2$ less than 70
- Respiratory acidosis with metabolic compensation
- Inappropriate and sudden daytime somnolence
- Sleep apnea
- Hypoxia

## Cardiovascular
- Cardiac output is increased primarily due to increases in stroke volume.
- It is estimated that C.O. increases by 0.1 L per minute for each kilogram of weight that is adipose.
- Pulmonary hypertension is common, most likely reflecting arterial hypoxemia increased pulmonary blood volume or both.
- Risk of ischemic heart disease is doubled in the obese patient.
- Risk of CAD, MI, and sudden death was increased among the obese of both sexes (Framingham Heart Study, Circulation 1983).

- Although association of high blood pressure and obesity is well established, there is no proven cause and effect relationship.
- Increases in work load caused by the increases in demand on the myocardium, result in increases in $O_2$ consumption, increased $CO_2$ production, leading to chronically elevated cardiac output.
- As these demands persist, stroke volumes increase, the heart starts to enlarge, with atrial and biventricular dilation, as hypertrophy ensues.
- The results are hypertension and eventual CHF.

**Gastrointestinal**
- Fatty liver infiltrates and abnormal LFTs are frequent findings.
- Vaughn et al. (Anesthesiology) found in 56 healthy obese patients in comparison to an equal number of average weight patients, 86% had gastric fluid volume exceeding 25 mL, and pH <2.5 (mean 1.7).
- There is a threefold risk of GB and biliary disease, perhaps reflecting abnormal cholesterol metabolism.
- Non alcoholic fatty liver disease (NAFLD), is strongly associated with obesity.
- The pathogenesis of this disease is related to insulin resistance and frequently found in central obesity and diabetics.
- "In the obese patients, mortality rate from liver cirrhosis is 1.5–2.5 times higher than in non-obese persons."

**Metabolic**
- There is resistance to the effects of insulin in the presence of adipose tissue.
- Oxygen consumption and carbon dioxide production are both increased.
- Lipid abnormalities, including hypercholesterolemia and hypertriglyceridemia may also be present.
- "The risk of type 2 diabetes increases linearly with BMI."
- Obese individuals may also have a pro-thrombotic and pro-inflammatory state.
- "Obese men may experience decreased libido or impotence indicative of hypogonadism." This is reflected by reductions in serum FSH and testosterone."

**Pediatric Obesity**
- This is a growing problem among US children, indicated by a 2004 study from the National Center of Health Statistics showing 20% of children and adolescents ages 2–19 years of age are overweight.
- Obese adolescents have a 70–80% chance of becoming obese adults.
- "Being overweight as young as age 18 could be the strongest predictor of future hip replacements secondary to osteoarthritis".

**Maternal Obesity**
- Obesity is a known risk factor for developing gestational HTN or PIH, preeclampsia, gestational DM, pre-term labor, infection, c-section delivery (40%), macrosomic infants, and hydramnios.
- Deliveries may be complicated by difficult epidural placement, difficult airway, increased post-op complications, increased blood loss and DVTs.
- As with their non-pregnant counterparts, using a ramp, with blankets under their head and neck is helpful in achieving a "sniff" position.

## Surgical Management

Surgical management of obesity is superior to medical management [1]. Despite perioperative complications, surgical patients experience faster, more substantial weight loss, resulting in improved comorbidity control. This decreases morbidity and mortality compared to diet, exercise and medication alone. Bariatric surgery has evolved since the original jejunoileal bypass, a malabsorptive procedure with high morbidity, was performed in 1954. There are currently five procedures endorsed by the American Society for

Metabolic and Bariatric Surgery (ASMBS), indicated for patients with a BMI greater than 40 kg/m$^2$ or 35–40 kg/m$^2$ with comorbidities. They include laparoscopic roux-en-y gastric bypass, duodenal switch, sleeve gastrectomy, adjustable gastric banding, and re-operative procedures, while the vertically banded gastroplasty is under review for approval [2]. The resulting gastrointestinal rearrangements lead to caloric restriction, malabsorption or both, promoting weight loss.

## Surgical Procedures

### Roux-En-Y Gastric Bypass

The roux-en-y gastric bypass was introduced by Mason in 1966 [3], and as of 2003, accounted for over 80% of all bariatric procedures performed in the United States [4]. This combined restrictive-malabsorptive procedure is the "gold-standard" of bariatric surgery. First, a 20–30 mL stomach pouch is created, separating it from the body of the stomach and avoiding inclusion of the fundus. This restrictive pouch promotes satiety. Next, the jejunum is separated from the proximal small bowel below the ligament of Treitz and connected to the gastric pouch, creating the Roux limb. Finally, the free end of the duodenum and proximal jejunum are reconnected to the small bowel 75–250 cm beyond the gastrojejunostomy, creating the biliopancreatic limb. This rearrangement decreases caloric absorption by bypassing the proximal digestive limb and mixing stomach acid and digestive enzymes with food distally. Gut hormones are also altered, promoting appetite suppression and satiety.

The average patient loses 60–80% of excess weight, maintains 50% excess weight loss [5], and has more than 75% control of comorbidities [6]. An expected side effect of the procedure is vitamin and mineral deficiencies, especially vitamin B12, vitamin D, iron, calcium and folate. Routine laboratory monitoring and supplementation minimizes critical deficiencies. The most common early complications include wound infection, anastomotic leak, gastrointestinal hemorrhage, bowel obstruction and pulmonary embolus. The most common late complications include stomal stenosis, bowel obstruction, and incisional hernia.

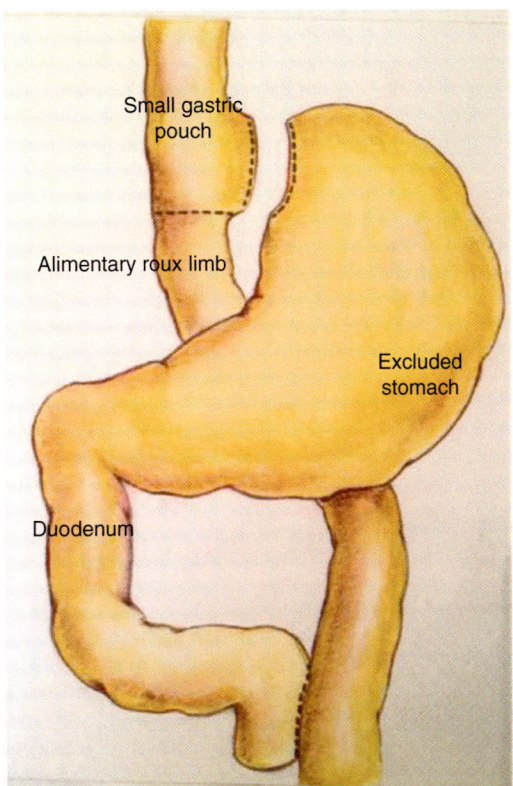

**Fig. 81.3** Roux-en-y gastric bypass

Both case series and prospective, randomized trials report similar weight loss for laparoscopic and open surgical approaches [7]. The conversion rate from laparoscopic to open procedure is 2.2%, most often for hepatomegaly [8]. Laparoscopic procedures are associated with increased rates of bowel obstruction, intestinal hemorrhage and stomal stenosis [9], but have decreased rates of wound infection, incisional hernia, perioperative mortality (0.1% vs. 0.3% open), and readmission (2.6% vs. 4.7% open) [10] at 30 days.

Patients report improvement in both gastroesophageal reflux disease (GERD) and dysphagia after roux-en-y bypass, as compared with vertical sleeve gastrectomy and duodenal switch, where severe restrictive changes worsen symptoms [11].

## Vertical Sleeve Gastrectomy (VSG)

Hess first performed the open VSG in 1988 as part of a duodenal switch procedure [12]. It evolved into a stand-alone, purely restrictive laparoscopic procedure. Multiple techniques are described; most involve 75–80% excision of the greater curvature of the stomach. Dissection begins 5–10 cm proximal to the pylorus, and the greater curvature and posterior stomach are mobilized. A bougie is inserted and positioned along the lesser curvature distal to the planned staple line, creating a gastric tube. A stapler separates the permanent gastric tube from the portion of the stomach to be excised, making sure not to leave behind a large posterior stomach or injure the esophagus. The surgeon reinforces the staple line with buttress staples or by oversewing it to minimize leaks and bleeding. Finally a gastroscope is inserted and the staple line is evaluated for leaks [13].

Advantages of the gastric sleeve include rapid, substantial weight loss, typical of those observed with gastric bypass and more significant than gastric banding. Patients typically lose and maintain greater than 50% of excess weight [14]. Initially, it was thought decreased gastric size increased satiety and decreased caloric intake. Evidence now suggests the mechanism for weight loss is a combination of this restriction along with favorable hormonal changes. Ghrelin, a peptide hormone predominately produced in the fundus of the stomach, promotes hunger. By resecting the fundus, ghrelin levels plummet and patients report satiety. This likely explains why gastric sleeve patients experience more weight loss than gastric band patients, who have a similar restriction in gastric size but no change in hormone levels [15].

While nutritional deficiencies occur, especially with dietary noncompliance, the risk is lower than gastric bypass. There is an increased risk for GERD, reported in 20% of patients during the first year and decreasing to 3% at 3 years. More serious complications include staple line leaks (1–4%), bleeding (1.2%) and stenosis or stricture (0.6%) [16]. The VSG is not reversible.

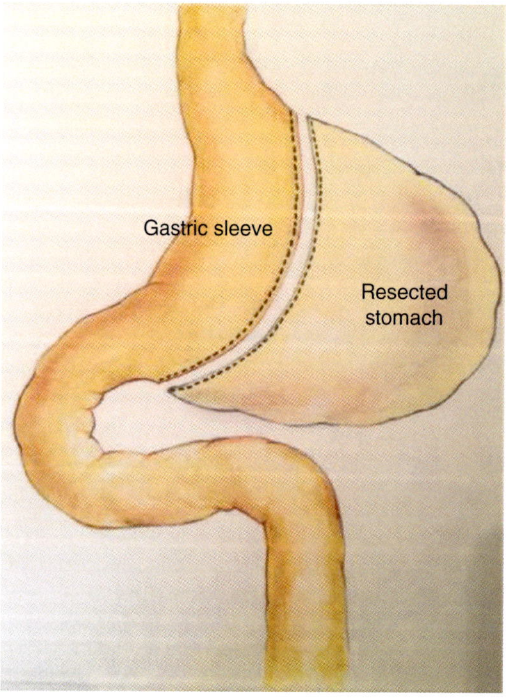

**Fig. 81.4** Vertical sleeve gastrectomy

## Biliopancreatic Diversion with Duodenal Switch (BPD/DS)

Biliopancreatic diversion, a combined restrictive, malabsorptive first performed by Scoparino, has evolved since 1979. In today's standard approach, a restrictive tubular stomach is created via sleeve gastrectomy. Next, the duodenum is divided distal to the pylorus. The pylorus is left intact to reduce the chance of ulceration. The ileum is divided 250 cm proximal to the ileocecal valve, and the distal bowel is anastomosed with tubular stomach to complete the alimentary limb, bypassing 75% of normal intestinal absorption. The free proximal end of the ileum is reattached approximately 100 cm from the ileocecal valve. Bile and pancreatic enzymes mix with food further along the digestive tract, increasing malabsorption [17].

Patients experience the greatest weight loss and comorbidity control versus other bariatric procedures. At 18 months 75–85% excess weight

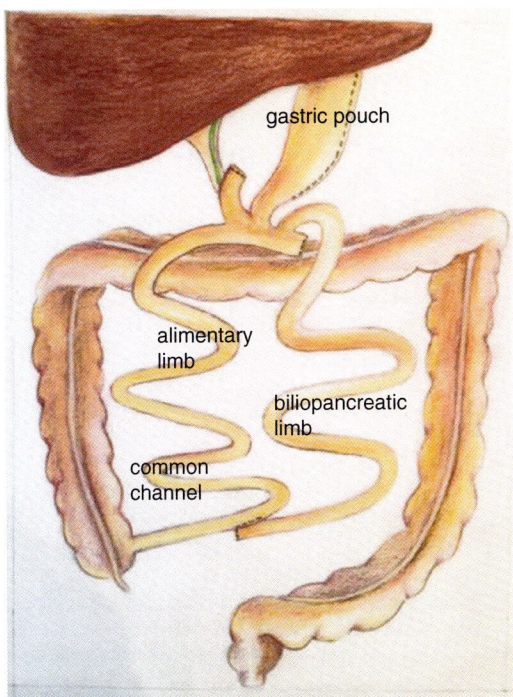

**Fig. 81.5** Biliopancreatic diversion with duodenal switch

## Adjustable Gastric Band (AGB)

The first gastric band was placed in 1986 via laparotomy, then performed laparoscopically in 1992 which continues to be the popular approach today [23]. Two devices have been approved for use in this restrictive procedure, the Lap-Band (Apollo) and the Realize Band (Ethicon). With the patient supine in modified lithotomy, the stomach is decompressed with an orogastric tube and trocars are placed. The pars flaccida approach is preferred over the perigastric approach due to decreased band slippage [24]. In this technique, the liver is retracted and a retrogastric tunnel is created between the pars flaccida and the angle of His. A calibration balloon is inserted into the stomach transorally and filled with 15–25 mL of saline. The band is fastened distal to this pouch through the newly created tunnel [25]. A port attached to the band is secured under the skin, which allows the opening of the stomach to be decreased over time by incrementally injecting saline [26].

is lost with 60–70% maintenance at 5 years [18]. Although patients must eat smaller meals initially, over time they can resume near normal consumption, unlike other bariatric procedures that mandate smaller portions indefinitely. Similar to gastric bypass and sleeve gastrectomy, favorable changes in gut hormones are observed, decreasing hunger and increasing satiety [19].

Morbidity and mortality have been significantly reduced since the original procedure was performed; yet still rank the highest when compared to other bariatric procedures. Because this procedure is often reserved for the most severe obese patients, their pre-existing conditions likely confound the increased complication rate. Thirty-day mortality ranges between 0.29 and 2.7% [20]. Common complications include diarrhea and protein, vitamin and mineral deficiencies. Patients require a longer hospital stay than other bariatric procedures [21]. Serious complications include anastomotic leak, duodenal stump leak, intra-abdominal infection, hemorrhage, venous thromboembolism, and bowel obstruction, incarceration or stricture [22].

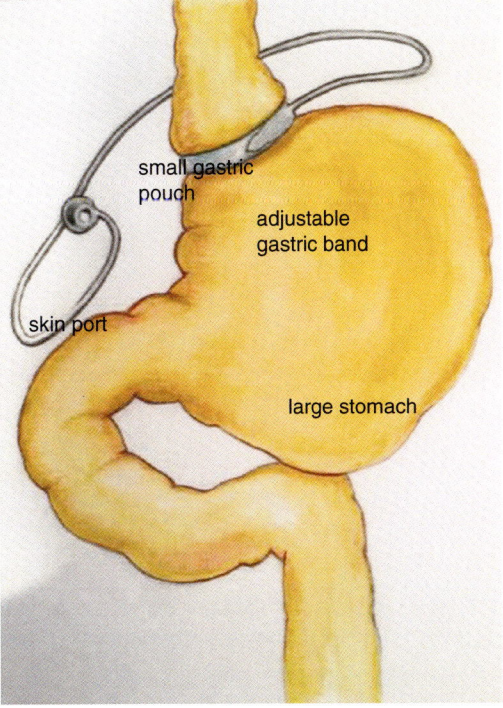

**Fig. 81.6** Adjustable gastric band

Weight loss after gastric banding is superior to medical therapy alone, but less significant and slower compared to gastric sleeve or bypass. At 6 months, the average excess body weight loss is 35%, at 12 months 40% and at 2 years 50% [27]. However, up to a quarter of patients fail to lose 50% of excess weight at 5 years [28].

The procedure is generally well tolerated and sometimes even performed as outpatient surgery. This procedure is fully reversible and patients have fewer vitamin and mineral deficiencies versus other bariatric procedures. Because there are no anastomoses or staple lines, patients are not at risk for leaks or anastomotic failure. Complications include band slippage or erosion, the need for pouch or esophageal dilation, and port-site complications [29].

## Additional Bariatric Procedures

In addition to the ASMBS endorsed procedures, there are several FDA approved devices for weight loss. Most are inserted endoscopically under light sedation while another involves laparoscopy and general anesthesia with minimal GI manipulation. Consequently, most are performed as outpatient procedures.

The AspireAssist (Aspire Bariatrics for patients with BMI 35–55 kg/m$^2$) connects a drain from the stomach to a skin port draining approximately 30% of calories after consumption but prior to absorption. Two balloon systems indicated for patients with BMI 30–40 kg/m$^2$, the ORBERA Intragastric Balloon System (Apollo Endosurgery) and ReShape Integrated Dual Balloon System (ReShape Medical Inc.), involve endoscopically inserting balloons in the stomach and inflating them with saline. Both devices are temporary with recommended removal after 6 months. The Maestro Rechargeable System (EnteroMedics, indicated for BMI 40–45 kg/m$^2$ or 35–39 kg/m$^2$ with comorbidities) is a vagus nerve stimulator. It is laparoscopically inserted into the abdomen and interferes with signaling from the stomach to the brain, promoting the sensation of fullness. Because this procedure is performed laparoscopically, it is performed under general anesthesia.

## Complications

In addition to procedure specific complications, bariatric surgery patients are at risk for deep venous embolism and pulmonary embolism. Malnutrition and vitamin deficiencies cause severe osteoporosis, placing patients at risk for non-traumatic fractures. Cholelithiasis and nephrolithiasis risks increase. Massive weight loss leaves patients with sagging skin. This causes physical discomfort, inhibits physical activity, risks cellulitis or ulceration, and is physically displeasing to patients.

## Anesthetic Management

### Airway Management

- Airway management of the obese patient begins with a thorough preoperative evaluation. While obesity is a poor predictor, neck circumference greater than 43 cm has 92% sensitivity and 84% specificity for difficult airway. Neck circumference and Mallampati score are the most important factors in the obese population [30]. History is equally important; characteristics such as pharyngeal tissue redundancy increase risk of airway difficulty but are difficult to identify on physical exam. Personal history of difficult airway or obstructive sleep apnea should alert a provider to the potential for difficult ventilation or intubation.
- The method chosen to secure the airway is at the discretion of an experienced anesthesia provider. It must account for both the patient assessment and an individual provider's unique strengths. Direct laryngoscopy, video laryngoscopy, and fiberoptic intubation are commonly selected techniques. Regardless which is chosen, difficult airway equipment should be immediately available, an experienced provider should be present to assist with airway management, and a surgeon capable of performing emergency cricothyroidotomy should be available.
- If a fiberoptic intubation is selected, good topicalization of the airway is superior to sedative

hypnotics and anxiolytics in accomplishing the goal.
- Decreased FRC and increased oxygen consumption cause rapid oxygen desaturation during periods of apnea in obese patients. Preoxygenation is essential, and four vital capacity breaths demonstrated superiority over 3 min of tidal volume breathing in the obese [31].
- Rapid sequence induction is often utilized, to reduce the risk of pulmonary aspiration; this must be balanced with the risk for difficult airway. These patients often require antacids or H2 blockers as pre-medications.
- Placement of a "log roll" or a "ramp", under the patients shoulders, may enhance the laryngoscopic view of the trachea.
- Obese patients will more likely require intubation rather than an LMA, especially if the procedure planned will be done laparoscopically.
- During positive pressure ventilation an LMA may not maintain a seal at higher airway pressures needed for obese patients; the safety and use of supraglottic devices (LMAs), has remained a matter of debate.

**Ventilation**

- Controlled ventilation versus spontaneous is preferred to prevent hypoventilation.
- Based on available evidence and expert opinion, low tidal volumes (6–8 mL/kg IBW), low levels of oxygen concentrations ($FiO_2$ 0.5–0.8) to prevent resorption atelectasis and oxygen toxicity, PEEP 10–15 cm $H_2O$, and recruitment maneuvers (RM) are best suited for the obese patients.
- Maintain reverse Trendelenburg (head up) position whenever possible.
- In a 2012 meta-analysis of ventilation strategies, comparing pressure-controlled or volume-controlled ventilation, tidal volumes, PEEP, or Rescue Maneuvers (RMs), in obese patients, RMs added to PEEP improved intraoperative oxygenation and compliance, compared with PEEP alone; there was no increase in adverse effects and no difference between pressure-controlled and volume-controlled ventilation.

**Monitoring and Access**

- Standard ASA monitors are appropriate to continuously assess oxygenation, ventilation, circulation and temperature. It can be difficult to achieve a good fit with blood pressure cuffs. For accurate reading, the cuff must encircle a minimum of 75% of the upper arm. Too small of a cuff reports too high of a pressure. Even an appropriate sized cuff can be inaccurate if excess adipose tissue creates a poor fit. Blood pressure cuffs can be placed on the wrist or ankle when unable to obtain accurate readings using the upper arm [32]. Invasive blood pressure monitoring is not required, though indicated if a non-invasive blood pressure cuff does not fit properly or for significant cardiopulmonary disease. Peripheral venous access is sufficient for most patients. Central venous access is reserved for patients in whom peripheral access is difficult to obtain or those with comorbidities that justify central venous pressure monitoring or pulmonary artery catheterization and monitoring.

**Positioning**

- Strategic positioning facilitates both airway and surgical management, and promotes patient safety. The operating room table must accommodate the weight of the patient. Beanbags, foot-rests and straps help prevent sliding. Padding minimizes pressure sores and nerve injuries, which are more common in this population. Compartment syndrome and rhabdomyolysis are uncommon but severe consequences of poorly positioned patients.
- When laryngoscopy is planned, the *head elevated laryngoscopy position* (HELP) increases the success rate in morbidly obese patients [33]. The head, neck, and shoulders are elevated, aligning the external auditory meatus with the sternal notch. This facilitates alignment of the pharyngeal, laryngeal and oral axis, improving success with intubation. Making a ramp with blankets or using a specially designed pillow or inflatable wedge achieves this position.

- Positioning may be difficult, and the prone or Trendelenberg positions may further reduce chest wall compliance, thus contributing to high peak pressures and hypoxia.

**Pharmacology**

- "Although volume of distribution ($V_d$) is the primary determinant in dosing, $V_d$ is largely dependent on the physiochemical properties of a drug and varies with plasma protein binding and tissue blood flow. These changes are not consistent for all drugs in each category, and in many cases have not been determined."
- Drug clearance is generally higher in obese, this being largely controlled by hepatic and renal physiology, and increases in cardiac output.
- "Obesity affects hepatic metabolic pathways in different ways, with some only slightly and others significantly enhanced."
- Elimination half-life ($t_{1/2}$) impacts dosing intervals and dosing of continuous infusions.
- The $t_{1/2}$ of a drug varies directly with $V_d$, and inversely with clearance, both of which are altered in obesity.
- Highly lipid soluble drugs will likely have a prolonged elimination half-life, like sufentanyl, for example.
- Dosing of meds requires some extra thought, keeping in mind the significant increase in the volume of distribution, or $V_d$, present in the obese.
- The easiest way to think of dosing is, if a drug is lipid soluble dosing should be increased due to the increased $V_d$.
- Water soluble drugs, like most muscle relaxants should be dosed using ideal body weight.
- Pharmacokinetics, including absorption, distribution, metabolism and elimination, describe how the body affects a drug and are impacted by obesity. Pharmacodynamics describe how the drug affects the body. While difficult to predict, pharmacodynamic changes occur in obese individuals; for instance, therapeutic windows may be narrowed or side-effects exaggerated. Because morbidly obese patients are often excluded from clinical drug trials, an understanding of pharmacokinetics and pharmacodynamics must be combined with clinical judgment to determine drug selection and dosing.
- Drug **dosing** is weight based. Weight is described as total, lean or ideal body weight.
  - **Total body weight** (TBW) is the patients measured weight.
  - **Lean body weight** (LBW) based on the James Formula[1] [34]

$$Men = 1.1 \times weight(kg) - 128(weight(kg)/height(cm))^2$$
$$Women = 1.07 \times weight(kg) - 148(weight(kg)/height(cm))^2$$

  - **Ideal body weight** (IBW) based on the JD Robinson Formula[1] [35]

$$Men = 52\,kg + 1.9\,kg\,per\,inch\ over\ 5ft$$
$$Women = 49\,kg + 1.7\,kg\,per\,inch\ over\ 5ft$$

- Drug **dosing** is weight based, though application of the appropriate scale: TBW, IBW, or LBW, is important to achieve therapeutic levels without overdose. Relying on TBW can lead to overdose, as adipose tissue accounts for a greater percentage of body composition. Using IBW is also problematic because it assumes every patient of the same height and gender requires the same dose, risking subtherapeutic drug levels. Obese patients have increased adipose and lean mass, and LBW formulas adjust to account for the 20–40% excess weight due to increased lean mass [36]. LBW also correlates with cardiac output, which increases with obesity and is a major factor in early distribution pharmacokinetics. LBW is generally the optimal anesthetic scale, with specific recommendations for individual drugs listed.
- Deciding which dosing scale to use also depends on whether a loading or maintenance

---

[1] Multiple formulas exist for each calculation, though they share relative agreement.

dose is administered. **Volume of distribution** ($V_d$) is important when administering a **loading dose**. Adipose tissue, lean mass, blood volume, and cardiac output are all increased in the obese. If a drug is distributed to lean tissue, the loading dose should be calculated based on LBW. If a drug is distributed to both the lean and adipose tissue, the loading dose should be based on TBW. **Maintenance** doses depend more on **drug clearance**. When a drug has similar clearance times in obese and lean patients, drug dosing is based on LBW; when clearance increases with weight dosages are based on TBW [37].

- Drug **selection** also requires clinical judgment, with consideration of a patient's medical history, the institution's available resources, and the intraoperative variations unique to each facility including surgical length of time and procedural steps. Premedication with oral or 1–2 mg of intravenous midazolam provides anxiolysis with minimal respiratory depression in most patients. Standard intravenous induction medications are appropriate. Succinylcholine is an excellent neuromuscular relaxant to facilitate airway management due to its rapid onset and short duration. Maintenance is achieved with numerous combinations of inhaled and intravenous medications. Volatile anesthetics are titrated to similar minimum alveolar concentration (MAC) values obese and lean patients. The low blood: gas partition coefficient of desflurane allows for rapid, predictable recovery [38], and is suggested as the inhaled anesthetic of choice for obese patients. Sevoflurane has been identified as advantageous over isoflurane due to rapid recovery, good hemodynamic control, low incidence of nausea and vomiting, and low cost [39]. Intravenous medications are used either for total intravenous anesthesia or as part of a balanced technique with inhaled agents. Dexmedetomidine, propofol, and remifentanil can all be titrated with relative ease, each offering unique advantages. Muscle relaxation facilitates ventilation and ideal laparoscopic surgical conditions.

## Intravenous Medications

**Sedative Hypnotics** facilitate induction and airway management; propofol and dexmedetomidine are also used for maintenance.

- **Propofol.** Induction: LBW, Maintenance: TBW
  Propofol is the most common induction agent for bariatric surgery. It has a rapid onset and rapid redistribution from the plasma to the peripheral tissues, resulting in a short duration of action. It is highly lipophilic, resulting in increased $V_d$. The increase in $V_d$ is offset by increased clearance. Lean patients receiving TBW induction doses had similar times to loss of consciousness as obese patients receiving LBW doses in controlled trials; consequently LBW is appropriate for induction [40]. Maintenance doses are derived from TBW calculations because the increased $V_d$ is proportional to the increased clearance, offsetting each other at steady state [41]. However, like any anesthetic, maintenance doses are titrated to the desired effect.
- **Etomidate.** Induction: LBW
  Etomidate has similar properties to propofol: it is lipophilic and the duration depends on redistribution. It is dosed on LBW and offers the advantage of a stable hemodynamic profile.
- **Dexmedetomidine.** TBW
  This selective α-2 adrenergic agonist has sedative, analgesic, and sympatholytic properties. It causes minimal respiratory depression and is ideally suited to facilitate fiberoptic airway management. It is also an adjuvant for maintenance, and intraoperative infusions improve hemodynamic stability and reduce intraoperative and postoperative opioid requirements [42]. Infusions are titrated to 0.2–0.7 μg/kg/h TBW [43].

**Opioids.** Obese patients are susceptible to respiratory depression and airway obstruction; 48% of ASA closed claims reports of adverse respiratory events associated with opioid use occur in obese patients [44]. Underlying respiratory dysfunction such as obstructive sleep apnea and obesity hypoventilation syndrome exacerbate opioid induced hypoventilation and airway obstruction. Continuous capnography or pulse oximetry is appropriate when parenteral opioids are administered to obese patients.

- **Fentanyl.** LBW

    Fentanyl is administered in bolus doses 0.5–1.5 mcg/kg LBW with titration to effect. Increased cardiac output reduces plasma fentanyl levels and clearance increases nonlinearly with obesity, best correlating to LBW. Peak onset is 5 min. Use of an infusion is unpopular during bariatric surgery due to the long, unpredictable context-sensitive half-life [45].

- **Sufentanil.** TBW: BMI <30–39.9 kg/m$^2$, LBW: BMI >40 kg/m$^2$

    Sufentanil is highly lipophilic with an onset similar to fentanyl and ten times greater potency. Obese patients have an increased $V_d$ and elimination half-life that correlates with the degree of obesity, though similar clearance when compared to lean patients [46]. Small studies conclude that the pharmacokinetics derived from normal-weight subjects predicts plasma sufentanil concentrations in obese patients [47]. These results were based on obese patients with BMI 30–39.9 kg/m$^2$ but were not validated in patients with a BMI greater than 40. TBW is used until BMI exceeds 40 kg/m$^2$, then LBW is appropriate. With either scale, close observation and titration to desired effect are essential.

- **Remifentanil.** LBW

    Due to remifentanil's rapid onset and elimination it is usually administered via infusion. Peak effect occurs at 1 min and metabolism by organ-independent plasma esterases occurs 5 min after discontinuation. Very little accumulation occurs even with prolonged exposure due to the short context-sensitive half-life, and long acting analgesics are necessary for post-operative pain management. Obese patients administered doses based on LBW had similar plasma concentrations to normal weight subjects who received doses based on TBW [48]. 0.1–1 mcg/kg/min LBW is titrated to effect as an adjuvant to inhalational or intravenous sedatives.

- **Morphine.** IBW

    Individual variability has been observed with morphine administration in the obese; genetics, absorption, clearance and pain perception interplay, resulting in variable clinical responses [49]. Morphine use in the obese is associated with a higher incidence of PACU respiratory events compared with normal weight patients. Obese patients using PCA also reported a higher incidence of postoperative nausea and vomiting [50]. Retrospective data suggests obese and normal weight patients report similar improvements in pain scores after administration of a fixed dose of morphine [51]. Fixed doses should be administered with monitoring for adverse events.

**Nonopioid Analgesics.** Pain control after surgery improves patient satisfaction and facilitates hospital discharge. Fear of adverse opioid effects risks under-treatment. Inadequate analgesia leads to its own set of complications: hypoventilation and consequently atelectasis, hypoxemia and pneumonia; delayed ambulation, and delayed discharge. By targeting multiple receptors, individual doses can be reduced, decreasing adverse events without compromising analgesia. Choice of adjuvant therapy varies by institution, physician preference, and patient indications. Analgesics include gabapentin/pregabalin, acetaminophen (oral, rectal and IV), short-term use of NSAIDs, ketamine, dexmedetomidine and tramadol. Transversus abdominis plane block or local infiltration at surgical sites complements intravenous analgesics with low risk.

- **Ketamine**.

    Ketamine is an N-Methyl-D-aspartate antagonist and phencyclidine derivative with analgesic properties. It is synergistic with opioids, improving analgesia without respiratory depression. Patients administered a pre-induction infusion of ketamine and clonidine before biliopancreatic diversion had shorter time to extubation and decreased postoperative analgesic requirements [52]. Small doses of 0.2 mg/kg provide analgesia.

- **Acetaminophen.** IBW
  Acetaminophen offers effective analgesia without respiratory depression, platelet dysfunction or gastrointestinal side effects. Dosing based on IBW avoids hepatotoxicity, as metabolic enzymes do not increase with obesity [53].
- **NSAIDs.** IBW
  Inhibition of cyclo-oxygenase inhibits thromboxane and prostaglandin synthesis, resulting in anti-inflammatory and analgesic effects without respiratory depression. NSAID use remains controversial after bariatric surgery, as long-term use increases the risk of anastomotic ulceration. However, short-term (24 h) use of ketorolac after laparoscopic gastric bypass leads to earlier PACU discharge and improved pain scores without any increase in renal dysfunction or hemostatic complications when compared with remifentanil infusion [54].

**Neuromuscular Blocking Agents.** Neuromuscular blockade facilitates laryngoscopic airway management and improves surgical conditions.

- **Succinylcholine.** TBW
  This depolarizing muscle relaxant is ideal for airway management due to its rapid onset and short duration. Obese patients have increased levels of pseudocholinesterase [55] and an increased volume of extracellular fluid [56], decreasing succinylcholine's duration of action. To prevent underdosing, it should be dosed based on TBW. Induction doses of 1 mg/kg TBW improved intubating conditions compared to the same dose using IBW or LBW [57]. Postoperative myalgias are uncommon in obese patients [58].
- **Rocuronium.** IBW
  Rocuronium, a highly ionized, weakly lipophilic, aminosteroid nondepolarizing neuromuscular relaxant, is distributed mostly to the extracellular fluid. Despite the increased extracellular fluid volume in the obese, the impact on dosing is minimal. The duration of action of rocuronium in obese patients receiving 0.6 mg/kg TBW exceeded twice the duration (55 min) of obese patients dosed on IBW (22 min) and lean patients dosed on TBW (25 min) [59]. While conflicting data exists, it is reasonable to dose rocuronium based on IBW while monitoring twitches and titrating to desired effect.
- **Vecuronium.** IBW
  Vecuronium is an aminosteroid nondepolarizing neuromuscular relaxant. Elimination is primarily hepatic, though recovery from small doses is the result of redistribution. When a 0.1 mg/kg bolus dose was administered in obese and non-obese patients, the obese group had prolonged recovery times [60]. This is attributed to delayed hepatic clearance and increased time for redistribution. It is recommended to dose based on IBW to avoid prolonged muscle relaxation.
- **Atracurium.** LBW
  This benzylisoquinoline is eliminated by Hoffman degradation, independent of renal and liver metabolism. Conflicting data exists regarding how to dose atracurium in the obese. Some support TBW to dosing, arguing that $V_d$, clearance and elimination are unchanged. This is supported by a study finding similar recovery times between obese and lean patients receiving 0.5 mg/kg TBW atracurium [61]. However, there is also data supporting prolonged duration of action in the obese when dosing based on TBW [62]. Until more evidence is available, it is reasonable to use LBW with twitch monitoring to titrate to effect.
- **Cisatracurium.** LBW
  Similar to atracurium, this benzylisoquinoline neuromuscular relaxant is eliminated by Hoffman degradation. Obese women receiving 0.2 mg/kg TBW of cisatracurium had delayed recovery times, compared to IBW doses in obese women or TBW doses in normal weight women [63]. Use of LBW to dose cisatracurium avoids overdose.

**Inhaled Anesthetics**
- **Desflurane.** Desflurane has been suggested to be the inhaled anesthetic of choice for bariatric

surgery. It has a low blood: gas coefficient, resulting in a more rapid onset and elimination compared to other halogenated anesthetics. Time to emergence, extubation, and orientation after bariatric surgery was shorter with desflurane when compared with isoflurane or propofol. Episodes of hypoxia in the PACU were less frequent. Additionally, patients were more able to move themselves from the bed to the stretcher after desflurane, important for both patient and staff safety [64]. While desflurane is considered the preferred agent, comparative studies between desflurane and sevoflurane are still needed.
- **Sevoflurane.** Sevoflurane is a cost-effective alternative to desflurane. In a randomized trial of 30 patients undergoing laparoscopic gastric band placement, those exposed to sevoflurane had shorter emergence, extubation, and PACU discharge times when compared with isoflurane [65]. In another study of 90 patients with BMI greater than 45 kg/m² for biliopancreatic diversion, the sevoflurane group had improved level of consciousness, oxygen saturation, respiration, blood pressure and activity in the first 10 min in the PACU compared with the isoflurane group, though subsequent scores were similar [66]. Hemodynamic parameters and adverse events were similar with both agents in both studies.
- **Isoflurane.** Isoflurane has been associated with increased time to emergence and extubation, and increased oxygen desaturation in the recovery phase. However, comparison studies enrolled a small number of patients and utilized rigid titration guidelines, such that sevoflurane and isoflurane were administered with equivalent concentrations and discontinued at similar times during the procedure. Under such conditions, it would be expected that patients receiving isoflurane would take longer to emerge. Judicious titration of isoflurane by a skilled anesthesia provider would likely result in acceptable conditions. Hemodynamic parameters and adverse events were no different from sevoflurane [67].
- **Nitrous oxide.** While nitrous oxide offers analgesia and rapid elimination, it is at the cost of decreased oxygen availability in patients with increased oxygen consumption [68]. It causes bowel distention, limiting visibility during laparoscopy, and increases postoperative nausea and vomiting. These adverse effects worsen when the duration of exposure to nitrous oxide is prolonged [69]. Because of these effects, and the broad availability of alternatives, its use is limited in bariatric surgery.

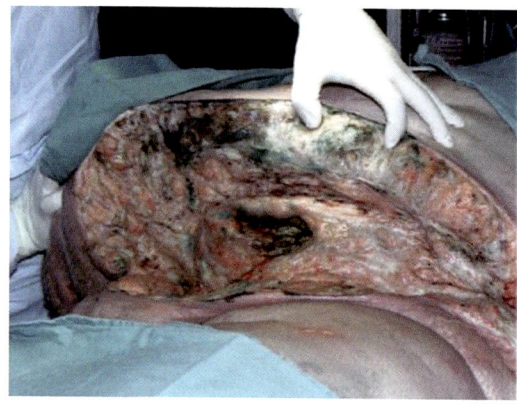

**Fig. 81.7** Example of a postoperative wound infection in a morbidly obese patient

## Postoperative Complications and PACU Management

- Postop morbidity and mortality is increased in the obese patient compared to their non-obese counterparts.
- Wound infection is twice as common.
- Deep vein thrombosis and pulmonary emboli occur with greater frequency in this population.
- A semi-sitting position, or 45° of head elevation may reduce the likelihood of postoperative hypoxemia.
- Supplemental O2 is helpful in transporting these patients to the recovery room area.
- Most problems the obese patient faces in the PACU are respiratory and ventilatory.
- Some may be slower to emerge and should remain intubated until they are fully awake and meet standard extubation criteria.

- An arterial blood gas is the best assessment for suspected hypoventilation.
- Post-operative obese patients have relative hypoxia compared to non-obese due to physiologic changes
- Position these patients in head up (sitting or semi-sitting), or laterally if surgically acceptable.
- Administration of $O_2$ is a priority, upon arrival to the recovery unit.
- "Despite concern that aspiration of air during CPAP treatment may cause disruption of new anastomotic suture lines following intestinal surgery, PACU studies have not shown an increased risk for anastomotic leak."

### Conclusion

Bariatric surgery is becoming increasingly popular and readily available in multiple health centers across the world. Various options are available to the patients and some degree of due diligence is required on the patients part regarding the selection process and willingness to maintain a lifestyle, which will keep their weight in check. Great diligence is required on the part of the anesthesiologist or nurse anesthetist, in the care of these patients, and airway management plays an extremely important role in the safe management of these special individuals.

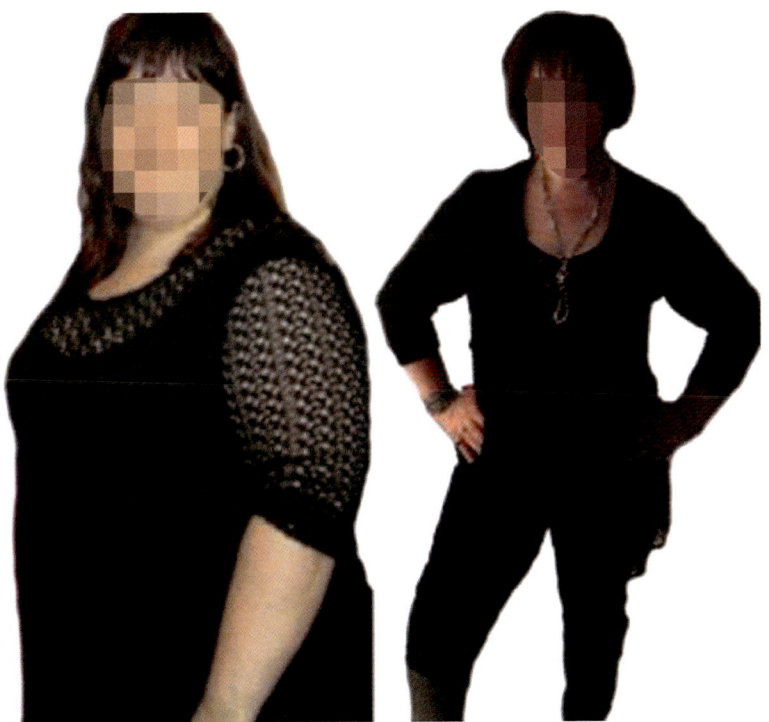

**Fig. 81.8** Patient Gina Taylor pre-gastric sleeve and 14 months post-procedure

| Plan/preparation/adverse events | Anesthetic management |
|---|---|
| Pre-operative evaluation<br>Airway: Mallampati, neck circumference<br>Pulmonary: OSA, obesity hypovent syndrome ↓ FRC, VC, TLC, ERV, inspiratory capacity<br>Cardiac: ↑ CO, ? valvulopathy/CAD<br>GI: fatty liver, GERD<br>Metabolic: DM<br>Psych: motivation/expectations<br>Social: smoking, EtOH, recreational drug use | Airway evaluation and patient history should guide airway management planning. A skilled assistant and backup equipment/planning should be in place prior to induction. ↓ FRC leads to rapid oxygen desaturation demanding adequate preoxygenation<br>Comorbidities should be evaluated and treated, pt should have realistic expectations, and smoking cessation is necessary |
| Position—supine<br>Laparoscopic—often reverse Trendelenberg<br>Intubation—*HELP* | Beanbags, footrests, and straps help prevent sliding. Padding decreases nerve injuries<br>Ventilation and hemodynamic considerations of Trendelenberg or reverse Trendelenberg position<br>*HELP* aligns oropharyngeal, laryngeal, and tracheal axis to facilitate intubation |
| IV access—peripheral<br>Monitoring—standard noninvasive monitoring of oxygenation, ventilation, circulation, temperature | Peripheral IV access and noninvasive BP monitoring are adequate unless body habitus precludes their placement or pt comorbidities justify invasive access/monitoring |
| GA with ETT<br>  Inhalational agent<br>  Intravenous sedative/analgesic<br>  Muscle relaxant | TBW, LBW and IBW should be calculated<br>The appropriate dosing scalar should be applied to each drug based on available evidence |
| Postoperative Considerations<br>  Pain<br>  Hypoxia/hypoventilation<br>  Nausea/vomiting | Multimodal analgesia including opioids, nonopioid intravenous agents, and local anesthetics decrease risk of respiratory depression and airway obstruction<br>Multimodal antiemetic therapy is often appropriate<br>Consider noninvasive positive pressure ventilation |
| Complications<br>  Hypoventilation/hypoxia<br>  DVT/PE<br>  Wound infection<br>  Procedure specific complications: leak, bowel obstruction/incarceration/stricture | VTE prophylaxis<br>Pre-procedure antibiotics<br>Procedure specific complication rate decreases after surgeon completes 70 laparoscopic gastric bypass procedures |

# References

1. Guidelines for clinical application of laparoscopic bariatric surgery—a SAGES guideline. 2008. https://www.sages.org/publications/guidelines/guidelines-for-clinical-application-of-laparoscopic-bariatric-surgery. Accessed 17 Mar 2017.
2. Approved procedures. 2016. http://asmbs.org/resources/approved-procedures. Accessed 17 Mar 2017.
3. Mason EE, Ito C. Gastric bypass in obesity. Surg Clin North Am. 1967;47:1345–51.
4. Santry HP, Gillen DL, Lauderdale DS. Trends in bariatric surgical procedures. JAMA. 2005;294(15):1909–17.
5. Bariatric surgery procedures—ASMBS. https://asmbs.org/patients/bariatric-surgery-procedures. Accessed 17 Mar 2017.
6. Guidelines for clinical application of laparoscopic bariatric surgery—a SAGES guideline. 2008. https://www.sages.org/publications/guidelines/guidelines-for-clinical-application-of-laparoscopic-bariatric-surgery. Accessed 17 Mar 2017.
7. Westling A, Gustavsson S. Laparoscopic vs open Roux-en-Y gastric bypass: a prospective, randomized trial. Obes Surg. 2001;11(3):284–92.
8. Podnos YD, Jimenez JC, Wilson SE, et al. Complications after laparoscopic gastric bypass: a review of 3464 cases. Arch Surg. 2003;138(9):957–61.
9. Podnos YD, Jimenez JC, Wilson SE, et al. Complications after laparoscopic gastric bypass: a review of 3464 cases. Arch Surg. 2003;138(9):957–61.
10. Dorman RB, Ikramuddin S. Surgical treatment of obesity and metabolic syndrome, scientific American surgery 9/2012.
11. Dorman RB, Ikramuddin S. Surgical treatment of obesity and metabolic syndrome, scientific American surgery 9/2012.
12. Jossart GH, Anthone G. The history of the sleeve gastrectomy. Bariatric Times. 2010;7(2):9–10.
13. Karmali S, Schauer P, Birch D, Sharma A, Sherman V. Laparoscopic sleeve gastrectomy, an innovative new tool in the battle against obesity in Canada. Can J Surg. 2010;53(2):126–32.
14. Bariatric Surgery Procedures—ASMBS. https://asmbs.org/patients/bariatric-surgery-procedures. Accessed 17 Mar 2017.

15. Karmali S, Schauer P, Birch D, Sharma A, Sherman V. Laparoscopic sleeve gastrectomy, an innovative new tool in the battle against obesity in Canada. Can J Surg. 2010;53(2):126–32.
16. Himpens J, Dapri G, Cadiere GB. A prospective randomized study between laparoscopic gastric banding and laparoscopic isolated sleeve gastrectomy: results after 1 and 3 years. Obes Surg. 2006;16(11):1450–6.
17. Guidelines for clinical application of laparoscopic bariatric surgery—A SAGES Guideline. 2008. https://www.sages.org/publications/guidelines/guidelines-for-clinical-application-of-laparoscopic-bariatric-surgery. Accessed 17 Mar 2017.
18. Bariatric surgery procedures—ASMBS. https://asmbs.org/patients/bariatric-surgery-procedures. Accessed 17 Mar 2017.
19. Bariatric surgery procedures—ASMBS. https://asmbs.org/patients/bariatric-surgery-procedures. Accessed 17 Mar 2017.
20. Anderson B, Gill R, deGara C, Karmali S, Gagner M. Biliopancreatic diversion: the effectiveness of duodenal switch and its limitations. Gastroenterol Res Pract. 2013;2013:1–7.
21. Bariatric surgery procedures—ASMBS. https://asmbs.org/patients/bariatric-surgery-procedures. Accessed 17 Mar 2017.
22. Guidelines for clinical application of laparoscopic bariatric surgery—a SAGES guideline. 2008. https://www.sages.org/publications/guidelines/guidelines-for-clinical-application-of-laparoscopic-bariatric-surgery. Accessed 17 Mar 2017.
23. Sabharwal A, Christelis N. Anesthesia for bariatric surgery. Contin Educ Anaesth Crit Care Pain. 2010;10(4):99–103.
24. Guidelines for clinical application of laparoscopic bariatric surgery—a SAGES guideline. 2008. https://www.sages.org/publications/guidelines/guidelines-for-clinical-application-of-laparoscopic-bariatric-surgery. Accessed 17 Mar 2017.
25. Guidelines for clinical application of laparoscopic bariatric surgery—a SAGES guideline. 2008. https://www.sages.org/publications/guidelines/guidelines-for-clinical-application-of-laparoscopic-bariatric-surgery. Accessed 17 Mar 2017.
26. Bariatric surgery procedures—ASMBS. https://asmbs.org/patients/bariatric-surgery-procedures. Accessed 17 Mar 2017.
27. O'Brien PE, McPhail T, Chaston TB, Dixon JB. Systematic review of medium-term weight loss after bariatric operations. Obes Surg. 2006;16(8):1032–40.
28. Angrisani L, Di Lorenzo N, Favretti F, et al. The Italian group for LAP-BAND: predictive value of initial body mass index for weight loss after 5 years of follow-up. Surg Endosc. 2004;18(10):1524–7.
29. Suter M, Giusti V, Worreth M, Heraief E, Calmes JM. Laparoscopic gastric banding: a prospective, randomized study comparing the LAP BAND and the SAGB: early results. Ann Surg. 2005;241(1):55–62.
30. Gonzalez H, Minville V, Delanoue K, Mazerolles M, Concina D, Fourcade O. The importance of increased neck circumference to intubation difficulties in obese patients. Anesth Analg. 2008;106(4):1132–6.
31. Goldberg ME, Norris MC, Larijani GE, Marr AT, Seltzer JL. Preoxygenation in the morbidly obese: a comparison of two techniques. Anesth Analg. 1989;68:520–2.
32. Ogunnaike BO, Jones SB, Jones DB, Provost D, Whitten CW. Anesthetic considerations for bariatric surgery. Anesth Analg. 2002;95:1793–805.
33. Levitan RM, Mechem CC, Ochroch EA, Shofer SF, Hollander JE. Head-elevated laryngoscopy position: improving laryngeal exposure during laryngoscopy by increasing head elevation. Ann Emerg Med. 2003;41(3):322–30.
34. Absalom AR, Mani V, De Smet T, Struys MM. Pharmacokinetic models for propofol—defining and illuminating the devil in the detail. Br J Anaesth. 2009;103:26–37.
35. Robinson JD, Lupkiewicz SM, Palenik L, Lopez LM, Ariet M. Determination of ideal body weight for drug dosage calculations. Am J Hosp Pharm. 1983;40(6):1016–9.
36. Ingrande J, Lemmens HJM. Dose adjustment of anaesthetics in the morbidly obese. Br J Anaesth. 2010;105(1):16–23.
37. Barash P, Cullen B, Stoelting R, Cahalan M, Stock MC. Clinical anesthesia. 6th ed. Philadelphia: Lippincott Williams & Wilkins; 2009. p. 1236–45.
38. Juvin P, Vadam M, Malek L, Dupont H, Marmuse JP, Desmonts JM. Postoperative recovery after desflurane, propofol or isflurane anesthesia among morbidly obese patients: a prospective randomized study. Anesth Analg. 2000;91(3):714–9.
39. Torri G, Casati A, Albertin A, Comotti L, Bignami E, Scarioni M, Paganelli M. Randomized comparison of isoflurane and sevoflurane for laparoscopic gastric banding in morbidly obese patients. J Clin Anesth. 2001;13:565–70.
40. Ingrande J, Brodsky JB, Lemmens HJ. Lean body weight scalar for the anesthetic induction dose of propofol in morbidly obese subjects. Anesth Analg. 2011;113(1):57–62.
41. Servin F, Farinotti R, Haberer JP, Desmonts JM. Propofol infusion for maintenance of anesthesia in morbidly obese patients receiving nitrous oxide. A clinical and pharmacokinetic study. Anesthesiology. 1993;78:657–65.
42. Bakhamees HS, El-Halafawy YM, El-Kerdawy HM, Gouda NM, Altemyatt S. Effects of dexmedetomidine in morbidly obese patients undergoing laparoscopic gastric bypass. Middle East J Anesthesiol. 2007;19(3):537–51.
43. Ramsay M. Bariatric surgery: the role of dexmedetomidine. Semin Anesth Periper Med Pain. 2006;25(2):51–6.
44. Bird M. Acute pain management: a new area of liability for anesthesiologist. ASA Newsl. 2007;71:7–9.
45. Ingrande J, Lemmens HJ. Dose adjustment of anaesthetics in the morbidly obese. Br J Anaesth. 2010;105(1):16–23.
46. Ingrande J, Lemmens HJ. Dose adjustment of anaesthetics in the morbidly obese. Br J Anaesth. 2010;105(1):16–23.

47. Slepchenko G, Simon N, Goubaux B, Levron JC, LeMoing JP, Raucoules-Aime M. Performance of target-controlled sufentanil infusion in obese patients. Anesthesiology. 2003;98:65–73.
48. Egan TD, Huizinga B, Gupta SK, Jaarsma RL, Sperry RJ, Yee JB, Muir KT. Remifentanil pharmacokinetics in obese versus lean patients. Anesthesiology. 1998;89:562–73.
49. Linares CL, Decleves X, Oppert JM, Basdevant A, Clement K, Bardin C, Scherrmann JM, Lepine JP, Bergmann JF, Mouly S. Pharmacology of morphine in obese patients. Clin Pharmacokinet. 2009;48(10):635–51.
50. Linares CL, Decleves X, Oppert JM, Basdevant A, Clement K, Bardin C, Scherrmann JM, Lepine JP, Bergmann JF, Mouly S. Pharmacology of morphine in obese patients. Clin Pharmacokinet. 2009;48(10):635–51.
51. Patanwala AE, Holmes KL, Erstad BL. Analgesic response to morphine in obese and morbidly obese patients in the emergency department. Emerg Med J. 2014;31(2):139–42.
52. Sollazzi L, Modesti C, Vitale F, Sacco T, Ciocchetti P, Idra AS, Tacchino RM, Perilli V. Preinductive use of clonidine and ketamine improves recovery and reduces postoperative pain after bariatric surgery. Surg Obes Relat Dis. 2009;5(1):67–71.
53. Rumack B. Acetaminophen misconceptions. Hepatology. 2004;40(1):10–5.
54. Govindarajan R, Ghosh B, Sathyamoorthy MK, Kodali NS, Raza A, Aronsohn J, Rajpal S, Ramaswamy C, Abadir A. Efficacy of ketorolac in lieu of narcotics in the operative management of laparoscopic surgery for morbid obesity. Surg Obes Relat Dis. 2005;1(6):530–5.
55. Viby-Mogensen J. Correlation of succinylcholine duration of action with plasma cholinesterase activity in subjects with the genotypically normal enzyme. Anesthesiology. 1980;53:517–20.
56. Bentley JB, Borel JD, Vaughan RW, Gandolfi AJ. Weight, pseudocholinesterase activity, and succinylcholine requirement. Anesthesiology. 1982;57:48–9.
57. Lemmens HJ, Brodsky JB. The dose of succinylcholine in morbid obesity. Anesth Analg. 2006;102:438.
58. Lemmens HJ, Brodsky JB. The dose of succinylcholine in morbid obesity. Anesth Analg. 2006;102:438.
59. Leykin Y, Pellis T, Lucca M, Lomangino G, Marzano B, Gullo A. The pharmacodynamic effects of rocuronium when dosed according to real body weight or ideal body weight in morbidly obese patients. Anesth Analg. 2004;99(4):1086–9.
60. Weinstein JA, Matteo RS, Ornstein E, Schwartz AE, Goldstoff M, Thal G. Pharmacodynamics of vecuronium and atracurium in the obese surgical patient. Anesth Analg. 1988;67:1149–53.
61. Weinstein JA, Matteo RS, Ornstein E, Schwartz AE, Goldstoff M, Thal G. Pharmacodynamics of vecuronium and atracurium in the obese surgical patient. Anesth Analg. 1988;67:1149–53.
62. Kirkegaard-Nielsen H, Helbo-Hansen HS, Lindholm P, Severinsen IK, Pedersen HS. Anthropometric variables as predictors for duration of action of atracurium-induced neuromuscular block. Anesth Analg. 1996;83(5):1076–80.
63. Leykin Y, Pellis T, Lucca M, Lomangino G, Marzano B, Gullo A. The effects of cisatracurium on morbidly obese women. Anesth Analg. 2004;99(4):1090–4.
64. Golembiewski J. Considerations in selecting an inhaled anesthetic agent: case studies. Am J Health Syst Pharm. 2004;61(20):S10–7.
65. Torri G, Casati A, Albertin A, Comotti L, Bignami E, Scarioni M, Paganelli M. Randomized comparison of isoflurane and sevoflurane for laparoscopic gastric banding in morbidly obese patients. J Clin Anesth. 2001;13:565–70.
66. Sollazzi L, Perilli V, Modesti C, Annetta G, Ranieri R, Maria Taccino R, Proietti R. Volatile anesthesia in bariatric surgery. Obes Surg. 2001;11:623–6.
67. Torri G, Casati A, Albertin A, Comotti L, Bignami E, Scarioni M, Paganelli M. Randomized comparison of isoflurane and sevoflurane for laparoscopic gastric banding in morbidly obese patients. J Clin Anesth. 2001;13:565–70.
68. Ogunnaike BO, Jones SB, Jones DB, Provost D, Whitten CW. Anesthetic considerations for bariatric surgery. Anesth Analg. 2002;95:1793–805.
69. Peyton PJ, Wu CY. Nitrous oxide–related postoperative nausea and vomiting depends on duration of exposure. Anesthesiology. 2014;120(5):1137–45.

# Anesthesia for TURP

Maimouna Bah and Michael Stuart Green

## Introduction

Transurethral Resection of the prostate (TURP) is a common urological procedure that is considered the "gold standard" for the treatments of patients with symptomatic urinary obstruction related to benign prostatic hypertrophy (BPH). The prostate consists of four integrated zones that is divided and named based on their location; the anterior, peripheral, central, and preprostatic zones. Each zone consists of secretory, smooth muscle, and fibrotic tissues that are enclosed in one capsule rich in blood supply. In BPH the smooth muscle and epithelial cells proliferate within the transition zone of the prostate, in which the middle and posterior lobes are the ones commonly involved [1]. The result of this proliferation is a bladder outlet obstruction due to increased muscle tone. TURP is still considered the main treatment modality for BPH, however due to the significant side effect that can occur with the procedure, the development of other treatment options have resulted in the steady decline of it use. Other options include transurethral needle ablation of the prostate (TUNA) and transurethral microwave thermotherapy (TUMT) [2].

## Surgical Technique

Transurethral resection of the prostate (TURP) is performed by inserting a resectoscope through the urethra into the prostate to resect layers of the prostate tissue while preserving the prostatic capsule. If the capsule is penetrated a significant risk of large amounts of irrigation solution being absorbed into the circulation is realized [3]. The resectoscope uses either an electrically powered cutting coagulating metal loop or a laser vaporizer. The coagulation can be accomplished with either a monopolar TURP (M-TURP) technique, which transmits a high energy electrocautery current from a single electrode or bipolar TURP (B-TURP) technique, which utilized electrodes with continuous bidirectional flow of current [3]. There been several studies that have shown lower rates of complications with bipolar techniques compared to monopolar. In contrast to either of these techniques the laser vaporization resectoscope allows the sealing of prostatic veins during the resection [4]. The laser can vaporize tissue in millimeter cuts, therefore compared to electrocautery, laser significantly reduces surgical complication, procedure time, and overall hospital length of stay [4].

M. Bah, M.S., M.D.
Department of Anesthesiology and Perioperative Medicine, Drexel University College of Medicine, Hahnemann University Hospital, Philadelphia, PA, USA

M. S. Green, D.O., M.B.A. (✉)
Department of Anesthesiology and Perioperative Medicine, Drexel University College of Medicine, Philadelphia, PA, USA
e-mail: Michael.Green@Drexelmed.edu

TURP requires continuous use of fluid for visualization, distention, and irrigation of the bladder and prostate. Ideally, the irrigation solution should be a transparent isotonic and nontoxic solute that is inexpensive. However, that solution does not exist. When the available solution is examined, distilled water for example, it is inexpensive but is hypotonic and when large contents is absorbed into the circulation it result into hemolysis, shock, and renal failure. Crystalloids, including Lactate ringer's and normal saline, are highly ionized which could result in disbursement of electric current to the surrounding tissue. Commonly used solutions are glycine 1.2 and 1.5%, mannitol 3–5%, glucose 2.5–4%, sorbitol 3.5%, Cytal (a mixture of sorbitol 2.7%, and mannitol 0.54%), and urea 1% [5]. These solutions are moderately hypotonic to preserve their transparency and do not result in hemolysis and excessive absorption. However, if significant amounts of these solutes are absorbs, the patient will experience specific adverse effects. For example, glycine can cause cardiac and retinal toxic effects, mannitol will rapidly expands the blood volume resulting in pulmonary edema with worsening CHF in cardiac patients, and glucose causes severe hyperglycemia specifically in diabetic patients [5].

## Anesthetic Concerns

The patient population that undergo TURP are generally older and have significant coexisting medical conditions such as coronary artery disease, congestive heart failure, cerebrovascular disease, chronic obstructive pulmonary diseases, obstructive sleep apnea, and renal impairment. The development of deep vein thrombosis is a significant risk due advanced age, presence of malignancy, varicose veins, and obesity. Therefore, a comprehensive preoperative medical evaluation with history and physical exam is required with the goal of optimizing patients to minimize and prevent complications. Due to the complications associated with the procedure these patients must be constantly monitored for hemodynamic changes. Routine monitoring includes electrocardiogram, noninvasive blood pressure, pulse oximetry, and capnography. In addition, emergency drugs and intubation equipment should remain ready available.

## General Anesthesia Versus Regional Anesthesia

Anesthesia for TURP can be accomplished via either general or neuraxial techniques. Sensation from the prostate and bladder is transmitted by afferent parasympathetic nerve fibers from the second and third sacral roots and by sympathetic nerves of the hypogastric plexus which is derived from nerve roots extending inferiorly from T11 to L2 [6]. In order to obtain satisfactory regional anesthesia for TURP, a block level that interrupts sensory transmission from the prostate and bladder neck is required therefore anesthesia about T10 is ideal. Sensory levels block above T9 is undesirable due to the pain resulting from the prostatic capsule perforation which would then not be apparent to the patient.

Spinal anesthesia has been the most frequently used anesthetic for TURP in the United States. Spinal provides adequate anesthesia for the patient with good relaxation of the pelvic floor and perineum, and allows the early recognition of symptoms of water intoxication and fluid overload since the patient is awake. A change in the patient's mental status is an early indicator of excess absorption of irrigation fluid and complications may ensue.

Other advantages of regional anesthesia over general anesthesia is that regional has been shown to be associated with a decreased in incidence of deep vein thrombosis and operative blood loss due to decrease in systemic blood pressure secondary to the sympathetic blockade resulting in decrease in peripheral and central venous pressure and therefore blood loss during prostate surgery. Regional anesthesia also decreased analgesics requirement in the immediate postoperative period compared with general anesthesia. A study by Wang et al. showed low dose bupivacaine spinal anesthesia with intrathecal sufentanil resulted in an effective spinal sensory blockade with less motor blockade and provided hemodynamic stability in elderly patients. It also helped decrease postoperative pain and reduced the need for other analgesic medication [7].

Spinal is preferred over a continuous epidural for several reasons. Compared to epidural spinal is technically easier to perform in elderly patients, incomplete block of sacral nerve roots is avoided, and the short duration of the procedure. Bladder perforation is also recognized more frequently if the spinal level is limited to T10. General anesthesia however may be necessary in patients who require ventilatory or hemodynamic support, have a contraindication to regional anesthesia, or refuse regional anesthesia.

## Positioning

TURP is performed in the lithotomy position with the patient placed in slight trendelenburg. Trendelenburg positioning result in numerous physiological changes. Increase in cardiac preload due to increase in venous return, decrease in pulmonary blood volume and pulmonary compliance due to cephalad shift of the diaphragm, and a decrease in lung volume parameters including residual volume, functional residual volume, tidal volume, and vital capacity all occur. Nerve injuries to the common peroneal, sciatic, and femoral nerves can occur. Patients in the lithotomy position are also at high risk for development of deep vein thrombosis (DVT) due to polling and stagnant nature of the blood in the lower extremities [8].

## Ammonia and Glycine Toxicity

Visual disturbances have been associated with TURP. This has been found to be related to the systemic absorption of glycine. Visual symptoms can include halos, loss of light perception, blurred vision, and transient blindness. The pupils are usually dilated and unresponsive to stimulation, but the fundoscopic examination and intraocular pressure are normal. Symptoms can last several hours after the resection. Glycine is an amino acid that is an inhibitory neurotransmitter within the central nervous system. Normal plasma glycine levels are 13–17 mg/L. A case report showed that glycine levels of 1029 mg/L were measured during one episode of blindness. Twelve hours later, the glycine level in this case had declined to 143 mg/L, by which time vision had returned to preoperative status. However, an overall correlation between plasma glycine levels and CNS toxicity has not been established [9]. Glycine can also become oxidized into ammonia, leading to CNS toxicity. The ammonia causes suppression of norepinephrine and dopamine in the CNS resulting in encephalopathy. Ammonia toxicity usually presents within the first hour with nausea and vomiting, and progress rapidly to coma. Glycine has also has been implicated in myocardial depression and hemodynamic changes associated with TURP syndrome.

## Perforations

Another common complication of TURP is perforation of the bladder. This may occur due to difficult placing instruments and bladder over distension with irrigation fluid. Perforations usually occur during difficult resections in which the cutting loop or knife electrode comes in contact with the bladder wall. Most perforations are extra-peritoneal, and in a conscious patient result in pain in the periumbilical, inguinal, or suprapubic regions. The surgeon may also note an irregular return of irrigating fluid. If the perforation extends into the peritoneum the patient may experience pain in the generalized upper part of the abdomen or it may be referred to the diaphragm, precordial region, and/or shoulders. Other signs and symptoms include pallor, bradycardia, hypotension, restlessness, diaphoresis, nausea, vomiting, abdominal pain, abdominal rigidity, dyspnea, shoulder pain, and hiccups. The severity of symptoms depends on the location, size of the perforation, and the type of irrigating fluid.

## Coagulopathies

The prostate is highly vascular and has an extensive plexus of venous sinuses that can be opened during the procedure. As a result there is a significant risk of bleeding both during the procedure and in the postoperative time period. It is difficult to adequately estimate blood loss due to the blood being mixed with ample quantities of irrigation fluid. Therefore patient's vital signs and serial hematocrit values should be monitored to assess the blood loss and need for transfusion. Factors that influence blood loss are the vascularity, size of the gland, the duration of surgery, and sinuses opened during resection. The resection of prostate causes release of urokinase and plasminogen activator tissue causing local fibrinolysis and bleeding of the surrounding tissue [10]. Thromboplastin is also released and can enter the circulation resulting in disseminated intravascular coagulation (DIC) and systemic coagulopathy [10]. If bleeding becomes uncontrollable, the procedure should be terminated and a Foley catheter placed into the bladder with traction applied allowing for the exertion of pressure on the prostatic bed reducing bleeding. Bleeding requiring transfusion occurs in approximately 2.5% of TURP procedures [11]. Fibrinolysis can be treated with aminocaproic acid.

## Hypothermia

Irrigation fluids are usually stored at room temperature and during the TURP procedure a patient can receive several liters; this may result in a loss of a significant amount of heat. The absorption of this fluid also leads to a decrease in the patient's body temperature causing shivering. About 1 °C per hour is estimated to be lost with the irrigation fluid. The use of warmed irrigating solutions has been shown to be efficacious in reducing heat loss, however this practice is not widely followed due to concerns regarding warmed fluids yielding increased bleeding due to the vasodilation effects, which have not been proven.

## TURP Syndrome

TURP syndrome is a clinical diagnosis that presents with concerning cardiovascular and/or neurological symptoms caused by excessive absorption of the irrigating fluid. This syndrome can be diagnosed through the first postoperative day and should remain on the differential if changes are noted. TURP syndrome results in severe CNS derangements associated with extreme hyponatremia, such as convulsions and coma. Due to the degree of vascularity of the prostate gland a significant amount of irrigation solution can potentially be absorbed. Factors that significantly affect the amount absorb are hydrostatic pressures of the irrigant and the time length of the resection. On average, 20 mL/min of fluid is absorbed with a total of greater than 6 L absorbed in procedures lasting up to 2 h [12]. Additional factors include heavier tissue resection and use of monopolar resectoscope. Violation of the prostate capsule during the resection can lead to solution entering peritoneal and retroperitoneal spaces and therefore the circulation. The type of absorbed fluid determines the sequela the patient presents with. Currently, the two most commonly used fluids are glycine and Cytal. Therefore, previously common complications such as hemolysis or hyponatremia have been significantly reduced [13]. Fluid overload/over hydration does still remain a challenge. About 20–30% of absorbed solution remains in the intravascular space with the remaining entering the interstitial space. These result in increased capillary leak, pulmonary edema, cardiovascular overload, cerebral edema, and possibly death (see Table 82.1).

Extracellular sodium concentration must be in the physiologic range for depolarization of excitable cells and production of the action potential to occur, which is 135–145 mEq/L. Hyponatremia is serum sodium below 135 mEq/L. Symptoms ranges from nausea, malaise, irritability, apprehension, confusion, and headache. These may present early even with mild to moderate hyponatremia. Neurological symptoms are most often observed with levels <115 mEq/L. This includes seizures and coma [13]. Cardiovascular

**Table 82.1** Signs and symptoms of TURP syndrome

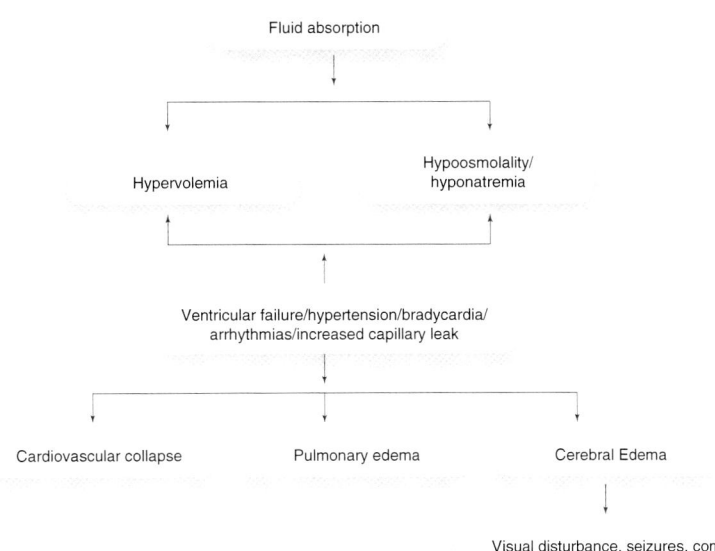

symptoms are a result of negative inotropy with causes dysrhythmias, electrocardiogram changes including QRS widening, U waves, ST-segment elevation. Cardiovascular symptoms are usually seen around the same sodium levels (less than 115 mEq/L) [13].

## Treatment of Transurethral Resection of the Prostate Syndrome

Management of TURP syndrome is initiated with supportive care. It is very important to ensure appropriate oxygenation, ventilation, and circulatory assistance if needed. It should include fluid restriction and possible diuretic administration such as furosemide if indicated to promote excretion of free water. Seizures are treated with anticonvulsants such as benzodiazepines. Patients with severe hyponatremia 3% hypertonic saline can be initiated slowly (less than 100 mL/h) to avoid worsening cerebral edema and central pontine myelinolysis.

### Conclusion

TURP is associated with significant risk that can cause a short procedure to become life threatening. Patents are in a dynamic state and need careful monitoring. General and neuraxial anesthesia have advantages and disadvantages related to each. Spinal or epidural anesthesia allows the patient's subjective judgment to contribute to assessment of their condition during surgery. Bleeding is very common during TURP which can be easily controlled, however when large venous sinuses are opened hemostasis can be difficult to obtain [14]. Mortality rates are similar in patients receiving regional anesthesia or general anesthesia.

## References

1. Azar I. Transurethral resection of prostate. In: Malhotra V, editor. Anesthesia for renal and genitourinary surgery. New York: McGraw-Hill; 1996. p. 93–109.
2. Feng F, Chen Z, Cromer J, et al. Anesthetic concerns for patients undergoing a transurethral resection of the prostate (TURP). Urol Nurs. 2016;36(2):75–81.
3. Omar MI, Lam TB, Alexander CE, et al. Systematic review and meta-analysis of the clinical effectiveness of bipolar compared with monopolar trans-

urethral resection of the prostate (TURP). BJU Int. 2014;113(1):24–35. https://doi.org/10.1111/bju.12281.
4. Engeler DS, Schwab C, Neyer M, Grun T, Reissigl A, Schmid HP. Bipolar versus monopolar TURP: a prospective controlled study at two urology centers. Prostate Cancer Prostatic Dis. 2010;13(3):285–91.
5. Miller RD. Miller's anesthesia. 7th ed. Philadelphia, PA: Churchill Livingstone/Elsevier; 2010.
6. Barash PG, Cullen BF, Stoelting RK, et al. Clinical anesthesia. 6th ed. Philadelphia: Lippincott Williams & Wilkins; 2009.
7. Wang J, Pang L, Han W, Li G, Wang N. Effect of preemptive intravenous oxycodone on low dose bupivacaine spinal anesthesia with intrathecal sufentanil. Saudi Med J. 2015;36(4):437–41.
8. Rice KR, Brassell SA, McLeod DG. Venous thromboembolism in urologic surgery: prophylaxis, diagnosis, and treatment. Rev Urol. 2010;12(2–3):e111–24.
9. Ovassapian A, Joshi CW, Brunner EA. Visual disturbance: an unusual symptom of transurethral prostatic resection reaction. Anesthesiology. 1982;57:332–4.
10. Fujiwara A, Nakahira J, Sawai T, Inamoto T, Minami T. Prediction of clinical manifestations of transurethral resection syndrome by preoperative ultrasonographic estimation of prostate weight. Bio Med Central Urol. 2014;16(14):67.
11. Thomas AZ, Thomas AA, Conlon P, Hickey D, Little DM. Benign prostatic hyperplasia presenting with renal failure—what is the role for transurethral resection of the prostate (TURP)? Ir Med J. 2009;102(2):43–4.
12. Seitz M, Soljanik I, Stanislaus P, Sroka R, Stief C. Explosive gas formation during transurethral resection of the prostate (TURP). Eur J Med Res. 2008;13(8):399–400.
13. Aziz W, Ather MH. Frequency of electrolyte derangement after transurethral resection of prostate: need for postoperative electrolyte monitoring. Adv Urol. 2015;2015:415735.
14. Bach T, Geavlete B, Pfeiffer D, Wendt-Nordahl G, Michel MS, Gross AJ. TURP in patients with biopsy-proven prostate cancer: sensitivity for cancer detection. Urology. 2009;73(1):100–4.

# Anesthesia for Major Joint Surgery

Scott R. Coleman and Michael Stuart Green

## Introduction

With an aging population, joint replacement surgery is becoming more common [1]. More than one million arthroplasties are done each year worldwide, and these numbers are expected to continue to rise [2]. Major orthopedic joint surgery offers a few unique challenges an anesthesiologist should be aware of when formulating an anesthetic plan. Pain is a major complication of these surgeries that needs to be addressed to improve patient satisfaction and outcomes [3–5]. A major cause of morbidity and mortality of these surgeries to be mindful of is deep vein thrombosis [6]. The physiologic changes that occur when using pneumatic tourniquets and bone cement also need to be considered. All of this will be discussed in the context of total shoulder, hip, and knee arthroplasty in this chapter.

S. R. Coleman, D.O. · M. S. Green, D.O., M.B.A. (✉)
Department of Anesthesiology and Perioperative Medicine, Drexel University College of Medicine/ Hahnemann University Hospital, Philadelphia, PA, USA
e-mail: Michael.Green@Drexelmed.edu

## Surgical Technique

### Shoulder Arthroplasty

Shoulder arthroplasty is commonly performed in beach chair position. Access to the joint is typically done via an anterior incision and medial reflection of the subscapularis muscle. The humeral head is then anteriorly dislocated. Internal rotation of the arm should be restricted post-operatively to allow the subscapularis muscle to heal. Total shoulder replacement exchanges both the humeral head and glenoid portion of the scapula. Hemiarthroplasty of the joint is replacement of only the humeral head and is indicated when a concomitant rotator cuff tear is present. A typical case lasts 2–5 h and blood loss can vary from 200 to 1000 mL [7].

### Hip Arthroplasty

Position for hip arthroplasty is typically supine or lateral decubitus with the operative side up. The incision can be on the anterior, lateral, or posterior portion of the hip. The joint is dislocated and the femoral head and neck are excised to allow for replacement. Unipolar arthroplasty replaces the femur and bipolar replaces both the femur and acetabulum. A typical case lasts 2–3 h and can have an estimated blood loss of 250–750 mL [7].

## Knee Arthroplasty

Knee arthroplasty is performed with the patient in the supine position. The incision is typically over the anterior to medial portion of the knee. The femur, patella, and tibia are all exposed. Cartilage is removed, and a bone saw is used to create space for the prosthesis. Replacement can involve both sides of the joint or it can be unicompartmental and replace only the medial or lateral side. A typical case takes approximately 2 h and estimated blood loss can range from 300 to 500 mL [7].

## Pre-operative Evaluation

### Patient Evaluation

A standard, thorough pre-operative evaluation should be performed for all patients including past medical history, allergies, medications, past anesthesia history, airway and cardiopulmonary examination, and functional status. Because blood loss can be significant in these surgeries, a CBC and type and screen are judicious tests to collect prior to entering the operating room. Additional labs and testing should be based on patient co-morbidities, i.e. a basic chemistry for a diabetic or dialysis patient. Risk of adverse events can be evaluated in patients using the American College of Surgery National Surgery Quality Improvement Program (ACS NSQIP) [8].

### Common Comorbidities

Joint replacements surgeries are common for elderly and obese patients due to increased 'wear and tear' of the joints. Obese patients present additional challenges for many reasons. Obtaining intravenous access and regional anesthesia is often more challenging. Mask ventilation and intubation can be more difficult as well. Obese patients desaturate quicker due to increased metabolic consumption of oxygen and a diminished functional residual capacity [9]. Other common co-morbidities in this patient population include anxiety, depression and rheumatoid arthritis [1].

If a patient with rheumatoid arthritis is encountered, other complications of this disease should be considered. Range of motion of the neck should be evaluated, as well as inquiring about any cervical or lumbar radiculopathy. Rheumatoid patients also have an increased risk of pericardial and pleural effusions. Care should be taken prior to and during direct laryngoscopy of these patients due to the increased risk of atlanto-axial instability [10]. Additionally, more patients undergoing these procedures have diabetes, renal disease, cerebrovascular disease, and heart failure than in the past. [1] Each of these co-morbidities requires further investigation by the anesthesia provider prior to surgery.

## Choosing an Anesthetic Approach

Total shoulder arthroplasty can be done with general anesthesia, regional anesthesia, or a combination of the two. In addition to general and regional anesthesia for hip and knee replacement, neuraxial anesthesia can also be used. The reasons for increased use of neuraxial and regional techniques will be discussed in detail below.

### General Anesthesia

Traditionally, major orthopedic procedures were done under general anesthesia. However, neuraxial anesthesia is being used more frequently as studies are showing improved patient satisfaction and decreased complications [11]. General anesthesia is also associated with increased risk of unplanned intubation and extended ventilator use [12]. Shoulder replacements are still commonly done with general anesthesia. The use of an endotracheal tube versus supraglottic device depends upon airway examination, patient body habitus, operative time, and ultimately, provider comfort.

### Neuraxial Anesthesia

Neuraxial anesthesia, which includes epidural and spinal anesthesia, can be used for total hip and knee replacement surgery. When comparing neuraxial versus general anesthesia, studies have found a number of significant differences. When compared to general anesthesia, neuraxial techniques decrease length of hospital stay, operative time, estimated blood loss, need for transfusions, risk of stroke, and risk of cardiac arrest [12–14]. Concerns that neuraxial techniques prolong operating room time due to added time needed to perform the block or increased surgical difficulty resulting from absence of muscle relaxation have not been validated [12]. Neuraxial anesthesia has not increased surgical site infections or nerve injury compared to general anesthesia [13]. However, epidural and spinal anesthesia may lead to urinary retention, leg weakness, and hypotension [15]. Of note, deep venous thrombosis and pulmonary embolism are less likely with epidural anesthesia compared to general anesthesia. However, in these studies, chemical prophylaxis was not used. When chemical prophylaxis is used, the difference in rate of thrombotic complication is not statistically significant [12, 13]. Therefore, the need for chemical prophylaxis is likely paramount to using a neuraxial technique in preventing thrombotic sequelae. The contraindications for these techniques based on thromboprophylaxis will be discussed in detail below.

## Peripheral Nerve Blocks

Peripheral nerve blocks can be used as a sole anesthetic for major joint surgery. However, more commonly, they are the first line choice for analgesia after such procedures. Post-operative pain is a prominent issue for these patients. The most significant pain occurs immediately after surgery, which nerve blocks can help reduce tremendously [5, 16]. When pain is better controlled, patients are more satisfied and have increased mobility. Increased mobility will allow for quicker rehabilitation time and decrease the risk of deep vein thrombosis and pulmonary embolism. Nerve blocks have been shown to control pain better than patient controlled morphine infusions [5]. Blocks can be done before or after surgery. However, pre-operative placement is likely more beneficial as it decreases the nervous system's sensitization to painful stimuli [3].

## Perineural Catheters

During the localization of the peripheral nerve a catheter may be left in place to provide analgesia for a longer duration. These catheters have minimal risk of bleeding, infection, and nerve injury [17]. While epidural catheters can also be used for longer analgesic duration, patients with lumbar plexus catheters have shorter hospital stays, less opioid use, and are able to ambulate sooner. The side effects of urinary retention and hypotension are also avoided with a perineural catheter [15].

## Regional Anesthesia for the Shoulder

For patients undergoing shoulder replacement, an interscalene block can help with post-operative pain. This block provides anesthesia to both the shoulder and upper arm. Use of this technique in conjunction with general anesthesia decreases opioid use, post-operative nausea and vomiting, recovery room time, and hospital length of stay [18]. However, this block does not come without risk. Ipsilateral diaphragm paralysis, pneumothorax, intrathecal injection, and injection into the vertebral artery are potential complications [18].

## Regional Anesthesia for the Hip

The preferred regional technique for total hip arthoplasty is a lumbar plexus block. This is considered a deep plexus block and is performed via a posterior approach. The injection is done lateral and inferior to the L4 spinous process. This will anesthetize the anterolateral and medial thigh as well as the knee. Potential complications of this block include intrathecal injection, nerve injury, and renal and retroperitoneal hematoma [19]. Although this is quite rare, significant bleeding in an area that is not easily compressed may lead to devastating outcomes [17]. Therefore, clinical

Table 83.1 ASRA guidelines regarding DVT prophylaxis and neuraxial/regional anesthesia [20]

| Medication | Procedure | ASRA recommendation |
|---|---|---|
| Aspirin/NSAIDs | Neuraxial or regional anesthetic | No restrictions |
| Heparin DVT prophylaxis (BID/TID daily dosing) | Neuraxial/deep peripheral block | Hold 4–6 h before; restart without delay |
| | Catheter removal | Hold 4–6 h before; restart without delay |
| Enoxaparin (daily prophylactic dosing) | Neuraxial/deep peripheral block | Hold 10 h before; restart 12 h after surgery |
| | Catheter removal | Hold 12 h before; restart 4 h after removal |
| Enoxaparin (BID prophylactic dosing) | Neuraxial/deep peripheral block | Hold 10 h prior; restart 12 h after surgery |
| | Catheter removal | Must remove catheter before 1st dose after surgery; restart 4 h after removal |
| Enoxaparin therapeutic dose | Neuraxial/deep peripheral block | Hold 24 h prior to block |
| | Catheter removal | Catheters should be removed before restarting regimen |
| Warfarin/Coumadin | Neuraxial/deep peripheral block | Hold 4–5 days prior and confirm normal INR |
| | After procedure | Restart without delay |
| | Catheter removal | INR <1.5 to remove catheter; 24 h neurologic checks after removal |
| Direct thrombin inhibitors | Neuraxial/deep peripheral block | Avoid procedure |
| Direct Xa inhibitors | Neuraxial/deep peripheral block | Hold 3 days before; restart 6 h after block |
| | Catheter removal | Hold 3 days before; restart 6 h after removal |
| Platelet ADP inhibitors | Neuraxial/deep peripheral block | Hold 10–12 h before; restart 6–8 h after block |
| | Catheter removal | Hold 10 h before; restart 2 h after removal |
| Thrombolytics | Neuraxial/deep peripheral block | Avoid procedure |

judgment should be used in patients at risk for bleeding. See Table 83.1 for details about performing this block in anticoagulated patients.

## Regional Anesthesia for the Knee

The knee can be blocked with a lumbar plexus block as mentioned above. However, femoral and sciatic nerve blocks are more commonly used due to decreased risk of intrathecal injection and because they are not a deep block [19]. Adductor canal blocks cover the anterior knee without causing the quadriceps weakness seen with femoral blocks. However, some degree of weakness will occur. This can help expedite discharge from the hospital and post-operative rehabilitation [4]. The adductor canal is located with ultrasonography.

In obese patients, this block becomes increasingly difficult, and a femoral block may be more prudent to ensure post-operative pain relief.

## Deep Venous Thrombosis Prophylaxis

The risk of deep venous thrombosis (DVT) after major orthopedic surgery is significantly increased. For patients without prophylaxis, the rates are increased by as much as 80%. Risk factors for DVT include obesity, age greater than 60, use of a tourniquet, fractures, and length of case more than 30 min [20]. Total hip and knee arthroplasty are high-risk surgeries for DVT formation [21]. The hypercoaguable response to surgery along with venous stasis contributes to the formation of

DVTs. Long-term complications of DVTs include post-thrombotic syndrome, recurrence of clots, and chronic thromboembolic pulmonary hypertension [21]. Unless contraindicated, pneumatic compression devices should be placed on the lower extremity. Pharmacologic prophylaxis is also strongly recommended unless contraindicated and should be started 12 h prior to or 12–24 h after surgery depending upon bleeding risk [20, 21]. Both neuraxial and general anesthesia have been found to decrease the risk of DVTs. This is likely due to the sympathectomy that occurs, which leads to increased venous flow [6].

## American Society of Regional Anesthesia Guidelines

Thromboprophylactic medications contraindicated for neuraxial technique include thrombolytics, direct thrombin inhibitors, anti-platelet agents (except aspirin), and low-molecular weight heparin (LMWH) in therapeutic doses. If a patient's total daily dose of subcutaneous heparin is 10,000 units or less, neuraxial techniques can be safely performed. LMWH can be combined with neuraxial anesthesia in a few instances. If once daily dosing of LMWH is used, neuraxial techniques can be done safely 10 h after the last dose and 4 h before the next dose. However, if twice daily dosing will be used, even with prophylactic dosing, any catheter (epidural or peripheral) should be removed 2 h prior to starting the regimen. The evidence regarding anti-coagulation and peripheral nerve blocks is sparse. Therefore, current recommendations for deep blocks are the same as for neuraxial techniques and there are no recommendations for superficial blocks [20]. See Table 83.1 for full details about the compatibility of regional anesthesia and anti-coagulants.

## Intraoperative Considerations

### Patient Positioning

As with all patients, pressure points should be padded to prevent nerve injury and pressure ulcers during these cases, which typically last multiple hours. Beach chair position, which is commonly used for shoulder replacement, provides unique challenges. Most importantly, cerebral perfusion can be compromised if the anesthesia provider is not vigilant. Cerebral perfusion pressure is the difference between mean arterial pressure (MAP) and intracranial pressure (ICP). Therefore, maintain the MAP and minimizing the ICP are important. Often, blood pressure measurements are collected from an arm or leg of the patient. However, this measurement is higher than the blood pressure in the circle of Willis. The anesthesia provider must be aware that for every 2.5 cm difference in height, the blood pressure varies by approximately 2 mmHg. For example, a blood pressure of 100/60 mmHg measured in an upper extremity that is 25 cm below the circle of Willis, correlates with a blood pressure of 80/40 mmHg in the brain [22]. Placement of an arterial line to monitor blood pressure closely can be justified based on other patient characteristics. In this situation, the transducer can be placed at the level of Circle of Willis to measure cerebral blood pressure.

### Tourniquet Use

Tourniquets are pneumatic cuffs inflated on an extremity above the patient's systolic blood pressure to create a bloodless surgical field. While this strategy helps reduce blood loss and improves visualization for the surgeon, it does have complications [23]. Tourniquet pain can occur despite adequate anesthesia via neuraxial, peripheral nerve blocks, or general anesthesia. Tourniquet pain manifests as a severe, dull ache in an awake patient and as diaphoresis, hypertension, and tachycardia in the anesthetized patient. Increasing depth of anesthetic and administering opioids may help initially, but will eventually lose efficacy [24]. However, patients with neuraxial and peripheral nerve blocks have a lower frequency of this phenomenon than those under general anesthesia [25]. Ultimately, the pain will not resolve until the tourniquet is released. Administering magnesium sulfate in awake patients has shown to reduce the pain via NMDA receptor activation [26]. Release of the tourniquet also has significant hemodynamic implications, one of which is hypotension. The etiology of the hypotension is multifactorial. Carbon dioxide, lactate, and potassium are metabolites of anaerobic metabolism that are released into the systemic circulation leading to vasodilation. Additionally, the blood re-enters the exsanguinated limb, leading to a drop in blood pressure. The risk of deep venous thrombosis is also increased, which may contribute to hypotension and hypoxia when the tourniquet is released and the clots migrate toward the pulmonary circulation. Arrhythmias are also rare, but a concern [27]. There have also been reports of rhabdomyolysis associated with tourniquet use [23].

## Bone Cement

Bone cement (polymethylmethacrylate) is used to enhance the adhesion between prosthetic material and native bone. However, it is also associated with bone cement implantation syndrome. Cement can be avoided in a younger, healthier patient where new bone growth can help adhere the new joint. However, in elderly patients, cement may be needed to maintain the integrity of the new joint. As the cement is prepared it produces heat and expands as part of an exothermic reaction. The heat and expansion leads to intramedullary hypertension. This elevated pressure within the bone can cause embolization of fat, bone marrow, and air [28]. Additionally, cement can be absorbed systemically leading to vasodilation and hypotension. Signs of bone cement implantation syndrome include hypoxia secondary to increased pulmonary shunting, pulmonary hypertension, cardiac arrhythmias, and hypotension [29]. Treatment is supportive management. Preventive measures include maintaining euvolemia, increasing the fraction of inspired oxygen prior to cementing, creating a hole in the distal femur to relieve the intramedullary pressure, and only using cement when needed [28]. An additional concern with bone cement is the risk to pregnant women. Research about the teratogenicity of methylmethacrylate is sparse and limited to animal studies. To date, the evidence is conflicting with some studies showing no effect with exposure while others showed early fetal deaths and skeletal abnormalities in exposed rats [30].

## Fat Embolism Syndrome

When there is disruption to the integrity of a bone, particularly a long bone, fat embolism syndrome is possible. This typically occurs 1–3 days after the inciting event. The classic presentation includes hypoxia, neurologic changes, and petechiae on the thorax, neck, and axillae. Thrombocytopenia, anemia, and disseminated intravascular coagulation are possible as well. Neurologic symptoms range from confusion and lethargy to focal defects and coma. Damage to the pulmonary tissue can progress to adult respiratory distress syndrome. Signs in a patient under general anesthesia include decreased oxygen saturation, decreased end-tidal carbon dioxide, and possibly ST segment changes on EKG. The most widely accepted postulation of its pathogenesis is the release of fat cells from bone that initiates an inflammatory and thrombotic response. Another theory is that the breakdown of bone marrow fat releases toxic fatty acids and glycerol, which can lead to end-organ damage. Treatment is supportive. Heparin and other forms of anticoagulation have been theorized to help, but there is no data to support this treatment. Mortality can be as high as 10%, but in most cases the symptoms completely resolve as the clot burden is decreased [31].

## Blood Loss

Blood loss can be significant during major orthopedic procedures [32]. Closely monitoring temperature is also important because hypothermia leads to coagulopathy, increased bleeding, and increased transfusions [33]. Prior to the case, calculating maximum allowable blood loss (MABL) may be helpful. This is done via the following equation: MABL = [Estimated Blood

Volume × (Initial hematocrit − Final hematocrit)]/Initial hematocrit [34].

## Enhanced Recovery Pathways

Enhanced recovery after surgery (ERAS) has become a popular topic in perioperative medicine. The goal is to reduce length of hospital stay, complications, and eventually cost. This requires a multidisciplinary approach to patient care before, during, and after surgery. ERAS is well established in colorectal surgery, but has only started to be applied to major orthopedic surgery. Preoperatively, patient education results in greater satisfaction and decreased length of stay. Pain control should be multimodal and opioid sparing. Oral analgesics before surgery, NSAIDs, and acetaminophen should all be used to reduce opioid requirements post-operatively. The ideal anesthetic technique appears to avoid general anesthesia as it leads to increased complications and post-operative pain. Oral intake before surgery can also be optimized. In fact, 300 mL of a clear drink with a carbohydrate load 2–3 h prior to surgery helps hasten recovery. Patients should still wait 2 h after clear liquids and 6 h after solid food before having anesthesia. Infection, blood loss, and coagulopathy can be improved with normothermia, goal directed fluid therapy, preoperative correction of anemia, and tranexamic acid. Post-operative thrombotic events are reduced with early mobilization and chemical and mechanical prophylaxis [35].

## References

1. Singh J, Lewallen D. Increasing obesity and comorbidity in patients undergoing primary total hip arthroplasty in the U.S.: a 13-year study of time trends. BMC Musculoskelet Disord. 2014;15:441. https://doi.org/10.1186/1471-2474-14-441.
2. Pivec R, Johnson A, Mears S, Mont M. Hip arthroplasty. Lancet. 2012;380:1768–77.
3. Horlocker T, Kopp S, Pagnano M, Hebl J. Analgesia for total hip and knee arthroplasty: a multimodal pathway featuring peripheral nerve block. J Am Acad Orthop Surg. 2006;14:126–35.
4. Vora M, Nicholas T, Kassel C, Grant S. Adductor canal block for knee surgical procedures: review article. J Clin Anesth. 2016;35:295–303.
5. Singelyn F, Deyaert M, Joris D, Pendeville E, Gouverneur J. Effects of intravenous patient-controlled analgesia with morphine, continuous epidural analgesia, and continuous three-in-one block on postoperative pain and knee rehabilitation after unilateral total knee arthroplasty. Anesth Analg. 1998;87:88–92.
6. Modig J, Borg T, Karlstrom G, Maripuu E, Sahlstedt B. Thromboembolism after total hip replacement. Anesth Analg. 1983;62:174–80.
7. Jaffe R, Schmiesing C, Golianu B. Anesthesiologist's manual of surgical procedures. 5th ed. Philadelphia: Lippincott Williams & Wilkins; 2014.
8. Bilimoria K, Liu Y, Paruch J, Zhou L, Kmiecik T, Ko C, Cohen M. Development and evaluation of the universal ACS NSQIP surgical risk calculator: a decision aid and informed consent tool for patients and surgeons. J Am Coll Surg. 2013;217:833–42.
9. Littleton S. Impact of obesity on respiratory function. Respirology. 2011;17:43–9.
10. Lisowska B, Rutkowska-Sak L, Maldyk P, Cwiek R. Anaesthesiological problems in patients with rheumatoid arthritis undergoing orthopaedic surgeries. Clin Rheumatol. 2008;27:553–6.
11. Cozowicz C, Poeran J, Zubizarreta N, Mazumdar M, Memtsoudis S. Trends in the use of regional anesthesia. Reg Anesth Pain Med. 2016;41:43–9.
12. Mauermann W, Shilling A, Zuo Z. A comparison of neuraxial block versus general anesthesia for elective total hip replacement: a meta-analysis. Anesth Analg. 2006;103:1018–25.
13. Johnson R, Kopp S, Burkle C, Duncan C, Jacob A, Erwin P, Murad M, Mantilla C. Neuraxial versus general anaesthesia for total hip and total knee arthroplasty. Surv Anesthesiol. 2016;60:200–2.
14. Basques B, Toy J, Bohl D, Golinvaux N, Graucr J. General compared with spinal anesthesia for total hip arthroplasty. J Bone Joint Surg Am. 2015;97:455–61.
15. Wilson S, Wolf B, Algendy A, Sealy C, Demos H, McSwain J. Comparison of lumbar epidurals and lumbar plexus nerve blocks for analgesia following primary total hip arthroplasty: a restrospective analysis. J Arthroplasty. 2017;32:635–40.
16. Jenstrup M, Jaeger P, Lund J, Fomsgaard J, Bache S, Mathiesen O, Larsen T, Dahl J. Effects of adductor-canal-blockade on pain and ambulation after total knee arthroplasty: a randomized study. Acta Anaesthesiol Scand. 2012;56:357–64.
17. Njathi C, Johnson R, Laughlin R, Schroeder D, Jacob A, Kopp S. Complications after continuous posterior lumbar plexus blockade for total hip arthroplasty. Reg Anesth Pain Med. 2017;42:446–50.
18. Abdallah F, Halpern S, Aoyama K, Brull R. Will the real benefits of a single-shot interscalene block please stand up? A systematic review and meta-analysis. Surv Anesthesiol. 2015;59:288–9.

19. Capdevila X, Coimbra C, Choquet O. Approaches to the lumbar plexus: success, risks, and outcome. Pain Med. 2005;30:150–62.
20. (ASRA Guidelines) Horlocker T, Wedel D, Rowlingson J et al. (2010) Regional anesthesia in the patient receiving antithrombotic or thrombolytic therapy. Reg Anesth Pain Med 35:64–101.
21. Eymin G, Jaffer A. Thromboprophylaxis in major knee and hip replacement surgery: a review. J Thromb Thrombolysis. 2012;34:518–25.
22. Kotha R, Orebaugh S. Shoulder surgery in the beach chair position. Adv Anesth. 2014;32:37–57.
23. Palmer S, Graham G. Tourniquet-induced rhabdomyolysis after total knee replacement. Ann R Coll Surg Engl. 1994;76:416–7.
24. Allee J, Muzaffar A, Tobias J. Dexmedetomidine controls the hemodynamic manifestations of tourniquet pain. Am J Ther. 2011;18:35–9.
25. Valli H, Guerrerosantos J. Arterial hypertension associated with the use of a tourniquet with either general or regional anesthesia. Plast Reconstr Surg. 1988;82:1112.
26. Satsumae T, Yamaguchi H, Inomata S, Tanaka M. Magnesium sulfate attenuates tourniquet pain in healthy volunteers. J Anesth. 2012;27:231–5.
27. Parmet J, Horrow J, Berman A, Harding S. Thromboembolism coincident with tourniquet deflation during total knee arthroplasty. Lancet. 1993;341:1057–8.
28. Byrick R. Cement implantation syndrome: a time limited embolic phenomenon. Can J Anaesth. 1997;44:107–11.
29. Donaldson AJ, Thomson HE, Harper NJ, Kenny NW. Bone cement implantation syndrome. Br J Anaesth. 2009;102(1):12–22.
30. Linehan C, Gioe T. Serum and breast milk levels of methylmethacrylate following surgeon exposure during arthroplasty. J Bone Joint Surg Am. 2006;88:1957–61.
31. Kosova E, Bergmark B, Piazza G. Fat embolism syndrome. Circulation. 2015;131:317–20.
32. Sculco T. Global blood management in orthopaedic surgery. Clin Orthop Relat Res. 1998;357:43–9.
33. Schmied H, Reiter A, Kurz A, Sessler D, Kozek S. Mild hypothermia increases blood loss and transfusion requirements during total hip arthroplasty. Lancet. 1996;347:289–92.
34. Gross J. Estimating allowable blood loss. Anesthesiology. 1983;58:277–80.
35. Soffin E, YaDeau J. Enhanced recovery after surgery for primary hip and knee arthroplasty: a review of the evidence. Br J Anaesth. 2016;117:iii62–72.

# Index

**A**

Abdominal aortic aneurysms (AAA)
   diameter, 615, 616
   emergent *vs.* elective repair, 616
   incidence, 615
   intraoperative management
      general anesthesia, 609
      induction and maintenance, 610
      MAC, 609
      monitoring, 610
      preparation, 610
   mortality, 607
   open (*see* Open abdominal aortic aneurysms)
   postoperative care, 610, 611
   preoperative evaluation
      cardiac, 608, 609
      COPD, 609
      renal function, 609
   risk factor, 615
Abdominal compartment syndrome (ACS), 396, 399, 401
Abdominal wall defect, 395, 400
Acetaminophen, 93, 124, 128, 137, 309, 336, 338, 341, 347, 349, 352, 355, 357, 400, 407, 426, 439, 448–449, 769, 839, 857
Achalasia, 275, 276, 278, 280, 281
Acquired asphyxiating chondrodystrophy, 436
Acute anemia, 203
Acute coronary syndrome (ACS), 608, 617
Acute kidney injury (AKI), 94, 640
Acute lung injury (ALI), 103, 758
Acute respiratory distress syndrome (ARDS), 36, 758
Adaptive autoregulatory displacement, 573
Adjustable Gastric Band (AGB), 833–834
Adolescent idiopathic scoliosis (AIS), 329, 331, 333
Adrenocorticotropic hormone (ACTH), 805
Adult respiratory distress syndrome (ARDS), 737, 856
Advanced Trauma Life Support (ATLS), 667, 669, 670, 672
Age-related arterial endothelial dysfunction, 796
Aging, 795–799
   cardiovascular
      age related valvular changes, 799
      anti-coagulants, 800
      anti-platelet agents, 800
      beta blockers, 800
      calcium channel blockers, 800
      calcium sensitizing drugs, 800
      diastolic dysfunction, 797
      fluid therapy, 798–799
      general anesthesia, 798
      induction agents, 800
      meticulous evaluation, 798
      pathophysiological changes, 795–797
      rhythm abnormalities, 799
      rhythm disturbances, 798
      stiffness, 796
      vascular system, 796
      vasopressor therapy, 799
   central nervous system
      cognitive abilities, 809–810
      cognitive assessment, 808–809
      cognitive function, 806
      frailty, 808
      functional status, 808
      hydration, 807
      mood/depression, 810
      neuronal function, 806
      nutritional status, 807
      sarcopenia, 808
      vertibro-basilar insufficiency, 806
   endocrine system
      ACTH stimulation, 805
      age-related changes, 805
      diabetes mellitus, 805–806
      growth hormone stimulation, 805
      insulin resistance, 805
   gastrointestinal tract, 804
   liver, 804
   respiratory system, 802
      age related changes, 800
      airway management, 801
      asthma, 802
      bronchodilators, 801
      COPD (*see* Chronic obstructive pulmonary disease (COPD))
      lung function, 801
      obstructive sleep apnea, 802
      pneumonia, 802
      postoperative pulmonary complications, 803
      pre-anesthetic evaluation, 801

Aging (cont.)
　　pulmonary function testing, 801
　　6 minute walk test, 801
　　snoring, 801
　　upper airway, 800
Air embolism, 36, 146, 278
Air trapping, 211, 802, 803
Airway compromise, 62, 98, 109, 110, 150, 182, 202, 208, 218, 249, 557, 560, 594, 652, 693
Airway management, 834–835
Airway Management on Placental Support (AMPS), 473
Airway management, trachea, 115
Airway obstruction, 278, 768
Alert, Verbal, Painful, Unresponsive (AVPU), 669
Alfentanil, 206, 236, 277, 549, 663, 694
Alpha blockade, 682, 684–686
Amantadine, 590
American Society for gastrointestinal endoscopy (ASGE) guidelines, 180
American Society of Regional Anesthesia and Pain Management (ASRA), 732
Ammonia toxicity, 847
Ampulla of Vater, 176
Anemia, 16, 79, 126, 206, 273, 275, 369, 373, 423, 510, 659, 702, 710, 732, 748, 767
Anesthesia considerations in patients, 240
Anesthesia related maternal mortality, 494
Aneurysm repairs, 78
Angiotensin converting enzyme inhibitors (ACEI), 316, 627, 628, 804
Angiotensin receptor blockers (ARBs), 627, 628, 658, 804
Ano-rectal malformations, 413
Antepartum hemorrhage (APH)
　　incidence, 517
　　placenta abruption, 518
　　placenta previa, 517, 518
　　uterine rupture, 518–519
Anterior mediastinoscopy, 108, 109
Anterograde cerebral perfusion (ACP), 80
Anticholinergics, 236, 590
Anticoagulants
　　atrial fibrillation, 815
　　comorbidities, 816
　　indications, 815
　　inherent bleeding risk, 816
　　kidney function, 816
　　newer anticoagulation agents, 816
　　pharmacology, 816
　　valvular heart disease, 815
Anticoagulation medications, 279, 280, 316, 549
Antidiuretic hormone (ADH), 760
Antifibrinolytic therapy, 301, 673, 736
Anxiolysis, 205, 223, 224, 248, 257, 318, 553, 585, 653, 663, 769, 837
Aortic aneurysms, 75, 76, 80, 611, 615, 616, 618, 667
Aortic arch aneurysms, 75, 611
Aortic dissection, 75, 540, 541
Aortic regurgitation, 17, 18
Aortic rupture, 75, 82, 143, 145

Aortic stenosis, 17, 24
　hemodynamic management
　　afterload, 327
　　contractility, 326
　　heart rate, 325–326
　　preload, 326
　　sinus rhythm, 327
　neonatal critical aortic stenosis, 324–325
　pathophysiology, 324
　subvalvular aortic stenosis, 323
　supravalvular aortic stenosis, 323
　treatment, 324
　valvular aortic stenosis, 324
Aortic surgery
　anesthetic and surgical management
　　ACP/RCP, 80
　　arch, 78
　　arterial line placement, 78
　　ascending, 78
　　comorbid conditions, 78
　　CSF drainage, 79
　　descending, 78, 80
　　dissection point, 78
　　EEG/BIS/cerebral oximetry, 79
　　hypothermia, 78
　　LA-FA bypass, 81
　　large bore and central intravenous access, 79
　　MEP, 80
　　monitors/regional epidural cooling, 79, 80
　　multiple central venous catheters, 79
　　near infrared spectrophotometry, 79
　　pulmonary artery catheters, 79
　　shunts/cardiopulmonary bypass, 80
　　SSEP, 80
　　TEE probe, 78
　　temperature management, 79
　CPB separation/post CPB, 82
　DeBakey System, 75
　diagnostic laboratory tests, 75, 76
　double lumen endotracheal tube, 82
　etomidate, 81
　general anesthesia, 81
　imaging studies, 76
　incidence, 75
　intraoperative phase
　　barbiturates, 82
　　corticosteroid, 82
　　naloxone infusion, 82
　modified RSI, 81
　opioids, 81
　preoperative assessment
　　cardiac index values, 77
　　clevidipine, 77
　　esmolol, 77
　　fenoldapam, 77
　　heart rate control, 77
　　IV dihydropyridine calcium channel blocker, 77
　　labetalol, 77
　　lowering ejection velocity, 77
　　nicardipine, 77

nitroglycerin, 77
nitroprusside, 77
vasodilating medications, 77
propofol, 81, 82
remifentanil infusions, 82
signs/symptoms, 75, 76
single lumen endotracheal tubes, 82
Stanford system, 76
TEVAR, 83
Aortic transection/dissection, 145
Apnea-Hypopnea Index (AHI), 720
Apomorphine, 590
Appendicitis, 413, 418
Aprepitant, 128, 269
Arnold Chiari malformations, 298
Arnold–Chiari II malformation, 334
Arrhythmias, 27, 36, 227
Arterial blood gas (ABG), 617
Arterial lines, 16, 338, 746, 761, 783
Arteriovenous (AV) fistula surgery
   goal, 657
   intraoperative management
      general anesthesia, 661–662
      medication management, 663
      regional anesthesia/local infiltration, 662, 663
   postoperative management, medication management, 663, 664
   preoperative assessment
      cardiovascular disease, 658, 659
      diabetes mellitus, 660
      gastrointestinal function, 660, 661
      hematology, 659
      pulmonary evaluation, 659
      renal function, 659, 660
   procedure, 658
Arteriovenous malformations (AVM)
   ICH, 573–574
   intraoperative management
      anesthetic technique, 575, 576
      brain protection, 576, 577
      emergence from anesthesia, 578, 579
      fluid management, 577
      hemodynamic control, 578
      hypothermia, 578
      monitoring and vascular access, 575
   pathophysiology, 573
   postoperative period, 579
   preoperative management, 575
   risk assessment, 574
   treatment, 574
Artery of Adamkiewicz, 83, 612, 618
Artificial pneumothorax, 438
Ascending aneurysm, 75, 611
Asleep-Awake-Asleep (SAS) technique, 585
AspireAssist, 834
Atracurium, 839
Atrial contraction, 799
Atrial fibrillation, 94
Atrial fibrillation (AF), 799, 815
Atrial kick, 797
Atrial septal defects, 22
Automated Implantable Cardioverter-defibrillators (AICD), 232, 594
Awake craniotomy (AC)
   anesthetic technique, 583
   complications
      airway complications, 586
      cerebral oedema, 586
      nausea and vomiting, 586
      pain, 586
      seizure, 586
   definition, 581
   dexmedetomidine, 585
   emergency drugs and equipments, 583
   final phase, 581
   initial phase, 581
   MAC
      advantages, 585
      definition, 585
      disadvantages, 585
      SAS, 585
   monitoring, 583
   patient selection, 582
   preoperative evaluation
      anesthetic assessment, 582
      patient selection, 582
   propofol, 585
   remifentanil, 585
   scalp block, 583
      auriculotemporal nerve, 584
      drugs, 583
      greater auricular nerve, 585
      greater occipital nerve, 585
      lesser occipital nerve, 584, 585
      supraorbital nerve, 583
      supratrochlear nerve, 584
      zygomaticotemporal nerve, 584
   second phase, 581
   theatre layout, 583
Awake extubation, 426
Axillary block, 663

**B**

Balloon-expandable valves, 59
Bare metal stent (BMS), 608
BCIS, *see* Bone cement implantation syndrome (BCIS)
Beckwith-Wiedemann syndrome, 399
Belsey technique, 122
Benign prostatic hypertrophy (BPH), 743
Benzocaine, 185, 277
Benzodiazepines, 189, 192, 217, 233, 236, 267, 813
Berlin questionnaire, 721
Beta-blockers, 235, 537, 541, 683
Bicaval anastomosis, 699
Bicaval technique, 699
Bicuspid aortic valve (BAV), 24
Bilateral sequential single lung transplantation (BSSLT), 35

Bilateral thoracoscopy with carbon dioxide insufflation, 439
Biliopancreatic diversion with duodenal switch (BPD/DS), 832–833
Biotransformation, 811–812
Bipolar electrocautery, 70, 781
Bipolar transurethral resection of prostate (B-TURP) technique, 845
Bispectral index (BIS), 116, 192
Biventricular pacemaker, 67, 155
Bladder perforation, 847
Blood products, 33
Blunt chest trauma, 143
Blunt force trauma, 141, 145
Body mass index (BMI), definition of, 827
Bone cement, 736, 851, 856
Bone cement implantation syndrome (BCIS), 736
Brachytherapy, 260
Bradyarrhythmias, 787
Brain edema, 575, 577
Brain Trauma Foundation, 599–601
Brain tumors, 298–299, 547, 549, 560
Brain tumor surgery
   cerebral perfusion pressure, 551
   diuretics, 551
   emergence from anesthesia
      delayed awakening, 551–552
      hypothermia, 553
      medications and anesthetic agents, 552
      postoperative stress, 552
      side effects, 552
   inhalational and intravenous anesthetics, 550, 551
   monitoring, 551
   patient position, 550
   VAE, 550
Breech delivery, 501, 503
Broncheoalveolar lavage (BAL), 200, 201
Bronchopleural fistula (BPF), 131, 134, 135
Bronchopulmonary dysplasia (BPD), 466
Bronchoscopic procedure
   airway devices
      ETT, 208
      LMA, 207, 208
      rigid bronchoscope, 208
   airway exam, 200
   CBC, 203
   coagulopathy, 203
   conscious sedation, 205
   diagnostic procedure
      BAL, 200, 201
      EBUS-FNA, 201
      EMN, 201
      pleuroscopy, 201, 202
      TBNA, 201
   electrolyte, 203
   general anesthesia
      depth of anesthesia monitoring, 207
      factors, 206
      $FiO_2$, 207
      muscle relaxants, 206
      TIVA, 206
   historical perspective, 199, 200
   interventional bronchoscopy suite, 211, 212
   interventional pulmonary procedures, complication with
      airway obstruction, 211
      airway reactivity, 210
      bleeding, 210
      hypercapnia, 211
      hypercarbia, 211
      hypoxemia, 211
   MAC, 206
   modes of ventilation
      assisted ventilation, 209
      handheld Jet ventilation, 209
      high frequency mechanical jet ventilation, 210
      NIV, 209
      positive pressure ventilation, 209
      spontaneous ventilation, 208, 209
   post-procedure care, 211
   pre-procedural evaluation
      airway assessment, 202
      cardiovascular system assessment, 203
      dental assessment, 202
      respiratory system assessment, 202
   renal and liver function, 203
   therapeutic interventional pulmonary procedures, 202
   topical anesthesia
      ester and amide local anesthetics, 204
      mouth and oropharynx, 204
      nasal mucosa and nasopharynx, 204
      RLN, 205
      side effects of local anesthetics, 204
      SLN, 205
   type and screen, 203
Burns
   acetaminophen, 769
   anxiolysis, 769
   continuous IV infusions, 769
   dexmedetomidine, 769
   gabapentin, 769
   ketamine, 769
   local anesthetics, 769
   management
      airway, 770
      fluid, 770, 771
      monitoring, 771–772
      nutrition, 772
      pharmacologic, 771
      vascular access, 771
   non opioid analgesia, 769
   NSAID, 769
   opioids, 769
   pain control, 769
   patient-controlled analgesia, 769
   physiology
      direct thermal injury, 768
      ebb phase, 766

full thickness, 765
hypermetabolic (flow) phase, 766, 767
infections, 769
inhalation injury, 768
partial thickness, 765
shock, 766–767
superficial, 765
pregabalin, 769
reconstruction, 772
regional anesthesia, 769, 770
Butorphanol, 179

## C
Carbamazepine, 334
Carbidopa, 590
Cardiac arrhythmias, 162, 439
Cardiac contusion, 143, 145
Cardiac evaluation, 335, 437, 619, 767
Cardiac implantable electronic devices (CIEDs), 745
Cardiac output (CO), 373
Cardiac resynchronization therapy (CRT), 67
Cardiac rupture, 143
Cardiac tamponade, 142, 143, 145
Cardiac transplantation, 155, 156, 158, 159
Cardiopulmonary bypass (CPB), 6, 637, 639–641
fluid restriction, 7
initiation of, 7, 8
separation from, 9
Cardiopulmonary complications, 195
Cardiopulmonary dysfunction, 435
Cardiovascular aging
age related valvular changes, 799
anti-coagulants, 800
anti-platelet agents, 800
beta blockers, 800
calcium channel blockers, 800
calcium sensitizing drugs, 800
diastolic dysfunction, 797
fluid therapy, 798–799
general anesthesia, 798
induction agents, 800
meticulous evaluation, 798
pathophysiological changes, 795–797
rhythm abnormalities, 799
rhythm disturbances, 798
stiffness, 796
systemic blood pressure, 796–797
vascular system, 796
vasopressor therapy, 799
Cardiovascular disease, 191
Cardiovascular implantable electronic devices (CIEDs), 246
AAI, 69
cardiac interventions, 73
check patient device card, 73
chest x-ray, 73
DDD mode, 68–69
defibrillators, 68

device manufacturer, 73
DOO pacing, 69
examining medical records, 73
intraoperative considerations
bipolar electrocautery, 70
cardioversion/defibrillation, 72
continuous EKG/rhythm strip, 70
EMI, 70–72
harmonic scalpel, 70
monopolar electrocautery, 70–72
peripheral pulse monitoring, 70
reprogramming, 72
loop recorders, 68
NASPE/BPEG code, 68
pacemakers, 67
pacer spikes, 73
postoperative management, 72
preoperative considerations, 69–70
VVI, 69
Cardiovascular system, 203, 757–758
Cardioversion
anticipated adverse events, 217, 218
electrical cardioversion
direct current cardioversion, 215
indications for, 215
patient assessment, 216
monophasic and biphasic waveforms, 216
off site anesthetics, 217
preoperative management, 216
TEE, 217
volatile anesthetics, 217
Carotid endarterectomy (CEA), 645, 651
anesthetic plan, 646
awake patient, 648
carotid arteries (*see* Carotid stenosis)
cerebral ischemia monitoring, 647, 648
cervical epidural anesthesia, 652
deep cervical plexus block, 651, 652
electroencephalography, 648
general anesthesia techniques, 650
general *vs.* regional anesthesia, 649, 650
hemodynamic management, 650, 651
NIRS, 649
postoperative conditions, 652
preoperative evaluation, 647
regional anesthesia, local infiltration, 651
SSEPs, 648–649
superficial cervical plexus block, 651
TCD, 649
Carotid Revascularization Endarterectomy versus Stenting Trial (CREST), 645, 649, 652
Carotid stenosis (CAS), carotid arteries
anatomy, 645, 646
atherosclerosis, 646, 647
imaging, 647
physiology, 646
Catecholamines, 679–686
Catecholamine storm, 757, 770

Centers for Disease Control and
    Prevention (CDC), 221
Central nervous system
    cognitive abilities, 809–810
    cognitive assessment, 808–809
    cognitive function, 806
    frailty, 808
    functional status, 808
    hydration, 807
    mood/depression, 810
    neuronal function, 806
    nutritional status, 807
    sarcopenia, 808
    vertibro-basilar insufficiency, 806
Central venous catheters (CVC), 631
Central venous pressure (CVP), 575, 761
Cerclage
    anesthesia management, 505–506
    definition, 503
    surgical considerations, 504, 505
Cerebral and extremity ischemia, 110
Cerebral aneurysms surgery, 568
    epidemiology, 563
    investigation and management, 563
    preoperative assessment
        cardiovascular function, 568
        investigation, 568
        neurological examination, 568
        optimisation, 568
        renal function, 568
        respiratory, 568
    presentation, 563
    prognosis, 563
Cerebral autoregulation, 551
Cerebral blood flow (CBF), 294, 547, 549–551
Cerebral dys-autoregulation, 573
Cerebral hyperemia, 573
Cerebral metabolic rate, 547, 549–551
Cerebral metabolic rate for oxygen ($CMRO_2$), 293
Cerebral oedema, 560, 586, 600, 602
Cerebral oximetry, 17, 375
Cerebral palsy (CP)
    airway management, 432
    anesthesia considerations in children, 430
    antenatal associations, 430
    anticonvulsants, 431, 432
    anti-epileptic medications, 431
    cerebral motor cortex, 429
    clinical manifestations, 429, 431
    CNS syndromes and lesions, 431
    description, 429
    diagnosis, 431
    epidural catheters, 432
    epidural/spinal needle placement, 432
    fetal/immature brain, 429
    heat loss, general anesthesia, 433
    heat redistribution, 433
    history and physical examination, 431
    induction of anesthesia, 432
    intraoperative and postoperative pain management, 433
    intraoperative hyperthermia, 433
    medical and surgical history, 431
    mild motor impairment, 431
    motor defect, 431
    motor related issues, 429
    nerve compression, 433
    neuraxial anesthetics, 432
    neurocognitive dysfunction, 433
    neuroimaging tests, 431
    operative procedures, 432
    orthopedic and neurosurgical interventions, 431
    perinatal injury, 430
    perioperative concerns, 429
    peripheral nerve catheters, 432
    positioning, 433
    post-operative complications, 433
    preoperative anxiety, 432
    preoperative considerations, 431
    surgical interventions, 429
    treatment, 431
    vecuronium resistance, 432
Cerebral perfusion pressure (CPP), 295, 547–549, 551
Cerebro vascular accident (CVA), 550
Cervical dilation, 529, 530
Cervical insufficiency, 503, 504, 507
Cervical mediastinoscopy, 108, 109
Cervical ripening, 529
Cervical teratoma, 473
Cesarean delivery
    anesthesia considerations, 488
    arrest of labor, 487
    epidural local anesthetics, 490
    general anesthesia, 490–492, 494
    history and physical examination, 488
    intrathecal local anesthetics, 489
    non-reassuring fetal heart tones, 487
    NPO guidelines, 489
    primary, 487
    subjective indications, 487
Chamberlain's procedure, 108
Chemoreceptor Trigger Zone, 586
Chest wall infusion, 309
Chest wall/pleural cavity surgery
    anesthetic options, 133
    blood pressure and temperature, 133
    cancer incidence, 131
    cardiac testing, 132
    electrocardiogram, 133
    end-tidal capnography, 133
    history and physical examination, 132
    intraoperative complications, 134, 135
    intravenous anesthesia agents, 133
    invasive hemodynamic monitors, 133
    local infiltration of local anesthetics, 137
    lung isolation, 134
    opiate medications, 137
    positioning, 134
    post-operative complications, 138
    postoperative pain control, 135, 136
    preoperative studies, 132

Index 865

pre-surgical baseline with oxygenation
or ventilation, 132
pulmonary and cardiac complications, 133
pulse oximetry, 133
restrictive lung defects, 132
routine monitoring, 133
tumor invasion, 131
Chiari malformations, infants with, 334, 335
Child life specialist, 454
Chloral hydrate, 224, 225, 249
Chronic obstructive pulmonary disease (COPD), 617
cigarette smoking, 802
definition, 802
diagnosis, 802
endotracheal intubation, 802
extra-pulmonary systemic effects, 802
general anesthesia, 802
intermittent positive pressure ventilation, 802
pathophysiology, 802
pharmacological management, 802
Chronic rhinosinusitis, 351
Chronic thromboembolic pulmonary hypertension (CTEPH), 41
Circle of Willis, 646, 648
Cirrhosis, 689–693, 700–703, 705
Cirrhotic cardiomyopathy, 691, 701
Cisatracurium, weight reduction surgery, 839
Citrate Phosphate Dextrose Adenine (CPDA), 44
Claggett's procedures, 131, 133
Clevidipine, 77, 236, 541
Clinical Randomization of an Antifibrinolytic in Significant Hemorrhage-2 (CRASH2) Trial, 673
Coagulation status, 762
Coagulation studies, 33
Coagulopathy, 520, 521, 848
Coarctation of aorta, 24, 25
Cocaine, 199, 233, 351, 564
Cognitive abilities, 809–810
Cognitive assessment, 808–809
Cognitive behavioral therapy (CBT), 454
Cognitive function, 193, 223, 224, 806, 808, 809
Collis-Belsey technique, 122
Colloid oncotic pressure (COP), 577
Colloids, 7, 297, 370, 378, 416, 492, 551, 577, 672, 694, 758
Colonoscopy
anesthesia involvement, 189
depth of sedation, 189, 190
intraoperative concerns
abdominal pain/discomfort, 195
benzodiazepine, 192
depth of sedation, 192
dexmedetomidine, 193
difficult colonoscopy, 194
gas explosion, 195
hemorrhage, 195
ketamine, 193
monitoring, 192
nitrous oxide, 194
opiates, 192

perforation, 195
prophylactic antibiotics, 191
propofol, 192, 193, 195
remifentanil, 193
splenic injury, 195
preoperative assessment
aspiration, 190
bowel preparation, 190
cardiovascular disease, 191
mask ventilation concerns, 191
sedation expectations, 191
Color flow Doppler (CFD), 45
Combined spinal-epidural anesthesia, 492
Complex lesions, Ebstein's malformation, 25
Comprehensive geriatric assessment (CGA), 819
Computed tomography (CT)
anesthesia considerations in patients, 240
anesthesia equipment, 252
anesthesia techniques, 252, 253
contrast enhancement, 251, 252
indications for, 252
physics and radiation, 251
safety, 251
Congenital aganglionic megacolon, 415
Congenital aortic stenosis, 24, 325
Congenital diaphragmatic hernia (CDH), 473, 481
anesthetic management
intraoperative assessment, 390, 391
perioperative assessment, 392
postoperative assessment, 391
pre-operative assessment, 389, 390
definition, 387
diagnosis and testing
comorbidities, 388
postnatal, 389
prenatal, 388, 389
embryology, 387, 388
genetics, 388
Congenital heart disease (CHD), 21, 23, 25
complex lesions (see Complex lesions)
non-cardiac surgery
arrhythmias, 27
cyanosis, 28
incidence, 27
intraoperative management, 27
postoperative management, 28
preoperative assessment, 27
pulmonary hypertension, 27–28
prevalence (see Right-to-left shunting)
shunt lesions (see Shunt lesions)
single ventricle physiology, 26
stenotic lesions (see Stenotic lesions)
TOF, 25, 26
Connective tissue disorders, 435
Conscious sedation, 189, 205, 223
Continuous positive airway pressure (CPAP), 92, 93, 268, 355
Continuous renal replacement therapy (CRRT), 702
Continuous spinal anesthetics, 492
Contrast-induced nephropathy (CIN), 609, 611
Corneal or conjunctival edema, 782

Coronary artery bypass grafting (CABG)
   anesthetic management, 10
   cardiopulmonary bypass, 6
   CPB
      initiation of, 7, 8
      separation from, 9
   induction and maintenance of anesthesia, 6
   intraoperative management, 7
   management, principles of, 4
   monitoring, 4, 5
   on-pump anesthetic management, 8, 9
   operative revascularization, ideal candidates for, 4
   oxygen supply and demand, 5, 6
   postoperative management and complications, 10
   OPCAB (*see* Off-pump coronary artery bypass grafting (OPCAB))
   preoperative anesthetic management, 6
   preoperative risk reduction, 3, 4
   surgical principles, 7
Coronary artery disease (CAD), 3, 60, 608
Coronary artery perfusion, 327
Cortical mapping, 581
Craniofacial surgery
   anesthetic concerns
      airway evaluation, 345
      cardiac and pulmonary evaluation, 345
      communication, 345
      hemorrhage, 347
      induction, 346
      intraoperative management, 345
      monitoring, 346
      nausea and vomiting, 347
      neurologic evaluation, 345
      neuromonitoring, 346
      pain management, 347
      positioning, 346
      postoperative, 347
      temperature regulation, 346
   cranial vault deformities, 344, 345
   sagittal synostosis, 344
   Spring assisted cranioplasty, 344
   timing of surgery, 343
Craniosynostosis, 300
   associated features and anesthetic concerns, 342, 344
   cranium, suture lines of, 342, 343
   types of, 342, 343
Crawford classification system, 607, 608
Critical limb ischemia (CLI), 625
Cushing's reflex, 548
Cyanosis, 28, 185, 312–314, 389, 466, 789
Cyanotic heart disease, 311–313
   nitrous oxide, 319
   postoperative recovery location, 320
   respiratory infections, 316
   surgical positioning of patients, 320
   Tetralogy of Fallot, 313
   total anomalous pulmonary venous return, 314
   transposition of great arteries, 314
   tricuspid valve abnormality, 314
   truncus arteriosus, 314

Cystectomy, 749
Cystenterostomy, 274, 280, 281
Cystgastrostomy, 274–278
Cystic fibrosis (CF), 414, 415

**D**
Da Vinci® Surgical System, 778
DeBakey System, 75
Decortication surgeries, 131, 135
Deep brain stimulation (DBS)
   awake technique, 593
   components, 591
   general anesthesia, 593, 594
   intra-operative complications, 594
   mechanism of action, 591
   non-DBS related surgery, 594, 595 (*see also* Parkinson's disease (PD))
   post-operative complications, 594
   pre-operative evaluation, 592–593
   STN, 590
   surgical technique, 591, 592
Deep cervical plexus block, 651, 652
Deep hypothermic circulatory arrest (DHCA), 43–47
Deep sedation, 223, 279
Deep venous thrombosis (DVT), 846
   general anesthesia, 855
   long-term complications, 855
   neuraxial technique, 854, 855
   pharmacologic, 855
   regional anesthesia, 854, 855
   risk factors, 854
Defibrillators, 33, 68, 168, 191, 218, 245, 566
Demerol, 225
Dental injury, 279, 281
Dental procedures
   anesthesia considerations, 227
   anesthesia, pharmacology of, 224, 225
   arrhythmias, 227
   dental anatomy, 221, 222
   dental identification
      Palmer Notation system, 222, 223
      Universal Numbering system, 222
   dental procedures, 223
   general anesthesia, 225, 226
   incubation techniques, 226
   local anesthetic selection, 225
   SBE, 226, 227
   sedation and analgesia, level of, 224
      deep sedation, 223
      general anesthesia, 224
      minimal sedation, 223
      moderate sedation, 223
      monitoring and emergency equipment, 224
Depression
   incidence, 810
   prevalence, 810
Desflurane, 289, 365, 839
Destination therapy (DT), 159
Device thrombosis, 165–167

Dexmedetomidine, 193, 206, 237, 249, 259, 277, 333, 356, 585, 769, 837
Diabetes insipidus (DI), 299, 761
Diabetes mellitus, 805–806
Dialysis outcomes and practice patterns study (DOPPS), 657
Diastolic dysfunction, 324, 658, 662, 701, 709, 797, 798
Difficult colonoscopy, 194
Dilated cardiomyopathy, 423
Dilation and curettage (D&C), 528–530
    anesthetic management, 508, 509
    definition, 507
    surgical considerations, 508
Dilation and evacuation (D&E), *see* Dilation and curettage (D&C)
Dilation and extraction (D&X), 530
Diltiazem, 236, 541, 552
Disseminated intravascular coagulation (DIC), 848
Dobutamine, 9, 17, 18, 34, 461, 787
Donation after brain-death (DBD), 756
Donation after cardiac death (DCD), 707, 756–757
Dopamine-b-hydroxylase (DBH), 681
Double lumen endotracheal tube (DLETT), 82, 89, 90, 100–102
Down's syndrome, 414
Drug-eluting stent (DES), 608
Drug induced sleep endoscopy (DISE), 356
Dual anti-platelet therapy (DAPT), 608, 628, 629
Dual chamber pacemakers, 67, 69
Duct of Wirsung, *see* Pancreatic duct
Duodenal atresia, 413, 414
Dystrophic epidermolysis bullosa (DEB), 422, 423

**E**
Ear surgery
    cochlear implantation
        anesthetic considerations, 350, 351
        ECAP, 350
        ESRT, 350
        internal electrodes, 350
        PET, 349
Ebb phase, 766
Ebstein's anomaly, 313–315
Ebstein's malformation, 21, 25
Echothiophate, 365
ECT, *see* Electroconvulsive therapy (ECT)
Ehlers-Danlos syndrome, 435, 436
Eisenmenger's reaction, 22, 23, 27
Elderly, 810–816, 818–821
    anticoagulants
        atrial fibrillation, 815
        comorbidities, 816
        indications, 815
        inherent bleeding risk, 816
        kidney function, 816
        newer anticoagulation agents, 816
        pharmacology, 816
        valvular heart disease, 815
    central neuraxial blockade, 822
    general anesthesia, 822
    pharmacokinetics and pharmacodynamics
        biotransformation, 811–812
        body compartments, 810–811
        dose adjustments, 812
        drug distribution, 810–811
        inhaled anaesthetics, 812, 813
        intravenous anaesthetics, 813–814
        local anaesthetics, 814, 815
        neuromuscular blocking drugs, 814
        protein binding, 811
    preoperative assessment
        ASA physical status classification, 819
        comprehensive geriatric assessment, 819
        effective pre-anaesthetic evaluation, 821
        history and nutritional assessment, 820
        informed consent, 820
        METs, 818–819
        physical examination, 821
        POSSUM, 819
        vs. older adults, 820
    pre-operative investigations, 821
    regional anesthesia, 821, 822
    renal system, 804–805
    *See also* Aging
Electroconvulsive therapy (ECT)
    anticoagulated patients, 233
    applications, 229
    BP cuff technique, 234
    children and adolescents, 233
    complications/adverse events, 236, 237
    drug-drug interactions, 234
    mechanism of action, 229–231
    methohexital, 234
    pathophysiological responses
        cardiovascular effects, 231, 232
        cerebral effects, 232
        hyperglycemia, 232
    patient considerations, 232
    patients with cerebral aneurysms and intracranial masses, 234
    patients with pacemakers/AICD, 232
    perioperative anesthesia considerations and plans, 230–231
    pharmacologic considerations
        analgesics, 236
        benzodiazepines, 236
        hemodynamic modulation, 235, 236
        induction agents, 234, 235
        neuromuscular blocking agents, 235
    pregnant patient, 233
    stimulus electrodes, 234
Electrocorticography (ECoG), 297
Electrolyte homeostasis, 804
Electrolytes, 762
Electromagnetic interference (EMI), 69–72, 745
Electromagnetic navigation guided lung biopsy (EMN), 201
Elicited Compound Action Potential (ECAP), 350
Elicited Stapedius Reflex Threshold (ESRT), 350

Eloesser flaps, 131, 133
Embolic stroke, 80, 218
Emergency undocking, 783, 784, 788–790
Emphysema, 89, 94, 132, 134, 135, 280, 281, 469, 668, 710, 789, 802
Empyema, 131–133, 135
End-diastolic pulmonary artery pressure, 458
End-diastolic pulmonary artery pressure, 458
Endoaortic occlusion balloon (EOAB), 53
Endobronchial ultrasound guided fine needle aspiration (EBUS-FNA), 200
Endobronchial ultrasound/transbronchial lymph node biopsy (EBUS-FNA), 201
Endocardial cushion defects, 23
Endocrine system
    ACTH stimulation, 805
    age-related changes, 805
    corticosteroid, 760
    diabetes mellitus, 805–806
    growth hormone stimulation, 805
    HPA dysfunction, 759
    insulin, 760
    insulin resistance, 805
    thyroid hormone, 761
    vasopressin, 760
Endocrinology evaluation, 295
Endoleak, 611
Endoscopic airway techniques, 352–354
Endoscopic cystenterostomy, 280, 281
Endoscopic necrosectomy, 274, 280
Endoscopic retrograde cholangiopancreatography (ERCP), 176–182
    airway emergencies, 184
    anesthetic considerations
        anesthesia providers, 182
        prone/semi prone positioning, 182
        safety issues, 181
    benefits of, 175
    Benzocaine, 185
    biochemical investigations, 180, 181
    deep sedation, 184
    ETT, 183, 185, 186
    glucagon, 185
    hepato-pancreato biliary tract
        neurovascular supply, 178, 179
        pancreaticobiliary drainage system, 176–178
    limitation of, 175
    methemoglobinemia, 185
    postoprative and post-discharge considerations, 186
    preoperative evaluation, risk estimation strategies, 179, 180
    procedure/operating room preparation, 182, 183
    propofol, 184, 185
Endoscopic ultrasound (EUS), 273
    general anesthesia, 280
    patient safety, 279
    patients positioning, 277
    sedation level, 276
Endotracheal intubation, 183, 185, 186
Endotracheal tube (ETT), 208, 383–385
Endourology procedures, 742, 743

Endovascular aneurysm repair (EVAR), 607, 611
    AAA (*see* Abdominal aortic aneurysms (AAA))
    TEVAR (*see* Thoracic endovascular aortic repair (TEVAR))
Endovascular aortic aneurysm repair (EVAR), 616
    advantages, 607
    complications, 611
    mortality, 607
    surgical considerations, 607
End-stage liver disease (ESLD), 691, 693, 697, 700, 702–704
End-stage renal disease (ESRD), 658–661
    AV fistula
        diabetes mellitus, 660, 661
        electrolyte abnormalities, 660
        general anesthesia, 661
        hypertension, 658, 659
        preoperative questions, 659
        statins and beta-blockers, 658
    definition, 657
    incidence, 657
    medication management, 663
    morbidity and mortality, 657
End tidal anesthetic monitoring, 494
Enhanced recovery after surgery (ERAS), 93, 749, 750, 857
Epidermolysis bullosa (EB), 423
    airway management, 423, 426, 427
    anesthesia induction, 424, 425
    communication, 424
    dental and wound care, 421
    dental rehabilitation, 424
    esophageal balloon dilation, 424
    incidence, 421
    junctional, 421
    mental health, 421
    monitoring and protective measures, 424
    monitors, 423
    nasotracheal intubation, 425
    non-invasive blood pressure monitoring, 424
    non-invasive monitors, 425
    nutrition, 421
    pain management, 421
    patient management, 423
    perioperative algorithm, 427
    perioperative analgesia, 426, 427
    perioperative management, 423, 424, 426
    phenotypes, 421
    postoperative management, 426
    prevalence, 421
    pseudosyndactyly, 424
    recessive dystrophic, 421
    structural proteins, 421
    subtypes, 421
    types, 421
    vascular access, 423
    wound care, 424
Epidermolysis bullosa simplex (EBS), 421, 422
Epidural abscess, 494
Epidural anesthesia, 490
Epidural catheters, 750

Epidural pain management techniques, 453, 454
Epiglottis, 359, 360
Epinephrine, 345
Erythrocytosis, 313
Esmolol, 236
Esophageal atresia (EA), 381
Esophageal contractions, 804
Esophageal surgeries and procedures, 120, 122
  anesthetic considerations, 128
  congenital lesions repair, 120
  EGDs (see Esophagogastroduodenoscopy (EGD))
  fundoplication/hiatal hernia repair (see Fundoplication/hiatal hernia repair)
  gastroesophageal reflux, 120
  neoplasm resection, 120
  postoperative considerations and management, 127, 128
Esophagectomy
  adjuvant/neoadjuvant chemotherapy, 125
  incisions and surgical techniques, 124
  incision sites, 125
  intraoperative and postoperative analgesia, 125, 126
  intraoperative management, 126, 127
  intravenous access, 125
  neoplastic disease resection, 124
  pathologic regions, 124
  perioperative factors, 125
  preoperative pulmonary function testing, 125
  radiation therapy, 125
  solid unassisted pulmonary mechanics and gas exchange, 126
  surgical population, 126
  surgical targets, 125
Esophagogastroduodenoscopy (EGD), 273, 275
  general anesthesia, 276, 280
  moderate sedation for, 276
  patient positioning, 277
  patient safety, 279
  procedural complications, 281
  sedation level, 276
  with stenting surgery
    awake fiberoptic intubation, 121
    baseline considerations, 120
    conservative NPO management, 121
    endotracheal tube placement, 121
    esophageal narrowing or dysmotility, 121
    esophageal perforation, 120
    fluid management, 121
    hemodynamic stability, 121
    intraoperative management, 121
    mean arterial pressure, 121
    opioid administration, 121
    opioid sparing therapies, 121
    preoperative evaluation, 120, 121
    prophylactic pharmacotherapy, 121
    single lumen endotracheal tube placement, 121
Esophagus
  abdominal esophagus, 119
  anatomy, 119
  azygos and gastric veins, 120
  cervical esophagus, 119
  lower esophageal sphincter, 119
  mid esophagus, 119
  muscularis propia, 119
  neurovascular supply, 120
  portal hypertension, 120
  postpharyngeal foregut, 119
  thoracic aorta, 120
  thoracic esophagus, 119
  upper esophageal sphincter, 119, 120
Etomidate, 235, 319, 837
European Carotid Surgery Trial, 645
Euro-Therm trial, 602
Ex utero intrapartum treatment (EXIT), 290, 291, 480
  airway management, 478
  airway procedure, 474
  antenatal diagnosis, 482
  case blood transfusion, 478
  CHAOS, 476, 478
  congenital diaphragmatic hernia, 482
  congenital heart diseases, 482
  congenital high airway obstruction syndrome, 482
  extracorporeal membrane oxygenation procedure, 474
  fetal neck masses, 482
  fetal oxygenation, 475
  fetoplacental circulation, 473
  general anesthesia, 475, 479, 482
  indications, 473, 474, 482
  inhalational agents, 482
  inhaled anesthetic agents, 475
  intraoperative considerations
    anesthesia induction, 479
    anesthetic principles, 480
    aortocaval compression, 479
    combined spinal epidural anesthesia, 479
    fetal bradycardia, 479
    nitroglycerin, 479
    phenylephrine infusion, 480
    placental circulation, 480
    procedure, 478, 479
    sugammadex reversal of rocuronium, 479
    volatile anesthetics, 479
  intrathoracic pressure, 476
  large neck masses, 476
  lung and mediastinal masses, 482
  maternal complications, 482
  maternal laparotomy and hysterotomy, 476
  maternal physiological hemodynamic changes, 475
  maternal risks, 477
  maternofetal physiology, 475
  morphologic and genetic diagnosis, 476
  multidisciplinary team, 477
  neonatal carbon dioxide colorimetric device, 475
  non-depolarizing muscle relaxants, 482
  postpartum hemorrhage, 478
  prenatal diagnosis, 476
  preoperative case conference, 477
  procedures, 510
  rapid sequence induction, 482
  resection procedure, 474
  separation procedure, 474

Ex utero intrapartum treatment (EXIT) (cont.)
    strategic planning, 473, 476, 483
    therapeutic interventions, fetus, 473
    tracheal occlusion, fetus, 473
    in twin pregnancy, 474
    uterine relaxation, 492
    uteroplacental circulation, 473, 477
    vs. cesarean delivery, 476
    vs. cesarean section, 478
Expiratory reserve volume (ERV), 691
External beam radiotherapy
    intra-procedure, 258, 259
    monitoring, 259
    post-procedure, 259
    pre-procedure, 258
External cephalic version (ECV)
    anesthetic management, 502, 503
    risks, 501
    surgical considerations, 501
External ventricular drain (EVD), 299, 601
Extracorporeal membrane oxygenation (ECMO), 46, 389–392
Extra-thoracic injuries, 143

**F**
Face, legs, activity, cry, consolability (FLACC) scale, 446, 447
Faces Pain Scale-Revised, 447
Failure of regional technique, 493
Fat embolism syndrome (FES), 737, 856
Fentanyl, 192
    pharmacokinetics and pharmacodynamics, 813
    weight reduction surgery, 838
Fetal anesthesia, 480, 481
Fetal complications, 482
Fetal heart rate (FHR), 288
Fetal magnetic resonance imaging scan, 477
Fetal malformations, 482
Fetal resuscitation equipment, 480, 481
Fetal therapy
    fetal anesthetic considerations, 287, 288
    intraoperative anesthetic management
        EXIT procedure, 290, 291
        minimally invasive procedures, 288, 289
        open midgestation procedure, 289, 290
    maternal anesthetic considerations, 287
    MMC, 335
    postoperative maternal management, 291
    preoperative evaluation, 288
Fetal thyroid teratoma, 477
Fetal tracheostomy, 474
Fibrinolysis, 736, 848
Fisher grading, 564, 565
Flail chest, 141, 143, 146
Flexible fiberoptic bronchoscopy, 353
Flexible fiberoptic laryngoscopy, 352
Fluid resuscitation, 758
Fluid therapy, 798–799
Flumazenil, 192, 224

Focused Assessment with Sonography for Trauma (FAST) exam, 669
Fontan circulation, 22, 26, 27
Forced duction test, 366
Fraction Inspired Oxygen ($FiO_2$), 207
Frailty, 741, 807, 808
Frank-Starling Law, 807
Fresh frozen plasma (FFP), 642, 673
Fronto-Orbital advancement and reconstruction, 344
Functional endoscopic sinus surgery (FESS), 351, 352
Functional reserve capacity (FRC), 691
Functional residual capacity (FRC), 233, 476
Functional status (FS), 808
Fundoplication/hiatal hernia repair, 122–124
Fusiform aneurysm, 76

**G**
Gas explosion, 195
Gastroesophageal (GE) varices, 689
Gastroesophageal reflux disease (GERD), 122–124, 489
Gastrointestinal (GI) endoscopy, 175
Gastroschisis
    anesthetic considerations, 401
    definition, 395, 399
    diagnosis, 400
    post-operative care and outcomes, 401
    treatment, 400
Gastrostomy, 384
General anesthesia (GA), 224–226, 259, 260, 276, 280
General endotracheal anesthesia (GETA), 168, 280, 641
General movement assessment (GMA), 431
Generalized intermediate epidermolysis bullosa simplex, 422
Generalized severe epidermolysis bullosa simplex, 422
Genital trauma, 519, 520
Geographic location, 31
Germinal matrix hemorrhage (GMH), 463
Glasgow Coma Scale (GCS), 142, 598, 669, 670
Glomerular filtration rate (GFR), 702, 804
Glucagon, 185
Glycine toxicity, 847
Glycopyrrolate, 236
Goal directed therapy (GDT), 631
Goldenhaar syndromes, 342
Great vessel injury, 143
Growth hormone (GH), stimulation, 805

**H**
Haller index, 436, 437
Heart failure (HF), 155
    AHA Heart Disease and Stroke Statistics Update, 155
    cardiac transplantation, 155
    classification, 155
    medical therapy and LVADs, 156
    stages of, 155
    VADs (see Ventricular assist devices (VADs))
Heart transplantation
    intraoperative management
        induction, 34

maintenance, 34
    primary graft dysfunction, 37
    right ventricular failure, 37–38
    surgical considerations, 36
    ventilation strategy, 34, 35
  postoperative management, 38–39
  preoperative management
    blood products, 33
    cardiac echocardiography, 33
    coagulation studies, 33
    donation, 31–32
    electrolyte abnormalities, 33
    evaluation and management, 33–34
    geographic location, 31
    liver function tests, 33
    recipient evaluation, 32–33
Heart valve replacement and repair
  anesthesia monitoring, 16, 17
  intraoperative management, 18, 19
  intraoperative physiologic considerations
    aortic regurgitation, 17–18
    aortic stenosis, 17
    mitral regurgitation, 18
    mitral stenosis, 18
  postoperative management, 19
  preoperative evaluation, 15, 16
  valvular heart disease, 15
  valvular lesions, etiologies of, 15, 16
Hematocrit, 7, 44, 98, 296, 320, 325, 372, 481, 519, 675, 704, 761, 766, 771, 848, 857
Hematologic system, 759
Hemifacial microsomia, 342
Hemodialysis (HD), 658, 659, 710, 712, 713
Hemodynamic instability, 757
    aortic dissection or rupture, 64
    coronary artery obstruction, 64
    paravalvular leak, 64
    rhythm disturbances, 63
    valve malposition, 64
Hemodynamic, robot-assisted surgery, 786–787
Hemoglobin, 761
Hemolysis, elevated liver enzymes, and low platelet count (HELLP) syndrome, 520
Hemorrhage, 195, 278
Hemorrhagic shock, 669, 672–674
Hemorrhagic stroke, 165
Hemothorax, 135, 138
Hepatic pressure venous gradient (HPVG), 689, 692
Hepatopulmonary syndrome (HPS), 701
Hepatorenal syndrome (HRS), 690, 701, 702, 714
Heyde's syndrome, 191
Hiatal hernia, 122–124
    classification, 122
    definition, 122
    randomized control trial, 122
    supportive phrenoesophageal ligament, 122
    surgical repair, 122
High block/total spinal anesthesia, 493
Hip arthroplasty, 851
Hirschsprung's disease (HD), 413, 415
Home sleep testing, 720

Hudson face mask, 585, 586
Hurricaine®, 185
Hydration, 24, 397, 415, 418, 557, 611, 807, 821, 848
Hydrocephalus, 299, 300
Hydroxyethyl starch (HES), 758
Hydroxyzine, 225
Hyoscine-N-butyl bromide (HBB), 179
Hypercapnia, 132, 202, 209, 211, 268, 301, 459, 547, 551, 553, 719, 802, 803
Hypercarbia, 23, 27, 35, 37, 44, 54, 90, 134, 169, 203, 211, 320, 364, 460, 538, 586, 600, 670, 747, 803
Hypercortisolaemeia, 809
Hyperglycemia, 9, 232
Hypermetabolic (flow) phase, 766, 767
Hypertension, 537–540
    acute postoperative hypertension, 542
    aortic dissection, 540, 541
    definition, 535
    ICH, 541
    intraoperative emergency
        BP changes, 537, 538
            causes and complications, 538–539
            pharmacological treatment, 539, 540
    pheochromocytoma, 541, 542
    preoperative evaluation, 535–537
Hyperthermia, 79, 223, 265, 275, 302, 331, 371, 433, 570
Hypertrophic pyloric stenosis (HPS)
    aspiration risk management, 406
    atropine sulphate, 405
    biochemical derangement, 403
    biochemical derangement and dehydration, 405
    blood chemistry, 406
    diagnosis, 403
    gastric obstruction, 403
    genetic and environmental factors, 404
    genomic variation in neuronal NOS coding, 404
    impaired emptying, 403
    inhalation induction, 406
    inhalational anesthesia, 407
    intraoperative and post-operative analgesia, 407
    ketamine, 407
    maternal factors, 404
    nitric oxide synthase, 404
    opiate usage, 409
    pathophysiological cause, 403
    perioperative considerations, 409
    physical examination, 403
    pre-operative treatments, 405
    progressive hypertrophy, 403
    propofol, 407
    pyloromyotomy, 403
    regional anesthesia, 409
    regional techniques, 407, 408
    rocuronium, 407
    sedation and paralysis on induction, 407
    systemic analgesics, 407
    ultrasound imaging, 403
Hyperventilation, 236
Hypervolemia, 267–269, 567, 712, 798
Hypocarbia, 600

Hypochloremia, 405
Hypochloremic alkalosis, 414
Hypokalemia, 405
Hyponatremia, 203, 347, 370, 468, 551, 553, 636, 702, 848
Hypotension, 599
Hypothalamic-pituitary-adrenal axis (HPA), 759, 809
Hypothermia, 371, 418, 467, 667, 668, 670, 673, 675, 848
Hypovolemia, 459, 798
Hypovolemic shock, 671
Hypoxemia, 186, 195, 211, 312
Hypoxia, 36, 278, 599
Hypoxic pulmonary vasoconstriction (HPV), 91, 103

## I

Immediate induction of labor (IOL), 502
Imperforate anus, 413, 414
In utero pulmonary vascular resistance, 464
Incarcerated hernias, 413, 419
Indirect inguinal hernias, 419
Inflammatory cytokines, 759
Informed consent, 533, 731, 820
Infraclavicular block, 663
Infrahepatic vena cava (IHVC), 699, 700
Infra-tentorial fossa, see Posterior fossa surgery
Infratentorial tumors, 299
Inhalation injury, 768
Inhaled anesthetics, 839
Inhaled nitric oxide (iNO), 37, 390–392
Inherited bleeding disorders, 520
Inherited mechanobullous diseases, 421
In-line stabilization, 667
Innominate artery compression, 110
Inotropic support, 34
Intercostal nerve blocks, 136
Intermediate-term circulatory support device, 159
Intermittent positive pressure ventilation (IPPV), 802
Internal globus pallidus (GPi), 590
Internal mammary artery (IMA), 7
Internal pulse generator (IPG), 591
International Subarachnoid Aneurysm Trial (ISAT), 565
Interscalene block, 663
Intestinal lymphadenopathy, 416
Intestinal obstruction
 care, guide to, 417
 causes, 413
 in children, 413
 clinical presentations, 419
 congenital, 413
 electrolyte optimization, 413
 extubation, 418
 in infants, 413
  atresia, 415
  bowel necrosis, 416
  embryologic aberrancy, 415
  intussusception, 413, 415, 416
  ischemia, 415
  malrotation, bowel, 415
 in newborns (see Neonatal)
 malrotation and/with volvulus, 413, 415
 midgut volvulus, 415
 pathologies, 419
 pathophysiology, 413, 419
 postoperative management, 418
 preoperative and intraoperative anesthetic management, 416, 417
 principles of care, 419
 principles of care in children, 419
Intestinal obstruction
 etiologies, 413
 fluid status, 413
Intestinal oximetry, 375
Intra-atrial re-entrant tachycardia (IART), 27
Intracardiac injuries, 142
Intracranial aneurysms clipping
 BP and CSF, 568
 emergency, 570
 induction, 569
 invasive arterial monitoring, 568
 maintenance
  brain relaxation, 569
  cerebral protection, 569
  generic neuroprotective measures, 569
  intraoperative rupture, 569, 570
  positioning, 569
 neurophysiological monitoring, 569
 post operative period, 570
 radiological coiling, 570
Intracranial hemorrhage (ICH), 541
Intracranial pressure (ICP), 232, 293–295, 298, 299, 301, 547–550
Intracranial volume, 293, 294, 346, 548
Intraocular pressure (IOP), 364, 782
Intraoperative radiation therapy (IORT), 260, 261
Intravascular pulmonary vasodilations (IVPD), 691
Intravenous patient controlled analgesia (PCA), 309, 530, 821
Intravenous sedation, 530, 532
Intraventricular hemorrhage (IVH), 463
In-utero tracheal clip application during pregnancy, 473
Investigation of Nontransplant-Eligible Patients Who Are Inotrope-Dependent (INTREPID) trial, 155–156
Ischemia-reperfusion (IR) injury, 35
Ischemic stroke, 218
Isoflurane, weight reduction surgery, 840
Ivor Lewis approach, 125

## J

Jejunoileal atresia (JIA), 413, 414
Junctional epidermolysis bullosa (JEB), 422

## K

Ketamine, 193, 225, 259, 267, 277, 319, 365, 769, 838
Ketofol, 267
Kidney Disease Outcomes Quality Initiative, 659
Knee arthroplasty, 852

## L

Labetalol, 77, 235, 552, 594
Lambert-Eaton Syndrome, 109, 110
Laminaria, 529
Large volume paracentesis (LVP), 691
Laryngeal cleft defects, 357
Laryngeal cleft repair, 357, 359
Laryngeal mask airway (LMA), 207, 208, 585, 770
Laryngomalacia, 357, 383
Laser vaporization resectoscope, 845
Left internal mammary artery (LIMA) graft, 612
Left subclavian artery stent (LSA), 612
Left ventricular (LV) assist devices (LVADs), 156, 159, 170
Lidocaine, 204, 277
Light amplification by stimulated emission of radiation (LASERs), 359
Limb tourniquets, 737
Liposomal-bupivicaine (Exparel) TAP blocks, 750
Liposuction, 266–268
Lithotripsy, 745
Liver function tests, 33
Liver transplantation
    anhepatic phase, 699
        bicaval technique, 699
        piggyback technique, 699, 700
    dissection phase, 698, 699
    intraoperative considerations
        anhepatic phase, 704
        dissection phase, 703, 704
        neohepatic phase, 704
        pre-incision, 703
    neohepatic phase, 699, 700
    preoperative evaluation
        CAD, 701, 702
        gastrointestinal failure, 703
        hematology, 702
        hepatic failure, 702, 703
        neurology, 700
        renal failure, 702
        respiratory, 701
Local anaesthetic scalp block, 583
Local anesthetic systemic toxicity (LAST), 493
Localized epidermolysis bullosa simplex, 422
Loop recorders, 67, 68
Lower extremity bypass surgery
    comorbid disease management
        CAD, 626
        diabetes, 627
        hypertension, 626, 627
        peripheral arterial disease, 626
        tobacco abuse, 627
    intraoperative management
        anesthetic technique, 630, 631
        intra-operative events, 632
        intravenous access and monitoring, 631
    medication on surgery day
        ACEI and ARBS, 627, 628
        beta-blockers, 628
        DAPT, 628–629
        statin therapy, 628
    nervous system, 630
    post-operative management, 632
    pre-operative evaluation, 625, 626
    vasculature, 629, 630
Lower limb and spinal surgeries, 433
Lung isolation/single lung ventilation, 144
Lung-protective ventilation strategies, 758
Lung resection surgery
    airway management, 89, 90
    anatomical considerations, 86
    anesthetic agents, 88–89
    ERAS, 93
    hemodynamic management, 88, 89
    hypoxemia on OLV, 91, 92
    intraoperative concerns, 88
    OLV, 90, 91
    pain management, 92, 93
    patient positioning, 88
    postoperative considerations, 93–94
    preoperative evaluation, 86, 87
    surgical considerations, 85, 86
    volume administration, 88
Lung transplantation
    evaluation and management, 33
    intraoperative management
        induction, 34
        maintenance, 34
        primary graft dysfunction, 36–37
        right ventricular failure, 37–38
        surgical considerations, 35–36
        ventilation strategy, 34, 35
    postoperative management, 38–39
    preoperative management
        blood products, 33
        cardiac echocardiography, 33
        coagulation studies, 33
        donation, 31
        electrolyte abnormalities, 33
        geographic location, 31
        liver function tests, 33
        recipient evaluation, 32–33
Lymphangioma, 482

## M

Maestro Rechargeable System, 834
Magnesium sulfate, 287, 542, 685, 855
Magnetic resonance imaging (MRI)
    anesthesia techniques, 248, 249
        cardiovascular MRI, 250
        general anesthesia, 249, 250
        implant immobilizers, 250
        in patients, 240
        monitored anesthesia care/sedation, 249
    anesthesia equipment, 247, 248
    Faraday cage continuity, 242
    gradient magnetic field, 241
    indications for, 248
    intraoperative, 250
    nuclear magnetic resonance, 241
    properties of tissue measurement, 241

Magnetic resonance imaging (MRI) (cont.)
  quenching, 242
  radiofrequency field, 241
  resonant frequency, 241
  RF pulses, 241
  safety, 243, 244
    acoustic noise, 246
    CIEDs, 246
    contrast enhancement, 246, 247
    effects on patients, 244
    emergency, 245
    implanted medical devices, 245
    occupational safety, 246
    pregnancy, 246
    projectiles/missile effects, 245
    temperature and burns, 244, 245
  static field, 241
  Zones, 242
Magnets, 72, 241
Major adverse cardiac events (MACE), 180, 647
Major joint surgery
  comorbidities, 852
  deep venous thrombosis, 854–855
  general anesthesia, 852
  hip arthroplasty, 851
  intraoperative considerations
    blood loss, 856
    bone cement, 856
    enhanced recovery after surgery, 857
    fat embolism syndrome, 856
    patient positioning, 855
    tourniquets use, 855
  knee arthroplasty, 852
  neuraxial anesthesia, 852, 853
  patient evaluation, 852
  peripheral nerve blocks
    hip, 853–854
    knee, 854
    perineural catheters, 853
    shoulder, 853
  shoulder arthroplasty, 851
Malnutrition, 261, 422, 423, 557, 747, 772, 807, 808, 820, 834
Malnutrition Universal Screening Tool (MUST), 807
Marfan syndrome, 24, 75, 435, 436
Massive hemothorax, 143
Massive intraoperative hemorrhage, 788
Massive transfusion protocols (MTP), 642, 673–675
Maternal complications, 481
Maternal hemodynamics, 476
Maternal hemorrhage, 517, 518, 521, 522
Maternal hypotension, 492, 493
Maternal massive transfusion protocol (MTP), 522, 523
Maternal mortality rate (MMR), 517
Mayo System, 598
McKeown approach, 125
Mean arterial pressure (MAP), 547, 548, 551, 600
Mean pulmonary artery pressure (mPAP), 457, 458

Mechanical circulatory support systems, generation of, 163
Meckel's diverticulum, 416
Meconium ileus (MI), 414, 415
Mediastinal surgery, see Mediastinoscopy
Mediastinoscopy
  anesthesia considerations, 108
  anesthesia maintenance, 110
  anterior mediastinal masses, 109
  arterial blood pressure monitoring, 110
  bronchogenic carcinoma, 107
  complications
    autonomic reflexes, 111
    esophageal injury and chylothorax, 111
    phrenic/recurrent laryngeal nerve injuries, 111
    pneumothorax, 111
    stroke, 111
  contraindications, 108–109
  general endotracheal anesthesia, 110
  indications, 108
  induction for GETA, 110
  intraoperative complications
    major hemorrhage, 110, 111
    venous air embolism, 111
  muscle relaxation, 110
  open thoracotomy, 107
  peripheral venous access, 110
  postoperative care, 111, 112
  preoperative considerations, 109, 110
  procedure, 109
  video-assisted thoracoscopy, 107
Mediastinum, anatomy, 107, 108
MELD score, 697
Meningitis, 350, 494
Meperidine (Pethidine), 179, 277, 814
Metabolic alkalosis, 405
Metabolic equivalents (METs), 626, 818–819
METEOR trial, 729
Methemoglobinemia, 185, 204
Methohexital, 233–235
Methotrexate, 528
Metyrosine (methyl-tyrosine), 683, 685
Midazolam, 192, 224
Milrinone, 9, 18, 28, 34, 36, 37, 46, 167, 169, 320, 458, 461
Mini Mental State Examination (MMSE), 809
Minimal alveolar concentration (MAC), 479
Minimally invasive approach to aortic valve replacement ("Mini"-AVR), 50–53, 56
Minimally invasive cardiac surgery (MICS)
  MIDCAB, 49, 50
  MIMVS, 52–54
  "mini"-AVR, 50–53, 56
  patient selection and and optimization, 54
Minimally invasive coronary artery bypass (MIDCAB), 49
Minimally invasive mitral valve surgery (MIMVS), 52–54
Minimally invasive thoracic surgical (MITS), 97

Minimum alveolar concentration (MAC), 491, 552, 672
Mini-Nutritional Assessment, 807
Misoprostol, 528, 529
Mitral regurgitation, 18, 65
Mitral stenosis, 18
Mitral valve, 65
Mivacurium, 235
Model for End-stage Liver Disease (MELD), 697
Moderate sedation, 276
Modified Mallampati (MMP) scoring, 180
Monitored anesthesia care (MAC), 166, 168, 206, 658
Monoamine oxidase (MAO) B inhibitors, 590
Monopolar electrocautery, 70–72
Monopolar resectoscope, 848
Monopolar transurethral resection of prostate (M-TURP) technique, 845
Monro-Kellie hypothesis, 548
Mood and anxiety disorders, 435
Morphine
    pharmacokinetics and pharmacodynamics, 813
    weight reduction surgery, 838
Motor evoked potentials (MEP), 79, 80, 558, 612
Moyamoya disease, 301
Muscle relaxants, 206, 814
Myasthenia gravis, 147, 148, 151
Myelodysplasia, 334
Myelomeningocele (MMC), 329, 334
    etiology/pathogenesis, 334, 335
    intraoperative considerations, 335, 336
    postoperative considerations, 336
    preanesthetic preparation, 335
    spina bifida, 334
    syringomyelia, 334
    tethered cord, 334
    ventriculoperitoneal shunting is, 334
Myocardial contusion, 142
Myocardial infarction (MI), 142, 180, 649
Myocardial ischemia, 3, 5–7, 24, 76, 77, 88, 133, 179, 217, 236, 324, 325, 327, 535, 538, 542, 610, 616, 620, 720, 799

**N**
Naloxone, 179, 192
Narcotics, 250
Nasal surgery, 351–352
Nasotracheal fiberoptic intubation, 426
National EB Registry (NEBR), 421
Near infrared spectrophotometry (NIRS), 79
Near-infrared spectroscopy (NIRS), 297, 370, 649
Necrotizing enterocolitis (NEC), 374
Neonatal emergencies
    continuous invasive venous saturation, 374
    glucose and fluid management, 369–371
    intraoperative considerations, 377, 378
    neonatal ICU, 378, 379
    NIRS, 375, 376
    oxygen consumption, 374
    oxygen delivery and extraction, 374
    perioperative monitoring, 372, 373
    postoperative considerations, 379
    preoperative assessment, 376, 377
    temperature regulation, 371
    transfusion considerations, 372
Neonatal Infant Pain Scale (NIPS), 446
Neonatal intensive care unit, 378, 379
Neonatal intestinal obstruction
    anesthetic management, 414
    causes, 413, 414
    congenital, 413
    delay in diagnosis, 413
    enterotomy, 415
    etiology, 413
    gastric decompression and intravenous fluids, 414
    incidence, 413, 414
    intraabdominal repair, 414
    metabolic status, 413
    perioperative and anesthetic care, 413
    radiographs, 414
    surgical correction, 415
    surgical intervention, 413, 415
    surgical treatment, 414
    symptoms and signs, 413
    treatment, 414
Neonatal outcome, 481, 482
Nephrectomy
    CPB, 641
    hemorrhage, 641
    indication, 747
    intraoperative and postoperative bleeding, 748
    intraoperative embolization, 641
    intraoperative management, 748–749
        analgesia, 642
        dissection phase, 642
        fluid resuscitation, 642
        IVC clamping, 642
        monitors and access, 641, 642
        post operative care, 642, 643
    partial, 748
    surgical treatment, 747
    thrombus with TEE, 640, 641
    vascular clamping, 641
    venovenous bypass, 641
Nephrogenesis, 466
Nerve block, 137
Neuraxial anesthesia, 168, 260, 320, 492, 852, 853
Neuraxial blockade, 799
Neuraxial techniques for cesarean delivery, 494
Neurologic disease, TAVR, 61
Neurologic injury, 494
Neuromuscular blockers, 814
Neuromuscular blocking agents (NMBA), 549, 839
Neuromuscular blocking drugs, 814
Neuromuscular disorders, 432, 801
Neuromuscular paralysis, 491
Neuromuscular system, 759
Neuronal function, 806

Neurosurgical procedure, 298–302
   developmental considerations, 293–295
   disease states and surgeries
      Arnold Chiari malformations, 298
      congenital anomalies, 298
      craniosynostosis, 300
      hydrocephalus, 299, 300
      hypercapnia and hypocapnia, 301
      Moyamoya disease, 301
      neuroimaging, 301
      neurotrauma, 301, 302
      perioperative ischemia, 301
      pial synangiosis, 301
      seizures, 300
      tumors, 298, 299
      vascular anomalies, 301
   intraoperative management, 297, 298
   neuroanatomy, 293–295
   neurophysiology, 293–295
   postoperative management, 297, 298
   preoperative evaluation, 294–296
Neurovascular supply, 178, 179
Nicardipine, 77, 236
Nitroglycerin, 77, 290, 479, 506, 509, 621, 684
Nitrous oxide, 225, 840
Nocturnal oximetry, 720
Non-delivery obstetric procedures, 497, 500, 503, 507, 510, 511
   cerclage (*see* Cerclage)
   D&C and D&E (*see* Dilation and curettage (D&C))
   external cephalic version (*see* External cephalic version (ECV))
   fetal procedure
      anesthetic management, 510, 511
      antenatal diagnosis, 510
      surgical considerations, 510
   tubal sterilization (*see* Postpartum tubal sterilization)
Non-heart-beating cadaver donors (NHBCDs), 756
Non-invasive positive pressure ventilation (NIV), 209
Non-operating room anesthesia (NORA), 239, 240, 265
Nonopioid analgesics, weight reduction surgery, 838
Non-small cell lung cancer (NSCLC), 99
Non-steroidal anti-inflammatory (NSAID), 103, 236, 769, 839
Norepinephrine, 6, 17, 453, 681, 682, 693, 704, 713, 786, 847
Normal perfusion pressure breakthrough (NPPB), 573
Normothermia, 34, 288, 399, 552, 603, 610, 857
Normovolemia, 551, 576, 577
North American Symptomatic Endarterectomy Trial, 645
Nuclear magnetic resonance, 241
Nuss procedures, 133–137
   anesthesia-mediated Valsalva maneuver, 439
   anesthetic monitoring, 438
   carbon dioxide insufflation, 438
   cardiac arrhythmias, 438
   complications, 438
   deep extubation, 439
   endotracheal anesthesia, 438
   epidural placement, 438
   foley catheter, 438
   hemothorax, 438
   hypotension, 438
   intravenous access, 438
   liver perforation, 438
   lung parenchymal laceration, 438
   patient positioning, 438
   patient's vital signs, 438
   perioperative transesophageal ECHO, 438
   postoperative pain management, 438
   residual pneumothorax, 438
   right ventricular perforation, 438
   3-lead EKG and pulse oximetry, 438
   vascular injuries, 438
   vs. Ravitch procedure, 438

## O

Obesity, 194, 828–834
   definition, 827
   medical conditions, 828
   morbidity, 827
   paradox, 730
   physiologic abnormalities
      cardiovascular, 829
      gastrointestinal, 830
      maternal, 830
      metabolic, 828, 830
      obesity hypoventilation syndrome, 829
      OSA, 829
      pediatric, 830
      pulmonary, 828
   prevalence, 827
   statistics, 827
   surgery (*see* Weight reduction surgery)
   surgical management, 830
Obesity hypoventilation syndrome, 829
Obstetric anesthesia practice, 475
Obstetric hemorrhage, 517, 519, 521, 522, 524
   anesthetic management
      for cesarean delivery, 524
      neuraxial *vs.* general anesthesia, 524
      for vaginal delivery, 524
   APH (*see* Antepartum hemorrhage (APH))
   incidence, 517, 518
   morbidity and mortality prevention
      bleeding prevention, 521, 522
      blood loss, 521
      preparation, 522
      risk assessment, 521
   obstetric management, 522
   PPH (*see* Postpartum hemorrhage (PPH))
Obstructive sleep apnea (OSA), 268, 829
   anesthetic considerations, 355, 356
   clinical diagnosis, 720
   comorbidities, 720
   peri-operative considerations, 722, 724
   polysomnography, 355
   postoperative adverse events and complications, 720
   post-operative management, 723–725

preoperative assessment, 722–724
prevalence, 355, 720
risk-mitigation strategies, 724
screening, 721
upper airway, 719
Oculocardiac reflex
    anesthetic implications, 364
    physiology, 364
Office based anesthesia (OBA)
    anesthetic management and technique, 266–268
    definition, 265
    office facilities, 265, 266
    OSA, 268
    patient safety, 269
    patient selection, 265
    PONV, 269
    procedure, 266
    pulmonary embolism and deep vein thrombosis prophylaxis, 269
Off-pump coronary artery bypass grafting (OPCAB)
    ideal surgical candidates, selection of, 11
    intraoperative anesthetic management, 10–12
    surgical principles, 10, 11
Omphalocele
    anesthetic considerations, 398, 399
    definition, 395
    diagnosis, 395, 397
    post-operative care and outcomes, 399
    treatment
        bowel decompression, 397
        C-section, 397
        preoperative care, 397
        silo chimney/prosthesis, 398
One-lung ventilation (OLV), 91–93
On-pump anesthetic management, 8, 9
Open abdominal aortic aneurysms (AAA)
    intraoperative management
        anesthetic considerations, 620
        aortic clamping, 621
        aortic unclamping, 622
        emergence, 622
        induction, 619, 620
        maintenance, 620
        renal protection, 620, 621
        surgical dissection, 621
        temperature management, 620
    open vs. endovascular repair, 616
    postoperative considerations, 622, 623
    preoperative evaluation, 616
        CAD, 616, 617
        COPD, 617, 618
        endocrine, 618, 619
        neurology, 618
        renal disease, 618
    preoperative management, 619
Open aortic repair (OAR), 616
Open Nissen fundoplication, 122
Open pneumothorax, 143
Open Ravitch approach, 438
Operation on placental support (OOPS), 473

Ophthalmic surgery
    eye
        anatomy, 363
        anesthetic implications, 364
        physiology, 364
    oculocardiac reflex
        anesthetic implications, 364
        physiology, 364
    pharmacology
        anesthetic implications, 365
        medications, 364, 365
    ROP
        anesthetic considerations, 367
        pathology, 366, 367
    ruptured globe, 366
    strabismus
        anesthetic considerations, 366
        pathology, 365
Opiates, 189, 192, 612
Opioid-based balanced technique, 297
Opioid pharmacokinetics, 813
Opioids, 6, 236, 837
Optimal cerebral perfusion pressure, 576
Oral midazolam, 296
ORBERA Intragastric Balloon System, 834
Orbital hypertelorism, 341
Organ Care System (OCS), 32
Organ procurement organizations (OPOs), 759–761
    cardiovascular system, 757–758
    DBD, 756
    DCD, 756–757
    endocrine system
        corticosteroid, 760
        HPA dysfunction, 759
        insulin, 760
        thyroid hormone, 761
        vasopressin, 760
    equipment and monitoring, 761
    ethics, 757
    hematologic system, 759
    neuromuscular system, 759
    organ-type allocation, 755
    pulmonary system, 758, 759
Orthognathic surgery, 342
Orthopedic surgery
    hip surgery, 730
    intraoperative care
        hip surgery, 734
        knee surgery, 734–735
        neuraxial anesthesia, 733
        peripheral nerve blocks, 734
        shoulder surgery, 735
    knee surgery, 730
    operating room preparation
        BCIS, 736
        FES, 737
        limb tourniquets, 737
        patient position, 735, 736
        TXA, 736

Orthopedic surgery (cont.)
    pelvic fracture, 730
    postoperative analgesic planning, 732
    postoperative care, 738
    preoperative evaluation
        airway management, 731
        cardiovascular and pulmonary management, 731
        chronic pain, 732
        hematologic assessment, 732
        neurology and musculoskeletal assessment, 731
    regional vs. general anesthesia, 729, 730
    VTE, 737
Otoplasty, 341
OUCHER scale, 446–447
Oxygen delivery ($DO_2$), 374

**P**

Pacemakers, 33, 34, 67–71, 191, 232, 246, 594
Pacer spikes, 73
Packed red blood cells (PRBCs), 642
Pain management, in children, see Pediatric pain management
Palmer notation system, 222, 223
Panama classification system, 457
Pancreatic duct, 176
Pancreatic necrosectomy, 273, 278
Pancreaticobiliary drainage system, 176–178
Paracervical block, 529, 530, 532
Paraesophageal hernia, 122
Paragangliomas (PGL)
    alpha-antagonists, 682
    definition, 679
    genetic mutations, 680
    postoperative management, 685
    surgical approach, 685
Paraneoplastic manifestations, lung cancer, 109
Paravertebral blocks, 309
Paravertebral nerve blocks (PVB), 136
Parkinson's disease (PD)
    clinical features, 589
    diagnosis, 589
    pathophysiology, 590
    peri-operative implications, 590, 591
    pharmacological treatment, 590
    prevalence, 589
Partial thromboplastin time (PTT), 710
Patent ductus arteriosus (PDA), 23, 465
Patient controlled analgesia (PCA), 333, 350, 769
Pectoralis plane infiltration, 135
Pectus excavatum, 436
    adjuvants, 440
    aesthetic defect, 435
    analgesic modality, 439
    anesthesia considerations, 441
    autosomal recessive trait, 435
    bilateral paravertebral blocks, 440
    cardiac arrhythmias, 435
    cardiopulmonary symptoms, 436
    chest wall deformities, 435
    during adolescence and puberty, 436
    embryonic developmental defects, 435
    epidural analgesia, 440
    epidural opioids, 440
    hypnosis, 439
    intercostal nerve blocks, 440
    ketamine, 439
    multimodal therapy, 440
    non-steroidal anti-inflammatory agents, 439
    Nuss procedure (see Nuss procedure)
    outcomes after repair, 440
    pain management, 439
    paravertebral blocks, 440
    patient-controlled analgesia, 439
    physical manifestations, 436
    preoperative assessment, 437
    prevalence, 435
    psychological issues, 436
    regional anesthesia, 439
    restrictive ventilator defects, 435
    ropivacaine and adjuvants, 440
    severe and progressive deformity, 437
    severity, 436
    sloped ribs, 435
    surgical repair, 435–437
    symptoms, 436
    systemic opioids, 439
    treatment, 435
    ventricular compression, 435
Pediatric pain management
    alpha-2 adrenergic agonists, 453
    analgesic adjuvants, 452
    analgesic pharmacotherapy, 448
    anatomic and physiologic nociceptive pathways, 445
    assessment scales, 446
    behavioral and physiological measures, 446
    behavioral strategies, 454
    clonidine, 453
    codeine, 451
    cognitive strategies, 454
    coping behaviors, 448
    developmental plasticity, 445
    distraction techniques, 454
    fentanyl, 451
    gabapentin, 452
    hydromorphone, 451, 454
    intensity, 446
    morphine, 450, 454
    neurobiology, 445
    neurotransmitters, 445
    non-opioid analgesics, 448
    non-pharmacological pain treatments, 454
    nonsteroidal anti-inflammatory drugs, 449
    NSAIDs, 450
    opioids, 450
    pain rating, 448
    patient controlled analgesia pumps, 451, 452
    pharmacokinetics, 448
    pregabalin, 452
    self-report pain, 446

# Index

single shot caudal epidural injection, 453
tramadol, 451
untreated painful stimuli, 445
Pediatric Perioperative Cardiac Arrest (POCA) registry, 315
Pediatric plastic surgery procedures
    cleft lip and palate, 342
    hemifacial microsomia, 342
    midface surgery, 342
    orbital hypertelorism, 341
    orthognathic surgery, 342
    otoplasty, 341
    syndactyly, 341
    trauma, 341
Penetrating injuries, 141
Percutaneous coronary intervention (PCI), 3, 60
Percutaneous fetal endoluminal tracheal occlusion (FETO), 389
Perioperative anticoagulation, 799
Perioperative ischemia, 301
Perioperative Ischemia Randomized Anesthesia Trial (PIRAT), 630
Periotoneal dialysis (PD), 657
Peripheral and central intravenous (IV) access, 761
Peripheral arterial disease (PAD), 626–628
Peripheral nerve blocks
    perineural catheters, 853
    regional anesthesia
        hip, 853–854
        knee, 854
        shoulder, 853
Peripherally inserted central catheter (PICC), 397–398
Per oral endoscopic myotomy (POEM), 274
    achalasia, 275
    procedural complications, 281
    sedation level, 276
    spine position, 277
Pfannenstiel skin incision, 487
Pharmacodynamics
    biotransformation, 811–812
    body compartments, 810–811
    dose adjustments, 812
    drug distribution, 810–811
    inhaled anaesthetics, 812, 813
    intravenous anaesthetics, 813–814
    local anaesthetics, 814, 815
    neuromuscular blocking drugs, 814
    protein binding, 811
Pharmacokinetics
    biotransformation, 811–812
    body compartments, 810–811
    dose adjustments, 812
    drug distribution, 810–811
    inhaled anaesthetics, 812, 813
    intravenous anaesthetics, 813–814
    local anaesthetics, 814, 815
    neuromuscular blocking drugs, 814
    protein binding, 811
Pharmacologic prophylaxis, 855
Phenoxybenzamine (PBZ), 682, 686
Phenylephrine, 17, 19, 23, 43, 169, 204, 290, 365, 480, 492, 628, 642, 693, 694, 799
Phenylephrine eye drops, 365
Phenylethanolamine N-methyltransferase (PNMT), 681, 682
Pheochromocytomas (PCCs), 541, 542
    clinical presentation, 680
    definition, 679
    diagnosis, 681
    differential diagnosis, 681
    genetic mutations, 680
    incidence, 679
    intraoperative management/surgical technique, 684, 685
    pathophysiology, 681, 682
    pharmacology, 682, 683
    postoperative management and complications, 685
    preoperative evaluation and optimization, 683, 684
    research, 685, 686
    signs and symptoms, 680
Phosphodiesterase type 3 inhibitors, 787
PH-targeted medical therapy, 458
Physiological and Operative Severity Score for the enUmeration of Mortality and morbidity (POSSUM), 819
Pial synangiosis, 301
Pickwickian syndrome, 829
Piggyback technique, 699, 700
Placenta accreta, 520
Placental abruption, 518
Placenta previa, 517, 518
Plethysmography, 373
Pleurodesis, 131, 135
Pleuroscopy, 201, 202
Pneumocephalus, 560
Pneumoperitoneum, 782
Pneumothorax, 789
Polycythemia, 28, 44, 47, 312, 829
Polyhydramnios, 414, 478
Polymethylmethacrylate (PMMA), 736, 856
Polysomnography, 720
Portal hypertension, 689, 690, 692
Portopulmonary hypertension (POPH), 691, 700–702
Positive end expiratory pressure (PEEP), 46, 47, 559
Post-anesthesia care unit (PACU), 505, 694, 713
Post-anesthesia recovery unit (PACU), 642
Post dural puncture headache (PDPH), 493, 494
Posterior cranial vault reconstruction, 345
Posterior fossa surgery
    advanced monitoring, 558, 559
    anatomy, 555, 556
    brainstem, 556
    complications
        haemorrhage, 560
        macroglossia, 559–560
        pneumocephalus, 560
        VAE, 559
    indications, 555
    paediatric considerations, 560, 561
    pathology, 556
    position

Posterior fossa surgery (*cont.*)
    lateral/park-bench, 558
    prone, 557–558
    sitting, 557
    supine, 557
  postoperative care, 560
  pre-operative assessment, 556, 557
  routine monitoring, 558
Postoperative cognitive dysfunction (POCD), 809
Postoperative nausea and vomiting (PONV), 269, 352
Postoperative pulmonary complications (PPC), 803
Post-operative residual neuro-muscular block (PRNB), 814
Postpartum hemorrhage (PPH), 481
  coagulopathy, 520–521
  definition, 519
  genital trauma, 520
  placenta accreta, 520
  retained placenta, 520
  uterine atony, 519
  uterine inversion, 520
Postpartum tubal sterilization
  anesthetic management
    epidural anesthesia, 498–499
    general anesthesia, 499, 500
    preoperative evaluation, 498
    spinal anesthesia, 499
  sterilization failure, 497
  surgical considerations, 497, 498
Pragmatic Randomized Optimal Platelet and Plasma Ratios (PROPPR) Trial, 673
Pre-albumin, 807
Precordial Doppler, 550, 559
Preeclampsia, 487, 491, 508, 520, 536, 830
Preemies, *see* Preterm infants (preemies)
Prenatal imaging techniques, 482
Preoperative cognitive dysfunction, 808
Pressure equalization tube (PET), 349
Preterm infants (preemies)
  anesthesia circuits
    drug administration, 469, 470
    mechanical ventilation, 468
    types, 468
    ventilator adaptations, 469
  cardiac factors
    PDA, 465
    probe placement, 465
    reversal to transitional circulation, 464, 465
  catheter sizes, 468
  classification, 463
  endotracheal tube, 468
  ETT length, 468
  extremely low birth weight, 463
  extremely preterm, 463
  fluid distribution and requirements, 467
  fluid requirements, 467
  hematologic factors, 467
  hepatic function and albumin synthesis, 467
  low birth weight, 463
  mild preterm, 463
  neurologic factors
    bradycardia, 464
    intracranial hemorrhage, 463
    pain, 463, 464
    post-operative apnea, 464
    respiratory drive, 464
    ROP, 464
    ventilatory control systems, 464
  renal factors, 466
  respiratory factors, 466
  superficial peripheral veins, 468
  thermoneutral environment, 467
  tracheal intubation, 468
  vascular access, 467
  very low birth weight, 463
  very preterm, 463
Primary graft dysfunction (PGD)
  heart transplantation, 37
  lung transplantation, 36–37
Products of conception (POC), 530
Prophylactic tocolytic therapy, 233
Propofol, 182–185, 190, 192–195, 217, 225, 235, 249, 259, 263, 277, 279, 319, 356, 585, 784, 837
Prospective, Observational, Multicenter, Major Trauma Transfusion (PROMMTT) Study, 673
Prostatectomy
  complications, 747
  edema, 747
  indication, 746
  intraoperative management, 746–747
  pneumoperitoneum, 747
  preoperative evaluation, 746
  Steep Trendelenburg position, 746
  vs. open vs. laparoscopic, 746
Prothrombin time (PT/INR), 710
Proton beam therapy (PBT), 258
P-SAP score, 721
Pseudosyndactyly, 422
Pulmonary arterial steal, 46
Pulmonary artery catheter (PAC), 79, 619, 761
Pulmonary artery hypertension-targeted therapy, 458
Pulmonary compliance, 787
Pulmonary contusion, 143, 146
Pulmonary disease, 61
Pulmonary endarterectomy (PEA)
  bypass initiation, 45
  clinical manifestations, 42
  CTEPH
    epidemiology, 41, 42
    pathophysiology, 41, 42
  definition, 41
  DHCA, 45
  guiding principles, 43
  induction, 43, 44
  lines and monitors, 44
  post-bypass period, 46
  post-operative complications, 46
  pre-operative preparation, 43
  rewarming, 45, 46
  seperation from CPB, 45, 46
  TEE, 44, 45

Pulmonary function studies, 437
Pulmonary function testing (PFT), 98, 617, 710, 801
Pulmonary hypertension (PH), 313
    assessment and management, 457
    calcium channel blockers, 458
    care, 460
    dexmedetomidine, 459
    diagnostic procedures, 459–460
    disease pathomechanisms, 457
    echocardiography, 458
    etomidate, 459
    hypercarbia, 460
    hypoventilation/airway obstruction, 460
    induction of anesthesia, 459
    inhalation induction, 459
    inhalational induction, 459
    intraoperative monitoring, 459
    ketamine, 459
    long-term medications, 458
    nitrous oxide, 459
    opioids, 459
    preoperative tests, 458
    pulmonary vasculature, 457
    resting mean pulmonary artery pressure, 457
    right heart catheterization, 458
    risk stratification, 458
    surgical procedures, 460
    treatment, 458
    volatile anesthetics, 459
Pulmonary hypertensive crisis, 460, 461
Pulmonary laceration, 143
Pulmonary system, 758, 759
Pulmonary vascular hypertensive disease (PVHD), 457
Pulmonary vascular injury, 457
Pulmonary vascular resistance (PVR), 311, 314, 457, 459, 461, 700, 702
Pulmonary vascular resistance index (PVRI), 457–458
Pulse oximetry probe placement, 465, 466
Pulse pressure variability (PPV), 641, 761
Pyloric stenosis, 413
Pyloromyotomy, 409
    carbon dioxide pneumoperitoneum, 404
    complications, 405
    description, 404
    intraoperative inflation pressures, 404
    by laparoscopic surgery, 404
    microlaparoscopic pyloromyotomy, 404
    perioperative management, pyloric stenosis, 408
    single incision laparoscopic techniques, 404
Pyridostigmine, 150

# R

Radiation therapy
    analgesia, 258
    anesthesia
        advantages and disadvantages, 261
        brachytherapy, 260
        general anesthesia, 260
        IORT, 260, 261
        anxiolysis, 257
    childhood cancers, 255
    external beam radiotherapy
        intra-procedure, 258, 259
        monitoring, 259
        post-procedure, 259
        pre-procedure, 258
    immobility, 258
    immobilization, 256, 257
    radiation safety
        complications, 262, 263
        healthcare providers, 261, 262
    repeated sedation, 261
    sedation, 257
    therapeutic radiation, 256
    treatment planning and delivery, 256
Randomized Evaluation of Mechanical Assistance for the Treatment of Congestive Heart Failure (REMATCH) trial, 155
Rapid sequence induction (RSI), 81, 121, 141, 406
Rapid sequence intubation (RSI), 549, 671
Rebleeding, 567
Recessive (RDEB), 422, 423
Recurrent laryngeal nerve block (RLN), 205
Regional anesthesia, 168, 260, 320
Regional wall motion abnormalities (RMWAs), 7
Remifentanil, 193, 236, 277, 350, 581, 585, 784, 838
Remifentanyl, pharmacokinetics and pharmacodynamics, 814
Renal cancer, smoking, 748
Renal cell carcinoma (RCC)
    incidence, 635
    post-operative complications, 640
    preoperative evaluation, 636, 637
    preoperative imaging, 636
    surgical anatomy, 637, 638
    surgical technique, 638, 639
Renal disease, 61, 167, 252, 618, 692
Renal oximetry, 375
Renal transplantation
    combined liver-kidney transplantation, 714
    intraoperative management
        anesthetic technique, 711, 712
        fluid management, 712
        medication management, 712–713
        monitoring and access, 712
    living donors, 707
    post-operative care, 713, 714
    preoperative management
        diabetes mellitus, 710, 711
        ESRD, 709
        hematology, 710
        pulmonary disease, 710
        renal disease, 710
    single donor, 714
    surgical technique, 707–709
Renin-angiotensin-aldosterone system (RAAS), 804
Reperfusion pulmonary edema (RPE), 46, 47
Resection, trachea, *see* Tracheal resection and reconstruction
ReShape Integrated Dual Balloon System, 834

Respiratory distress syndrome (RDS), 463, 465, 466
Respiratory system, 802
　age related changes, 800
　airway management, 801
　asthma, 802
　bronchodilators, 801
　COPD (*see* Chronic obstructive pulmonary disease (COPD))
　lung function, 801
　obstructive sleep apnea, 802
　pneumonia, 802
　postoperative pulmonary complications, 803
　pre-anesthetic evaluation, 801
　pulmonary function testing, 801
　6 minute walk test, 801
　snoring, 801
　upper airway, 800
Resuscitation, 672–674
Retained placenta, 519, 520
Retinopathy of prematurity (ROP)
　anesthetic considerations, 367
　pathology, 366, 367
Retinopathy of prematurity (ROP), 464
Retrograde cerebral perfusion (RCP), 80
Revised cardiac risk index (RCRI), 179, 180, 608, 628, 658, 742
Rewarming, 45
Rhythm abnormalities, 799
Rhythm disturbances, 798
Rib resections, 131
Right ventricular coronary perfusion, 459
Right ventricular hypertrophy, 459
Right ventricular outflow tract (RVOT), 26
Right ventricular outflow tract obstruction (RVOTO), 312, 314
Right ventricular (RV) failure, 163
Right ventricular systolic function, 458
Right ventricular systolic pressure (RVSP), 458, 702
Right-to-left shunting
　cyanotic CHD lesions
　　Tetralogy of Fallot, 313
　　total anomalous pulmonary venous return, 314
　　transposition of great arteries, 314
　　tricuspid valve abnormality, 314, 315
　　truncus arteriosus, 314
　intraoperative management
　　induction of anesthesia, 318, 319
　　maintenance of anesthesia, 319, 320
　　patient monitoring, 318
　pathophysiology, 311–313
　perioperative anesthetic considerations
　　available resources, 318
　　cardiac anesthesia specialized care, 318
　　cardiac medications, 316, 317
　　cardiovascular status, 316
　　for children, 315
　　imaging, 317
　　intravenous access, 317
　　laboratory studies, 317
　　neurological status, 315
　　physical exam, 317
　　premedication, 318
　　respiratory infections, 316
　　spontaneous bacterial endocarditis prophylaxis, 317
　perioperative anesthetic considerations for children, 315–316
　postoperative management, 320
Rigid bronchoscope, 208, 383
Robot-assisted surgery, 780–785, 788–790
　advantages, 780
　cholecystectomy, 778
　Da Vinci® Surgical System, 778
　disadvantages, 780
　emergence, 787–788
　emergency undocking, 783
　gynecological procedures, 777
　hemodynamic changes, 786–787
　history, 778
　intraoperative emergencies
　　emergency undocking, 790
　　massive intraoperative hemorrhage, 788
　　mechanical and pharmacologic prophylaxis, 789
　　pneumothorax, 789
　　robotic malfunction, 789–790
　　venous gas embolism, 788–789
　　venous thromboembolism, 789
　MONA, 778
　patient positioning, 782
　　emergency undocking, 784
　　head and shoulder, 785
　　induction of anesthesia, 782–784
　　neuromuscular blocking agent, 785
　　oral or nasal pharyngeal temperature probe, 785
　　surgical procedure, 785
　pneumoperitoneum, 780
　postoperative analgesia, 788
　pre-operative assessment, 780
　　cardiovascular, 780–781
　　intracranial, 781
　　intraocular pressure, 782
　　pulmonary, 781
　　renal, 782
　ventilation, 787
Robotic malfunction, 789–790
Robotic mitral valve surgery, 52, 53, 56
Rocuronium, 235, 839
Rotigotine, 590
Roux-en-Y gastric bypass (RYGB), 186, 831
Ruptured diaphragm, 143
Ruptured globe, 366


**S**
Saccular aneurysm, 76
Sarcopenia, 807, 808
Scalp block, 583
Scoliosis
　intraoperative management
　　airway management, 331
　　hemodynamic monitoring, 332

Index 883

induction of anesthesia, 331
intraoperative neurophysiologic monitoring, 332, 333
perioperative management
  cardiac status, 330
  hematologic status, 330
  nutritional status, 330
  pulmonary status, 330
postoperative management, 333
Secondary brain injury prevention
  cerebral metabolic rate, 600, 601
  CPP maintenance, 599, 600
  endocrine considerations, 601
  hypo and hypercarbia, 600
  hypotension, 599
  hypoxia, 599
  ICP control, 601, 602
  randomised controlled trials, 599
  treatment, 602
Sedation related adverse events (SAE), 180
Sedative hypnotics, 837
Seizures, 229, 231, 234, 300
Selective Dorsal Rhizotomy, 298
Self-expanding valves, 59
Septoplasty, 351
Serious Complication Repository Project, 494
Sevoflurane, 193, 233, 235, 365, 840
Shock, 766–767
Shock wave lithotripsy (SWL), 745
Short-term circulatory support devices, 158–162
Shoulder arthroplasty, 851
Shunt fraction, 22
Shunt lesions
  atrial septal defects, 22
  endocardial cushion defects, 23
  patent ductus arteriosus, 23
  ventricular septal defects, 22, 23
Sievert, 262
Single chamber pacemakers, 67
Single lumen endotracheal tube (SLT), 82, 89
Single shot spinal anesthesia, 491
Single ventricle physiology, 26
Sliding hiatal hernia, 122
Small airway inflammation, 802
Society of Thoracic Surgeons National Database (STS database), 52
Somatic oximetry, 376
Somatosensory evoked potentials (SSEPs), 79, 80, 331–333, 558, 612, 648, 649
Spastic cerebral palsy, 431
Spetzler-Martin grading scale, 574
Spina bifida, 298, 334, 337
Spinal anesthesia, 489, 490, 846, 847
Spinal cord injuries, 142
Spinal cord ischemia, 611–613, 618, 622–623
Spinal dysraphism, 298
Splanchnic oximetry, 375
Splenic injury, 195
Spring assisted cranioplasty, 344
SpyGlass® system, 175

Squamous cell carcinoma, 423, 424
Staged closure, 399
Stanford System, 76
Starling curve, 691
Statin therapy, 628
ST-elevation myocardial infarction (STEMI), 4
Stenotic lesions
  aortic stenosis, 24
  coarctation of aorta, 24, 25
  pulmonary stenosis, 25
Stereotactic surgery, 589
Sternal and scapula fractures, 143
STOP-Bang questionnaire, 721
Strabismus
  anesthetic considerations, 366
  pathology, 365
Strip craniectomy, 344
Subacute bacterial endocarditis (SBE), 226, 227
Subarachnoid haemorrhage (SAH)
  coiling *vs.* clipping, 565, 566
  complications, 565, 566
  epidemiology, 564
  Fisher grading, 564, 565
  investigation and diagnosis, 564
  management, 565
  presentation, 564
  prognosis, 567, 568
  rebleeding, 567
  vasospasm, 566, 567
  WFNS grading, 564
Subclavian/axillary artery access, 63
Substantia nigra, 590
Subthalamic nucleus (STN), 590
Subvalvular aortic stenosis, 323
Succinylcholine, 365, 366, 839
Sufentanil, 332, 489, 490, 620, 783, 838, 847
Sugammadex, 235
Suicidal ideation, 435
Superficial cervical plexus block, 651
Superior laryngeal nerve (SLN), 205
Superior vena cava (SVC) syndrome, 99, 109, 147
Supraclavicular block, 663
Supraglottoplasty, 357–359
Suprahepatic vena cava (SHVC), 699, 700
Supratentorial masses
  pathophysiology, 547, 548
  preoperative assessment, 549
Supravalvular aortic stenosis, 323, 327
Sympathetic nervous system hormones, 809
SYNAPSE trail, 602
Synaptogenesis, 288
Syndactyly, 341
Synthetic opioid, 319
Syringomyelia, 334
Systemic blood pressure, 796–797
Systemic coagulopathy, 848
Systemic corticosteroid therapy, 351
Systemic inflammatory response syndrome (SIRS), 818
Systemic vascular resistance (SVR), 311
Systolic blood pressure (SBP), 535–537, 541, 542

Systolic pressure variability (SPV), 641
Systolic pulmonary artery pressure (sPAP), 458

**T**
Tachyarrhythmias, 26, 313, 494, 787
Tachyphylaxis, 261, 262
Target controlled infusion (TCI), 558, 585, 603
Tension pneumothorax, 143, 145, 146
Termination of pregnancy, 529–531
    abortion complications, 531, 532
    anesthesia controversies, 528, 532, 533
    anesthesia risks, 533
    first trimester, 530
    incidence, 527
    late gestational age
        definition, 531
        post-abortion care, 531
    preoperative considerations
        antibiotic prophylaxis, 529
        cervical dilation, 529
        cervical ripening, 529
        counselling, 529
        laboratory tests, 529
        medication-induced abortion, 529, 530
        ultrasound, 529
    prevalence, 527
    second trimester, 530–531
Tethered cord syndrome (TCS)
    cause of, 336, 337
    diagnosis of, 336
    intraoperative considerations, 338
    postoperative considerations, 338
    preoperative considerations, 338
    signs and symptoms, 337
Tethered cord (TC), 336
Tetralogy of Fallot (TOF), 25, 26, 313
Thiopentone, 407, 800, 813
Thoracic aortic aneurysms, 75
Thoracic endovascular aortic repair (TEVAR)
    aortic surgery, 83
    complications, 611
    intraoperative management
        induction and maintenance, 612, 613
        monitoring, 612
    postoperative care, 613
    preoperative consideration
        imaging, 612
        LSA, 612
        medical optimization, 612
Thoracic epidural analgesia (TEA), 136, 137, 309
Thoracic epidurals, 440
Thoracic outlet syndrome, 99
Thoracic surgery
    carbon dioxide insufflation, 308
    induction and management of anesthesia, 306
    one-lung ventilation
        bronchial blockers, 307
        double lumen endotracheal tubes, 308
        endobronchial intubation, 307
        evaluation and correction of hypoxemia, 308, 309
    perioperative monitoring, 306
    positioning and ventilation for thoracotomy, 306, 307
    postoperative analgesia, 309
    preoperative evaluation, 305
Thoracic trauma, 142, 143
    ABCDE of, 141
    airway, 141
    calmness and equanimity, 143
    causes of death, 141
    definitive airway, 143
    euvolemia, 144
    fluid management, 145
    5 lead ECG, 144
    hypoventilation, 141
    hypoxia, 141
    in-line capnography, 144
    intraoperative transesophageal echocardiography, 144
    intravenous anesthetics, 144
    intubation, 143
    neurologic injury
        CT scan, head, 142
        level of consciousness and arousal, 142
        radiographic imaging, 143
        supportive therapy, 142
    NIBP, 144
    peripheral circulation, 142
    pulse oximetry, 144
    radiological/ultrasonography procedures, 143
    resuscitation, 144
    surgical interventions, 143
    ventilation, 141
    ventilatory principles, 144
Thoracoabdominal aneurysm repair (TAAA), 79
Thoracoabdominal aortic aneurysms, 607
Throat surgery
    airway foreign bodies aspiration, 354, 355
    DISE, 356
    endoscopic airway techniques, 352–354
    epiglottis, 359, 360
    laryngeal cleft repair and supraglottoplasty, 357–359
    LASERs, 359
    MRI, 356
    OSA
        anesthetic considerations, 355, 356
        pediatric, 355
        polysomnography, 355
        prevalence of, 355
    tonsillectomy, 356, 357
Thrombelastography (TEG), 619
Thrombocytopenia, 34, 203, 313, 330, 692, 702, 710
Thromboelastography, 603, 675
Thromboembolization, 218
Thymectomy
    anesthetic management, 150, 151
    myasthenia gravis, 147–148
    outcomes, 151–152
    preoperative evaluation
        physical evaluation, 149
        radiographic evaluation, 149
        risk assessment and optimization, 149, 150
    thymoma, 148

Thymoma, 148
Thyroid hormone, 761
Timolol, 365
Tonsillectomy, 356–358
Topicalization, 277
Total calvarial reconstruction, 344
Total hip arthroplasty (THA), 729–732, 737
Total intra venous anesthesia (TIVA) technique, 6, 82, 103, 121, 206, 247, 259, 331, 350, 359, 551, 558, 569, 585, 610
Total knee replacement (TKR), 729, 732, 737
Totally endoscopic coronary artery bypass (TECAB), 49–51
Toxicity
    ammonia, 847
    glycine, 847
Tracheal anatomy
    imaging, 115
    surgical resection and reconstruction, 113
Tracheal obstruction, 114, 115
Tracheal perfusion, 113
Tracheal reconstruction, *see* Tracheal resection and reconstruction
Tracheal resection and reconstruction, 114, 115
    airway anatomy, 113
    airway patency, 116
    anatomy, 113
    anesthesia maintenance, 116
    anesthesia, patients, 116, 117
    anesthesiology and surgery teams communication, 113
    blood loss estimation, 116
    brachiocephalic compression, 115
    cardiopulmonary bypass, 116
    central venous access, 115
    endotracheal tube cuff, 114
    endotracheal tubes, 116, 118
    extracorporeal membrane oxygenation, 116
    flow-volume loops, 115
    fluid goals, 116
    hemodynamic goals, 116
    indications, 113
    inhaled volatile anesthetics, 116
    intra- and post-operative management, 113
    lung ventilation, 116
    median sternotomy, 116
    monitoring and intravenous access, 115
    non-invasive blood pressure, 115
    pathological process, 113
    patient extubation, 116
    patient selection, 113
    postoperative complications, 117
    preoperative evaluation, 113
        bronchoscopy, 115
        contraindications, 114
        CT, 115
        head and neck radiation therapy, 114
        imaging tests, 115
        medical conditions, 114
        patient's airway history, 114
        physical examination, 114
        pulmonary dysfunction, 114
        pulmonary function tests, 115
        steroid usage, 114
        ventilator dependence, 114
    preoperative sedation, 116
    pulse oximeter, 115
    right thoracotomy incision, 116
    rigid bronchoscopy, 116
    surgical procedure, 113
    trans-tracheal jet ventilation, 116
Tracheobronchial disruption, 146
Tracheobronchial injury, 143
Tracheoesophageal fistula (TEF), 382–385
    anesthetic management
        airway management, 383
        gastrostomy, 384
        open thoracotomy repair, 384, 385
        preoperative preparation, 382
        thoracoscopic repair, 385
    clinical features, 381, 382
    Gross type C, 381
    pathophysiology, 381, 382
    plan of anesthesia, 381, 382
    postoperative complications, 385
Train-of-four (TOF) ratio, 711
Tramadol, 179, 451, 814, 838
Tranexamic acid (TXA), 736
Trans esopahgeal echocardiography (TEE), 6, 550
Transaortic/direct aortic access, 62
Transapical approach, 62
Trans-bronchial aspiration (TBNA), 201
Transcarotid approach, 62
Transcatheter aortic valve replacement (TAVR)
    active valve surgery, 59
    anesthetic management, 66
    catheterization programs, 59
    co-morbid conditions, 59
        coronary artery disease, 60
        decreased ejection fraction, 61
        mixed valvular disease, 61
        neurologic disease, 61
        pulmonary disease, 61
        renal disease, 61
        vascular disease, 62
    general anesthesia, 59, 60
    hemodynamic instability
        aortic dissection/rupture, 64
        coronary artery obstruction, 64
        paravalvular leak, 64
        rhythm disturbances, 63
        valve malposition, 64
    medications, 59
    mitral valve, 65
    monitored anesthesia care with local, 60
    neurologic complications, 63
    post-procedure care, 65
    preoperative assessment, 59
    pulmonic valve, 66
    sedation techniques, 60
    tricuspid valve, 65
    valves, 59
    vascular complications, 63
    vs. SAVR, 59

Transcatheter mitral valve repair or replacement (TMVR), 65
Transcatheter pulmonic valve replacement (TPVR), 66
Transcatheter tricuspid valve repair/replacement (TTVR), 65
Transcaval approach, 62
Transcranial doppler (TCD), 649
Transcranial motor evoked potentials (TcMEPs), 331–333
Transcutaneous electrical nerve stimulator (TENS) therapy, 750
Transesophageal echocardiography (TEE), 17, 19, 44, 45, 217, 610, 619
Transhiatal approach, 125, 126
Transient neurologic injury, 494
Transient neurologic symptoms (TNS), 489, 506, 530
Transjugular intrahepatic portosystemic shunt (TIPS)
    anatomy, 689, 690
    contraindications, 690
    indications, 690
    intraoperative management
        anesthesia types, 692, 693
        anesthetic and medications, 693, 694
        fluids, 694
        post-operative care, 694, 695
    pathophysiology, 689
    patient preparation, 692
    preoperative evaluation
        cardiovascular function, 690, 691
        coagulation, 691, 692
        neurologic function, 691
        pulmonary function, 691
        renal disease, 692
Transsphenoidal approach, 299
Transthoracic/thoracotomy approach, 123
Transurethral microwave thermotherapy (TUMT), 845
Transurethral needle ablation of the prostate (TUNA), 845
Transurethral resection of the prostate (TURP)
    advantages, 744
    ammonia toxicity, 847
    BPH, 743
    coagulopathies, 848
    complications, 744
    disadvantages, 744
    general vs. regional anesthesia, 846–847
    glycine toxicity, 847
    hypothermia, 848
    integrated zones, 845
    management, 849
    neuraxial anesthesia, 744
    perforation, 847
    routine monitoring, 846
    signs and symptoms, 745, 848
    surgical technique, 845–846
    symptoms, 745
    syndrome, 848
    trendelenburg positioning, 847
    visual disturbances, 847
    water intoxication, 846
Trauma, 341
Trauma anesthesia
    initial assessment
        airway, 667, 668
        breathing, 668
        disability/neurologic assessment, 669, 670
        exposure/environmental control, 670
        hemorrhage control, 668, 669
        oxygenation, 668
        secondary and tertiary survey, 670
        ventilation, 668
    operating room
        airway management, 671, 672
        anesthetic maintenance, 672
        arrival preparation, 671
        burns, 675
        emergency surgery, 670
        head injury, 675
        induction of anesthesia, 671
        laboratory monitoring, 675
        post-operative care, 675, 676
        pre-arrival preparation, 671
        resuscitation, 672–674
        vasopressors, 673, 675
    roles, 667
Traumatic brain injury (TBI), 301, 302
    causes, 597, 598
    classification systems, 598
    epidemiology, 597
    future developments, 603
    history, 602, 603
    induction, 603
    investigations, 603
    Mayo System, 598
    pathophysiology, 597, 598
    post-op, 603
Treacher Collins, 342
Tricuspid valve abnormality, 314, 315
Triple H therapy (THT), 566, 567
Truncus arteriosus, 314
Tubal sterilization, 497, 498, 500
Tumescent anesthesia, 267
Turbinectomy, 351
Twin-twin transfusion syndrome (TTTS), 510
Two-lung ventilation (TLV), 90
Tympanostomy tubes, see Pressure equalization tube (PET)

U

Ultrasound-guided transverse abdominis plane (TAP) block, 419
Uniform Determination of Death Act, 757
United Network for Organ Sharing (UNOS), 697
United States Preventive Services Task Force (USPSTF), 615
United States Supreme Court upheld the Partial Birth Abortion Ban Act of 2003, 531

Universal Numbering system, 222
Upper gastrointestinal (GI) endoscopy
  adverse events and post pocedure complications, 281
  anesthetic considerations
    adverse events, prevention and management, 278
    monitoring and supplies, 276, 277
    patient positioning, 277
    sedation requirements, 276
    sedative medications, 277
  cystenterostomy, 274
  deep sedation, 279
  EGDs, 273
  EUS, 273
  general anesthesia, 280
  necrosectomy, 274
  patient safety, 279
  POEM, 274
  positive pressure ventilation, 280
  preoperative evaluation and optimization, 274, 275
  primary cystenterostomy and necrosectomy, 280
  propofol, 279
Ureteroneocystostomy, 708
Urolithiasis, 745
Urologic procedures
  cystectomy, 749
  endourology, 742, 743
  enhanced recovery after surgery, 749, 750
  lithotripsy, 745
  nephrectomy
    indication, 747
    intraoperative management, 748–749
    partial, 748
    postoperative bleeding, 748
    surgical treatment, 747
  perioperative assessment, 742
  pre-operative evaluation
    chest radiograph, 742
    electrocardiogram, 741, 742
    laboratory testing, 742
    revised cardiac risk index, 742
  prostatectomy
    indication, 746
    intraoperative management, 746–747
    open vs. laparoscopic, 746
    preoperative evaluation, 746
  transurethral resection of the prostate
    advantages, 744
    BPH, 743
    complications, 744
    disadvantages, 744
    neuraxial anesthesia, 744
    signs, 745
    symptoms, 745
Urological oncology, 746
Uterine atony, 481, 482, 519
Uterine incision, 480
Uterine inversion, 520
Uterine relaxation, 477, 482
Uterine rupture, 518, 519
Uterotonic drugs, 519

## V

Vacuum bell therapy, 437
Vaginal birth after cesarean section (VBAC), 487
Valproate, 21, 334
Valvular disorders, 61, 799
Valvular heart disease, 815
Vanillylmandelic acid (VMA), 681
Vascular access, burns, 771
Vascular anomalies, 301
Vascular clamping, 641
Vascular disease
  subclavian/axillary artery access, 63
  transaortic/direct aortic access, 62
  transapical approach, 62
  transcarotid approach, 62
  transcaval approach, 62
Vasoactive support, 34
Vasopressin, 758
Vasopressin in Traumatic Hemorrhagic Shock Study Trial, 673
Vasopressor therapy, 799
Vasopressors, 600, 673, 675
Vasospasm, 566
Vecuronium, 379, 432, 480, 662, 694, 814, 839
Vena cava thrombectomy, 640
Venous access, 783
Venous air embolism (VAE), 297, 347, 550, 557, 559
Venous gas embolism (VGE), 788
Venous thromboembolism (VTE), 737, 789
Venovenous bypass (VVB), 641, 699
Ventilation, robot-assisted surgery, 787
Ventilator associated pneumonia (VAP), 758
Ventilator-induced lung injury (VILI), 758
Ventralis intermedius nucleus (Vim), 590
Ventricular arrhythmias, 162
Ventricular assist devices (VADs)
  anatomy of, 157
  early complications
    arrhythmias, 162
    bleeding, 162
    end-organ failure, 164
    infection, 162
    neurological complications, 165
    RV failure, 163
    suction events, 164
  indications for, 157, 158
  intraoperative anesthetic considerations
    cardiac arrest, 170
    general anesthesia with endotracheal intubation, 168, 169
    hemodynamic monitoring, 167
    MAC, 168
    neuraxial anesthesia, 168
    power, 167
    power infection prophylaxis, 167
    preload and right ventricular function, 169
    regional anesthesia, 168
    reverse Trendelenburg position, 169
    VAD monitor, 169

Ventricular assist devices (VADs) (cont.)
　late complications
　　aortic valve degeneration, 165
　　device thrombosis, 165
　　gastrointestinal bleeding, 165
　physiological changes, 161
　postoperative and post-discharge considerations, 170
　preoperative evaluation and considerations, 166
　　airway assessment/aspiration risk, 166
　　anticoagulation requirements, 167
　　cardiovascular assessment, 166
　　hepatic and renal assessment, 166
　　medications, 167
　types of, 158–160, 165
Ventricular septal defects (VSD), 22, 23, 314
Ventriculoperitoneal shunting, 334
Verbal numeric scale, 447
Vertical skin and uterine incisions, 487
Vertical sleeve gastrectomy (VSG), 832
Veterans Administration Cooperative Trial, 645
Video-assisted thoracoscopic surgery (VATS)
　double lumen endotracheal tubes, 100–102
　emergence, 104
　evolution, 97
　fluid management, 103, 104
　intraoperative management, 99
　lung isolation technique, 100
　one lung physiology, 102, 103
　outcomes, 104
　pain control, 103
　patient positioning, 102
　preoperative evaluation, 98–99
　TIVA, 103
Visual analog scale (VAS), 447
Visual disturbances, 847

Volatile agents, 250
von Willebrand disease, 520

## W

Waste circumference, 827
Weight reduction surgery
　AGB, 833–834
　anesthetic management
　　airway management, 834–835
　　inhaled anesthetics, 839
　　intravenous medications, 837–839
　　monitoring and access, 835
　　PACU management, 840–842
　　pharmacology, 836–837
　　positioning, 835–836
　　postoperative complications, 840–842
　　Ventilation, 835
　ASMBS endorsed procedures, 834
　BPD/DS, 832–833
　complications, 828, 834
　high risk stratification, 828
　mobility and psychological status, 828
　patient selection, 827
　roux-en-y gastric bypass, 831
　VSG, 832
White coat hypertension, 536
Williams's syndrome, 327
Wong-Baker Faces pain scale, 446, 447
World Federation of Neurosurgeons (WFNS) grading, 564

## Z

Zeus® Robotic Surgical System (ZRSS), 778